P9-AGE-086

Sheehy's

Emergency Nursing

Principles and Practice

Sheehy's
Emergency
Nursing

Principles and Practice

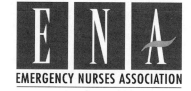

EMERGENCY NURSES ASSOCIATION

Sixth Edition

Edited by

Patricia Kunz Howard, PhD, RN, CEN, FAEN
Operations Manager
Emergency and Trauma Services
University of Kentucky Chandler Medical Center
Lexington, Kentucky

Rebecca A. Steinmann, RN, APN, CEN, CPEN, CCRN, CCNS
Clinical Educator
Emergency Department
Edward Hospital
Naperville, Illinois

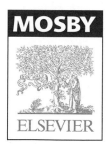

MOSBY

ELSEVIER

MOSBY
ELSEVIER

11830 Westline Industrial Drive
St. Louis, Missouri 63146

Notice

Previous editions copyrighted 1981, 1985, 1992, 1998, and 2003

ISBN 13   978-0-323-05585-7

Managing Editor: Maureen Iannuzzi
Developmental Editor: Laurie Sparks
Publishing Services Manager: Anne Altepeter
Senior Project Manager: Beth Hayes
Designer: Charles Seibel

Printed in the United States of America

Last digit is the print number: 9 8 7 6 5 4 3 2 1

Contributors

Sherri-Lynne Almeida, RN, DrPH, MSN, MEd, CEN, FAEN
Director
Cardinal Health
Center for Safety and Clinical Excellence
Houston, Texas

Knox Andress, RN, BA, AD, FAEN
Emergency Preparedness and Education Director
Louisiana Poison Center
Louisiana State University Health Sciences Center – Shreveport
Shreveport, Louisiana

Vicki Bacidore, RN, MSN, ACNP, CEN
Emergency Department
Loyola University Medical Center
Maywood, Illinois

Autumne Bailey Mayfield, MSN, RN
Assistant Manager
Children's Emergency Department
Monroe Carell Jr. Children's Hospital at Vanderbilt
Nashville, Tennessee

Susan Barnason, PhD, APRN-CS, CEN, CCRN
University of Nebraska Medical Center
College of Nursing, Lincoln Division
Lincoln, Nebraska

Cynthia S. Baxter, RN, MSN, ACNS-BC, CNA-BC, CEN, CCRN
Clinical Nurse Specialist
Critical Care and Emergency Department
Veterans Administration Medical Center
Lexington, Kentucky

Angela Black, BSN, MSN, RN, CPN
Manager of Pediatrics
Pediatric Intensive Care Unit, Outpatient Pediatrics,
  and Pediatric Emergency Department
Children's Memorial at Central DuPage Hospital
Winfield, Illinois

Nancy Bonalumi, RN, MS, CEN
Senior Consultant
Blue Jay Consulting, LLC
University of California Davis Medical Center
Davis, California

Heidi Bresee, CRNP, FNE A/P
Clinical Instructor
School of Nursing
University of Maryland
Baltimore, Maryland
Coordinator
Sexual Abuse and Assault Center
Shady Grove Adventist Hospital
Rockville, Maryland

Beth Broering, MSN, RN, CEN, CPEN, CCRN
Independent Consultant in Emergency Education
  and Trauma Programs
Nashville, Tennessee

Edith Ann Brous, RN, BSN, MS, MPH, JD
Nurse Attorney
Bar Admissions in New York, New Jersey, and Pennsylvania
Edie Brous, RN, Esq.
New York, New York

Amy Brown, MSN, APRN
Assistant Professor of Nursing
Associate Degree Nursing Program
Morehead State University
Morehead, Kentucky

Lori Carpenter, AAS, RRT
Respiratory Therapist
Shock Trauma Unit
Intermountain Medical Center
Lead Respiratory Therapist
Intermountain Life Flight
Salt Lake City, Utah

Mary Jo Cerepani, RN, MSN, CRNP, CEN
Nurse Practitioner
Emergency Department
University of Pittsburgh Medical Center
Emergency Resource Management, Inc.
Pittsburgh, Pennsylvania

Garrett K. Chan, APRN, PhD, CEN, FAEN
Lead Advanced Practice Nurse
Emergency Department Clinical Decision Area
Stanford Hospital and Clinics
Stanford, California
Assistant Clinical Professor
Critical Care/Trauma Graduate Program
University of California, San Francisco
San Francisco, California

Kate Copeland, RN, BSN
Assistant Nurse Manager
Monroe Carell Jr. Children's Hospital at Vanderbilt
Nashville, Tennessee

Nancy J. Denke, RN, MSN, FNP-C, CCRN
Trauma Nurse Practitioner
Trauma Services
Scottsdale Healthcare – Osborn
Scottsdale, Arizona

Nancy Stephens Donatelli, RN, MS, CEN, NE-BC
Staff Nurse
Emergency Department
University of Pittsburgh Medical Center – Horizon
Farrell, Pennsylvania

Darcy Egging, MS, RN, ANP, CEN
Nurse Practitioner
Valley Emergency Care, Inc.
Emergency Department
Delnor Hospital
Geneva, Illinois

John Fazio, MS, RN, FAEN
Clinical Nurse Specialist
Emergency Department
San Francisco General Hospital
Assistant Clinical Professor
Department of Physiological Nursing
University of California, San Francisco
San Francisco, California

Kathleen Flarity, ARNP, PhD, CFRN, CEN, FAEN
Flight Nurse
Airlift Northwest
Wenatchee, Washington
Lieutenant Colonel, Consultant to the Director
  of Air Force Nursing
HQ USAF, Office of the Surgeon General
United States Air Force Reserves
Nurse Practitioner
Wenatchee Valley Medical Center
Wenatchee, Washington

Lynne Gagnon, BSN, MS, CPHQ
Director of Patient Care Services
Mayo Regional Hospital
Dover-Foxcroft, Maine

Nicki Gilboy, RN, MS, CEN, FAEN
Nurse Educator, Emergency Department
Brigham and Women's Hospital
Boston, Massachusetts

Chris M. Gisness, RN, MSN, FNP
Nurse Practitioner
Emory Department of Emergency Medicine
Grady Memorial Hospital
Atlanta, Georgia

Sharon A. Graunke, RN, APN-CNS, MS, CEN, TNS
Clinical Nurse Specialist
Emergency Department/Pediatric Emergency Department
Northwest Community Hospital
Arlington Heights, Illinois
Nursing Editor (Consultant)
Education
Emergency Nurses Association
Des Plaines, Illinois

Colin Grissom, MD, FCCM, FCCP
Associate Professor of Medicine
University of Utah
Associate Medical Director
Shock Trauma Intensive Care Unit
Intermountain Medical Center
Assistant Medical Director for Critical Care
Life Flight, Intermountain Healthcare
Intermountain Medical Center
Murray, Utah

Amy Herrington, RN, MSN, CEN
Patient Care Manager
Emergency Department
University of Kentucky Chandle Medical Center
Lexington, Kentucky

Reneé Semonin Holleran, RN, PhD, CEN, CCRN, CFRN, CTRN, FAEN
Manager Adult Transport Services
Intermountain Life Flight
Salt Lake City, Utah

Patricia Kunz Howard, PhD, RN, CEN, FAEN
Operations Manager, Emergency and Trauma Services
University of Kentucky Chandler Medical Center
Lexington, Kentucky

Mary Jagim, RN, BSN, CEN, FAEN
Client Engagement Manager
Intelligent Insites, Inc.
Fargo, North Dakota

Kathleen Sanders Jordan, RN, MS, FNP-BC, SANE-P
Nurse Practitioner
Mid-Atlantic Emergency Medicine Associates
Charlotte, North Carolina
Pat's Place Pediatric Resource Center
Carolinas Health Care System
Charlotte, North Carolina

Vicki A. Keough, RN, PhD, ACNP, CCRN
Loyola University Chicago
Niehoff School of Nursing
Chicago, Illinois

Diana King, MSN, RN
Assistant Professor of Nursing
Associate Degree Nursing Program
Morehead State University
Morehead Kentucky

Jennifer Kingsnorth-Hinrichs, RN, MSN, CCRN
Clinical Manager
Emergency Medicine and Trauma Services
Children's National Medical Center
Washington, D.C.

Betty Kuiper, MSN, ARNP-CNS, CEN
Clinical Nurse Specialist, Critical Care Units
Western Baptist Hospital
Paducah, Kentucky
Adjunct Instructor
Murray State University
Murray, Kentucky

Donna L. Mason, RN, MS, CEN
Senior Consultant
Bluejay Consulting, LLC
Nashville, Tennessee

Nancy L. Mecham, APRN, FNP, CEN
Clinical Nurse Specialist
Emergency Department and Rapid Treatment Unit
Primary Children's Medical Center
Salt Lake City, Utah

Colette M. Morey, MSN, RN, CEN
Nursing School Instructor
School of Nursing
Truckee Meadows Community College
Reno, Nevada

Katherine R. Nash, MSN, RN, FNE-A/P, SANE-A, D-ABMDI
Johns Hopkins University School of Nursing
Baltimore, Maryland
Sexual Abuse and Assault Center
Shady Grove Adventist Hospital
Rockville, Maryland

Elizabeth Gaudet Nolan, RN, MA, CEN
Staff Development
University of Kentucky Medical Center
Lexington, Kentucky

Vicki C. Patrick, MS, APRN, ACNP, CS, CEN, FAEN
Instructor/Lead Teacher
Acute Care and Emergency Nurse Practitioner Programs
The University of Texas at Arlington
Arlington, Texas

CDR Christopher J. Reddin, RN, MSN, CEN
U.S. Navy Nurse Corps
Head, Staff Education and Training
Naval Hospital Corps School
Great Lakes, Illinois

Cynthia Blank-Reid, RN, MSN, CEN
Trauma Clinical Nurse Specialist
Department of Trauma
Temple University Hosptial
Philadelphia, Pennsylvania

Paul C. Reid, Sr, RN, MSN, CEN
Clinical Care Manager
Department of Emergency Medicine
Lourdes Medical Center of Burlington County
Willingboro, New Jersey
Clinical Nurse (per diem)
Department of Emergency Medicine
Hospital of the University of Pennsylvania
Philadelphia, Pennsylvania

Terri McGowan Repasky, RN, MSN, CEN, EMTP
Clinical Nurse Specialist
Emergency Services
Tallahassee Memorial Hospital
Tallahassee, Florida

Carol Rhoades, RN, BSN, CFRN, CTRN
Flight Nurse
Intermountain Flight Operations Center
Salt Lake City, Utah

Kathy S. Robinson, RN
Program Advisor
National Association of State EMS Officials
Falls Church, Virginia

Anita Ruiz-Contreras, RN, MSN, CEN, MICN, SANE-A, FAEN
Emergency Staff Developer
Santa Clara Valley Medical Center
San Jose, California

S. Kay Sedlak, RN, MS, CEN
Faculty/Laboratory Coordinator
Western Nevada College
Carson City, Nevada

Daniel J. Sheridan, PhD, RN, FNE-A, FAAN
Associate Professor
Johns Hopkins University School of Nursing
Baltimore, Maryland

Daun A. Smith, RN, MS
Professor, Nursing
River Valley Community College
Claremont, New Hampshire
Per Diem Staff Nurse
Emergency Department
Dartmouth Hitchcock Medical Center
Lebanon, New Hampshire

Rebecca A. Steinmann, RN, APN, CEN, CPEN, CCRN, CCNS
Clinical Educator
Emergency Department
Edward Hospital
Naperville, Illinois

Patty Sturt, RN, MSN, CEN
Emergency Department Manager
St. Joseph Berea Hospital
St. Joseph Health System
Berea, Kentucky

Paula Tanabe, PhD, RN, MPH
Research Assistant Professor
Department of Emergency Medicine
  and the Institute for Healthcare Studies
Feinberg School of Medicine
Northwestern University
Chicago, Illinois

Jennifer Wilbeck, MSN, ACNP, FNP, CEN
Assistant Professor and ED NP Program Coordinator
Vanderbilt University School of Nursing
Nashville, Tennessee

Darleen A. Williams, RN, MSN, CEN, CCNS, EMT-P
Clinical Nurse Specialist for Emergency Services
Orlando Regional Medical Center
Orlando, Florida

Paula Works, RN, MSN, ARNP, FNP
Charge Nurse Emergency and Trauma Services
Capital Medical Group
Frankfort, Kentucky

Cheryl Wraa, RN, MSN
Trauma Program Manager
University of California Davis Medical Center
Davis, California

Reviewers

Debra Marie Backus, MS, RN, CNAA
Assistant Professor of Nursing
State University of New York – Canton
Canton, New York

Darlene Baker, RN, MSN
Nursing Faculty
Green Country Technology Center
Okmulgee, Oklahoma

Everett H. Bayliss, Jr, RN
Nursing Consultant
Grove City, Ohio

Christopher A Bridgers, PharmD
Clinical Pharmacist
Saint Joseph's Hospital
Atlanta, Georgia

Beth Broering, MSN, RN, CEN, CPEN, CCRN
Independent Consultant in Emergency Education
  and Trauma Programs
Nashville, Tennessee

Patricia L. Clutter, RN Med, CEN, FAEN
Staff Nurse
Freelance Educator/Journalist
St. John's Hospital
Lebanon, Missouri
St. John's Regional Health Center
Springfield, Missouri

Laura R. Favand, RN, MS, CEN
67th Forward Surgical Team
United States Army
Miesaw, Germany

Joyce Foresman-Capuzzi, BSN, RN, CEN, CCRN, CPN, CTRN, CPEN, SANE-A, EMT-P
Clinical Nurse Educator
Emergency Department
The Lankenau Hospital, Main Line Health System
Wynnewood, Pennsylvania

Stephanie C. Greer, RN, MSN
Associate Degree Nursing Instructor
Southwest Mississippi Community College
Summit, Mississippi

Angela Hackenschmidt, RN, MS, CEN
Clinical Nurse Specialist, Emergency Services
San Francisco General Hospital
San Francisco, California

Dianne Husbands, BA, RN, BScN, MN, ENC(c)
Nurse Manager
Department of Endoscopy, Firestone Clinic, and ENT Clinic
St. Joseph's Healthcare
Hamilton, Ontario, Canada

Karen Lumsden, RGN, Bsc (Hons) NP, PGCLT (HE)
Senior Lecturer in Emergency and Critical Care
Canterbury Christchurch University
Canterbury, Kent, United Kingdom

Susie McGregor-Huyer, RN, MSN, CHPN, CLNC
MH Consultants
Mahtomedi, Minnesota

Linda Murray, RN, CEN
Staff Development Instructor
Emergency Department
University of Kentucky Chandler Medical Center
Lexington, Kentucky

Maureen Phillips, BSN, RN, CSPI
California Poison Control System – San Diego Division
University of California San Diego School of Pharmacy
San Diego, California

Maureen Quigley, MS, FNP
Clinical Program Director, Bariatric Surgery
General Surgery Clinic
Dartmouth Hitchcock Medical Center
Lebanon, New Hampshire

Bettina M. Stopford, RN, FAEN
Assistant Vice President, SAIC
McLean, Virginia

Linda Yoder, RN, MBA, PhD, AOCN, FAAN
Associate Professor
Director, Nursing Administration and Healthcare Systems
Management
Luci Baines Johnson Fellow in Nursing
School of Nursing
University of Texas at Austin
Austin, Texas

In memory of Lorene Newberry —
a friend to many, a teacher to all,
and a wonderful nurse to her patients.
She is missed.

Preface

The sixth edition of *Sheehy's Emergency Nursing: Principles and Practice* continues the tradition of defining emergency nursing practice. The authors of this edition have synthesized evidence and clinical guidelines to provide you with a resource that reflects best practices in emergency care. They have shared their knowledge to enhance the clinical outcomes of the patients for whom you care. The expertise of these professionals represents geographic diversity and spans all emergency nursing practice arenas.

The sixth edition retains the organization of the previous editions. Clinical information builds on information presented in the earlier Clinical Foundations. A separate unit on Special Patient Populations provides the information essential to treat members of these groups.

New to this edition are chapters on *Family Presence During Resuscitation; Management of the Critical Care Patient in the Emergency Department; Influenza: Seasonal, Avian, and Pandemic;* and *Forensics*. A new chapter on Evidence-Based Practice replaces Outcomes Management. In response to the dynamic and evolving nature of emergency nursing practice, significant enhancements have been made to all chapters. The chapters on *Emergency Operations Preparedness; Nuclear, Biologic, and Chemical Agents of Mass Destruction;* and *Communicable Diseases* have been expanded to reflect global changes in our environment. To help the nurse deal effectively with the increased number of patients seeking care in the emergency department, the *Triage* chapter has been extensively revised and reorganized, with new information on five-level triage systems, infection control, and special populations. Information on shock and sepsis is contained in the new chapter, *Management of the Critical Care Patient in the Emergency Department,* to assist nurses in caring for an increased number of critical care patients in the emergency department. In recognition of the fact that many emergencies are psychiatric in nature, Chapter 51, *Behavioral Health Emergencies,* contains expanded and updated information on conditions such as agitation, substance abuse, and suicide prevention, to assist the nurse in dealing with psychotic, violent, and delusional behaviors. Many chapters have been streamlined to focus on the unique challenges and practices of emergency nursing, nursing diagnoses have been moved to an appendix, and new illustrations have been added throughout the text.

It is our hope that the sixth edition will facilitate the very best in clinical outcomes for your patients.

Patricia Kunz Howard

Rebecca A. Steinmann

Acknowledgments

We were honored to be asked to co-edit the sixth edition of this well-respected text on emergency nursing. It seems only fitting that we acknowledge the original work of Sue Sheehy and her generosity in giving this text to the Emergency Nurses Association. Many individuals made this edition a reality: chapter authors, reviewers, Emergency Nurses Association staff, and Elsevier staff. Without the efforts of each of these individuals this edition could not have been written.

Authors, we applaud your perseverance. We asked you to meet challenging deadlines, repeatedly, and you each rose to the challenge. Your willingness to write, edit, and rewrite will be remembered for years to come as a gift to your emergency nursing colleagues, both present and future.

Much like in the emergency department, where a highly functioning team makes a difference, that has been true on this project as well. The team of staff members from both the Emergency Nurses Association and Elsevier were integral to the success of this project. We thank each of you for all of your work on this text.

Finally, we would like to acknowledge our co-workers who have tolerated our multitasking and attempts to do it all. Your support has meant a lot to each of us and we thank you for tolerating and working with us the past 2 years. Most important, we recognize the time we have taken away from those closest to us—our friends, family, and especially our patient husbands, Andy and Michael. We are humbled by your constant willingness to let us do things that will benefit others.

We hope the information in this edition gives each of you what you need in your daily practice to deliver the highest quality care.

Becca and Patti

Contents

UNIT I

Foundations of Emergency Nursing

CHAPTER 1

Emergency Nursing: A Historical Perspective

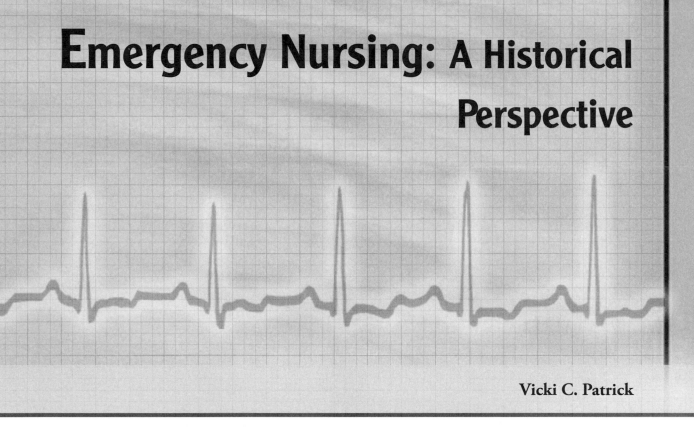

Vicki C. Patrick

ORIGINS OF EMERGENCY NURSING

Episodic illness and injury are part of the human experience. To care for one another is the essence of nursing. Thus nursing as an emergent caring experience is deeply rooted in history. Some of our earliest recordings chronicle the history of mankind, which is marked by reports of disasters, wars, and plagues. Throughout history's pages we find accounts of people caring for one another. Traditionally women in the family were the caregivers. Those who developed a propensity for caring were designated as nurses. As the art and science of nursing grew, so did the formation of the profession. Much of the profession's experiences are recorded as stories about the responses to emergent major events in history.

Early in civilization, as individual family units developed into societies, Hippocrates wrote of medical details we now call nursing tasks.[9] From one generation to the next, technical aspects of medicine and nursing were passed on, usually through oral teachings and direct observation. In European history, accounts of establishing hospitals for the ill and injured occur in the twelfth century and describe categories of nursing staff. Although accounts of specialized training do not exist, it can be assumed that some training existed in a more coordinated process. Greek history provides reports of emergent care during wars of the fourteenth and fifteenth centuries.[16] Other commentaries from this era describe nursing care delivered by monks and nuns. By the 1600s the French Sisters of Mercy was one of the first organized nursing orders that responded to care for epidemic victims.[8]

At the beginning of the nineteenth century the first reports of organized trauma care during the Napoleonic wars were described. Casualties were treated in the field, and a system of evacuation by ambulances was created.[15] Within this new military medical model, an organization of caregivers also had to be created from male soldiers, who were assigned to the work. Later in the century, in reporting the American Civil War, many sources cite the role of Clara Barton and Dorothea Dix in organizing voluntary nurses to care for wounded solders. Barton's nursing experiences on the front lines of battle are well chronicled.[6,13] Less than 10 years earlier, Florence Nightingale had led her nurses to the Crimea to support the British Army. Throughout her career, Nightingale recognized the foundation of the nursing role: individualized attention to the ill and injured, cleanliness, provision of good food and water, pain relief, and the importance of human caring touch. It was Nightingale who defined modern nursing with scientific process, quality control measures, and formal education.[6]

MODERN AMERICAN NURSING

In the early twentieth century American nursing was becoming organized and recognized as a profession. Hospital-based schools of nursing, based on Nightingale's design, combined the art of nursing with developing scientific principles. Wars and epidemics continued to give nurses the experience of caring for the emergently ill and injured. Over 23,000 nurses served in World War I according to the Red Cross.[17] As the war ended and the Spanish influenza pandemic increased, the Red Cross nurses transitioned from caring for the wounded to caring for victims of the influenza disaster.[1] In World War II professional nurses became part of the military, and specific training programs on caring for the injured were taught to nurses. The Vietnam War led to further recognition of trauma as a leading cause of death and disability. Experiences gained from advances in trauma care, development of antibiotics, and improvement of triage contributed to better postwar civilian emergency care.[6]

A NEW SPECIALTY: EMERGENCY CARE

After World War II the practice of medicine and the focus of hospitals were changing. Because most of the care was delivered in the community and prehospital care was ill defined at the time, private hospital emergency departments (EDs) were underutilized and staffed on an "as-needed" basis. Only public hospitals that served predominately indigent patients devoted staff resources to their EDs. Interns and resident physicians in training provided a majority of the medical care. During the 15 to 30 years after World War II, the increase in use of EDs was due to the changing dynamics of health care. The prewar medical practice of the "family doctor" primary care provider model was changing into a more specialty-based model, which led to less availability of primary care providers. The practice of medical providers being available continuously to their patients changed into directing patients to EDs for after-hours care. Hospitals were changing into community sources of help and information instead of institutions only for the seriously ill and injured.[18] As more patients arrived in EDs, hospitals were forced to assign increasing numbers of nursing staff to provide care. Even though the role was not well defined, only the most experienced nurses were selected for ED "duty" because of the unexpected, episodic nature and acuity of patient care.

At the same time as EDs were becoming more recognized as prominent care delivery areas in hospitals, transport of patients to hospitals for care was also gaining attention. Community leaders and the medical community realized that the lessons learned from World War II and the Korean conflict about triage, field care, and rapid transport could be translated into civilian practice. The military had developed training programs for field medics to initiate care and had refined transport strategies. In addition to ground ambulances, helicopter transport of injured soldiers was initiated in Korea. Legislation was created in the 1960s to establish community and educational programs leading to modern emergency medical services. Development of space-age technology, such as telemetry and portable defibrillators, also contributed to the growth of emergency care. As a result of these historical dynamics, emergency medicine and nursing became recognized specialties.

A NEW NURSING SPECIALTY: DEFINING THE SCOPE OF PRACTICE

By definition, emergency nursing is the care of individuals of all ages with perceived or actual physical or emotional alterations of health that are undiagnosed or require further interventions. Emergency nursing care is episodic, primary, usually acute and occurs in a variety of settings.[2]

Alliance or affiliation with a specific body system, disease process, care setting, age-group, or population defines most specialty nursing groups. In contrast, emergency nursing is defined by diversity of knowledge, patients, and disease processes. Emergency nurses care for all ages and populations across a broad spectrum of diseases and injury prevention, lifesaving, and limb-saving measures. Emergency nursing practice requires a unique blend of generalized *and* specialized assessment, intervention, and management skills. The multiple dimensions of emergency nursing specify roles, behaviors, and processes inherent in the practice and delineate characteristics unique to the specialty. Practice area, patient population, and the variety of those who provide care are as diverse in emergency nursing as in the nursing profession as a whole. Emergency nursing practice is systematic and includes nursing process, nursing diagnosis, decision making, and analytic and scientific thinking and inquiry. Professional behaviors inherent in emergency nursing practice require acquisition and application of a specialized body of knowledge and skills, accountability and responsibility, communication, autonomy, and collaborative relationships with others.

The scope of emergency nursing practice encompasses assessment, diagnosis, treatment, and evaluation. Resolution of problems may require minimal care or advanced life support measures, patient and/or family education, appropriate referral, and knowledge of legal implications. Care delivery occurs where the consumer lives, works, plays, and goes to school. Box 1-1 identifies multiple practice areas for emergency nursing.

Emergency nursing is multidimensional, requiring knowledge of various body systems, disease processes, and age-groups common to other nursing specialties. Processes unique to emergency nursing, such as triage and emergency operations preparedness, are discussed in later chapters. In addition to these recognized processes, emergency nursing is governed by a unique set of unwritten rules that developed as an outcome of the environment and the care of patients (Box 1-2).

Box 1-1	EMERGENCY NURSING PRACTICE SETTINGS

Hospital emergency department (ED)
Free-standing ED
Prehospital
Air and ground transport units
Military
Urgent care center
Health clinic
Health maintenance organization
Ambulatory services
Schools and universities
Business/Industry
Correctional institution
Occupational health clinics
Clinical decision units

Box 1-2	EMERGENCY NURSING ENVIRONMENT

Unplanned situations that require immediate intervention
Allocation of limited resources
Need for immediate care perceived by the patient or others
Geographic variables
Unpredictable numbers of patients
Unknown patient severity, urgency, and diagnosis
Cultural diversity

Box 1-3	HISTORY OF THE EMERGENCY NURSES ASSOCIATION

In 1968, Anita M. Dorr, RN, and Judith C. Kelleher, RN, working at opposite sides of the United States, perceived a need for nurses involved in emergency health care to pool their resources in order to set standards and develop improved methods of effective emergency nursing practice. In addition, they wished to provide continuing education programs for emergency nurses as well as a united voice for nurses involved in emergency care. By 1970, Ms. Dorr had formed the Emergency Room Nurses Organization on the east coast and Ms. Kelleher had formed the Emergency Department Nurses Association on the West Coast. The two groups joined forces and the Association was initially incorporated as the Emergency Department Nurses Association (EDNA) in Rochester, New York, on December 1, 1970. The first National Association meeting was held in New York in 1971.

From Emergency Nurses Association: *History of ENA.* Retrieved August 28, 2007, from http://www.ena.org.

Nursing roles include patient care, research, management, education, consultation, and advocacy. Emergency nursing practice is defined through specific role functions as delineated in the Emergency Nurses Association's (ENA's) *Standards of Emergency Nursing Practice, Scope of Practice Statement,* and *Emergency Nursing Core Curriculum.*[2,12]

EMERGENCY NURSING AND EDNA/ENA

The Growing Years: Late 1960s Through the 1970s

The development of emergency nursing as a specialty is intertwined with the rich history of the Emergency Department Nurses Association (EDNA) (later the Emergency Nurses Association), which was chartered in 1970 (Box 1-3 and Figure 1-1). Rapid growth of association membership, interest in defining emergency nursing, and recognition from community, medical, and legislative groups led to many initiatives. Within 5 years of its inception, EDNA developed a core curriculum for emergency nurse education, taught emergency nurse courses, and participated in every major program dealing with emergency care throughout the country.[11] In the mid-1970s emergency nursing's status in the nursing community continued to grow. EDNA published seminal works, the first *Core Curriculum, Standards of Emergency Nursing Practice* (with the American Nurses Association),

and the *Journal of Emergency Nursing.* By 1978 EDNA had determined that independent management for the organization was essential and established its own office with dedicated staff in Chicago. At the end of this busy decade, EDNA continued to validate the specialty of emergency nursing by funding a certification committee to begin the development process for a national certification credential.[4] ED nurses were beginning to further define their roles in flight nursing, mobile intensive care nursing, and advanced practice. Master of science in nursing programs with an emergency nursing major were established for specializing in advanced practice, administration, education, and providing much-needed research.

Success, Adversity, and Leadership: The 1980s

July 19, 1980, was a landmark day in emergency nursing history as 1400 nurses took the first certified emergency nurse examination. Although continuing to grow, the association was experiencing serious financial problems. It was time to stabilize the association, and leadership formed the first blue ribbon commission to focus on long-range planning. The commission's recommendations led to changes in the bylaws and decentralized leadership, emphasizing more involvement from the membership.

In 1985 the association name was changed to Emergency Nurses Association, recognizing the practice of emergency nursing as role-specific rather than site-specific. The *Standards of Emergency Nursing Practice* were updated, and the certification committee evolved into the Board of Certification for Emergency Nursing.[7] Another important educational program, the Trauma Nursing Core Course (TNCC), was developed, which standardized the core level of knowledge needed in implementing the trauma nursing process. TNCC became one of ENA's most successful programs, creating

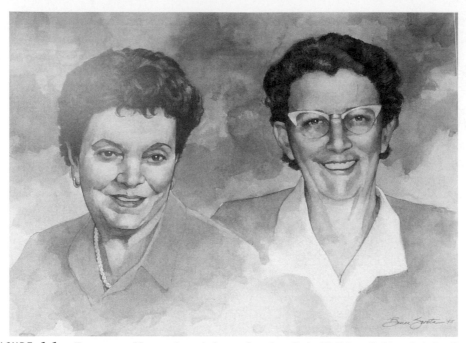

FIGURE **1-1.** Emergency Nurses Association cofounders Judy Kelleher *(left)* and Anita Dorr *(right)*. (*ENA Archives,* artwork by Bruce Sereta [brucesereta.com].)

a model for measuring competency. As other countries adopted TNCC, ENA established liaisons with other emergency nursing organizations internationally. In the latter part of the decade, ENA created Emergency Nurses Day and began to explore the formation of an Emergency Nursing Foundation for the purpose of education and research. It was a noteworthy decade, with the association working on many fronts to survive financial crisis, redefine the association, and support coalitions and collaborations with many other nursing, health care, and policy organizations toward common goals.[10]

Innovation: The 1990s

The decade of the 1990s was characterized by innovation and leadership. The Emergency Nurses Association Foundation (ENAF) was established to promote emergency nursing through research and scholarships. Guidelines were published to support emergency nursing and patient care: *Prehospital Nursing Guidelines, Patient Classification Systems Manual for Emergency Departments, Guidelines for Clinical Nurse Specialists,* and *Guidelines for Family Presence During Resuscitation.* ENA supported nursing practice by assisting legislators with mandating that institutions provide employees universal protective equipment. Educational innovations continued with the new Emergency Nursing Pediatric Course, Leadership Challenge, and development of a standardized orientation program for hospital-based emergency nurses. ENA commissioned a national survey, "Prevalence of Violence in U.S. Emergency Departments," which defined workplace violence, and identified contributing factors to violence, as well as preventive measures, to ensure workplace safety. ENA began working in cooperation with the National Highway Traffic

Safety Administration to develop national public and professional education programs. With an increasing emphasis on research, ENA initiated the LUNAR Project (Learning and Using New Approaches to Research), the first national multisite emergency nursing research study.[5] By the twenty-fifth anniversary of ENA in 1995, the association enjoyed a proven 25-year record as an enduring and influential nursing organization. The scope of emergency nursing practice expanded into injury prevention, and another milestone was reached when ENCARE (a safety education organization) merged with ENA. ENCARE (now the ENA Injury Prevention Institute/ ENCARE) has grown to a national organization of injury prevention providers and instructors whose goals are to decrease unintentional injuries through injury and violence prevention programs for health care professionals and communities. Also during the 1990s the important professional practice issues of cultural diversity, patient advocacy, government relations and public policy, organizational competency and strength, public awareness, and informational technology were addressed through nationally published position papers.[14]

The New Millennium: 2000 and Beyond

As emergency nursing entered the twenty-first century, practice problems of ED crowding, holding patients, rising costs, safety in the workplace, and nursing shortage continued. In addition to EDs, new practice areas included urgent care centers, clinical decision units, and occupational care. Protecting and providing resources to emergency nurses was a major focus of ENA. Internet technology expedited communication and resource acquisition. Important new education programs, Geriatric Emergency Nursing Education (GENE) and Key Concepts in Emergency Department Management, were introduced. After the events of 9/11, bioterrorism and weapons of mass destruction became new professional and educational initiatives for emergency nurses and the emergency care community. In addition, the topics of five-level triage and staffing and productivity in EDs were among the many issues addressed by position statements.[3] To meet future challenges, ENA once again examined itself and reorganized around the core competencies of administration, advocacy, membership, professional development, research, and practice.

Originally aimed at teaching and networking, the organization has evolved into an authority, advocate, lobbyist, and voice for emergency nursing. The Emergency Nurses Association continues to grow, with members representing over 32 countries around the world.

SUMMARY

Emergency nursing continues to become more complex and demanding. An increasing demand for emergency care, particularly for critically ill patients, requires innovations in care methodology and technology. As emergency nurses care for more critical patients for longer periods, the need for sophisticated monitoring equipment increases. Technology previously reserved for the critical care unit is now commonplace in the ED. As care becomes more complex, the emergency nurse's knowledge must continue to expand to make increasingly complex decisions about patient care.

With an aging population, health care needs continue to be diverse. Preventive medicine is prohibitively expensive for the indigent and most elders. Patients are discharged earlier after surgery, myocardial infarction, and many other conditions. Unfortunately, it means patients are sicker when they arrive in the ED and they stay longer. Emergency nurses serve increasingly demanding consumers. The public expects the latest technology and sophistication without loss of "high-touch" care. Insurance companies, employers, and the government are looking for the lowest health care cost available. Faced with reimbursement restrictions, health care administrators have tightened their budgetary belts, asking fewer to do more with less.

In the first decade of the new millennium, a hallmark issue has been the most significant nursing shortage in the past 20 years. Many issues will affect nursing as the health care system undergoes radical change. The nursing profession and how it is perceived will continue to evolve. As nursing becomes more active in the decision-making process and speaks with a single voice, these changes in health care become shining opportunities. Emergency nurses must continue to join together with new energy, speak with inspired voices, and maintain their prominence as partners in the emergency health care arena.

REFERENCES

1. American Red Cross: *World war accomplishments of the American Red Cross.* Retrieved September 1, 2007, from http://www.redcross.org/museum/history/ww1a.asp.
2. Emergency Nurses Association: *Scope of emergency nursing practice*, Des Plaines, Ill, 1999, The Association.
3. Emergency Nurses Association: The new millennium, *ENA Connection* 29(9):1, 2005.
4. Fadale J: The growing years, *ENA Connection* 29(4):1, 2005.
5. Fadale J: ENA gains prominence and builds for the future: years of innovation—1990-1994, *ENA Connection* 29(7):1, 2005.
6. Gebbie KM, Qureshi KA: A historical challenge: nurses and emergencies, *Online J Issues Nurs* 11:3, 2006.
7. Gurney D: Success despite adversity, *ENA Connection* 29(5):1, 2005.
8. Hjorth PS: Pioneers of modern nursing—a brief timeline, April 20, 2006, *History of European nursing.* Retrieved July 30, 2007, from http://nursinghistory.dk/html/content/articles/pioneers_of_modern_nursing.html.
9. Jones SR: Ancient nursing, In *Hippocrates*, vol 2, 1923, Loeb Classical Library, London, 1923, Heinemann.
10. Jordan JJ: Grassroots to leadership: years of change from 1985-1989, *ENA Connection* 29(6):1, 2005.
11. Kelleher J: In the beginning we were "roadrunners," *ENA Connection* 29(3):1, 2005.
12. McPhail E: Overview of emergency nursing. In Newberry L, editor: *Sheehy's emergency nursing,* ed 5, St. Louis, 2003, Mosby.
13. National Park Service: *Clara Barton: angel of the battlefield.* Retrieved August 15, 2007, from http://www.nps.gov/archive/anti/clara.gov.
14. Patton H: ENA prepares for the new millennium: the growing years, *ENA Connection* 29(8):1, 2005.
15. Pearce RL: War and medicine in the nineteenth century, *ADF Health* 3:88, September 2002.
16. Sapountzi-Krepia D: European nursing history: nursing care provision and nursing training in Greece from ancient times until the creation of the modern Greek state, *ICUS Nurs Web J* 18:1, April-June 2004.
17. Schreiber C: World War I: nurses volunteer for service, *Nurseweek*, September 29, 1999. Retrieved September 1, 2007, from http://www.nurseweek.com/features/99-12/ww1.html.
18. Weinerman ER, Edwards HR: "Triage" system shows promise in the management of emergency department load, *Hospitals* 38(22):55, 1964.

CHAPTER 2

Emergency Nursing Practice

John Fazio

DEFINITION OF NURSING

Since nursing's earliest beginnings, concepts central to the focus of nursing have included person, health, environment, and nursing.[13] Florence Nightingale defined nursing as an art and a science that would take charge of the personal health of the person.[14] She emphasized the importance of the interrelationship between the individual and the environment, astute observation, proper communication skills, and accurate record keeping. This perspective has contributed to the foundation of a knowledge base unique to nursing and continues to be relevant today.

This historical orientation is maintained within the American Nurses Association's (ANA's) landmark document *Nursing: A Social Policy Statement.*[1] The document delineates the nature and scope of nursing practice and the characteristics of nursing specialization. It is further used as a framework for understanding nursing's relationship with society and nursing's obligation to those receiving nursing care. The policy statement was revised in 1995 to represent clinical nursing practice as it has evolved and to set directions for the future. Some values and assumptions that serve as the underpinnings of this document were named: (1) humans manifest an essential unity of mind, body, and spirit; (2) human experience is contextually and culturally defined; (3) health and illness are human experiences; and (4) the presence of illness does not preclude health, nor does optimal health preclude illness.[2]

The most recent revision, *Nursing's Social Policy Statement,* provides the contemporary definition of nursing: *Nursing is the protection, promotion, and optimization of health and abilities, prevention of illness and injury, alleviation of suffering through the diagnosis and treatment of human response, and advocacy in the care of individuals, families, and populations.*[3] Nursing care is provided in many care settings and includes professional responsibilities such as patient assessment, nursing diagnosis, outcome identification, care planning, implementation of the plan, and outcome evaluation. Of all the members of the health care team, emergency nurses frequently have the most intensive and extensive contact with the patient. Emergency nurses also function in the role of patient advocate and coordinator of the multidisciplinary team.

SCOPE OF NURSING PRACTICE

Nursing's scope of practice is dynamic and evolves with changes in the phenomena of concern, in an expanding knowledge base about various patient interventions, and in political, legal, and cultural patterns in society.[2] Although nursing and medicine share many concepts such as illness and helping, unique phenomena vary according to the focus and applied practice of each discipline. Phenomena are observable events or facts, able to be explained or predicted through systematic observation.[2] The phenomena of central concern for nursing are human responses to illness or injury (e.g., dyspnea, pain, and alteration in consciousness).

This approach to practice is reflected in the use of the nursing process, which serves as an organizing framework for nursing practice in a variety of care settings. Although all nurses are responsible for practicing in accordance with this framework, the application may vary because nursing is practiced by nurses who are generalists, nurses who are specialists, and nurses in both basic and advanced practice. With each level, nurses are able to perform at the continuum from novice to expert.[5] In addition, emergency nurses have chosen to develop expertise in the specialty practice of emergency care.

SPECIALIZATION OF EMERGENCY NURSING

The specialty practice of emergency nursing emerged within the past 35 years. Emergency nursing is distinct due to the characteristics of the emergency patients, environment, and specific body of knowledge required.[12] Reflecting the emphasis on and need for emergency nursing care, the Emergency Department Nurses Association (EDNA) was chartered in December, 1970, primarily by the organizing efforts of two emergency nurses, Anita Dorr in New York and Judith Kelleher in California. In 1985 the association name was changed to the Emergency Nurses Association (ENA).

NURSING PRACTICE MISSION AND VALUES

The specialty practice of emergency nursing is guided by the association's vision and mission statement: "ENA leads the way in knowledge, resources, and responsiveness for emergency nurses, their patients and families."[8] The vision and mission are accomplished by directing the association's members to do the following:
- Promote the specialty of emergency nursing
- Promote the interests of ENA members and improve the professional environment of the emergency nurse through education and public awareness
- Promote ethical principles as defined by the ENA Code of Ethics for Emergency Nurses and the American Nurses Association Code of Ethics
- Actively collaborate with other health-related organizations to improve emergency care
- Be the primary resource for emergency nursing leadership, education, and research
- Define standards that serve as a basis for emergency nursing practice
- Develop, disseminate, and evaluate emergency nursing education and research
- Encourage interaction and mentorship among emergency nurses

- Identify and disseminate information on key trends affecting and pertinent to emergency nursing
- Serve as an advocate for the public regarding emergency care

Furthermore, the ENA Code of Ethics expects the emergency nurse to do the following[8]:
- Act with compassion and respect for human dignity and the uniqueness of the individual
- Maintain competence within, and accountability for, emergency nursing practice
- Act to protect the individual when health care and safety are threatened by incompetent, unethical, or illegal practice
- Exercise sound judgment in responsibility, delegating, and seeking consultation
- Respect the individual's right to privacy and confidentiality
- Work to improve public health and secure access to health care for all

DEFINING EMERGENCY NURSING PRACTICE

The first edition of the *Core Curriculum for Emergency Nursing,* published in 1975, identified a body of knowledge necessary for emergency nursing practice. Emergency nurses must possess a broad scope of knowledge and skills to care for those with a variety of health problems. *Standards of Emergency Nursing Practice* (1983) provided a foundation for the growth of emergency nursing. In 1991 ANA published *Standards of Clinical Nursing Practice.*[4] These practice and professional performance standards helped clarify and support the ability to define nursing practice in all areas where nursing care was delivered.

During the 1990s these standards shaped nursing practice and provided a framework for emergency nurses and ANA to foster a collaborative approach to defining the practice of nursing. In 1992 practice standards from the ANA were incorporated into the *Standards of Emergency Nursing Practice* to further delineate the role and function of the emergency nurse, enhance the quality and consistency of emergency nursing care, and provide criteria to evaluate the quality of emergency nursing practice. The ENA adapted the ANA definition of nursing found in *Nursing: A Social Policy Statement* to include the diagnosis and treatment of human responses to actual or potential, sudden or urgent, physical or psychosocial problems that are primarily episodic and acute in nature.

STANDARDS OF EMERGENCY NURSING PRACTICE

The following standards of emergency nursing practice are authoritative statements developed by the ENA that (1) reflect the values and priorities for emergency nurses, (2) provide direction for professional emergency nursing practice, and (3) provide a framework for evaluation of the practice.[12]

- The emergency nurse initiates accurate and ongoing assessment of physical, psychologic, and social problems of patients within the emergency care setting.
- The emergency nurse analyzes assessment data to identify patient problems.
- The emergency nurse identifies expected outcomes individualized to the emergency patient based on the patient's assessment, identified problems, and cultural diversity.
- The emergency nurse formulates a plan of care for the emergency patient based on assessment, patient problems, and expected outcomes.
- The emergency nurse implements a plan of care based on the assessment, patient problems, and expected outcomes.
- The emergency nurse evaluates and modifies the plan of care based on observable patient responses and attainment of expected outcomes.
- The emergency nurse evaluates the quality and effectiveness of emergency nursing practice.
- The emergency nurse adheres to established standards of emergency nursing practice, including behaviors that characterize professional status.
- The emergency nurse recognizes self-learning needs and is accountable for maximizing professional development and optimal emergency nursing practice.
- The emergency nurse engages in activities and behaviors that characterize a professional.
- The emergency nurse provides care based on philosophical and ethical concepts. These concepts include reverence for life; respect for the inherent dignity, worth, autonomy, and individuality of each human being; and acknowledging the beliefs of other people.
- The emergency nurse ensures open and timely communication with emergency patients, significant others, and other health care providers through professional collaboration.
- The emergency nurse recognizes, values, and uses research and quality improvement findings to enhance the practice of emergency nursing.
- The emergency nurse collaborates with other health care providers to deliver patient-centered care in a manner consistent with safe, efficient, and cost-effective use of resources.

COLLABORATIVE PRACTICE

Emergency nursing does not occur in a vacuum. Collaborative practice brings together health care professionals with distinct and complementary knowledge and skills (e.g., prehospital providers, emergency department physicians and nurses, trauma surgeons, respiratory therapists, radiologists, and pharmacists) to enhance the delivery of emergency care. This practice can address complex patient needs within a framework of quality, cost, and access. The primary commitment is to the patient, family, groups, and the community.[11] This commitment is directed to clinicians, managers, and health care organizations through ENA's position statement, *Autonomous Emergency Nursing Practice*[9]:

- Emergency nurses must facilitate open and timely communication with other health care providers through professional collaboration and interdependent practice.
- Emergency health care should be jointly coordinated by nurses and physicians with mutual respect for professional autonomy in both management and clinical practice.
- Health care organizations should ensure that nurse leaders are part of the policy-making bodies of their institutions and have the authority to collaborate on an equal basis with their institutions' medical leaders.

COALITION BUILDING

Coalitions are fundamental for creating successful changes within patients, families, groups, and communities. Commonly a joint purpose or activity or clinical dilemma may result in the formation of a permanent or temporary team that is likely to embrace collaborative practice. Coalitions may be built around any issue and on any scale, from neighborhood to national impact. The Emergency Nurses Association's *Procedural Sedation Consensus Statement* was successfully drafted following the formation of a coalition of professional organizations.[9] Successful coalition building is more likely to occur when the following are present[15]:

- Goals are similar and compatible.
- Working together enhances the ability of all to reach their goals.
- Benefits of coalescing are greater than costs.

COMMUNITY EDUCATION

Emergency nurses are actively involved in community education programs because they serve to reduce the risk and consequences of disease, illness, and injury. The ultimate outcome is achieved through primary, secondary, and tertiary prevention.[9]

- Primary prevention attempts to avert disease or injury by reducing risk factor levels (e.g., child safety seat distribution and education).
- Secondary prevention aims to detect disease early to control or limit its effects (e.g., human immunodeficiency virus [HIV] and sexually transmitted infection [STI] testing for those with risky behaviors).
- Tertiary prevention focuses on treating disease and injury in an effort to reduce disability and preserve function (e.g., referral to treatment programs for substance use).

The Emergency Nurses Association Institute for Injury Prevention/ENCARE (Emergency Nurses CARE) offers emergency nurses professional training and the opportunity to be active with established programs[10]:

- Alcohol Prevention Education
  - Choices for Living
- Safety Education
  - Bike and Helmet Safety
  - Child Passenger Safety
  - Gun Safety: It's NO Accident

- Healthy Aging Education
  - SAFER Medication Use
  - Stand Strong for Life

ENA and ENCARE are committed to reducing the number of preventable injuries through public education, professional training courses, and legislative advocacy.

POSITION STATEMENTS

The Emergency Nurses Association provides national and international leadership in emergency nursing care by identifying the standards of quality care. This leadership is set forth in the form of position statements, which are used to support the improvement of patient care at all levels. The position statements listed in Box 2-1 represent the organization's official stand on a variety of issues; the full listing may be accessed at http://ena.org.[9]

CORE MEASURES

Through the hospital accrediting process, emergency care is evaluated and further directed by The Joint Commission core measures. The Joint Commission has developed a process of identification, testing, and implementation of core performance measures to improve patient care. The Joint Commission is an independent, not-for-profit organization that has established standards for health care settings since 1951. Their comprehensive accreditation process is recognized as a symbol of quality and a hospital's commitment to meeting performance standards. Some of the core performance measure sets for hospitals include the following[17]:

- Acute myocardial infarction
- Heart failure
- Pneumonia
- Pregnancy and related conditions
- Surgical infection prevention

The use of the core performance measures has evolved over time. In addition to being used for internal quality improvement activities, core measures are now being used to focus the onsite survey visit. In 2004 The Joint Commission initiated public reporting of core measure data displayed against national and state comparative data. Core measures in the reporting are defined as National Quality Improvement Goals. Data may be accessed at http://www.qualitycheck.org. Additional performance measures are scheduled to be added.

PATIENT SAFETY CONCEPTS

The Joint Commission's Board of Commissioners publishes and updates annually a list of National Patient Safety Goals (NPSG). The NPSG are developed following a systematic review of the literature and available databases by patient safety experts and clinicians in a variety of health care settings. Emergency nurses integrate these safety goals into the care delivered to their emergency department patients. Table 2-1 lists the approved 2009 NPSG for hospitals.

DEVELOPING A SCIENCE IN NURSING

Nursing is a scientific discipline, as well as a profession. Nursing science is a domain of knowledge concerned with the adaptation of individuals to actual or potential health problems, the environments that influence health, and the therapeutic interventions that promote health and affect the consequences of illness.[16] The emphasis of nursing science is the health of whole human beings in relation to their environments.[6] Nurses use critical thinking skills and integrate the patient's subjective experience with the objective data of patients. The phenomena of concern are conceptualized as holistic, requiring a humanistic approach. Emergency nursing is clearly one area of specialization in which there are specific clusters of phenomena of concern. Some of the phenomena that have emerged within the emergency care setting await further delineation and exploration. Since Nightingale, recurrent themes that nurse scholars use to explain the domain of nursing suggest boundaries of an area for systematic inquiry and knowledge development. Nursing's knowledge will be developed from nursing's unique perspective, which guides the questioning and viewing of phenomena. These boundaries are concerned with principles and laws that govern the following: the life processes; the well-being and optimum functioning of human beings, sick or well; the patterning of human behavior in interaction with the environment in critical life situations; and the processes by which positive changes in health status are affected.[6] The knowledge required for nursing can be seen as a synthesis of what is known about the person, environment, health, and nursing. Therefore the discipline has a unique perspective, a distinct way of viewing all phenomena, which ultimately defines the limits and nature of its inquiry and knowledge.

Box 2-1	**ENA Position Statements**

Access to Health Care (February, 2006)
Advanced Practice in Emergency Nursing (March 2007)
Alcohol Screening and Brief Intervention (July 2004)
Autonomous Emergency Nursing Practice (March 2005)
End-of-Life Care in the Emergency Department (March 2005)
Family Presence at the Bedside During Invasive Procedures and/or Resuscitation (October 2005)
Holding Patients in the Emergency Department (May 2006)
Intimate Partner and Family Violence, Maltreatment, and Neglect (December 2006)
Mandatory Overtime (May 2006)
Procedural Sedation (July 2005)
Violence in the Emergency Care Setting (April 2006)

Table 2-1. 2009 NATIONAL PATIENT SAFETY GOALS

Goal 1	**Improve the accuracy of patient identification.**
NPSG.01.01.01	Use at least two patient identifiers when providing care, treatment, or services.
NPSG.01.03.01	Eliminate transfusion errors related to patient misidentification.
Goal 2	**Improve the effectiveness of communication among caregivers.**
NPSG.02.01.01	For verbal or telephone orders or for telephonic reporting of critical test results, verify the complete order or test result by having the person receiving the information record and "read back" the complete order or test result.
NPSG.02.02.01	There is a standardized list of abbreviations, acronyms, symbols, and dose designations that are not to be used throughout the organization.
NPSG.02.03.01	The organization measures, assesses, and, if needed, takes action to improve the timeliness of reporting, and the timeliness of critical tests, and critical results and values by the responsible licensed caregiver.
NPSG.02.05.01	Implement a standardized approach to "hand off" communications, including an opportunity to ask and respond to questions.
Goal 3	**Improve the safety of using medications.**
NPSG.03.03.01	Identify and, at a minimum, annually review a list of look-alike/sound-alike drugs used by the organization, and take action to prevent errors involving the interchange of these drugs.
NPSG.03.04.01	Label all medications, medication containers (for example, syringes, medicine cups, basins), or other solutions on and off the sterile field.
NPSG.03.05.01	Reduce the likelihood of patient harm associated with the use of anticoagulation therapy.
Goal 7	**Reduce the risk of health care–associated infections.**
NPSG.07.01.01	Comply with current World Health Organization (WHO) hand hygiene guidelines or Centers for Disease Control and Prevention (CDC) hand hygiene guidelines.
NPSG.07.02.01	Manage as sentinel events all identified cases of unanticipated death or major permanent loss of function associated with a health care–associated infection.
NPSG.07.03.01	Implement evidence-based practices to prevent health care–associated infections due to multiple drug–resistant organisms in acute care hospitals.
NPSG.07.04.01	Implement best practices or evidence-based guidelines to prevent central line–associated bloodstream infections.
NPSG.07.05.01	Implement best practices for preventing surgical site infections.
Goal 8	**Accurately and completely reconcile medications across the continuum of care.**
NPSG.08.01.01	A process exists for comparing the patient's current medications with those ordered for the patient while under the care of the organization.
NPSG.08.02.01	When a patient is referred or transferred from one organization to another, the complete and reconciled list of medications is communicated to the next provider of service and the communication is documented. Alternatively, when a patient leaves the organization's care directly to his or her home, the complete and reconciled list of medications is provided to the patient's known primary care provider, or the original referring provider, or a known next provider of service.
NPSG.08.03.01	When a patient leaves the organization's care, a complete and reconciled list of the patient's medications is provided directly to the patient, and the patient's family as needed, and the list is explained to the patient and/or family.
NPSG.08.04.01	In settings where medications are used minimally, or prescribed for a short duration, modified medication reconciliation processes are performed.
Goal 9	**Reduce the risk of patient harm resulting from falls.**
NPSG.09.02.01	The organization implements a fall reduction program that includes an evaluation of the effectiveness of the program.
Goal 10	**Reduce the risk of influenza and pneumococcal disease in institutionalized older adults.**
NPSG.10.01.01	The organization develops and implements protocols for administration of the flu vaccine.
NPSG.10.02.01	The organization develops and implements protocols for administration of the pneumococcus vaccine.
NPSG.10.03.01	The organization develops and implements protocols to identify new cases of influenza and to manage outbreaks.
Goal 11	**Reduce the risk of surgical fires.**
NPSG.11.01.01	The organization educates staff, including licensed independent practitioners who are involved with surgical procedures and anesthesia providers, on how to control heat sources, how to manage fuels while maintaining enough time for patient preparation, and establish guidelines to minimize oxygen concentration under drapes.
Goal 13	**Encourage patients' active involvement in their own care as a patient safety strategy.**
NPSG.13.01.01	Identify the ways in which the patient and his or her family can report concerns about safety and encourage them to do so.
Goal 14	**Prevent health care–associated pressure ulcers (decubitus ulcers).**
Goal 15	**The organization identifies safety risks inherent in its patient population.**
NPSG.15.01.01	The organization identifies patients at risk for suicide.

Table 2-1.	**2009 NATIONAL PATIENT SAFETY GOALS—CONT'D**
Goal 16	**Improve recognition and response to changes in a patient's condition.**
NPSG16.01.01	The organization selects a suitable method that enables health care staff members to directly request additional assistance from a specially trained individual(s) when the patient's condition appears to be worsening.
Universal Protocol	**The organization meets the expectations of the Universal Protocol.**
UP.01.01.01	Conduct a preprocedure verification process.
UP.01.02.01	Mark the procedure site.
UP.01.03.01	A time-out is performed immediately prior to starting procedures.

Modified from The Joint Commission: *Patient safety.* Retrieved August 15, 2008, from http://www.jointcommission.org/patientsafety/nationalpatientsafetygoals.

VALIDATION OF KNOWLEDGE THROUGH CERTIFICATION

One means of validating emergency nursing knowledge is through certification. The opportunity for certification in a nursing specialty dates back to 1945, when the American Association of Nurse Anesthetists first initiated certification. Most certifications in nursing, however, were established within the last three decades. An increase in the number of nursing specialty organizations has been a major factor in the proliferation of nursing certifications.

Overview of Certification

The primary purpose of certification is to assure society that an individual has acquired a specific body of knowledge. The Board of Certification for Emergency Nursing (BCEN) identifies an additional purpose, which is to validate, based on predetermined standards, an individual's qualifications and knowledge for practice in a defined functional or clinical area of nursing.[7]

Consequently, the certification process benefits both the individual nurse and the employer while serving society's interest. Achieving certification may lead to greater respect from employers and colleagues, salary increases, and perhaps greater self-esteem and a sense of professional pride. Employers and potential employers also benefit from nursing certification. Certification provides an objective measure of an employee's knowledge base, as well as valuable information about prospective employees.

The nursing profession as a whole benefits from certification. Because of the certification process, bodies of specialty nursing knowledge are defined and examined. Certification demonstrates to other health care disciplines that nurses are able to articulate a defined body of knowledge and establish levels of specialty competence based on that knowledge. An individual's preparation for the certification examination also benefits nursing. Successful certification requires thorough study of the body of knowledge of the specialty. Certification renewal encourages the practicing nurse to remain current in all aspects of specialty nursing practice.

There are three ways to obtain certification. One method is certification by a state or government agency. State certification represents legal endorsement of a nurse's ability to function in certain expanded nursing roles. Certification by a state usually refers to a specific aspect of nursing practice beyond the level addressed in a state board examination for registration. State certification is often based on prior certification by a nurse certification body, completion of an educational program, or both. In some instances a certifying examination is administered by a state agency. Requirements for state certification vary, so certification by one state may not be recognized by another. Examples of state certifications include emergency communications registered nurse (ECRN), mobile intensive care nurse (MICN), and trauma nurse specialist (TNS).

Certification may also occur through an institution. The institution may be a health care facility or an educational system. This type of certification is usually based on successful completion of an educational offering, often varying in length and characteristics. Most often the state or profession does not control content or requisites for such certification. Because of program variability and lack of oversight by a national body, this type of certification may have limited appeal or applicability outside the particular certifying institution.

The most common way to obtain certification in a nursing specialty is through a professional organization. Many types of certifications are offered by the American Nurses Credentialing Center (ANCC). Most nursing specialty organizations have also developed, or are in the process of developing, a certification process in their specialty. These efforts are testimony to the belief that knowledge beyond the level of safe basic nursing practice is required for specialty nursing practice.

Specialty Certification

Nursing certification organizations have various requirements for certification and renewal of certification. Requirements for nursing specialty certification may have the following categories: education, practice, demonstration of knowledge, and renewal mechanisms.

All nursing specialty certification organizations require that candidates be registered nurses. This requirement assumes successful completion of the initial licensure examination of nursing. Some specialties require a bachelor's degree as the minimum for certification eligibility; certification in emergency nursing (CEN) does not. Completion of a master's degree is a requirement for initial eligibility for ANCC's advanced practice certification examinations. The ANCC and other certifying organizations also require specific courses and clinical experience for certifications such as clinical nurse specialist, nurse practitioner, and nurse midwife. Some certifications have practice requirements in addition to educational requirements. To be eligible to take the certification examination, the nurse must have spent a minimum number of hours in specialty practice. In areas such as emergency nursing certification, the practice component of the certification process is a strong recommendation, rather than a requirement.

For initial certification, all nursing specialty certifications require the applicant to demonstrate mastery of the body of specialty nursing knowledge by written examination. Certification examinations vary in length and format, but all are sufficient to broadly examine the applicant's knowledge base in the specialty. Written examinations (including computer-based examinations) provide the most objective measure of mastery of core knowledge of the specialty. Practical or psychomotor examinations measure the application and attainment of requisite knowledge; however, most certifying agencies find these examinations too cumbersome to conduct with the consistency, objectivity, and integrity necessary for the examination process.

The final component of the certification process common to all is the renewal of certification. In nearly all cases, certification is granted for a limited time, with the usual range 3 to 5 years. This finite period of certification recognizes the dynamic and evolving state of nursing knowledge. Thus the certified nurse's continued mastery of the knowledge base of the specialty must be verified at regular intervals. The mechanism by which certification is renewed varies with the certifying body. Some require candidates to retake the examination, whereas others choose mandatory continuing education hours. Possible approaches to renewal of certification have broadened considerably in the past several years with such options as portfolio and open-book examinations. Regardless of the method used, the purpose of recertification is to ensure competence.

Emergency Nursing Certification

The first emergency nursing certification examination was administered in 1980. The examination was composed of 250 questions, all of which were calculated into the score. The correct number necessary for a passing score and certification was consistent at 175. Over time, the certification examination has evolved into a more sophisticated measure of emergency nursing knowledge. All question-and-answer sets are now pretested on actual examinations for accuracy, clarity, and reliability before inclusion into the test bank. This process tests the validity and reliability of the proposed certification examination questions. Items being pretested

are not included in scoring of the examination. Currently each examination contains 25 pretest items and 150 scored items. The American Board of Nursing Specialties (ABNS) has 17 standards that must be met for a certification to be accredited. In February 2002, ABNS approved the CEN certification for accreditation.

Examination Content for Certification in Emergency Nursing

To ensure the certification examination reflects current emergency nursing practice, three role delineation studies (RDS) have been completed by the BCEN. The first RDS was conducted from 1989 to 1990. Analysis of that study's findings indicated considerable concurrence between content of the emergency nursing certification examination and emergency nursing practice. Changes were made so the examination closely reflected information from the RDS. A second RDS in 1994 found a high degree of consistency between emergency nursing practice and certification examination content. The most recent RDS was completed at the end of 2006 with similar results.

Minor adjustments to the content blueprint for the certification examination have been made over time as a result of practice changes reflected in the analysis of responses to the latest RDS and changes made in the examination process. The blueprint for the examination is based on clinical categories and is summarized in Table 2-2. Within each of those categories, questions may focus on aspects of assessment, analysis/diagnosis, intervention, or evaluation.

Certification and Renewal

The BCEN is responsible for receiving and approving all applications for the CEN examination. Successful examination candidates will receive a card and certificate that are valid for 4 years. These individuals may use the certification mark

Table 2-2. CEN EXAMINATION CONTENT AREAS BY NUMBER OF ITEMS

Number of Items	Content Area
21	Cardiovascular tasks
9	Gastrointestinal tasks
10	Genitourinary, gynecologic, obstetric tasks
6	Maxillofacial/Ocular tasks
15	Neurologic tasks
13	Orthopedic/Wound tasks
6	Psychologic/Social tasks
18	Respiratory tasks
9	Patient care management tasks
10	Substance abuse/Toxicologic/Environmental tasks
11	Shock/Multisystem tasks
15	Medical emergency tasks
7	Professional issue tasks

CEN, Certification in emergency nursing.

"CEN." Unsuccessful candidates are eligible to reapply for the examination 3 months after the initial date of testing. CEN certification renewal may be achieved by one of three different options: (1) examination—successfully passing the computer-based test offered through the network of testing centers, (2) continuing education—submitting a log listing 100 continuing education hours with a minimum of 75 hours of clinical content, or (3) Internet-based testing—successfully passing the online test with 150 multiple-choice questions following the outline of the CEN examination. More information on CEN certification, as well as the certified flight registered nurse (CFRN), the certified transport registered nurse (CTRN) certification, and the newly developed certified pediatric emergency nurse, is available at http://www.ena.org/bcen.

SUMMARY

Emergency nursing practices are congruent with nursing's humanistic approach to health care. Nursing has formally defined the scope of practice and specialization in the ANA social policy statement. Emergency nursing is one area of specialization in which specific clusters of phenomena of concern emerge. Some of these phenomena await further delineation and exploration by our profession. The practice of emergency nursing results in an empowerment of our discipline to significantly affect the health needs of society.

REFERENCES

1. American Nurses Association: *Nursing: a social policy statement*, Kansas City, Mo, 1980, The Association.
2. American Nurses Association: *Nursing's social policy statement*, Washington, DC, 1995, The Association.
3. American Nurses Association: *Nursing's social policy statement*, ed 2, Washington, DC, 2003, Nursesbooks.org.
4. American Nurses Association: *Nursing: scopes and standards of practice*, Silver Spring, Md, 2004, The Association.
5. Benner P: *From novice to expert: excellence and power in clinical nursing practice*, Reading, Mass, 1984, Addison-Wesley.
6. Donaldson SK, Crowley DM: The discipline of nursing, *Nurs Outlook* 26:113, 1978.
7. Emergency Nurses Association: *Board of Certification for Emergency Nursing*. Retrieved January 5, 2008, from http://www.ena.org/bcen.
8. Emergency Nurses Association: *ENA mission and values*. Retrieved July 25, 2008, from http://www.ena.org/about/mission.
9. Emergency Nurses Association: *ENA position statements*. Retrieved August 14, 2008, from http://www.ena.org/about/position.
10. Emergency Nurses Association: *Injury Prevention Institute*. Retrieved August 14, 2008, from http://www.ena.org/ipinstitute/institute.
11. Emergency Nurses Association: *Scope of emergency nursing practice*, Des Plaines, Ill, 1999, The Association.
12. Emergency Nurses Association: *Standards of emergency nursing practice*, Des Plaines, Ill, 1999, The Association.
13. Fawcett J: *Analysis and evaluation of conceptual models of nursing*, Philadelphia, 1984, Davis.
14. Nightingale F: *Notes on nursing: what it is and what it is not*, London, 1859, Harrison & Sons.
15. Spangler B: *Coalition building beyond intractability*. Retrieved August 14, 2008, from http://www.beyondintractability.org/essay/coalition_building.
16. Stevenson JS, Woods NF: Nursing science and contemporary science: emerging paradigms. In G. E. Sorensen (Ed.), *Setting the agenda for the year 2000: knowledge development in nursing,* Kansas City, Mo, 1986, American Academy of Nursing.
17. The Joint Commission: *Performance measurements*. Retrieved January 5, 2008, from http://www.jointcommission.org/performancemeasurement.

CHAPTER 3

Legal and Regulatory Constructs

Edith Ann Brous

Health care in the United States is shaped by complex regulation at all levels. Federal, state, and local laws govern practice. Administrative agencies and private organizations oversee professionals and health care organizations. In 1997 University of Rochester health economist Charles Phelps stated, "[T]he U.S. health care system, while among the most 'market oriented' in the industrialized world, remains the most intensively regulated sector of the U.S. economy."[37] This is certainly truer today as billions of dollars are spent on health care regulation.[16] Indeed, it is claimed that the net burden of health services regulation exceeds what it would cost to provide coverage to the 44 million uninsured Americans.[16] Emergency nurses must understand the regulatory environment in which they work.

SOURCES OF LAW AND REGULATION

To prevent abuse and maintain a balance of power, the U.S. Constitution divides the federal government into three branches: the legislative branch to write laws,[47] the executive branch to execute laws,[48] and the judicial branch to interpret laws.[49] The legislative branch is Congress, divided into the House of Representatives and the Senate. The executive branch consists of the president and administration. The judicial branch is composed of the court systems. Each branch plays a constitutionally determined role in determining the law and is prevented from becoming too powerful by the checks and balances provided by the other two. Each state system mirrors that of the federal system with its governor, legislature, and court system.

At the federal level, Congress proposes laws that, once enacted, become statutes that are controlling throughout the nation. The statutes may be accompanied by federal funding, such as the Homeland Security Act or Medicare and Medicaid, or they may be "unfunded mandates" such as the Emergency Medical Treatment and Active Labor Act (EMTALA) and the Health Insurance Portability and Accountability Act of 1996 (HIPAA). State legislatures propose and enact state laws in the same manner.

The president and governors are responsible for enforcing the laws, and such enforcement is performed in large part through administrative agencies. Often referred to as the "fourth branch of government" because of their considerable political power, administrative agencies promulgate, interpret, and enforce agency rules and, as such, have quasi-executive, quasi-legislative, and quasi-judicial authority.

Federal agencies such as the Centers for Medicare and Medicaid Services (CMS) (formerly called the Health Care Financing Administration, or HCFA), the Occupational Safety and Health Administration (OSHA), the National Labor Relations Board (NLRB), and the Food and Drug Administration (FDA) are responsible for oversight of issues

Type of Law	Source or Origin	Content or Focus	Examples
Supreme law	U.S. Constitution	Individual rights Checks and balances of authority	Right to free speech Balance of powers HIPAA
Statute	Congress or state legislature	Focus varies but state law cannot be less stringent than federal law	State privacy laws
Common law	Judicial branch	Judge-interpreted laws that evolve as society and its laws change—case law	Individual lawsuits
Regulations	Executive branch of federal and state government Administrative agencies	Enforce federal and state laws	CMS—EMTALA State boards of nursing—professional licensure

Table 3-1. SOURCES OF LAW AND REGULATION

CMS, Centers for Medicare and Medicaid Services; *EMTALA*, Emergency Medical Treatment and Active Labor Act; *HIPAA*, Health Insurance Portability and Accountability Act.

that affect emergency departments (EDs). At the state level, state licensing boards, state health departments, offices of the attorney general, and child protective services are examples of state agencies regulating many issues that affect emergency nursing.

The judicial system is divided into federal and state courts. The federal courts resolve disputes regarding federal law or the U.S. Constitution and are divided into district courts sitting in each state. Each district court's decisions may be appealed to one of 10 respective circuit courts. The U.S. Supreme Court is the final authority for circuit court conflicts.[50] Again, the state systems mirror that of the federal system, with trial, appellate, and final appeals courts. State courts hear disputes regarding state laws, including civil cases such as medical malpractice (Table 3-1).

COMMUNICATION

The mission of Department of Health and Human Services (HHS) is to improve the health and well-being of all people affected by its programs. The Office for Civil Rights (OCR), is responsible for ensuring that people have equal access and opportunity to participate in and receive services from all HHS programs without facing unlawful discrimination and that the privacy of their health information is protected while ensuring access to care. OCR safeguards federal funds by ensuring that HHS-financed programs do not support unlawful discrimination.

Among others, OCR enforces Title VII of the Civil Rights Act of 1964, prohibiting discrimination on the basis of race, color, and national origin; Section 504 of the Rehabilitation Act of 1973, prohibiting discrimination on the basis of disability by recipients of financial assistance; and Title II of the Americans with Disabilities Act as it applies to health and human service activities of state and local governments.[19]

OCR requires hospitals to communicate effectively with patients, family members, and visitors who are deaf or hard-of-hearing and to take reasonable steps to provide meaningful access to their programs for persons who have limited English proficiency. These laws are further supported by Joint Commission standards, which also require hospitals to collect information about patients' language and communications needs.

Under OCR guidelines EDs must (1) promptly assess the communication needs of deaf and hard-of-hearing patients, (2) secure the services of qualified interpreters as quickly as possible, and (3) use other aids to augment effective communication with deaf and hard-of-hearing patients.[34] "Qualified sign language interpreter," "oral interpreter," or "interpreter" means a person who is able to interpret competently, accurately, and impartially, both receptively and expressively, using any specialized terminology necessary for effective communication in a medical setting to a deaf or hard-of-hearing patient or companion. Use of volunteers or family members as translators may not meet the required standards *and may violate privacy laws.*

For patients with limited English proficiency (LEP), hospitals must (1) assess the language needs of the population, (2) write policies addressing language access, (3) train staff in the policies, and (4) oversee the language assistance program.[34] The Department of Justice (DOJ) has specifically defined appropriate auxiliary aids and services and outlined services for which interpreters are deemed critical.[43] They are listed in Box 3-1.

Patients who think the hospital has violated antidiscrimination laws can make formal complaints to the DOJ. The DOJ investigates complaints and can file enforcement lawsuits in federal court. Alternatively, the DOJ can negotiate settlement agreements for corrective action plans and assess financial penalties. A noncompliant hospital can be fined up to $55,000 for a first violation and up to $110,000 for subsequent violations. In addition, a hospital may be ordered to pay damages to the complainant.[21]

MEDICAL RECORDS

In addition to communication among providers, written records of patient care are kept to meet legal, regulatory, managed care, and billing requirements. In the event of

<table>
<tr><td>

Box 3-1 CIRCUMSTANCES UNDER WHICH INTERPRETERS ARE REQUIRED

The following list of circumstances is neither exhaustive nor mandatory and shall not imply that there are not other circumstances when it may be appropriate to provide interpreters for effective communication or that an interpreter must always be provided in these circumstances.

- Determination of a patient's medical history or description of ailment or injury
- Provision of patients' rights, informed consent, or permission for treatment
- Determination and explanation of patient's diagnosis or prognosis and current condition
- Explanation of procedures, tests, treatment, treatment options, or surgery
- Religious services and spiritual counseling
- Explanation of living wills or powers of attorney (or their availability)
- Diagnosis or prognosis of ailments or injuries
- Explanation of medications prescribed (such as dosage, instructions for how and when the medication is to be taken, and side effects or food or drug interactions)
- Determination of any condition or allergy of patient that may affect choice of medication
- Explanation regarding follow-up treatments, therapies, test results, or recovery
- Blood donations or apheresis (removal of blood components)
- Discharge planning and discharge instructions
- Provision of mental health evaluations, group or individual therapy, counseling and other therapeutic activities, including but not limited to grief counseling and crisis intervention
- Explanation of complex billing or insurance issues that may arise
- Educational presentations, such as classes concerning birthing, nutrition, cardiopulmonary resuscitation, and weight management
- Any other circumstance in which a qualified sign language interpreter is necessary to ensure a patient's rights provided by law

</td></tr>
</table>

a malpractice lawsuit, the medical record is also used as evidence of the care provided.

ED records must be legible and clearly demonstrate the chronology of treatment. Every entry must be dated, timed, and signed. Dates must be complete, including the year; times must be complete, including military time or AM/PM; signatures must be complete and include status—RN, LPN, etc. Triage notes must indicate level of distress and duration of complaint to justify classification.

Providers must be identified by last name. Entries such as "MD aware," "supervisor notified," and "report to floor" do not adequately indicate that information has been transmitted. Policy and procedure manuals must reflect current practice and provide guidance in documentation methods.

Chart audits should be performed on a regular basis to ensure compliance with regulatory standards and best documentation practices. Abbreviations are error prone and should be restricted to those on the institution's approved list. Those that are specifically on the "Do Not Use" list must be avoided completely.

Electronic Medical Records

The use of electronic medical records (EMRs), electronic health records (EHRs), or electronic data interchange (EDI) allows organizations to meet regulatory standards and patient needs more effectively than traditional paper systems. The Joint Commission has been recommending the adoption of EMR since 1996.[27] Interoperable systems streamline information flow, reduce medical errors, eliminate illegibility, allow EDs to be compliant with regulatory and Joint Commission standards, facilitate data collection for quality improvement, interconnect clinical data, provide biosurveillance capability, and save provider time.[14] They may also reduce health care costs, enhance liability protection, and inform clinical practice.[15]

Compared with other industries, health care has been slow to adopt electronic, computerized systems. On May 6, 2004, President Bush appointed Dr. David J. Brailer to a newly created position of national coordinator for health information technology (HIT) and charged him with achieving widespread deployment of electronic HIT within 10 years. In a December 2004 address to the American Medical Association, Dr. Brailer advised, "[T]he answer for health care is the same as it is for every other industry. Information, automation, and standardization can support the central role of the consumer and the professional."[33]

In his February 2005 address to the Healthcare Information and Management Systems Society (HIMSS), Dr. Brailer stated, "[W]ithout EHRs in place, there is little chance of gaining significant improvements in quality and cost-effectiveness and of unifying the clinical process around the consumer."[10] He articulated four goals: (1) inform clinical practice, (2) interconnect clinicians, (3) personalize care, and (4) improve population health.

Implementation of an EMR requires careful planning and involvement of the institution's HIPAA compliance officer to address privacy concerns, as discussed below. Frontline personnel are crucial in the planning stages, because the expertise of the end users is necessary in design. It may be necessary to phase in the system with flexible implementation timelines. Significant time may be required for education because productivity can be affected by long learning curves. Staff readiness should be carefully assessed before going live with the EMR system. Postimplementation assessment is necessary to detect problems, revise the system, and support staff.

In a press release issued August 27, 2007, the Health Resources and Services Administration (HRSA) announced $31.4 million in grants to assist health centers with implementing EHRs and other HIT goals.[18] In an interview with

HealthCare Financial Management, Dr. Brailer said, "[T]he electronic health record is losing a little ground as being optional. It's becoming necessary. The evidence that it improves health status, reduces errors, and improves patient safety is so overwhelming that it's very hard to say to your customers, your insurers, your market, and your hospital leader that you're not going to do this."[9]

Whether using traditional paper systems or EMR, the ED records are hospital property, but patients have the right to review and make copies of their own charts and to make corrections in the records.[7] Each hospital must have a policy and procedure for responding to patient requests for their records.

HEALTH INSURANCE PORTABILITY AND ACCOUNTABILITY ACT

Congress had concerns about health care fraud and abuse, the portability of health insurance, and the potential for compromising patient privacy regarding personal medical information through the use of electronic media for collecting claims data and payments. In response to these concerns, Congress enacted the Health Insurance Portability and Accountability Act of 1996 on August 21, 1996.

HIPAA required HHS to develop rules for ensuring standardization of electronic patient health information, including administrative and financial data; unique health identifiers for individuals, employers, health plans, and health care providers; and security standards protecting the confidentiality and integrity of "individually identifiable health information," past, present, or future.

Pursuant to HIPAA's mandate, HHS was to promulgate rules to be effective in February of 1998 with compliance required by 2000. The rules underwent many revisions, however, and the final version of the privacy regulations was not issued until December 2000. They went into effect on April 14, 2001, with compliance not required until April 14, 2003.

HIPAA's privacy regulations require that covered entities protect personal health information (PHI) from disclosure and that access to PHI be limited to authorized entities with access restricted to the information necessary. Covered entities are health care providers conducting certain transactions in electronic form, health care clearinghouses, and health plans.

HIPAA provides patients with the right to access and make changes in their medical records while restricting access by others. Patients also have the right to information regarding how their records have been accessed. Formal notices of an institution's privacy practices are required. In addition, covered entities are required to assign a privacy officer who is responsible for administering the institutional privacy program and ensuring compliance. Covered entities are also required to educate all workers on privacy policies and procedures and to discipline infractions of those policies and procedures.

Hospitals are required to update their systems so PHI is protected. When instituting EMR, it is necessary to design computerized systems in a manner that limits medical record access to authorized persons. Password protection or data encryption may be necessary. Policies and procedures must be developed to protect e-mailed and faxed data. The Federal Communications Commission requires every page of every facsimile to have identifying information, including name of the business sending the fax, the date, the time, and the telephone number of the sending machine.[8] Computers should have the hard drives reformatted before recycling to prevent the inadvertent transmission of PHI. Confidentiality statements should be included in all e-mail or fax transmissions. Security measures must be instituted to verify users.

HIPAA does not create a private right of action, meaning that patients cannot directly sue providers for HIPAA violations.[23] The law does create both criminal and civil sanctions, however, for improper use or disclosure of PHI. Patients may make formal complaints to OCR. OCR reviews evidence about the complaint and may determine that there was no Privacy Rule violation. If the evidence indicates that there was a violation, OCR attempts to resolve the complaint by obtaining voluntary compliance, a corrective action plan, or a resolution agreement.

OCR may refer complaints to the DOJ for criminal investigation in cases involving the knowing disclosure or obtaining of PHI. Noncompliant organizations can be fined up to $100 per violation and up to $25,000 in a calendar year.[5] "Knowingly" obtaining or disclosing PHI can lead to fines up to $50,000, as well as 1 year in prison. Using false pretenses to commit offenses can allow for penalties up to $100,000 in fines and up to 5 years in prison. Committing offenses with the intent to sell, transfer, or use PHI for commercial advantage, personal gain, or malicious harm can allow for fines of $250,000 and up to 10 years in prison.[41]

Between April 14, 2003, when the law went into effect, and July 31, 2007, a total of 29,276 complaints were made, 79% of which were resolved. There have only been four criminal prosecutions since the law went into effect.[44] The compliance issues investigated most frequently were impermissible uses and disclosures of PHI, lack of safeguards of PHI, lack of patient access to PHI, uses or disclosures of more than the minimum necessary PHI, and lack of or invalid authorizations for uses and disclosures of PHI.

Confusion and misinterpretation of the Privacy Rule have resulted in the inappropriate withholding of information.[35,45] HIPAA does not prohibit the disclosure of PHI in all circumstances and explicitly allows disclosure when required by law and for health oversight, law enforcement, crime reporting, military and veterans' activities, national security and intelligence activities, organ and tissue donation, abuse and neglect reporting, judicial and administrative proceedings, public health surveillance, public health and safety, public benefits programs, treatment, payment, health care fraud reporting, health plan audits, health care operations, and certain research purposes.[6]

The U.S. Constitution specifically dictates that when there is conflict between federal and state law, federal law prevails when preemption is the clear and manifest purpose of Congress.[38] As federal law, HIPAA supersedes state privacy statutes. However, HIPAA only establishes minimum privacy protections and outlines basic principles for protecting PHI while recognizing that state law may impose more stringent requirements. State privacy laws are not preempted by HIPAA when the state law offers greater privacy protection or when the state law requires reporting.[4]

CONSENT

The law recognizes that an adult with intact mental capacity has the right to be autonomous in making health care decisions and to be free from unauthorized touching. To that end, providers must provide patients with adequate information to make informed decisions. Informed consent means the patient understands the risks, benefits, and alternatives to the proposed treatment. The patient has been given the opportunity to ask questions, and those questions have been answered to the patient's satisfaction. Consent forms should be designed to indicate this understanding. Patients should not be given consent forms to sign that contain blanks or are undated. Generally the emergency physician is responsible for explaining risks, benefits, and alternatives, although nurses may be called upon to witness the patient's signature. In the absence of consent, treatment may be considered assault or battery even if clinically appropriate.

Generally, if the patient is an unemancipated minor, consent must be obtained from the minor's parents or legal guardians. Other responsible adults, such as school officials acting with parental permission or child welfare authorities, may have legal authority to authorize treatment for minors. Simply being underage, however, does not always indicate that an individual lacks legal capacity to consent to medical treatment. The law also recognizes that minors are often mature enough to understand the implications of their health care decisions and that fear of parental retaliation may delay or prevent necessary treatment. As such, there are exceptions to the need for parental consent in the treatment of minors. These exceptions include emancipated minors, mature minors, and emergency situations.

An emancipated minor is considered an adult for consent purposes and may authorize treatment without parental consent or notification. Each state identifies criteria for emancipation, but general considerations include marital status, membership in the armed forces, living apart from one's parents, financial independence, pregnancy/parenthood, etc. In addition, a minor may be certified as emancipated by a court. This judicial certification emancipates the minor as a matter of law.

The "mature minor doctrine" exists in some states either by statute or court decisions. The doctrine states that providers can provide treatment in the absence of parental consent to minors who are mature enough to appreciate the consequences of their actions and exercise the judgment of an adult. The physician makes determinations on a case-by-case basis that the minor is mature enough to understand the risks associated with consenting to or refusing to consent to treatment.

In the absence of emancipation, minors may still be allowed to consent to some testing and treatment without parental consent or notification. The laws differ in each state, and the ED nurse must be aware of the law in the state in which he or she practices. Many states allow minors to be tested and/or treated for sexually transmitted infections, human immunodeficiency virus (HIV), communicable diseases, contraception, pregnancy, abortion, vaccinations, alcohol or chemical dependency, and mental health services without parental notification. Indeed, parental notification may violate the patient's privacy rights.

The doctrine of implied consent removes liability for the treatment of life-, limb-, or organ-threatening conditions.[38] In an emergency situation an incapacitated person or minor may be treated under the assumption that a reasonable person would consent to care. Second opinions regarding the need for immediate intervention may provide further protection. Court orders for treatment may be obtained when time permits.

In *In Re Estate of Allen*,[25] Ms. Allen was arrested for driving under the influence of drugs and taken by the police to the hospital. Although she did consent to treatment, she did not consent to a toxicology screen. The ED physician determined she was incompetent to withhold consent and ordered that blood and urine be obtained by force. When she brought a claim against the hospital for battery, the hospital claimed it was acting under the doctrine of implied consent. The court held that, ". . . [T]here are four essential elements required to establish that the common-law emergency exception applies: (1) there was a medical emergency; (2) treatment was required in order to protect the patient's health; (3) it was impossible or impractical to obtain consent from either the patient or someone authorized to consent for the patient; and (4) there was no reason to believe that the patient would decline the treatment, given the opportunity to consent." The court remanded the case for trial, finding that there was an issue as to whether or not it was impossible or impractical to obtain consent from someone else on Allen's behalf.

Parents may not refuse life-, limb-, or organ-saving treatment on behalf of their children for religious reasons. In 1944 the United States Supreme Court held, "[P]arents may be free to become martyrs themselves. But it does not follow they are free, in identical circumstances, to make martyrs of their children before they have reached the age of full and legal discretion when they can make that choice for themselves."[40]

Adults without capacity are unable to consent to treatment. Capacity can be lacking from unconsciousness, altered consciousness, mental illness, or chemical influences. In the absence of an emergency, consent must be obtained from the next of kin, legal guardian, health care proxy, or person with durable power of attorney for health care decisions. Court orders can also be obtained for treatment. Psychiatric consultation can be helpful in determining capacity.

Advance directive information must be obtained upon admission and do-not-resuscitate requests honored. The Patient Self-Determination Act (PSDA) of 1990 requires Medicare and Medicaid providers to obtain advance directive information upon admission.[2] If health care proxies and living wills are available, a copy is requested for the chart. If not, the patient is offered the opportunity to discuss advance directives and assistance in preparing them.

PSDA also requires that the patient be given information about rights under state law, including the right to participate in and direct his or her own health care decisions, the right to accept or refuse medical or surgical treatment, the right to prepare an advance directive, and information on the provider's policies that govern the exercise of these rights. Institutions are prohibited from discriminating against patients without advance directives. Institutions are required to document patient information and provide staff and community education on advance directives.

EDs must have policies and procedures regarding consent for law enforcement evidence collections and photographs, as well as refusal of treatment and leaving against medical advice (AMA). Documentation for AMAs must include a discussion and the patient's understanding of the risks of leaving before formal discharge. Patients who elope, or leave the ED without informing providers that they are leaving, may need to be recalled, and the ED must have a policy for determining when this is necessary and how it is performed. EMTALA, discussed below, also mandates ED responsibilities with AMAs:

[V]oluntary Withdrawal. If an individual chooses to withdraw his or her request for examination or treatment at the presenting hospital, a hospital must perform the following: (1) offer the individual further medical examination and treatment within the staff and facilities available at the hospital as may be required to identify and stabilize an emergency medical condition; (2) inform the individual of the risks and benefits of such examination and treatment, and of the risks and benefits of withdrawal prior to receiving such examination and treatment; and (3) take all reasonable steps to secure the individual's written informed consent to refuse such examination and treatment. The medical record should contain a description of the examination, treatment, or both, if applicable, that was refused.[20]

EMERGENCY MEDICAL TREATMENT AND ACTIVE LABOR ACT

EMTALA is an amendment to the larger Consolidated Omnibus Budget Reconciliation Act (COBRA). Enacted in 1985, the statute was intended to address patient "dumping" or "economic triage" in which uninsured patients were refused care or transferred to other facilities while clinically unstable. As part of the U.S. Code governing Medicare, EMTALA is enforced by the CMS. "Participating hospitals" are those that have EDs and have provider agreements to

receive funding from HHS, although the statute expressly states that it applies to all patients whether eligible or not for Medicare benefits.[3]

EMTALA states that any patient who "comes to the emergency department" requesting "examination or treatment for a medical condition" must be provided with "an appropriate medical screening examination" to determine if he or she is suffering from an "emergency medical condition." If he or she is, the hospital must either provide the patient with treatment until he or she is stable or transfer the patient to another hospital as per the statute's directives. There are no restrictions on transferring patients without emergency medical conditions.

To transfer an unstable patient, the following criteria must be met: the transferring hospital has stabilized the patient to the extent possible within its capacity; the patient requires the services of the receiving facility; the medical benefits outweigh medical risks of transfer; the risk/benefit analysis is documented in a medical certificate by a physician; the receiving hospital has accepted the transfer and has the facilities and personnel to provide the necessary treatment; and the patient is escorted in transfer by all required equipment and personnel, as well as treatment records from the transferring hospital.

Physicians signing the medical certificate for transfer are subject to EMTALA's penalties if they knew or should have known that the benefits of transfer were in fact outweighed by the risks of transfer and in so knowing misrepresented the patient's condition or the ED's obligations under the law. On-call physicians who refuse to appear when called by the ED may also be liable under EMTALA and may subject the hospital to a penalty in the process.

Some courts have held that EMTALA does not apply just to EDs but requires an emergency medical screening examination be provided to an individual requesting emergency care, regardless of where he or she presents in the hospital.[39] In *McIntyre v Schick*[32] the plaintiff brought an EMTALA claim as part of a wrongful death action. The uninsured mother arrived at the birthing center of the hospital and, despite almost 12 hours of labor with nonreassuring fetal heart tones, was discharged to home. She returned 16 hours later and was transferred to another hospital for an emergency cesarean section. The baby died a few days after birth. In its defense, the transferring hospital claimed EMTALA did not apply because the mother did not present to the ED. The court ruled that her EMTALA claim could go forward, stating, "[T]he rationale behind the COBRA patient anti-dumping statute is not based upon the door of the hospital through which a patient enters, but rather upon the notion of proper medical care for those persons suffering medical emergencies, whenever such emergencies occur at a participating hospital. Indeed, it is a ridiculous distinction, one which places form over substance, to state that the care a patient receives depends on the door through which the patient walks."

Other courts interpret EMTALA's screening requirement as applying only to hospital EDs. In *Rodriguez v American*

International Insurance Company, et al,[26] a cyanotic 5-month-old infant with congenital cardiovascular defects was taken to the ED of a freestanding regional diagnostic and treatment center, not attached to a hospital. She was intubated in the ED and transferred to a medical center 7 hours later. She died after arriving at the medical center. The U.S. Court of Appeals for the First Circuit distinguished between hospitals and outpatient centers and held, "[I]t is clear that EMTALA does not apply to all health care facilities; it applies only to participating hospitals with emergency departments. Further, the screening requirement under EMTALA only applies to patients seeking treatment at the emergency room, not elsewhere in a hospital."

The statute prohibits examination and treatment delays caused by insurance inquiries. As such, many legal authorities advise the ED to triage patients before registration, thus avoiding the appearance of determining payer status before performing medical screening examinations. Similarly, medical screening examinations cannot be delayed in obtaining preauthorizations from managed care organizations (MCOs).

In 1997 the Balanced Budget Act prohibited ED preauthorization requirements for Medicare and Medicaid plans. In recognizing that the preauthorization requirements of MCOs were creating compliance problems with EMTALA, HSS stated in 1998, "[I]nvestigations of allegations of the anti-dumping statute violations across the country have persuaded the OIG [Office of the Inspector General] and HCFA that managed care patients may be at risk of being discharged or transferred without receiving a medical screening examination, largely because of the problems inherent in seeking 'prior authorization.'"[51]

The OIG's and HCFA's view of the legal requirements of the antidumping statute in this situation is as follows:

> Notwithstanding the terms of any managed care agreements between plans and hospitals, the anti-dumping statute continues to govern the obligations of hospitals to screen and provide stabilizing medical treatment to individuals who come to the hospital seeking emergency services regardless of the individual's ability to pay. While managed care plans have a financial interest in controlling the kinds of services for which they will pay, and while they may have a legitimate interest in deterring their enrollees from overutilizing emergency services, no contract between a hospital and a managed care plan can excuse the hospital from its anti-dumping statute obligations. Once a managed care enrollee comes to a hospital that offers emergency services, the hospital must provide the services required under the anti-dumping statute without regard for the patient's insurance status or any prior authorization requirement of such insurance.[20]

Hospitals with "specialized capabilities or facilities" such as burn units, shock-trauma units, neonatal intensive care units, or "regional referral centers" may not refuse to accept a transfer if they have the capacity to treat the patient; "the receiving hospital will be obligated to accept the transfer in most cases, so long as it has the ability to treat the patient and its capabilities exceed those of the referring hospital, even if only because of overcrowding or temporary unavailability of personnel."[3] Receiving hospitals must also report EMTALA violations when receiving patients transferred in unstable condition.[1]

Initially under EMTALA, hospital-owned ambulances were required to transport patients to that particular hospital, regardless of another hospital's proximity. In 2003 the regulations were amended to allow hospital-owned ambulances to transport patients to a different facility as long they are integrated within the emergency medical services (EMS). EMTALA allows hospitals to deny access to patients in non–hospital-owned ambulances while the ED is on diversion for staffing or facility inadequacies. Even if there has been radio or telephone contact with the ED, EMTALA does not consider the patient in a non–hospital-owned ambulance to have "come to the emergency department."

Monetary penalties for EMTALA violations differ, depending on hospital bed size. A hospital with 100 or more beds can be fined up to $50,000 per violation. Hospitals with fewer than 100 beds can be fined up to $25,000 per violation. More alarmingly, a hospital's Medicare provider agreement can be revoked regardless of size. Unlike HIPAA, EMTALA does allow for a civil right of action, meaning patients may directly sue hospitals for EMTALA violations. The statute establishes two types of "dumping" claims: "(1) failure to conduct an appropriate medical screening examination to determine the existence of an emergency medical condition, and (2) failure to stabilize the emergency condition or to provide an appropriate transfer."[42] There are no limits on such claims unless liability caps are established by state law. The statute of limitations for an EMTALA claim is 2 years. Courts have held that EMTALA's private right of action allows patients to sue hospitals but not individual physicians for EMTALA violations.[22, 28]

Notwithstanding contrary individual state law, hospitals are required to be compliant with EMTALA. In a 1994 case the court even held that this obliged the hospital to provide medically futile care. In *Matter of Baby K,* the court found that EMTALA required the hospital to intubate and mechanically ventilate an anencephalic infant. The Commonwealth of Virginia's medical ethics and standards of care recognized the treatment of anencephaly as futile and unethical, yet the U.S. Court of Appeals for the Fourth Circuit held that EMTALA's obligations prevailed. Despite recognizing that the infant "lacks a cerebrum, she is permanently unconscious. Thus, she has no cognitive abilities or awareness. She cannot see, hear, or otherwise interact with her environment" and that "aggressive treatment would serve no therapeutic or palliative purpose," the court interpreted EMTALA's requirements as being absolute and ruled that "stabilization of her condition requires the Hospital to provide respiratory support through the use of a respirator or other means necessary to ensure adequate ventilation. In sum, a straightforward application of the statute obligates the Hospital to provide respiratory support to Baby K when she arrives at the emergency department of the Hospital in respiratory distress and treatment is requested on her behalf."[31] Subsequent rulings have narrowly interpreted *Baby*

K to require stabilizing treatment only within the context of transfer.[39]

EDs must carefully screen for medical emergencies associated with intoxication and psychiatric illness.[13] Intoxication may mask head injuries, which must be ruled out. A psychiatric patient is considered stable for purposes of discharge under EMTALA when he or she is no longer considered to be a threat to himself or herself or others.[46]

Table 3-2 lists definitions of key EMTALA provisions as they are stated in the statute and have evolved through case law interpretation.

NEGLIGENCE AND MALPRACTICE

Negligence is the failure to act in a manner in which a reasonably prudent person would act in same or similar circumstances. Expert witnesses are generally not required in negligence lawsuits because reasonably intelligent laypeople are able to anticipate the consequences of negligent behavior. Negligence does require foreseeability. *In Lane v St. Joseph's Regional Medical Center*,[29] Mae Belle Lane was an ED patient. While she was sitting in the waiting room, a teenage boy struck her on her right arm and shoulder.

Table 3-2. KEY EMTALA PROVISIONS

Provision	Description/Definition
Participating hospitals	Hospitals with emergency departments and Medicare provider agreements.
Medical screening	Performed by a "qualified medical provider" as determined by hospital bylaws, policies, and procedures to determine if an emergency medical condition exists. **NOTE: Triage does not constitute a medical screening examination. Triage determines in what order a patient is seen by a physician, not if he or she is seen by one.**
Emergency medical condition	"A medical condition manifesting itself by acute symptoms of sufficient severity (including severe pain) such that the absence of immediate medical attention could reasonably be expected to result in— placing the health of the individual (or, with respect to a pregnant woman, the health of the woman or her unborn child) in serious jeopardy, serious impairment to bodily functions, or serious dysfunction of any bodily organ or part, or With respect to a pregnant woman who is having contractions— that there is inadequate time to effect a safe transfer to another hospital before delivery, or that the transfer may pose a threat to the health or safety of the woman or her unborn child."[2]
Stabilize	Provide treatment for emergency medical conditions to ensure, within a reasonable degree of medical certainty, that no material deterioration of the patient's condition is likely to result from the transfer or is likely to occur during the transfer. Provide treatment for patients in active labor until the infant and the placenta have been delivered.
Transfer	Movement, including discharge, of an individual outside a hospital's facilities at the direction of any person employed by or associated with the hospital. Does not include movement of a dead individual or an individual who leaves the facility without permission.
"Appropriate" transfer	The patient has been treated at the transferring hospital and stabilized as far as possible within the limits of its capabilities. The patient needs treatment at the receiving facility, and the medical risks of transferring him or her are outweighed by the medical benefits of the transfer; the weighing process as described above is certified in writing by a physician; the receiving hospital has been contacted and agrees to accept the transfer and has the facilities to provide the necessary treatment to him or her; the patient is accompanied by copies of his or her medical records from the transferring hospital; the transfer is effected with the use of qualified personnel and transportation equipment, as required by the circumstances, including the use of necessary and medically appropriate life support measures during the transfer. The receiving facility has available space, qualified personnel, and agrees to accept the patient in transfer.
Patient refusal	A hospital has met the requirement of a medical screening if: • It offers the patient further medical examination and treatment; • It informs the patient or another on his or her behalf "of the risks and benefits of the offered examination and treatment"; • The patient or person acting on his or her behalf refuses to consent to the examination and treatment; • The medical record contains a description of the examination and/or treatment which was refused; • The hospital must take all reasonable steps to secure the refusal in writing; and • The document signed by the patient states that the patient or person acting on his or her behalf has been informed "of the risks and benefits of examination or treatment."
Physician certification	A physician is required to certify that medical benefits outweigh the risks of the transfer. Certification must contain a summary of risks and benefits upon which certification is based.

Continued

Table 3-2.	KEY EMTALA PROVISIONS—cont'd
Provision	**Description/Definition**
Transfer records	All available medical records pertaining to the individual's emergency condition, including copies of the H&P, observation notes, preliminary diagnosis, results of diagnostic studies, treatment and response to treatment, informed written consent of the individual or his or her designated representative, written physician certification, name and address of any on-call practitioner who refused or failed to appear within a reasonable time to provide necessary stabilizing treatment after being requested to do so by the emergency physician or by the treating physician.
	Any records not available at the time of transfer are sent as soon as possible.
	Vital signs are recorded on the transfer form immediately before transfer.
Nondiscrimination	A participating hospital with specialized capabilities or facilities shall not refuse to accept an appropriate transfer of an individual who requires such specialized capabilities or facilities if the hospital has the capacity to treat the individual.
EMTALA statute of limitations	A claim must be brought within 2 years of the alleged violation.
Financial inquiries	A participating hospital may not delay appropriate medical screening examinations in order to inquire about the individual's method of payment or insurance status or to seek MCO preauthorization. Stabilization must begin before financial inquiries.

EMTALA, Emergency Medical Treatment and Active Labor Act; *H&P,* history and physical; *MCO,* managed care organization.

Table 3-3.	ELEMENTS OF NURSING MALPRACTICE
Element	**Description**
Duty	In a provider–patient relationship the nurse provides care as per professional standards.
Breach of duty	Departure from the standard of care, failure to act as a reasonably prudent nurse would act in same or similar circumstances.
Substantial factor	The nurse's departure from the standard of care was, more likely than not, a substantial factor in the patient's injury.
Proximate cause	The injury would not have occurred but for the departure from the standards of practice.
Damages	Compensation for physical, emotional, and/or financial losses, as well as pain and suffering. Punitive damages are allowed in some jurisdictions for particularly egregious or willful injuries.

The attack stopped when her son-in-law struck the teenager and knocked him to the floor. She suffered some injuries from the attack and sued the hospital for failing to protect her from the criminal acts of the teenager.

The Indiana Court of Appeals concluded, "[T]here can be little dispute that a hospital's emergency room can be the scene of violent and criminal behavior. Violent and intoxicated individuals, those involved in crimes, and people injured in domestic disputes are routinely brought to the emergency room for treatment. In some cases, the violence spills into the emergency room itself and measures must be taken to control the situation. . . . [A] duty to maintain protection for patients of an emergency room exists. Thus, the Center had the duty to implement and maintain reasonable measures to protect emergency room patients from criminal acts of third parties."

Unlike simple negligence, malpractice is a form of negligence that does require expert witness testimony because it pertains to professional standards. To successfully prosecute a medical or nursing malpractice claim, the plaintiff must establish four elements: duty, breach, proximate cause, and harm (Table 3-3). Expert witnesses are necessary to prove that the provider being sued departed from the standards of practice and that it is that departure which caused the injury. In some states, only nurses can testify as to the standard of practice for nursing. In other states, however, physicians can be used as "expert witnesses" for nursing practice.

Although most malpractice lawsuits are against physicians, surgeons, and institutions and not nurses, claims against nurses do occur. Common causes of lawsuits against emergency nurses include medication errors, failure to observe and report, failure to rescue, and falls. Emergency nurses are sued as employees of the hospital, and as such the hospital has vicarious liability for the nurse's action under a theory of liability called *respondeat superior.* Generally the employee must be acting within the normal course of employment and acting as an agent of the employer for the institution to be liable for his or her actions.

The plaintiff's expert uses multiple sources to determine the standards of practice. The policy and procedure manuals of the ED are routinely demanded as part of discovery. It is critical that the policy and procedure manuals be regularly updated to reflect current practice. Policies must be clear enough to provide guidance, yet flexible enough to allow compliance and be amended when practice standards change.

In *Hillcrest Baptist Med v Wade*,[24] a 38-year-old woman presented to the ED at 3:45 AM with complaints of a cough and chest pain. The triage nurse documented that she smoked a pack of cigarettes a day but did not document a positive family history of coronary artery disease. Approximately 30 minutes after the patient was triaged, another nurse assessed the patient but did not place her on a cardiac monitor. The ED physician did not evaluate her until 5:07 AM, and an electrocardiogram (ECG) was not performed until 5:26 AM. She was subsequently placed on a monitor, the hospital's acute myocardial infarction (AMI) protocol was initiated, and she was placed on a nitroglycerine drip, which relieved her pain. Cardiology did not examine her until 11:10 AM. A cardiac catheterization performed at 12:00 PM demonstrated 100% occlusion of the left anterior descending coronary artery. Angioplasty was performed and a stent inserted. Ms. Wade filed suit against the hospital, alleging negligence by its nursing staff. She claimed she had significantly impaired cardiac ejection fraction, required an implantable cardioverter/defibrillator, and would possibly require a heart transplant in the future.

The plaintiff's nursing expert stated that the triage nurse departed from the standard of care in not recognizing a possible AMI, placing the patient on a cardiac monitor, immediately performing an ECG, and notifying the physician. It was her opinion the treating nurse also departed from the standard of care in not requesting Cardiology.

The court stated, "[T]he care a patient receives in a hospital does not occur in a vacuum, but rather is a collaborative effort involving doctors, nurses, and other health care providers. There was at least a seven hour delay in Wade's receiving cardiology care. We believe that a delay is a delay. [Nursing's] expert report establishes that the specific conduct of Hillcrest's nursing staff that breached the accepted standards of nursing care delayed Wade from receiving necessary cardiology care. [Expert physician] reports establish that the delay in Wade's receiving necessary cardiology care resulted in permanent and severe compromise of her cardiac output function with a future heart transplant highly likely. These physician expert reports clearly established the pathophysiologic basis explaining the causal relationship between the delay in Wade's receiving cardiology care and her injuries."

In another failure to observe and report case, *Matheny v Fairmont General Hospital*,[30] Ronald L. Matheny presented to the ED complaining of right hip pain. While in the ED, his temperature rose 3 full degrees, but his diagnosis was limited to "hip injury/severe arthritis" and he was discharged. No attempt was made to determine the source of his fever or to treat it. When his condition worsened after discharge, he returned to the hospital and was admitted. He was diagnosed with a *Staphylococcus aureus* infection in his right hip. Because it had been untreated, it progressed into a serious abscess. He remained in the hospital for several days, suffering complications, and was left with very little function in his right hip and an inability to walk without a cane.

The lawsuit claimed that although the nursing staff had recorded the dramatic rise in temperature during his visit to the ED, nurses failed to alert a physician, thereby contributing to the failure to diagnose the infection and its progression to the very serious abscess stage. The jury returned a defense verdict, but this was appealed on grounds that the jury instructions were improper and the case was remanded for a new trial.

SUMMARY

In the regulatory and litigious environment in which ED nurses work, it is essential to stay abreast of the legal aspects of practice. Standards of practice evolve and require constant vigilance for the nurse to remain current. Fast-paced, rapidly changing practice settings are often stressful, and ED nurses are at high risk for compassion fatigue. The best liability protection, however, comes from interpersonal skills. Patients sue providers when they are angry, when they feel they have been treated without respect, or when they have been ignored in an impersonal, fragmented system. The nurse with good communication skills and the ability to make the patient feel dignity and human worth is less likely to be named in a lawsuit or reported to the board of nursing in a complaint.

REFERENCES

1. 42 CFR 489.20(m).
2. 42 USC 1395dd(a).
3. 42 USC 1395dd(g); 42 CFR 489.24(f).
4. 45 CFR Part 160, subpart B: Preemption of state law.
5. 45 CFR 160, subpart D: Imposition of civil money penalties.
6. 45 CFR 164.512: Uses and disclosures for which an authorization or opportunity to agree or object is not required.
7. 45 CFR 164.524: Access of individuals to protected health information.
8. 47 USC, chapter 5, subchapter II, part I, section 227: Restrictions on use of telephone equipment.
9. Bolster C: National health IT initiative moves into action: an interview with David Brailer, *Healthc Financ Manage* 59(7):92, 2005. Retrieved October 12, 2007, from http://findarticles.com/p/articles/mi_m3257/is_7_59/ai_n14817854.
10. Brailer D: *Remarks by David Brailer, MD, PhD, National Coordinator for Health Information Technology, HIMSS* 2005. Retrieved October 12, 2007, from http://www.providersedge.com/ehdocs/ehr_articles/David-BrailerRemarksHIMSS2005.pdf.
11. *Bryan v Rectors of the Univ of Virginia*, 95 F3d 349, 352 (4th Cir 1996).
12. *Bryant v Adventist Health Systems/West*, 289 F3d 1162 (9th Cir 2002).
13. *Carlisle v Frisbie Mem Hosp*, 888 A2d 405 (NH Sup 2005).
14. Committee on Quality of Health Care in America, Institute of Medicine: *To err is human: building a safer health system*, Washington, DC, 2000, National Academies Press.

15. Committee on Quality of Health Care in America, Institute of Medicine: *Crossing the quality chasm: a new health system for the 21st century*, Washington, DC, 2001, National Academies Press.
16. Conover C: *Testimony before the Committee on Health, Education, Labor and Pensions of the U.S. Senate at a Jan 28, 2004 hearing on what's driving health care costs and the uninsured?* Retrieved October 12, 2007, from http://jec.senate.gov/Documents/Hearings/conovertestimony13may2004.pdf.
17. *Delaney v Cade*, 986 F2d 387 (10th Cir 1993).
18. Department of Health and Human Services: *HRSA awards $31.4 million to expand use of health information technology at health centers*, August 27, 2007. Retrieved October 12, 2007, from http://newsroom.hrsa.gov/releases/2007/HITgrantsAugust.htm.
19. Department of Health and Human Services, Office for Civil Rights, Hospitals and Effective Communication. Retrieved October 12, 2007, from http://www.hhs.gov/ocr/hospitalcommunication.html#law.
20. Department of Health and Human Services Office of Inspector General and Health Care Financing Administration: *Solicitation of comments on the OIG/HCFA special advisory bulletin on the patient anti-dumping statute: notice of proposed special advisory bulletin*, November 24, 1998. Retrieved October 12, 2007, from http://www.emtala.com/oblig.txt.
21. *Department of Justice status report, July-September*, 2006. Retrieved October 12, 2007, from http://www.usdoj.gov/crt/ada/julysep06.pdf.
22. *Eberhardt v City of Los Angeles*, 62 F3d 1253 (9th Cir 1995).
23. *Fed Regist* 65(250):82566, December 28, 2000. Retrieved October 12, 2007, from http://www.hhs.gov/ocr/part3.pdf.
24. *Hillcrest Baptist Med v Wade*, 172 SW3d 55 (Tex App 10th Dist 2005).
25. *In Re Estate of Allen*, 365 Ill App3d 378, 386, 393 (2006).
26. *Joan Rodriguez; Domingo Diaz Rojas; Conjugal Partnership Diaz-Rodriguez v American International Insurance Company of Puerto Rico; Corporacion De Servicios Integrales De Salud Del Area De Barranquitas, Corozal, Naranjito Y Orocovis*, 402 F3d 45, 48 (1st Cir, 2005).
27. Joint Commission on Accreditation of Healthcare Organizations: *Information management/information technology standards*, Oakbrook Terrace, Ill, 1996, The Joint Commission.
28. *King of Ahrens*, 16 F3d 265 (8th Cir 1994).
29. *Lane v St. Joseph's Reg Med Center*, 817 NE2d 266, 273 (Ind App 2004).
30. *Matheny v Fairmont General Hospital*, 212 WVa 740 (2002).
31. *Matter of Baby K*, 16 F3d 590, 592 (4th Cir 1994).
32. *McIntyre v Schick, MD, and Virginia Beach General Hospital*, 795 F Supp 777, 782 (US Dist Ct, ED VA 1992).
33. Moran M: AMA urged to make electronic records policy priority, *Psychiatr News* 40(2), 2005. Retrieved October 12, 2007, from http://pn.psychiatryonline.org/cgi/content/full/40/2/1-b.
34. National Center for Law and Economic Justice: *Recent HHS Office of Civil Rights Guidance—assuring that those with limited-English proficiency have access to federally-funded programs*. Retrieved October 12, 2007, from http://www.nclej.org/key-issues-civil-rights-programs.php.
35. National Committee on Vital and Health Statistics: Letter to HSS, June 21, 2007. Retrieved October 12, 2007, from http://www.ncvhs.hhs.gov/070621lt1.pdf.
36. Patient Self-Determination Act of 1990, 42 USC 1395cc(a). Retrieved October 12, 2007, from http://www.fha.org/acrobat/Patient%20Self%20Determination%20Act%201990.pdf.
37. Phelps CE: *Health economics*, ed 2, 1997, Reading, Mass, Addison-Wesley, p 539.
38. Pozgar GD: *Legal aspects of health care administration*, ed 10, Boston, 2007, Jones & Bartlett.
39. *Preston v Meriter Hosp, Inc*, 271 Wis2d 721, 734 (2004), "We are not persuaded that *In re Baby 'K'* remains viable precedent in the Fourth Circuit.... Contrary to its ordinary meaning, the term 'to stabilize' in §13955dd(b)(1)(A) has a narrow definition that only applies in connection with the transfer of an emergency room patient."
40. *Prince v Massachusetts*, 321 US 158 (1944).
41. *Scope of criminal enforcement under 42 USC §1320d-6*, memorandum opinion for the General Counsel Department of Health and Human Services and the Senior Counsel to the Deputy Attorney General, June 1, 2005. Retrieved October 12, 2007, from http://www.usdoj.gov/olc/hipaa_final.htm.
42. *Scott v Dauterive Hosp*, 851 So2d 1152:1165. (La App 3 Cir, 2003.
43. *Settlement agreement between the United States and Norwegian American Hospital under the Americans with Disabilities Act*. Retrieved October 12, 2007, from http://www.ada.gov/norwegian.htm.
44. Smith DeWaall IC: Successfully prosecuting Health Insurance Portability and Accountability Act medical privacy violations against noncovered entities, *United States Attorneys's Bulletin* 55(4), 2007. Retrieved October 12, 2007, from http://www.usdoj.gov/usao/eousa/foia_reading_room/usab5504.pdf.
45. *The federal update, call for changes to FERPA and HIPAA in wake of Virginia Tech shootings*, June 15, 2007. Retrieved October 12, 2007, from http://www.cde.ca.gov/re/lr/ga/june1507.asp.
46. *Thomas v Christ Hosp and Medical Center*, 328 F3d 890, 893, (7th Cir 2003).
47. U.S. Constitution, art I, sec 1.
48. U.S. Constitution, art II, sec 1.
49. U.S. Constitution, art III, sec 1.
50. U.S. Constitution, art VI, cl 2.
51. http://www.oig.hhs.gov/fraud/docs/alertsandbulletins/patientdump.htm.

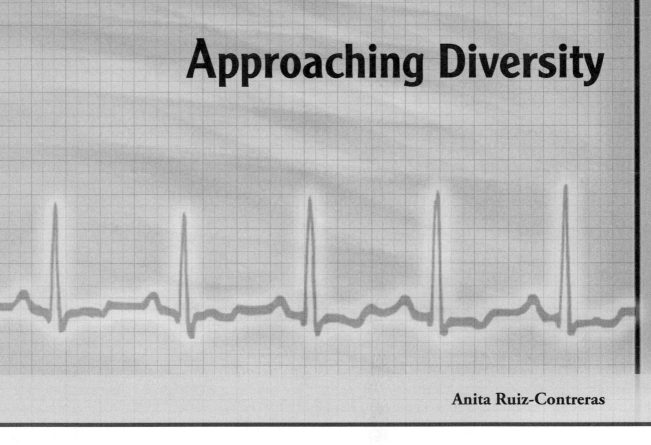

CHAPTER 4

Approaching Diversity

Anita Ruiz-Contreras

A s human beings, we are all diverse—each one of us is different from the other. As health care professionals, we care for patients who have recently arrived in this country and others whose families have been here for generations. We may or may not share attributes with our patients and fellow staff members. We may identify with a group that is not the dominant society. Many health care professionals have taken cultural sensitivity courses and learned basic information about different cultural or ethnic groups. Most likely, some of the learned information did not fit for all members of those groups. It is impossible to know everything about all the groups (patient populations) we serve. There is often as much diversity within groups as there is between them. Some individuals will identify closely with their country of origin or religion, whereas others will not. Health care professionals have an obligation to address and respect issues of diversity. A health care professional's response to a patient's individuality should not be one of shock or anger. There is always an opportunity to learn from patients and colleagues. As a way to begin, it is important for all health care professionals to examine their own beliefs and attitudes regarding diversity.

Diversity has been defined as the fact or quality of being diverse, differing one from another, made up of differences, or composed of distinct characteristics, qualities, and elements.[1] The Emergency Nurses Association Diversity Task Force defined diversity simply as the ways in which people differ.[1] These differences include invisible value and belief patterns, as well as characteristics such as age, class, culture, ethnicity, gender, nationality, race, religion, sexual orientation, and marginalization. It is important that health care professionals recognize and accept the differences in themselves and in us all.

AREAS OF DIVERSITY

When asking questions related to a patient's diversity, it is imperative to "ask the questions that need to be asked." These are questions that seek information needed to further assess the patient's condition and the patient's ability to complete the needed treatment. Questions that show a bias or that are derogatory can only hamper the patient-staff relationship. "Why" questions such as "Why are you homeless?" will not assist in determining if a patient can follow a plan of care or other needed treatment. Outlining the plan in a nonjudgmental, objective manner and enlisting the patient's help in ascertaining if the care plan is feasible based on his or her individual circumstances would be more beneficial.

A thorough patient assessment includes a diversity assessment. The diversity assessment seeks to identify the patient's language preference, information about who may assist the patient in decision making, and what the patient believes are his or her most pressing medical needs. During this assessment the health care professional should be keenly aware of the impact of nonverbal communication. Eye contact, personal space issues, and tone of voice may directly affect the ability of the patient to trust the health care professional. All the areas of diversity have unique characteristics that may or may not identify an individual patient as a member of that particular group.

Age

Age is a period of existence.[8] There are obvious anatomic, physiologic, and behavioral changes at every stage of life. The health care plan needs to be based on the impact of these stages and how these will affect the patient's response. The Joint Commission[4] requires hospitals and health care organizations to provide ongoing education, training, and competency validation to ensure safe and effective age-specific and culturally sensitive patient care.

Staff attitudes can affect the quality of care available to the older adult. The Age Discrimination Act of 1975 is a national law that prohibits discrimination on the basis of age in any program that receives federal financial assistance.[7]

Generational differences can explain a patient's need for care and reaction to that care. Advancing age is commonly associated with comorbidities; infants are completely dependent on caregivers for meeting their self-care needs. The older adult may have greater expectations of common courtesy, such as expecting staff members to knock before entering and to introduce themselves. Younger adults are more likely to be involved in traumatic events. When caring for pediatric patients, there can be increased anxiety within the family and staff.

Class

Class identifies a group of people whose members share the same attributes, such as social rank or socioeconomic status, and adhere to traditional roles and principles.[8] Socioeconomic status may have more to do with how individuals are judged by others than any other area of diversity. Socioeconomic status is a strong predictor of health. Race and culture are often blamed when socioeconomic status or poverty is actually the causative factor. Differences commonly seen with patients living in poverty directly affect access to care, transportation, and the ability to provide self-care when needed. Poverty is a fact of life for every racial/ethnic group.[6] Many people have come to the United States to escape war or long-time military rule. Poverty was the way of life in their home countries. They may arrive here with minimal resources or education.

Culture

Culture includes patterns of behavior and thinking that persons living in social groups learn and share.[1] Culture is closely related to the identified ethnic background. Culture may affect the way a patient responds to health concerns, such as in response to crisis or grief. Negative attributes

are often associated with being part of one's culture, when actually the effects of a lower socioeconomic status cause violence and/or criminal activities.

Culture is handed down from generation to generation. You may see one age-group that follows their parents' culture more closely than another, younger group might. Culture can also be self-identified. A patient may identify more with a culture because of an affinity for the group's traits. Asking open-ended questions about culture, without judgment, can aid in understanding.

Ethnicity

A person's ethnicity can be seen as a conscious choice of his or her identity based on beliefs, values, practices, and loyalty to a certain group or groups.[1] Ethnicity is generally related to heritage or country of origin of one's ancestors. An individual's ethnic identity may be an area of invisible diversity to someone not of that group. Statements such as "You don't look like someone from that ethnic group" are perceived as ignorant and unkind. Not all people from each group look alike. All ethnic groups have variations in skin color, hair color, and the color of their eyes. Some groups have pronounced features that may or may not be easily identified. There are, of course, many people whose mother and father come from different ethnicities. Such an individual may or may not identify with either or both groups. A patient's or staff member's last name may not be one normally identified as part of a particular ethnic group. It is also not appropriate to tell the patient or staff member that he or she has a name that does not "fit" for the group the person identifies with. If information about ethnicity is pertinent, the health care professional should ask open-ended questions without making initial assumptions. If the health care professional finds it necessary to identify a person according to his or her ethnicity, it is most appropriate to ask the patient what he or she prefers. Table 4-1 lists terms used by certain groups that may or may not be used as identifiers by all members of those groups.

Gender

Gender is a described identity, male or female.[1] This seems to be an easy question to answer, but it may not always be apparent. The use of a form that asks basic demographic information with a gender checkbox is helpful. Transgender patients identify with a gender other than the one that was applied to them at birth. Transgender patients may or may not have had reassignment surgery, but this does not change the fact that the patients identify their own gender. The name and gender the patient describes should be used as identifiers.

There continue to be stereotypic presentations that pertain to gender. A health care professional is less likely to expect a male sexual assault victim than a female. Heart disease can be misdiagnosed in women who do not present with the classic signs and symptoms. The health care professional needs to take into account gender issues and how they affect the care of a patient.

Table 4-1.   TERMS USED TO DESCRIBE GROUPS (ALWAYS ASK WHAT THE PERSON WOULD PREFER)

African-American	Black, African-American, Afro-American, colored (older people)
Arab	Arab, Middle Eastern, by country of origin *When asked about country of origin, some may respond with the city they were born in.*
Chinese	Chinese or Chinese American
Puerto Rican	Puerto Rican, Puertorriqueño(a), Boricua
Japanese	Japanese American
Mexican	Mexican, Mexican-American, Latino(a), Chicano(a) *Acculturated Mexican Americans may prefer American.*
American Indians	Tribal names are often used: Chippewa, Hopi, Seneed, Colulle, Native Americans, American Indians *Tribal affiliation names such as Navaho are not the real names.*
Vietnamese	Vietnamese (English speakers), ngŏi, Viet Nam *It is derogatory to use the term* refugee.

Data from Lipson JG, Dibble SL, editors: *Culture and clinical care,* San Francisco, 2005, UCFS Nursing Press

Sexual Orientation

Sexual orientation is one's identity based on sexual expression.[1] Health care professionals may unintentionally offend a gay or lesbian patient by assuming that he or she is heterosexual.[2] This would include assuming that a woman is possibly pregnant even though she states there is no chance of pregnancy. A better routine question when information about sexual activity is needed would be "Are you sexual with others—are they male, female, or both?"[2] All questions should be asked in an open, nonjudgmental manner.

Nationality

Nationality is defined as belonging to a particular nation by birth, family origin, or naturalization.[1] Nationality is often confused with race and ethnicity. In the United States, 10% of the population is foreign born.[6] The identified race and ethnic background may not have anything to do with the person's county of origin. Many people born in the United States identify with an ethnic background of their ancestors.

Race

Race is defined as a group of people united or classified together on the basis of common history, nationality, or geographic distribution.[6] Other definitions of race include characteristics that are visible and identifiable to that group. These definitions include skin color and facial feature similarities. There is much debate about what constitutes a race. Often race and ethnicity are used interchangeably.

Anthropologists in the seventeenth and eighteenth centuries proposed racial classifications based on observable characteristics such as skin color, hair type, body proportions, and skull measurements. The traditional terms for these populations are *Caucasoid, Mongoloid,* and *Negroid.* In certain circumstances the use of these terms is seen as offensive. Current-day anthropologists now consider race to be more a social construct than an objective biologic fact.

Religion

Religion is an organized or unorganized belief system.[1] Patients may identify a religion even if they do not actively participate in that religion. Staff should not impose their own religious beliefs but should take their cues from what the patient or family wishes. It is not uncommon for staff and patients to have religious beliefs in conflict. This is particularly true when the patient's religious belief prohibits the planned health intervention. Staff must remember that the patient has the right to consent or decline care even if his or her decision is not what the staff believes to be prudent. Issues where conflict may occur include use of contraception, organ donation, blood administration, and decisions regarding death. Staff members should discuss concerns they have with their management if there are religious issues that may affect their ability to care for certain patient groups. Managers should make provisions for staff to switch assignments or have another staff member care for that particular patient.

Marginalization

Individuals seen as possessing relatively little social power are of a marginalized status.[1] Hence these are people whose diversity is assumed to be "wrong" or "unworthy" by some members of the dominant society. Individuals who perform criminal acts or are incarcerated are often viewed as dispensable. Overweight individuals pose a challenge for health care professionals; the additional needs of the overweight patient can elicit ill feelings in staff members. A homeless person may be viewed as someone who chooses his or her lifestyle and thus is not deserving of services. Health care professionals may feel that a homeless patient misuses emergency services for non–health-care-related issues such as food or shelter. A patient with a history of mental illness may have difficulty articulating his or her medical concerns and therefore is categorized as just a "psych" patient. Frequently these patients are discharged or referred to psychiatric services only to return to the emergency department with a medical condition that was overlooked. A developmentally delayed individual may be seen as a difficult patient because of communication barriers and self-care issues. The patient's caregiver can be instrumental in assessing baseline status and the patient's ability to assist with the health care plan.

The impact of a marginalized status must be recognized. There needs to be an objective review of how the marginalized status affects the plan of care. The health care professional must examine any bias he or she may have and ensure that it does not negatively affect patient care.

THE DIVERSITY PRACTICE MODEL

There must be a realization that the delivery of quality health care includes an appreciation and respect for patient and staff diversity. Caring for diverse populations in a sensitive manner implies that there is recognition of differences and those individual differences are not seen as wrong or unworthy of respect.[3] Health care professionals should ask those questions that need to be asked because they are pertinent to the medical plan of care. These would be questions that further understanding and assist in formulating the patient care plan.

The Diversity Practice Model (Table 4-2) was developed by the Emergency Nurses Association Diversity Task Force to provide a framework to use when discussing diversity issues.[1] The model uses an ABCDE mnemonic to guide relevant ideas and questions.[1]

The Diversity Practice Model can be used to discuss sensitive issues or when presenting case review. Any staff member can initiate the Diversity Practice Model by saying, "Let's start with A." This acknowledges that there is an issue pertaining to a patient's or staff member's diversity that needs to be discussed. Table 4-3 contains the fundamental questions to ask when using the model. The model begins with staff examining their assumptions about the patient. Assumptions are ideas or thoughts, which may or may not be true and are usually based on little factual information. This is a time in the discussion to recognize that everyone makes assumptions. It is what we do with those assumptions and how they can negatively affect patient care that needs to be examined.

The model then moves to an examination of beliefs. Beliefs are long-held ideals and may be based on assumption. In the professional health care arena, facilities have belief statements or mission statements that outline the organizational

philosophy. These documents can be helpful to show how those initial assumptions may be incongruent with the beliefs of the organization. Generally there is a statement of the fundamental rights of patients and how they should be treated equally regardless of their diversity. In one example, we can look to the forefathers of the United States and relate the beliefs of the preamble of the Declaration of Independence: "We hold these truths to be self-evident, that all men are created equal, that they are endowed by their Creator with certain unalienable Rights, that among these are Life, Liberty and the pursuit of Happiness."[5]

If one believes that all men and women are created equal, then the standard of health care has to be the same for everyone. This belief, whether it be from a governmental document, a facility mission statement, or a group consensus, should override any implied negative assumptions.

The third step of the model involves a discussion of communication, which is the transfer of information from a sender to a receiver. It is imperative that we know if our communication has been received and understood. When obtaining informed consent, diversity issues need to be considered. Table 4-4 gives some general information on how different groups may approach consent.

A patient must have an avenue to ask questions, and in turn the patient must be able to understand the answers. The goal when discussing communication is to ensure that the patient understands the plan of care. In hospitals, certified translators should be used whenever a patient requests or a staff member determines that a translator is needed to facilitate communication. Translators should be trained and their fluency in the identified language(s) evaluated. When using a translator, the health care professional should always be present. The health care professional should direct his or her questions to the patient. Even if the words are not understood, a caring tone and professional manner of speech assist the patient in trusting the health care professional.

Table 4-2.	DIVERSITY PRACTICE MODEL	
A	Assumptions	The act of taking for granted or supposing that a thought or idea about a group is true.
B	Beliefs	Beliefs are shared ideas about how a group operates.
C	Communication	The two-way sharing of information that results in an understanding between the receiver and the sender.
D	Diversity	The ways in which people differ and the effect that these differences have on health perception and health care.
E	Education	The act of attaining knowledge about diversity.

Table 4-3.	PERTINENT QUESTIONS WHEN DISCUSSING DIVERSITY	
Assumptions	What assumptions do you have regarding this patient situation?
Beliefs/Behavior	What are your organizational beliefs? How are they different from your assumptions?
Communication	What are the communication issues?
Diversity	Which aspects of diversity are present? Reminder: age, class, culture, ethnicity, gender, nationality, race, religion, sexual orientation, and marginalization
Education	What educational recommendations do you have?

The model continues with a focus on the patient's areas of diversity. The health care professional can ask questions such as "What do you believe caused your illness?" This may encourage the patient to discuss his or her views on health. The patient's view may be rooted in his or her cultural/ethnic background. Another question may be "What have you done to treat yourself?" The patient may then disclose the use of folk medicine practices. This may include the use of herbs or rituals. When the patient is asked, "What is most important in your ability to recover from this illness?" the response may reveal a strong religious or spiritual belief or give the health care professional more information about the patient's family structure. Family structure is extremely important when communicating about serious illness.

Table 4-4. CONSIDERATIONS WHEN OBTAINING CONSENT

African-American	Avoid using medical jargon. Elicit feedback to check understanding. Involve the family in the consent process.
Arabic	Written consent may be problematic. Verbal consent based on trust is more acceptable. There is a dislike to listening to all possible complications before the procedure. Explain the need for written consent while emphasizing positive consequences.
Chinese	Involve oldest male family member during consent explanations, especially if the patient is a young girl or woman.
Puerto Rican	Prefer verbal consent to signed consent if feasible. Nodding affirmatively may not necessarily mean agreement or understanding. Provide an option for language preference for either verbal or written information. Allow time for the reading of material or the sharing of information with other family members.
Japanese	Explain procedure clearly. Stop to elicit feedback and understanding. Patients may be uncomfortable asking questions. Nisei may be more likely to consent than Sansei and Yonsei because of the recommendation of the health care professional.
Mexican	Undocumented immigrants tend to be suspicious of any type of consent, especially written consent. A latino health care provider may be helpful in obtaining consent. Language preference and reading level must be considered. Important decisions may require consultation among entire family.
American Indians	Discuss consent with the patient while explaining the roles of all involved including the family. Ask if the patient needs to consult anyone before consenting. Some individuals may be unwilling to sign written consents based on political and personal history of documents being misused.
Vietnamese	The patient may nod affirmatively although not understand or approve of what is said. May not ask questions publicly; allow for private time with the patient. Assess understanding by asking the patient to verbalize what was discussed. Allow patient to discuss forms with spouse or trusted friend.

Data from Lipson JG, Dibble SL, editors: *Culture and clinical care,* San Francisco, 2005, UCSF Nursing Press.

Table 4-5. PATIENT/FAMILY RESPONSE TO SERIOUS ILLNESS

African-American	Have a family conference or talk with a family elder or family-identified minister. Patient may have an older relative reveal a poor prognosis.
Arabic	Family members buffer the sick person from knowing the whole truth about his or her health situation. Discuss with the family spokesperson about the best way to provide information to the patient. Accommodate family needs for the gradual and prolonged disclosure of information.
Chinese	Some families may prefer to be present when discussing serious illness. The head of household should be involved.
Puerto Rican	Terminal illness often kept secret from the patient. Family does this as a protective mechanism to provide the best quality of life for the patient. On admission, ask the patient if someone else has the responsibility for health care decisions.
Japanese	Family may filter information for the non–English-speaking patient. Families may be reluctant to divulge a terminal diagnosis. Consult with family members.
Mexican	Clinician should inform patient and family together and as soon as possible. Ask patient who should be included in the discussion.
American Indians	The health care team may suggest a family meeting to discuss condition and course of treatment.
Vietnamese	The family may not want the patient informed without consulting the head of the family. It is believed that the patient will experience more stress and worry.

Data from Lipson JG, Dibble SL, editors: *Culture and clinical care,* San Francisco, 2005, UCSF Nursing Press.

Table 4-5 identifies how families and patients may respond to discussions about serious illness. It is interesting that most of the described groups respond in a similar manner. Most of the families would prefer not to tell a patient about a serious illness or diagnosis. This would not be congruent with the health care practice of informing a patient. This is an area where the health care professional needs to work with the family/patient to discover a common ground that allows all parties to fully participate in the health care plan.

Identifying the pertinent areas of diversity and how those areas affect care is vital. Is there conflict with the staff because of a misunderstood gesture? Does that conflict have to do with the staff's not understanding how the area of diversity (age, class, culture, ethnicity, gender, nationality, race, religion, sexual orientation, and marginalization) directly affects care?

Health care professionals should be prepared to address the differences between them and their patients. The goal is harmony and better understanding for all.

The model ends with a plan for education. Staff members may decide that formal presentations are needed and invite representatives from a particular group to speak. A needs assessment can be performed to assess staff response to diversity issues. It may highlight areas that require further staff education, such as religious groups and their wishes to refuse blood transfusion. Questions can be geared to reveal bias, such as toward individuals who are not able to pay their medical bills. Staff can then receive additional information (e.g., about poverty and government or hospital programs that can assist patients with payment) to help overcome those biases.

There are many ways that staff can share information with each other. One might document a case study in a newsletter or e-mail format to let other staff members benefit from the discussion session on a diversity issue. Even a potluck meal with foods from different regions can serve to celebrate diversity.

SUMMARY

The delivery of competent care is enhanced by an appreciation and understanding of those qualities that define us as individuals, as well as those qualities we share. Regardless of personal views, each patient should be treated with dignity and respect. Ethnocentrism, prejudice, bias, stereotypes, and ignorance of cultural differences negatively affect relationships with both our patients and our colleagues. Approaching diversity in a positive, nonjudgmental, and sensitive manner will only aid in our ability to deliver quality patient care.

The author wishes to acknowledge the valuable contributions of the following members of the Emergency Nurses Association Diversity Task Force:

Doreen K. Begley, RN, BS, CEN

John Fazio, RN, MS, CEN

Deborah St. Germaine, RN, MN, CEN

Ivy Buddha-Henry, RN, BSN, CEN

Reneé Semonin-Holleran, RN, PhD, CEN, CFRN

Anita Ruiz-Contreras, RN, MSN, CEN

Nancy Stonis, RN, BSN, CEN (ENA Staff Liaison)

REFERENCES

1. Emergency Nurses Association Diversity Task Force: *Approaching diversity: an interactive journey*, unpublished work, 1996-1998.
2. Lipson JS, Dibble SL, Minarik PA: *Culture and nursing care: a pocket guide*, San Francisco, 1996, UCSF Nursing Press.
3. Newberry L, Criddle L: *Sheehy's manual of emergency care*, ed 6, St. Louis, 2005, Mosby.
4. The Joint Commission: *Requirements related to the provision of culturally and linguistically appropriate health care*, 2007. Retrieved August 15, 2007, from http://www.jointcommission.org/NR/rdonlyres/1401C2EF-62F0-4715-B28A-7CE7F0F20E2D/0/hlc_jc_stds.pdf.
5. *United States Declaration of Independence: annotated text of the declaration*. Retrieved September 4, 2007, from http://en.wikipedia.org/wiki/.
6. U.S. Census Bureau: Adding Diversity from Abroad. Accessed September 2, 2007, from http://www.census.gov/population/pop-profile/2000/chap17.pdf
7. U.S. Department of Health and Human Services: *OCR fact sheet: your rights under the Age Discrimination Act (in federally funded health and human service programs)*. Retrieved December 7, 2007, from http://www.hhs.gov/specificpopulations/index.shtml
8. *Webster's II New College Dictionary*, New York, 2001, Houghton Mifflin.

SUGGESTED READING

Emergency Nurses Association: *Position statement: diversity in emergency care*, 2003. Retrieved September 15, 2008, from http://www.ena.org/about/position/PDFs/Diversity-in-Emergency-Care.PDF.

UNIT II

PROFESSIONAL PRACTICE

CHAPTER 5

Evidence-Based Practice

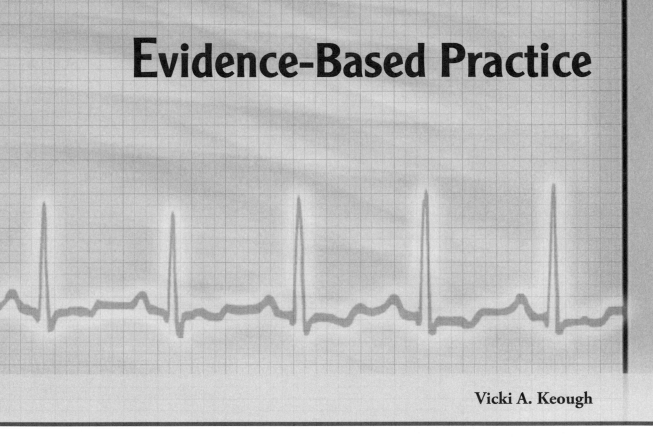

Vicki A. Keough

Every nurse can be proud to know that evidence-based practice (EBP) began with the founder of professional nursing practice, Florence Nightingale.[24,25] When she threw open the windows of the home hospitals during the Crimean war and insisted that nurses use clean linens to dress wounds and then started keeping a record of the results of her practice, evidence-based nursing practice was born. More than 100 years later, nurses are still asking important questions regarding their clinical practice. Nurses want to know that their interventions make a difference in patient outcomes. But what is evidence? What is quality evidence? What evidence is necessary before a practice can be changed? These questions continue to constitute much of the work of bedside nurses, nurse leaders, nurse researchers, and nurse scholars. Nurses, along with physicians and practitioners in the health care arena, are clearly still in the beginning stages of developing a practice based on evidence.[30]

Some popular recent actions taken by nurses as a result of using an EBP model are the use of saline flushes instead of heparin flushes for peripheral intravenous (IV) lines; discontinuing the common practice of placing patients in Trendelenburg's position for hypotension, highlighting the fact that volume, supine position, and keeping the head of the bed flat are the most beneficial interventions for patients with hypovolemia; and discontinuing the common practice of administering syrup of ipecac for patients coming to the emergency department (ED) with ingestions.[1,5,18]

When early goal-directed therapy (EGDT) for sepsis became the standard of care for all septic patients in EDs across the country,[6] the number of patients treated early for sepsis in the ED dramatically increased. This initiative came from nurses and physicians who asked the important question, Does EGDT truly decrease the mortality and morbidity of these patients?[1] To effectively use evidence to guide practice, nurses need a very specialized set of skills. This chapter will provide a brief overview of how ED nurses can use EBP to enhance their individual and collective nursing practice and leadership skills.

WHAT IS EVIDENCE-BASED PRACTICE?
Definitions

One of the most prolific authors and leaders in the use of EBP is David Sackett from the University of Oxford, England. He describes EBP as "the conscious, explicit and judicious use of current best evidence in making decisions about the care of individual patients."[29] Nurses are asking for research-based evidence to guide their practice. Evidence consists of both knowledge gained from clinical experience and knowledge gained from scientific studies. The blending of clinical experience and science provides a solid foundation from which care decisions can be made.[32] Many believe that evidence must be derived only from large, randomized control trials (RCTs) that use sophisticated research techniques to propose changes to practice. However, clinicians know that often these recommendations are either not useful or not practical for their patient population or for their clinical practice setting. This is where the art of nursing enters the arena of EPB. EPB is not just the review and critique of research and translation of these findings into practice, but the integration of all knowledge, clinical experience, and research findings to help nurses make the best decisions for their patients.[8,19,31,35] ED nurses are looking for evidence that demonstrates to patients and the public that they are receiving the best possible care within the best-designed health systems. Once the use of EBP is developed, it becomes a lifelong commitment to excellence and a commitment to a continual search for knowledge. If EBP is to be a lifelong commitment, then nurses must understand the importance of developing an organized and thoughtful approach to developing a practice based on evidence. There are several models that guide health care providers to developing EBP routines that will ensure best practices and optimal patient outcomes.

Evidence-Based Practice Models

Although there are many models for conducting EPB, four models will be presented in this section. The first is a model proposed by Sackett as a guideline for clinicians to use to implement EBP.[29] He proposed a five-step approach (Box 5-1). Sackett suggests that first clinicians must recognize specific problems within their practice and come up with a question that can be researched. Then they search the literature for any research or publications focusing on the question proposed. The clinicians will then conduct a critique of the literature and decide whether the findings would be applicable to their practice. Once a conclusion has been made based on the evaluation of the evidence and applicability to practice, a change in practice is implemented and then evaluated.

The University of Iowa Hospitals and Clinics has developed a similar model; however, the Iowa model proposes a team approach to EBP (Figure 5-1).[35] The model suggests that a research question must come from problem "triggers." These triggers can come from actual problems that have been identified through practice or from knowledge such as new research findings or new philosophies in health care. Once these problem triggers have been identified, a team decides whether or not the problem is a priority for the organization. If the team decides that this problem is a priority, the team will then review the current research and literature available on the topic, critique the research and literature, and if needed, develop a plan for a change in practice. This plan may include collection of further data, conducting research, designing new guidelines, or a modification of current guidelines. The team then determines whether or not the recommendations are appropriate for the

Box 5-1	**SACKETT'S FIVE-STEP APPROACH TO CONDUCTING EVIDENCE-BASED PRACTICE**[29]

1 Convert the need for clinically important information regarding practice decisions concerning diagnosis, prognosis, therapy and other health care issues into answerable questions.
2 Track down the best evidence to answer the question.
3 Critically appraise the evidence for validity and clinical applicability.
4 Integrate the appraisal with clinical expertise, and apply to practice.
5 Evaluate the results.

From Sackett DL: Evidence-based medicine, *Semin Perinatol* 21:3, 1997.

current practice environment and if so, the change is implemented and evaluated. This model is designed to be used within an organizational type of environment, rather than a private practitioner–based environment, where the Sackett model may be more appropriate. An important aspect of the Iowa model is the recognized need for support staff and organizational support as an integral part of the model. For example, resources such as librarians, risk management information, financial data, and benchmarking data are integral to the success of this model.

Rosswurm and Larrabee[28] (Figure 5-2) developed a model for nurses using an approach based on theories of EBP, research utilization, standardized nursing language, and change theory. Step 1 of this model uses important concepts of change theory by assessing the need for change among stakeholders. Stakeholders can be patients, nurses, administrators, interdisciplinary team members, administrators, etc. The stakeholders then take control of the investigation and come together as a team to collect internal data about the current problem or practice to be challenged and compare the results of the internal data findings with published data. The team of stakeholders then clearly identifies the problem and makes a commitment to develop an evidence-based change. Step 2 links the problem with practice by using standard classification systems of Nursing Outcomes Classification (NOC) and Nursing Interventions Classification (NIC), which allow nurses to link patient problems with nursing activities. The use of standardized language allows nurses to communicate more effectively, determines the effectiveness and cost of care, and helps to identify nursing resources. In step 3 the findings from the research and literature review are synthesized and critiqued. In step 4 a change in practice is designed. Step 5 focuses on implementing and evaluating the change in practice. Finally, step 6 involves integrating and maintaining change in practice by using a strategic approach to change. Having an open and ongoing relationship with the stakeholders, administrative support, and a clear dissemination of the findings of the research will enhance acceptance of the new protocol.

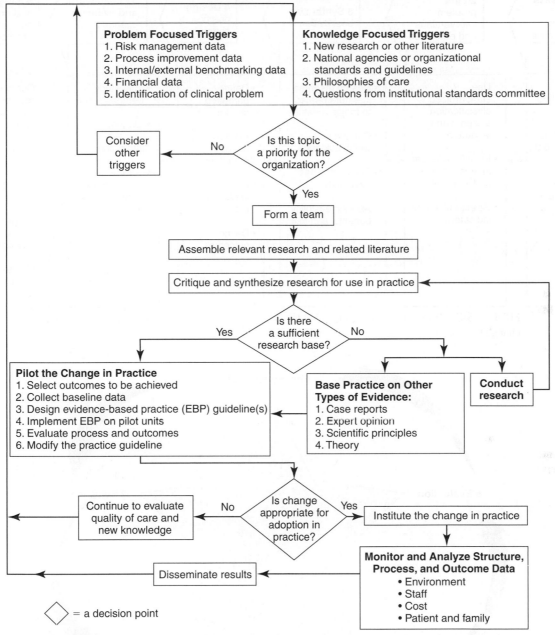

FIGURE 5-1. Iowa Model of Evidence-Based Practice to Promote Quality Care. (From Titler MG, Kleiber C, Steelman VJ et al: The Iowa Model of Evidence-Based Practice to Promote Quality Care, *Crit Care Nurs Clin North Am* 13:497, 2001.)

Finally, the ACE Star Model of Knowledge Transformation is a simplified model to help transform evidence into practice (Figure 5-3).[3,27,33] The value of this model is that it is very easy to remember and provides a practical approach to clinical practice. The ACE Star Model uses the five points of the star to represent the five stages of knowledge transformation. The top of the star represents knowledge discovery, followed by evidence synthesis, translation into practice recommendation, implementation into practice, and finally evaluation.

FINDING THE EVIDENCE
What Is Evidence?

Once a clinical question or problem has been identified, whether by a nurse at the bedside or by a team within the institution, the identification and revelation of the evidence related to the problem is the next step in finding a solution to the problem. There has been much discussion about what type of information can be considered as evidence. Evidence can range from very scientific research publications such as

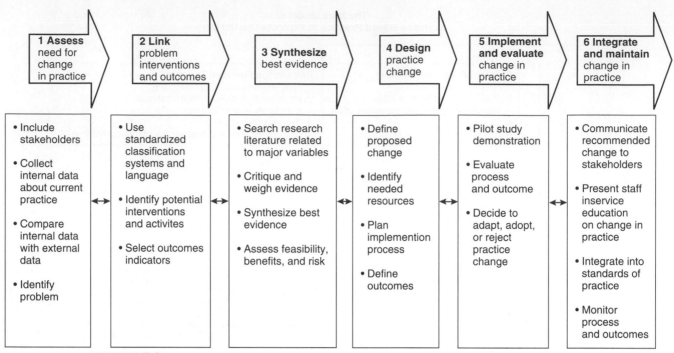

FIGURE **5-2.** Rosswurm and Larabee model. (From Rosswurm MA, Larrabee JH: A model for change to evidence-based practice, *Image J Nurs Sch* 31:317, 1999.)

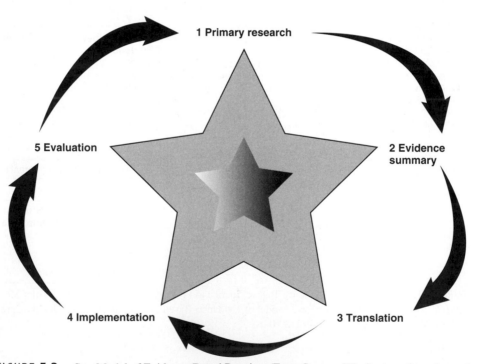

FIGURE **5-3.** Star Model of Evidence-Based Practice. (From Stevens KR: Systematic reviews: the heart of evidence-based practice, *AACN Clin Issues* 12:529, 2001.)

RCTs, survey research, and cohort studies to case studies of interesting or unusual cases, expert opinions, or consensus conference recommendations.[12,26,29,36] RCTs are generally large experimental research studies designed to randomly assign patients to experimental and nonexperimental groups and compare the results of one form of treatment against a control group, which generally receives the current standard of care. The researchers then determine if the new experimental treatment is more effective than the current treatment. The "gold standard" for evidence used to guide practice is clearly RCTs, systematic reviews, and meta-analyses.[29,32,33,38] Systematic reviews and meta-analyses are types of research whereby the authors review multiple studies on a particular topic, separate the best research, critically analyze the research, and then make practice recommendations based on the findings.[17,33,38] These very carefully and systematically designed research trials have the greatest ability to inform clinicians about the best practices based on research. It is unrealistic to think that individual nurses or physicians have the skill, knowledge, or time to conduct systematic reviews of every question they have regarding their practice[38]; therefore systematic reviews or meta-analyses can be very useful to the health care provider. The Cochrane Collaboration is an international organization that was initiated in an effort to promote the accessibility of systematic reviews on the effects of health care interventions.[14] When a topic is chosen by the Cochrane Collaboration to undergo a systematic analysis, a rigorous standardized review process is undertaken by a group of experts on the topic. Once the review is completed, recommendations for practice are published. Cochrane reviews have been found to be more rigorous than either systematic reviews or meta-analyses published in peer-reviewed journals.[13] For more information on interpretation of systematic reviews, the journal *Archives of Pediatric & Adolescent Medicine* has published an excellent three-part guide for interpreting systematic reviews.[15,17,20]

Although RCTs, systematic reviews, and meta-analyses are the gold standard for providing evidence, many topics do not have an RCT, systematic review, or meta-analysis of the data available to help guide the clinician. Therefore it is important for the nurse to examine the available data on cohort studies, smaller experimental studies, qualitative studies, or case studies. Although it is clear that this type of research represents a less rigorous research design and is rated lower on the hierarchy of evidence, it is still very important information that will alert the nurse to trends or problems in current practice that need to be identified and examined. Most large trials result from a compilation of smaller studies that alert the scientists to the need for larger studies. Case studies are excellent means of highlighting a problem or issue that needs to be addressed by the health care community. A case study generally highlights an unusual or interesting case a practitioner has encountered. Although this is not considered scientific evidence, it may represent an interesting finding or a future trend in health care.

How to Search for the Evidence

Conducting a literature review takes time, a great deal of research knowledge, and mastery of the art of reviews. Many health care organizations employ research librarians who can be an invaluable resource to nurses conducting a search for evidence. The review must be conducted in an organized and systematic manner. The first step of the literature review is to formulate a question that provides clear direction for the literature search. For example, What is the best treatment for croup? can clearly be researched, as opposed to a question that is nebulous and difficult to search such as, How can patients live with croup?

Once the question has been formulated, a search can begin. The first step is to conduct a computer-generated search on the keywords involved in the topic. Common keywords can often be found within databases. Common databases used by nurse researchers include CINAHL (Cumulative Index to Nursing and Allied Health Literature), MEDLINE (Medical Literature Analysis and Retrieval System Online), CANCERLIT (cancer literature), and PsycINFO (psychology information).[26,33]

When beginning to conduct a literature search, a nurse must first understand the difference between primary research and secondary sources. A simplified explanation of these two concepts is that primary research studies are studies published by the researchers who actually conducted the study. Secondary sources are authors who publish papers about research conducted by others. Because secondary sources generally report, critique, and evaluate the research of primary studies, they are providing their interpretation of the research and do not provide a detailed account of the original research.[26]

Finding the best research or secondary sources that evaluate the research takes skill and practice. It is not good enough to simply find all the research and literature published on a specific topic; it is necessary to find "evidence that matters." Evidence that matters refers to finding evidence that has implications to change a patient's "overall prognosis and outcome and quality of life."[38] An acronym exemplifying this concept was coined in 1994 by Slawson and Shaughnessey—POEM, patient-oriented evidence that matters.[38] This concept was developed by a group of clinicians in England that publishes monthly findings of POEM research. They also have an active web site (http://www. infopoems.com) with monthly updates on current reviews. Before the evidence on a particular topic can be considered for a possible change in practice, the evidence has to meet the following three criteria (http://www.infopoems.com/index.cfm):

- It addresses a question that faces clinicians.
- It measures outcomes that clinicians and patients care about (i.e., symptoms, morbidity, quality of life, and mortality).
- It has the potential to change practice.

Searching for systematic reviews can also be conducted using a search of systematic review sources. Some of the sources that publish systematic reviews are listed in Table 5-1 and are available online, either free or with a yearly subscription. Journals can also be a rich source of systematic reviews, and a list of journals dedicated to publishing systematic reviews is included in Table 5-1.[22,26,33,38]

Evidence can also be found by reviewing the bibliography of a research article that is focusing on the topic of interest. A nurse can find a rich source of similar studies and reports that discuss issues relevant to the topic at hand by reviewing the bibliographies of articles on the topic of interest.

Finally, evidence can be found by attending local, regional, national, and international conferences. Often landmark studies are revealed at large conferences where there are groups of interested health care providers who converge from many geographic areas to learn about the latest findings within their specialty area.

Table 5-1. SYSTEMATIC REVIEWS	
Name	**Web Address: http://www.**
SYSTEMATIC REVIEWS	
Cochrane Database of Systematic Reviews	cochrane.org
BMJ Evidence Center	clinicalevidence.com
DynaMed	dynamicmedical.com
First Consult	firstconsult.com
SUMSearch	sumsearch.uthscsa.edu
InfoRetriever	infopoems.com
TRIP Database	tripdatabase.com
The York Database of Abstracts of Reviews of Effects (DARE)	crd.york.ac.uk/crdweb/
Agency for Healthcare Research and Quality (AHRQ)	ahrq.gov
US Preventive Services Task Force	ahrq.gov/clinic/uspstfab.htm
The Joanna Briggs Institute	joannabriggs.edu.au
The Ontario Ministry of Health and Long-Term Care's Effective Public Health Practice Project (EPHPP)	oldhamilton.ca/phcs/ephpp/ReviewsPortal.asp
JOURNALS	
ACP Journal Club	acpjc.org
American Family Physician	aafp.org/afp
Bandolier	medicine.ox.ac.uk/bandolier/journal.html
Evidence-Based Nursing	evidencebasednursing.com
The Journal of Family Practice	jfponline.org

Data from Morrisey LJ, DeBourgh GA: Finding evidence: refining literature searching skills for the advanced practice nurse, *AACN Clin Issues* 12:560, 2001; Polit DF, Beck CT: *Nursing research: generating and assessing evidence for nursing practice*, New York, 2008, Lippincott Williams & Wilkins; Stevens KR: Systematic reviews: the heart of evidence-based practice, *AACN Clin Issues* 12:529, 2001; and White B: Making evidence-based medicine doable in everyday practice, *Fam Pract Manag* 11:51, 2004.

Once the evidence is collected and read for applicability and considered of high enough quality and relevance to the topic, the evidence must be evaluated and summarized.

EVALUATING THE EVIDENCE
Levels of Evidence

There are several strategies for evaluating evidence found in research. The most commonly used hierarchy for evaluating evidence is found in Figure 5-4.[26] This hierarchy is based on the rigor of the findings. The validity, reliability, and generalizability of the studies are factored into the hierarchy. There are seven different levels of research designs included in the hierarchy, with level I being the very best evidence and level VII being the lowest level of validity and reliability. The type of research that is considered to be at the top of the hierarchy is first, systematic reviews of RCTs and next, systematic reviews of nonrandomized trials. The type of research that is considered to be at the bottom rung of the hierarchy, although still important, is opinions of authors, case studies, and reports from expert committees.

Once the evidence is collected on a specific topic, it is then evaluated for scientific rigor and each study is critiqued and analyzed for applicability to the current topic. Determining where the research sits on the hierarchy of evidence scale is an important first step. There are several other factors that need to be considered when evaluating the current science of a particular topic. Understanding statistical reporting is a very important skill that nurses must acquire to evaluate research. The next section will focus on some important statistical measures nurses need to know to correctly interpret and evaluate the evidence.

Statistical Significance

A basic understanding of common statistical references is important in evaluating the evidence. The first number the nurse should pay attention to is the number of subjects involved in the study. It makes sense that a study involving a small number of subjects in a single setting is not going to be as valid and reliable as a study that looks at large numbers of subjects from across the country. The number of subjects will vary depending on the design. For descriptive, qualitative studies, the number of subjects in the study is generally small; however, for RCTs the numbers have to be large enough to allow for randomization, a control group, and for the variables and variances found in the study.[26] If there are too few subjects in the study, there may not be enough subjects to show any difference between those who received the intervention and those who did not. Many studies are published with subjects of 100 or less; however, at least 400 subjects is generally considered the minimum for an RCT study.[9]

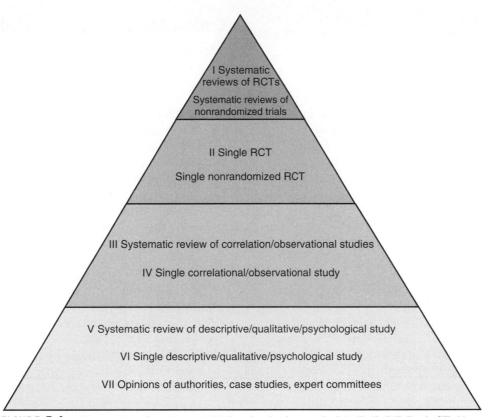

FIGURE **5-4.** Hierarchies of evidence. *RCT,* Randomized control trial. (Polit DF, Beck CT: *Nursing research: generating and assessing evidence for nursing practice*, New York, 2008, Lippincott Williams & Wilkins.)

Although statistical data can be very intimidating to most nurses, there are only a few statistics that will be critical to evaluation. This section will give a brief overview of five important statistics that are integral in evaluating research: (1) the alpha statistic (*p*-value), (2) relative risk reduction (RRR), (3) absolute risk reduction (ARR), (4) number needed to treat, and (5) confidence intervals.

p Value

The *p*-value, represented by the Greek letter alpha (α) and indicating significance, informs the researcher of the probability that the results found in the study are due only to chance and have nothing to do with the intervention (type I error). A *p*-value reported as <0.05 means that there is less than 5% chance that the reported results are incorrect and a 95% chance that the results reported are correct. Of course, most clinicians want a *p*-value of less than 0.00001, meaning that the probability is less than 1 out of 100,000 that the finding is due purely to chance. In reality, most scientists accept a *p*-value of less than 0.05 as being a statistically significant finding.[26] Of course, if an intervention has life-threatening implications, a much lower *p*-value will be required before the findings are used to change practice. For example, if a drug is being examined that has a life threat, the clinician will want to have a *p*-value much lower than 0.05, meaning that fewer than 5 out of 100 people may be

at risk for death from the drug. Therefore the acceptable *p*-value is directly tied to the life-threatening implications of the study. Because many studies are not dealing with life-and-death matters, a *p*-value of less than 0.05 is generally accepted as representing a statistically significant finding. A *p*-value greater than 0.05 means that, although the information may be interesting, there is no statistically significant difference found between the experimental group and the control group.

Relative Risk Reduction

RRR is the percentage reduction in the measured outcome between the experimental and control groups in relative terms (e.g., a significant 35% percent reduction in prostate cancer mortality was found among subjects who were treated with the experimental drug).[2,9,26] This statistic can be a little misleading because it can make small differences seem very large. For example, a study examines 2 groups of 100 subjects treated for skin cancer. The experimental group is given drug A and the control group is given standard therapy, which is drug B. If 75 people in the experimental group did not have a recurrence in cancer, and 50 people given drug B did not have a recurrence of cancer, one would report a 33% reduction in cancer with drug A. This number is arrived at by dividing the difference between those successfully treated with drug A and those successfully treated with drug B (75 − 50) by the total number successfully treated with drug A, which is 75. Therefore the mathematical problem would be $25 \div 75 = 0.333$, or 33%. The RRR would therefore be 33%.

Absolute Risk Reduction

ARR, also known as the risk difference, is the mathematical difference in outcome between the control group and the experimental group.[2,9,26] For example, using the same experimental group as described above, there is a 75% reduction in cancer with drug A; however, there is a 50% reduction in cancer with drug B. To calculate the ARR you would subtract the outcome reported in Group A from the outcome reported in Group B, and your ARR would be 25% (75% − 50%), giving you the true value of drug A. Thus drug A was actually 25% more effective in reducing cancer than drug B. As one can see, the ARR is a more accurate indication of the actual effect of the experimental drug or event.

Number Needed to Treat

Number needed to treat (NNT) is a very clinically useful statistic. NNT is the number of patients that must be treated to prevent one patient from having an adverse outcome over a given period of time.[2,9,26] Another way to look at this is to indicate how many patients would need to be treated with the experimental therapy to achieve benefit over the standard care. This is actually the inverse of the ARR statistic. Using our example above, if 25% of the people benefited from therapy from drug A, NNT is $\frac{1}{25}$%, or $\frac{1}{0.25}$, or 4. This indicates that 4 patients would need to be treated with Drug A to have 1 positive outcome. The most enviable NNT for an experimental study is 1, meaning that every time you treated a patient with Drug A there was a cure. In most circles, an NNT of 10 or less is considered acceptable.[9]

Confidence Intervals

The confidence interval (CI) informs the reader about the degree of precision that is involved in the findings and the degree within which the true difference in treatment would occur.,[21] Another way to put it is the degree for which the researcher is sure of making a correct assumption.[26] For example, with a confidence interval of 95%, the reader would know that the probability that the experiment reported correct findings is 95%. This means that there would be a 5% chance that the findings are wrong. Most clinicians require a CI of 95% to 99% for them to consider using the intervention espoused by the study.[26] The second piece to reporting the confidence interval is to report the range in which the reported findings reach 95% accuracy. When confidence intervals are reported, two numbers are generally reported with the confidence and these numbers represent the lowest and highest range the 95% confidence interval represents. For example, consider a study that reports findings of incidence of lead poisoning among 200 inner city children. The report states that lead poisoning was found among 33 inner city children, (95% CI, 20, 50). This means that the number of children with lead poisoning that fell within the 95% confidence ranged between 20 and 50.

Critical Appraisal of the Evidence

Once the evidence has been gathered and interpreted, the nurse will have to make a decision as to the overall meaning of the evidence. There are many facets to interpreting scientific reports, and depending on the needs of the interpreter, findings may have different meaning. McAlister et al[19] examined the quality of evidence cited to support cardiovascular risk management recommendations and found that the results of internally valid RCTs were not always applicable to the populations, interventions, or outcomes specified in a guideline recommendation. This study highlights the importance of evaluating the evidence for overall quality and applicability to one's setting.

One way to organize information is to make a grid that succinctly summarizes the evidence. The grid should serve as a brief overview of the studies and reviews and give the clinician a bird's-eye view of the findings. See Table 5-2 for an example of how to organize the evidence in a table format.

Questions to ask when appraising the overall value of the evidence include the following[10,22,38]:

- Is the study design appropriate to the research questions?
- How does the scientific rigor compare with standards?
- What is the number of subjects in the study?
- Are the numbers sufficient?
- Are the studies published in a peer-reviewed journal?
- What are the qualifications of the researchers?
- Is the study population similar to the population in which the results will be implemented?
- Is the treatment feasible in one's practice setting?
- Are the study findings realistic, are they too costly, or is the regimen too difficult for patients to adhere to?
- Where was the study conducted, and is the geographic difference a problem?
- Would the outcome matter to one's patient population?
- How do these results compare with practice guidelines?

Once the critical appraisal of the research is complete, the nurse or the team of health care workers translates the findings into practice recommendations.

TRANSLATION

Translation is taking the knowledge gained from a critical appraisal of the research and literature within a certain topic and translating these findings into recommendations for change in practice.[3] In making these recommendations, one must take into consideration change theories, applicability to the practice setting, acceptance by the stakeholders, and cost and timeliness of the intervention.[3] Deriving a plan for a systematic way to implement change is integral to the success of the project. For example, take the study cited in this chapter regarding treatment of hypovolemia with Trendelenburg's position. The findings indicate that there are very effective treatments for hypovolemia such as fluid restoration, supine positioning, and laying the head flat and that the old standard of placing patients in Trendelenburg's position is not effective.[5] This knowledge must now be disseminated

Table 5-2. **REVIEW GRID**				
Title/Author/Journal/ Date	Design	No. of Subjects	Significant Findings Related to Topic	Limitations/Notes

among the staff that will be expected to make the change, policies and protocols need to be rewritten, education of all professional and nonprofessional staff must take place, and finally, a process for evaluating the success of the interventions must be established.

Doran and Sidani[7] developed a useful framework for knowledge translation related to patient outcomes improvement. This framework incorporates four components for translating research into practice. The first step in their model is to collect accurate data on patient outcomes. Next, best-practice guidelines are reviewed in light of current tools available for disseminating this information. The team must also be very clear about patient satisfaction and patient needs, and finally, there must be advanced practice nurses who embrace the change and provide leadership for the change to occur. Below are components involved in the framework:
1. Patient outcomes measurement and real-time feedback about outcomes achievement
2. Best-practice guidelines, embedded in decision support tools that deliver key messages in response to patient assessment data
3. Clarification of patients' preferences for care
4. Facilitation by advanced practice nurses and nurse leaders

Once evidence-based changes have been made, the changes must be evaluated for efficacy and satisfaction. The next section will discuss the importance of evaluating the changes implemented.

EVALUATION

Was the change that was implemented as a result of the EBP study helpful to patients and staff? Was the change effective? Are patients and staff satisfied with the change? Evaluation is just as important as the critique and implementation phase of EBP.

Evaluation must elicit reviews from the stakeholders and be instrumental in the decision to adapt, adopt, or reject the change based on feedback. The change should be evaluated for feasibility, usability, satisfaction, and risk/benefit analyses. Quality improvement and cost data must also be evaluated.[28] Along with the plan for evaluation, there must be a plan for disseminating the results of the evaluation and a plan for ongoing assessment and change.

USING EVIDENCE TO BENCHMARK

Benchmarking is a way to compare performance or outcomes of a particular measure to a given standard. This standard can be a regional or national standard, past performance, or a specific unit or organizational goal that one is attempting to achieve.

For example, to determine if one's institutional length of time patients spend in the ED waiting for admission to a floor bed was above the national standards, one would examine the national standards for ED wait times and compare the time of one's own institution with the national standard. Patients may not be the only people interested in how units and institutions compare with national standards. Agencies that have an interest in benchmarking are The Joint Commission, national councils, government agencies, insurance agencies, and other agencies providing service or payment to the organization.[4] Of course, the most common benchmarking tool and the one that is most widely discussed at hospital meetings is patient satisfaction scores. Using EBP to evaluate benchmarking data is an excellent way to approach a clinical or administrative issue. Because benchmarking relies on accurate interpretation of data such as number of ED visits, number of admissions from the ED, return visits to the ED, length of time in the ED,[4] and patient satisfaction with

ED care, it is essential that the data be collected, analyzed, and evaluated using EBP techniques described throughout this chapter. By marrying the concept of benchmarking and the skills of conducting, analyzing, evaluating, and implementing EBP, health care providers and organizations can improve their performance.[37]

The Joint Commission[34] began asking hospitals across the nation to demonstrate their outcomes and performance measurement data in 1997 by reporting evidence related to performance measures. The Joint Commission asked hospitals to look at the evidence that provided information about quality care and outcome performance around five core measures: acute myocardial infarction, heart failure, pneumonia, pregnancy and related conditions, and surgical care. Under each of the core measures, The Joint Commission identified several questions that could provide evidence that the core measures were being evaluated. For example, under the core measure of acute myocardial infarction, The Joint Commission wanted hospitals to report on items such as whether or not aspirin was given upon arrival, if acetylsalicylic acid (ASA) was prescribed at discharge, if the patient was prescribed an angiotension-converting enzyme inhibitor, if the patient received a beta-blocker, and how long it took the patient to receive fibrinolytics or percutaneous intervention. In order for these questions to be addressed, hospitals were required to track specific data related to the core measures. As a result of this initiative, health care providers now have access to large volumes of data that provide a rich source of evidence-based information and allow health care providers to track the progress of health care as a nation and as individual units. This initiative has also provided opportunities for individual hospitals and health care organizations to design automated systems that can assist in the management, collection, and analysis of large volumes of data.

SUMMARY

Using evidence to help lead the way to better practice provides for a win-win relationship between research and practice. Before 2004, when early goal-directed therapy for treating sepsis was introduced,[6] patients across the country were being treated for sepsis in the ED according to individual physician or organizational criteria. Survival rates and morbidity rates were discouraging. Once the evidence-based guidelines were introduced and a national campaign was begun to educate health care workers across the country, dramatic changes in survival and morbidity rates for septic patients were realized.[11,16,23] Nurses have a responsibility to maintain currency in their practice. The only way to accomplish this is to understand the rigor that is involved in interpreting and evaluating research and to develop the skills needed to take the findings from the research and translate the science into practice. Nurses have always been good about asking the hard questions. Now the onus is on the nurse to couch the questions in a manner that can lead to responsible investigation, to understand the importance of interpreting and evaluating the research, and to take this information to the patients, the units, the community, and other health care workers. By acquiring the necessary knowledge and skills to design, analyze, and translate research and by using evidence to guide decisions, nurses can continue to be responsible leaders within the health care arena.

REFERENCES

1. Ahrens T: Evidenced-based practice: priorities and implementation strategies, *AACN Clin Issues* 16:36, 2005.
2. Barratt A, Wyer PC, Hatala R: Tips for learners of evidence-based medicine: 1. Relative risk reduction, absolute risk reduction and number needed to treat, *CMAJ* 171:353, 2004.
3. Bonis S, Taft L, Wendler MC: Strategies to promote success on the NCLEX-RN: an evidence-based approach using the ACE Star Model of Knowledge Transformation, *Nurs Educ Perspect* 28:82, 2007.
4. Burch MG, Kozeny D: Outcomes management, In Newberry L, editor: *Sheehy's emergency nursing: principles and practice,* ed 5, Philadelphia, 2003, Elsevier.
5. DeBourgh GA: Champions for evidence-based practice: a critical role for advanced practice nurses, *AACN Clin Issues* 12:491, 2001.
6. Dellinger RP, Carlet JM, Masur H et al: Surviving sepsis campaign guidelines for management of severe sepsis and septic shock [published correction of dosage error in text appears in *Crit Care Med* 32(6):1448, 2004], *Crit Care Med* 32:858, 2004.
7. Doran DM, Sidani S: Outcomes-focused knowledge translation: a framework for knowledge translation and patient outcomes improvement, *Worldviews Evid Based Nurs* 4:3, 2007.
8. Fisher CG, Wood KB: Introduction to and techniques of evidence-based medicine, *Spine* 32:S66, 2007.
9. Flaherty RJ: A simple method for evaluating the clinical literature, *Fam Pract Manag* 11:47, 2004.
10. Glasziou P, Guyatt GH, Dans AL: Applying the results of trials and systematic reviews to individual patients, *ACP J Club* 129:A15, 1998.
11. Huang DT, Clermont G, Dremsizov T T et al: Implementation of early goal-directed therapy for severe sepsis and septic shock: a decision analysis, *Crit Care Med* 35:2090, 2007.
12. Humphris D: Disturbance and resilience: an overview of evidence based practice, *J Tissue Viability* 8:16, 1998.
13. Jadad AR, Cook DJ, Jones A et al: Methodology and reports of systematic reviews and meta-analyses: a comparison of Cochrane reviews with articles published in paper-based journals, *JAMA* 280:278, 1998.
14. Jadad AR, Haynes RB: The Cochrane Collaboration—advances and challenges in improving evidence-based decision making, *Med Decis Making* 18:2, 1998.
15. Jadad AR, Moher D, Klassen TP: Guides for reading and interpreting systematic reviews. II, How did the authors find the studies and assess their quality? *Arch Pediatr Adolesc Med* 152:812, 1998.

16. Jones AE, Focht A, Horton JM et al: Prospective external validation of the clinical effectiveness of an emergency department–based early goal-directed therapy protocol for severe sepsis and septic shock, *Chest* 132:425, 2007.

17. Klassen TP, Jadad AR, Moher D: Guides for reading and interpreting systematic reviews. I, Getting started, *Arch Pediatr Adolesc Med* 152:700, 1998.

18. Manoguerra AS, Cobaugh DJ, Guidelines for the Management of Poisoning Consensus Panel: Guideline on the use of ipecac syrup in the out-of-hospital management of ingested poisons, *Clin Toxicol* 43:1, 2005.

19. McAlister FAet al, van Diepen S, Padwal RS et al: How evidence-based are the recommendations in evidence-based guidelines? *PLoS Med* 4:e250, 2007.

20. Moher D, Jadad AR, Klassen TP: Guides for reading and interpreting systematic reviews. III, How did the authors synthesize the data and make their conclusions? *Arch Pediatr Adolesc Med* 152:915, 1998.

21. Montori VM, Kleinbart J, Newman TB et al: Tips for learners of evidence-based medicine. II, Measures of precision (confidence intervals), *CMAJ* 171:611, 2004.

22. Morrisey LJ, DeBourgh GA: Finding evidence: refining literature searching skills for the advanced practice nurse, *AACN Clin Issues* 12:560, 2001.

23. Nguyen HB, Corbett SW, Steele R et al: Implementation of a bundle of quality indicators for the early management of severe sepsis and septic shock is associated with decreased mortality, *Crit Care Med* 35:1105, 2007.

24. Nightingale F: *Observation of the evidence contained in the statistical reports submitted by her to the Royal Commission on the Sanitary State of the Army in India*, London, 1863, Edward Stanford.

25. Nightingale F: Notes on nursing, *Am J Nurs* 47:508, 1947.

26. Polit DF, Beck CT: *Nursing research: generating and assessing evidence for nursing practice*, New York, 2008, Lippincott Williams & Wilkins.

27. Reeves K: The importance of utilizing evidence-based practice, *Medsurg Nurs* 15:329, 2006.

28. Rosswurm MA, Larrabee JH: A model for change to evidence-based practice, *Image J Nurs Sch* 31:317, 1999.

29. Sackett DL: Evidence-based medicine, *Semin Perinatol* 21:3, 1997.

30. Sackett DL, Richardson SW, Rosenberg WR et al: *Evidence-based medicine: how to practice and teach EBM*, London, 1997, Churchill Livingstone.

31. Sackett DL, Rosenberg WM, Gray JA et al: Evidence based medicine: what it is and what it isn't, *BMJ* 312:71, 1996.

32. Sackett DL, Rosenberg WM, Gray JA et al: Evidence based medicine: what it is and what it isn't, 1996, *Clin Orthop Relat Res* 455:3, 2007.

33. Stevens KR: Systematic reviews: the heart of evidence-based practice, *AACN Clin Issues* 12:529, 2001.

34. The Joint Commission: *Facts about ORYX for hospitals, core measures and hospital quality measures*, Retrieved November 22, 2008. http://www.joint commission.org/AccreditationPrograms/Hospitals/ORYX.

35. Titler MG, Kleiber C, Steelman VJ et al: The Iowa Model of Evidence-Based Practice to Promote Quality Care, *Crit Care Nurs Clin North Am* 13:497, 2001.

36. Titler MG, Mentes JC, Rakel BA et al: From book to bedside: putting evidence to use in the care of the elderly, *Jt Comm J Qual Improv* 25:545, 1999.

37. Vassallo ML: Benchmarking and evidence-based practice: complementary approaches to achieving quality process improvement, *Semin Perioper Nurs* 9:121, 2000.

38. White B: Making evidence-based medicine doable in everyday practice, *Fam Pract Manag* 11:51, 2004.

CHAPTER 6

Research

Susan Barnason

The continual infusion of new information gleaned from research findings and integrated into clinical nursing practice is an expectation in health care today. Clinical practice and patient care improvements emerge from the development, evaluation, and expansion of nursing knowledge resulting from research. The staff nurse is a critical link in bringing research-based changes into clinical practice. The focus of this chapter is to provide an overview of the research process as a basis for emergency nurses to become better consumers of research and to understand how research can be incorporated into clinical practice.

BRINGING RESEARCH TO CLINICAL PRACTICE

Bridging the gap between theory, research, and practice is essential to bringing innovations and advances from nursing research to practical application at the bedside. A theory-practice gap exists when research findings fail to be integrated into practice.[3] This can result from the lack of knowledge regarding research findings or from the perception that research findings are irrelevant to clinical practice.[25] Research is a systematic investigation that is designed to develop or contribute to generalizable knowledge.[22] Research findings are the foundation for problem solving to improve clinical practice and lead to evidence-based nursing practices.[20]

Clinical decisions using the best available research evidence, clinicians' clinical expertise, pathophysiologic knowledge, and patient preferences are the components of evidence-based nursing practices.[12,21,29,31,36] To integrate research into clinical practice and develop evidence-based practices, nurses need to develop an expertise for interpreting and using research. The gap between research findings and application to the clinical setting can be closed by nurses who have an informed understanding of the research process.[24]

Using Research in Clinical Practice: Comparison of Research Utilization, Evidence-Based Practice, and Quality Improvement

The use of research in clinical practice does not just refer to research utilization, nor is it synonymous with evidence-based practice.[9] Although use of research findings is an important component of both evidence-based practice and research utilization, both have limitations related to use in clinical practice. Research utilization was originally intended to be the application of a portion of the research in a way that was not related to the original research study.[26] Research utilization models include a synthesis of research literature on a given topic to summarize research-based knowledge that can be used in clinical practice.[13,17] The degree to which

Table 6-1.   COMPONENTS OF THE RESEARCH STUDY

Components of a Research Study	Overview of the Components
Problem identification	Identifies the "problem" that will be answered by the research study.
Literature review	Synthesizes current literature and state of the art to summarize how current study can contribute to current body of literature on the topic.
Theoretic or conceptual framework	In theoretically driven studies, sets the context for the propositions or relationships related to the variables in the study.
Purpose and research questions or hypotheses	What the study intends to accomplish.
Methodology • Design • Sampling • Data collection • Data measurement • Data analysis	The methods section communicates what approaches will be or were used by the researcher to answer the research questions or hypotheses.
Results	• Reports the results obtained in the analyses of data.
Discussion of the findings • Conclusions • Limitations • Recommendations	• Discussion of the findings includes the drawing of conclusions based on what the results mean, explaining why results were obtained, and how results can be used in practice.

research utilization is integrated into practice can vary along a continuum.[4,9,13] At one end of the continuum is the initial conceptualization of the literature (referred to as *conceptual utilization*).[2] The next step of research utilization is thinking about research ideas and findings on a given topic (referred to as *knowledge creep*). The next level of research utilization is taking action to move to a decision about the implications of research synthesis (referred to as *decision accretion*), and finally, at the other end of the research utilization continuum is the implementation of research into clinical practice (referred to as *instrumental utilization*).

Evidence-based practice uses the best available evidence, which includes an individual's expertise and other external clinical evidence from systematic research.[22] Research is a key component in delineating evidence-based nursing practices. The strongest source of evidence for evaluating interventions is from systematic reviews.[34] These reviews include an appraisal of individual studies, and when these individual studies are combined, they provide a meta-analysis of the effectiveness of an intervention. However, the reality is that nursing, like other health care disciplines, lacks a comprehensive body of research to support all interventions performed in nursing practice. Therefore when there is insufficient or no research available, clinicians need to use other resources and sources of data to augment their problem solving. Other recommended sources of "evidence" include benchmarking data, clinical expertise, patient preferences, infection control data, standards (international, national, and local standards), quality improvement and risk data, retrospective or concurrent chart review, pathophysiology, and analysis of cost-effectiveness.[11]

Regardless of the source of data upon which to build evidence-based practices, it is essential to take into consideration the level of evidence or the strength of the scientific evidence.[32] The Agency for Healthcare Research and Quality (AHRQ)[1] summarized the published reports on how to determine or grade the strength of evidence. The AHRQ report concluded that for any system grading the strength of the evidence, three elements should be included: quality, quantity, and consistency. Quality refers to the extent to which studies minimize bias and are valid studies. Quantity is the number of studies and total number of subjects in the study. Consistency refers to the extent to which findings are similar between different studies on the same topic. There is no one best method for determining the level of evidence; the process of evaluating evidence should employ the most relevant levels of an evidence grading system for the topic or type of procedure being assessed.[5,7]

Quality improvement initiatives are a rich source of "evidence" reflecting clinical expertise, patient preferences, and local context. Nowadays quality improvement is an inherent part of "best care" for patients.[16] It is assumed that clinicians will use data from their own clinical practice to improve practice.[22] Furthermore, accrediting and certifying bodies expect that quality improvement initiatives are an intrinsic part of an organization's patient care delivery. Quality improvement initiatives often arise from health care professionals' experiences and insights. Analyzing aggregate patient population data is necessary to determine potential changes in processes and interventions needed for improved patient care.[16] In summary, the types of research sources and ways in which to integrate research findings into clinical practice will vary along a continuum.

APPRAISAL OF RESEARCH

In evaluating the merits of published research studies, nurses should proceed through a series of well-defined, logical steps to determine the merits of a research study. The key components of a research study, delineated in Table 6-1 and further summarized below, can guide the appraisal or critique of a research study's quality.

Problem Identification

The initial step of the research process is defining the research question or research problem.[15] The research question or problem reflects an identified problem related to patient care, nursing education, nursing administration, or any issue of nursing interest. Patient care or nursing practice problems generally address practice differences and what is ideal or desirable. Researchable questions often reflect clinical experiences, such as (1) How effective is triage in prioritizing patient acuity? (2) What type of pain management can be used for pediatric patients undergoing procedures in the emergency department (ED)? and (3) How effective are discharge instructions for ED patients? Researchers may also derive their research question based on focuses or problems identified in the nursing literature itself.[2] Research studies often make recommendations for future studies when summarizing implications of the current study. Researchable questions or clinical problems yet to be addressed are often identified when reviewing several research articles on the current state of the science. In addition, several nursing and federal organizations have published recommendations for future research studies. The Emergency Nurses Association, American Association of Critical Care Nurses, American Nurses Association, Sigma Theta Tau International, and National Institutes of Health are examples of organizations that have identified research priorities.

Literature Review

The purpose of the literature review is to explore work conducted in a particular area of interest to further formulate or clarify the research problem. After critiquing previous research in a particular area, the researcher summarizes what has been previously studied and delineates how a proposed study will contribute to the state of the science. A good literature review critiques and summarizes other studies to see how they fit into the scope of the study being conducted. A thorough review reinforces the need for the study in light of what has already been done. A written literature review should include summaries of articles that differ from the proposed point of view. This indicates that the author conducted an exhaustive review of available knowledge.[2]

Information sources for literature reviews include both primary and secondary resources.[17] A primary source of information is the description of an investigation written by the person who conducted it. A secondary source is a description of a study prepared by someone other than the original researcher. Literature reviews are very useful for examining the body of evidence for best clinical practices, as well as for identifying the existing gaps in a given area of content.

Theoretical and Conceptual Frameworks

Theories and conceptual frameworks provide a structure or blueprint to guide the study of clinical problems. A theoretical framework defines the concepts and proposes relationships between those concepts to provide a systematic view of a phenomenon.[15] It further enables the researcher to link the findings to a body of knowledge. This framework consists of the definition of concepts and propositions about the relationships of those concepts, a way to organize rules or beliefs about what is observed, and a systematic method to organize information about a particular aspect of interest in a research study.[15]

Two components of a theory are concepts and propositions. Concepts, the building blocks of a theory, are abstract characteristics, categories, or labels of things, persons, or events. Examples of nursing concepts are health, stress, adaptation, caring, and pain. Propositions are statements that define the relationships among concepts. A set of propositions may state that one concept is associated with another or is contingent upon another. Examples of theories used in nursing are psychoanalytic theory, the theory of relativity, the theory of evolution, the theory of gravity, learning theory, systems theory, and the theory of homeostasis. The power of theories lies in their ability to explain the relationship of variables.[2] Theories can stimulate research by giving direction. Questions and ideas formulated about what will occur in specific situations are called hypotheses. In research, hypotheses are tested to determine whether the information fits the theory.[15]

Conceptual frameworks represent a less formal, less well developed system for organizing phenomena. They contain concepts that represent a common theme but lack the deductive system of propositions that identify the relationship among concepts. Conceptual frameworks are more or less a map for the proposed study.[15] The groundwork for more formal theories often evolves from conceptual frameworks.

Research Questions or Hypotheses

Before a problem is researched, it must be narrowed, refined, and made feasible for study. The research interest can be stated as a research question or a hypothesis. The research question in a study should identify key independent and dependent variables. An independent variable is what is assumed to cause or thought to be associated with the dependent variable. Changes in the dependent variable are presumed to depend on the effects of the independent variable. The dependent variable is what a researcher wants to explain or understand. Research questions should be specific and not attempt to measure too much, because data analysis may be complex and be confusing to interpret.[2] For example, a research question might be, What effect does the presence of the parent in the child's room have on the child's experience of pain during fracture reduction? The dependent variable is the child's pain experience and the independent variable is the presence of the parent in the room. The dependent variable is explained through its relationship with the independent variable. It is known that many factors affect a child's perception of pain, but only one independent variable (parent's presence) is intended to be measured in the proposed research question.

Often the dependent variable can have multiple causes. A study may be designed to examine several factors and their influence on a phenomenon. For example, a researcher may want to know whether experience with triage or an educational program concerning triage influences ability to accurately perform triage. Both independent variables (education and experience) can influence triage performance ability (dependent variable).[2]

Several dependent variables can be designated as measures of treatment effectiveness. An example of multiple dependent variables identified in a research question is, Does a comprehensive triage system have an influence on length of stay in the ED, patient satisfaction, and patient outcome? Length of stay, patient satisfaction, and patient outcome are all dependent variables by which triage effectiveness is measured.[2]

A hypothesis expands upon a research question, because it is a prediction of the relationship or differences between two or more variables.[15,17] This prediction of expected outcomes is the basis of the research process. Hypotheses, which often stem from theories, are possible solutions or answers to research problems. The hypothesis is a prediction of the nature of the relationship between several variables that is intended to be identified before the initiation of the research study. For example, one hypothesis might be that pediatric patients who are promised a reward at the end of a suturing procedure will cooperate and be more compliant than pediatric patients who are not promised a reward. In this example, the researcher is not only delineating whether a relationship between rewards and behavior exists but is also predicting outcomes from this relationship. The null hypothesis indicates that the two populations (samples) have the same mean. The null hypothesis plays a major role in testing the significance of differences between the treatment and control groups. The assumption at the outset of the experiment is that no difference exists between the two groups (for the variable being compared). Therefore the null hypothesis, stated as "there will be no relationship between" or "there will be no difference in …," is often generated for statistical purposes, data analysis, and discussion.[2,15,17]

Methodology

The methods section of a research study reflects how the researcher plans to or did implement the research study to answer the research questions or hypotheses. The components of the methodology section include research design, subjects, measures used to collect data, and study procedures. There are two major categories of research designs: quantitative and qualitative (Tables 6-2 and 6-3). In the context of this chapter, the focus will be quantitative studies.[2]

Sampling

Subjects sampled for a research study will depend on the population to be studied and the estimated number of subjects needed to demonstrate a significant difference between experimental and control groups. The definition of a population is not restricted to human subjects. A population can consist of records, blood samples, actions, words, organizations, numbers, or animals. Regardless of the unit to be studied or sampled, a population is always made up of specific elements of interest. Often it is not feasible to include large populations due to expense and time involved for data collection. Generally a study limits the population sampled to a representative sample. Samples should typify a portion of the entire population to be studied to ensure that the sample is "representative" of that population. The sample should mirror the population to be studied to avoid sampling bias. Sampling error can result from sampling bias, which is the tendency to select a sample that has particular characteristics, rather than the sample's being representative of the population to be studied.

Researchers use probability and nonprobability sampling techniques when designing studies. Probability sampling is the use of some form of random selection to choose the subjects or units to be sampled. Statistical measures, known as "power analyses," can be used by researchers to estimate the sample size needed. Nonprobability sampling is a method based on convenience. Three types of nonprobability sampling are accidental, quota, and purposive sampling. Accidental samples are based on convenience of gathering subjects, such as surveying the first 100 patients in the ED on a particular day. Quota samples are used when a researcher knows an element of the population and bases sampling on the known representativeness within the population. For example, if a researcher knows that 25% of the nurses in the ED setting are males, the researcher makes sure that males constitute 25% of the sample of ED nurses. This increases the representativeness of the population. Purposive sampling occurs when a researcher "handpicks" cases to be included in the sample that represent the "typical" subjects within a given population. A study may use purposive sampling to ensure a wide variety of responses or because the choices are judged to be typical of the population. In general, it is recommended that a sample size of 30 be selected for each subset of data or "cell" of the design.[2,15,17]

Institutional Review Board Approval

Institutional Review Board (IRB) approval of the research study is a necessity. The purpose of IRB study approval is to safeguard the rights and welfare of subjects, ensure appropriate procedures for informed consent, and allow subjects to make independent decisions about risks and benefits.[2] Box 6-1 delineates the components to be included in a consent form. There are circumstances when emergency consent is needed, without having the prior approval of the IRB.[27,31] The determinants of the waiver to informed consent for emergency research are listed in Box 6-2.

Data Collection and Data Measurement

Data collection simply refers to a description of the processes used to implement the study and gather data. The key to successful data collection is using appropriate measures that accurately describe the variables in the study. Measurement tools have some common characteristics: (1) they are objective, (2) they are standardized measures (uniform items, response, and scoring), (3) items of measurement should be unambiguous, (4) types of items on any one test should have a limited number

Table 6-2. OVERVIEW OF COMMON TYPES OF QUANTITATIVE RESEARCH DESIGNS

Research Design	Characteristics of Research Design
EXPERIMENTAL AND QUASI-EXPERIMENTAL	
Experimental	
Examples of experimental research designs: • Nonequivalent control • After-only nonequivalent group • One-group (pretest-posttest)	• Manipulation of independent variable • Randomization of subjects (subjects randomly assigned to control and experimental groups) • Control or comparison group (one of groups in study does not receive "experimental" treatment but receives normal or routine care)
Quasi-Experimental	
Examples of quasi-experimental research designs: • Nonequivalent control • After-only nonequivalent group • One-group (pretest-posttest) • Time-series	• Manipulation of independent variable • Lacks control group or randomization
NONEXPERIMENTAL	
Survey	
Examples of survey nonexperimental research designs: • Descriptive • Exploratory • Comparative	• Collect and describe existing data • Helps to describe the characteristics of subjects or a group • No intervention is performed • May identify trends and possibly help to identify future needs
Relationship/Differences	
Examples of relationship/differences nonexperimental research designs: • Correlational • Developmental • Cross-sectional • Longitudinal and prospective • Retrospective and ex post facto	• Overall goal is to determine if there is a relationship or difference between variables *Correlational* • Examining the relationship between two or more variables • *Cannot* imply causal relationships • Able to determine the "strength" of a relationship between variables *Cross-sectional* • Examines data at one point in time *Longitudinal and prospective* • Collects data from the same group at different time points *Retrospective and ex post facto* • Variations of independent variable in the natural course of events • This type of design also referred to as explanatory, causal-comparative, or comparative
OTHER TYPES OF QUANTITATIVE RESEARCH DESIGNS	
Methodological	• A controlled investigation related to ways of obtaining or organizing data • Addresses development, validation, and evaluation of research tools or techniques
Meta-analysis	• Analyzes the results from many studies on a specific topic • Combines data from many studies, usually randomized control clinical trials • Synthesizes findings and statistically summarizes data to obtain a precise estimate of the treatment effectiveness (effect size) and statistical significance

Table 6-3. OVERVIEW OF COMMON TYPES OF QUALITATIVE RESEARCH DESIGNS

Research Design	Characteristics of Research Design
Phenomenological	• Learning occurs through dialogue with persons representative of the population of interest to be studied • Construct meaning from the "lived" experience
Grounded theory	• Goal is to derive a theory about social processes • Uses inductive reasoning approaches, with theory arising from the data to reflect the social processes being studied
Ethnographic	• Goal is to understand, scientifically describe, and interpret cultural or social groups and systems
Case study	• Overall goal is to study the uniqueness and commonalities of a specific case • Natural conditions are studied and variables related to history, current characteristics, interactions, or problems • Usually focuses on why the subject feels, thinks, and behaves in a particular manner
Historical	• An approach used to understand the past through a critical appraisal of facts

---

Box 6-1   KEY COMPONENTS OF AN INFORMED CONSENT FORM FOR RESEARCH

• Statement involving research, explanation of purposes of the research, delineation of expected duration of subject's participation, description of procedures to be expected and identification of any procedures that are experimental

• Description of any reasonably foreseeable risks or discomforts to the subject

• Description of any benefits to the subject or to others that may reasonably be expected from the research

• Disclosure of appropriate alternative procedures or courses of treatment, if any, that may be advantageous to the subject

• A statement describing to what extent, if any, confidentiality of records identifying the subject will be maintained

• For research involving more than minimal risk, an explanation as to whether any medical treatments are available if injury occurs and if so, what they consist of or where further information may be obtained

• An explanation of whom to contact for answers to pertinent questions about the research and the subject's rights and whom to contact in the event of a research-related injury to the subject

• A statement that participation is voluntary, refusal to participate will not involve any penalty or loss of benefits to which the subject is otherwise entitled, and the subject may discontinue participation at any time without any penalty or loss of otherwise entitled benefits

---

Box 6-2   KEY COMPONENTS OF INFORMED CONSENT WAIVER

• The patient has a life-threatening condition.

• Available treatments are unsatisfactory or unproven.

• The patient is not capable of giving informed consent (due to his or her medical condition), or the patient's legal representative is not available.

• Participation in the research may have direct benefit to the patient.

• The research could not feasibly be carried out without the waiver of informed consent.

• The investigator defines the length of therapeutic window and how the investigator will attempt to contact the legal representative.
  · This includes summarizing the efforts to contact the patient's legal representative.

• Other provisions:
  · The Institutional Review Board had reviewed and approved the informed consent.
  · There has been community consultation regarding the proposed research study.
  · Public disclosure has occurred.
  · There is an independent data monitoring committee.

---

of variations, (5) items should not provide irrelevant cues, (6) measures requiring complex operations are avoided, (7) the measurement tool should encompass the defined variable, and (8) the measure must demonstrate a relationship between performance on the tool and a subject's behavior.[2,15,17]

Some of the more common types of data collection measures include (1) physiologic and biophysical measurements, (2) observational measurements, (3) interviews and questionnaires, (4) scales, and (5) records or available data. Physiologic measurements are those used to measure characteristics of subjects being studied such as temperature, weight, height, cardiac output, muscle

strength, and biochemical levels (e.g., hemoglobin, blood glucose, and potassium). Advantages of physiologic measurements are objectivity, preciseness, and sensitivity because the data are not influenced by the person performing the study.

When researchers observe the research aspect of interest, direct observation measurements are used. For example, a researcher wants to observe the response of parents to casting or suturing procedures performed on their children. The observation method is most useful for entities difficult to measure, such as interactions, nursing process, changes in behavior, or group processes.

A third type of data collection is the use of interviews and questionnaires, which allows subjects to report data for or about themselves. The purpose of questioning participants is to seek direct data, such as age, religion, or marital status, or indirect data, such as level of intelligence, anxiety, and pain.

Measurement scales can be used to make distinctions among subjects concerning the degree to which they possess a certain trait, attitude, or emotion. Scales also permit comparisons in dimensions of interest. For example, a researcher interested in knowing whether a nerve block or a local injection of anesthetic is more effective for relieving pain during fracture reduction would use a pain scale to measure pain. Finally, use of records or available data refers to the researcher collecting data from existing databases, such as the electronic patient record.

Data Measurement Validity and Reliability

When instruments or tools are used for measuring subjects, the validity and reliability of tools need to be addressed by the researcher.[2,15,17] Validity is the degree to which an instrument measures what it is intended to measure. Validity is content, construct, or criterion related. Although an instrument may appear to measure some aspect of a construct or element, the instrument must be evaluated to determine whether it really does provide such measurement. Content validity is the degree to which an instrument measures the universe of content that it is said to represent or measure. Content validity is often determined by a panel of experts in the field to be evaluated. If a researcher wanted to measure bereavement behaviors in the ED, social workers, members of the clergy, and emergency nurses might be asked to review the instrument to be used to measure bereavement behavior.

Construct validity is the degree to which a tool measures the construct in the study. A construct is an abstraction developed for a scientific purpose. Construct validity is usually determined over time after data from research studies support the construct to a greater degree or question it further. An example might be if a research study was implemented to determine the sense of hope in trauma patients' families. The researcher's instrument must discriminate between families who possess hope and families who do not possess hope to ensure construct validity.

Criterion-related validity consists of both predictive validity and concurrent validity. The subject's performance on one measure is used to infer the likely response on another measure. Predictive validity is a measure used to predict future performance. For example, a nurse's score on a content knowledge test in emergency nursing predicts how well he or she will perform in practice. Concurrent validity is the degree to which an instrument can distinguish subjects who differ on a certain criterion measured at the same time.

Reliability of a measure or an instrument refers to its ability to consistently and accurately measure a criterion. A test of reliability is whether the tool produces the same measurement when a measurement is repeated several times. The less an instrument varies in repeated measurements, the greater the reliability of the instrument. An example for a physiologic measure might be a thermometer that measures a temperature as 98° F and upon repeat measurement obtains the same reading; this would demonstrate a measuring instrument with high reliability.[2,15,17]

Data Analysis

After completing data collection, the researcher summarizes the data through statistical procedures. The purpose of analysis is to answer the study questions or hypotheses. Researchers who use quantitative methods for data collection should also have a data analysis plan in place before beginning data collection. Statistical tests give meaning to quantitative data because they reduce, summarize, organize, evaluate, interpret, and communicate numeric data. One does not need to know how to conduct all of the statistical tests to understand the common principle of data analysis. Specifically, it is more important to be able to determine if the findings are statistically significant. This means the findings are probably valid and replicable with a new sample of subjects. The level of statistical significance is an index of the probability of reliability of the findings. For example, if a study indicates findings are significant at the 0.05 level, this means that 5 out of 100 times there is a risk that the result would be different from the reported finding, or possibly due to chance; in other words, 95 out of 100 times the findings would be the same.

Statistical tests are referred to as either descriptive or inferential. Descriptive statistics describe and summarize data. Examples are mode, median, mean, average, percentage, and frequency. Inferential statistics are used to draw conclusions about a large population based on a sample from a study, to make judgments, and to generalize information. Inferential statistics are then used to test the hypotheses to determine whether they are correct.

Two categories of inferential statistics are nonparametric and parametric. Most statistical tests are parametric tests, which focus on population parameters, require measurements on at least one interval or ratio scale, and make assumptions about distribution of the variables.[2] Nonparametric tests are used when measured variables are nominal or ordinal. These tests do not make assumptions about distribution of variables. Table 6-4 provides an overview of commonly performed statistical tests, both nonparametric and parametric, based on the level of measurement and variables in the study. Nurses often collaborate with biostatisticians to determine the appropriate statistical analyses to be used and obtain assistance with the data analyses for the research studies they undertake.

Results, Conclusions, and Recommendations

Results of the study are often organized by the research aims or hypotheses of the study. Results are often reported in the form of tables and graphs. Data summarized in graphs and tables can be more easily interpreted and compared with research questions or hypotheses and theoretical framework. Based on the findings of the study, the researcher draws conclusions. Study conclusions provide the foundation for the discussion section of the research report or manuscript.

Table 6-4.	COMMONLY USED STATISTICAL TESTS	
Parametric Test	**Example of an Equivalent Nonparametric Test**	**Purpose of the Statistical Test**
Two-sample (unpaired) t-test	Mann-Whitney U-test	Compares two independent samples drawn from the same population
One-sample (paired) t-test	Wilcoxon matched pairs test	Compares two sets of observations on a single sample
One-way analysis of variance (F-test) using total sum of squares	Kruskall-Wallis analysis of variance by ranks	Effectively, a generalization of the paired t-test or Wilcoxon matched pairs test where three or more sets of observations are made on a single sample
Two-way analysis of variance	Two-way analysis of variance by ranks	Effectively, a generalization of the paired t-test or Wilcoxon matched pairs test where three or more sets of observations are made on a single sample; tests the influence and interaction of two different covariates
Chi-square (χ^2)	Fisher's exact test	Tests the null hypothesis that the distribution of the discontinuous variable is the same in two (or more) independent samples
Pearson's r (product moment correlation coefficient)	Spearman's rank correlation coefficient	Assesses the strength of the straight line association between two continuous variables
Regression by least squares method	Nonparametric regression	Describes the numerical relation between two quantitative variables allowing one value to be predicted from the other
Multiple regression by least squares method	Nonparametric regression	Describes the numerical relation between a dependent variable and several predictor variables (covariates)

The researcher should attempt to give meaning to "why" the findings occurred by interweaving previous studies that have been done related to the study topic. Recommendations stem from changes the researcher plans in sample, design, or analysis if the study is repeated. Other explanations for results should be discussed so progress can be made in future studies of the research problem. Implications of research, such as how findings can be used to improve nursing or how to advance knowledge through additional research, should be provided.[2,15,17]

USING RESEARCH FINDINGS IN PRACTICE
Factors Promoting Research in the Clinical Setting

Multiple factors have been identified as critical to the integration of research and evidence-based practices into the clinical setting. At the individual nurse level, a key determinant is the nurse's attitude toward research or research utilization.[6] Attitudes and perceptions toward research utilization can be enhanced through both organizational characteristics[6] and the organizational environment[8] factors. Factors associated with higher rates of research utilization were related to an organization's actual hospital size or number of staffed beds, with larger hospitals demonstrating more research utilization.[6]

Within the organizational environment, research utilization increases when there is clear support from nursing leadership and administration for the integration of research and evidence-based practices, creating a "culture" within the environment that thrives on the infusion of research.[12,23] Strategies that promote an organizational environment conducive to research utilization include support by administration and key stakeholders (including delineation of resources such as access to research-based journals, computer access, and dedicated time to support these efforts),[12,14] having formal roles for nurses that include use of research in practice, engaging clinical staff nurses to identify variations in practices and process that affect patient care,[12] marketing or communicating to staff about the available resources to support research-based activities,[14] supporting clinical staff to make important patient care and work decisions,[33] having multidisciplinary committee structures to prioritize clinical practice issues and provide facilitation for research utilization initiatives,[35] and implementing organization-wide initiatives to maintain the enthusiasm and value of the importance of integrating research into practice. Supportive research utilization environments are enhanced by organizational committee structure and provision of resources to support the necessary preparation and research on specific clinical topics.[14,29] Barriers include lack of perceived control by nurses over having the authority to change practice.[21]

Other major determinants of research utilization in clinical practice revolve around staff education and skill

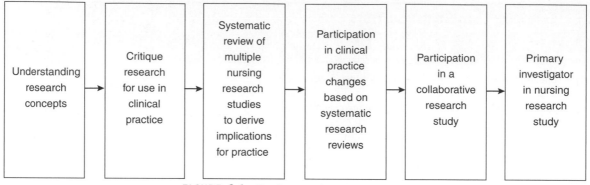

FIGURE 6-1. Continuum of nursing research.

development, as well as the actual efforts that go into the implementation of relevant research and evidence-based practices.* A key strategy is the implementation of an educational plan to update the nurses' skill sets related to research using a variety of formats (e.g., continuing education, self-paced modules, and web-based tutorials).[8,13] It is recommended that the education include both a dissemination component (e.g., sharing and dialoguing about benefits of research for practice) and implementation strategies to update the nurses' skill set related to use of research (e.g., reading the research literature, understanding and appraising the research findings, and conducting systematic reviews).[23] In addition to the education component to promote research utilization, additional strategies include using collaborative teams that use cooperative learning approaches, providing opportunities for nurse-to-nurse collaboration, and having role models and mentors to support research utilization efforts by staff nurses (e.g., clinical nurse specialists).† Specifically finding ways to incorporate the process of research into day-to-day practices is another key strategy. Approaches can include patient rounds to discuss supporting research and evidence for treatment interventions and decisions,[8] using "teachable" moments on the nursing unit for problem solving, establishing protocols, using consistent methods to systematically review and appraise research,[20] collecting information and data in daily work, and having staff lead practice reviews.

The other major research utilization issue to be addressed is designing a consistent method for implementing practice changes. Once staff begin generating practice changes based on research utilization, it is vital that changes be made in a consistent manner that will promote adoption and sustain the practice change. Useful strategies include planning the implementation, pilot testing in the clinical setting, reevaluating the effectiveness of the implementation plan, and modification of the processes to implement the recommended clinical practice changes throughout all clinical settings in the organization.[10]

SUMMARY

This chapter has provided an overview of nursing research processes and the importance of integrating research findings into clinical practice. Nurses' participation in the research process can vary along a continuum. At one end, participation can be reflected by a nurse's understanding of research concepts, whereas at the other end of the spectrum participation is exemplified by the nurse being a primary investigator in a research study. The overview of the continuum of nursing research participation is depicted in Figure 6-1. Regardless of the level of participation, all nurses have the opportunity to participate in research. The key role for all nurses is to strive for more integration of research into clinical practice.

References

1. Agency for Healthcare Research and Quality: *Systems to rate the strength of scientific evidence,* Evidence reports/technology assessment No. 47, AHRQ publication No. 02-E015, Department of Health and Human Services, 2002, Rockville, Md, 2002.
2. Barnason S: Research. In Newberry L, editor: *Sheehy's emergency nursing: principles and practice*, ed 5, St. Louis, 2003, Mosby.
3. Billings DM, Kowalski K: Bridging the theory-practice gap with evidence-based practice, *J Contin Educ Nurs* 27(6):248, 2006.
4. Cummings GG, Estabrooks CA, Midodzi WK et al: Influence of organizational characteristics and context on research utilization, *Nurs Res* 56(4 suppl):S24, 2007.
5. Ebell MH, Siwek J, Weiss BD et al: Strength of recommendation taxonomy (SORT): a patient-centered approach to grading evidence in the medical literature, *J Am Board Fam Pract* 17:59, 2004.
6. Estabrooks CA, Midodzi WK, Cummings GG et al: Predicting research use in nursing organizations, *Nurs Res* 56(4 suppl):S7, 2007.
7. Evans D: Hierarchy of evidence: a framework for ranking evidence evaluating healthcare interventions, *J Clin Nurs* 12:77, 2003.

---

*References 8, 18, 19, 25, 35, 36.
†References 4, 9, 10, 18, 25, 36.

8. Fineout-Overholt E, Levin RF, Melnyk BM: Strategies for advancing evidence-based practice in clinical settings, *J N Y State Nurses Assoc* 35(2):28, 2004.

9. Fineout-Overholt E, Melnyk BM, Schultz A: Transforming health care from the inside out: advancing evidence-based practice in the 21st century, *J Prof Nurs* 21(6):335, 2005.

10. French B: Contextual factors influencing research use in nursing, *Worldviews Evid Based Nurs* 2(4):172, 2005.

11. Goode CJ: What constitutes the "evidence" in evidence-based practice? *Appl Nurs Res* 13(4):222, 2000.

12. Hockenberry M, Walden M, Brown T et al: Creating an evidence-based practice environment, *J Nurs Care Q* 22(33):222, 2007.

13. Kajermo KN, Nordstrom G, Krusebrant A et al: Nurses' experience of research utilization within the framework of an educational programme, *J Clin Nurs* 10:671, 2001.

14. Larrabee JH, Sions J, Fanning M et al: Evaluation of a program to increase evidence-based practice change, *J Nurs Adm* 37(6):302, 2007.

15. LoBiondo-Wood G, Haber J: *Nursing research: methods and critical appraisal for evidence-based practice*, ed 6, Philadelphia, 2005, Mosby.

16. Lynn J, Bally MA, Bottrell M et al: The ethics of using quality improvement methods in health care, *Ann Intern Med* 146:666, 2007.

17. Macnee CL, McCabe S: *Understanding nursing research*, ed 2, Philadelphia, 2007, Lippincott Williams & Wilkins.

18. Melnyk BM: Finding and appraising systematic reviews of clinical interventions: critical skills for evidence-based practice, *Pediatr Nurs* 29(2):147, 2003.

19. Melnyk BM: Integrating levels of evidence into clinical decision making, *Pediatr Nurs* 30(4):323, 2004.

20. Melnyk BM, Fineout-Overholt E: Rapid critical appraisal of randomized controlled trials (RCTs): an essential skill for evidence-based practice (EBP), *Pediatr Nurs* 31(1):50, 2005.

21. Micevski V, Sarkissian S, Byrne J et al: Identification of barriers and facilitators to utilizing research in nursing practice, *Worldviews Evid Based Nurs* 1(4):229, 2004.

22. Newhouse RP: Diffusing confusion among evidence-based practice, quality improvement and research, *J Nurs Adm* 37(10):432, 2007.

23. Ockene JK, Zapka JG: Provider education to promote implementation for clinical practice guidelines, *Chest* 118(2 suppl):33S, 2000.

24. Panik A: Research on the frontlines of health care: a cooperative learning approach, *Nurs Res* 55(2 suppl):S3, 2006.

25. Paramonczyk A: Barriers to implementing research in clinical practice, *Can Nurse* 101(3):12, 2005.

26. Polit D, Beck C: *Essentials of nursing research: methods, appraisal and utilization*, Philadelphia, 2005, Lippincott Williams & Wilkins.

27. Raju TNK: Waiver of informed consent for emergency research and community disclosures and consultations, *J Investig Med* 52(2):109, 2004.

28. Ritter B: Considering evidence-based practice, *Nurse Pract* 26(5):63, 2001.

29. Rycroft-Malone J, Harvey G, Seers K et al: An exploration of the factors that influence the implementation of evidence into practice, *Issues Clin Nurs* 13:913, 2004.

30. Sackett DL, Straus EE, Richardson WS et al: *Evidence-based medicine: how to practice and teach EBM*, London, 2000, Churchill Livingstone.

31. Sugarman J: Examining the provisions for research without consent in the emergency setting, *Hastings Cent Rep* 37(1):12, 2007.

32. Thomas BH, Ciliska D, Dobbins M et al: A process for systematically reviewing the literature: providing the research evidence for public health nursing interventions, *Worldviews Evid Based Nurs* 1(3):176, 2004.

33. Titler M, Everett LQ, Adams S: Implications for implementation science, *Nurs Res* 56(4 suppl):S53, 2007.

34. Upton J: Research evidence: finding it and using it, *Practice Nurse* 34(4):8, 2007.

35. Vratny A, Shriver D: A conceptual model for growing evidence-based practice, *Nurs Adm Q* 31(2):162, 2007.

36. Welk DS: How to read, interpret, and understand evidence-based literature statistics, *Nurse Educ* 32(1):16, 2007.

UNIT III

CLINICAL FOUNDATIONS OF EMERGENCY NURSING

CHAPTER 7

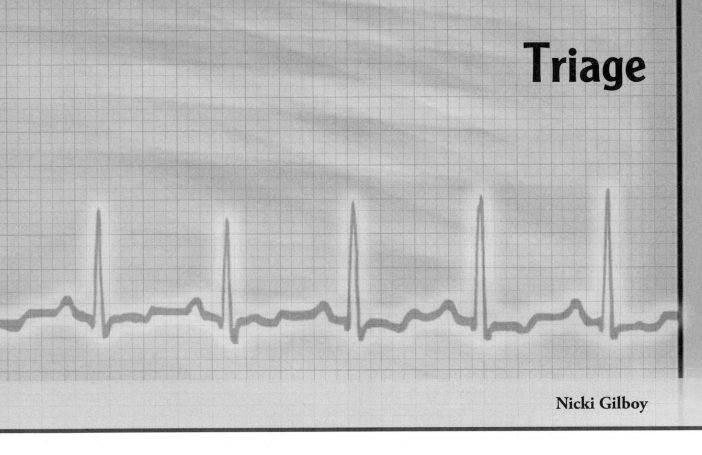

Triage

Nicki Gilboy

The number of patients seeking care in emergency departments (EDs) is increasing, while the number of EDs continues to decrease.[19] EDs are busier with about 50% reporting they are "at" or "over" capacity.[1] As a result, continuing ED crowding has placed even greater importance on the triage function and the role of the triage nurse.

Triage is the process of sorting patients as they present to the ED for care. The triage nurse must quickly identify those patients who need to be seen immediately and those patients who are safe to wait for care. This important decision needs to be based on a brief patient assessment that enables the triage nurse to assign an acuity rating. In many EDs the triage nurse will also decide in which area of the ED the patient will be seen. The overall goal of triage is to place the right patient in the right place at the right time for the right reason.

The word *triage* is derived from the French verb *trier,* which means to sort or to choose. Triage dates back to the French military, which used the word to designate a "clearing hospital" for wounded soldiers. The U.S. military used triage to describe a sorting station where injured soldiers were distributed from the battlefield to distant support hospitals. After World War II, triage came to mean the process used to identify those most likely to return to battle after medical intervention. This process allowed concentration of medical resources on soldiers who could fight again. During the Korean War, Vietnam War, and subsequent military conflicts, triage was refined to accomplish the "greatest good for the greatest number of wounded or injured men."[28]

Most U.S. EDs use some sort of triage process to sort incoming patients. In the event of a catastrophic occurrence, when the number of incoming patients exceeds the capabilities of a department, a system of disaster triage is activated. Disaster triage begins at the scene, and patients are retriaged upon presentation to the ED. It is similar to military triage in that the goal is the greatest good for the greatest number of ill or injured. In a disaster the triage process is very rapid and includes a brief assessment of airway, breathing, perfusion, and mental status. Patients are assigned to one of four categories, and there is recognition that there are limited resources and some patients are not salvageable (see Chapter 17).

The concept of triage was first introduced into U.S. EDs in the 1950s when the volume of patients seeking emergency care increased. Many of these patients were presenting with nonurgent problems, and the process of seeing patients by time of arrival was no longer feasible. ED staff with a military background brought the concept of triage to the civilian EDs. At the same time physicians were moving away from solo practice and forming group practices with regular office hours. Patients seeking care during off-hours were referred to the local ED. The role of the ED as a provider of care at all times was established.[17]

The number of U.S. ED visits in 2005 was 115.3 million.[19] Between 1995 and 2005 there was a 20% increase in ED visits, while the number of hospital EDs decreased 9% from 4,176 to 3,795.[19] Reasons cited for the increase in visits include the growing older adult population, an increase in the number of uninsured persons, and poor access to primary care or urgent care.[17] Because U.S. EDs are seeing an increase in number of patients seeking emergency care, a system for rapid, accurate triage upon presentation is critical to patient safety.

TRIAGE SYSTEMS

There is no single type of triage system used by all EDs in the United States. Three types of triage systems have been described in the literature. The simplest triage system is called traffic director.[17,26] In this type of system a nonclinical person is stationed at the ED entrance to greet patients upon presentation. Based on his or her initial impression, this nonclinical person decides if the patient should go to the waiting room or go to an open ED bed. Another system used by EDs with a lower volume of visits is called spot-check triage. For these departments it is not cost-effective to staff triage with a registered nurse (RN) 24 hours a day. Instead, the RN is notified when a patient presents. The RN does a quick look or brief assessment and then assigns a triage acuity.[17,26]

Comprehensive triage, the most advanced system, is performed by an RN and is the system recommended by the Emergency Nurses Association (ENA).[17] ENA's *Standards of Emergency Nursing Practice* state: "The ED RN triages every patient and determines priority of care based on physical, developmental, and psychosocial needs as well as factors influencing flow through the emergency care system."[10] Based on this assessment, the RN will assign an acuity rating. There are many advantages to comprehensive triage, as follows:

- The triage process is conducted by an experienced ED RN whose competency has been validated.
- The RN is able to rapidly identify those patients in need of immediate care.
- Laboratory studies, x-ray examinations, and electrocardiograms can be initiated using triage protocols.
- The RN is able to provide reassurance to patients and families.
- First aid and comfort measures can be provided (in some EDs this may include medications for fever control and pain).
- Patient teaching can be initiated.
- Reassessment can be done.
- The RN can advocate for patients and work with the charge nurse to get patients to care.
- Patients in the waiting room are safe to wait.[13]

The ENA recommends that the triage encounter take no more than 2 to 5 minutes.[31] Travers[27] found that this was met only 22% of the time and the time frame was extended with patient age. The average time spent on comprehensive triage of the pediatric patient was 7 minutes.[18]

Many EDs are using comprehensive triage, but some are struggling with how to manage the rapid influx of patients at various points in the day. Patients are waiting an unacceptably long period of time from entry into the ED (time of arrival) to actual triage time. Some EDs have addressed this issue by choosing to use a greeter as the first contact with ambulatory patients. Their role is to greet the patient, document time of arrival, and keep a list of the patients waiting for triage. Other EDs ask the patient or family member to write their name and reason for the visit on a list or card. The triage nurse uses this initial information from the greeter or from a list to determine the order in which patients are triaged. However, this system is not perfect and delays in care can occur. Delay may be due to the patient giving a vague description of why he or she came to the ED or the patient putting an incorrect label on his or her problem. For example, a patient tells the greeter, "I have a migraine," when he or she is in fact having a stroke. To prevent this potential problem, some hospitals have adopted a two-tiered triage process or system.

Two-Tiered Triage Systems

In a two-tiered triage system the patient enters the ED and is greeted by an experienced ED RN who determines the chief complaint and conducts a rapid visual assessment to determine if this patient needs to be seen immediately or is safe to proceed to step two of the triage process. The first nurse initiates documentation. Those patients identified as needing to be seen immediately are taken to an open bed and registered at the bedside. Those patients identified as safe to wait are seen by the second triage nurse, who completes and documents a comprehensive triage assessment. The patient is then registered, and care may be initiated using triage protocols.

The advantage of a two-tier triage system is that an experienced ED nurse immediately screens all patients when they enter the ED. The patient with symptoms of a possible stroke, myocardial infarction, or other serious problem will be immediately identified and taken directly to a bed. EDs are faced with many quality measures with time parameters, such as a door-to-balloon time of 90 minutes, that the two-tiered system can help meet.[21] In a two-tiered system these patients are immediately identified upon arrival.

TRIAGE ACUITY RATING SYSTEMS

Based on an "across-the-room assessment," brief interview, and focused examination, the triage nurse assigns an acuity rating. Historically a three-level acuity rating system has been used by most EDs.[13] The three levels are emergent, urgent, and nonurgent (Table 7-1). In an effort to better sort incoming patients, some hospitals added a fourth level to relieve the number of patients who were assigned to the middle or urgent level.

A number of published research studies demonstrate the poor interrater reliability of the three-level triage acuity

Table 7-1. URGENCY CATEGORIES

Category	Description
Emergent	Immediate care required; condition is threat to life, limb, or vision; "severe"
Urgent	Care required as soon as possible; condition presents danger if not treated; "acute" but not "severe"
Nonurgent	Routine care required; condition minor; care can be delayed

Thompson J, Dains J: *Comprehensive triage: a manual for developing and implementing a nursing care system,* Reston, Va, 1982, Reston.

rating system.[16,29,30] Interrater reliability is the level of agreement or consistency among users of the system. As triage has evolved, there has been an increasing recognition that high interrater reliability is a necessary characteristic of an effective triage acuity rating system.

With the publication of research questioning the reliability of a three-level acuity rating system and concerns about ED crowding, the American College of Emergency Physicians (ACEP) and the ENA convened a five-level triage task force to review the evidence on five-level triage scales. The following statement was developed by the task force and approved by the boards of directors of both ENA and ACEP:

> ACEP and ENA believe that quality of patient care would benefit from implementing a standardized emergency department (ED) triage scale and acuity categorization process. Based on expert consensus of currently available evidence, ACEP and ENA support the adoption of a reliable, valid five-level triage scale.[14]

As a result of this effort the Five-Level Triage Task Force recommended the use of either the Canadian Triage and Acuity Scale (CTAS) or the Emergency Severity Index (ESI).[15]

The CTAS, which is based on the Australasian Triage Scale, was developed by a group of Canadian emergency physicians working with the National Emergency Nurses Association (Canada).[2,3] All Canadian EDs use this five-level acuity rating system. The system mandates that every patient presenting for care should be at least visually assessed within 10 minutes of presentation. For each triage level there is a list of presenting complaints or conditions. The ED RN assigns acuity based on chief complaint and a focused subjective and objective assessment. CTAS identifies time to physician for each triage level but recognizes that meeting this time objective 100% of the time is not realistic. Accordingly, fractile response time, or the percentage of patient visits for a given triage level in which the patient should be seen within the CTAS time frame, is identified.[3] Reassessment times are identified for each of the five triage levels. Training materials are available from the Canadian Association of Emergency Physicians, http://www.caep.ca.

Two ED physicians, Richard Wuerz and David Eitel, developed the original concept for the Emergency Severity Index (ESI). Working with a group of emergency physicians

and nurses, they made further refinements to the original algorithm based on research. The ESI is a five-level triage scale that categorizes patients initially by acuity and then by expected resource consumption (Figure 7-1). The algorithm is straightforward to use and allows for the rapid sorting of patients into one of five categories. Research has demonstrated that it is a valid and reliable system. Training materials that include the implementation handbook and training DVD are available free of charge from the Agency for Healthcare Research and Quality, http://www.ahrq.gov/research/esi, or call 1-800-358-9295.17.[23,24,30]

THE TRIAGE PROCESS

The triage process is the rapid collection of relevant subjective and objective data in order for the triage nurse to assign an accurate acuity rating. It should be brief and occur soon after the patient arrives in the ED. The triage process begins with an across-the-room assessment. The triage nurse uses his or her sense of sight, hearing, and smell to gather vital information (Table 7-2) and form a general impression of the patient's health status.[11-13] Occasionally the patient is so ill or injured that the nurse will recognize the patient needs to be seen immediately. At that point the triage process is over, and the patient is taken directly to the treatment area. This occurs in a small number of patients, and usually the triage process continues.

In a two-tiered triage system the first nurse is performing an across-the-room assessment, as well as determining the patient's chief complaint. Based on this information, the first triage nurse decides whether this patient needs to be taken directly to the patient care area or is stable enough to go to step two of the triage process.

The Triage Interview

The patient is brought to a triage room or area where the triage interview can be conducted. The purpose of the interview is to gather additional information about the patient's illness or injury. The triage interview should begin with the nurse confirming the patient's identity, introducing himself or herself to the patient, and explaining to the patient the purpose of the triage process. For example, "Mr. Smith, my name is Sue. I am one of the emergency department nurses. I need to ask you a few questions about what brought you here today. Please have a seat, and take off your coat." A friendly greeting and smile can go a long way to developing rapport with the patient and his or her family. Many are anxious and concerned about the patient, and a few words of reassurance will be appreciated.

The patient's chief complaint should be documented in his or her own words and in quotation marks. Some patients need to be asked directly, "What made you come to the emergency department today?" "What made you call the ambulance?" Once the chief complaint has been determined, the triage nurse can proceed with a brief interview to elicit information about the chief complaint and relevant signs and symptoms.

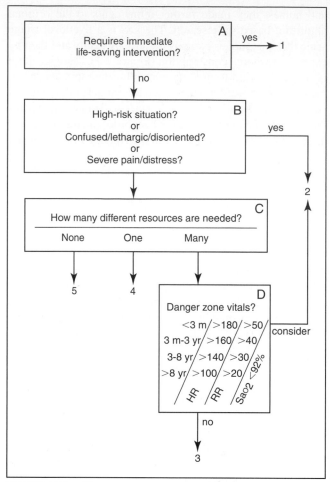

FIGURE 7-1. The Emergency Severity Index conceptual algorithm. (© ESI Triage Research Team, 2004. Used with permission.)

Gathering appropriate subjective information is vital to making the right triage acuity rating decision. If the triage nurse does not clearly understand what the patient is trying to say, follow-up questions and clarification are needed. Obtaining information can be a challenge when the patient provides vague or global reasons for the visit: "I've been so sick," or "My doctor told me to come here." The triage nurse must focus his or her investigation on the history of the complaint and related symptoms and signs. The PQRST mnemonic is one example of a systematic approach to patient assessment (Tables 7-3 and 7-4).

The triage nurse should use a variety of open (i.e., eliciting feelings and perceptions) and closed (i.e., "yes/no," factual) questions to obtain information. Closed-ended questions are helpful for obtaining basic information such as, Do you have any allergies? To elicit details, open-ended questions are more effective. Restating, verbalizing observations, sharing information, actively listening, and summarizing are important communication strategies. The nurse's style will vary with each patient and situation.

A medical interpreter should be used when the patient does not speak English or is more comfortable speaking in his or her native language. Many hospitals have medical interpreters on staff for non–English-speaking patients or have access to interpreters on call or via the telephone system such as the AT&T language line. Using family members can be problematic because you are asking the patient to share personal information with family members, and in addition, the family member may not understand exactly what you are asking. The triage nurse should document when an interpreter or family member was used to gather the history.

The triage process should take between 2 and 5 minutes. The triage nurse needs to be organized and efficient. It is important for the triage nurse to multitask or delegate to ancillary personnel specific tasks.

When sufficient information has been obtained about the chief complaint and related symptoms, the triage nurse may then obtain information about medications, past medical history, allergies, last menstrual period, and immunizations. Medication usage will include prescribed medications, over-the-counter drugs, herbal preparations, and home remedies.

At this point the triage nurse will perform a brief, focused physical examination based on the patient's current injury or illness. The purpose of the examination is to gather additional information to support the triage nurse's decision that this patient is safe to wait for care. The primary nurse will do a more in-depth assessment when the patient is taken to a treatment area. The triage examination is brief and should not require the patient to undress. It is not a head-to-toe assessment or a systems assessment but is a brief focused examination (Table 7-5).

Vital Signs and Triage

EDs have traditionally required a full set of vital signs on all patients as part of the triage process. Patients identified as unstable and in need of immediate care should be taken directly to an open treatment area. Care should never be delayed because a full set of vital signs has not been obtained. In some situations, vital signs may provide the triage nurse with additional information that will influence the acuity rating decision. Some EDs have chosen to assess and document a full set of vital signs on all lower acuity patients. Documentation of stable vital signs provides additional data to support the triage acuity rating. In one study of over 14,000 patients, vital signs changed the level of triage acuity in only 8% of cases.[6] Vital signs were found to be an important part of the triage process in the pediatric patient age 2 or younger, older adults, and those with communication issues.[6] The triage nurse needs to know normal parameters for age, the effect of medications, and certain disease processes (Table 7-6).

Triage Acuity Rating

Based on the information obtained from the across-the-room assessment, chief complaint, patient interview, and focused physical examination, the triage nurse then

Table 7-2. ACROSS-THE-ROOM ASSESSMENT

Sense	Category	Examples or Specifics
Sight	Sick or not sick	
	Obvious deformities/amputations	Child with a craniofacial abnormality
		Severe kyphosis
	Method of arrival	Walked in
		Carried, wheelchair
	Body habitus	Tall, short
		Cachectic, thin, obese
	Dress	Appropriate
		Clean, disheveled
	Chronic illness	Bald due to chemotherapy
		Pursed-lip breathing from COPD
	Activity level	Walking with no difficulty
		Walking bent over, holding abdomen
		Using an assistive device (e.g., cane)
	Obvious blood on clothing, skin	
	Breathing	Obvious respiratory distress, working hard
		Using home oxygen
	Skin color	Severe jaundice
	Level of consciousness	Crying, moaning, laughing, talking, lethargic
Hearing	Breathing	Wheezing, stridor, grunting
	Speech	Tone, cadence, volume
		Language spoken, slurred
Smell	Stool, urine, vomit	Incontinence, illness related
	Ketones	Diabetic
	Alcohol, cigarettes	
	Poor hygiene	Living situation may need assessment
	Pus	Infection
	Chemicals	Exposure—skin, clothing

COPD, Chronic obstructive pulmonary disease.

Table 7-3. PQRST MNEMONIC

Component	Sample Questions
P (provokes)	What provokes the symptom? What makes it better? What makes it worse?
Q (quality)	What does it feel like?
R (radiation)	Where is it? Where does it go? Is it in one or more spots?
S (severity)	If we gave it a number from 0 to 10, with 0 being none and 10 being the worst you can imagine, what is your rating?
T (time)	How long have you had the symptom? When did it start? When did it end? How long did it last? Does it come and go?

Table 7-4. INTERVIEWING A PATIENT WITH AN INJURY AT TRIAGE

Event	Triage Questioning
Minor burn	Cause or mechanism of the burn
	Location and depth of the burn
	Extent of the burn
	Treatment before arrival
Motor vehicle collision, not life-threatening	When did the event occur?
	Ambulatory at the scene?
	Speed of the vehicle
	Driver, passenger front or back
	Seat belt use, airbag deployed
	Vehicle damage
	Current complaints
Fall	When did this occur?
	Current complaints
	Fall—from what onto what?
	Why do you think you fell? (e.g., dizzy before fall)
Sports-related injury	Describe what happened
	Were you wearing a helmet or other protective equipment?
	Loss of consciousness?
	Ambulatory at the scene?
	Current complaints

assigns an acuity rating. This is a critical decision that has implications for patient safety. If the patient is assigned a lower acuity, his or her care may be delayed; if the patient is overtriaged or assigned a higher acuity rating, then the patient may take priority over someone who needs care more quickly.

Table 7-5.	FOCUSED PHYSICAL ASSESSMENT AT TRIAGE
Chief Complaint	**Focused Assessment**
Short of breath	Respiratory rate, depth, effort
	Accessory muscle use
	Skin color
	Oxygen saturation
	Peak flow
	Level of consciousness
	Position
	Ability to talk in full sentences
	Abnormal sounds
Injured arm	Deformity, angulation
	Color, capillary refill, pulse
	Sensation
	Movement—ROM
Finger laceration	Wound length, depth, location
	Shape, swelling
	CSM, tendon involvement
	Evidence of foreign material
	Bleeding, bruising
Itchy eyes	Signs of inflammation, drainage
	Tearing, photophobia
	Visual acuity
Arm weakness	Level of consciousness
	Glasgow Coma Scale
	Facial symmetry
	Pronator drift
	Speech clarity and articulation
	Hand grasp strength
	Pupils—size and reaction

CSM, Circulation, sensation, and motor; *ROM,* range of motion.

It is important that every patient be assigned a triage acuity rating even if the patient bypasses the triage process and goes directly to a treatment area. Use of a valid and reliable triage acuity rating system provides ED leadership with triage data that can be used for many purposes. For example, EDs typically use the average number of patients seen per day or per year to describe their patient population. Review of acuity data, volume, and types of patients most commonly seen will be more reflective of the ED population. Case mix or percentage of patients in each triage category may also provide a more accurate description of the ED demographics. ED leadership can use triage acuity and case mix information to identify internal trends or benchmark with other similar facilities.

Triage Care

The extent of care provided at triage varies from one ED to another and often depends upon the availability of an available treatment area. Certain hospitals have gone back to the original concept of triage as a mechanism to sort incoming patients when no emergency treatment area is available.[20] Some facilities have instituted triage bypass when there is an available emergency treatment area. The patient is taken directly to the treatment area, registered at the bedside, and seen by the care team, which collects the necessary patient information. The triage process will begin when all available treatment spaces are in use and patients will need to wait to be seen.

The triage nurse will often need to provide initial interventions to patients such as ice, elevation, and immobilization of an injured extremity. The triage nurse has the opportunity to educate the patient and family as to why these measures are important. Patients often present with a bloody cloth wrapped around an injury or wound. The triage nurse needs to remove the makeshift dressing, assess the extent of the wound, and then apply a sterile dressing.

Table 7-6.	VITAL SIGNS BY AGE		
Age	**Respiratory Rate/Minute**	**Heart Rate/Minute**	**Systolic Blood Pressure (mm Hg)**
Preterm newborn	55-65	120-180	40-60
Term newborn	40-60	90-170	52-92
1 month	30-50	110-180	60-104
6 months	25-35	110-180	65-125
1 year	20-30	80-160	70-118
2 years	20-30	80-130	73-117
4 years	20-30	80-120	65-117
6 years	18-24	75-115	76-116
8 years	18-22	70-110	76-119
10 years	16-20	70-110	82-122
12 years	16-20	60-110	84-128
14 years	16-20	60-105	85-136

Modified from Proehl JA: Secondary survey. In Proehl JA, editor: *Emergency nursing procedures,* ed 2, Philadelphia, 1999, WB Saunders.

Many EDs have triage protocols or standing orders in place that allow nurses to initiate care at triage. Protocols can include diagnostic testing (laboratory, radiographs, and electrocardiograms) or can be for the administration of medications for fever or pain if the patient meets certain criteria. Triage protocols are developed by the department and approved by the medical staff. Once a patient has been triaged, the triage nurse may choose to implement the appropriate protocol to initiate care. The goal of protocols is to decrease the patient's length of stay, increase patient and staff satisfaction, and decrease the number of patients who choose to leave without being seen.[31]

SPECIAL POPULATIONS
The Pediatric Patient

The majority of infants and children brought to an ED have nonurgent problems. The triage nurse needs to be able to rapidly and accurately identify the other 5% of children who are in need of immediate care.[11] Infants and children are small and portable, so when they are seriously ill or injured, many are brought to the ED by car rather than by ambulance.[11]

For a variety of reasons emergency nurses often feel uncomfortable triaging children, which can lead to either overtriage or undertriage. To triage this population, the triage nurse needs to know about normal growth and development to quickly identify deviations from normal. For example, an 8-month-old who does not cry when a stranger picks him or her up or a 7-year-old carried into the ED warrants further investigation. Knowledge of developmental milestones will assist the nurse with both the subjective and objective assessment. A school-age child can tell the nurse if he or she is having pain. An adolescent can give the triage nurse a detailed history. The triage nurse needs to be familiar with illnesses or injuries that are prevalent in the pediatric age-group, such as pyloric stenosis or bronchiolitis.

The ENA Emergency Nursing Pediatric Course (ENPC) outlines the components of comprehensive pediatric triage. This includes the pediatric assessment triangle, the history, and physical examination.[11]

The pediatric assessment triangle is the first step of the assessment process and is a more clearly defined across-the-room assessment. The triage nurse uses his or her senses, forms a general impression, and then assesses work of breathing and circulation to the skin (Table 7-7). This quick assessment is used to decide whether the child needs to go directly to a treatment area or is stable and the triage process may continue. This across-the-room assessment is done without the child being aware that he or she is being observed.

If no life-threatening emergencies are identified using the pediatric assessment triangle, the triage nurse will begin the subjective and objective assessment. The ENPC identifies the components for the history, primary assessment, and secondary assessment. The mnemonic for history is CIAMPEDS (Table 7-8).[11] The triage nurse needs to be familiar with common pediatric red flags that indicate a serious problem when found during the triage assessment (Box 7-1). The history is obtained from the parent or caregiver who knows the infant or child best and can share with the triage nurse his or her concerns and impressions. For the child with disabilities, it is the caregiver who is most likely to notice subtle signs or changes that can suggest a problem. The verbal child can answer specific questions posed by the triage nurse such as, What happened? or Does it hurt?

Before assigning a triage acuity, the triage nurse needs to look at the infant's or child's vital signs and question whether they are within the normal range for this infant or child. If they are abnormal, can the variation be readily explained?

Table 7-7.	THE PEDIATRIC ASSESSMENT TRIANGLE
General impression	Does the child look ill?
	Is the child playful?
	Is the child aware of surroundings?
	Is the child alert? Crying? Sleepy or unresponsive?
	What is the child's interaction with the environment and caregiver?
Work of breathing	What is the position of comfort to facilitate air entry?
	Are there audible airway sounds? Is the child coughing? Drooling?
	How is the child breathing? Is the respiratory rate slow, normal, or rapid for age?
	Are there signs of accessory muscle use?
Circulation to skin	Is the child's skin color pale, dusky, cyanotic, mottled, or flushed?
	Is here any obvious bleeding?
	Is the child diaphoretic?

Table 7-8.	COMPONENTS OF BASIC PEDIATRIC ASSESSMENT (CIAMPEDS)	
C	Chief complaint	Reason for the child's ED visit and duration of complaint (e.g., fever for past 2 days)
I	Immunizations	Evaluation of the child's current immunization status: • The completion of all scheduled immunizations for the child's age should be evaluated. • If the child has not received immunizations because of religious or cultural beliefs, document this information.
	Isolation	Evaluation of the child's exposure to communicable diseases (e.g., meningitis, chickenpox, shingles, whooping cough, tuberculosis): • A child with active disease or who is potentially infectious must be placed in respiratory isolation on arrival to the ED. • Other exposures that may be evaluated include exposure to meningitis and scabies.
A	Allergies	Evaluation of the child's previous allergic or hypersensitivity reactions: • Document reactions to medications, foods, products (e.g., latex), and environmental allergens. The type of reaction must also be documented.
M	Medications	Evaluation of the child's current medication regimen, including prescription and over-the-counter medications, herbal and dietary supplements: • Dose administered. • Time of last dose. • Duration of use.

P	Past medical history	A review of the child's health status, including prior illnesses, injuries, hospitalizations, surgeries, and chronic physical and psychiatric illnesses. Use of alcohol, tobacco, drugs, or other substances of abuse should be evaluated, as appropriate:
		 • The past medical history of the neonate should include the prenatal and birth history:
		  • Maternal complications during pregnancy or delivery.
		  • Infant's gestational age and birth weight.
		  • Number of days infant remained in hospital following birth.
		 • The past medical history of the menarcheal female should include the date and description of her last menstrual period.
		 • The past medical history for sexually active patients should include the following:
		  • Type of birth control used.
		  • Barrier protection.
		  • Prior treatment for sexually transmitted diseases.
		  • Gravida (pregnancies) and para (births, miscarriages, abortions, living children).

	Parent's/ Caregiver's impression of the child's condition	• Identify the child's primary caregiver. • Consider cultural differences that may affect the caregiver's impressions. • Evaluation of the caregiver's concerns and observations of the child's condition: • Especially significant in evaluating the special needs child.

E	Events surrounding the illness or injury	Evaluation of the onset of the illness or circumstances and mechanism of injury:
		 • Illness:
		  • Length of illness, including date and day of onset and sequence of symptoms.
		  • Treatment provided before ED visit.
		 • Injury:
		  • Time and date injury occurred.
		  • M: Mechanism of injury, including the use of protective devices (seat belts, helmets).
		  • I: Injuries suspected.
		  • V: Vital signs in prehospital environment.
		  • T: Treatment by prehospital providers.
		  • Description of circumstances leading to injury.
		  • Witnessed or unwitnessed.

D	Diet	• Assessment of the child's recent oral intake and changes in eating patterns related to the illness or injury:
		  • Changes in eating patterns or fluid intake.
		  • Time of last meal and last fluid intake.
		  • Regular diet: breast milk, type of formula, solid foods, diet for age and developmental level, cultural differences.
		  • Special diet or diet restrictions.

Table 7-8.	COMPONENTS OF BASIC PEDIATRIC ASSESSMENT (CIAMPEDS)—CONT'D	
	Diapers	Assessment of the child's urine and stool output: • Frequency of urination over last 24 hours; changes in frequency. • Time of last void. • Changes in odor or color of urine. • Last bowel movement; color and consistency of stool. • Change in frequency of bowel movements.
S	Symptoms associated with the illness or injury	Identification of symptoms and progression of symptoms since the time of onset of the illness or injury event.

ED, Emergency department.

Box 7-1   PEDIATRIC RED FLAGS

In addition to abnormal vital signs, the triage nurse should be aware of the following pediatric red flags:
• Abnormal airway sounds such as stridor
• Grunting
• Increased work of breathing (using accessory muscles or retracting)
• Capillary refill greater than 2 seconds
• Sunken or bulging fontanel
• Change in level of consciousness
• Severe pain or distress
• Petechiae

For example, a heart rate of 160 beats per minute is normal in a neonate, but this same rate in a toddler who fell off a slide is a major concern.

The Geriatric Patient

People age 65 and older make up about 13% of the U.S. population but account for nearly 15% of all ED visits.[19,22] Over one third of older adults are brought to the ED by ambulance. The average life expectancy for both males and females is continuing to increase, and many are living with chronic medical problems and taking multiple medications. Of all hospitalized, 57% are admitted through the ED.[19] Research has shown that the triage process can take longer with the geriatric patient.[27] The ED length of stay for these patients has been shown to be 20% longer than for younger patients, and older patients consume more resources.[22]
• The triage interview may be more difficult. The patient may have multiple complaints, vague complaints, or may not be able to tell the triage nurse why someone called the ambulance. Additional information should be obtained from emergency medical services (EMS), the sending facility, or the family.
• The patient may have a list of medications he or she is supposed to be taking. It is important to determine what medications the patient is actually taking.
• The effect of medications on vital signs must be considered.

• Admission to the ED provides the triage nurse with the opportunity to evaluate the patient's interactions with his or her family. EMS may provide the triage nurse with valuable information about the patient's living conditions and ability to manage his or her activities of daily living. It is also an opportunity to screen for elder abuse and neglect.
• Older adults will often present with atypical signs and symptoms of common medical problems. For example, a change in level of consciousness may be the first sign of a urinary or respiratory tract infection.[22]

The Psychiatric Patient

Patients with a psychiatric history or new onset of symptoms usually present to the ED when their coping mechanisms fail. They may self-present or be brought in by family, friends, or the police. Occasionally the patient is brought in handcuffed or restrained to an ambulance stretcher. This patient bypasses triage and goes directly to a secure treatment area.

Triage of the psychiatric patient begins with the across-the-room assessment, which can provide the triage nurse important information. Bizarre dress, loud rapid speech, odor of alcohol, demeanor, and activity level can be determined. Based on the across-the-room assessment, the triage nurse decides if the patient goes directly to a treatment area or if the patient can go through the triage process. The priority concern with this patient is staff and patient safety: Is this patient a danger to himself or herself, others, or the environment? The experienced triage nurse will have security on standby in the ED, quickly establish rapport with the patient, and assess for both patient and staff safety. Questions may include the following:
• What brought you here today?
• Have you thought about hurting yourself or others? If the answer is yes, determine if the patient has a plan and whether the patient has the means to carry out the plan.
• Do you have anything with you that can hurt you or me?
• Have you ever been hospitalized for any medical or emotional problems?
• What medications do you take, and are you taking them?
• Assess for alcohol and drug use—How much? How often? Last used or last drink? Occasionally patients presenting to the ED decided to stop drinking or using drugs and

may already be tachycardic and showing signs of withdrawal.

- When the triage nurse suspects that the patient is having auditory, tactile, or visual hallucinations, it is important to ask the patient if this is indeed what is going on.
- Is the patient making any paranoid statements?
- During the triage assessment describe the patient's appearance, behavior, motor activity, and speech. For example, is the patient making eye contact and answering your questions appropriately?[12]

AMBULANCE TRIAGE

In 2005 about 15% of patients seen in U.S. EDs were transported by ambulance.[19] Most EDs have a separate ambulance triage area. The triage process for ambulance patients should be exactly the same as it is for "walk-in" patients: an across-the-room assessment, followed by a brief subjective and objective assessment, and assignment of an acuity rating. The triage nurse should assess the ambulance patient who does not need to be seen immediately and decide if it would be appropriate for the patient to wait in the waiting room. Method of transportation to an ED should not determine how quickly the patient is seen.

TRIAGE DOCUMENTATION

How much information should the triage nurse gather and document about each patient? This is a question that many EDs are struggling with because they are being asked to do increased screening of patients when they present to the ED for care. This includes screening for fall risk, smoking, drug and alcohol use, and domestic violence. Every ED should have a documentation policy or guideline that details what elements are required by the department. At a minimum, the triage nurse should document enough information to support the triage acuity rating assigned to the patient. The general elements of triage documentation must include the following:

- Time and date of triage interview
- Two patient identifiers (patient name, date of birth, or medical record number)
- Chief complaint
- Brief subjective and objective assessment
- Vital signs for lower acuity patients
- Triage acuity rating
- Interventions initiated
- Assessment of pain
- RN signature

This is an example of poor documentation for a trauma patient who walks into triage: "27-year-old male presents to triage ambulatory stating, 'I got shot,' and pointing to his abdomen. To trauma 1 via wheelchair. Skin cool and clammy." This note is brief, no vital signs were taken, and no other information was gathered by the triage nurse.

For stable, patients who do not need to go directly to a treatment area, the triage nurse may gather more detailed information. This may include the following:

- Weight
- Last menstrual period
- Allergies
- Medications—including prescriptions, over-the-counter, and herbals; medication reconciliation may begin at triage
- Past medical history
- Immunization status
- Medications administered at triage per protocol
- Diagnostic tests initiated (laboratory, radiographs, electrocardiogram)
- Mode of arrival
- Bedside glucose level determination or other point-of-care testing

It is important that the triage nurse document if the history was obtained from someone other than the patient. Was it the mother or the caregiver or from EMS? If the patient is non–English-speaking, who served as the interpreter? Was family, the hospital medical language interpreter, or the AT&T language line used?

If a paper record is being used for triage, it is imperative that the form contain as many check boxes as possible to save time in the documentation process. Check boxes also serve as reminders to busy triage nurses that they need to gather certain information. Triage documentation may be standardized through the use of an electronic medical record. This method may eliminate duplication of information because the data flows throughout the continuum of care. Electronic documentation may force entry of certain data elements to be able to advance to the next screen. Regardless of the system, triage documentation provides a "snapshot" of the patient's chief complaint, appearance, and acuity. Figure 7-2 is an example of triage documentation.

INFECTION CONTROL

The Joint Commission 2009 National Patient Safety Goals focus on reduction of the risk for health care–associated infections.[25] Infection control begins at triage with strict adherence to hand hygiene guidelines. Hand hygiene with soap and water or an alcohol-based hand rub is essential before and after every patient contact. Many EDs have placed signs at the entrance to the ED with dispensers of an alcohol-based hand rub to educate patients and visitors on preventing the spread of infections through appropriate hand hygiene.

To prevent the spread of any respiratory infection the Centers for Disease Control and Prevention recommends that any patient presenting to the ED with a cough should be asked to wear a surgical or procedure mask to prevent the spread of droplets to others.[4] In addition to hand hygiene, respiratory hygiene and cough etiquette need to be emphasized. The waiting room needs to have tissues available for patients and visitors and a place to dispose of them. Waiting rooms with toys for children must have a system in place for cleaning the toys to prevent the spread of infection.

ARRIVAL TIME

BRIGHAM AND WOMEN'S HOSPITAL
A Teaching Affiliate of Harvard Medical School
75 Francis Street, Boston, Massachusetts 02115

EMERGENCY DEPARTMENT
NURSING RECORD

CC:		ESI ☐1 ☐2 ☐3 ☐4 ☐5	
Current Pain:	CAP	☐I D Screening completed ☐Mask applied	Behavioral Risk Assessment ☐N/A ☐Completed - see note
Last Name:	First Name:		Age:
Arrived Via: ☐Car ☐Ambulance ☐Other			D.O.B.
☐Arrives C-spine immobilized	IV		LMP:
Primary Language: ☐English ☐Spanish ☐Other Interpreter: ☐Professional ☐Family ☐Employee			TD:

ARRIVAL TIME

PTA VS:	P	R	BP	SpO_2	O_2	T
Triage VS:	P	R	BP	SpO_2	O_2	T

PMH: ☐Reports none	Meds: ☐None	Allergies: ☐None known
		NPO☐Y ☐N

Triage Note:

Signature RN I.D. #

Recheck time: Signature RN I.D. #

FIGURE **7-2.** Emergency department nursing record. (Courtesy Brigham and Women's Hospital, Boston.)

Infectious disease screening is a routine part of any triage assessment. Does this person potentially have an infection that could be easily transmitted to other patients, staff, or visitors? Does the patient have symptoms of tuberculosis? Does the patient have a cough, fever, and diarrhea or a rash that could be communicable? Has the patient been traveling out of the country recently or exposed to anyone else who has a communicable disease? One role of the triage nurse is to identify the patient with a potential infectious disease, institute the appropriate infection control measures, document the situation, and then work with the charge nurse to get the patient to an appropriate treatment area. Some ED patients are immunosuppressed from chemotherapy, radiation, or a disease process that makes them more prone to infection. Every effort should be made to protect them and isolate them from patients in the general waiting room. They should be separated from potentially ill patients and taken as quickly as possible to a positive pressure treatment room.

THE PATIENT LIAISON

The patient liaison is a role being used by some EDs to facilitate communication between patients, families, and visitors in the waiting room. The role requires the individual to have well-developed communication and customer service skills. Stationed in the waiting room, the patient liaison is focused on answering patient, family, and visitor questions. They are able to go into the treatment area to determine patient status and if the patient can have a visitor. The goal of the role is to improve the patient and family experience in the ED.

SECURITY

Few data exist on the actual incidence of violence in the ED, but crowded EDs, long waiting times, pain, alcohol and drug abuse, psychiatric issues, and gang-related violence all contribute to the risk for violence.[9] EDs need to have safety measures in place to protect patients, staff, and visitors. These may include the following:

- Visible, uniformed security guards with a commanding presence.
- Limited department access.
- Visitors policy with visitor passes or badges.
- Continuous surveillance with closed-circuit cameras in strategic locations such as ED entrances, waiting rooms, and triage rooms.
- Panic buttons and other methods for RNs and other personnel to call for immediate security assistance.
- Metal detectors.
- Staff training in crisis intervention. ED staff need to be able to recognize an escalating situation and to intervene appropriately. Early identification and early intervention can effectively defuse most situations and prevent violence.

LEGAL ISSUES

Emergency Medical Treatment and Active Labor Act

In 1986 the U.S. Congress passed the Emergency Medical Treatment and Labor Act (EMTALA) to ensure access to emergency care regardless of an individual's ability to pay.[5]

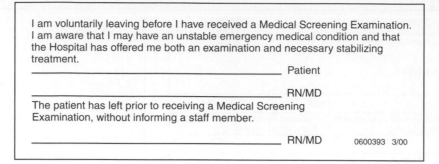

I am voluntarily leaving before I have received a Medical Screening Examination. I am aware that I may have an unstable emergency medical condition and that the Hospital has offered me both an examination and necessary stabilizing treatment.

_____ Patient

_____ RN/MD

The patient has left prior to receiving a Medical Screening Examination, without informing a staff member.

_____ RN/MD   0600393 3/00

FIGURE **7-3.** Left without being seen sticker. (Courtesy of Brigham and Women's Hospital, Boston.)

This legislation was enacted in response to reports of hospitals "dumping" or transferring patients to other facilities because of their inability to pay for care. EMTALA obligates hospitals that participate in Medicare to provide a medical screening examination (MSE) to every patient presenting for care to determine if an emergency medical condition exists. If an emergency condition is identified, then the patient must be stabilized within the facility's capabilities before transfer. If the patient cannot be stabilized and is in need of care beyond the hospital's capabilities or the patient requests a transfer, an appropriate transfer can be arranged. This federal mandate applies to every hospital with an ED. Facility bylaws must clearly identify individuals approved to complete the MSE. The Centers for Medicare and Medicaid Services (CMS) has stated that the triage process is not a medical screening examination.[5] If a hospital does not see children and a mother presents to the ED stating her daughter is sick, the patient needs to be triaged, registered, and an MSE done by an independent practitioner. If further care is needed, the child should be transferred to an appropriate facility in compliance with EMTALA.

Left Without Being Seen

In 2005 over 2 million patients triaged and registered into an ED left without being seen (LWBS) by a licensed independent practitioner, accounting for about 2% of all ED visits and a reflection of an overburdened emergency care system.[19] The percentage of LWBS is believed to be higher in larger hospitals, teaching hospitals, and in hospitals that treat a disproportionate number of patients with no insurance.[7] Patients who leave without being seen are often frustrated by the long wait times. Research has shown that a significant portion of the patients who leave are in need of medical care.[7] Most EDs track their LWBS rate over time because these patients are seen as lost opportunities.

EDs need to have a policy and procedure in place to guide the triage nurse's actions when a patient reports that he or she is leaving. The nurse can talk with the patient and family to encourage them to stay and determine the reason for their decision. If the patient has a significant injury or illness, the charge nurse and physician should be notified. Patients who insist on leaving should be asked to sign a statement saying they are leaving before receiving an MSE (Figure 7-3). Some patients walk out without notifying ED staff of their intent to leave. Standard practice is that patients whose names have been called in the waiting room three times approximately 15 minutes apart should be classified as LWBS.

TRIAGE REASSESSMENT

In this era of crowded EDs with longer wait times, EDs need to have a recheck or reassessment protocol to ensure that patients waiting have not had a change in acuity. When the waiting room is full, the department is busy; a triage reassessment policy that says all patients will be reassessed every so often may be unrealistic.[20] Each ED should have in place some method of rechecking and documenting on patients waiting to be seen.

TELEPHONE ADVICE

Telephone calls eliciting medical advice are problematic for EDs because evaluation of patients by telephone is difficult.[8] Most EDs have a strict policy that directs the staff to inform the caller that if this is a life-threatening emergency the person should hang up and dial 9-1-1. For other questions the caller should be politely informed that the ED does not give out any medical advice over the telephone and they are welcome to come to the ED to be seen. The ENA position statement on telephone triage states: "Nurses working in facilities with no established telephone triage program should not offer medical advice over the phone. In extreme situations the triage nurse may instruct the caller in lifesaving techniques such as CPR and how to access the emergency medical system."[8]

TRIAGE NURSE QUALIFICATIONS

The triage nurse is a vital member of the ED health care team who serves as the gatekeeper to the ED. Based on a brief triage assessment, the triage nurse determines who goes directly to care and who waits to be seen. This decision has patient safety implications: overtriage can take a bed away from someone who really needs it, and undertriage can delay care. Therefore the triage nurse must have the knowledge, experience, temperament, and qualifications necessary to function in this high-stress role.

Triage is usually a chaotic and demanding assignment that can be very stressful when the department is at or over capacity. The triage nurse must remain professional at all times and manage multiple tasks simultaneously while communicating with patients, visitors, staff, and the charge nurse. The triage nurse is usually the first health care professional that the patient and family/caregiver encounter in the ED. The triage nurse has the opportunity to provide reassurance, begin to address the patient and family's/caregiver's concerns, and set expectations about time to treatment. To function effectively the triage nurse must possess expert assessment skills, demonstrate competent interview and organizational skills, maintain an extensive knowledge base of diseases and injuries, and use past experiences to identify subtle clues to patient acuity. Patients with an obvious critical condition do not present the greatest challenge to the triage nurse. The true test of a competent triage nurse is his or her ability to think critically and recognize the subtle signs and symptoms of a low-volume but high-risk presentation.

The complexity of the triage role led to the recommendation from the ENA that a nurse have at least 6 months of emergency nursing experience before being oriented to the triage role. The emergency nurse functioning in the triage role should have successfully completed Basic Life Support, Advanced Cardiac Life Support, the Trauma Nurse Core Course, and the Emergency Nursing Pediatric Course. In addition, obtaining the certified emergency nurse credential is preferred.[12]

Triage is not just another nursing staff assignment in the ED. It is a specialized area that requires a formal orientation program that includes a didactic and clinical component. Anecdotal information suggests that formal triage orientation and special training improve the triage nurse's effectiveness and comfort in the role. Written protocols to assist decision making and a clinical orientation with a preceptor gives the novice triage nurse the opportunity to ask questions, review cases, and become comfortable with the role.

PERFORMANCE IMPROVEMENT AND TRIAGE

EDs should closely examine their intake or "front-end" process to ensure that it provides for patient and staff safety while maximizing efficiency. Delays at triage can lead to a longer patient length of stay.

ED leadership needs to measure and evaluate the following parameters:

- Arrival time—when the patient enters the ED.
- Arrival time to triage time. What is an acceptable time frame for each facility?
- Are patients presenting for chest pain having an electrocardiogram performed within 10 minutes?
- Is the LWBS rate increasing? Who are the people who are leaving? Should a call-back system be put into place?
- Triage acuity rating—are ratings accurate?
- Where are the bottlenecks in the department?

Every ED needs to continually look at each step of its entry process for ways to increase efficiency and facilitate flow of patients into the department.

SUMMARY

EDs have become the safety net of the U.S. health care system. As an increasing number of patients use the ED for primary care, the role of the triage nurse will continue to be vital to safety and efficiency. The triage nurse remains the initial contact for the patient and family in their emergency experience and, more important, can directly affect patient outcome. Although approaches vary, the common ingredient of a successful program requires an experienced, competent ED RN.

REFERENCES

1. American Hospital Association: *The 2007 state of America's hospitals: taking the pulse,* 2007. Retrieved August 26, 2007, from http://www.aha.org/aha/content/2007/PowerPoint/StateofHospitalsChartPack2007.ppt.
2. Beveridge R, Ducharme J, James L et al: Reliability of the Canadian emergency department triage and acuity scale: interrater agreement, *Ann Emerg Med* 34(2):155, 1999.
3. Canadian Association of Emergency Physicians: *Canadian Triage and Acuity Scale.* Retrieved August 15, 2007, from http://www.caep.ca.
4. Centers for Disease Control and Prevention: *Hand hygiene guidelines fact sheet.* Retrieved August 28, 2007, from http://www.cdc.gov/od/oc/media/pressrel/fs021025.htm.
5. Centers for Medicare and Medicaid Services: *EMTALA overview.* Retrieved August 27, 2007, from http://www.cms.hhs.gov/EMTALA/.
6. Cooper R, Flaherty H, Lin E et al: Effect of vital signs on triage decisions, *Ann Emerg Med* 39(3):223, 2002.
7. Ding R, McCarthy M, Li G et al: Patients who leave without being seen: their characteristics and history of emergency department use, *Ann Emerg Med* 48(6):686, 2006.
8. Emergency Nurses Association: *Emergency Nurses Association position statement: telephone advice.* Retrieved August 26, 2007, from http://www.ena.org/about/position.
9. Emergency Nurses Association: *Emergency Nurses Association position statement: violence in the emergency care setting.* Retrieved August 26, 2007, from http://www.ena.org/about/position.
10. Emergency Nurses Association: *Standards of emergency nursing practice,* ed 4, Des Plaines Ill, 2001, The Association.
11. Emergency Nurses Association: *Emergency nursing pediatric course,* ed 3, Des Plaines, Ill, 2004, The Association.

12. Emergency Nurses Association: *Emergency nursing core curriculum*, ed 6, Philadelphia, 2006, WB Saunders.

13. Emergency Nurses Association: *Sheehy's manual of emergency care*, ed 6, St. Louis, 2006, Elsevier.

14. Emergency Nurses Association and American College of Emergency Physicians: *Standardized ED triage scale and acuity categorization: joint ENA/ACEP statement.* Retrieved August 26, 2007, from http://www.ena.org/about/position.

15. Fernandes C, Tanabe P, Gilboy N et al: Five-level triage: a report from the ACEP/ENA Five-Level Triage Task Force, *J Emerg Nurs* 31(1):39, 2005.

16. Fernandes CMB, Wuerz R, Clark S et al: How reliable is emergency department triage? *Ann Emerg Med* 34(2):141, 1999.

17. Gilboy N, Tanabe P, Travers DA et al: *Emergency Severity Index, version 4: implementation handbook,* AHRQ publication No. *05-0046-2*, Rockville, Md, 2005, Agency for Healthcare Research and Quality.

18. Keddington RK: A triage vital sign policy for a children's hospital emergency department, *J Emerg Nurs* 24(2):189, 1998.

19. Nawar E, Niska R, Xu J: National Hospital Ambulatory Medical Care Survey: 2005 emergency department summary, *Adv Data* 386:1, 2007.

20. Pate B, Pete D: *Solving emergency department overcrowding: successful approaches to a chronic problem,* Marblehead, Mass, 2004, HCPro, Inc.

21. Ryan TJ, Antman EM, Brooks NH et al: ACC/AHA guidelines for the management of patients with acute myocardial infarction: a report of the American College of Cardiology/American Heart Association Task Force on Practice Guidelines (Committee on Management of Myocardial Infarction), *J Am Coll Cardiol* 34:890, 1999.

22. Sanders A, editor: Geriatric Emergency Medicine Task Force: *Emergency care of the elder person*, St. Louis, 1996, Beverly Cracom Publications.

23. Tanabe P, Gimbel R, Yarnold PR et al: Reliability and validity of scores on the Emergency Severity Index version 3, *Acad Emerg Med* 11:1, 2004.

24. Tanabe P, Travers DA, Gilboy N et al: Refining Emergency Severity Index criteria, ESI v4, *Acad Emerg Med* 12:6, 2005.

25. The Joint Commission: *2009 Hospital National Patient Safety Goals: hospital program.* Retrieved August 28, 2007, from http://www.jointcommission.org/PatientSafety/NationalPatientSafetyGoals/08_hap_npsgs.htm.

26. Thompson J, Dains J: *Comprehensive triage: a manual for developing and implementing a nursing care system, Reston, Va.* 1982, Reston.

27. Travers D: Triage: how long does it take? How long should it take? *J Emerg Nurs* 25(3):238, 1999.

28. U.S. Department of Defense: *Emergency war surgery*, Washington, DC, 1975, U.S. Government Printing Office.

29. Wuerz R, Fernandes CMB, Alarcon J: Inconsistency of emergency department triage, *Ann Emerg Med* 32(4):431, 1998.

30. Wuerz RC, Milne LW, Eitel DR et al: Reliability and validity of a new five-level triage instrument, *Acad Emerg Med* 7(3):236, 2000.

31. Zimmermann PG, Herr R: *Triage nursing secrets*, St. Louis, 2006, Mosby.

CHAPTER 8

Patient Assessment

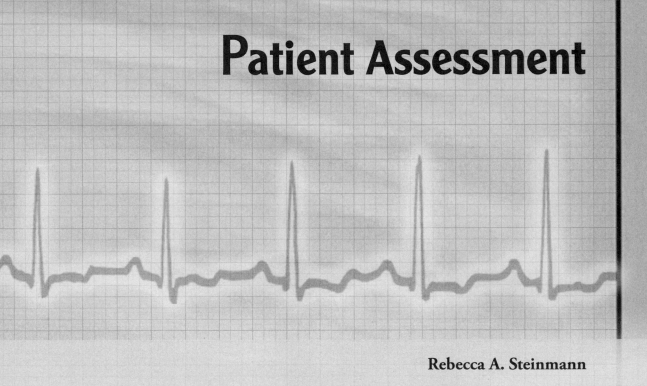

Rebecca A. Steinmann

Patients present to the emergency department (ED) with every possible medical, surgical, traumatic, social, and behavioral health condition. Not only do emergency nurses need to be capable of managing a broad spectrum of illnesses and injuries, but they must also be comfortable in caring for patients who span the age spectrum, from newborns to centenarians. The competent emergency nurse must be a "jack-of-all-trades, master of most." Accurate, appropriate, and ongoing assessment is the basis of all patient care. Assessment is not only the first step in the nursing process but also the key to identifying the nature of each patient's presenting illness or injury, the severity of that problem, and the patient's need for and response to intervention. A systematic approach to the evaluation of each patient is essential for immediate recognition of life-threatening conditions, identification of signs/symptoms of specific illness and/or injury, and determination of priorities of care. Box 8-1 describes a standardized approach to initial assessment using the A-to-I mnemonic.[10]

Two types of information are routinely collected during the assessment process: subjective and objective. Subjective data is the information provided verbally by the patient, family, or significant other. This information reflects the person's perception of the problem and the information the patient or family member has chosen to impart (e.g., a patient presenting with chest pain may or may not volunteer that the pain was precipitated by cocaine use, critical information

that facilitates identification and management of the underlying condition). Objective data are considered factual, findings that can be observed or measured. This information is obtained from the physical assessment process—inspection, auscultation, palpation, percussion, smell—and from physiologic measurements, laboratory tests, and other diagnostic studies. Many objective signs are manifestations of specific illnesses and disorders indicating the need for a specific focused assessment. Gathering objective data provides an opportunity to clinically validate the patient's subjective information. Essential assessment tools for the emergency nurse include interpersonal skills, knowledge of anatomy and physiology, physical assessment skills, the ability to apply critical thinking to each patient's unique situation, and common sense.

The purpose of this chapter is to provide general guidelines that can be applied to every patient encounter. Detailed assessment and management considerations for specific patient problems can be found in the corresponding chapters of this text.

INITIAL ASSESSMENT

Initial assessment is divided into two phases, the primary and secondary assessments. The purpose of the primary assessment is to ensure that potentially life-threatening conditions are immediately identified and addressed through sequential evaluation of airway, breathing, circulation, disability, and exposure of the patient (the ABCDE mnemonic). The goal of the secondary assessment is to identify all clinical indicators of illness or injury (the FGHI portion of the mnemonic). Both the primary and secondary assessment can be completed within minutes unless resuscitative measures are required.

Primary Assessment

A general impression of the patient is formed ("sick" or "not sick") in the first seconds of the initial contact based on observations of the patient's general appearance (manner of dress, hygiene, color of skin, facial expression), posture and motor activity, quality of speech (normal, slurred, silent, unable to speak), affect and mood, and apparent degree of distress. Any unusual odors should be reported; certain conditions are associated with specific odors such as the smell of ketones on the breath of patients with diabetic ketoacidosis, the smell of a patient with a *Pseudomonas* infection, or

the "bitter almonds" odor associated with cyanide exposure. Components of the primary assessment are summarized in Table 8-1.

Airway

Evaluation of airway patency includes assessment for vocalization or sounds appropriate for age; observing for tongue obstruction; presence of foreign material visible in the oropharynx (blood, vomitus, secretions, foreign objects, debris—loose teeth/dentures); edema of the lips, mouth, oropharynx, or neck; drooling; dysphagia and abnormal airway sounds (i.e., stridor). If the airway is partially or totally obstructed, immediate intervention to restore airway patency is required. Interventions may include manually opening the airway with a head tilt–chin lift (in the absence of trauma) or jaw thrust, suctioning, insertion of an airway adjunct, and preparation for endotracheal intubation. Any life-threatening compromise in airway patency must be addressed before proceeding to assessment of breathing. Spinal protection (i.e., providing manual in-line stabilization until placement of a rigid cervical collar and/or stabilizing devices are secured) is required if cervical spine injury is suspected. In such cases, all airway maneuvers must be accomplished while maintaining the cervical spine in neutral alignment.

Breathing

Evaluation of breathing includes assessment for the presence of spontaneous breathing, rate and pattern of breathing, symmetrical chest rise and fall, increased work of breathing (nasal flaring, retractions), use of accessory muscles, chest wall integrity, and skin color. Bilateral breath sounds may be assessed if breathing appears significantly compromised or deferred to the secondary assessment. If breathing is absent or ineffective, assisted ventilation using a bag-mask device is required. Supplemental oxygen, positioning the patient to maximize ventilation, occluding open chest wounds, and interventions to relieve tension pneumothoraces may be instituted to support breathing effectiveness. Any life-threatening

---

Box 8-1	COMPONENTS OF THE INITIAL ASSESSMENT

PRIMARY ASSESSMENT

A Airway with simultaneous cervical spine protection for trauma patients
B Breathing effectiveness
C Circulation effectiveness
D Disability (brief neurologic assessment)
E Exposure/environmental control

SECONDARY ASSESSMENT

F Full set of vitals, focused adjuncts (cardiac monitor, continuous pulse oximetry), facilitate family presence
G Give comfort measures
H History and head-to-toe assessment
I Inspect posterior surfaces

Table 8-1. ASSESSMENT OF THE ABCDs

Component	Description	Action
Airway	Appraise airway patency.	Identify and remove any partial or complete airway obstruction; position airway to maintain patency; insert oropharyngeal or nasopharyngeal airway; protect cervical spine.
Breathing	Determine presence and effectiveness of respiratory efforts. Identify other abnormalities in breathing (e.g., abnormal pattern, abnormal sounds, break in chest wall integrity).	Assist breathing with oxygen therapy, mouth-to-mask ventilation, or bag-mask ventilation; intubate when necessary.
Circulation	Evaluate pulse presence and quality, character, and equality; assess capillary refill, skin color and temperature, and the presence of diaphoresis.	Initiate chest compressions, defibrillation, synchronized cardioversion and medications as indicated; treat dysrhythmias, control bleeding, establish intravenous access, replace lost volume with isotonic crystalloids or blood products.
Disability	Determine level of consciousness.	Identify potential cause of altered level of consciousness, and treat as indicated; assess pupil size and reactivity.

compromise to ventilation must be addressed before proceeding to assessment of circulation.

Circulation

Initial evaluation of circulation includes assessing for skin color, temperature, and moisture; capillary refill (assess centrally on forehead or chest[10]); and uncontrolled external bleeding (trauma). Palpation of central and peripheral pulses for rate and quality may be performed if circulation appears compromised or deferred to the secondary assessment. If circulation is ineffective, cardiac monitoring and vascular access should be established. If no pulse is present, resuscitative measures, including basic and advanced life support, should be initiated.

Disability

A brief neurologic assessment is conducted to determine the patient's level of consciousness. The AVPU mnemonic is a simple, rapid screening tool:

A Alert: Patient is awake, alert, and responsive to voice and is oriented to person, time, and place.

V Verbal: Patient responds to voice but is not fully oriented to person, time, or place.

P Pain: Patient does not respond to voice but does respond to a painful stimulus.

U Unresponsive: Patient does not respond to voice or painful stimulus.

If an altered level of consciousness is noted, pupils should be assessed for size, equality, and reactivity to light. Any alteration in consciousness requires further investigation during the secondary assessment.

Exposure and Environmental Control

The patient's clothing should be removed to examine and identify any underlying signs of illness or injury. Covering the patient maintains privacy and prevents heat loss.

Secondary Assessment

Once emergent threats are addressed, a secondary assessment can be completed (the FGHI components of the A-to-I mnemonic). This phase includes measurement of vital signs, pain assessment, history, and a head-to-toe assessment, including assessment of the posterior surfaces.

Full Set of Vital Signs

Vital signs are indicators of the patient's present physiologic status. Temperature, pulse and respiratory rates, blood pressure (BP), oxygen saturation, and weight are objectively measured. Vital signs may be obtained before the secondary assessment phase, especially when a team of providers is simultaneously involved in providing care to a seriously ill or injured patient. Recognizing subtle and significant alterations in vital signs is an important part of analyzing the assessment data. All vital signs must be taken and evaluated serially. The patient's condition is a continuum that can be assessed only through constant monitoring. Whenever therapy

is instituted, appropriate vital signs should be reevaluated to assess efficacy of treatment. Vital signs should be repeated when abnormal and before a decision is made about disposition of the patient from the ED (discharged, admitted, or transferred to another facility).

TEMPERATURE. Body temperature is affected by activity, certain disease conditions (e.g., hypothyroidism/hyperthyroidism), environmental factors (e.g., hypothermia/hyperthermia), inflammation, infection, and injury. Temperature measurement is mandatory for all ED patients because deviation from normal temperature may be the only clue of a significant medical problem. Temperature measurement is most commonly performed at the oral, tympanic, temporal artery, axillary, or rectal sites. Institutional preference and the patient's age and condition should be considered when choosing an appropriate measurement site. Some situations necessitate core temperature measurement; urinary catheter thermistors, esophageal probes, and temporal artery and tympanic thermometers correlate highly with pulmonary artery temperature, considered the "gold standard." An abnormally high or low temperature reading should always be confirmed by an alternate route, thermometer, or observer.

PULSE. Assessment of the pulse involves determination of the heart rate and rhythm (regular or irregular), as well as the quality (bounding, normal, weak and thready, or absent) and equality of central and peripheral pulses. Increased dependence on electronic technology has decreased tactile assessment of the pulse. The electronically monitored pulse rate gives no indication of quality and other characteristics of the pulse. Equally important are rhythm disturbances that may not be identified unless these changes are seen on the cardiac monitor. Premature beats may be felt on palpation as missing beats or beats with less amplitude than preceding ones. Irregular rhythms, even subtle ones, can be felt as a chaotic rhythm with varying intensity. In context with other physical findings, the pulse is an important indicator of cardiovascular function. A change in pulse rate is often the first sign that compensatory mechanisms are being used to maintain homeostasis. In early volume depletion, a healthy person with an intact autonomic nervous system can maintain normal systolic pressures with only one subtle change—a slight increase in pulse rate. Any deviation from the normal range for the patient's age that cannot be related to psychologic or environmental factors should be considered an indication of an abnormal physiologic condition until proven otherwise.

RESPIRATIONS. Assess the rate, rhythm and depth of respirations, and work of breathing. To determine an accurate respiratory rate and pattern, breathing should be measured for a full minute. Generally a healthy person does not require any extra effort to breathe: airway noise is absent, nasal cartilage is quiet, and sternocleidomastoid or intercostal muscles are not required to lift the chest cage. Signs of increased respiratory effort include tracheal tugging; nasal flaring; suprasternal, intercostal, or substernal retractions; accessory muscle use (neck and abdominal muscles); an inability to speak in complete sentences; and the presence of adventitious sounds. With inspiration the chest should expand symmetrically on both sides. When pulmonary or chest wall conditions exist, the chest may rise asymmetrically during ventilation. This asymmetry can be observed with the chest exposed and can also be palpated during inspiration. Increased anteroposterior diameter can generally be seen on casual observation and indicates chronic alveolar distension. Other changes in chest contour include funnel chest, pigeon chest, kyphosis, and kyphoscoliosis. These particular anatomic changes in contour may interfere with normal lung inflation and exacerbate respiratory conditions. The patient's tidal volume can be estimated by observing the rise and fall of the chest during ventilation. Depth of ventilations is described as shallow, normal, or deep. A normal adult moves 300 to 500 mL of air at rest and as much as 2000 mL during exercise, with a corresponding increase in rate. A fast rate is not necessarily indicative of moving more volume, nor is a slow rate necessarily indicative of moving less volume.

OXYGEN SATURATION. Measurement of oxygen saturation with a pulse oximeter is essential for patients with respiratory or hemodynamic compromise, an altered level of consciousness, or serious illness/injury. Knowledge of the patient's baseline is helpful in determining severity of the situation or response to therapy. To ensure accuracy of readings, it is important to position the sensor with the two light sources directly opposite the photo detector; the pulse reading on the oximeter should be compared with the radial or apical pulse rate. Inaccurate readings may occur with hypotension, anemia, extreme peripheral vasoconstriction, hypothermia, carbon monoxide poisoning, and methemoglobinemia. Readings may also be affected by ambient light sources in the room (e.g., fluorescent lights and infrared heating lamps) and artificial nails and nail polish, particularly with blue, red, or bright polish. The oximetry reading should always be correlated with the patient's clinical presentation.

BLOOD PRESSURE. BP is a complex parameter reflecting cardiac contractility, heart rate, circulating volume, and peripheral vascular resistance. Systolic pressure is a function of cardiac output; diastolic pressure is a measure of peripheral vascular resistance. Pulse pressure (the difference between systolic and diastolic pressures) represents approximate stroke volume. A narrowing pulse pressure indicates a drop in cardiac output and a compensatory rise in peripheral vascular resistance (vasoconstriction). Pulse pressure is much more sensitive than systolic BP to hypovolemic changes in early shock.[8]

BP can be obtained by auscultation, palpation, noninvasive BP monitors, or through Doppler ultrasound. Proper cuff size is essential to obtaining accurate measurements—a cuff that is too small leads to falsely elevated readings, whereas a cuff that is too large results in erroneously low readings. The method used for assessment should be communicated so that other providers use the same method, allowing hemodynamic status to be trended over time. A single BP recording yields little or no information. Normal pressures measured in the ED are not necessarily an indication that all is well. A healthy person may not demonstrate a drop in systolic

BP despite significant volume loss until all compensatory mechanisms (i.e., the ability to increase heart rate and vasoconstrict) have been exhausted. If the patient is undergoing antihypertensive therapy, the values obtained during the ED visit may represent a significant deviation relative to the patient's "normally abnormal" pressure.

Orthostatic Vital Signs. Orthostatic vital signs evaluate the BP and pulse rate in two or three positions: lying, sitting, or standing. Orthostatic vital signs may be obtained in patients presenting with syncopal episodes or suspected volume depletion, although the value of these measurements in reliably predicting volume status has been questioned.[5] When evaluating patients for orthostatic changes, BP and pulse rate are recorded after the patient has been supine for 2 to 3 minutes; BP, pulse, and symptoms are then recorded after the patient has been sitting for 1 minute; the patient is assisted to a standing position, and after 1 minute the BP, pulse, and symptoms are again reassessed.[7] The test is considered positive if pulse rate increases 30 beats/min or more in an adult and symptoms suggesting cerebral hypoperfusion with position change (i.e., dizziness or syncope) occur. A supine-to-standing measurement is more accurate than a supine-to-sitting measurement.[7]

WEIGHT, HEIGHT, AND HEAD CIRCUMFERENCE. Pediatric patients should be weighed with each ED visit to obtain an accurate measurement. Because fluid resuscitation and most pediatric medications are dosed by kilogram of body weight, weight should always be recorded in kilograms. Weights may or may not be measured on all adult patients, depending on institutional policy. Reported weights are subject to error; however, unless the patient requires weight-based medications (e.g., vasopressors or heparin infusions), this subjective measure may be adequate. Measurement of height may be necessary to calculate expected peak expiratory flow rates or determine body surface area. The Joint Commission requires evaluation of head circumference on all patients less than 2 years of age, *as appropriate*. Indications for measurement of head circumference in the ED include children who have obvious cranial abnormality and children presenting with suspected ventriculoperitoneal shunt malfunction.[8]

Give Comfort Measures

Pain is commonly referred to as "the fifth vital sign." Although pain is a subjective experience, all patients presenting to the ED should be queried about the presence of pain during the initial assessment, noting any self-reports or behavioral cues suggesting discomfort. The PQRST mnemonic is frequently used to characterize pain by focusing on essential elements of pain assessment (i.e., provoking factors, quality, radiation, severity, and timing in terms of onset and duration). An age-appropriate standardized tool such as a numeric rating scale (0 to 10), FACES Pain Rating Scale, or observational pain rating scale such as the face, legs, activity, cry, and consolability (FLACC) scale should be used to quantify the severity of pain or discomfort for both the initial and all subsequent pain assessments.

Comfort measures should be initiated based on the patient's chief complaint and obvious injury. Simple non-pharmacologic comfort measures include reassurance, positioning the patient to minimize discomfort, covering open wounds, stabilizing suspected fractures, and applying cold or warm packs. Refer to Chapter 12 for a detailed discussion of pain assessment and management.

History

Obtaining a relevant history is an important component of the patient assessment. The patient interview is often conducted simultaneously with the head-to-toe survey. Historical data include the patient's chief complaint, history of the present illness or injury, past medical history, current medications (prescription, over-the-counter, herbal supplements, and recreational substances), and allergies. The key to obtaining information about the chief complaint—why the patient came to the ED—is to listen to what the patient says in trying to tell you what is wrong. The chief complaint should

not be recorded as a diagnosis ("possible fractured left arm") but exactly as the patient describes the problem ("fell from stepladder, now pain and swelling in left arm"). Sometimes patients cannot describe their symptoms or reason for coming to the ED (e.g., a patient who is unresponsive or a preverbal child). Attempts should be made to contact someone who can reliably relate the history of the present complaint. The AMPLE mnemonic is helpful for organizing and obtaining an adequate history. Table 8-2 summarizes pertinent historical data to be obtained using the AMPLE mnemonic. The questions, although open ended, should be directed by the chief complaint and build on information offered by the patient. As time permits, a family and social history may be elicited. Special communication needs related to vision, hearing, or language should be identified and addressed.

If the patient initially presents to the triage area and is physically able to proceed through the triage process, history can be completed in the triage area. If the patient enters the ED by ambulance or other vehicle and cannot be processed

Table 8-2.	PERTINENT HISTORICAL DATA USING THE AMPLE MNEMONIC	
	Description	**Interview Questions**
A	Allergies	Is the patient allergic to any medications? (record type and severity of reaction)
		Any adverse reactions to medications?
		Food allergies?
		Environmental allergies?
M	Medications	Current medications (prescribed or unprescribed, over-the-counter, herbals, and recreational)
		When was medication last taken?
P	Past health history	Pertinent medical history
		Has this problem ever occurred before?
		If so, was a medical diagnosis made? What was it?
		Has the patient ever had surgery? For what reason? What was the result?
		Is there any family medical history that may influence the patient's present complaint?
		Are there psychosocial factors that may be influencing the patient's condition?
		Does the patient have a private physician? (Obtain full name and where the physician practices if possible)
		When was the last tetanus immunization? (if open wounds/eye injuries involved)
		When was the last normal menstrual period (females)?
		Any possibility of pregnancy?
L	Last meal eaten	History of dietary intake?
		Last ingestion of fluids? Solids?
		Last void? Last bowel movement?
E	Events leading to the illness/injury	History of present illness or injury
		How and when injury or illness first occurred
		Influencing factors
		Travel within days or weeks of symptom onset
		Illness of household contacts
		Symptom chronology and duration
		Related symptoms
		Location of pain or discomfort
		What, if anything, the patient has done about the symptoms

through triage, the nurse managing the patient in the treatment area will obtain the history and whatever information prehospital personnel may have regarding status or treatment before arrival. If the patient can respond to questions, any history obtained from others should be validated by the patient. Previous medical records may be helpful, if available; with expanded use of computerized medical records these records are often immediately accessible. Treatment should never be delayed until history is available. An additional source of information is health care providers who have previously interacted with the patient (e.g., private physician, home care nurses, health care workers in clinics, and hospital staff who have provided frequent or long-term care for a patient). These care providers may offer valuable information not necessarily documented anywhere but known from frequent interactions with the patient.

In addition to the data described, many facilities employ a variety of screening tools as part of the assessment process for stable patients. Patients may be asked a series of questions regarding immunization status and signs and symptoms of tuberculosis or exposure to other communicable diseases (e.g., chickenpox). Screening for interpersonal violence, suicidal ideation, alcohol and tobacco use, and obstructive sleep apnea may be performed.

Head-to-Toe Assessment

A complete head-to-toe assessment is necessary for all critically ill or injured patients. For patients presenting with minor illness or injury or symptoms isolated to one body system, clinicians may rapidly and systematically complete the various components of the head-to-toe evaluation, then focus the assessment on the specific problem.

HEAD AND FACE. The head and face should be inspected and palpated for any signs of surface trauma (e.g., lacerations, abrasions, avulsions, puncture wounds, foreign objects, or burns), rashes, ecchymosis, or edema. Any discharge from the nose, ears, or eyes should be noted. The bones of the head and face should be palpated, noting any bony deformity or crepitus, asymmetry, and tenderness. The oral mucosa is assessed for color, hydration status, inflammation, swelling, and bleeding; malocclusion and loose or missing teeth should be noted. The eyes and lids should also be observed for ptosis, exophthalmos, subconjunctival hemorrhage, excessive tearing or blinking, or any redness, and the patient should be questioned about any recent visual changes. Visual acuity should be measured for patients presenting with ocular complaints. The integrity of extraocular muscles should be assessed if orbital trauma is suspected. The symmetry of facial features and expressions should be noted.

For patients presenting with neurologic complaints or deficits (e.g., headache, dizziness, seizure, altered mental status, loss of consciousness, or syncope), a focused neurologic assessment should be performed. The most important indicator of cerebral function is the patient's level of consciousness. Box 8-2 offers a mnemonic for investigating potential causes of an altered level of consciousness.

The patient's orientation to time, place, person, and situation is evaluated. When the cerebral hemispheres become dysfunctional for any reason, level of consciousness and degree of orientation begin to deteriorate. It may be necessary to apply noxious or painful stimuli (e.g., a squeeze of the trapezius muscle) to elicit a response if the patient does not react to verbal commands. Changes may initially be extremely subtle. Unless orientation and level of consciousness are tested in the same way each time, subtle changes may be overlooked. The Glasgow Coma Scale (GCS) and the National Institutes of Health (NIH) stroke scale are standardized tools used to measure and communicate neurologic status and provide trending over time. Pupil size, shape, and reactivity should be evaluated. More detailed neurologic assessment includes evaluation of muscle strength and tone, sensation, and cranial nerve function.

NECK. The neck should be observed for any signs of soft-tissue injury, bony deformity or crepitus, edema, rashes, lesions, and masses. The appearance of jugular veins is evaluated. The neck is palpated to determine tracheal position, signs of subcutaneous emphysema, and areas of tenderness. The cervical spine should be palpated for the presence of point tenderness, bony crepitus, or step-offs. Complaints of dysphagia (difficulty swallowing) and hoarseness should be noted.

CHEST. Assessment of the chest involves clinical evaluation of both pulmonary and cardiac function. Respiratory rate and depth, degree of effort, symmetry of chest wall expansion, use of accessory or abdominal muscles, and any paradoxical chest wall movement should be recorded. The anterior and lateral chest walls should be observed for lacerations, abrasions, contusions, lesions, rashes, puncture wounds, impaled objects, ecchymosis, swelling, scars, and the presence of central venous access devices, pacemakers, implantable cardioverter-defibrillators (ICDs), and medication patches. The chest should be palpated for bony deformity, crepitus, tenderness, and subcutaneous emphysema. Breath sounds should be auscultated for bilateral equality (normal, decreased, or absent) noting any adventitious sounds such as wheezes, crackles, and rhonchi. Further assessment is required for patients with dyspnea and abnormal breath sounds. Heart sounds provide information about the

---

Box 8 -2 CAUSES OF ALTERED LEVEL OF CONSCIOUSNESS: AEIOU-TIPPS

A Alcohol
E Epilepsy/electrolytes
I Insulin (hypoglycemia or hyperglycemia)
O Opiates
U Uremia
T Trauma
I Infection
P Poison
P Psychosis
S Syncope

integrity of heart valves, atrial and ventricular muscles, and the conduction system. Heart rate, rhythm, muffled sounds, and presence of abnormal sounds such as murmurs, gallops, and friction rub are assessed using auscultation. Patients presenting with suspected ischemic chest pain require further assessment, including continuous cardiac monitoring and a 12-lead electrocardiogram.

ABDOMEN. The contour of the abdomen should be inspected, documenting distention, ascites, lacerations, abrasions, contusions, rashes, masses, pulsations, impaled objects, ecchymosis, scars from healed surgical incisions, feeding tubes, and stomas. The presence or absence and character of bowel sounds should be assessed. All four quadrants of the abdomen are gently palpated for rigidity, tenderness, and guarding. Palpation of the abdomen should always be initiated away from the site of any reported pain or tenderness. Rebound tenderness, sharp pain elicited by sudden removal of your fingers, suggests peritoneal irritation. Emesis or stool should be tested for blood and other laboratory diagnostics performed as ordered by the physician. Patient complaints of constipation, diarrhea, nausea, vomiting, indigestion, abdominal pain, and gastrointestinal bleeding require further evaluation.

PELVIS/PERINEUM. The pelvis and perineal area should be observed for lacerations, abrasions, rashes, lesions, edema, or bleeding from the meatus. Drainage or discharge from the vagina or penis should be described in patients presenting with genital concerns. If vaginal bleeding is noted, the character and amount of blood loss should be reported (a saturated pad/tampon holds 20 to 30 mL of blood).[8] Priapism, if present, is indicative of pathologic conditions such as sickle cell crisis or spinal cord injury. The pelvis is palpated for bony stability; anal sphincter tone may be evaluated. Patients presenting with urinary complaints should be queried about pain or burning with urination, frequency, hematuria, decreased urination, dribbling, and flank tenderness. A urine sample should be obtained for analysis. For female patients of reproductive age, the possibility of an unknown pregnancy should be considered and a careful menstrual history obtained; a urine pregnancy test may be performed. If the patient is pregnant, fetal heart tones (first heard with Doppler ultrasonography at around 10 to 12 weeks' gestation) are assessed for presence, location, and rate.

EXTREMITIES. All four extremities should be assessed for redness, edema, rashes, lesions, scars; pulse quality, movement, and sensation should be noted. Limbs should

be carefully inspected and palpated for pain or tenderness, angulation, deformity, open wounds with evidence of protruding bone fragments, puncture wounds, and other signs of surface trauma. Neurovascular status distal to the site of injury requires evaluation of pulse quality and skin temperature (injured extremity compared to the uninjured site), capillary refill, sensation, and movement.

POSTERIOR SURFACES. The patient's back and posterior aspects of the arms and legs should be evaluated for the presence of bleeding, abrasions, wounds, hematomas, ecchymosis, rashes, lesions, and edema. Patterned injuries or injuries in various stages of healing are suggestive of maltreatment requiring further investigation. The vertebral column is palpated for tenderness and deformity. A rectal examination may be performed to determine rectal tone, character of any stool, and presence of blood.

ONGOING ASSESSMENT

Ongoing assessment is indicated to identify the individual patient's response to interventions and to determine improvement or deterioration in patient status. No definitive rules govern how often repeat assessment should be completed; reassessment intervals should be based on the patient's clinical status. Facility protocols may offer guidelines for specific situations, such as trauma score calculation on arrival and 1 hour after presentation; repeat vital sign measurements and neurologic assessment every 15 minutes for patients receiving fibrinolytic therapy; and reassessment of pain score 30 minutes after parenteral opioids have been administered. A high index of suspicion guides the experienced nurse in determining which follow-up measurements to obtain and the appropriate intervals for doing so.

SPECIAL PATIENT POPULATIONS

Children and elders have unique anatomic and physiologic characteristics that must be considered in the assessment process because of their extremes in age. Obstetric and bariatric patients pose assessment challenges because of their change in body habitus. Attention to these variables can enhance the assessment process and optimize patient outcomes. Table 8-3 describes assessment considerations for these populations. Refer to specific chapters in this book on pediatric, obstetric, and geriatric emergencies for additional information.

Table 8-3.	ASSESSMENT CONSIDERATIONS FOR SPECIAL POPULATIONS			
	Pediatric[2,10]	**Geriatric[4,8]**	**Obstetric[4,6]**	**Bariatric[1,11]**
Airway	Infants <3 months of age are obligate nose breathers—assess patency of nares Proportionally large tongue Large occiput of young child may cause hyperflexion of airway and cervical spine when supine—place padding under shoulders/trunk to achieve "sniffing" position Upper and lower airways smaller—more easily occluded Uncuffed tubes generally used for intubation in children <8 years of age	Loose partial plates or dentures may cause airway obstruction	Capillary engorgement of mucosal lining of airway predisposes to nosebleeds and airway obstruction Prostaglandin release, as well as tocolytics, make the patient prone to airway swelling Increased risk for aspiration due to pressure of enlarged uterus on diaphragm/chest contents and delayed gastric emptying	Large neck circumference, limited neck mobility, and small oropharyngeal opening may make effective bag-mask ventilation difficult Excess tissue and inability to identify normal landmarks contributes to difficulty with intubation Obstructive sleep apnea affects 5% of obese patients
Breathing	Infants/young children are predominately abdominal breathers Thin chest wall—breath sounds easily transmitted from one side to the opposite side—auscultate breath sounds at both axillae Increased work of breathing assessed by observing for nasal flaring, retractions, head bobbing, expiratory grunting, accessory muscle use	Increased anteroposterior chest diameter Senile kyphosis Limited chest excursion Diminished breath sounds particularly at bases Decreased pulmonary reserve Decreased respiratory muscle strength Reduced cough reflex Decreased resting oxygen tension	Decreased functional pulmonary reserve Increased maternal oxygen consumption and diminished oxygen reserve increase risk for hypoxia Normal ABGs demonstrate compensated respiratory alkalosis, hypocapnia	Increased load on respiratory muscles leads to increased work of breathing Diminished breath sounds common Position patient on side or in reverse Trendelenburg's position to maximize breathing effectiveness
Circulation	Child's circulating volume is proportionally greater than an adult (90 mL/kg infant; 80 mL/kg child; 70 mL/kg adult)—volume losses can produce hypovolemia more quickly Younger child's heart can not increase contractility—cardiac output maintained by increasing heart rate Excellent sympathetic compensatory mechanisms—increase heart rate and vasoconstrict to maintain systolic blood pressure—skin perfusion a better indicator of shock than blood pressure	Reduction in cardiac output at rest Atherosclerotic changes of blood vessels—arterial pulses more pronounced Pedal pulses often not detectable Color and temperature changes in extremities Slowed response to catecholamines Cardiac dysrhythmias more common Abnormal heart sounds may result from valvular rigidity Decreased amplitude of QRS complex and lengthening of PR, QRS, and QT intervals	Pregnancy is a hyperdynamic, hypervolemic state— blood volume increases 40%-50% by 28 weeks' gestation After 20 weeks' gestation, the weight of the fetus, uterus, placenta, and amniotic fluid compress the vena cava, decreasing blood pressure when patient is supine—position on side (left side preferred) Pregnancy is a hypercoagulable state—increased risk for deep venous thrombosis and pulmonary embolism	Obesity is a hyperdynamic, hypervolemic state— persistent increase in cardiac output required to perfuse additional adipose tissue Hypertension, coronary artery disease, and congestive heart failure are frequent comorbidities Muffled heart tones Decreased amplitude of QRS complex Increased risk for deep venous thrombosis and pulmonary embolism

Table 8-3.	ASSESSMENT CONSIDERATIONS FOR SPECIAL POPULATIONS—CONT'D			
	Pediatric[2,10]	**Geriatric[4,8]**	**Obstetric[4,6]**	**Bariatric[1,11]**
Disability/ neurologic status	Assess fontanels in children ≤18 months of age Child's activity level and ability to recognize caregivers is an important indicator of neurologic function in preverbal children Pediatric Glasgow Coma Scale used	Cerebral atrophy Decreased cerebral blood flow Nerve transmission slows Decrease in cerebral neurotransmitter content—repetitive movements, tremors Changes in gait and ambulation Slowing/altered sensory reception and motor response Baseline neurologic function confirmed by family/friends	Any change in level of consciousness is an abnormal finding	Increased risk for stroke with elevated body mass index Idiopathic intracranial hypertension may be exacerbated by head injury/positioning Daytime somnolence may be related to obstructive sleep apnea
Vital signs	Heart rate and respiratory rate decrease with age Minimal acceptable blood pressure = 70 + (2× child's age in years) Hypotension is a late sign of shock Length-based resuscitation tapes may be needed to estimate weight	Heart rate often affected by beta-blocker or calcium channel blocker therapy Respiratory rate declines as metabolic rate slows Elevated systolic BP common; diastolic BP may also rise—does patient know his or her baseline readings?	Heart rate increases 10-20 beats/min above baseline Respirations become more rapid and shallow as pregnancy progresses Diastolic BP drops 5-10 mm Hg in second trimester, returns to baseline in third trimester; minimal change in systolic BP throughout pregnancy Assessment of fetal heart tones is included in measurement of mother's vital signs	Increased resting heart rate resulting from increased cardiac workload Respiratory rate increases 25%-40% Appropriate size cuff necessary to obtain accurate BP reading
Other	Assess birth history in young infants as part of past medical history Assess immunization status Must consider child's developmental stage—perform more obtrusive aspects of assessment last Gastric distention common from air swallowed by crying Ineffective temperature regulation—prone to hypothermia Limited glycogen stores—prone to hypoglycemia when stressed Bones flexible, significant force required to fracture, significant underlying injuries can occur without fractures	Often atypical presentation of illness/injury Comorbidities and polypharmacy common Abdominal protrusion, muscle flabbiness Decreased intestinal peristalsis Ineffective temperature regulation—prone to hypothermia Decreased bone and muscle mass Increased capillary fragility—bruising Skin tears common Assess skin carefully for pressure sores	Fundal height is evaluated during abdominal examination Perineal assessment should report presence of bleeding/amniotic fluid in vaginal vault Pertinent history should include questions regarding date of confinement, prenatal care, and pregnancy complications	Comorbidities common Cyanosis/ruddiness of face/neck Dermatitis frequently occurs in deep skin folds under breast, abdomen, and perineum Perineal irritation—skin breakdown from inability to perform proper cleansing Chronic venous insufficiency noted in lower extremities—edema, hyperkeratosis, ulcers Pressure sores discovered in unusual locations Biomechanical/gait changes with increasing weight

ABG, Arterial blood gas; *BP*, blood pressure.

SUMMARY

This chapter describes the essential components of the initial assessment of the ED patient. Although the majority of patients present with nonresuscitative conditions, a systematic approach to evaluation is needed to ensure that life threats are immediately identified in the primary assessment (ABCDE portion of the A-to-I mnemonic) and that all indicators of illness/injury are identified in the secondary assessment (FGHI portion of the A-to-I mnemonic). The extent of evaluation is the decision of the emergency nurse based on the patient's condition at that time, chief complaint, and environmental factors. Priority setting through knowledgeable assessment and appropriate intervention contributes significantly to decreasing mortality and morbidity. This is particularly true for the early moments of the patient's visit, but it is also valid for the patient's entire stay in the ED.

REFERENCES

1. Barth MM, Jenson CE: Postoperative nursing care of gastric bypass patients, *Am J Crit Care* 15(4):378, 2006.
2. Emergency Nurses Association: Initial assessment, In Hawkins H, editor: *Emergency nursing pediatric course provider manual*, ed 3, Des Plaines, Ill, 2004, The Association.
3. Emergency Nurses Association: Initial assessment. In *Trauma nursing core course provider manual*, ed 6, Des Plaines, Ill, 2007, The Association.
4. Emergency Nurses Association: Special populations: pregnant, pediatric and older adult trauma patients. In *Trauma nursing core course provider manual*, ed 6, Des Plaines, Ill, 2007, The Association.
5. Garmel GM: Approach to the ED patient. In Garmel GM, Mahadervant SV, editors: *An introduction to clinical emergency medicine*, Cambridge, 2005, Cambridge University Press.
6. Kerr MS: Obstetric trauma. In Newbury L, Criddle LM, editors: *Sheehy's manual of emergency care*, ed 6, Philadelphia, 2005, Mosby.
7. Layman ME, Quigley MT: Measuring postural vital signs. In Proehl JA, editor: *Emergency nursing procedures*, ed 3, St. Louis, 2004, Saunders.
8. Lombardo D: Patient assessment. In Newbury L, Criddle LM, editors: *Sheehy's manual of emergency care*, ed 6, Philadelphia, 2005, Mosby.
9. Novak A: Geriatric trauma. In Newbury L, Criddle LM, editors: *Sheehy's manual of emergency care*, ed 6, Philadelphia, 2005, Mosby.
10. Proehl JA: Nursing assessment and resuscitation. In *Emergency nursing core curriculum*, ed 6, Philadelphia, 2007, Saunders.
11. Solheim J: Pediatric trauma. In Newbury L, Criddle LM, editors: *Sheehy's manual of emergency care*, ed 6, Philadelphia, 2005, Mosby.
12. Uwaido GI, Arioglu E: Obesity, *eMedicine,* June 19, 2006. Retrieved July 20, 2007, from http://www.emedicine.com/med/topic1653.htm.

CHAPTER 9

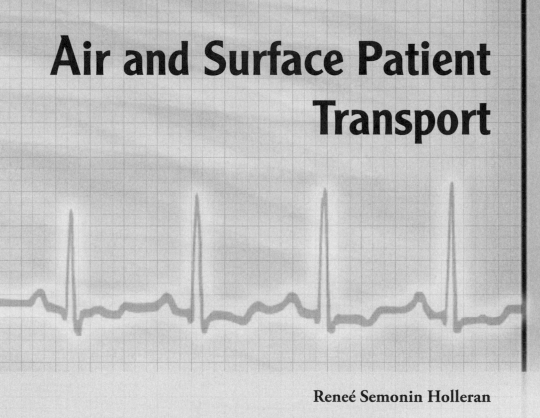

Air and Surface Patient Transport

Reneé Semonin Holleran

P atient transport is an integral part of all emergency departments (EDs). Whether a patient must be transferred to another care facility, moved from the ED for diagnostic testing, or transported within the hospital for admission, patients will be moved. Transport nursing has evolved into a specialty that involves detailed education and training.[13] Emergency nurses are generally involved with patient preparation and stabilization before transport. This requires that the emergency nurse be familiar with indications for transport, how the practice of nursing and medicine differ in the transport environment, preparation for transfer and transport, how transport can affect the patient, and the legal issues related to patient transport.

Transport teams are staffed with a variety of personnel, including nurses, physicians, paramedics, respiratory therapists, and emergency medical technicians (EMTs). Patient transport levels can vary from basic life support (BLS) to critical care. The condition and needs of the patient must dictate the type of team needed.

Transport vehicles include modular and van type of ground ambulances, fixed-wing aircraft, and helicopters (Figure 9-1). The condition of the patient, the timely need

for further care, the location of the patient, the weather, and availability of specific transport services may influence the type of vehicle used to transport the patient.

The overriding concept of any patient transport should always be safety. This includes patient safety, transport team safety, and the safety of anyone who interacts with the transport team and the vehicle used.

The quality and competency of the transport team, the vehicles, the equipment, and the training of the personnel should always be considered when choosing a transport team. The Commission on Accreditation of Medical Transport Systems (CAMTS) (http://www.camts.org) accreditation provides support that the transport program has met a set of standards that ensures the patient will receive organized, safe, and expert care before and during the transport process.

HISTORICAL PERSPECTIVE

Transferring patients from one location to another is not a new concept, and nurses have played a role in many of the historical landmarks related to transport. Florence Nightingale assisted in the transport of injured soldiers during the Crimean War.[8] Throughout the ages, soldiers on the battlefield have been transported in all types of moving conveyances. Dominique Larrey, Napoleon's private physician, developed an organized system to triage and transport injured soldiers from the battlefield in carts.

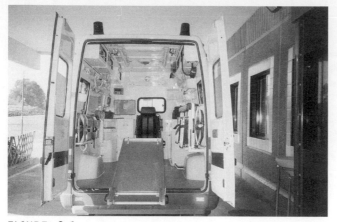

FIGURE **9-1.** An example of a ground transport vehicle. (© Marek Pawluczuk.)

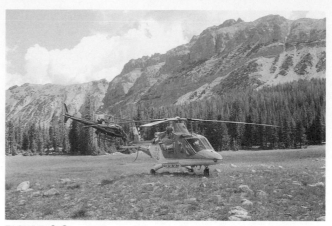

FIGURE **9-2.**   Helicopter transport. (© Arlene Jean Gee.)

The first hospital-based ambulance service was started in Cincinnati, Ohio, in 1865. Unfortunately, patient transport continued to develop in parallel with war. In 1945 the first helicopter rescue was recorded in the jungles of Burma.[4] In the twentieth century the use of air medical transport expanded.

The Korean War, Vietnam conflict, and the wars in the Middle East have demonstrated the effectiveness of helicopter transport in the care of the injured from the battlefield. The first hospital-based helicopter programs began in the early 1970s in Colorado and California. Today there are over 270 civilian-based helicopters transporting patients all over the United States and the world including Europe, Africa, Australia, and New Zealand.

During the 1960s and 1970s, Congress enacted numerous pieces of legislation addressing emergency medical care and transport. The Emergency Medical Treatment and Active Labor Act (EMTALA) was established to clarify guidelines for transfer and transport of patients. The discussion about legal regulations related to emergency nursing practice and patient transport is in Chapter 3.

TYPES OF TRANSPORT

Patient transport occurs in two distinct environments: on the surface by ambulance or in the air by a rotor-wing vehicle (helicopter) or fixed-wing vehicle (airplane). Air and surface transport have both advantages and disadvantages; therefore an informed decision to use air or surface transport must be made on the basis of many factors, such as patient condition, out-of-hospital time, weather, terrain, work space, equipment, personnel, and proximity of a landing site.

Surface Transport

Surface transport is most often accomplished using a modular type of vehicle (Figure 9-2). Patient access is generally easier in most surface vehicles. These vehicles can also accommodate larger pieces of equipment such as isolettes,

ventilators, and intraaortic balloon pumps. The level of care during transport varies with the education and training of the transport personnel, from BLS to critical care transport. There are also critical care transport teams and vehicles available in many parts of the United States that provide transport of critically ill and injured patients who require complex physiologic support. In choosing a transport vehicle, the referring center must remember that legally the quality and level of care cannot diminish during the transport. In addition, the sending/transferring physician maintains accountability for the level of care provided during the transfer of the patient.

Adverse weather conditions influence the transport decision. When roads are impassable, air transport is usually the only alternative. When weather has grounded air transport vehicles, surface transport is the only option. Another important transport consideration is transit time. For many critically ill or injured patients the shorter the out-of-hospital time, the better the patient's chance for survival. Finally, choice of a transport vehicle depends on needs of the community. Some isolated rural areas have only one surface ambulance for a largely scattered population base. If this vehicle is taken out of service for an interfacility transport, the community is left without coverage for the duration of the transport.

Air Transport

Air transport should not be chosen indiscriminately. In many parts of the United States, air medical transport should be considered an adjunct to, and not a replacement for, surface-based services. However, in rural and frontier areas of the country, it may be the most cost-effective and safest way to transport patients. Research remains inconclusive as to the advantage of rotor-wing transport over surface transport. Some of the reasons that a helicopter may be chosen over a surface vehicle include time or length of transport and the critical care capabilities of the medical crew. However, there are critical care teams available in some areas of the country that only perform ground transport.[14]

Rotor-wing aircraft provide rapid point-to-point transport. Helicopters can reach most areas, bypassing difficult terrain. Landing zones can be made at or near the patient to prevent lengthy surface transport time. Most helicopters operate within 150 miles of their base station to allow routine flights without refueling. One disadvantage of helicopters is that their use depends on minimum weather conditions, without which flights can be delayed or canceled. Helicopter cabin size and configuration can restrict access to the patient and limit in-flight interventions. Weight limitations restrict the number of passengers and amount of equipment on board. When transferring by rotor-wing vehicles, comprehensive patient stabilization may be required before transport.

The advantage of fixed-wing transport is the ability to travel long distances. Care is provided in a pressurized cabin with sophisticated on-board medical equipment. Many fixed-wing aircraft can transport multiple patients. All-weather navigational equipment allows for transfer during inclement weather. Fixed-wing transport requires suitable airfields to ensure safety of the crew and patient. Accessibility to such fields may be a problem in isolated areas.

TRANSPORT PROCESS

Patient transport today requires an organized process. There are multiple elements to the transport process, and in order to make it smooth and time-effective these components should be put in place before a transport is required.

This process continues to vary throughout the United States and throughout the world. Multiple organizations, including prehospital, emergency, and critical specialties, have published recommendations on how to perform patient transport. However, the National Guideline Clearinghouse[11] has published guidelines for the interhospital and intrahospital transport of critically ill patients. Using evidence-based research, these guidelines provide information about pretransport coordination and communication, transport personnel, monitoring during transport, and documentation.

Prehospital Transport

In most parts of the country, prehospital transport can be initiated by laypersons through the 9-1-1 and enhanced 9-1-1 emergency access numbers. Sophisticated prehospital emergency medical services (EMS) provide patient transport to the nearest appropriate medical care facility. Emergency nurses possess the knowledge to function as prehospital care providers, but their ability to function in this role varies from state to state. Surface transport can also be initiated for interfacility transport of patients with medical needs that exceed the capabilities of the local hospital.

The use of helicopters in the prehospital transport environment (scene responses) may be governed by local EMS or other state agencies. The National Association of EMS Physicians[15] and the American College of Emergency Physicians[2] have proposed guidelines for the use of air medical transport from the field. These are summarized in Box 9-1.

Box 9-1	**INDICATIONS FOR THE USE OF AIR MEDICAL TRANSPORT FROM THE OUT-OF-HOSPITAL SETTING**

Timely need for specific interventions, for example, bleeding control in an operating suite

Injuries that result in unstable vital signs requiring transport to the most appropriate center for care

Need to be transported by a team with more advanced intervention skills, for example, chest tube insertion

Location of the patient makes air medical transport a more reasonable mode of transportation

Distance of the patient to definitive care

Trauma score <12

Significant trauma in patients <12 years of age and >55 years of age

Pregnant patient with trauma or prenatal complications

Multisystem injuries

Ejection from a vehicle

Pedestrian or a cyclist struck by a vehicle

Crush injury to the head, chest, or abdomen

Glasgow Coma Scale score <10

Spinal cord injury

Significant abdominal pain

Presence of a "seat belt" sign

Flail chest

Amputations (specialty hospital need)

Major burns based on the American Burn Association criteria

Interfacility Transfers

Every emergency nurse has the potential to become involved with organizing and implementing an interfacility transfer. Effective organization includes assessment and understanding of the referring facility's capabilities and an in-depth knowledge of available EMS and transport systems. Implementation of the transport process is expedited if this knowledge is part of a proactive referral strategy developed well in advance.

Emergency nurses must be aware of the potential role they may be asked to play in patient transport. Today there are few places in the United States where a transport team may not be available. If an emergency nurse or any other nurse is asked to accompany a transport team on a patient transfer, he or she must be aware of the type of equipment accessible in the transport vehicle, how to operate it, the skills level of the team that is accompanying the patient. The safety of the nurse is also an important component of the transfer process. Appropriate restraint devices should be present in the transport vehicle. A safety briefing should also be given and the nurse provided with any other information that would assist in providing a safe transport.

Development of transfer strategies begins with objective assessment of the referring institution's personnel and facilities. Qualifications and availability of physicians and nurses to care for all patients who come to the ED must be examined. Specific areas that should be considered include the critical care unit; the operating suites; and pediatric,

BOX 9-2	**DETERMINING WHETHER A PATIENT SHOULD BE TRANSFERRED AND THE MOST APPROPRIATE MODE OF TRANSPORT**

- Does the patient's condition require minimal time out of the hospital during transport?
- Does the patient require time-sensitive evaluation or treatment not available at the referring facility?
- Is the patient located in a place where surface transport may pose a problem?
- What is the current and predicted weather along the transport route?
- Is there a helipad or an airport available to the referring facility?
- What is the weight and size of the patient?
- What type of equipment must accompany the patient?
- What type of team does the patient require? For example, critical care, pediatric, neonatal?
- Would the use of a surface vehicle leave the referring facility or community without adequate emergency services?
- Is there a specialty ground service available to the referring facility?
- Is rotor- or fixed-wing service available to the patient?
- If the patient requires international transport, is there a service available for the patient's medical needs?

Modified from Thomson D, Thomas S: Guidelines for air medical dispatch, *Prehosp Emerg Care* 7(2):265, 2003.

obstetric, neonatal, and psychiatric units. Ability to perform advanced diagnostic testing and provide adequate blood and blood products must also be analyzed. All these factors influence the level of care available to sick or injured patients.

Understanding the capabilities of the receiving institution is an inherent responsibility of the referring institution. Trauma patients are best cared for in facilities designated by the American College of Surgeons Committee on Trauma as trauma centers. High-risk neonates benefit from care in a neonatal intensive care unit. Other areas of advanced specialized care include stroke centers, burn centers, limb replantation centers, pediatric centers, high-risk obstetric centers, open-heart centers, and hyperbaric centers.

The act of transferring a patient from one facility to another should be well documented and fall within legal guidelines identified by each institution. Determining the appropriate mode and type of team is one of the most important roles of the referring facility. Choices must be made using federal mandates (i.e., EMTALA). If a patient is unable to give consent because of his or her medical condition, and no family is located, a patient may be transferred under the implied consent law. The patient, a family member, or a representative of the referring facility should sign a consent form for the transport. Box 9-2 contains some questions that may assist the referring center with determining what type of patient should be transferred and the appropriate transport mode.[15,16]

Communication

There should be nurse-to-nurse communication from the referring facility to the receiving facility. If this cannot be accomplished, a member of the transport team may provide a report. A copy of the medical record and relevant laboratory and radiographic studies must accompany the patient. Technology in some areas of the country may allow these studies to be transmitted ahead of the patient. Preparation of documents should never delay patient transport. If time is of the essence, critical information will need to be communicated verbally. Policies and procedures should exist within transport programs that assist in directing how communication will be initiated and followed up between the referring and receiving facilities. Health Insurance Portability and Accountability Act (HIPAA) guidelines must be followed when communicating protected health care information.

Transport Team Members

The team members that accompany a patient will be determined by the condition and level of care that the patient requires. CAMTS standards[7] outline the required team members for BLS, advanced life support (ALS), and critical care transport. Two team members at a minimum along with the vehicle operator should accompany the patient. For critical care transports CAMTS recommends that one member of the team be an appropriately educated and competent registered nurse. Other members of the team may include a physician, paramedic, respiratory therapist, or another registered nurse. All should be competent in the transport process.

If a physician is not part of the transport team, the team should operate using protocols and have the ability to communicate with a command physician to provide medical direction if there is a variation from protocol or a problem develops.

Transport team configurations are many and varied. Transport nursing has developed into a subspecialty of emergency and critical care nursing. Transport nurses now go through specific and rigorous training before joining a transport team. The Air Surface Transport Nurses Association (ASTNA), formerly the National Flight Nurses Association, has developed a flight and ground transport nursing core curriculum to provide standardized education and training in such areas as flight physiology, stabilization, communications, and medicolegal issues.[6] Initial training should include classroom and clinical experiences, including advanced airway management, invasive skills, and critical and emergency care. Preceptor programs are frequently used to allow the new transport nurse exposure to the transport environment. Recurrent training is needed to maintain skills, update information regarding current therapies, and review policies and procedures. Monthly transport reviews provide performance improvement opportunities and promote shared learning experiences among staff. Continuous performance improvement should be one of the guiding principles of transport nursing practice.

Nurses should be advanced cardiac life support (ACLS) verified with training and continuous evaluation of advanced airway management skills and other invasive skills such as chest tube insertion, needle thoracostomy techniques, and intraosseous needle insertion. Depending on the capabilities of the program, additional education should include invasive line management and intraaortic balloon pumps. Many programs also require advanced trauma life support (ATLS) credentials. Development of the Transport Nurse Advanced Trauma Course (TNATC) demonstrates ASTNA's commitment to improving educational opportunities available to transport nurses. Development of the certified flight nurse examination encourages flight nurses to achieve certification in flight nursing (CFRN). In addition, there is now a certified ground transport nurse (CTRN) for those transport nurses who provide critical care transport by ground.

Some states require additional credentials for nurses who work in the prehospital environment. This may include the need to become an EMT or an EMT-paramedic (EMT-P). It is the professional responsibility of transport nurses to be aware of the regulations that may dictate their practice within the states in which they perform transports.

Specialty teams are required for the transport of the obstetric, pediatric, or neonatal patient. These teams undergo specific training to provide care for these patients. The American Academy of Pediatrics offers guidelines for the education, training, and the specific equipment required to stabilize, manage and transport pediatric and neonatal patients.[17]

Transport team members work under a unique set of circumstances. Interactions with the patient are short and often rushed. The patients who are transported are at an increased risk for further injury or death because of circumstances necessitating transport. Transport personnel must remember that they are often the only contact the family has with the receiving hospital. The team should try to make contact with the family, explaining interventions and other procedures that may be needed for transport. Maintaining contact and follow-up with referring personnel also provides the transport team with opportunities to communicate patient status. Fostering collegial relationships instills a sense of commitment and pride in the transport nurse role, as well as providing an opportunity to improve patient care.

Transport Equipment

State regulations generally dictate what equipment should be on both surface and air transport vehicles. However, there are some general guidelines recommended by CAMTS, the National Association of Emergency Medical Services Physicians (NAEMSP), the American College of Emergency Physicians (ACEP), the American Academy of Pediatrics, and the American College of Surgeons for equipment that should be available for transport.[2,7,15,17]

The mission, size of the transport vehicle, and patient clinical condition are factors that influence the equipment carried during transport. General equipment should include equipment used to monitor and manage airway, oxygenation, and vital signs, as well as devices necessary for resuscitation and stabilization such as a defibrillator and external pacemaker. Medications for advanced life support and pain management should also be included.

All equipment should be routinely evaluated to see if it functions properly. Annual preventive maintenance checks should be dated and visible for team members to view. Medications must be checked for expiration and stored at the appropriate temperature. Policies and procedures must be in place to ensure that team members receive the proper education and training as to how to use the equipment. There should be an established method of removing and replacing malfunctioning equipment. Documentation of this process is imperative.

As technology continues to advance, many pieces of equipment are becoming multifunctional and longer lasting. In addition, advanced procedures such as extracorporal perfusion can now be continued during transport. Box 9-3 contains a sum-mary of some of the equipment that may be used during transport.

Preparation for Transport

Preparation for transfer of an ill or injured patient depends on the specific illness, injury, and age of the patient. The mode of transport and the size and capabilities of the transport vehicle will also assist in determining how to prepare the patient for transport. Potential problems during transport must be identified before departure, and proper interventions must be undertaken at the scene or the referring hospital.

The referring EMS agency (scene transports) and the referring hospital (interfacility) can help in reducing the time it may take to prepare the patient by beginning the appropriate evaluation and stabilization within their resources and personnel available. Unnecessary procedures and diagnostic tests should be avoided so that once the transport team arrives, the patient can be quickly and safely packaged and moved.

AIRWAY AND BREATHING. Airway patency during transport is of greatest importance. Potential airway compromise must be anticipated before transport so that proper interventions can be accomplished under controlled circumstances rather than during transport. Endotracheal intubation should be considered in patients who might aspirate, have difficulty with chest expansion, or need ventilatory support (e.g., patients with altered level of consciousness, facial fractures, airway obstruction, or inhalation burns). The interior size of the transport vehicle and location of the transport team within the vehicle may also contribute to the decision to stabilize the airway before transport.

Patients with chest wall injury, spinal cord injury, or neurologic dysfunction may also require ventilatory assistance. Chest tube placement for a possible pneumothorax or hemothorax should be done before transport. A closed drainage system or flutter valve should be in place to avoid recurrence of a pneumothorax.

HEMODYNAMIC STABILIZATION. Interventions to maintain an adequate pulse rate and blood pressure should be initiated before transport. These include control of bleeding, correction of hypovolemia, insertion of a urinary catheter, and institution of cardiac monitoring. Control of external bleeding sites with pressure or wound closure may be necessary. Splints for long-bone fractures or the pneumatic anti-shock garment (PASG) or other pelvic stabilization devices

---

BOX 9-3 RECOMMENDED EQUIPMENT FOR PATIENT TRANSPORT*

AIRWAY AND VENTILATION

Portable and fixed suction device

Large-bore suction catheter

Suction catheters (varied sizes depending on the patients transported)

Laryngoscope handles with extra batteries and bulbs (age-related handles)

Laryngoscope blades (sizes depending on the types of patients transported)

Endotracheal tubes (cuffed and uncuffed depending on age of patients transported)

Syringes

Magill forceps (size dependent on ages of patient transported)

Lubricating jelly

Gastric tubes (depending on ages transported)

End-tidal CO_2 devices

Bag-mask device

    Hand-operated, self-inflating (age-appropriate sizes)

Alternative airways as approved for use by medical direction or state or local regulations

Nebulizer

Pulse oximeter with age-appropriate probes

Portable ventilator

CARDIAC

Portable, battery-operated monitor, defibrillator, and external pacemaker

VASCULAR ACCESS

Intravenous catheters (age-appropriate)

Intravenous access equipment either in packets or separate components

Crystalloid solutions

Intravenous administration sets

Intravenous pumps or solution monitors

Intraosseous access equipment

MEDICATIONS

Cardiovascular medications

Antidysrhythmics

Epinephrine

Nitroglycerin

Aspirin

Vasopressors

Respiratory medications

Albuterol

Analgesics

Narcotic

Nonnarcotic

Antiepileptics

Sedation or other intubation adjuncts

Neuromuscular blocking agents

Glucometer and glucagon or $D_{50}W$

IMMOBILIZATION DEVICES

Rigid cervical collars (appropriate for patient age and size)

Head immobilization device

Lower extremity traction device

Splints

Radiolucent backboard

BANDAGES

Burn pack

Triangular bandages

Dressing supplies

Gauze rolls

Elastic bandages

Occlusive dressing

Tape (various sizes)

Large dressing

COMMUNICATION

Two-way radio communication

Cell phone

OBSTETRIC

Delivery pack

Bulb suctions

Thermal absorbent and head cover

Appropriate heat source

MISCELLANEOUS

Depends on local protocols, state regulations, or mission of the transport team

*Note that this is a suggested list and may vary as noted.

---

for pelvic injuries stabilize fractures and control bleeding. When applied, air pressure in the PASG should be monitored carefully during flight—air volume increases with altitude increases.

Proper intravenous (IV) access is needed to replace fluid loss. Large-caliber IV catheters with blood tubing provide rapid fluid resuscitation routes. Presence of two or more IV access points during transport obviates the need for restart in a moving vehicle. Use of plastic fluid bags allows for the use of pressure bags. Blood replacement products prepared for transport and placed in a proper container may accompany the patient.

Patients requiring fluid management should have a urinary catheter (if not contraindicated) attached to a device to properly measure urinary output. In addition to measuring output, bladder drainage decreases patient discomfort during a long transport.

All IV access lines should be checked for patency and should be secured. When there are multiple lines, labeling can decrease the risk for using the wrong line to administer medications during transport. If a subclavian or internal jugular line has been inserted, a chest radiograph should be obtained to rule out the presence of a pneumothorax before air transport.

Medications should be placed on infusion pumps or monitoring devices based on transport protocols. Most transport teams at a minimum will place all vasoactive medications on a pump or infuser. Medications not on monitors need to be carefully watched during transport.

The cardiac status of the patient must be determined before transport. An electrocardiogram may need to be obtained before departure to determine the need for any intervention before transport. Continuous monitoring should take place during transport.

CENTRAL NERVOUS SYSTEM STABILIZATION. All attempts should be made to stabilize the patient's neurologic condition (i.e., maintain normal intracranial pressure, control seizure activity, and preserve integrity of the spinal cord).

Maintenance of cerebral perfusion pressure in the head-injured patient includes measures to control increased intracranial pressure. The receiving neurologist or neurosurgeon should be consulted to decide what therapeutics, such as medications (i.e., mannitol, sedation, and neuromuscular blocking agents), fluid resuscitation, patient position, and ventilation settings, need to continue during transport.

Whether prophylactic medications are needed to reduce the risk for seizures during transport should be determined during the physician-to-physician consultation. Any patient at risk for seizure activity who has received neuromuscular blocking agents should receive antiseizure prophylaxis as directed by medical control.

A patient with a suspected or documented spinal cord injury should be placed in a rigid cervical collar and then secured on a backboard with head blocks to prevent movement of the spinal column. Long transport times are not uncommon, and preventive measures should be undertaken to reduce risk for pressure sore development. Padding of bony areas or the use of a vacuum splint may better serve the patient.

MUSCULOSKELETAL STABILIZATION. Care of the patient with musculoskeletal injuries should include prevention of blood loss, fracture immobilization, wound care, and administration of analgesia.

Splints should permit assessment of distal pulses as well as observation of increased swelling or bleeding during transport. Air splints respond to pressure changes during air transport and should not be used in this environment. Pelvic fractures may be stabilized with a PASG or other approved pelvic stabilization devices. Traction splints for femur fractures can be used in transport; however, length of the splint must be kept to a minimum so that the transport vehicle door can be closed properly. Free-swinging traction weights are avoided in transport because of risk to medical crew members.

Patients transferred for limb replantation need special care. Wrapping the amputated part in saline-moistened gauze and placing it in a plastic bag should preserve the affected part. The plastic bag should be placed in a sealed container on ice inside a cooler. The part should not be allowed to freeze—this causes tissue destruction and prevents replantation.

Wound care before transport may be limited to control of bleeding, initial cleansing, and the application of a sterile dressing. The transport team member should note if tetanus prophylaxis has been given before leaving.

Burn care includes calculation of the percentage of body surface area burned and fluid resuscitation (see Chapter 26). Fluid resuscitation must be continued throughout transport. The transport team must ensure that an adequate supply of fluid is available in the transport vehicle. The patient must be kept warm, which may require running a heater in the transport vehicle even during the summertime. Constricting rings, necklaces, and clothing should be removed. If circulation impairment is present, escharotomy must be performed before transport under the direction of medical control.

EMOTIONAL AND PSYCHOSOCIAL SUPPORT OF THE PATIENT AND FAMILY. The patient who will be transferred has many physical, emotional, and psychosocial needs. Emergency and transport nurses can address these needs by recognizing the patient's fears and answering any questions.

Removing patients from their homes, family, and a familiar environment increases patient stress. Patients that need to be transported by air may have a fear of flying. The patient and the family may be angry, with their anger directed at the referring hospital for being unable to care for them. The need for transport is often translated in a patient's or family's minds to mean he or she is dying. The stresses of transport may produce anxiety, causing increased heart rate and respiratory rate, diaphoresis, nausea, vomiting, and a general worsening of condition.

Personnel from the referring hospital and the transport team can work together to alleviate the patient's fears by thoroughly explaining all procedures, noises, and reasons for the transport. Transport personnel should work to instill confidence in the patient concerning the referring hospital. This confidence is important because, if the patient survives, he or she will be returning to the home community and will be cared for by the referring hospital in the future.

Research has shown that families have specific needs when a patient is to be transported to another hospital.[3,9,10,12] Families want to feel that the transport team truly cares for their loved ones. They want to know specific facts about the patient's condition, including the prognosis, especially whether the patient will live or die; to have procedures and treatments explained in terms that they can understand; to have questions answered honestly; and at a minimum to feel there is some hope as to a positive outcome. This information should always be given so that the family's reaction can be evaluated. Working with a family may appear to be a time-consuming activity, but it is an important part of transport care.

The patient's family also has tremendous fears. If the patient is acutely ill or injured, this interaction may be the last they have with their loved one. The family may not understand the need for the transport. Time must be taken to explain the necessity for immediate transfer. The family may also have what is called the "Mecca syndrome," an inflated idea of what can be done for the patient at the receiving facility. The family may believe the receiving hospital will save the life of a patient, when in fact that may not happen.

A family member may want to accompany the patient. In helicopter transports, this option may not be possible because of space and weight limitations.[3,9] However, depending on the type of surface ambulance or fixed-wing aircraft, room may be available for a family member. Transport personnel should make the decision whether to allow the family member to come with the patient during a surface transport, but the final decision in air transport is the responsibility of the pilot in command. The family member's presence may alleviate some of the patient's anxiety, especially when the patient is a child. The decision should not be made until the time of the transport, because the patient's condition may change and promises cannot always be kept.

To alleviate family anxiety, provide as much information as possible about the receiving hospital. Maps, plans for patient admission, and a telephone contact give them some direction after the patient departs. The family should be informed of the estimated length of transport and expected time of arrival at the receiving hospital. This time should be calculated taking into consideration weather, unexpected delays, changes in time zone, and other factors. Overestimation of time is always best—if the transport is completed sooner than anticipated, the family will feel relief. On the other hand, if the transport takes longer than expected, the family may fear the outcome of the transport itself.

One of the last things that should be done before departure is to allow the family time with the patient. The last remarks and the last kiss goodbye may be the most important few minutes of the transport.

Documentation

Documentation of the transfer is essential. It confirms adherence to legal mandates, ensures compliance with established standards of care, and protects the caregiver in potential litigious situations. Documentation of prehospital care includes mechanism of injury, time of injury, time of EMS arrival, care provided in the field and during transport, and protocols or orders used during transfer. Documentation related to interfacility transfer includes the prehospital record, the ED record, and documentation of care during the transfer. Consent for transport form and an indication for transport form should be included with the documentation. The content of these forms may vary from one health care system to another.

Care During Transport

During transport, at a minimum, monitoring of the patient's oxygenation through continuous pulse oximetry, electrocardiograph monitoring, and regular measurement of the blood pressure and respiratory rate should be performed.[11]

Transport personnel must be prepared to implement interventions to maintain patient stability. Protocols and physician orders regarding specific interventions clarify expectations for the transporting team. Interventions that may be needed during transport include securing the airway,

suctioning, administering fluids, performing emergency thoracotomy, administering medications, and performing ALS measures. In unforeseen emergencies when sophisticated medical equipment and personnel are critical, diversion to a closer facility may be necessary. The location of these facilities should be identified before transport to prevent unnecessary delays.

Appropriately trained personnel should manage any equipment that is not usually used by the transport team, for example a left ventricular assist device or an intraaortic balloon pump (IABP). Any additional persons who accompany the transport team must receive an orientation to the transport environment that includes safety and operational issues. They should also be clothed in uniforms and helmets if going by air.

All care during transport should be documented. A copy of the transport form should be inserted in the patient's chart at the receiving facility. Documentation should include patient assessment, interventions, and the patient's response to these interventions. Unusual events or effects of the transport on the patient's condition should also be noted.

Communication

Effective communication is an essential component of the entire transport process. When a call is placed to an emergency operations center, the dispatcher notifies appropriate units to respond. Radio communication is established, and pertinent information is transmitted. Depending on severity and local protocols, the mobile unit can be directly linked to the medical command center or the base station at the receiving hospital. Cell phone communication can also be used. Transmission of pertinent data is necessary so the transport team can receive specific protocols for intervention.

Successful communication includes a complete loop in which all parties are notified and aware of the patient's status. This begins with the physician-to-physician contact that establishes the transport process. Communication is ongoing and should focus on essential information for the transporting and receiving personnel.

Communication techniques, radio codes, and communication technology are too extensive to be included here. Emergency and transport nurses must be familiar with the communication centers and methods used in their area of service. Regardless of technology used, every effort should be made to protect patient confidentiality during any communication. Use of patient names or other identifying factors is discouraged. A standard reporting format may be developed by the transport program to ensure quality assurance for each communication.

Medical Control

Organization of medical control varies from system to system. Online medical control is direct communication between transport personnel and the physician (or physician-surrogate) via radio or telephone for the purpose of providing orders for patient care. Offline medical control includes those administrative functions necessary to ensure quality of care. Each medical control officer is a physician who is directly responsible for care provided in transport. It is the medical control officer's responsibility to ensure proper training, orientation, and continuing education for those people working under his or her control.[5]

Transfer of Care

While the patient is in transit, the referring and receiving facilities share responsibility for care of the patient. Only after arrival at the receiving facility is the referring hospital's legal responsibility terminated. Time of arrival at the receiving hospital should be noted in the copy of the chart that remains at the referring facility.

STRESSES OF TRANSPORT

Exposure to environmental factors occurs during transport of patients. Problems encountered depend on changes in atmospheric conditions, vehicle configurations, motion of the aircraft, and the patient's condition. Some of these can be detrimental to the patient, but with proper nursing care before and during transport, these harmful effects can be minimized or eliminated. It is also important to keep in mind these factors can cause stress to both the patient and the transfer team and interventions may be required for both the patient and the team members to complete a safe transport.

Effects of Altitude

Atmospheric changes occur when the aircraft's altitude changes. Ascending into the atmosphere from sea level causes a decrease in atmospheric pressure, which in turn causes a decrease in the partial pressure of gases, temperature, and expansion of gases. The opposite occurs during descent.

According to Boyle's law, the volume of gas is inversely proportional to its pressure. As an aircraft ascends, atmospheric pressure decreases and gas expands. One hundred milliliters of gas at sea level expands to 130 mL at an altitude of 6000 feet, 200 mL at 18,000 feet, and 400 mL at 34,000 feet. Gas expansion is a potential problem in all transports in which the aircraft ascends.

Patients with a pneumothorax, pneumopericardium, pneumomomediastinum, abdominal distention, or trapped gas or any equipment that may be affected by gas expansion, such as some mechanical ventilators, must be closely monitored for the effects of changes in barometric pressure. Interventions such as chest thoracotomy or insertion of a gastric tube must be done before transport.[1]

Fixed-wing and rotary-wing vehicles are designed according to different principles. Fixed-wing aircraft used in patient transport are pressurized, which allows for a comfortable cabin atmosphere when flying at high altitudes. Pressurization differentials allow for different cabin pressures at different atmospheres. Generally the lower the altitude

at which a plane is flying, the lower the cabin pressure that can be achieved. This ability to maintain a physiologically comfortable environment within the aircraft is a benefit when transporting patients who may be affected by atmospheric changes. Although pressurization allows for flights at high altitudes, even subtle changes in the environment may be harmful to a person whose condition is severely compromised.

If the pressurization system fails, pressurization within the cabin might be lost, causing a sudden change in atmospheric pressure. This rapid decompression causes the interior of the cabin to equalize with the pressures outside the cabin, resulting in sudden and often detrimental effects on the human body: rapid loss of oxygen, sudden drop in temperature, and expansion of gas. A healthy person may be able to withstand these changes, but the person in poor health may deteriorate rapidly. Those transporting patients should be aware of these effects and do everything possible before departure to minimize complications.

Rotary-wing vehicles are not pressurized; therefore these atmospheric changes are felt whenever the helicopter ascends and descends. As a result, patients transported by helicopter may be at greater risk than those transported by fixed-wing aircraft. If a higher altitude may be a problem for the patient, the transport nurse should ask the rotor-wing pilot to fly as low as safely possible.

Hypoxia

Many patients transported by air are hypoxic as a result of their condition. This hypoxic state is potentiated when changes in atmospheric pressure occur. There are four major types of hypoxia[1]:

- *Hypoxic hypoxia:* results from insufficient oxygen in the air breathed or when oxygen is prevented from diffusing from the lungs to the bloodstream
- *Hypemic hypoxia:* results from reduction in oxygen-carrying capacity in the blood
- *Stagnant hypoxia:* results from inadequate circulation
- *Histotoxic hypoxia:* results from interference with the use of oxygen by the body's tissues

When an aircraft ascends in altitude, the partial pressure of oxygen (PO_2) decreases and causes a decreased diffusion gradient for the oxygen molecule to cross the alveolar membrane.

Simple calculation of the diffusion gradient is accomplished by using the following formulas:

$$(\text{Atmospheric pressure} - \text{Water pressure}) \times (\text{Percentage of oxygen}) = PO_2$$

and

$$\text{Alveolar } PO_2 - \text{Venous } PO_2 = \text{Diffusion gradient}$$

Room air is 21% oxygen. If the patient is receiving oxygen, the fraction of inspired oxygen is used for the patient's oxygen therapy. Assuming that water pressure is equal to 47 mm Hg, the PO_2 at sea level is 150 mm Hg: (760 mm Hg atmospheric pressure − 47 mm Hg) × (0.21) = 150 mm Hg. At an altitude of 6000 feet the calculated PO_2 is 118 mm Hg: (609 mm Hg − 47 mm Hg) × (0.21) = 118 mm Hg.

The decrease in PO_2 that occurs in the respiratory tree is approximately 45 mm Hg; therefore at the alveolar level, the PaO_2 at sea level is approximately 105 mm Hg and the PaO_2 at 6000 feet is about 73 mm Hg. The PO_2 of venous blood is approximately 40 mm Hg; therefore the diffusion gradient at sea level is 65 mm Hg (105 − 40) and at 6000 feet is 22 mm Hg. Patients with disease-induced hypoxia are severely affected by this drop in diffusion gradient and are at increased risk for compromise during air medical transport. Patients at risk include those with heart failure, respiratory distress syndrome, carbon monoxide poisoning, hypovolemic shock, inadequate amount of circulating hemoglobin, and stagnant hypoxia induced by low-flow states such as hypothermia. Altitude-induced reduction in PO_2 causes further deterioration in these patients if interventions are not performed to correct the problems related to hypoxia. Risk for hypoxia is even greater when the patient smokes.

Signs and symptoms of hypoxia include changes in vital signs, tachycardia, pupillary constriction, confusion, disorientation, and lethargy. All of these signs may be caused by a number of other illnesses and injuries, making the diagnosis of hypoxia more difficult. Astute observation of the patient is necessary to detect and correct the problems related to hypoxia. Transporting patients by pressurized fixed-wing aircraft can limit complications secondary to this drop in PO_2. Most aircraft used for air transport are able to maintain a sea level cabin pressure when flying below 7000 to 10,000 feet. At higher altitudes, the cabin can be pressurized. Maximum cabin pressure altitude is generally maintained well below 9000 feet. When cabin pressures are controlled, atmospheric changes that occur are limited, controlled, and within a tolerable range.

Before the patient is transported, stabilization measures can be taken to reduce effects of atmospheric changes in oxygenation. Supplemental oxygen can be provided, and if the patient has previously required oxygen, the percentage of oxygen can be increased. This increase in oxygen delivery is prophylactic, a temporary measure during transport. When the patient arrives at the receiving institution, oxygen can be decreased or terminated pending outcome of arterial blood gas analysis.

Proper positioning of the patient combats the effects of hypoxia. Ensuring proper chest excursion by loosening chest restraints on the stretcher allows the patient to breathe easier. Elevation of the patient's head when not contraindicated may also assist with ventilation and oxygenation.

The hypovolemic patient may receive transfusions to increase hematocrit and oxygen-carrying capacity of the blood. Patients who are alert are generally anxious regarding their outcome, which increases respiratory rate and decreases oxygenation. Providing a calm environment and thoroughly explaining all procedures, noises, and equipment can reduce the patient's feeling of helplessness.

Level of consciousness, continuous pulse oximetry readings, and vital sign monitoring provide the best indicators of how a patient is tolerating the transport. During transport, all patients should receive oxygen.

Dehydration

Another problem encountered during an increase in altitude is a drop in ambient humidity. Loss of humidification is magnified in a pressurized fixed-wing aircraft, because recycling air and removing moisture from it achieve system pressurization. Patients who are dehydrated or diaphoretic are at increased risk for dehydration and possible fluid volume deficits. Supplemental IV fluids should be administered to prevent dehydration.

Other patients affected by dehydration include mouth breathers and those who are intubated. These patients have lost the natural respiratory humidification mechanisms, so secretions become tenacious and difficult to mobilize. Suction should be available to ensure that the airway remains patent.

Decreased Temperature

As altitude increases, temperature decreases. For each 1000-foot gain in altitude, temperature drops 2° C until it reaches −55° C. During ascent, this temperature drop cools the aircraft. Although transport vehicles are heated, the fuselage becomes quite cold and radiates cold into the cabin interior. Outside temperature changes will also affect the patient being transported by ground. The coldest area of all transport vehicles is against the outside walls. This cooling, although most significant during cold-weather months, is noticeable at all times of the year.

In addition to altitude-induced and outside temperature changes, a number of environmental conditions affect transport of patients. Of particular importance is a drop in environmental temperature. Interhospital transports require patient movement outside the hospital, transport outside to the helipad or into an ambulance for transfer to the airfield, and subsequent transfer into the transport vehicle. The opposite occurs at the receiving end of the transfer. These multiple transfers expose the patient to changing environmental conditions, including cold weather. A patient requiring transport, especially an infant or older adult patient, is less able to tolerate these stresses and can exhibit signs and symptoms of cold stress, including decreased level of consciousness, increased heart rate, and shivering. These symptoms increase the patient's oxygen demands, causing mild hypoxia to worsen significantly.

Awareness of an environmental drop in temperature allows adequate stabilization before the transport. Minimizing exposure to environmental conditions is of utmost importance. The interior temperature of the transport vehicle can be controlled in accordance with the patient's needs rather than needs of the transport crew. Maintaining an adequate supply of linen and wrapping the patient in a rescue blanket is useful in cold environments. A cap can be put on the patient's head to reduce radiated heat losses.[1]

Cold can also affect transport equipment. Transport teams should be aware of the temperature ranges that affect their equipment. Policies and procedures should be in place to monitor and replace anything that may become damaged.

Other problems that develop with cold environments include cooling IV solutions and crystallization of medications, most notably mannitol. A patient with cold stress resulting from changes in the environment requires warm IV fluids. Solutions stored in the aircraft or solutions exposed to the environment are quite cold and must be warmed before administration. If possible, solutions should be stored in the warmest spot in the cabin. Some transport vehicles have environmental drawers to manage medications.

Remember that medications such as neuromuscular blocking agents can interfere with the patient's ability to maintain his or her body temperature. The use of these types of medications dictates that the patient be closely monitored during transport. The patient should be covered at all times even when the transport team feels that the environment is comfortable for them.

Acceleration and Deceleration Forces

Acceleration forces occur during takeoff and "climb-out." Blood pools in dependent areas, most commonly the lower extremities, causing fluid shifts that may not be tolerated by the severely compromised patient. Restoration of intravascular volume and proper positioning of the patient can minimize the effects of these forces.

Deceleration forces occur during slowing, stopping, or rapid descent. For the patient lying head forward in an aircraft, deceleration forces cause blood to pool in the head and upper body. Pooling produces what is known as "redout" as blood rushes to the head, causing an increase in blood within the ocular cavity. Deceleration forces are most harmful to a patient with increased intracranial pressure. The phenomenon may also adversely affect a patient with congestive heart failure.

Effects of acceleration and deceleration forces vary with speed, angle, and duration. These forces are much more pronounced in a fixed-wing aircraft. In certain instances, pilots can control these effects as long as safety measures and regulations are met. If a patient is known to be severely ill or injured, transport personnel should discuss this problem with their flight crew. A slow descent is often an option. If the airfield is long enough, a longer landing roll can decrease some deceleration forces that occur as the aircraft is slowed to a stop.

Positioning of the patient is crucial to counter these forces. In many aircraft, stretcher restraints are not interchangeable; therefore the patient must be loaded head first into the cabin. If the patient can tolerate a head-elevated position, effects of these forces can be minimized, because fluid shifts would be centered at the core of the body rather than in the head.

Rotary-wing vehicles are also subject to acceleration and deceleration forces but to a lesser magnitude than fixed-wing aircraft. In addition to forward and rearward movement, helicopters are capable of lateral movement. Forces resulting from these movements are of little consequence. Because of confined space within the helicopter, positioning the patient to counteract these forces is usually more difficult, if not impossible. Fortunately, pilot control is much greater in the helicopter.

Motion Sickness

Changes in equilibrium caused by excessive motion can cause motion sickness either by air or ground transport. Nausea and vomiting may develop in the patient and transport personnel. Prophylactic premedication is the best intervention available to limit these complications.

Other causes of motion sickness include hypoxia; excessive visual stimuli, such as blinking lights on the aircraft control panel; stress; fear; unpleasant odors; heat; and poor diet. Gastric gas expansion occurring during ascent can worsen the problem. To prevent or limit these symptoms, transport personnel should provide adequate oxygenation, stare at a fixed visual reference, cool the cabin interior, attempt to limit stressors and fear, and have the patient lie in the supine position.

For crew members with motion sickness, premedication may be needed. Medications should be selected that do not cause drowsiness or interfere with the transport team member's ability to provide patient care and remain safe during the transport. Other preventive measures include eating ginger cookies and using acupressure bracelets. Crew members often "recover" from motion sickness when they focus their attention on the patient; however, residual symptoms may occur after the transport.

Noise

Transport vehicles are inherently noisy. Engine noises create a constant loud hum that not only is distracting but also increases stress. Reducing extraneous noise is often impossible, but limiting sound input can be accomplished by application of earplugs, headphones, or helmets. Unfortunately, use of noise reduction devices by the patient reduces communication so he or she is not able to hear. The patient may become increasingly agitated, believing the team is talking about him or her. It is essential to include the conscious patient in as much conversation as possible.

Noise also interferes with ability to hear breath sounds, heart sounds, and blood pressure. Doppler devices are available to assist with detecting blood pressure but are of little use for hearing breath or heart sounds. Other assessment techniques to ascertain adequate ventilation include observing for bilateral chest wall movement, using pulse oximetry, and placing the stethoscope over the trachea to listen for air movement.

The transport team may be familiar with noises of the aircraft or ground transport vehicle, but the patient should be warned ahead of time. Many aircraft have audible warning signals to prevent accidents, but to the patient these alarms may indicate the aircraft is in danger of crashing. Continual reminders to alleviate these fears should follow a preflight and transport briefing with the patient.

Long-term noise exposure is also a problem for the transport team. Protective earplugs or helmets should be used to minimize the deleterious effects of noise over time. Periodic hearing tests are recommended to monitor changes in hearing.

Vibration

As a result of vehicle design, aircraft vibrate. The effects of vibration are much more noticeable in a helicopter, especially during takeoff and landing. This constant motion can cause equipment to loosen and become a danger during flight. Federal Aviation Administration (FAA) regulations require that all equipment be secured during takeoff and landing. Equipment should be secured at all times in anticipation of unexpected turbulence.

The patient should be secured to the stretcher at all times. Before loading and unloading, stretcher restraints should be checked for proper fit. During transport, straps may be loosened to allow the patient to move; however, restraints should never be fully released.

Vibrations may affect equipment. Again, equipment should be routinely inspected to prevent any problems.

Immobilization

Long transport times combined with prolonged immobilization of the patient can lead to pressure sores and venous stasis. Space limitations and inability to change the patient's position exacerbate these problems. The patient at greatest risk is one with a suspected spinal injury who is secured to a backboard.

Before departure, all splints, casts, and pressure areas should be padded. A small towel or pad can be placed under the coccyx area of a patient with a suspected cervical spine injury who is secured to a backboard. In transport, proper positioning and assessment of range of motion should be performed within the space constraints. Assessing for areas of decreased perfusion should be part of assessment of vital signs.

Length of transport includes not only the time it takes to fly from the referring location to the receiving hospital, but also surface transport times, unexpected delays, and transfer times. For example, a patient injured in a motor vehicle crash at a remote site is secured to a backboard to protect the cervical spine. This patient is then transported by surface ambulance to the nearest hospital. After evaluation of injuries, it is determined that the patient requires care in a major trauma center. Radiographs of the cervical spine are inconclusive, so the patient must remain on the backboard during transport. Subsequently the patient is taken by surface ambulance to the nearest airport, flown to the receiving airfield, and again transferred by surface ambulance to the trauma center.

Consideration of injuries must take precedence during stabilization of the patient, but using padded splints, traction devices, and protecting bony prominences are a necessary follow-up, limiting preventable problems associated with immobilization.

TRANSPORT OF SELECTED PATIENT POPULATIONS

Transport of any patient can be challenging. Emergency and transport nurses need to be familiar with the entire process, but some patient populations offer more challenges than others. The following is a discussion of some of these special populations.

Patients With Respiratory Distress

A patient with a preexisting pulmonary problem needs to be carefully assessed and prepared for transport. If intubated, the position of the endotracheal tube must be confirmed. The endotracheal tube should be carefully secured.

Arterial blood gas levels may be obtained to determine patient oxygenation and if the fraction of inspired oxygen (FiO_2) has been appropriately adjusted.

Gas expansion within the pleural cavity can cause the size of a previously undetected pneumothorax to increase, which may lead to respiratory compromise. A flutter valve should be placed to reduce pressure within the chest cavity. If the patient had a chest tube placed before transport, the tube should never be clamped during flight. A one-way (Heimlich) valve can be placed between the chest tube and the drainage set to prevent reaccumulation of air in the chest cavity.

Pulmonary secretions become more tenacious with dehydration and decreased ambient humidity. Instillation of sterile saline before suctioning enhances removal of secretions. Hyperventilation can accompany cold stress or may be caused by excessive noise and vibration. Measures should be taken to warm the patient and allay any fears and anxieties.

Immobilizing the patient on the stretcher interferes with chest expansion and can lead to hypoventilation and subsequent atelectasis. Elevating the patient's head improves oxygenation and gas exchange and helps limit pulmonary congestion that occurs secondary to acceleration and deceleration forces.

Mechanical volume ventilators used in the transport environment should be constantly monitored for delivery of adequate tidal volumes, because gas expansion can affect volume of gas delivered. High oxygen flow rates of at least 15 L/min are required to operate some ventilators, which can rapidly decrease oxygen supply. The patient should be allowed a period of time to adjust to the transport ventilator. Some patients may require sedation in order to tolerate a ventilator during transport. Some patients may not be able to tolerate a transport ventilator at all, and alternative ventilation methods may need to be considered. Should the ventilator fail, a bag-valve device should be available to support the patient's ventilation.

Patients With Cardiovascular Conditions

Hypoxia presents the greatest risk for the cardiac patient during transport. It can lead to increased myocardial irritability and ventricular ectopy. Providing supplemental oxygen and positioning the patient for optimal gas exchange is imperative. Interventions to decrease oxygen demand include keeping the patient warm, allaying fears, and preventing motion sickness.

Placing a gastric tube can prevent decreased venous return caused by gastric distension. However, placement must be performed with caution because vagal stimulation and bradycardia can develop. The decision to place a gastric tube should be made on a patient-by-patient basis.

Acceleration forces cause pooling of blood in the lower extremities with subsequent poor cardiac return. The opposite effect develops as a result of deceleration forces, in which cardiac congestion and transient fluid overload develop. The patient with heart failure is severely affected by these factors.

Specialized equipment associated with cardiac patients needs special attention. Patients with pacemakers should be monitored for pacemaker malfunction that can occur as a result of radio and navigational equipment signals. Intraaortic balloon pumps may be used during transport. Only trained personnel should use these devices, because the risk for balloon dislodgment and equipment malfunction is increased in the transport environment. During transport, close monitoring of the patient and equipment is required.

Burn Victims

Burns of the face, head, and neck can cause massive swelling, reducing the airway size. Prophylactic intubation before transport eliminates the need for intubation in the poorly lit, cramped interior of a transport vehicle. Supplemental oxygen should be administered to all patients with suspected smoke inhalation to combat the effects of hypoxia.

Loss of the skin causes massive fluid shifts and loss of temperature regulation. Evaporative heat loss increases in the burned area, and the burn victim becomes increasingly dehydrated and cold. All wounds should be covered with absorbent dressings to control heat loss and limit contamination of the wounds. Dressings should not be moistened with saline solution or other fluids because this enhances hypothermia. The patient should be covered, and the vehicle's heater may be needed to provide additional warmth during transport.

Patients with burns require large amounts of fluids and dressings; therefore adequate supplies must be available throughout the transport of a burn victim. Escharotomies may become necessary to assure adequate ventilation when there are circumferential burns of the neck and chest. These should be performed only by qualified personnel and usually under the direction of medical control.

Pain management is an important component of burn care. Appropriate analgesia should be continued throughout the transport.

Patients With High-Risk Obstetric Conditions

Hypoxia and fluid shifts increase uterine irritability and can lead to premature labor. Hypoxia of short duration has little effect on the fetus, but prolonged maternal hypoxia can lead to fetal distress and subsequent fetal demise. Supplemental oxygen should be provided to the pregnant patient throughout transport.

Pressure from a distended stomach increases uterine irritability and increases pressure on the diaphragm, which leads to dyspnea. Gastric tube placement may be uncomfortable for the pregnant woman but is necessary to decompress the stomach and decrease the risk for aspiration from delayed gastric emptying.

Pregnancy increases blood volume in the third trimester by approximately 45% to 50%. This increased volume must be replaced if the woman is hypovolemic. Pregnant women can lose a significant portion of their circulating blood volume before hypovolemia is evident. Fluid shifts accompanying acceleration and deceleration forces can decrease uterine blood flow. Proper positioning is essential for the pregnant patient.

The pregnant patient should be placed in the left lateral decubitus position during transport. Safely securing the patient to the stretcher in this position is often difficult. The patient may have to be secured in the supine position during loading and unloading. The woman should be returned to the left lateral decubitus position as soon as the aircraft reaches cruising altitude or with signs of fetal distress. For the pregnant trauma patient, secure the woman to the backboard, and then tip the entire board to the left.

Pregnancy-induced hypertension (preeclampsia and eclampsia) increases nausea and vomiting associated with motion. These patients are also sensitive to extraneous stimulation; noise and vibration may increase blood pressure. Dim lighting and earplugs for the patient help prevent overstimulation.

All personnel who transport high-risk obstetric patients must be familiar with the techniques of childbirth and neonatal resuscitation. Equipment for delivery and resuscitation must be readily available. If delivery is imminent, the transport should reroute to the nearest hospital to avoid in-transport delivery regardless of final destination. Keeping a newly delivered infant warm, dry, and oxygenated is the priority for newborn care.

Pediatric Patients

Pediatric transport teams should be considered for the transport of the ill or injured pediatric patient. If a pediatric team is not available, the team performing the transport should have received additional education and training to ensure that they can safely and competently manage the ill or injured child during transport.

The problems associated with transport of children are similar to those for adults. However, interventions must take into account the unique anatomic and physiologic features of children. Because equipment of the appropriate size varies with age and weight of the child, the appropriate equipment must be available.

Pediatric patients are more prone to the effects of hypoxia. Children may not be able to tolerate or cooperate with application of an oxygen mask. In these cases the oxygen mask can be placed in front of the child's face and oxygen can be blown at the child. A family member accompanying the child can assist with administration of oxygen by holding the mask and encouraging the child to cooperate.

Because the gastric cavity of a child is small, the child has a greater tendency to develop complications from gastric gas expansion. Many gastric tubes for children do not have a sump port and should not be used, because absence of the sump port makes emptying the stomach more difficult.

The greater ratio of surface area to body mass in children makes them more susceptible to evaporative heat losses. The proportionally larger surface area of the head and neck also enhances radiated heat loss, which puts the child at great risk for hypothermia. A stocking cap and extra linen help keep the child warm.

Children should be secured and transported in age-appropriate equipment. Providing familiar items such as toys and security blankets helps alleviate the child's fear of the unknown.

If the child's condition is stable, including a family member in the transport may be advantageous. The family member can comfort the child, help explain procedures, and provide diversionary activities as warranted to keep the child occupied.

SAFETY

Safety before, during, and after transport should be the primary concern of all people involved. There are inherent risks with patient transport whether by air or ground, and all involved in the transport process need to be aware of how to keep themselves and their patients safe.

Transport team members should have recurrent training in handling the emergencies that may occur during transport. In addition, there should be a safety program that includes education of the personnel who use the transport service. Basic procedures that should be reviewed include how to assist the vehicle operator during an emergency (based on the type of vehicle), emergency oxygen shutoff, and how to prepare the patient. Communication should occur as to what to do after an emergency has occurred and should include where the team should assemble, how to contact help, and basic survival skills. The ASTNA has prepared an extensive document about safety during transport. This document can be obtained from http://www.astna.org.

Transport team members should always feel comfortable and be supported in refusing to participate in or tolerate unsafe practices. Each transport service must have a safety program that continuously evaluates the transport environment and provides a way to communicate safety.

Fixed-Wing Transports

All equipment must be secured in accordance with FAA regulations. Meeting stringent requirements ensures that flying objects do not injure passengers and crew during turbulence or if a crash occurs. Equipment not secured to the airframe itself should be kept in soft packs and placed on the floor during takeoff and landing. Equipment or extraneous items should never block emergency exits.

Ground personnel must be trained and briefed regarding aircraft safety. This briefing should include information on loading and unloading the patient. For instance, weight distribution is critical in the aircraft, but ground personnel may not be aware of these requirements. Also, ground personnel should be trained to avoid hazardous areas, such as propellers and the exhaust cowling on a jet engine. No one should approach the aircraft until the pilot in command or a designated member of the transport team has given approval to do so.

The pilot in command is responsible for safety of the aircraft at all times and may determine whether to cancel a flight because of weather conditions; however, all members of the team are responsible for safety. Most flight programs do not discuss severity of the patient's condition with the pilot until a decision has been made regarding weather. This relieves the pilot of undue stress when a life-or-death mission is being considered; the pilot should be able to make this decision without feelings of guilt or doubt affecting his or her judgment.

Everyone involved in the transport should be briefed before departure. Pilots should be informed of the patient's condition and specific needs related to takeoff and landing. For example, a short landing that results in shifts in internal organs and fluids adversely affects some patients. Family members should be briefed on the length of the flight, in-flight expectations, and the location and operation of emergency exits. Smoking is prohibited. Seat belts are required on landing and takeoff, although their use is preferred throughout the flight.

Fire extinguishers should be clearly marked, and all personnel must be trained in their use. Emergency procedures for rapid egress should be practiced on a regular basis.

Rotor-Wing Transports

Helicopter transports create a sense of drama. Many people assemble to watch a helicopter land and take off. Bystanders must be kept away from danger. A safe landing zone (LZ) should be established in a clearing that measures 100 feet × 100 feet up to 200 feet × 200 feet, depending on the size of the helicopter. All wires, trees, and possible hazards should be marked and described over the radio to the pilot. Smoke flares can be ignited to assist the pilot in locating the LZ. Flares are blown away from the helicopter during landing, which could ignite a fire. The patient, ground personnel, and bystanders should be at least 500 feet from the LZ and should turn their backs to the helicopter while it is landing. The rotor wash (wind created by the rotor blades) causes swirling dust, dirt, and gravel, which pose hazards to people on the ground.

Ground personnel should not approach the helicopter until the pilot or a designated transport team member gives the signal it is safe to do so and from the direction (front or side) as directed by the transport team. The helicopter should be approached from the downhill side, never the uphill side. Many injuries occur because people approach the helicopter while the blades are still rotating. When blade rotation slows down, the blades drop, which may cause unexpected injury. Each aircraft is different, so it is a good idea to be familiar

---

Box 9-4	GUIDELINES FOR HELICOPTER LANDING SAFETY

Landing zone (LZ) size ranges from 100 to 200 square feet, depending on size of the helicopter.

Select an LZ that is easily identifiable, as level as possible, and free of debris and overhead obstructions.

Mark one corner of the LZ with a smoke flare, so the pilot can estimate wind speed and direction.

Flashing emergency lights are difficult to see in daylight. Landmarks such as intersections, waterways, distinctive buildings, or baseball or football fields are much easier to find from the air.

Turn off unnecessary lights and white lights such as strobe lights or headlights at night. These lights interfere with the pilot's night vision. Never direct a spotlight at an approaching helicopter.

Flags, cones, safety tapes, ambulance mattresses, poles used for intravenous infusion, other loose equipment, sticks, stones, and broken glass can be drawn into rotor blades or thrown during landing and liftoff.

Only people such as firefighters with proper personal protection, including safety goggles, should be permitted in the vicinity of the LZ.

Assign personnel to guard the area. Prohibit smoking, and keep spectators at a safe distance.

Never approach the helicopter unless signaled to do so by the pilot or another air medical crew member. Keep low if the main rotor is still spinning.

Always approach the helicopter within the crew's line of sight and never from the rear or sloped side. If the aircraft is rear loading, approach cautiously with head down after being signaled by the pilot or crew.

Only transport team members should lock, unlock, or otherwise handle aircraft doors.

Assist the transport team only as requested. Never attempt to contact the pilot by radio during the helicopter's final approach unless an extreme emergency jeopardizes safety.

---

with those that provide service to the ED. A "hot" loading or unloading is one that is performed with rotor blades turning at idle power. Only in extreme circumstances and only by experienced personnel should this procedure be used. Additional guidelines for helicopter landing safety are listed in Box 9-4. This information should be reviewed frequently and be readily available for review when a helicopter transport is expected. Most transport programs are very happy to provide ongoing education to the departments that use them.

Surface Transports

Surface vehicles should be inspected and licensed by their local or state regulatory agencies. The location of the emergency oxygen shutoff valves and fire extinguishers should be known. Restraints should be available for all who ride in a surface vehicle and must be used. Equipment should be secured so that it does not injure transport team members or patients.

A policy for the use of lights and sirens should be in place. Just as with air transport, surface team members must feel comfortable and be supported in refusing a transport that may put themselves and their patients at risk.

Vehicle Accidents

Because many EDs are involved with both surface and air transport programs, they should be aware of the post-accident/incident plan (PAIP) that a program has in place and what role they may play in its implementation. Unfortunately, accidents, injuries, and deaths do occur, and in many areas the ED will be the place where the victims are brought. Some hospitals have specific codes that indicate that an accident may have occurred so that emergency personnel can prepare.

The PAIP should contain notification procedures, resources for staff and family, as well as how to manage the inevitable publicity and community concerns that are a part of any incident. For some EDs, vehicle accidents are incorporated within their disaster plans.

SUMMARY

Air and surface patient transport has improved outcomes for many. Proper stabilization procedures anticipate and plan for potential problems that may be encountered during transport. Employing specialized equipment and personnel trained in transporting patients ensures that the patient is provided with safe and competent care during the transport process.

Sophistication of air and surface transport is limited by the size and weight of most medical equipment. As miniaturization continues and transport equipment becomes lightweight and truly transportable, transporting patients will develop into an even more specialized aspect of nursing.

REFERENCES

1. Air and Surface Transport Nurses Association: *Transport nurse advanced trauma course (TNATC)*, Denver, 2006, The Association.
2. American College of Emergency Physicians: *Appropriate utilization of air medical transport in the out-of-hospital setting*, Dallas, 1999, The College.
3. Brown J, Tompkins K, Chaney E et al: Family member ride-alongs during interfacility transport, *Air Med J* 17(4):169, 1998.
4. Carter G, Couch R, O'Brien M: The evolution of air transport systems, *J Emerg Med* 6(6):499, 1988.
5. Carubba C: Role of the medical director in air medical transport, In Blumen I, Lemkin D, editors: *Principles and directions of air medical transport,* Salt Lake City, 2006, *Air Medical Physicians Association.*
6. Clark D, Stocking J, Johnson J: *Flight and ground transport nursing core curriculum,* Denver, 2006, Air and Surface Transport Nurses Association.
7. Commission on Accreditation of Medical Transport Systems: *Accreditation standards*, ed 7, Andersonville, SC, 2006, The Commission.
8. Donahue P: *Nursing: the finest art*, St. Louis, 1996, Mosby Year Book.
9. Holleran R, Dries D: The care of the family during transport, *Air Med J* 16(2):36, 1997.
10. Macnab A, Gagnon F, George S et al: The cost of family oriented communication before air medical interfacility transport, *Air Med J* 20(4):20, 2001.
11. National Guideline Clearinghouse: *Guidelines for the inter- and intrahospital transport of critically ill patients.* Retrieved September 2, 2007, from http://www.guideline.gov/summary/summary.aspx?ss=15&doc_id4912&nbr=3509.
12. Perez L, Alexander D, Lowell W: Interfacility transport of patients admitted to the ICU: perceived needs of family members, *Air Med J* 22(5):44, 2003.
13. Semonin Holleran R: Challenges in transport nursing, *Aust Emerg Nurs J* 5(1):7, 2002.
14. Svenson J, O'Connor J, Lindsay M: Is air transport faster? A comparison of air versus ground times for interfacility transfer in a regional referral system, *Air Med J* 24(5):170, 2005.
15. Thomson D, Thomas S: Guidelines for air medical dispatch,, *Prehosp Emerg Care* 2:265, 2003.
16. Warren J, Fromm RE, Orr RA et al: Guidelines for the inter-intrahospital transport of critically ill patients, *Crit Care Med* 32(1):256, 2004.
17. Woodward GA: *Guidelines for air and ground transport of neonatal and pediatric patients*, ed 3, Elk Grove, Ill, 2006, American Academy of Pediatrics.

CHAPTER 10

Vascular Access and Fluid Replacement

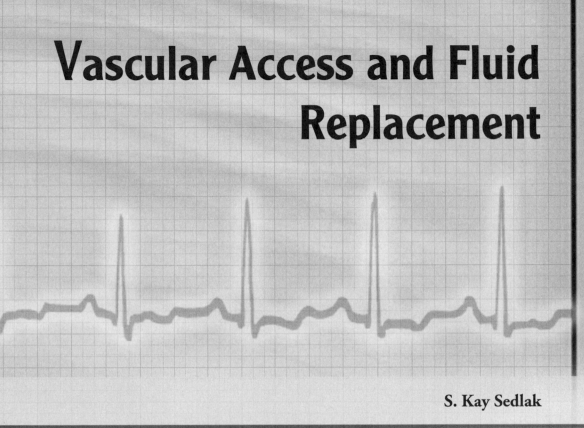

S. Kay Sedlak

Assessment of circulatory status and manipulation of the variables involved is a cornerstone of emergency department (ED) patient management, regardless of the presenting complaint or symptoms. Vascular access may be necessary for medication administration, fluid and electrolyte replacement, or transfusion of blood or blood products. Routine access involves inserting catheters into peripheral veins of hands and arms. Site selection depends on the urgency of the situation, the condition of the patient's veins, and the characteristics of the solution that will be infused into the line. Central veins may be used for invasive hemodynamic monitoring, to infuse certain concentrated solutions, or when peripheral access is not easily accomplished. Needle insertion into bone marrow (intraosseous insertion) is also used for emergency vascular access. Patients may have catheters or implanted ports for long-term therapies.

Fluid replacement is used for patients with subtle and overt volume losses. Solution, rate, and amount are determined by patient condition, underlying pathologic condition, and current fluid imbalance. Maintenance fluids are used for patients with little or no oral intake, whereas aggressive fluid replacement is indicated for patients with significant volume depletion. Patients with hematologic disorders, cancer, or hemorrhage may also require blood or blood product replacement. Vascular access options and various aspects of fluid replacement are described in the following sections.

ANATOMY AND PHYSIOLOGY

Low-pressure vessels located throughout the body receive blood from capillary beds and return it to the heart. Small venules flow into increasingly larger veins, which eventually flow into the inferior and superior vena cava. Vessel diameter varies among patients and with location in the body. Surface vessels in hands and arms are primary peripheral access points; however, vessels in the neck, legs, feet, and head may be used. Valves located within veins prevent backflow; therefore intravenous catheters must be inserted in the same direction as venous flow. Older adult patients lose collagen in vessel walls, which causes significant thinning over time. This may cause vessels to become fragile and "blow" when a catheter is inserted with a tourniquet in place. Vessels may also sclerose and become tortuous with aging.

Peripheral veins of the neck flow into the subclavian vein and can be used for vascular access (Figure 10-1). The external jugular vein is visible in most patients on the lateral aspect of the neck. The internal jugular vein is located beneath and medial to the external jugular. Subclavian veins are used for access to central circulation.

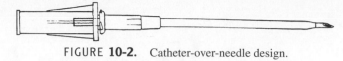

FIGURE **10-2.**   Catheter-over-needle design.

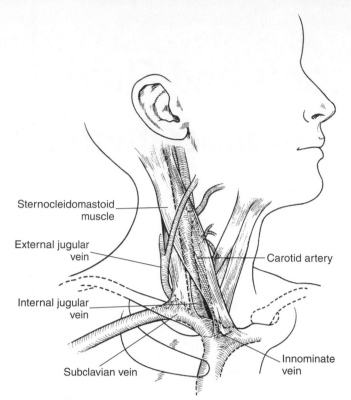

Sternocleidomastoid muscle

External jugular vein

Carotid artery

Internal jugular vein

Subclavian vein

Innominate vein

FIGURE **10-1.**   Veins in the neck. (Modified from Meeker MH, Rothrock JC: *Alexander's care of the patient in surgery,* ed 10, St. Louis, 1995, Mosby.)

VASCULAR ACCESS
Peripheral Venous Access

Inserting peripheral intravenous catheters is a routine skill for emergency nurses. Some agencies also allow nurses to insert central catheters, depending upon training and state regulations. This is not a basic skill for the majority of emergency nurses, however. Nurses assess, use, and maintain established vascular access sites. Catheters are usually inserted into peripheral veins of the hand, arm, or the external jugular veins of the neck. Vessels in the dorsal venous network of the foot and the saphenous vein are rarely used for routine vascular access in adults because of increased incidence of embolism and phlebitis, however, these veins are commonly used in infants.

Vascular access is obtained using aseptic technique. Initial insertion attempts should begin with distal veins and progress up the extremity. Proximal veins are not routinely used unless patients need immediate fluid replacement, such as trauma patients or patients in hypovolemic shock. During cardiac compressions, peripheral veins are used to avoid interruption in compressions, which upper-body central line insertion would require. To minimize the slower delivery of medications via this route, drug doses are followed by a rapid fluid bolus. Proximal peripheral veins are also used for patients receiving drugs that have an extremely short half-life and could become metabolized before reaching their target organ (e.g., adenosine) and for rapid boluses of contrast

media required for specific imaging studies (e.g., spiral chest computed tomography [CT]). Scalp veins have no valves, so fluid can be infused in either direction; they are also easily visualized, making them an ideal alternative in infants.

Insertion of intravenous catheters is not without risk to the patient and the emergency nurse. Potential complications for the patient include infiltration of fluid/medications; phlebitis; embolism of blood, air, or catheter fragments; infection; and cellulitis. Catheters that are inserted under emergent conditions should be assessed to determine if appropriate aseptic technique was used. If it was not, the catheter needs to be replaced as soon as possible. The emergency nurse risks exposure to potentially infectious blood through a needle stick or direct contact with blood or body fluids. Extreme care should be taken to minimize risks through use of standard precautions and appropriate disposal of needles.

Catheter Selection

The size and type of catheter are determined by urgency of need and patient size, age, and vasculature. Blood should flow easily around the catheter after insertion. Larger diameter catheters are used for administering significant volume, colloid solutions, or blood or blood products, whereas smaller diameter catheters are used for routine vascular access. The smallest size and shortest length catheter that will deliver the prescribed therapy should be selected to decrease the potential for developing phlebitis. Catheters that are too large for a vessel can impede flow around the catheter and cause damage to the surrounding vessel wall. Catheters used for peripheral access include a straight catheter-over-needle design (Figure 10-2) and a butterfly or winged catheter (Figure 10-3). Catheters over needles are ideal for aggressive fluid replacement but can present problems with stabilization, particularly in distal veins of the hand. Winged catheters are easily inserted and can be stabilized with minimal effort; however, these catheters are not ideal for rapid fluid replacement. Their availability in smaller sizes increases their usefulness for pediatric and older adult patients. Unfortunately, they may be more uncomfortable than other catheters. Dual-lumen peripheral catheters must be flushed before insertion to activate a hydrolytic lubricant on the outside of the catheter. Intravenous catheters with safety features such as self-capping needles and retracting needles are readily available to decrease the health care worker's potential exposure to bloodborne pathogens.

Insertion

Aseptic technique is essential to protect the patient from infection during intravenous catheter insertion. Gloves should be worn for site preparation and catheter insertion; additional

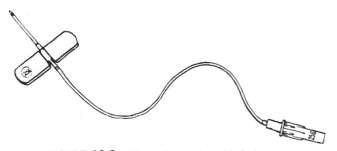

FIGURE **10-3.** Butterfly or winged infusion set.

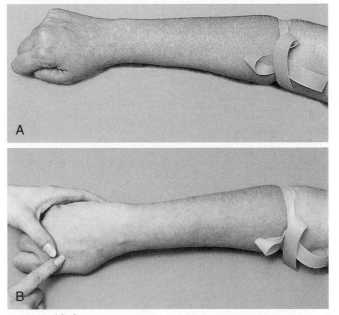

FIGURE **10-4.** **A,** Placement of tourniquet. **B,** Increased vessel size after application of warm towels. (From Potter PA, Perry AG: *Fundamentals of nursing,* ed 5, St. Louis, 2001, Mosby.)

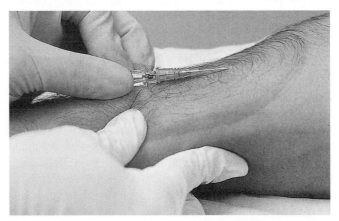

FIGURE **10-5.** Venipuncture. (From Potter PA, Perry AG: *Fundamentals of nursing,* ed 5, St. Louis, 2001, Mosby.).

precautions are required for central line insertion. The selected insertion site should have adequate circulation and be free of infection. Peripheral veins in hands and arms are the first choice for intravenous access. Other sites include veins of the lower extremities or the external jugular veins. The external jugular vein is accessible in most patients but requires turning the patient's neck for access. Lowering the patient's head distends the vein and decreases risk for air embolism during insertion. Use of the external jugular vein is not recommended for patients with suspected neck injury. Use of the internal jugular vein is contraindicated in these patients.

After an extremity site is selected, a tourniquet is placed proximally to distend vessels for easy insertion (Figure 10-4, *A*). Because veins may be more prominent in older adult patients, a tourniquet may not be required. Tourniquets may actually rupture vessels because of increased pressure in fragile veins. Gently tapping or rubbing vessels below the tourniquet increases vessel size by dilation. When vessels are not easily visualized or palpated, applying warm towels over the vein for 5 minutes causes vasodilation and can facilitate catheter insertion (Figure 10-4, *B*).

Skin preparation begins with initial cleansing using a 2% chlorhexidine-based solution.[1] Alcohol or povidone-iodine (Betadine) solution may be substituted if necessary. The solution is applied directly over the insertion site in a back-and-forth motion. Allow the antiseptic solution to air-dry on the selected site before catheter insertion.

Local anesthesia is not routinely used for catheter insertion when time is an issue. However, after site preparation, lidocaine 1% may be injected at the insertion site for immediate anesthetic effect. A topical anesthetic (EMLA, LMX-4) can be applied over the insertion site as an alternative to injection if time allows—depending on the agent used, 30 to 60 minutes is required to achieve an anesthetic effect. Vapocoolant sprays may also be used to decrease the discomfort associated with catheter insertion, depending on institutional protocol.

After the site is prepared, the catheter is inserted by stabilizing the vein to prevent movement during puncture. With the needle bevel up, skin is punctured using the smallest angle possible between skin and needle (Figure 10-5). Veins may be entered on the top or side. The catheter and needle are advanced slowly until blood flashes into the catheter, then the catheter is advanced over the needle into the vein. The tourniquet is removed, and intravenous tubing is

connected. One-way valves are recommended to prevent bleeding from the catheter during subsequent tubing changes. If fluid therapy is not required, catheters may be capped with a one-way valve and sterile cover. The catheter and tubing should be secured with tape according to hospital policy; however, tape should never be applied directly over the insertion site. A sterile, transparent, semipermeable dressing is recommended for application over the insertion site. Sites should be labeled with the date, time, catheter size, and initials of the person inserting the catheter.

Central Venous Access

The subclavian, internal jugular, and cephalic veins are used for short- and long-term vascular access. Short-term central venous access is indicated when peripheral access cannot be

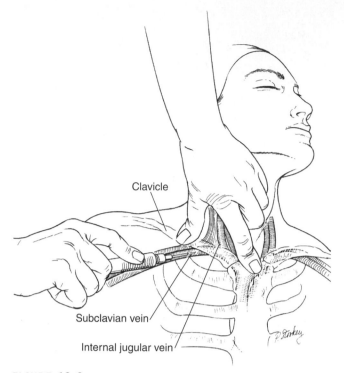

Clavicle

Subclavian vein

Internal jugular vein

FIGURE 10-6. Puncture of subclavian vein with needle inserted beneath middle third of clavicle at a 20- to 30-degree angle aiming medially. (From Daily EK, Schroeder JS: *Techniques in bedside hemodynamic monitoring,* ed 5, St. Louis, 1994, Mosby.)

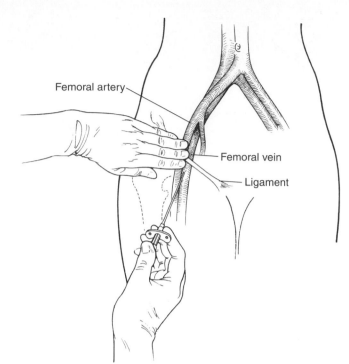

Femoral artery

Femoral vein

Ligament

FIGURE 10-7. Femoral vein. (Modified from Meeker MH, Rothrock JC: *Alexander's care of the patient in surgery,* ed 10, St. Louis, 1995, Mosby.)

obtained or when the patient's condition requires hemodynamic monitoring. Long-term vascular access is indicated for prolonged intravenous therapy, total parenteral nutrition, extended antibiotic therapy, or therapy with caustic drugs such as vancomycin, and in patients with debilitating diseases such as cancer or acquired immune deficiency syndrome. To decrease the patient's risk for developing a catheter-related infection, sterile surgical technique should be employed to insert these devices: the person inserting the line and the nurse assisting should be wearing sterile gloves and gown, mask, and cap with the patient draped from head to toe. In the ED, establishing central venous access is usually an emergent procedure that uses the subclavian or jugular veins. Figure 10-6 illustrates subclavian vein cannulization. Complications related to initial insertion include infection, hematoma, pneumothorax, and air embolism. The femoral vein located medial to the femoral artery may also be used for access to central circulation in some patients (Figure 10-7). The femoral vein is an excellent choice in cardiac arrest because cardiac compressions can continue during insertion. Access via the femoral vein also provides an opportunity for hemodynamic pressure monitoring. Complications associated with femoral vein access include hematoma and infection. Femoral sites should always be considered contaminated and replaced as soon as adequate alternative access can be obtained.

Most central venous access catheters are made of silicone or polyurethane and have a radiopaque strip. Silicone is less thrombogenic than other materials and becomes pliable with

moisture. Disadvantages of silicone include migration of the catheter tip and inability to withdraw blood over time as the catheter softens and collapses inward. Single-lumen and multiple-lumen catheters are available. Awareness of access ports and indications for each lumen is critical for appropriate management. The proximal lumen, which can be used for medication and blood component administration, can also be accessed for blood collection after infusates have been stopped for one full minute.[5] The distal port, which is generally larger, can be used to administer high-volume or viscous fluids, colloids, and medications. Some catheters have additional ports, which should be utilized according to manufacturer recommendations.

Patients may come to the ED with nonemergent, long-term access central lines in place. These include catheters that may be peripherally inserted, tunneled externally, or totally implanted (Table 10-1). Long catheters inserted peripherally in the cephalic or basilic vein can be left in place for 6 to 8 weeks.[2] The safe length of time to leave these catheters in place is steadily increasing. The midline catheter (MLC) ends just inside the subclavian vein, whereas a peripherally inserted central catheter (PICC) extends as far as the superior vena cava (Figure 10-8). Complications include infection and catheter migration. Tunneled external lines (Figure 10-9) and implanted ports (Figure 10-10) are used for long-term access, usually over months or even years. Implanted infusion ports are placed in the subcutaneous tissue, usually below the right clavicle or inner aspect of the upper arm. A catheter is threaded from the port through a large vein and into the superior vena

Table 10-1.   VENOUS ACCESS DEVICES

	Nontunneled	Tunneled	Implanted
Examples	Peripherally inserted central catheters (PICCs) and midline catheters (MLCs)	Hickman; Broviac	Hickman Port; Port-a-Cath; Norport; LifePort
Specific characteristics	Single lumen or multilumen; PICC lines are 60 cm long; MLC lines are 15-20 cm long	Single lumen or multilumen; Dacron cuff where tissue adheres helps ensure placement and decreases infection	Typically implanted in the chest wall; has a self-sealing septum; is accessed through skin with noncoring needle such as Huber needle to prevent damage to septum; special access catheter can be left in place, making repeated sticks unnecessary
Advantages	Does not require surgery for removal; easily removed or replaced	Unlimited use: painless when accessing; easily repaired when damaged; large gauge facilitates blood withdrawal	Less traumatic to body image; less maintenance; decreased chance of infection
Disadvantages	Activity restriction; no sutures so becomes dislodged easily; dressing needed at all times; maintenance costs are high because of frequent heparin flushing and injection cap changes	Mental and physical requirements for managing self-care; high maintenance cost; some patients cannot use this catheter because of body image (tube exiting the body)	High insertion costs; more painful in comparison with tunneled and nontunneled lines

NOTE: New access devices are continuously being developed.

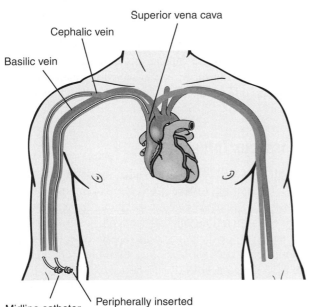

FIGURE **10-8.**   Placement of peripherally inserted central venous catheter and midline catheter. (Modified from Lewis SM, Heitkemper MM, Dirksen SR et al: *Medical-surgical nursing: assessment and management of clinical problems,* ed 7, St. Louis, 2007, Mosby.)

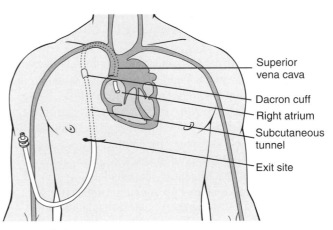

FIGURE **10-9.**   Tunneled catheter with exit in anterior chest wall. (Modified from Lewis SM, Heitkemper MM, Dirksen SR et al: *Medical-surgical nursing: assessment and management of clinical problems,* ed 7, St. Louis, 2007, Mosby.)

cava. Only noncoring (e.g., Huber) needles are used to access the port. These catheters and ports should be flushed after each use with saline and then heparin per hospital protocol.

Groshong catheters are a type of tunneled catheter with a unique slit that remains closed unless blood is withdrawn or

fluid or medications are given. The slit collapses during blood withdrawal but opens during fluid or medication administration. Because of this unique feature, heparin flush is not required for Groshong catheters.[6] The catheter is still flushed with saline solution after each use, however.

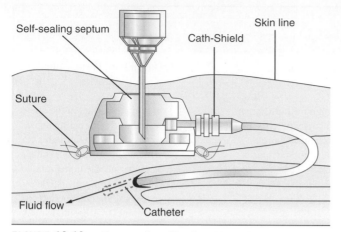

FIGURE 10-10. Cross-section of implantable port displaying access of port with Huber needle. Note deflected point of Huber needle that prevents coring of the port's septum. (Modified from Lewis SM, Heitkemper MM, Dirksen SR et al: *Medical-surgical nursing: assessment and management of clinical problems,* ed 7, St. Louis, 2007, Mosby.)

BOX 10-1   GUIDELINES FOR VENOUS ACCESS DEVICES

- Wear mask and gloves when accessing central access devices.
- Check insertion site for infection.
- Use infusion pump to infuse fluids through central lines.
- Use injection caps for all ports.
- Clamp lines if cap is removed (except for Groshong catheters).
- Clamps with teeth can damage the catheter.
- Phenytoin and diazepam precipitate in response to silicone and can cause the catheter to clot.
- Forceful irrigation may rupture the catheter because of increased pressure.
- Insert a noncoring needle into an implanted port until the posterior wall is felt.
- Use noncoring needles to prevent damage to septum of the port.

Venous access devices should be used according to manufacturer recommendations whenever these lines are available and patent. Many of these devices can be used for blood collection, as well as fluid replacement. Aseptic technique, masks, and gloves are essential when accessing central catheters to minimize risk for infection. Introduction of contaminants into the central circulation represents significant risk for patients with central venous access devices. Box 10-1 lists general guidelines for their use. Central venous catheters must be flushed appropriately after use to ensure patency. Inadequate flushing jeopardizes patency and leads to painful device replacement. The mnemonic SASH can be used to remember appropriate flushing order:

Saline—initial flush with saline

Administer—administer fluids, medication, or blood product as indicated

Saline—flush with saline to clear above contents from line

Heparin—deliver recommended concentration and amount of heparin to maintain line patency

Table 10-2 describes flushing guidelines for various central venous access devices. Manufacturer recommendations should always be consulted for appropriate volumes and concentrations of flush solutions for a specific catheter.

Problems related to central lines include venous occlusion from a lodged catheter tip, mural thrombus (found on or against the wall of the vessel), and fibrin sleeve formation. Symptoms of occlusion include pain in the insertion area or path of the catheter, facial edema, or edema at the insertion site. Superficial veins may become more pronounced as vascular workload increases around the occluded vessel. The catheter tip can also migrate or become lodged against the endocardium or vessel wall. This problem is usually identified when blood cannot be withdrawn or when the external marker is not in the appropriate location. Turning the patient to the side, raising the arm, or asking the patient to cough may help move the catheter back into proper position.

A fibrin sleeve can develop on the tip of the catheter and prevent blood withdrawal. The fibrin sleeve is confirmed with a chest radiograph. Treatment includes fibrinolytic administration with tissue plasminogen activator, also known as tPA, alteplase, or Cathflo Activase. Other conditions such as mechanical failure and deposits of lipids or medication precipitates can also cause catheter malfunction and should be ruled out before considering this therapy.[6] Specific protocols, including drug dose and catheter dwell times, are described in the drug package insert and hospital protocols.

Irritation of the intimal lining of the vessel wall by medications, friction from the catheter tip, or bacteria can lead to a mural thrombus in the vessel in which the catheter is inserted. When this occurs, blood cannot be withdrawn from the device.

Intraosseous Infusion

This method is used for rapid vascular access in both adults and children. An intraosseous needle, bone marrow aspiration needle, or spinal needle is inserted into the marrow cavity of the anterior tibia, medial malleolus, sternum, distal femur, humerus, or iliac crest. An 18-gauge needle is used for infants less than 3 months of age. For older children and adults a 15-gauge needle should be used. There is at least one device on the market for adult use that instills fluids into the sternum; however, its use is currently not widespread. Immediately after insertion, marrow may be withdrawn and used for some diagnostic studies. Fluids, blood and blood products, and medications can be safely infused into the intraosseous site. Manual pressure or an infusion device may be necessary for rapid fluid administration. The tibia is the preferred insertion site in children; the thin sternum should not be used. Figure 10-11 shows preferred sites. A needle should not be inserted through infected or burned tissue. Intraosseous infusion is contraindicated in a fractured extremity, cellulitis, and osteoporosis.[4] Complications related

Table 10-2. **FLUSHING GUIDELINES FOR VENOUS ACCESS DEVICES**

Flushing Type	Tunneled/Nontunneled Device	Groshong Catheter	Implanted Ports	PICC
General flushing	Heparin 10-100 units/mL; use 2.5-5 mL after use and/or every 12-24 hr	No heparin; 5 mL of saline after use or once per week	Flush one time per month (if not in use) with 500 units heparin (5 mL); use same amount each time	Heparin 10-100 units/mL; use 1-2.5 mL after use and/or once every 12 hr or according to manufacturer recommendations
After blood withdrawal	Stop infusion for 1 min before blood draw; withdraw and discard 10 mL of blood; draw blood for laboratory tests with syringe; flush with 5 mL saline before heparinizing as above	20 mL saline	Use 10 mL saline to flush port, followed by heparin	Flush with saline before heparin flush
Before medication administration	Flush with 5 mL saline before medication administration	5 mL saline	5 mL saline	
After medication administration	Flush with 5 mL saline before heparinizing	5 mL saline	10 mL saline followed by heparin	Flush with saline before heparin flush

PICC, Peripherally inserted central catheter.

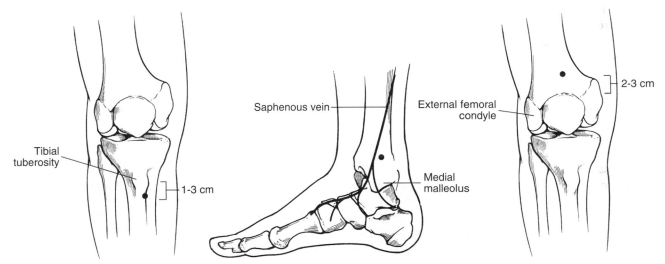

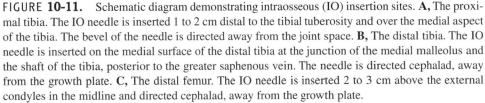

FIGURE **10-11.**   Schematic diagram demonstrating intraosseous (IO) insertion sites. **A,** The proximal tibia. The IO needle is inserted 1 to 2 cm distal to the tibial tuberosity and over the medial aspect of the tibia. The bevel of the needle is directed away from the joint space. **B,** The distal tibia. The IO needle is inserted on the medial surface of the distal tibia at the junction of the medial malleolus and the shaft of the tibia, posterior to the greater saphenous vein. The needle is directed cephalad, away from the growth plate. **C,** The distal femur. The IO needle is inserted 2 to 3 cm above the external condyles in the midline and directed cephalad, away from the growth plate.

to this technique include air or fat emboli, bone fracture, osteomyelitis, compartment syndrome, and subcutaneous abscess. Epiphyseal damage can occur in children. Alternative vascular access should be obtained as rapidly as possible, because it is undesirable to continue use of an intraosseous site for longer than 4 hours.

FLUID REPLACEMENT

Intravenous fluids may be given to maintain fluid requirements or in an effort to replace fluid losses. Normal metabolic processes in the body and insensible fluid losses through the skin and respiratory tract account for more than

1500 mL/day of fluid loss for the average adult. Calculation of basal fluid needs is based on patient size, calculated as body surface area. Box 10-2 provides formulas for maintenance fluids and for volume replacement. Isotonic, hypotonic, and hypertonic fluids may be used as maintenance fluids. Isotonic fluids are similar in composition to body fluids and provide greater intravascular volume because more fluid remains in the vascular space. Hypotonic fluids shift fluid into intracellular spaces and are more useful for preventing cellular dehydration. They deplete circulatory volume, and blood pressure may drop with their administration. Hypertonic fluids move fluid from cells to the extravascular space and may be used to replace electrolytes and promote diuresis. Table 10-3 gives examples and describes use of these maintenance fluids.

Crystalloid and colloid solutions are used for volume replacement. Crystalloid solutions increase intravascular volume through actual volume administered, whereas colloids pull fluid into the vascular space through osmosis. Synthetic and natural colloid solutions are available. Examples of crystalloid and colloid solutions and actions for each are presented in Table 10-4.

Blood and Blood Products

These naturally occurring colloid solutions are used to replace blood losses and replenish clotting factors. Blood loss depletes the body of blood cells and clotting factors, so whole blood replacement is ideal in frank blood loss. However, whole blood is expensive, not readily available, and has greater risk for transmission of infectious diseases. Blood may be separated, and only those components that are needed are administered. This preserves valuable components for other potential patients. Packed red blood cells (RBCs) are used most often for blood replacement. Other blood products used for component replacement include platelets, fresh frozen plasma, and albumin. Table 10-5 summarizes administration of these and other blood products in adults. Blood products are always administered using normal saline. A blood warmer is recommended for large-volume blood transfusions.

Before blood administration, a blood sample should be obtained for type and crossmatch. Two specimens should be obtained if large-volume replacement is anticipated. Ideally, complete type and crossmatch should be done on all blood before administration; however, this procedure can take 40 minutes or more. Additional time may be required if antibodies are found. Table 10-6 summarizes compatible types of plasma and RBCs for different donor types. Type-specific

blood or blood that is not completely crossmatched may be given to patients with critical blood loss. The physician must

---

Box 10-2	**FORMULAS FOR FLUID ADMINISTRATION**

BASAL FLUID MAINTENANCE

1500 mL/m^2 BSA/24 hr = 62.5mL/m^2 BSA/hr

General Guidelines

- Up to 10 kg = 4 mL/kg/hr
- 11-20 kg = 2 mL/kg/hr *plus* 4 mL/kg for first 10 kg
- >20 kg = 1 mL/kg/hr *plus* 2 mL/kg for each kg 11 through 20 *plus* 4 mL/kg for first 10 kg

VOLUME REPLACEMENT WITH CRYSTALLOIDS

Administer 3 mL for each mL lost. Fluid challenges/options are:

- IV bolus 20 mL/kg NS or LR in children
- IV bolus of 200-300 mL LR in adult surgical patients
- IV bolus of 200-300 mL NS in adult medical patients

VOLUME REPLACEMENT WITH COLLOIDS

Administer 1 mL for each mL lost

VOLUME REPLACEMENT FOR MEASURED LOSSES

- Gastric losses: Replace 1 mL for each mL lost every 4 hr. Use D5% 0.45% NS plus 30 mEq KCl
- Intestinal losses: Replace 1 mL for each mL lost every 4 hr. Use D5% LR
- Basal urine output
  - Newborn and infant up to 1 year: normal is 2 mL/kg/hr
  - Toddler: 1.5 mL/kg/hr
  - Older child: 1 mL/kg/hr during adolescence
  - Adult: 0.5 mL/kg/hr

Modified from Kidd PS, Sturt P, Fultz J: *Mosby's emergency nursing reference,* ed 2, St. Louis, 2000, Mosby.
BSA, Body surface area; *LR,* lactated Ringer's solution; *NS,* normal saline.

Table 10-3.	**MAINTENANCE IV FLUIDS**	
Solution Type	**Examples**	**Uses**
Isotonic	0.9% Normal saline (NS)	Expands intravascular volume. Used for dehydration (e.g., diabetic ketoacidosis, hyperosmolar nonketotic coma) and packed red blood cell administration.
	Lactated Ringer's solution	Expands intravascular volume. Used for maintenance fluid when patient is at risk for free water loss.
Hypotonic	NS 0.45%	Shifts water into intracellular spaces.
	NS 0.2%	Useful in preventing dehydration and assessing renal status.
	Dextrose 5% in water (D$_5$W)	D$_5$W may be used in adult patients for mixing some intravenous medications. Used for maintenance fluid when patient is at risk for free water loss.
Hypertonic	Dextrose 5% in NS	Shifts fluid from intracellular to extracellular space.
	Dextrose 10% in NS	Used in water intoxication states created by too much hypotonic fluid administration.
	Dextrose 10% in water	Used for maintenance fluid to promote diuresis.
	Dextrose 5% in 0.45 NS	
	Dextrose 20% in water	

Modified from Kidd PS, Sturt P, Fultz J: *Mosby's emergency nursing reference,* ed 2, St. Louis, 2000, Mosby.

Table 10-4. FLUID RESUSCITATION SUMMARY*

Crystalloids	Description/Indication	Action(s)
0.9% Normal saline†	Isotonic	• May produce fluid overload, hypernatremia, and hyperchloremia • 25% of volume administered remains in vascular space
0.45% Normal saline	Hypotonic, moves fluid from vascular space to interstitial and intracellular spaces	• Decreases blood viscosity • May promote hypovolemia • May promote cerebral edema
5% Dextrose	Hypotonic	• 7.5 mL /100 mL infused remains in vascular space • Inadequate for fluid resuscitation
Lactated Ringer's solution	Isotonic, contains multiple electrolytes and lactate	• May produce fluid overload • May promote lactic acidosis in prolonged hypoperfusion with decreased liver function • Lactate metabolizes to acetate, may produce metabolic alkalosis when large volumes are transfused
Hypertonic saline (7.5%)	Hypertonic, pulls fluid from interstitial and intracellular spaces into vascular space	• Requires smaller amount to restore blood volume • Increases cerebral oxygen drive while decreasing ICP • May promote hypernatremia • May promote intracellular dehydration • May promote osmotic diuresis • Controversial

Synthetic Colloids	Description	Action(s)
Dextran‡	(Comes in 40, 70, and 75 molecular weight)	• Associated with anaphylaxis • Reduces factor VIII, platelets, and fibrinogen function, so increases bleeding time • May interfere with blood type and crossmatch, glucose, and erythrocyte sedimentation level • Risk for fluid overload
Hetastarch‡		• May increase serum amylase levels • Associated with coagulopathy • Risk of fluid overload

Natural Colloids	Description	Action(s)
Fresh frozen plasma	Contains all clotting factors	• Potential to transmit bloodborne infection • Can cause hypersensitivity reaction • Blood volume expander
Plasma protein fraction (Plasmanate)	Does not contain clotting factors	• May cause hypersensitivity reaction • May cause hypotension with rapid infusion • Blood volume expander
Albumin‡	5% isooncotic 25% hyperoncotic "salt poor"	• Preferred as volume expander when risk from producing interstitial edema is great (e.g., pulmonary and heart disease) • Hypocalcemia
Whole blood	Can be administered without normal saline; reduces donor exposure	• Hyperkalemia, hypothermia, and hypocalcemia • May require greater amount than packed RBCs to increase oxygen-carrying capacity of blood • Rarely used, not cost-effective
Packed RBCs	Administer with normal saline	• Deficient in 2,3-diphosphoglycerate and may increase oxygen affinity for hemoglobin and decrease oxygen delivery to tissue • Hypothermia, hyperkalemia, and hypocalcemia

Experimental Agents	Description	Action(s)
Liposome encapsulated hemoglobin hypertonic saline (7.5%)	NOT APPROVED BY FDA	• Improves skeletal muscle oxygen tension • Expands vascular volume quickly • Improves tissue oxygenation
Hypertonic saline (7.5%) with dextran 70	Combined crystalloid and colloid therapy	• Promotes rapid expansion of blood volume and promotes retention of volume in vascular space • Controversial

Modified from Kidd PS, Sturt P, Fultz J: *Mosby's emergency nursing reference*, ed 2, St. Louis, 2000, Mosby.

FDA, Food and Drug Administration; *ICP*, intracranial pressure; *RBCs,* red blood cells.

*Dosages are not listed because of variability in patient response and need.

†Fluid overload using these agents may occur because of large amount required (3:1 ratio fluid to volume lost).

‡Fluid overload using these agents may occur in cases of preexisting pulmonary and/or heart disease.

Table 10-5. BLOOD COMPONENT ADMINISTRATION IN ADULTS

Blood Component	Uses	Blood Type	Infusion Rate	Filter	Volume	Comments
Whole blood	Acute or chronic anemia, aplastic anemia, bone marrow failure, heart failure, chronic renal failure, hepatic coma	Must be ABO compatible	2-4 hr; max: 4 hr	Required	500 mL	Rapid infusion if need is urgent. Clotting factors deteriorate after 24 hr.
Packed RBCs	Acute massive blood loss, hypovolemic shock	Must be ABO compatible	2-4 hr; max: 4 hr	Required	250 mL (may be variable)	Hgb rises 1 g/dL; Hct rises 3% after 1 unit.
Leukocyte-poor RBCs	Thrombocytopenia, platelet function abnormality	Need not be ABO compatible	2 hr	Required	Variable	
Fresh frozen plasma	Hypovolemia combined with hemorrhage caused by deficiencies	Must be ABO compatible	1-2 hr, rapidly if bleeding	Use component filter	250 mL	Notify blood bank—plasma takes 20 min to thaw; use within 6 hr of thawing. Do not use microaggregate filter.
Platelets	Hemophilia, von Willebrand's disease, hypofibrinogenemia, factor XIII deficiency	Need not be ABO compatible	Rapidly as patient tolerates	Use component filter	35-50 mL units	Usually 6-10 units are ordered. Request that blood bank pool all units. Do not use microaggregate filter.
Albumin	Shock caused by burns; maintains blood volume in patients with hypovolemia; hypoproteinemia	Need not be ABO compatible	1-2 mL/min in normovolemic patients	Special tubing	Varies	Comes in 5% and 25%; can increase intravascular volume quickly; infuse cautiously.
Cryoprecipitate	Repeated febrile reaction; reaction from leukocyte antibodies and patients who are candidates for organ transplants	Must be ABO compatible	30 min	Use component filter	10 mL units	Usually 6-10 units ordered; request that blood bank pool units. Unstable to heat and storage.
Granulocytes			2-4 hr	Use component filter	300-400 mL	VS every 15 min during infusion. Granulocytes have a short life span. Transfuse as soon after collection as possible.

Hct, Hematocrit; *Hgb,* hemoglobin; *RBCs,* red blood cells; *VS,* vital signs.

Table 10-6. BLOOD TYPE IDENTIFICATION

Patient	Compatible Transfusion
Type A	A or AB plasma
	A or O RBCs
Type B	B or AB plasma
	B or O RBCs
Type AB	AB plasma
	A, B, AB, or O RBCs
Type O	A, B, AB, or O plasma
	O RBCs
Rh−	Must receive Rh− blood
Rh+	Can receive Rh− or Rh+ blood
O−	Universal donor for RBCs
AB+	Universal donor for plasma

Modified from Elkin MK, Perry AG, Potter PA: *Nursing interventions and clinical skills,* ed 3, St. Louis, 2004, Mosby.
RBCs, Red blood cells.

acknowledge responsibility for potential adverse effects. Type O blood may be given for patients with extreme blood loss who cannot wait for type-specific blood. Type O-negative blood is given to females, and type O-positive blood is given to males. However, many facilities give type O-negative blood to both females and males.

Blood administration is not without risk. Blood processing procedures have reduced risk for transmission of infectious diseases; however, transfusion reactions can occur because of transfusion of incompatible blood, patient allergy, or depletion of clotting factors (Table 10-7). Unrecognized transfusion reactions represent a significant threat to the patient's life. Before transfusion, blood and patient identification should be checked carefully according to institutional policies. During the transfusion, the patient should be carefully monitored for signs of reaction, including fever, chills, urticaria, breathing difficulty, back pain, and hematuria.

Table 10-7. TRANSFUSION REACTIONS

Reaction	Cause	Prevention	Assessment	Intervention
Hemolytic	Blood incompatibility	Type and crossmatch; infuse first 50 mL slowly	Fever, chills, dyspnea, tachypnea, lumbar pain, fever, oliguria, hematuria, tightness in chest; collect blood and urine samples	Discontinue immediately; fatality may occur after 100 mL infused Start NS or LR Consider diuretics; monitor BUN, serum creatinine
Allergic	Antibody reaction to allergens	Screen donors for allergy; administer antihistamines before transfusion	Hypersensitivity, chills, hives, wheezing, vertigo, angioneurotic edema, allergic itching Anaphylaxis, dyspnea, bronchospasm, hypotension, decreased responsiveness, generalized edema	Stop infusion; give antihistamine, steroids, and antipyretics Stop infusion; give epinephrine, start NS; administer LR; anticipate intubation
Pyrogenic	Recipient antibodies to donor leukocytes; bacterial contamination; inflammatory cytokine release.	Screen donors; use aseptic technique in administration, use leukocyte-poor products for high-risk recipients	Fever, chills, nausea, lumbar pain	Stop infusion
Hypothermic	Infusing chilled blood	Give at room temperature; use warming coils for rapid infusion	Chills	Slow infusion; cover patient
Circulatory overload	Infusion of large amounts of blood, especially to patients with cardiac disease or extremes of age	Infuse slowly; check drip rate frequently	Pulmonary crackles, cough, dyspnea, cyanosis, pulmonary edema, increased CVP	Stop infusion; treat pulmonary edema
Air embolism	Entry of air into vein	Use proper infusion technique; avoid giving under pressure; check connections to tubings; avoid Y-tubes; use filter; use plastic containers	Chest pain, dyspnea, hypotension, venous distension	Stop infusion; position on left side; give oxygen; embolectomy may be performed
Hypocalcemic	Precipitate from acid citrate dextrose Calcium dilution with massive transfusions	Use blood immediately	Numbness, tingling in extremities May contribute to development of diffuse intravascular coagulation	Stop infusion; give calcium as ordered
Hyperkalemic	Hemolysis of red blood cells releases potassium	Use blood immediately	Nausea, vomiting, muscle weakness, bradycardia	Stop infusion

Modified from Barber J, Stokes L, Billings D: *Adult and child care: a client approach to nursing*, ed 2, St. Louis, 1977, Mosby.
BUN, Blood urea nitrogen; *CVP*, central venous pressure; *LR*, lactated Ringer's soulution; *NS*, normal saline.

Intravenous medications cannot be added to a blood transfusion. If the ordered medications cannot be delayed for the duration of the transfusion, an additional access site is required.

SUMMARY

Vascular access provides a route for administration of medications, fluids, blood, and blood products. This access and fluid replacement often saves the patient's life.

Unfortunately, it can also create significant threats to health if vigilance is not used with catheter insertion and fluid administration. Consistent use of standard precautions, sharps disposal, and aseptic technique protects the patient and the emergency nurse. Assessment and reassessment during fluid replacement can identify symptoms related to fluid overload, anaphylaxis, and other side effects.

REFERENCES

1. Centers for Disease Control and Prevention: *Guidelines for the prevention of intravascular catheter-related infections,* 2002, http://www.cdc.gov/mmwr/PDF/rr/rr5110.pdf
2. deWit SC: *Fundamental concepts and skills for nursing,* ed 2, Philadelphia, 2005, Elsevier.
3. Elkin MK, Perry AG, Potter PA: *Nursing interventions and clinical skills,* ed 3, St. Louis, 2004, Mosby.
4. Emergency Nurses Association: *ENPC provider manual,* ed 3, Des Plaines, Ill, 2004, The Association.
5. Josephson DL: *Intravenous infusion therapy for nurses: principles and practice,* ed 2, Clifton Park NY, 2004, Delmar Learning.
6. Proehl JA: *Emergency nursing procedures,* ed 3, St. Louis, 2004, Saunders.

CHAPTER 11

Wound Management

Nancy J. Denke

A wound is a disruption of the normal anatomic integrity and function of any tissue. It is a term usually applied to skin injuries resulting from the transfer of external mechanical forces. The goal of emergent wound management is to restore tissue integrity by wound closure and to restore function to damaged tissue. In the emergency department (ED), nurses encounter many simple and straightforward wounds; other wounds are complex and can greatly alter the appearance and function for those injured individuals. Unless life-threatening bleeding or neurovascular compromise is present, patients with skin wounds (surface trauma) are not a triage priority. Wound management in the ED includes careful assessment, cleansing, wound closure, and discharge care. Basic principles of wound care are promotion of optimal healing, prevention of infection, and reduction of scar formation.

ANATOMY AND PHYSIOLOGY

Skin is the largest organ of the body, receiving approximately one third of the circulating blood volume. It is one of the fastest-growing tissues, regenerating every 4 to 6 weeks[4] and plays an important role in homeostatic regulation of the body.[5] Skin is composed of three layers: epidermis, dermis, and subcutaneous tissue (Figure 11-1). The epidermis, or outer layer, provides protection against chemicals and microorganisms and generates cells that promote wound healing.

The epidermis is avascular and receives nutrients from underlying blood vessels in the dermis and subcutaneous tissues.[16] Thickness of the epidermis varies with location; it is significantly greater in the soles of the feet and palms of the hand than in the eyelids. Thickening of the epidermal layers (calluses) is caused by repeated pressure or friction, such as that seen with poorly fitted shoes, repetitive actions such as plucking guitar strings, or manual labor such as raking the yard.

The dermis lies below the epidermis and is composed of collagen and elastin fibers and provides strength, elasticity, and protection against external forces.[4] It is the thickest layer of the skin. The connective tissue of the dermis has a rich vascular supply, along with lymphatic vessels, nerves, and thermoreceptors. Collagen found in the dermis provides tensile strength, whereas elastin allows skin to resist deformation. Collagen is produced by fibroblasts, which become active during inflammatory conditions and wounding.[5] Sensory receptors for pain, touch, pressure, heat, and cold are also found in the dermis, whereas hair follicles and sweat glands are found between the epidermal and dermal layers of the skin.

The subcutaneous layer lies below the dermis and above the muscle tissue, providing body contour. It stores fat below the dermis and provides insulation against heat loss. In addition, the subcutaneous tissue provides protection against injury and acts as an energy storage site. Hypoperfusion of

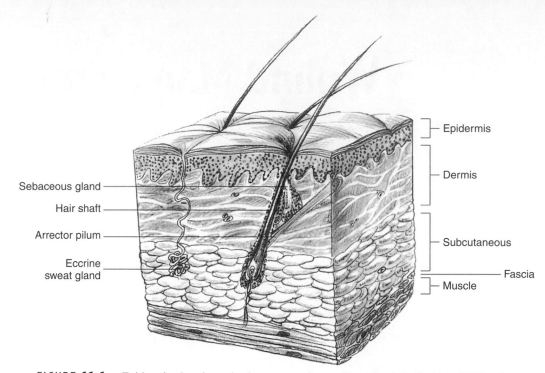

FIGURE 11-1.   Epidermis, dermis, and subcutaneous tissue. (From Davis P, Sheldon GF, Drucker WR I: *Surgery: a problem solving approach,* ed 2, St. Louis, 1995, Mosby.)

subcutaneous tissue negatively affects wound healing. Complications of impaired healing, such as infections, often have their origin in the subcutaneous tissue.[5]

Skin regulates body temperature through sweating and evaporation. Insensible fluid loss through the skin and lungs accounts for 450 to 600 mL/day or 12 to 16 calories/hr of heat loss.[7] Skin provides innate immunity because mast cells and Langerhans cells (macrophages) in the skin respond to antigens and pathogens. The normal skin flora (i.e., coagulase-positive and coagulase-negative staphylococci, streptococci, and diphtheroids) confer a line of defense against other microbes in the environment.

WOUND HEALING

Normal wound healing occurs in three overlapping phases: the inflammatory, proliferative, and remodeling (or maturation) phases. Each phase is sequential, creating the pathway for the next phase to occur.

Inflammatory Phase

The initial, or inflammatory, phase is a protective mechanism that begins immediately with tissue injury and lasts 3 to 5 days. The inflammatory phase begins with the coagulation cascade, platelets adhering to injured vessels to form a clot. It is a complex series of events consisting of cellular and histologic reactions in the affected blood vessels and adjacent tissues.[4] Macrophages (which produce growth factors and cytokines) are attracted to the area, and bacteria and debris are phagocytized and then removed as the body attempts to

repair itself. Beneath the clot a network of fibrinogen strands form to unite wound edges. Prostaglandins cause vasodilation, leading to increased capillary permeability, which allows plasma to leak into tissue surrounding the wound, forming "inflammatory exudates."[15] Scab formation begins within 2 hours to minimize fluid loss and prevent bacterial invasion.

Proliferative Phase

The proliferative phase can begin as early as 12 to 72 hours after injury and usually ends approximately 3 weeks later.[4] After scab formation begins, inflammatory processes begin, and the wound becomes painful and edematous. Vasodilation in injured tissues leads to protein leakage and antibody release, which creates a medium for white blood cells arriving at the site 6 hours after injury. White blood cells attack bacteria through phagocytosis by using neutrophils to surround and engulf bacteria, providing short-term defense against infection; monocytes provide long-term defense against infection. Macrophages recruit fibroblasts and create a network of collagen fibers, which in the presence of vitamin C and adequate oxygenation begin the granulation of tissue.[15]

During granulation, fibroblast activity peaks, forming new capillary beds, meshing with damaged tissue, and providing oxygen and proteins for tissue growth. During fibroblast activity, collagen is produced for dermal scar tissue. This scar tissue is initially translucent, grayish red, moist, and friable, leading it to bleed easily and become damaged with minimal force. Wound contraction begins following fibroblast formation, angiogenesis, and collagen synthesis and is stimulated

Table 11-1. FACTORS DELAYING WOUND HEALING

Factor	Effects on Wound Healing
Nutritional deficiencies	
Protein	Decreases supply of amino acids for tissue repair
Vitamin C	Delays formation of collagen fibers and capillary development
Zinc	Impairs epithelialization
Inadequate blood supply	Decreases supply of nutrients to injured area, decreases removal of exudative debris, inhibits inflammatory response
Corticosteroid drugs	Impair phagocytosis by WBCs, inhibit fibroblast proliferation and function, depress formation of granulation tissue, inhibit wound contraction
Infection	Increases inflammatory response and tissue destruction
Mechanical friction on wound	Destroys granulation tissue, prevents apposition of wound edges
Advanced age	Slows collagen synthesis by fibroblasts, impairs circulation, requires longer time for epithelialization of skin, alters phagocytic and immune responses
Obesity	Decreases blood supply in fatty tissue
Diabetes mellitus	Decreases collagen synthesis, retards early capillary growth, impairs phagocytosis (result of hyperglycemia)
Poor general health	Causes generalized absence of factors necessary to promote wound healing
Anemia	Supplies less oxygen at tissue level

From Lewis SM, Heitkemper MM, Dirksen SR et al: *Medical-surgical nursing: assessment and management of clinical problems,* ed 7, St. Louis, 2007, Mosby. *WBCs,* White blood cells.

by platelet growth factors, prostaglandins, bradykinins, and angiotensin. During contraction, myofibroblasts (fibroblast cells that attach to collagen fibers) pull wound edges closer together and decrease the size of the wound. This wound contraction and remodeling can continue for 6 to 18 months after injury.[5]

Remodeling Phase

This third and final phase of wound healing begins about 2 to 3 weeks after injury and can last up to 2 years.[4] Initially collagen fibers develop randomly. However, within 2 weeks these fibers reorganize into thick fibers along stress lines and increase in strength over weeks or months. At 2 weeks approximately 10% to 20% of the tensile strength has returned, whereas at 10 weeks approximately 80% of the preinjury tensile strength has returned.[14] Heredity, stress, and movement of the affected area determine the amount of scarring. Healing, with increasing collagen density and nerve regeneration, may actually take years.

Factors Affecting Wound Healing

Wound healing is significantly affected by preexisting conditions such as arterial/venous insufficiency, lymphedema, morbid obesity, neuropathy, neoplasms, sickle cell disease, infection, diabetes, and malnutrition.[9] Table 11-1 describes the effects of preexisting factors on wound healing. Another variable that may affect wound healing is the environment of the patient at the time of the injury. Bacterial contamination on the patient can increase the risk for infection, with wounds of the mouth, perineum, and web spaces of the feet hosting the highest concentration of resident flora.[14]

WOUND EVALUATION

Initial assessment of wounds follows assessment and stabilization of the airway, breathing, and circulation. Mechanisms of injury can provide clues to severity of injury. Wounds caused by small objects may be superficial, whereas crush injuries by a large dog's bite can cause significant deep tissue damage. Appearance of the wound provides clues to the difficulty of wound closure. Jagged edges require more skill to close and may not heal as well. The time elapsed since injury is critical because delayed care increases the risk for complications such as infection. Special closure techniques are required for wounds more than 12 hours old.

Patient age, physical condition, current health status, and occupation also affect wound healing. Medical conditions such as diabetes mellitus, secondary peripheral neuropathy, morbid obesity, malnutrition, or use of medications such as corticosteroids can delay wound healing. Aspirin and nonsteroidal antiinflammatory drugs affect coagulation and healing. Patient occupation may influence long-term wound management and compliance with wound care. Social factors should not be overlooked. Patients who smoke often exhibit a delayed wound healing process, thus increasing their risk for infection. Allergy history and immunization status should also be evaluated during initial assessment.

The patient should be assessed for associated injuries such as fractures, dislocations, or neurovascular compromise. Tendon or ligament injuries, presence of a foreign body, and peripheral nerve damage should also be considered and managed appropriately. Wounds that are heavily contaminated at the time of wounding are at an extreme risk for becoming infected. Farming-related accidents and human bites are representative of wounds that are usually heavily contaminated at the time of injury.[14]

SPECIFIC WOUNDS

Wounds are categorized into six basic types: abrasions, abscesses, avulsions, lacerations, puncture wounds, and bites. Their severity varies with the cause of injury and amount of tissue damaged. Wounds may be a minor inconvenience that do not alter lifestyle or affect work requirements. More severe wounds may cause significant discomfort and affect self-care, self-image, and work. In some cases, lifestyle is permanently altered. Prevention of a chronic wound caused by a treatable acute injury is always a major concern.

Abrasions

Abrasions occur when skin is rubbed or scraped against a hard surface. Friction removes the epithelial layer and can also remove part of the epidermis so deeper layers are exposed. Examples of abrasions are floor burns, carpet burns, road rash, or brush burns (Figure 11-2). Abrasions have the same physiologic effect as a partial-thickness burn; thus a significant risk for infection exists from loss of skin and its protective properties. Fluid loss also occurs with loss of surface area.

Foreign bodies left in the skin stain the epidermis and cause permanent scars or a "tattoo." Cleansing is critical in management of abrasions to prevent this complication. Local anesthesia by topical application or infiltration should be used for abrasions with heavy contamination. Topical antibiotic ointment and nonadherent dressings are used; however, abrasions may occasionally be left open to air. Dressings should be changed daily until eschar forms. Clothing or sunblock should be used for 6 months to prevent discoloration of fragile new tissue.

Abscesses

Localized collection of pus beneath the skin causes an abscess. Pus may eventually erupt; however, wound management does not include waiting for this to occur. The wound is cleaned, infiltrated with local anesthetic, and drained. An elliptical area of tissue may be removed to facilitate drainage, and then the wound is packed loosely with iodoform or similar material and covered with loose dressing. Antibiotics are indicated when the patient has a fever or when there is reoccurrence of abscess formation. Follow-up with a health care provider is imperative to closely monitor the patient and wound healing.

Avulsions

An avulsion is full-thickness skin loss in which approximation of wound edges is not possible. A degloving injury is a severe avulsion injury in which skin is peeled away from the hand, foot, or a greater portion of an extremity. Figure 11-3 shows a degloving injury of the scalp. Degloving injuries of the fingers are more common and involve injury to tendons and ligaments. Management includes local anesthesia by injection or topical application followed by irrigation and debridement of devitalized tissue. A split-thickness skin graft is often necessary with large avulsions. The wound should be covered with a bulky dressing to protect exposed tissue.

Contusions

Blunt trauma that does not alter skin integrity causes a contusion or bruise. Swelling, pain, and discoloration occur with extravasation of blood into damaged tissues. After assessment of neurovascular status, therapeutic interventions include cold packs and analgesia as necessary. Large wounds or those located in an extremity should be carefully observed for cellulitis or development of compartment syndrome.

Lacerations

Lacerations are open wounds caused by shearing forces through dermal layers. Superficial lacerations (Figure 11-4) involve the epidermis and dermis, whereas more severe injuries involve deeper layers, including subcutaneous tissue and

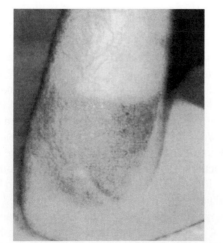

FIGURE 11-2. Abrasion. (From McSwain NE Jr, Paturas JL: *The basic EMT: comprehensive prehospital patient care*, ed 2, St. Louis, 2001, Mosby.)

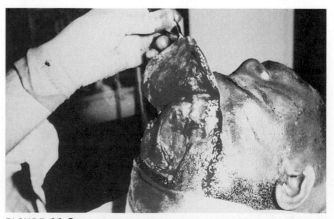

FIGURE 11-3. Degloving injury of the scalp. (From Auerbach P: *Wilderness medicine*, ed 4, St. Louis, 2001, Mosby.)

muscle (Figure 11-5). Initial interventions focus on controlling bleeding and assessing neurovascular function distal to the injury. Anesthetic should be used to facilitate removal of foreign bodies and excision of necrotic or devitalized tissue. Exploration is indicated when damage to underlying structures is possible. Wound closure involves approximation of edges followed by closure with a tape closure, staples, or sutures. Deeper wounds are closed in layers. After the wound is closed, a thin layer of antibiotic ointment may be applied followed by a nonadherent dressing.

Puncture Wounds

Puncture wounds are caused by tissue penetration with a sharp object such as a knife blade or injection from high-pressure nail guns or paint guns, which can exert pressures up to 2000 pounds per square inch (psi).[18] Injection injuries cause more severe damage to underlying tissues than indicated by the appearance of the surface wound. Lack of consistency in therapeutic approach can lead to serious complications in a substantial number of puncture wounds. Because puncture wounds do not have a dramatic appearance, the wounds are often undertreated. Regardless of appearance, the zone of injury and the wound's proximity to underlying structures should be assessed. Infection is reported in 10% to 15% of puncture wounds.

A greater risk for infection exists in wounds that are more than 6 hours old, large and deep, contaminated with foreign matter and debris, occur outdoors, penetrate through footwear, have osseous involvement, or occur in patients with underlying disease such as diabetes mellitus or immunosuppression.[18] Risk for wound contamination increases with high-pressure injuries. Management includes removal of necrotic tissue followed by drain placement and sterile dressing application. Injuries of this type are at a greater risk for being infected with an anaerobic organism. Morbidity and mortality rates are increased due to a delayed identification of the organisms and increased deep tissue necrosis. Impaled objects should be stabilized until safe removal is possible.

A foreign body can be removed if the object is small and if removal does not cause further damage. Plain radiographs may be helpful to identify the location of select embedded objects; however, standard films may not show objects such as small pieces of glass, wood, or plastic. In these cases, xeroradiography, ultrasonography, computed tomography, or magnetic resonance imaging can help locate the object. Fluoroscopy has also been used to successfully identify foreign bodies such as needles or wires. Some objects may be left in place or removed surgically.

Bites

Bites may be caused by animals or humans and involve contusions, avulsions, lacerations, and puncture wounds. Teeth can crush or tear tissue, causing extensive damage. An estimated 1 to 2 million people in the United States are bitten by animals each year; dog bites account for 80% to 90% of these injuries, whereas cat bites are reported in 5% to 18%. Exotic animals such as primates, felines, alligators, and camels also cause bite injuries. Regardless of the source, bite wounds are considered contaminated. Infection, abscess, cellulitis, septicemia, osteomyelitis, tenosynovitis, rabies, tetanus, and loss of body parts are potential complications of bite wounds.

Human bites usually result from fighting, sexual activity, or can be self-inflicted. Accidental bite injuries of the tongue, cheeks, and lips can occur during falls or seizures. Surgical closure may or may not be necessary. Infection is the greatest risk with human bites because human saliva contains 100,000,000 organisms per milliliter,[13] including *Staphylococcus aureus,* streptococci, *Proteus, Escherichia coli, Pseudomonas,* and *Klebsiellae* organisms.[13] More than 3% of these organisms are penicillin-resistant *S. aureus.* Hepatitis B virus may also be transmitted through human saliva; however, risk for human immunodeficiency virus infection appears to be low.[18] The most serious of these human

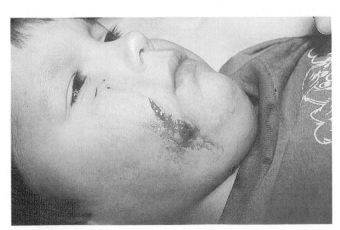

FIGURE **11-4.** Superficial laceration. (Courtesy Thomas Lintner, MD.)

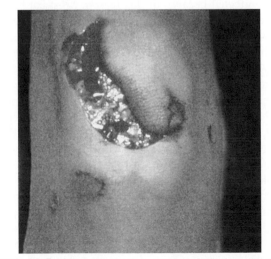

FIGURE **11-5.** Deep laceration. (From Roberts J, Hedges J: *Clinical procedures in emergency medicine,* ed 4, Philadelphia, 2004, WB Saunders.)

bites is the "fight-bite," in which there is penetration of the metacarpal joint capsule by a tooth. These "fight-bites" must be treated with antibiotics because of the high incidence of infection, and the hand must be immobilized to place the joint at rest and improve healing. Immobilization decreases the lymphatic flow and the flow of microflora.[10]

Management of human bite wounds includes neurovascular assessment, wound exploration, copious irrigation, debridement of devitalized tissue, and application of a bulky dressing. The wound is initially left open, except for those wounds on the face. Prophylactic antibiotics should be given within 3 hours of ED arrival. The use of penicillin plus a β-lactamase inhibitor (such as Augmentin) is the recommended antibiotic of choice for these bites. Alternative agents include cefoxitin or erythromycin.[6]

Animal bites carry the risk for infection, tetanus, and rabies. The Centers for Disease Control and Prevention estimates that as many as 4.5 million dog bites occur annually, with almost 800,000 requiring medical attention; 12% were seen in EDs.[2] Infection occurs in 5% to 15% of dog bite wounds and in a significant number of cat bite wounds. Up to 33 organisms have been identified in dog saliva. Cat saliva contains *Pasteurella multocida,* an extremely virulent organism that can lead to septic arthritis and bacteremia. An increased risk for infection exists in persons more than 50 years of age and in those with hand wounds, deep puncture wounds, and treatment delays of greater than 24 hours.

Dog bites frequently involve associated crush injury from compressive forces of the canine jaw—up to 400 psi in some breeds—with injury to underlying vessels, bones, and nerves. Most dog bites occur on the extremities, head, and neck, with fewer bites on the trunk. Children are more likely to have wounds on the head, face, and neck. Antibiotic use for dog bites is controversial because there is a very low rate of infection.[10] Of all cat bites, 57% to 86% are puncture wounds caused by the cat's long, slender fangs, which penetrate deeply into underlying tissue and inoculate the wound with bacteria; these wounds are hard to irrigate and tend to become infected because of this reason. Most cat bites are found on the arm, forearm, and hand. Children are more likely to have wounds on the head and trunk. Organisms commonly found in cat bites include *Staphylococcus* and *Streptococcus* species and most often *P. multocida.*[10]

Treatment for cat and dog bites is essentially the same: copious irrigation followed by cleaning, debridement, and wound closure for small wounds. It is useful to separate animal bites into high versus low risk when deciding to suture the wound or provide appropriate antibiotic coverage. Proponents of oral antibiotics have two different perspectives on the value of amoxicillin/clavulanate therapy versus amoxicillin and cephalexin therapy. Amoxicillin/clavulanate is assumed to cover staphylococci and *Pasteurella* species. A single medication taken 3 times a day should have good compliance. In contrast, two-drug therapy with amoxicillin and cephalexin may offer better coverage but may result in poorer compliance. Five days of prophylactic antibiotics is generally considered adequate.[2,6]

Although these are less effective options, patients who are allergic to penicillin may use one of the following:
- Cefuroxime (cat)
- Doxycycline (cat)
- Erythromycin
- Trimethoprim-sulfamethoxazole

Clindamycin plus ciprofloxacin (adults) or clindamycin plus trimethoprim-sulfamethoxazole (pediatrics) may provide better coverage. Azithromycin may be an effective alternative because of high tissue concentration.[2,6] High-risk wounds include all human and cat bites; hand and foot wounds; wounds surgically debrided; puncture wounds involving joints, ligaments, tendons, and bones; bites with delayed treatment more than 12 hours; and bites in immunocompromised patients. These wounds generally should not be sutured, but they do require antibiotics. Hand bites should also be splinted in a position of function and elevated. Low-risk wounds include bites involving the extremities, face, or body. These wounds are generally sutured and do not require antibiotic coverage unless already infected. Rabies and tetanus prophylaxis should be considered for all patients.

WOUND PREPARATION

There are two methods of wound cleaning used to remove bacteria and contamination with foreign material. High-pressure irrigation, the preferred method, is excellent in removing debris and decreasing the rate of infection. Appropriate personal protective equipment should be used because of probable exposure to splashing body fluids. Cleansing the wound by direct contact (such as using a soft brush) is effective in wound debridement but potentially destroys tissue. The wound can be cleansed with isotonic saline or other acceptable solutions (Table 11-2). Hydrogen peroxide should not be used because it causes absorption of oxygen in the wound and cell destruction and gives no protection against anaerobes. Soaps with strong cleaning agents or those containing alcohol may cause further tissue damage. Wounds with heavy contamination must be irrigated for a minimum of 5 minutes; at times lengthier irrigation may be needed. A wound culture may be obtained before or after irrigation if gross contamination is present.

Wound irrigation can be performed with the use of several different systems: a commercial pressurized irrigation device; a 35-ml syringe with an 18-gauge plastic tip of an intravenous catheter with a splash guard attached (the force of the stream depends on the pressure placed on the plunger by the user); or an even simpler method using a "squirt" bottle that is a new, sterile 1-liter bottle of normal saline with 8 to 12 holes placed in its lid. Figure 11-6 shows one type of irrigation device. The wound can be anesthetized with either a local anesthetic or a topical anesthetic before vigorous irrigation. Puncture wounds should be irrigated vigorously, because the ability to explore the wound is limited and it is important to remove any debris that may have become buried into the wound. Be sure to ask the patient whether the object that caused the puncture wound was removed intact

Table 11-2. ANTISEPTIC SOLUTIONS

Agents	Antimicrobial Activity	Mechanics of Action	Tissue Toxicity	Indications and Contraindications
Povidone-iodine solution (iodine complexes) (*Betadine*)	Available as 10% solution with polyvinylpyrrolidone (povidone) containing 1% free iodine with broad rapid-onset antimicrobial activity	Potent germicide in low concentrations	Decreases PMN migration and life span at concentration >1% May cause systemic toxicity at higher concentrations; questionable toxicity at 1% concentration	Probably safe and effective wound cleanser at 1% concentration 10% solution is effective to prepare skin around the wound
Povidone-iodine surgical scrub	Same as the solution	Same	Toxic to open wounds	Best as a hand cleanser; **never use in open wounds**
Nonionic detergents *Pluronic F-68* *Shur Clens*	Ethylene oxide is 80% of its molecular weight Has **no antimicrobial activity**	Wound cleanser	No toxicity to open wounds, eyes, or intravenous solutions	Appears to be an effective, safe wound cleanser
Hydrogen peroxide	3% solution in water has brief germicidal activity	Oxidizing agent that denatures protein	Toxic to open wounds	Should not be used on wounds after the initial cleaning; may be used to clean intact skin
Hexachlorophene (*pHisoHex*) (polychlorinated bis-phenol)	Bacteriostatic (2% to 5%) Greater activity against gram-positive organisms	Interruption of bacterial electron transport and disruption of membrane-bound enzymes	Little skin toxicity; the scrub form is damaging to open wounds	Never use scrub solution in open wounds Very good preoperative hand preparation
Alcohols	Low-potency antimicrobial most effective as 70% ethyl and 70% isopropyl alcohol solution	Denatures protein	Kills irreversibly and functions as a fixative	No role in routine care
Phenols	Bacteriostatic >0.2% Bactericidal >1% Fungicidal 1.3%	Denatures protein	Extensive tissue necrosis and systemic toxicity	Never use >2% aqueous phenol or >4% phenol plus glycerol

From Simon B, Hern HG Jr: Wound management. In Marx J, Hockberger R, Walls R: *Rosen's emergency medicine,* ed 6, St. Louis, 2006, Mosby.
PMN, Polymorponuclear neutrophil.

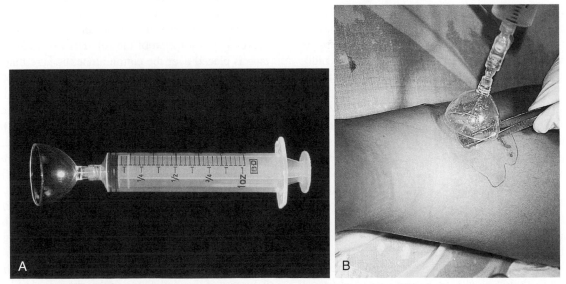

FIGURE **11-6.**   **A,** ZeroWet Splashield attached to the end of a syringe. This device is used in lieu of a needle. **B,** The shield is held near the skin, and the tip of the syringe directs the irrigating solution. (From Roberts JR, Hedges JR: *Clinical procedures in emergency medicine,* ed 4, Philadelphia, 2004, WB Saunders.)

Table 11-3. PRACTICAL ANESTHETIC AGENTS FOR EMERGENCY DEPARTMENT USE—LOCAL INFILTRATION

Agent	Concentration (%)	Maximum Dose*† Adult (mg)	Pediatric (mg/kg)	Onset (min)	Duration‡
Procaine	0.5-1	500§ (600)	7 (9)	2	15-45 min
Lidocaine	0.5-1	300 (500)	4.5 (7)∞	2	1-2 hr
Bupivacaine	0.25	175 (225)	2 (3)¶	2	4-8 hr

From Roberts JR, Hedges JR: *Clinical procedures in emergency medicine,* ed 4, Philadelphia, 2004, WB Saunders.

*These are conservative figures; see text for explanation.

†Higher dose for solutions containing epinephrine is in parentheses.

‡These values are for the agent alone; they can be extended considerably with the addition of epinephrine.

§Some authorities recommend up to 1000 mg or 14 mg/kg for procaine.

∞Some authorities recommend up to 7 mg/kg for plain lidocaine in children older than 1 year.

¶Because of lack of clinical trial experience, drug companies do not recommend the use of bupivacaine in children under the age of 12 years.

and if there were any contaminants that may have been on the object. There is no evidence to suggest that soaking puncture wounds with antiseptic solutions decreases the incidence of wound infection.

It is not necessary to shave the hair around a laceration before wound closure. Shaving destroys the hair follicles and increases the possibility of infection at the site. Clipping the hair instead of shaving is the preferred method. Eyebrows should never be shaved because hair in this area may not grow back in a cosmetically pleasing way, if it grows back at all. Eyebrows also function as landmarks for wound alignment and closure.

Nonviable injured tissue must be debrided before wound closure, and foreign bodies should be removed.[14] Wounds may be closed by primary, secondary, or tertiary intention. The type of closure depends on age of the wound, presence of infection, and amount of contamination present.

LOCAL ANESTHESIA

Local anesthesia is used to block pain when suturing or stapling, and sometimes for cleansing wounds, to minimize discomfort during these procedures. Table 11-3 highlights anesthetic agents commonly used for local infiltration. Lidocaine is the preferred agent for local and regional anesthesia because of greater potency, decreased irritation, and long-lasting anesthetic effect in comparison with other anesthetic agents. Epinephrine is commonly added to lidocaine to prolong the duration of local anesthesia, provide hemostasis, slow absorption of the anesthetic, and increase the level of anesthetic blockade. Lidocaine with epinephrine should only be used for lacerations in highly vascular areas. Epinephrine solutions should never be used in areas supplied by end arteries, including the nose, ears, digits, and penis.

Disadvantages of lidocaine are dose related and include the possibility of an allergic reaction. Central nervous system (CNS) stimulation, seizure, myocardial depression, and cardiac conduction blocks are the toxic reactions most commonly reported. Other anesthetic agents include procaine, mepivacaine (Carbocaine), bupivacaine (Marcaine or Sensorcaine), and tetracaine (Pontocaine). When deciding

on the practical agent for local infiltration, the duration of these agents is important: procaine has a duration of 15 to 45 minutes; lidocaine has a duration of 1 to 2 hours; and bupivacaine has a duration of 4 to 8 hours.[12] The duration of these agents will be extended considerably with the addition of epinephrine. Adding sodium bicarbonate 8.4% with any of these agents (warmed or at room temperature) decreases pain associated with infiltration.

Topical anesthetics are ideal for management of minor lacerations in children. Available solutions include Xylocaine, adrenalin, and Pontocaine (XAP); and lidocaine, epinephrine, and tetracaine (LET). Tetracaine, adrenalin, and cocaine (TAC) is in limited supply because many pharmacies have banned this cocaine-containing mixture. Cocaine solutions should be used cautiously because of potentially deleterious side effects such as CNS stimulation and vasomotor collapse. Topical anesthetics may obviate the need for needle infiltration but do require a minimum of 20 minutes for adequate anesthesia. A cotton ball is saturated with 2 to 3 mL of the anesthetic solution and applied directly to the laceration. A clear dressing, such as Tegaderm, may be applied directly over the cotton ball to hold it in place, while preventing absorption of the solution when tape is used. (If tape is placed over the cotton alone, be sure that a glove is used while holding it in place to prevent absorption of the anesthetic). The vasoconstrictive effect of epinephrine causes a white ring around the wound, indicating the area is anesthetized. Because of the epinephrine component, these solutions cannot be used in areas supplied by end arteries (nose, ears, digits, and penis). Infiltration of a local anesthetic agent may still be required if the desired anesthetic effect is not achieved. Anesthetic effect varies slightly with each solution because of duration of individual agents. Another topical anesthetic widely used is viscous lidocaine. This topical agent may be applied to abrasions before cleaning but is not used as an anesthetic for wound closure. Application of viscous lidocaine to large areas may result in lidocaine toxicity if enough of the medication is absorbed. Table 11-4 outlines topical anesthetic agents. Although anesthetic creams such as EMLA and LMX4 are commonly used to reduce procedural pain, these agents can be applied only to intact skin.

Table 11-4. PRACTICAL ANESTHETIC AGENTS FOR EMERGENCY DEPARTMENT USE—TOPICAL APPLICATION					
		Maximum Dosage*†			
Agent	Usual Concentration (%)	Adult (mg)	Pediatric (mg/kg)	Onset (min)	Duration (min)
Tetracaine	0.5	50	0.75	3-8	30-60
Lidocaine	2-10	250-300†	3-4†	2-5	15-45
Cocaine	4	200	2-3†	2-5	30-45

From Roberts JR, Hedges JR: *Clinical procedures in emergency medicine,* ed 4, Philadelphia, 2004, WB Saunders.
*These are conservative figures; see text for explanations.
†The lower dosage should be used for a maximum safe dose when feasible.

Local blocks can be very useful when evaluating alternative routes to wound infiltration. Local blocks require smaller amounts of anesthetic and can be more effective by blocking afferent sensory nerves of a specific region. A local nerve block, or digital block, is accomplished by injecting the anesthetic agent along the nerve innervating the wounded area to abolish afferent and efferent impulse conduction. The syringe is aspirated before each injection to prevent inadvertent parenteral lidocaine injection. Regional anesthesia, or Bier block, may be selected when a greater anesthetic effect is desired. A tourniquet is placed proximal to the wound, and then the anesthetic agent is injected distal to the injury. After wound repair, the tourniquet is released and the anesthetic agent is slowly absorbed.

One alternative to local and regional anesthesia is nitrous oxide. The patient inhales a 50% mixture of nitrous oxide and oxygen during short, painful procedures such as wound debridement. Self-administration limits the amount of nitrous oxide used while providing the appropriate level of anesthesia. The patient should be continuously monitored with a pulse oximeter.

WOUND CLOSURE

Wound healing occurs by primary, secondary, or tertiary intention (Figure 11-7). Primary intention is the healing that occurs when the wound edges of a clean laceration or surgical incision are approximated and underlying structures are aligned, eliminating dead space. Healing occurs through formation of new blood vessels, scar tissue, and epidermal repair.[4] Secondary intention is healing that occurs when extensive loss of tissue prevents the wound edges from being approximated and the wound is left open to heal by granulation, contraction, and epithelization. Delayed closure or tertiary intention is a combination of the first two types of healing when the wound is not considered clean enough to close, substantial edema is present, or all debris has not been removed. It is usually left open for 5 to 10 days and then is sutured to decrease the risk for infection.[15] Those wounds that cannot be closed with any of the above techniques may require a skin graft or flap closure.

Primary wound closure uses a tape closure (Steri Strips), sutures, staples, or wound adhesive. The technique chosen depends on wound size, depth, and location. Tape closure is used for superficial linear wounds under minimal tension or as an adjunct after suture removal in patients with thin, frail skin such as older adults or steroid-dependent patients. Tincture of benzoin is thinly applied to intact skin before application of tape to ensure adherence. A tape closure may also be used after deeper layers are closed with sutures. Dressings may or may not be applied over the tape closure. An anesthetic is not necessary with simple tape closures. Wounds closed with this method pose a lower risk for infection. Tape strips remain in place until they fall off. Figure 11-8 illustrates a wound managed with tape closure.

Sutures approximate and attach wound edges, which decreases infection, promotes wound healing, and minimizes scar formation. A local anesthetic applied by infiltration or topically is required for suturing. Different stitches are used to close various wounds depending on depth, location, and tension of the wound. Sutures may be absorbable or nonabsorbable, which means they are composed of natural or synthetic material, respectively. Essential qualities of suture material are security, strength, reaction, workability, and infectious potential. Table 11-5 describes these qualities for various suture materials. Ideal suture material is strong, easily secured, resistant to infection, and causes minimal local reaction. Sutures cause minimal discomfort after insertion; however, they also act as a foreign body and can cause local inflammation. A thin layer of antibiotic ointment is applied after suture application and then covered by a nonadherent dressing. Recommendations for suture removal vary with wound location. For wounds in areas of movement or increased surface tension, sutures should remain longer. Table 11-6 provides guidelines for suture removal.

Staples are a fast, economical alternative for closure of linear lacerations of the scalp, trunk, and extremities (Figure 11-9). Wounds closed with staples have a lower incidence of infection and tissue reactivity, but staples do not provide the same quality of closure as sutures. Scars are more pronounced; therefore staples are recommended only for areas where a scar is not apparent (e.g., scalp). Staples should not be used in areas of the scalp with permanent hair loss because of poor aesthetic results. Local anesthesia is optional when only one or two staples are required because pain from infiltration of anesthetic agents is greater than pain associated with insertion of one or two staples. Staples usually

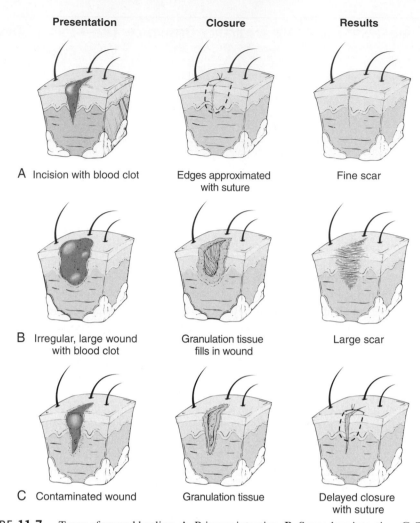

Presentation   Closure   Results

A Incision with blood clot   Edges approximated with suture   Fine scar

B Irregular, large wound with blood clot   Granulation tissue fills in wound   Large scar

C Contaminated wound   Granulation tissue   Delayed closure with suture

FIGURE **11-7.** Types of wound healing. **A,** Primary intention. **B,** Secondary intention. **C,** Tertiary intention. (Modified from Lewis SL, Heitkemper MM, Dirksen SR et al: *Medical-surgical nursing: assessment and management of clinical problems,* ed 7, St. Louis, 2007, Mosby.)

remain in place 7 to 10 days. A special staple remover (Figure 11-10) is required for removal.

Dermabond, the newest form of wound closure, is topical skin glue used to close skin edges that are easily approximated. This type of wound closure should not be used around the eyes, in high skin tension areas, or across areas of increased skin tension. Application of three thin layers, in a zigzag fashion, is more effective than a single thick layer; Dermabond dries within 2½ minutes. Discharge teaching should stress not applying liquid or ointment to the closed wound because these substances can weaken the glue, leading to dehiscence. Patients should also be instructed that the adhesive will slough naturally, usually within 5 to 10 days. If removal of Dermabond is necessary, petroleum jelly can be used.

WOUND DRESSINGS

A moisture-balanced wound environment promotes wound healing and can potentially increase the rate of wound re-epithelialization by 50%.[11] Modern wound dressings are designed to keep the wound moist, clean the wound or keep it clean, and protect the wound from physical trauma or bacterial invasion. Types of wound dressings are described in Table 11-7. Wounds to the face and ears may not require a dressing as long as the area is kept clean. Depending on the wound, a thin layer of antibiotic ointment (e.g., bacitracin, Polysporin, or Neosporin) may be applied before the dressing. Use of a silver-coated absorbent dressing is being explored for use with all types of wounds. Early studies show these silver-coated dressings have a much faster bactericidal action against broad-spectrum organisms than does a film dressing.

Wound pouching systems (e.g., KCI Wound Vac) are used for wounds that drain more than 50 mL of fluid a day or are associated with fluid that is especially damaging to skin.[8] These wound devices are based on eliminating exudates from the wound bed, reducing edema, and increasing blood flow. This treatment is not a replacement for antibiotic use but a therapy to manage excess exudates produced by wounds that are critically colonized or infected.[11]

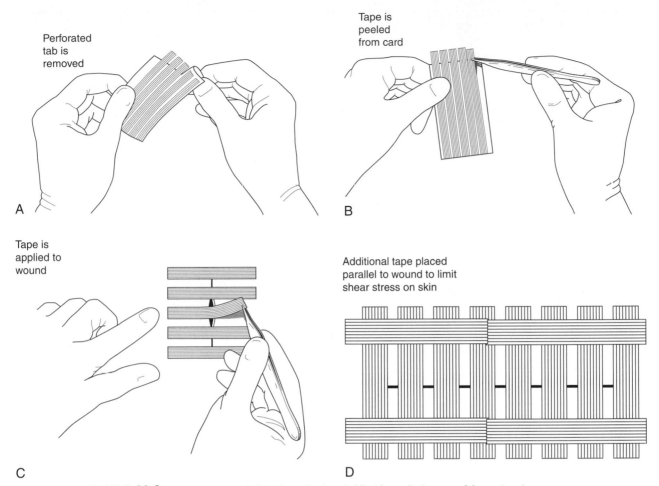

Perforated tab is removed

A

Tape is peeled from card

B

Tape is applied to wound

C

Additional tape placed parallel to wound to limit shear stress on skin

D

FIGURE **11-8.**   Tape closure **(A-D).** (From Rothrock JC: *Alexander's care of the patient in surgery,* ed 13, St. Louis, 2007, Mosby.)

WOUND PROPHYLAXIS

Wounds are at risk for local and systemic infection from contaminants, surface organisms, tetanus, and rabies. Protection against these infectious agents begins with cleansing and irrigation.

Tetanus Prophylaxis

Tetanus is a systemic infection caused by *Clostridium tetani,* a gram-positive, spore-forming, anaerobic bacillus. Once activated, the bacillus is extremely resistant to almost anything, including sterilization. The incubation period for tetanus is 2 days to 2 weeks or more. *C. tetani* spores are present in soil, garden moss, and anywhere animal and human excrement are found. Spores may contaminate wounds but remain dormant in tissue for years. After *C. tetani* enters the circulatory system, bacilli attach to cells in the CNS, causing depression of the respiratory center in the medulla. Symptoms may be mild or severe and include local joint stiffness and mild trismus or inability to open the jaw, which is where the term *lockjaw*

came from. Severe tetanus is characterized by severe trismus, back pain, penile pain, tachycardia, hypertension, dysrhythmias, hyperpyrexia, opisthotonos, and seizures.

Prevention of tetanus includes immunization and scrupulous wound care, particularly for tetanus-prone wounds (Box 11-1). The majority of patients who are not immunized are in the over-50 age-group; therefore tetanus must be considered in all patients no matter how severe the injury.[10] Tetanus immunization is part of the childhood immunization regimen that continues with regular tetanus immunizations in adults. Tetanus toxoid provides active immunization, whereas tetanus immune globulin (TIG) provides passive immunization. People who are inadequately immunized against tetanus should receive active and/or passive protection depending on the type of wound and their individual immunization status; when both TIG and a tetanus toxoid–containing vaccine are indicated, each product should be administered in a separate syringe at different anatomic sites.[3] Table 11-8 lists the recommendations for tetanus prophylaxis for clean and tetanus-prone wounds.[3] Prophylaxis should be given within 72 hours to decrease the risk for tetanus.

Table 11-5. SUTURE MATERIALS FOR WOUND CLOSURE

Type	Description	Security	Strength	Reaction	Workability	Infection	Comment
NONABSORBABLES							
Silk		++++	+	++++	++++	++	Suitable around mouth, nose, or nipples; too reactive and weak to be used universally
Mersilene	Braided synthetic	++++	++	+++	++++		Good tensile strength; some prefer for fascia repairs
Nylon	Monofilament	++	+++	++	++	+++	Good strength; decreased infection rate; knots tend to slip, especially the first throw
Prolene Polypropylene	Monofilament	+	++++	+	+	++++	Good resistance to infection; often difficult to work with; requires an extra throw
Ethibond	Braided, coated polyester	+++	++++	++$\frac{1}{2}$	+++	+++	Costly
Stainless steel wire	Monofilament	++++	++++	+	+	+	Hard to use; painful to patient; some prefer for tendons
ABSORBABLES							
Gut (plain)	From sheep intima	+	++	+++		+	Loses strength rapidly and quickly absorbed; rarely used today
Chromic (gut)	Plain gut treated with chromic salts	++	++	+++		+	Similar to plain gut; often used to close intraoral lacerations
Dexon	Braided copolymer of glycolic acid	++++	++++	+		++++	Braiding may cause it to "hang up" when tying knots
Vicryl	Braided polymer of lactide and glycolide	+++	++++	+		+++	Low reactivity with good strength; therefore, nice for subcutaneous healing; good in mucous membranes
Polydioxanone	Monofilament	++++	++++	+	Excellent	Unavailable	First available monofilament synthetic absorbable sutures; appears to be excellent

From Simon B, Hern HG Jr: Wound management. In Marx J, Hockberger R, Walls R: *Rosen's emergency medicine,* ed 6, St. Louis, 2006, Mosby.

Table 11-6. GUIDELINES FOR SUTURE REMOVAL

Location	Removal Date (days)
Eyelids	3-5
Eyebrows	4-5
Ear	4-6
Lip	3-5
Face	3-5
Scalp	7-10
Trunk	7-10
Hands and feet	7-10
Arms and legs	10-14
Over joints	14

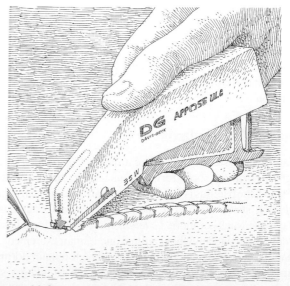

FIGURE **11-9.** Application of skin staples. Staples are centered over incision line, using locating arrow or guideline, and placed approximately ¼ inch apart. (From Rothrock JC: *Alexander's care of the patient in surgery,* ed 13, St. Louis, 2007, Mosby.)

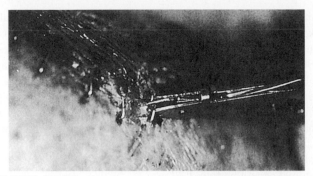

FIGURE **11-10.** Staple remover. (From Potter PA, Perry AG: *Fundamentals of nursing,* ed 6, St. Louis, 2008, Mosby.)

Rabies Prophylaxis

Rabies exposure can occur with bites from wild or domestic animals. Although rabies is rare in the United States, it should be considered when an animal attack was not provoked, involved a domestic animal not immunized against rabies, or involved a wild animal (such as a bat). Rabies is a neurotoxic virus found in saliva of some mammals. Incubation period is 4 to 8 weeks. After inoculation, the rabies virus travels by peripheral nerves to the CNS, causing encephalomyelitis, which is almost always fatal. Sources of rabies in wild and domestic animals are listed in Table 11-9. Carnivorous wild

Table 11-7. **TYPES OF WOUND DRESSINGS**		
Type	**Description**	**Examples**
Gauze	Provides absorption of exudate; supports debridement if applied and kept moist; can be used to maintain moist wound surface and as filler dressings in sinus tracts	Numerous products available
Nonadherent dressings	Woven or nonwoven dressings may be impregnated with saline, petrolatum, or antimicrobials; minimal absorbency	Adaptic Exu-Dry Sofsorb Telfa Vaseline gauze Xeroform
Transparent film	Semipermeable membrane permits gaseous exchange between wound bed and environment; minimally absorbent so fluid environment created in presence of exudate. Bacteria do not penetrate membrane. Used for dry, noninfected wounds or wounds with minimal drainage	Acu-Derm Bioclusive Blisterfilm OpSite Polyskin Tegaderm Transeal
Hydrocolloid	Occlusive dressing does not allow oxygen to diffuse from atmosphere to wound bed. Occlusion does not interfere with wound healing; not used in infected wounds; supports debridement and prevents secondary infections; used for superficial and partial-thickness wounds with light to moderate drainage	Comfeel DuoDerm Intact Intrasite Restore Tegasorb Ultec
Polyurethane foams	Moderate to heavy amounts of exudate can be absorbed; can be used on infected wounds; used for partial- or full-thickness wounds with minimal to heavy drainage	Allevyn Epi-Lock Hydrasorb Lyofoam Mitraflex Synthaderm
Absorption dressing	Large volumes of exudate can be absorbed; supports debridement; maintains moist wound surface; placed into wounds and can obliterate dead space; for partial- or full-thickness wounds or infected wounds	AlgiDERM Bard Absorption Debrisan DuoDerm Paste Hydragan Kaltostat Sorbsan
Hydrogel	Debridement because of moisturizing effects; maintains moist wound surface; provides limited absorption of exudate; available as sheet or gel; most require a secondary dressing. Used for partial- or full-thickness wounds, deep wounds with minimal drainage, and necrotic wounds	Vigilon Elasto-Gel Intrasite Gel Geliperm

Modified from Lewis SM, Heitkemper MM, Dirksen SR et al: *Medical-surgical nursing: assessment and management of clinical problems,* ed 7, St. Louis, 2007, Mosby.

animals are always considered rabid, so immediate rabies prophylaxis should be administered.

Risk assessment for rabies transmission should include the following: degree of exposure; circumstances of the bite; behavior of the animal; vaccination status of dogs, cats, and ferrets; and prevalence of rabies in the geographic area and/or in the animal species involved. Cage-raised pocket pets (e.g., hamsters, gerbils, and mice) have little or no opportunity to be exposed to rabies-infected animals and

therefore pose little if any risk. Unfortunately, wild animals kept as pets must be treated as wild animals; they must be sacrificed and their brains examined for evidence of rabies. Stray or unwanted dogs, cats, ferrets, or other animals may also be sacrificed for laboratory examination. Those animals that appear healthy are observed for 10 days, with prophylaxis required only if the animal exhibits signs of rabies. It has been well documented that dogs, cats, or ferrets will not shed rabies in their saliva more than 4 to 7 days before onset of clinical rabies.[13,17] Prophylaxis is always given when the animal cannot be found.

When should the rabies prophylaxis be started? Remember that this is a prophylactic treatment, not an emergency treatment, but the decision to treat must be made with some urgency, especially while in the ED. Bites with a high risk for rabies transmission may warrant immediate treatment, whereas bites with a lower risk can await the 10-day observation period or laboratory results. Much depends on the offending species, the general rabies risk in the area, and the ability to quickly obtain laboratory results from public health

---

Box 11-1 TETANUS-PRONE WOUNDS

More than 6 hours old
Stellate or avulsed
Caused by missile, crushing mechanism, heat, or cold
Obvious signs of infection
Devitalized tissue
Contaminants such as dirt, feces, soil, saliva

Table 11-8. GUIDE TO TETANUS PROPHYLAXIS IN ROUTINE WOUND MANAGEMENT

Characteristic	Clean, Minor Wound		All Other Wounds*	
History of Adsorbed Tetanus Toxoid (doses)	Tdap or Td[†]	TIG	Tdap or Td[†]	TIG
Unknown or <3	Yes	No	Yes	Yes
≥3	No[‡]	No	No[§]	No

Modified from Centers for Disease Control and Prevention: Preventing tetanus, diphtheria, and pertussis among adults: use of tetanus toxoid, reduced diphtheria toxoid and acellular pertussis vaccine, *MMWR Recomm Rep* 55(RR-17):1, 2006.
Td, Tetanus and diphtheria vaccine; *Tdap,* tetanus, diphtheria, pertussis vaccine; *TIG;* tetanus immune globulin.
*Includes wounds contaminated with dirt, feces, soil, and saliva; puncture wounds; avulsions; and wounds resulting from missiles, crushing, burns, and frostbite.
[†]Tdap is preferred to Td for children aged 11-18 years and adults aged 19-64 years who have never received Tdap. Td is preferred to Tdap or adults who received Tdap previously. Tdap is not licensed for use among adults aged ≥ 65 years.
[‡]Yes, if ≥10 years since the last tetanus toxoid–containing vaccine dose.
[§]Yes, if ≥5 years since the last tetanus toxoid–containing vaccine dose.

Table 11-9. SOURCES OF RABIES

Animal Type	Evaluation and Disposition of Animal	Postexposure Prophylaxis Recommendations
Dogs, cats, and ferrets	Healthy and available for 10 days' observation	People should not begin prophylaxis unless animal develops clinical signs of rabies*
	Rabid or suspected rabid	Immediately immunize
	Unknown (e.g., escaped)	Consult public health officials
Skunks, raccoons, foxes, and most other carnivores; bats	Regarded as rabid unless animal is proven negative for rabies by laboratory tests[†]	Consider immediate immunization
Livestock, small rodents, lagomorphs (rabbits and hares), large rodents (woodchucks and beavers), and other mammals	Consider individually	Consult public health officials; bites of squirrels, hamsters, guinea pigs, gerbils, chipmunks, rats, mice, other small rodents, rabbits, and hares almost never require antirabies postexposure prophylaxis

Modified from Centers for Disease Control and Prevention: Human rabies prevention—United States, 1999 recommendations of the Advisory Committee on Immunization Practices (ACIP), *MMWR Recomm Rep* 48(RR-1):1, 1999, http://www.cdc.gov/mmwr/preview/mmwrhtml/00056176.htm.
*During the 10-day observation period, begin postexposure prophylaxis at the first sign of rabies in a dog, cat, or ferret that has bitten someone. If the animal exhibits clinical signs of rabies, it should be euthanized immediately and tested.
[†]The animal should be euthanized and tested as soon as possible. Holding for observation is not recommended. Discontinue vaccine if immunofluorescence test results of the animal are negative.

laboratories. Consultations with local public health officials may be helpful in the decision-making process.[13,17]

One question that has become a topic of concern for clinicians is how to approach the care of persons who awaken to find a bat in their room or their child's room even though no bite is observed. The Advisory Committee on Immunization Policies has issued a recommendation stating: "PEP (postexposure prophylaxis) can be considered for persons who were in the same room as the bat and who might be unaware that a bite or direct contact had occurred (e.g., a sleeping person awakens to find a bat in the room or an adult witnesses a bat in the room with a previously unattended child, mentally disabled person, or intoxicated person) and rabies cannot be ruled out by testing the bat."[13]

Rabies immunization includes administration of rabies immune globulin (RIG) and human diploid cell vaccine (HDCV). RIG provides passive immunization, and HDCV provides active immunization.[1] Individuals who have received PEP in the past or who have undergone preexposure prophylaxis (veterinarians and their staff, animal control and wildlife workers, rabies researchers, and laboratory workers) should not receive rabies immune globulin but should receive two booster doses of vaccine on day 0 and day 3. The best defense against rabies continues to be prevention through vaccinating domestic animals and educating the public about the danger of handling wild animals, especially bats. Table 11-10 summarizes rabies immunization.

Use of Antibiotics for Acute Wounds

The use of antibiotics for all acute wounds is controversial. Uncomplicated minor wounds do not require prophylactic antibiotics. Meticulous wound care, debridement, and proper wound closure and dressings are the most important infection control factors indicated for these minor wounds. The use of prophylactic antibiotics is recommended in the following situations: open joint or open fracture, heavy contamination or major soft tissue injury, delay in care, the patient is immunocompromised, or the patient has special health problems (e.g., diabetes/cardiac valvular disease).[14]

SUMMARY

Skin is the first barrier between the body and the rest of the world. Loss of skin integrity affects ability to resist infection, retain fluids, and regulate body temperature. Changes caused by surface trauma such as scarring or tattooing affect body image and can cause significant anxiety for the patient. The emergency nurse plays a vital role in reducing potential wound complications through assessment, meticulous wound care, knowledge of the indications for tetanus immunization and antibiotic use, and detailed discharge teaching. The most effective intervention to decrease the risk for infection is thorough wound cleansing. Box 11-2 provides a summary of wound care management.

Table 11-10. RABIES POSTEXPOSURE PROPHYLAXIS SCHEDULE

Vaccination Status	Treatment	Regimen*
Not previously vaccinated	Wound cleansing	All postexposure treatment should begin with immediate thorough cleansing of all wounds with soap and water; if available, a virucidal agent such as a povidone-iodine solution should be used to irrigate wounds
	RIG	Administer 20 internation units/kg body weight; if anatomically feasible, the full dose should be infiltrated around the wound(s) and any remaining volume should be administered IM at an anatomic site distant from vaccine administration; also, RIG should not be administered in the same syringe as vaccine; because RIG might partially suppress active production of antibody, no more than the recommended dose should be given
	Vaccine	HDCV, RVA, or PCEC 1 mL, IM (deltoid†), one each on days 0‡, 3, 7, 14, and 28
Previously vaccinated§	Wound cleansing	All postexposure treatment should begin with immediate thorough cleansing of all wounds with soap and water; if available, a virucidal agent such as a povidone-iodine solution should be used to irrigate the wounds
	RIG	RIG should not be administered
	Vaccine	HDCV, RVA, or PCEC 1 mL, IM (deltoid area†), one each on days 0‡ and 3

Modified from Centers for Disease Control and Prevention: Human rabies prevention—United States, 1999 recommendations of the Advisory Committee on Immunization Practices (ACIP), *MMWR Recomm Rep* 48(RR-1):1, 1999, http://www.cdc.gov/mmwr/preview/mmwrhtml/00056176.htm.
HDCV, Human diploid cell vaccine; *IM,* intramuscular; *PCEC,* purified chick embryo cell vaccine; *RIG,* rabies immune globulin (human); *RVA,* rabies vaccine absorbed.
*These regimens are applicable for all age-groups, including children.
†The deltoid area is the only acceptable site of vaccination for adults and older children. For younger children, the outer aspect of the thigh may be used. The vaccine should never be administered in the gluteal area.
‡Day 0 is the day the first dose of vaccine is administered.
§Any person with a history of preexposure vaccination with HDCV, RVA, or PCEC; prior postexposure prophylaxis with HDCV, RVA, or PCEC; or previous vaccination with any other type of rabies vaccine and a documented history of antibody response to the prior vaccination.

Box 11-2	SUMMARY OF WOUND CARE

A. Stabilize the patient
B. History (be sure to include tetanus immunization status and allergies)
C. Physical examination
    a. Neurovascular examination
    b. Under sterile conditions (after the area is anesthetized, and a bloodless field is obtained) an exam of the anatomic structures, skin, nerves, tendons, vessels, muscles, fascia should be completed
    c. Consult to specialist as indicated
D. X-rays to detect injury to bone or presence of foreign bodies
E. Wound preparation
    a. Cut—do not shave—surrounding hair to decrease the risk for microscopic injuries to the skin
    b. Prepare surrounding skin with Betadine solution
    c. Sharp debridement of foreign matter and devitalized tissue
    d. High-pressure irrigation (i.e., 18-gauge needle on a 35-mL syringe) with saline, 1% povidone-iodine (Betadine) an antibiotic solution, or a nonionic solution

F. Wound closure
    a. Adhesive tape, sutures, or staples
    b. No use of subcutaneous sutures unless wound is under high tension
G. Antibiotics
    a. Apply topical antibiotics (i.e., triple antibiotic ointment)
    b. No systemic antibiotics unless wound is at high risk
H. Dress and immobilize
I. Wound care instructions to include:
    a. Signs of infection—redness, swelling, red streaks progressing up an extremity, increased pain and fever
    b. Elevation—use of sling when appropriate
    c. Cleansing of wound daily to remove debris and crusting with use of a dilute hydrogen peroxide
    d. Immobilization, if indicated, until sutures removed
    e. Wound check—for high risk (cat bites, "fight-bites") routinely at 48 hours
    f. Suture removal—may apply adhesive strips if sutures removed early

Modified from Simon B, Hern HG Jr: Wound management. In Marx J, Hockberger R, Walls R: Rosen's emergency medicine, ed 6, St. Louis, 2006, Mosby.

REFERENCES

1. Centers for Disease Control and Prevention: Human rabies prevention—United States, 1999 recommendations of the Advisory Committee on Immunization Practices (ACIP), *MMWR Recomm Rep* 48(RR-1):1, 1999, http://www.cdc.gov/mmwr/preview/mmwrhtml/00056176.htm.
2. Centers for Disease Control and Prevention: Nonfatal dog bite–related injuries treated in hospital emergency departments—United States, 2001, *MMWR Morb Mortal Wkly Rep* 52(26):605, 2003.
3. Centers for Disease Control and Prevention: Preventing tetanus, diphtheria, and pertussis among adults: use of tetanus toxoid, reduced diphtheria toxoid and acellular pertussis vaccine, *MMWR Recomm Rep* 55(RR-17):1, 2006.
4. Emergency Nurses Association: Course in advanced trauma nursing, II, A conceptual approach to injury and illness. Dubuque, Ia, 2003, Kendall/Hunt Publishing Co.
5. Flynn MD: Traumatic wounds. In McQuillan KA, Von Ruede KT, Hartsock RL et al, editors: *Traumatic nursing from resuscitation through rehabilitation*, ed 3, Philadelphia, 2002, Harcourt Health.
6. Gilbert DN, Moellering RC, Ellopoulos GM, et al: *Sandford guide to antimicrobial therapy*, ed 27, Sperryville, Va, 2007, Antimicrobial Therapy, Inc.
7. Guyton AC, Hall JE: *Textbook of medical physiology*, ed 10, Philadelphia, 2000, WB Saunders.
8. KCI Licensing, Inc: *VAC therapy, clinical guidelines*, January 2005. San Antonio, Tx.
9. Kidd PS, Sturt P: *Mosby emergency nursing reference*, ed 2, St. Louis, 2002, Mosby.
10. Marx J, Hockberger R, Walls R: *Rosen's emergency medicine*, ed 6, St. Louis, 2006, Mosby.
11. Okan D, Woo K, Ayello EA et al: The role of moisture balance in wound healing, *Adv Skin Wound Care* 20(1):39, 2007.
12. Roberts JR, Hedges JR: *Clinical procedures in emergency medicine*, ed 4, Philadelphia, 2004, WB Saunders.
13. Schlessinger J: Animal bites, *E-medicine.com*, May 25, 2007.
14. Stewart RM, Myers JG, Dent DL: Wounds, bites, and stings, In Moore E, Felician D, Mattox K, editors: *Trauma*, ed 5, New York, 2004, McGraw-Hill.
15. Stillman RM: Wound healing, *E-medicine.com*, January 4, 2007.
16. Stotts NA: Integumentary clinical physiology, In Kinney MK, Dunbar SB, Brooks-Brunn JA et al, editors: *AACN's clinical reference for critical care nursing*, ed 4, St. Louis, 1998, Mosby.
17. Stump J: Animal bites, *E-medicine.com*, February 2, 2006.
18. Tintinalli JE, Kelen GD, Stapczynski JS: *Emergency medicine: a comprehensive study guide*, ed 6, New York, 2003, McGraw-Hill Professional.

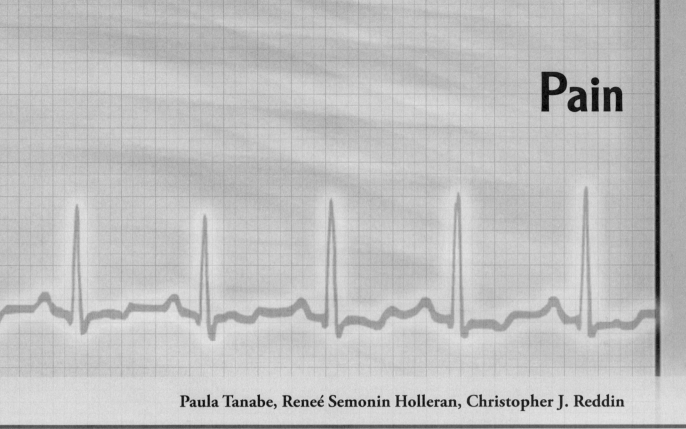

CHAPTER 12

Pain

Paula Tanabe, Reneé Semonin Holleran, Christopher J. Reddin

Pain is the most frequent complaint among emergency department (ED) patients, and traditionally pain has been inadequately treated for many patients.[24,47,111] In 2004 over 56% of ED patients in the United States presented with pain, 39% of these patients complained of either moderate or severe pain.[61] Over the past decade, research and efforts to improve pain management have proliferated and resulted in increased attention to ED pain management. Although many strides have been made, the opportunity for maximizing pain control for the individual ED patient remains great. The ED nurse can and should play a key role in ED pain management. The ED nurse is often the patient's primary advocate for achieving optimal control of pain. Emergency nurses are usually the first to assess and identify a patient in pain, can independently implement nonpharmacologic interventions, request analgesic orders from their physician colleagues, are primarily responsible for assessing the adequacy of any interventions, and have an opportunity to provide patient teaching at discharge to promote optimal management of pain at home. By taking a proactive role in pain management, emergency nurses have a unique opportunity to make a meaningful difference for the majority of the patients they care for.

This chapter will discuss the pathophysiology of pain, current definitions, and provide a detailed review of both adult and pediatric pain management specific to the ED.

DEFINITIONS AND CLASSIFICATIONS OF PAIN

The International Association for the Study of Pain has defined pain as "an unpleasant sensory and emotional experience associated with actual or potential tissue damage."[48] Pain has both a physiologic and an emotional component.[27] As more research has been conducted and with an additional understanding of pathophysiology, a continuum of pain has been identified.

Pain is classified as nociceptive or neuropathic. Neuropathic pain can result from trauma or diseases of the nerves. This causes abnormal processing of sensory impulses from the peripheral or central nervous systems. Nociceptive pain results from impulses that travel along normal nerve conduction pathways. Nociceptive pain may be stimulated by neurotransmitters contained in the soma and viscera. The pathophysiology of pain is discussed in the next section of this chapter.[48,87]

Acute pain is described as pain that results from potential or actual tissue damage. Acute pain occurs suddenly and should go away when the injury has healed or

Table 12-1. TYPES OF PAIN SEEN IN THE EMERGENCY DEPARTMENT

Type of Pain	Characteristics	Causes
Acute	Sudden onset	Trauma
	Warning	Surgery
	Protective	Procedures
	Transient in length	Fractures
	Able to identify area of pain	Illnesses such as pancreatitis
	Specific objective signs and symptoms	Infections
	Anxiety	
Chronic	State of existence	Mechanical low back pain
	Less able to differentiate where the pain is	Arthritis
	Prolonged—months to years	Migraine
	Difficult to treat	Pelvic pain
	Depression common	
Cancer	State of existence	Tumor
	May increase with treatment or changes	HIV/AIDS
	in the disease process	Chemotherapy
		Radiation therapy
Neuropathic	Burning	Primary lesion, dysfunction in the peripheral
	Numbness	or central nervous system
	Electrical jolts	
Visceral	Squeezing	Bowel obstruction
	Cramping	Venous occlusion
	Bloated feeling	Ischemia
	Stretching	
Somatic	Aching	Bone metastasis
	Throbbing	Degenerative joint disease

HIV/AIDS, Human immune deficiency virus/acquired immunodeficiency syndrome.

the illness resolved. Acute pain functions as a protective mechanism, warning the body of illness or injury. Defense mechanisms such as removal of the offending cause, for example a bee stinger, are initiated. Acute pain has both physiologic and emotional components. Most patients are able to describe its location and intensity, as well as identify what provides relief from the pain (pharmacologic and nonpharmacologic methods).[87] Acute pain continues to be one of the most common reasons why patients seek care in the ED.[111]

Chronic (cancer and noncancer) pain may be initiated by an acute event, or its source may be unknown. It is prolonged pain lasting longer than 3 months and in many cases continuing for months to years. The source of chronic pain is not always easily differentiated. It can be difficult to relate the amount and the patient's response to the pain. Examples of the types of chronic pain seen in the ED are mechanical low back pain and degenerative or inflammatory joint pain. More research is needed to understand the best methods to treat chronic pain in the ED.

A subtype of chronic pain is chronic noncancer pain. Patients with this type of pain report levels of pain that weakly correspond to identifiable levels of tissue abnormality. These patients respond poorly to standard treatments.[27]

Cancer pain is a form of chronic pain specifically related to the disease. Cancer pain may be attributed to the advance of the disease, pain associated with the treatment of the disease process (e.g., radiation or chemotherapy), or pain associated with preexisting medical problems. Cancer pain has been designated separately because treatment is generally focused on the management of the pain related to the disease process.

Pain is a multifaceted phenomenon. Table 12-1 contains a summary of some of the different types of pain that may be seen in the ED.[46,48,67,84,87] There are also multiple pain terms that emergency nurses should be familiar with when evaluating pain in the ED. Table 12-2 contains descriptions of some of these terms.[*]

PATHOPHYSIOLOGY OF PAIN

The pathophysiology of pain is complex, involving sensory, emotional, behavioral, and spiritual factors. The perception of pain is nociception and involves three pathways that transmit and modulate pain stimuli.[46,87] A theory that explains this phenomenon is the gate control theory. Nociceptors, or pain receptors, are located in the skin, muscles, joints, arteries, and the viscera. Nociceptors are stimulated by chemical, thermal, or mechanical stimuli. Examples of stimuli may include a laceration, heat that causes tissue damage, or stretch

---

[*]References 23, 25, 27, 30, 46, 48, 64, 67, 76, 84, 86, 87, 111.

Table 12-2.	**Pain Terminologies**
Terminology	**Definition/Description**
Allodynia	Pain due to stimulus that does not normally provoke pain. It involves a change in the quality of sensation. The stimulus does not normally cause pain, but the response is painful.
Analgesia	Absence of pain in response to a stimulus that should be painful.
Hyperalgesia	An increased response to a stimulus that is normally painful.
Hyperesthesia	Increased sensitivity to stimulation, excluding the special senses.
Neuralgia	Pain in the distribution of a nerve or nerves.
Neuritis	Inflammation of a nerve or nerves.
Neuropathy	A disturbance of function or pathologic change in a nerve.
Noxious stimulus	A noxious stimulus is one that is damaging to normal tissues.
Pain threshold	The least experience of pain that a patient can recognize.
Pain tolerance level	The greatest level of pain that a patient can tolerate.
Paresthesia	An abnormal sensation whether spontaneous or evoked.

of an abdominal muscle when there is inflammation or blood in the abdomen. Pain receptors are sensitive to multiple stimuli, but they are concentrated at various levels throughout the body. The skin has a higher concentration than the viscera, which makes sense because the skin is the first line of defense for the body.

When tissue is damaged, it releases neurotransmitters such as potassium, leukotrienes, bradykinins, serotonin, histamines, arachidonic acid, thromboxanes, substance P, and platelet activating factor. These chemicals not only play a role in acute pain, but also may be a factor in chronic pain. Prostaglandins are also released but do not directly stimulate nerve endings. Instead, they make the nerve endings more sensitive.[30]

Pain Fibers

The nerve action potentials of the nociceptors are transmitted by two fiber types (Figure 12-1). The myelinated A-delta fibers rapidly transmit the pain impulse (fast pain). This produces a sharp pain sensation. The unmyelinated C fibers are slower (slow pain) and are responsible for the diffuse burning or aching sensation of pain. C fibers also produce throbbing, deep visceral pain and the sensations associated with chronic pain. Both eventually terminate in the dorsal horn of the spinal cord. The majority of these transmissions terminate in the substantia gelatinosa.[46]

Spinal Cord

Many of the afferent fibers synapse with second-order neurons in the dorsal horn. There are three classes of second-order neurons in the dorsal horn. These are projection cells that will relay information to higher brain areas; excitatory interneurons, which relay nociceptive transmissions to other interneurons, other projection cells, or motor neurons involved with local reflexes; and inhibitory interneurons, which will modulate the transmission.[27,30,87] The connection between the cells of the primary- and secondary-order neurons located here compose the "pain gate." This gate postulated in the gate control theory regulates the transmission of pain impulses to the brain. It also helps to explain why many nonpharmacologic methods such as acupuncture and massage can assist in pain management.[46]

There are multiple pathways through the spinal cord that a pain impulse can go along to the brain, primarily the thalamus, which functions as the relay station for pain impulses. Two of these pathways are the neospinothalamic and the paleospinothalamic. The neospinothalamic is the primary pathway for the fast pain fibers. The fibers of this tract cross to the opposite side of the spinal cord and pass upward to the thalamus. This tract transmits the discriminating aspects of pain such as its location, intensity, and duration.[30]

The paleospinothalamic tract transmits the stimuli from the slower C fibers. Not all of these fibers cross over before ascending. The slower fibers make it more difficult to specifically localize pain sensations.[30] Substance P has been identified as the main neurotransmitter associated with slow pain sensations.

The Brain

The third-order neurons located in the thalamus, brain stem, and midbrain project to portions of the central nervous system (Figure 12-2).[46] The sensory homunculus, located on the postcentral gyrus of the parietal lobe, is thought to be involved in the discriminative and cognitive components of pain.[46] The frontal lobe also plays a role in pain perception and interpretation.

The limbic and the reticular tracts respond to pain signals. Stimulation of these areas of the brain will result in arousing the person to the danger, release of stress hormones, and emotional responses to pain.

Pain Modulation

The body has its own intrinsic means of managing pain. This occurs in the pain-inhibitory or antinociceptive response system. Afferent fibers stimulate the periaqueductal gray area, the magnus raphe nucleus, and the pain inhibitory complex in the anterior horn. This allows the body to manage debilitating pain and still survive. The gate control theory has assisted in explaining how pain can be modulated. There are sensory nerves within the dorsal horn that literally can compete with the pain sensory fibers to "modulate" their

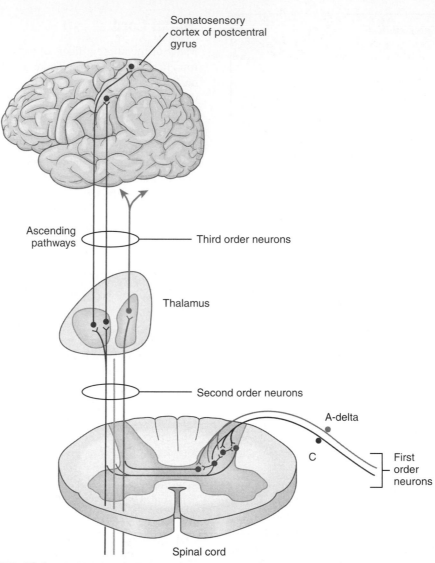

FIGURE 12-1. Nociception pathways. A-delta and C fibers constitute the primary, first-order sensory afferents coming into the gate at the posterior part of the spinal cord. Here we see second-order neurons crossing the cord (decussating) and ascending to the thalamus as part of the spino-thalamic tract. Third-order afferents project to higher brain centers of the limbic system, the frontal cortex, and the primary sensory cortex of the postcentral gyrus of the parietal lobe. (From McCance KL, Huether SE: *Pathophysiology: the biologic basis for disease in adults and children*, ed 5, St. Louis, 2006, Mosby.)

effect. Larger A-beta fibers in the dorsal horn can decrease the amplitude of the afferent pain fibers. This again explains how acupuncture, rubbing an injury, or the use of a topical medication can relieve pain.[30,46] Figure 12-3 illustrates pain modulation.[46]

Another method of modulating pain occurs through inhibitory neurotransmitters or antinociception response. When the nociceptors are stimulated by heat, toxic chemicals, or tissue injury, there is a threshold depolarization or a direct excitation. After the tissue is injured, the inflammatory response can initiate an indirect excitation.

The spinal cord, brain, and other areas of the body produce inhibitory neurotransmitters. Neurotransmitters that contribute to pain modulation, γ-aminobutyric acid (GABA)

and glycine, inhibit pain impulses in the brain and spinal cord. Norepinephrine and serotonin inhibit pain impulses in the medulla and pons.

Endogenous Opioids

The human body also has its own endogenous opioids. Endogenous opioids are neuropeptides that inhibit pain impulse transmission in the brain and spinal cord. The receptor sites for these neurotransmitters are also the sites where exogenously administered opioids act. The four types of opioid neuropeptides are enkephalins, endorphins, dynorphins, and endomorphins. Until the late 1970s with the discovery of these peptides, there was

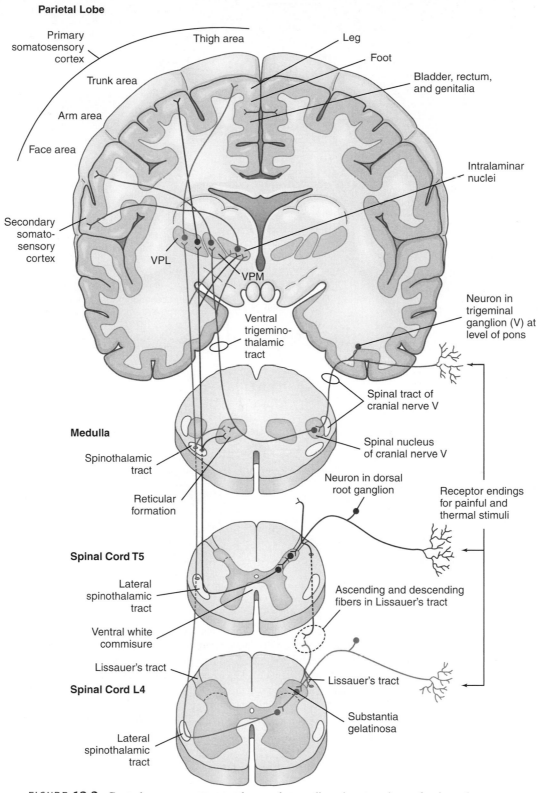

Parietal Lobe

Primary
somatosensory
cortex

Thigh area

Leg

Foot

Bladder, rectum,
and genitalia

Trunk area

Arm area

Face area

Intralaminar
nuclei

Secondary
somato-
sensory
cortex

VPL

VPM

Ventral
trigemino-
thalamic
tract

Neuron in
trigeminal
ganglion (V) at
level of pons

Medulla

Spinal tract of
cranial nerve V

Spinothalamic
tract

Spinal nucleus
of cranial nerve V

Reticular
formation

Neuron in dorsal
root ganglion

Receptor endings
for painful and
thermal stimuli

Spinal Cord T5

Lateral
spinothalamic
tract

Ascending and descending
fibers in Lissauer's tract

Ventral white
commisure

Lissauer's tract

Lissauer's tract

Spinal Cord L4

Substantia
gelatinosa

Lateral
spinothalamic
tract

FIGURE **12-2.** Central nervous system pathways that mediate the sensations of pain and temperature. *VPM,* Ventral posterior medial thalamic nuclei; *VPL,* ventral posterior lateral thalamic nuclei. (From McCance KL, Huether SE: *Pathophysiology: the biologic basis for disease in adults and children,* ed 5, St. Louis, 2006, Mosby.)

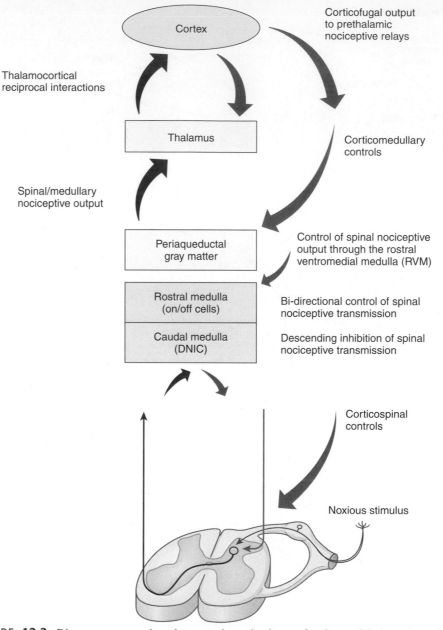

FIGURE 12-3. Diagram representing the central mechanisms of pain modulation. A noxious peripheral stimulus activates both segmental and bulbospinal heterosegmental modulatory mechanisms, which either accentuate or inhibit afferent pain transmission to the brain. The most important and widespread source of top-down (corticofugal) modulation arises from the cortex. Both thalamic and prethalamic nociceptive relays are under the influence of this corticofugal control. The dorsal horn of the spine is also under the influence of the caudal medulla through descending noxious inhibitory control (DNIC). (Modified from Villanueva L, Fields HL: *The pain system in normal and pathological states: a primer for clinicians,* Seattle, 2004, IASP Press. In McCance KL, Huether SE: *Pathophysiology: the biologic basis for disease in adults and children,* ed 5, St. Louis, 2006, Mosby.)

little understanding as to how pain medications work, and research and discovery still continues today. Enkephalins are weaker than endorphins but more powerful than morphine and last longer. Dynorphins will generally impede pain impulses, and endomorphins are primarily antinociceptive.[84]

The specific opioid sites where these neurotransmitters work throughout the body are the mu (μ) (with subtypes μ-1 and μ-2), kappa (κ), and delta (δ). Each of these receptor sites binds differently with distinctive types of opioids.[30,46] Mu receptors inhibit the release of excitatory neurotransmitters. Beta receptors interact with enkephalins to modulate pain impulses. Kappa receptors produce sedation and some analgesia.[23,84] Research has uncovered some other endogenous opioid peptides, as well as additional subtypes to the known opioid sites. A recently discovered opioid peptide is nociception/orphanin-FQ, which resembles the dynorphins.[23]

PAIN THEORIES

Pain is a protective mechanism, and understanding its physiology has led to theories about pain. Three specific theories have been proposed. The first is the gate control theory discussed earlier. Melzack and Wall proposed in 1965 that a "gate" could be opened and closed that would manage pain impulses. This could be done by either pharmacologic (e.g., local anesthetics) or nonpharmacologic (e.g., acupuncture) means that can "close" or slow the pain transmissions through the gate. As discussed previously, the body intrinsically "modulates" pain so that the organism can survive. Research continues to demonstrate the validity of this theory.[25]

René Descartes proposed that injury activates specific pain receptors. This is known as the specificity theory and is particularly useful in explaining acute pain and acute pain management.[25] However, chronic pain and the emotional components of pain cannot be completely clarified using this theory.

Chronic pain has become a common and difficult problem in today's society and EDs. All pain management requires a holistic approach; especially chronic pain.[86] The neuromatrix theory of pain expands the gate control theory to encompass chronic pain. Chronic pain is theorized to be a multidimensional experience caused by patterns of nerve impulses known as signatures. The impulses are generated in the brain by a widely distributed network called the body-self neuromatrix. This neuromatrix includes the individual and his or her feelings, experiences, and genetic predisposition. It is composed of centers and loops of neurons whose synapses are initially genetically determined but can be modified. It can be triggered by sensory inputs from the body or independently trigged by the brain. The output of one's neuromatrix generates the neurosignature pattern of pain. This assists in explaining some forms of chronic pain, such as phantom limb pain, where there is no specific or obvious cause of the pain. It also emphasizes differences in individual pain experiences and the need for individualized management tailored to the patient. Even patients with the same complaint (i.e., acute appendicitis) will not have the same pain experience.[46,64,84,86]

PHYSIOLOGIC CONSEQUENCES OF PAIN

Even though pain plays an important role in warning and protecting humans, it can also have detrimental consequences that must be recognized by the emergency nurse. There are multiple sources of pain that may be experienced by the patient in the ED, for example, physical pain from the illness or injury or pain produced by procedures required to manage the illness or injury. Psychosocial pain is often related to fear or anxiety, which can be caused or augmented by not understanding the ED treatment and separation from one's family. The ED environment can cause pain from such sources as noise from equipment, staff, and bright lighting. A lack of temperature control can cause or exacerbate a patient's pain. Finally, many patients suffer spiritual pain as victims of violence or discrimination when their symptoms are not even considered.

Pain generates many harmful effects on the body. The autonomic nervous system responds to pain by releasing "stress hormones" such as epinephrine and cortisol. These cause vasoconstriction, which may impede healing. The patient's heart rate will increase and cause an increase in cardiac output and oxygen consumption. The patient may splint his or her chest and decrease ventilations, which can lead to reduced pulmonary blood flow. This can contribute to atelectasis, pneumonia, and eventually sepsis and death. Pain can cause muscle contractions, spasms, and rigidity. Unrelieved pain will cause immune system suppression, physical changes, and psychologic injury. Pain can cause suffering.[76]

Pain remains the most common complaint that brings patients to the ED. Emergency nurses need to be familiar with the definitions of pain, its physiology, and its physiologic consequences. Pain must be viewed both holistically and individually so that appropriate compassionate care can be provided.

MYTHS AND BARRIERS TO PAIN MANAGEMENT

Traditionally many myths and barriers have precluded optimal pain management for all patients and include the following: (1) the perception that many patients are addicted to opioids or are drug seeking, (2) disparities in treatment of minorities and women, (3) fear of negative physiologic effects of opioid administration, (4) physician and nurse lack of education regarding pain management, (5) inadequate treatment of high-risk patients (older adults, cognitively impaired patients, non–English-speaking patients, and children), and (6) the belief that physiologic signs such as tachycardia and grimacing are more reliable than patient self-report.[49,60] Myths 2 to 6 will be briefly addressed, and the perception that many patients are drug seeking will be elaborated upon following this introduction to general myths.

Evidence documents that minorities and women receive inadequate analgesic management more frequently than whites and males. This is an important barrier to adequate analgesia in the ED, and emergency nurses can do much to avoid this barrier.[43,79,110] Nurses may be unjustifiably fearful of apnea and hypotension when administering opioids. Selection of the correct age-specific dose and route of analgesic combined with appropriate monitoring will allow nurses to safely administer opioids. Emergency clinicians may lack specific education in pain management. Increased knowledge will result in an increased comfort when providing analgesics and optimize the ability to provide optimal pain management. Emergency nurses should also have a high index of suspicion of unrelieved pain when caring for children, older adults, cognitively impaired patients, and non–English-speaking patients. If these patients present with a chief complaint that is usually associated with pain, emergency nurses should advocate for appropriate analgesic management. Special attention should be paid to age when recommending the selection of analgesic agents. Nonsteroidal antiinflammatory drugs (NSAIDs) should often be avoided in older adults because of their renal and gastrointestinal side effects, and opioid doses should be reduced.[83] An additional ED-specific barrier is the commonly held belief that treatment of pain cannot begin until a diagnosis is made, in particular for patients with abdominal pain and multiple trauma victims. This barrier will be discussed later in the chapter.

"Opiophobia" is likely the most important barrier to adequate pain management in the ED setting. With recent federal attention to the increasing incidence of prescription drug abuse, EDs have been the target of heightened concern, particularly in regard to prescription drug abuse.[50,117] Many emergency nurses and physicians are overly concerned that patients are really addicted to opioids and are drug seeking. This perception results from two facts: (1) the only valid indicator of pain is patient self-report, and nurses must believe the patient; and (2) it is nearly impossible to diagnose opioid addiction in the ED setting. In a study of EDs in Tennessee, 9% of patients tested positive for opioids (urine toxicologic results).[82] This study does not specify how many of these patients were using opioids for pain management. An emergency nurse who assumes a patient is addicted to opioids runs the risk of not treating a patient with pain. The ethical dilemma is clear; nurses will do more harm than good when assuming many ED patients are addicted.

Despite this, some patients with back pain, migraines, and abdominal pain may have frequent visits, and treatment with opioids may or may not be appropriate.[117] Individual care plans were developed in one ED for patients with six or more visits in 1 year with the above-mentioned chief complaints. Of the 45,000 total ED visits in the year the program was initiated, only 124 (0.002%) patients met the criteria.[16] Although the number of ED visits from these patients decreased in the following years of the program, long-term effectiveness for individual patients was not measured, and the "success" of the program cannot be evaluated. However, the use of individual care plans for patients with repeat visits for analgesic management may be beneficial. Individualized plans should be developed in collaboration with the primary care provider, the patient, and the ED staff. In particular, patients with cancer, back pain, headaches, and sickle cell disease may benefit. Establishing a standard care plan that can be easily accessed by emergency clinicians will allow for standardization of care, independent of the individual nurse or physician. The goal of the plans should be to improve patient-reported pain relief, not merely to reduce ED visits.

Definitions of Addiction, Tolerance, Physical Dependence, and Pseudoaddiction

One of the reasons emergency nurses may inaccurately categorize patients as addicted is a misunderstanding of the terms *addiction, tolerance, physical dependence,* and *pseudoaddiction.*[103] It is important to accurately use these terms to avoid further confusion and inappropriate categorization that results in stigmatization of patients. In 2001 the American Society of Addiction Medicine, the American Academy of Pain Medicine, and the American Pain Society recommended the following definitions.[1]

Tolerance

"Tolerance is a state of adaptation in which exposure to a drug induces changes that result in a diminution of one or more of the drug's effects over time." Opioid tolerance causes the need for higher doses to achieve the same analgesic effect in some patients who require chronic opioid use. This may result in the need for very high opioid doses to attain the desired analgesic affect. Tolerance to some side effects develops (e.g., respiratory depression), but not others (e.g., constipation).

Physical Dependence

"Physical dependence is a state of adaptation that often includes tolerance and is manifested by a drug class–specific withdrawal syndrome that can be produced by abrupt cessation, rapid dose reduction, decreasing blood level of the drug, and/or administration of an antagonist." Physical dependence occurs with many drug classes, including opioids, insulin, and beta-blockers; abrupt cessation causes withdrawal symptoms.

Addiction

"Addiction is a primary, chronic, neurobiological disease, with genetic, psychosocial, and environmental factors influencing its development and manifestations. It is characterized by behaviors that include one or more of the following: impaired control over drug use, compulsive use, continued use despite harm, and craving." There is no evidence reporting how many patients seen in the ED are addicted to opioids. As discussed above, it is extremely difficulty to diagnose addiction in the ED setting.

Pseudoaddiction

Pseudoaddiction is a related term and was defined in 1989 by Weissman.[116] Patients with pseudoaddiction exhibit behaviors of addiction (frequently asking for more analgesics or higher doses). These behaviors resolve when pain is adequately treated. Patients are often labeled as "drug-seeking." The treatment for pseudoaddiction is adequate analgesic management. Pseudoaddiction results in a crisis of mistrust between the patient and staff and threatens the ability to provide analgesic management. Pseudoaddiction is probably more common than addiction in the ED setting. Patients with acute exacerbations of pain episodes such as sickle cell disease often request specific opioids and doses. Emergency clinicians often perceive these patients as being addicted to opioids; yet, when other patients are able to report their medications and doses, we categorize these patients as educated.

A better understanding of these definitions can help emergency nurses differentiate between these commonly misunderstood terms, which can ultimately lead to inadequate analgesic management.

ADULT PAIN MANAGEMENT
Patient Expectations

Patients expect pain relief. In a study of adult ED patients with (n = 752) and without (n = 522) pain, patients reported the expectation that their pain would be reduced by 72%, and 18% of patients expected a 100% reduction in pain. There was no difference in expectation related to the severity of pain on arrival, age, or gender.[31,55] Expectations of pain relief between Hispanic and non-Hispanic white ED patients were compared, and no difference in pain-relief expectations was found; most patients expected a decrease in pain scores between 69 and 81 mm using a 100-mm visual analog scale.[55] In another study 48 patients with acute abdominal pain were interviewed; 44% expected complete pain relief while in the ED.[120]

Patients also expect rapid analgesic management. In a single-site study, upon arrival in the ED 620 adult patients were asked to report a "reasonable" time before receiving an analgesic. At discharge they were asked if their pain-relief needs were met and to rate their overall satisfaction with ED care. The average "reasonable" time to initial analgesic reported for the group was 23 minutes and did not vary by chief complaint. Patients who reported having their pain-relief needs met were more satisfied with their overall ED care.[33] In this era that has a strong focus on patient satisfaction, optimal pain management may help improve overall ED patient satisfaction scores. It is clear ED patients expect rapid and aggressive pain management.

Assessment: More Than a Pain Score

It is impossible to provide optimal pain relief without conducting an excellent pain assessment. Pain assessment guides the selection of intervention (pharmacologic versus nonpharmacologic), and reassessment is the key to ultimate pain relief or reduction of pain to meet the patient's desired goal. Pain assessment typically means obtaining a pain intensity score from the patient. The use of pain scales allows for the objective measurement of a subjective state. The numeric rating scale (0 to 10) is the most commonly used scale in the ED and has been validated for use with acute pain in the ED setting.[12] It is sufficient for many but not all adults.[49] Assessment tools should be age appropriate, and special consideration and scales, such as the face, legs, activity, cry, and consolability (FLACC) scale, should be given to assessing patients who are nonverbal. Although many assessment tools exist, it is not the intent of this chapter to review multiple tools but to present core principles of pain assessment. Many multidimensional tools are available and assess dimensions of pain other than pain intensity. Often their use is impractical in the ED setting. However, in addition to assessing pain intensity, the ED nurse should assess the chief complaint, type of pain (acute, chronic, cancer, and end-of-life pain), location of pain, duration, prehospital interventions, patient age, and cultural expression of pain.

Merely recording a pain score in the medical record does not provide pain relief. Nurses must believe the patient and initiate appropriate interventions aimed at reducing pain. A recent study reported that ED nurses underestimate the patient's report of pain. In a single-center study of ED nurses and patients, ED nurses were asked to rate the patients' pain, and nurses scored the patients' pain an average of 2.4 points lower than the patient-reported score.[78] Minimizing the patient-reported pain score may lead to inadequate interventions.

Establishing the link between pain assessment, pain management, and patient outcomes is critical.[34] Several studies have examined the effect of a designated space in the medical record to record a pain score. The impact of recording a pain score on the actual provision of analgesics has been mixed. Nelson et al[70] found a significantly larger proportion of patients received analgesics during the ED visit after a documentation education intervention (25% before and 36% after). In a study of trauma patients with high pain scores, documentation of a pain assessment was associated with a higher rate of analgesic administration (60%) when compared with patients without documentation of a pain score (33%).[93] In another ED, investigators implemented a chart template for nurse practitioners and physicians designed to improve pain assessment. Although documentation of pain assessments using the chart improved from 41% to 57% of patients, no difference in analgesic administration was noted and the number of analgesic prescriptions provided at discharge actually decreased.[7] In summary, documentation of pain scores is important; however, nurses must take the next step and assist in the selection of the appropriate intervention and reassessment of any intervention to make sure optimal pain management has been attained.

Management: Establishing a Pain Management Goal

Establishing the optimal and individualized pain management goal early in the ED visit is important. A pain score of 0 at discharge or reduction in pain score from admission to discharge may or may not be the right goal. Patients should be involved in determining the pain management goal whenever possible. Fosnocht et al[33] examined this issue and recorded arrival and discharge pain scores and asked patients to report overall pain relief during the ED stay. There was no difference in change in pain scores between patients who did and did not report pain relief at discharge. These data demonstrate that a change in pain score alone cannot be used to evaluate the effectiveness of ED pain management.

Although it is critical to involve the patient in the selection of the pain management goal and plan or care, should nurses assume patients will ask for pain medications? Recent data report that 98% of patients with abdominal pain reported pain to either the physician or nurse, but only 33% specifically requested analgesics.[120] Severity of pain intensity scores has also been found to be an unreliable indicator of whether or not patients requested analgesics.[14] These studies demonstrate that assessment cannot consist of recording a pain score alone. Emergency nurses have the opportunity to help establish a pain plan of care by actively engaging the patient in not only determining a pain management goal, but specifically inquiring if a patient would like analgesics.

General Pain Management Principles

The policy "Pain Management in the Emergency Department" written by the American College of Emergency Physicians outlines the following basic principles: pain management should begin rapidly and not be delayed by delays in diagnosis, opioids and nonopioids should be used, safety should be an important consideration, physician and patient education strategies should be developed, and ongoing research should be conducted.[3] These principles address fundamental points to guide pain management.

Nonpharmacologic Approaches

Nonpharmacologic interventions should be used as an adjunct when administering analgesics and, in some cases, may be sufficient in isolation. Some patients with mild pain may not require analgesic administration, and others may refuse analgesics; in one study, up to 15% of ED patients refused pain medications.[102] Many nonpharmacologic interventions are available; some are useful, and others may not be practical for use in EDs without specialized training (e.g., hypnosis). All nurses should be able to facilitate distraction, the use of physical therapies such as positioning and elevation of extremities, and the use of heat and cold therapies. Heat may be useful for chronic pain and patients with sickle cell pain episodes. Ice should always be used for acute pain caused by musculoskeletal injuries and is often useful for pain associated with acute back injuries. Distraction techniques include music therapy, reading materials, and conversation. It is important for emergency nursing leaders to ensure distraction materials are made available and are readily accessible to promote their use. Use of distraction techniques has been found to reduce pain scores in a sample of pediatric patients with minor musculoskeletal trauma, but not for adults.[104,107] In a single-site study, adult patients reported they were satisfied with their pain management and would like to have the option of music distraction in future ED visits, despite no change in pain scores.[107] Nonpharmacologic interventions play an important role in relieving pain for many ED patients.

Pharmacologic Approaches

Pharmacologic interventions are often required to meet the patient's pain management goal. The ED nurse can help suggest the best analgesic agent, dose, and route for the individual patient. The patient's chief complaint, age, medical history, allergies, pain history, and stated pain goal should help determine analgesic interventions.

Analgesics can be administered by several routes including oral, intravenous, subcutaneous, and patient-controlled analgesic pump. The use of intramuscular injections, especially when multiple doses will be required, is discouraged. Intramuscular injections are painful and associated with erratic absorption, tissue damage, and an increased risk for abscess development.[4] When oral analgesics are not sufficient or when the intravenous route is not available, the subcutaneous route should be used.[4] The subcutaneous route has a somewhat slower onset of action than intravenous, but it is equally effective and is commonly used with cancer and palliative care patients. The intravenous route is indicated for patients with severe pain who are receiving opioids, and it has a peak effect of 15 to 30 minutes for most agents.[4] Reassessment of pain and administration of additional doses should occur if the pain goal has not been met in 15 minutes. Although multiple priorities challenge the ED nurse, all efforts should be made to reassess pain 15 minutes after administration of an intravenous or subcutaneous agent and within 60 minutes of administering an oral agent. Additional oral agents cannot be provided for 2 hours after initial dose. Finally, patient-controlled analgesia (PCA) is an excellent method of providing opioid analgesics for patients who may require multiple and frequent doses. PCA provides patients with control over their pain management. Reports of use in the ED are limited. Nurses will require specific training, and the equipment and dosing cartridges should be made available in the department to promote use of PCA as a method of providing analgesia in the ED.

It is also important to select the correct analgesic agent. Acetaminophen, NSAIDs, and opioids are the mainstays of ED pain management. Acetaminophen is useful for the relief of mild to moderate pain without inflammatory components, can be administered orally or rectally, and does not irritate the gastric mucosa.[4] It is also included in many combination oral opioid analgesics, including codeine, oxycodone (Percocet), and hydrocodone (Norco and Vicodin). The maximum daily recommended dose of acetaminophen (4000 mg for normal healthy adults) often limits the number of oral acetaminophen-opioid medications that can be administered within 24 hours. Healthy patients who exceed 4000 mg of acetaminophen within 24 hours are at an increased risk for hepatic toxicity.[4] Emergency nurses have an opportunity to educate patients about the limitations of acetaminophen when patients are discharged with analgesic prescriptions that include acetaminophen.

NSAIDs are a second analgesic category frequently used in the ED setting and are indicated for patients with mild to moderate pain, including pain with an inflammatory component (e.g., sprains and strains). Ibuprofen is most commonly used in these situations. NSAIDS can also be used as adjunct therapy to opioids for patients with severe pain associated with an inflammatory component (e.g., renal colic, acute sickle cell pain episodes, and musculoskeletal trauma). In a systematic review of renal colic patients who received either an opioid or a NSAID, patients who received NSAIDs achieved greater reductions in pain scores.[44] However, NSAIDs alone are often not sufficient to manage renal colic pain. NSAIDs may also allow for administration of a smaller dose of opioid. When intravenous access is established, 15-mg doses of ketorolac (Toradol) may be administered intravenously every 6 hours.[4] Ketorolac can cause acute renal failure in dehydrated patients. All NSAIDs are associated with an increased risk for renal impairment, gastrointestinal bleeding due to inhibition of the enzyme cyclooxygenase (COX), and cardiovascular risks.[4] Careful consideration should be given before administering these agents to either the older adult patient or patients with a preexisting history of renal or gastrointestinal disease. At a minimum, the dose should be reduced for these patients. In 2005 the Food and Drug Administration instructed all manufacturers of NSAIDs to issue a box warning on all agents informing patients of the increased risk for gastrointestinal and cardiovascular complications, especially with long-term use.[113] Finally, NSAIDS have an analgesic ceiling effect, which means that additional doses beyond a certain level will not result in any increase in analgesic affects.

Theoretically, COX-2 selective NSAIDs provide gastrointestinal protection by selectively inhibiting the COX-2 enzyme responsible for inflammation and not inhibiting the COX-1 enzyme, which is protective of the gastrointestinal system. They do not offer renal or liver protection. COX-2 selective agents have been found to be beneficial for patients with osteoarthritis. However, COX-2 inhibitors have been found to be associated with an increased risk for myocardial infarction and stroke.[113] COX-2 selective agents are very expensive and should rarely be used or prescribed in an ED setting.

Opioids are indicated for patients with severe pain, and specific agents can be administered orally (e.g., codeine, hydrocodone, morphine, and oxycodone), intravenously (morphine, fentanyl, and hydromorphone), or by using a PCA pump. Unlike NSAIDS, opioids do not have an analgesic ceiling effect. Oral agents are frequently combined with acetaminophen and are indicated for moderate pain; they are often prescribed at discharge from the ED to help manage pain after discharge. Acetaminophen with codeine is frequently prescribed. Some patients report no pain relief when taking codeine because codeine is a pro-drug and not all persons are able to convert the drug to the active form.[9] Morphine and hydromorphone (Dilaudid) are the primary options for management of severe pain in the ED setting; morphine has traditionally been used as the gold standard. There is a liquid formulation of morphine sulfate (Roxanol) that can be administered sublingually or buccally when no other route is available. In a study by Chang et al[20] ED patients received either morphine 0.1 mg/kg or hydromorphone 0.015 mg/kg, equianalgesic doses. Both agents were found to be equally effective in reducing pain scores.[20] The incidence of nausea, vomiting, hypotension, and respiratory depression were similar for both agents.[20] The most frequent side effect of both agents was nausea and vomiting with up to 19% of subjects reporting these symptoms. ED nurses should be prepared to administer antiemetics to relieve these symptoms. In this study no patients experienced a respiratory rate less than 12 breaths per minute, one patient in each group experienced an

oxygen saturation less than 90%, and no patients required administration of naloxone.[20] The incidence of pruritus was reported less frequently with hydromorphone when compared with morphine.[20] Data support the use of either agent for severe pain in the ED. Nurses should not be concerned about a high incidence of respiratory depression or hypotension when administering opioids. However, nurses should assist with selecting the correct agent, dose, and route when assessing individual patient characteristics (age, mental status, weight, medications, and medical history).

Selection of the appropriate starting dose for morphine and hydromorphone is important. Data from a recent study of ED patients randomized to receive either 0.10 mg/kg or 0.15 mg/kg of morphine sulfate demonstrate no meaningful difference in pain-relief scores and stress the importance of reassessment and individualized dosing.[13] Emergency nurses may be unaware of the dosing and equianalgesic differences between morphine sulfate and hydromorphone dosing. Table 12-3 describes these differences.[58] A typical initial dose for intravenous morphine is 0.10 mg/kg, which equals hydromorphone 0.015 mg/kg in the healthy adult who is less than 60 years of age. For a 70-kg adult, this would roughly equal 7 mg of morphine or 1 mg of hydromorphone. Often nurses are reluctant to administer 7 mg of intravenous morphine but not hesitant to administer 1 mg of intravenous hydromorphone.[20] This phenomenon is most likely due to lack of familiarity with equianalgesic dosing principles and the comfort of believing 1 mg of hydromorphone is much less than 7 mg of morphine. Either dose is safe and should be used as a starting point. Nurses should become familiar and comfortable with hydromorphone administration because it offers an excellent option for treatment of severe pain in the ED setting.

Fentanyl is a third opioid that has specific indications for use in patients with severe pain in the ED. Fentanyl has a rapid onset (1 to 2 minutes) and a short duration of action, up to 60 minutes. It is useful for procedural sedation and short-term pain relief.[9] It may be particularly useful for trauma patients with an altered neurologic status or borderline hypotension because of its limited hemodynamic effect compared with other opioids and its short duration of action. Patients with the potential for altered mental status can be reevaluated in 30 to 60 minutes after the agent has worn off. Fentanyl is administered in micrograms, and 1 mcg/kg is a reasonable starting dose (70 mcg for a 70-kg adult).

Table 12-3. **EQUIANALGESIC DOSE CHART**

Opioid	Equianalgesic Dose (mg)	
	Oral	Parenteral
Morphine	30	10
Hydromorphone	7.5	1.5
Fentanyl	—	0.1
Oxycodone	20	—

From Max MB, Payne R, Edwards WT et al: *Principles of analgesic use in the treatment of acute pain and cancer pain,* ed 4, Glenview, Ill, 1999, American Pain Society.

No discussion of opioids is complete without mentioning meperidine (Demerol). The use of meperidine is discouraged due to its neurotoxic metabolite normeperidine, which is responsible for associated seizures and central nervous system toxicity.[4] Many other agents are available and for most patients equally effective. However, if an individual patient receives pain relief only from meperidine, its use should not be strictly prohibited. These cases should be rare.

Selection of the correct drug, dose, and route will help promote optimal pain management. The key to effective pain management is rapid assessment, treatment, reassessment, and titration of analgesic agents until the patient's pain goal has been met.

Nurse-Initiated Analgesic Protocols

Crowded EDs are the norm and may limit the emergency nurse's ability to provide rapid analgesic management. Crowding also presents an opportunity to implement physician/nurse-developed, nurse-initiated analgesic protocols (NIAPs). Support for NIAPs is evident in the literature.[5,32,97,108] NIAPs allow nurses, in particular triage nurses, to administer analgesics before a physician evaluation. This can promote rapid initial analgesic management[15,32,97]and an overall increase in analgesic use.[32,97] These protocols would be most beneficial for patients with mild to moderate pain who often wait longer for initial physician evaluation because of their lower triage acuity. NIAPs are not a new concept, and emergency nurses from Australia and the United Kingdom are the leaders in this area.[5,36,71]

NIAPs typically include interventions in any of three categories: (1) nonpharmacologic, (2) nonopioid, and (3) opioid. Nonpharmacologic interventions include the use of ice, elevation, and distraction, and these interventions should be encouraged. Nonopioid protocols include ibuprofen and acetaminophen for mild pain.[15,32,97] Protocols that include oral opioids most frequently allow administration of acetaminophen with codeine.[15,36] Other researchers have developed protocols that allow nurses to administer oxycodone with acetaminophen[17,68] or hydrocodone with acetaminophen.[32] Seguin[85] and colleagues developed a NIAP that allowed administration of morphine, hydromorphone, and oxycodone, and Seguin reports that the protocol was rarely used. Inclusion of stronger opioids such as morphine and hydromorphone would not be appropriate for administration at triage (unless it is possible to monitor the patient's response) but would be very appropriate in the treatment areas of the ED when a more thorough nursing assessment and adequate monitoring can occur, but physician assessment may be delayed. Colleagues from Australia have implemented protocols that allow nurses to administer morphine before physician evaluation. They have developed a comprehensive training packet and monitor the effect of the protocols on analgesic management and adverse outcomes. They have reported excellent success.[41,51] Patient satisfaction with NIAP at triage has been investigated, and patients who received interventions at triage aimed at decreasing pain reported being more satisfied with their overall ED care because of the immediate attention to pain relief at triage.[107] Interventions consisted of ice and elevation and either ibuprofen or distraction.

The following barriers to implementation of NIAPs exist: (1) concern over safety, (2) nurses may not follow the protocol, (3) nurse reluctance to use NIAPs, (4) patients will leave without being seen, and (5) "drug-seeking" patients. Concern over the safety of analgesics, in particular opioids, before physician evaluation is a frequent concern; however, data support the safety of this practice.[22,36] Another valid concern is that nurses will not follow the protocol and will expand its use beyond the original intent. Most NIAPs exclude patients with chest or abdominal pain. Fry et al[36] noted nurses did administer an oral opioid to 7 (3%) patients with abdominal pain who were excluded from the protocol; no adverse events occurred. In a very small study, Seguin[85] noted that the guidelines for obtaining vital signs after analgesic administration were not always followed. In the current era of medication safety the strongest argument against NIAPs will most likely be concern over the possibility that patients may leave before physician evaluation and that the "drug-seeking" patient will routinely present to the ED for oral opioids. In a prospective evaluation of 202 patients who received acetaminophen with codeine, 31 (15%) patients left before physician evaluation.[36] Although concern over liability for these patients is valid, many patients leave before physician evaluation, and the risk to patients after receiving an analgesic such as hydrocodone or codeine should be placed in perspective of the many other patients who also leave before physician evaluation. All patients that leave before physician evaluation pose a potential liability. Quality monitoring procedures should be in place to track patients who leave after receiving an oral opioid, and individual patients can be managed appropriately.[17] Institutional policies can state the NIAP will not apply to patients in the future if they at any point leave before physician evaluation.

In summary, NIAPs provide an opportunity to facilitate rapid analgesic management. The development of protocols will require a collaborative approach between emergency physicians, nurses, administrators, and hospital pharmacists. Adequate training, policy development, ongoing quality improvement monitoring, and attention to medication safety will be key elements in maintaining the balance between providing optimal analgesia and preventing abuse potential and adverse outcomes.

Specific Emergency Department Pain Management Challenges

Treating Abdominal and Trauma-Related Pain

Patients with abdominal pain or those with multiple trauma are at high risk for inadequate analgesic management in the ED setting. One of the most pervasive myths and important barriers to providing analgesia in the ED setting has been the inability to provide analgesics to a patient with abdominal pain until a diagnosis was made. This myth originates from the 1987 edition of *Cope's Early Diagnosis of the Acute Abdomen,* yet the more recent 2000 edition refutes this practice.[91,92] The myth has now been refuted with data from multiple studies.[57,80,109] Despite the research, controversy still exists and nurses who desire more information are referred to a 2006 editorial by Knopp and Dries.[54] Emergency nurses are encouraged to participate in developing protocols to manage abdominal pain with their emergency physician and surgical colleagues.

Multiple trauma patients are also at risk for undertreatment of pain. Recent data report a national increase in the administration of analgesics to patients with long bone fractures.[21,69,81] The only absolute contraindications to analgesic administration are respiratory depression, hemodynamic instability, and coma.[18] Hypotension can be minimized by carefully selecting agents with less negative cardiac effects (e.g., fentanyl), administering agents very slowly, and maintaining intravascular volume.[21] Analgesics should be administered to patients who are paralyzed and intubated because they may be unable to communicate but remain able to feel pain.

Sickle Cell Acute Pain Episodes

Many ED nurses and physicians express frustration and believe patients with sickle cell disease are opioid dependant, despite data to disprove this belief.[72,89,114] Patients with this chronic and often debilitating disease also express frustration with ED care.[59,73,112] Sickle cell disease is associated with many serious pathophysiologic complications (e.g., acute stroke, acute chest syndrome, cholecystitis, chronic hemolytic anemia, iron overload, pulmonary hypertension, end-organ failure, avascular necrosis of the joints, and chronic leg ulcers) and acute pain episodes which at times require ED analgesic management. An increasing frequency of pain episodes is associated with an increased risk for death.[75] Acute pain episodes should be treated as a high priority, and rapid analgesic management should occur.[8,75] The Emergency Severity Index, version 4, five-level triage system specifies patients with an acute pain episode associated with sickle cell disease should be triaged as a high priority, level 2 patient.[39] Despite this, recent data from a multicenter project report only 27% of patients received the correct triage score and patients waited a median time of 90 minutes before receiving an analgesic. There was no difference in time to initial analgesic based on the total number of visits for an individual patient during the 12-month study period.[105] It is possible that emergency clinicians may generalize their experiences with a few individual patients to all patients with sickle cell disease. At this time we do not understand the reasons why some patients with sickle cell disease have more frequent visits than others. It is possible that their disease is more severe, they experience more pain episodes, or other unknown sociocultural factors are responsible.

ED nurses are encouraged to initiate rapid, aggressive analgesic management for patients with an acute pain episode and sickle cell disease.[74] Guidelines recommend administration of intravenous morphine or hydromorphone within 15 minutes of ED arrival.[8] Although this may not be feasible in many cases, 90 minutes far exceeds the analgesia management recommendation. Patients with sickle cell disease represent another population at risk for inadequate analgesic management, and the ED nurse can play a crucial role in maximizing pain relief for these patients.

Health Care Worker–Induced Procedural Pain

Emergency nurses and other health care workers can cause pain by performing procedures including insertion of urethral and intravenous catheters and nasogastric tubes. Data support the topical administration of lidocaine jelly in males, but not females, before urethral catheterization.[90,106] A variety of analgesic approaches have been evaluated to decrease the pain associated with nasogastric tube insertion. The literature supports the use of lidocaine gel administered nasally, atomized nasopharyngeal and oropharyngeal lidocaine, and lidocaine and phenylephrine for the nose and tetracaine with benzocaine spray for the oropharynx.[26,94,118] Finally, nurses have an opportunity to decrease the pain associated with laceration repair by applying a pharmacy-prepared mixture of lidocaine, epinephrine, and tetracaine (LET) at triage. Application of LET is associated with less pain during injection of a local anesthetic.[95] Standing orders for this or similar preparations should exist in all EDs.

Discharge Teaching

Emergency nurses play a key role in providing discharge analgesic teaching. Recent data suggest pain scores at discharge remain moderate.[37,111] Many patients continue to experience pain up to 96 hours after discharge from the ED, and up to 78% of patients reported using the analgesics prescribed at discharge from the ED.[37] Analgesic discharge teaching should include a discussion of analgesic dosing, scheduling, side effects, and when appropriate, the need to avoid additional doses of either acetaminophen or NSAIDs. Patients should always be encouraged to contact a health care provider for unrelieved pain or return to the ED if necessary.

PEDIATRIC PAIN MANAGEMENT

Approximately one third of all ED visits each year are attributed to the care of children.[6] Although some of these encounters are caused by traumatic injuries such as fractures, lacerations, and blunt organ injury, chronic diseases such as cancer, bowel disorders, migraines, and acute exacerbation of diseases such as sickle cell and appendicitis all require developmentally appropriate pain assessment and management.[99] In addition, most of these injuries and disorders require painful and anxiety-provoking diagnostic and management procedures such as venipuncture, heel sticks, lumbar puncture, urethral catheterization, laceration repair, diagnostic imaging, or fracture reduction. As a patient advocate, it is the emergency nurse's responsibility to be knowledgeable and skilled in the use of developmentally appropriate assessment and pain management techniques. Principles of pediatric pain assessment and management are summarized in Table 12-4.

Pediatric-Specific Pain Management Myths and Barriers

Despite research-based advances in pediatric pain management and assessment, myths and barriers continue to influence practice[2,40,45,66,77] One of the most common myths is

---

Table 12-4. PROCEDURAL PAIN ASSESSMENT AND MANAGEMENT GUIDELINES

GENERAL PRINCIPLES:
1. All infants and children experience pain.
2. Failure to manage pain can produce negative short- and long-term effects.
3. Pain that can be predicted (procedural) should be treated prophylactically.
4. Assessment and management should be developmentally appropriate and use nonpharmacologic and pharmacologic interventions in conjunction.

Age	Assessment	Indication	Nonpharmacologic Interventions	Pharmacologic Interventions	Concerns
Newborn and infant (preverbal)	PIPP (Premature Infant Pain Profile): preterm–3 months; and FLACC (face, legs, activity, cry and consolability): 3 months–7 years	Heel sticks, lumbar puncture (LP), venipuncture, circumcision, urethral catheterization, immunizations and injections	Parental involvement; swaddling, touching, positioning, suckling	Oral sucrose drops and pacifier, LMX4, EMLA (eutectic mixture of lidocaine and prilocaine), vapocoolants	• TAC and LET should not be applied to fingertips, toes, or penis • Sucrose not advised in unstable newborns and NPO • Do not use EMLA with history of methemoglobinemia
Preschool (verbal and non-verbal)	FLACC, Oucher Scale, (visual analog scale (VAS), color analog scale (CAS), FACES Pain Scale, Poker Chip Tool	LP, venipuncture, urethral catheterization, diagnostic procedures, laceration repair, immunizations and injections	Parental involvement, blowing bubbles, distraction, play, TV/video, songs, praise, rewards, simple explanations	LMX4, EMLA, vapocoolants, TAC (tetracaine, adrenaline, and cocaine), LET (lidocaine, epinephrine, and tetracaine), S-Caine Patch (lidocaine and tetracaine), lidocaine	• LMX4, EMLA for intact skin only
School-age	Oucher Scale, VAS, CAS, FACES Pain Scale, Poker Chip Tool	LP, venipuncture, urethral catheterization, diagnostic procedures, laceration repair, immunizations and injections	Parental involvement (allow choice for older children), distraction, video games, trivia, deep breathing, music, praise, ice/hot pack	LMX4, EMLA, vapocoolants, TAC, LET, S-Caine Patch, lidocaine	
Adolescent	Self-report, verbal numeric scale, word graphic numeric scale, VAS	LP, venipuncture, urethral catheterization, diagnostic procedures, laceration repair, immunizations and injections	Allow choice of parental involvement, distraction, video games, trivia, deep breathing, guided imagery, music, praise, ice/hot pack	LMX4, EMLA, vapocoolants, TAC, LET, S-Caine Patch, lidocaine, buffered lidocaine, lidocaine iontophoresis	

Data from Bauman BH, McManus JG Jr: Pediatric pain management in the emergency department, *Emerg Med Clin North Am* 23(2):393, 2005; Hatfield L, Messner E, Lingg K: Evidence-based strategies for the pharmacological management of pediatric pain during minor procedures in the emergency department, *Top Emerg Med* 28(2):129, 2006; Mace S: Pain management and procedural sedation in pediatric patients. In Mace S, Durcharme J, Murphy M, editors: *Pain management and sedation,* New York, 2006, McGraw-Hill; and Merkel S, Voepel-Lewis T, Malviya S: Pain assessment in infants and young children: the FLACC scale, *Am J Nurs* 102(10):55, 2002.
NPO, Nothing by mouth.

that infants and children experience less pain than adults and retain no memory of the painful event. Infants are in fact hypersensitive to painful stimuli and exhibit extreme physiologic and hormonal responses to unmanaged pain.[56] This stress response increases oxygen demands and metabolism, delays healing, and contributes to morbidity and mortality.[38] When the pain response during circumcision was evaluated, unanesthetized newborns demonstrated greater pain responses than anesthetized newborns and greater distress during subsequent immunizations 4 to 6 months later.[100,101] Severe pain can lead to posttraumatic stress disorder, affecting future health care encounters as evidenced by avoidance behaviors, disproportionate pain and anxiety responses, nightmares, and needle phobias.[52] If pain is untreated, the ability to adequately manage subsequent painful procedures has been shown to be diminished.[115]

A second commonly held belief is that opioid administration is more dangerous in children and that it interferes with physical examination and diagnosis.[28] Although opioids are used more cautiously in neonates because of immature

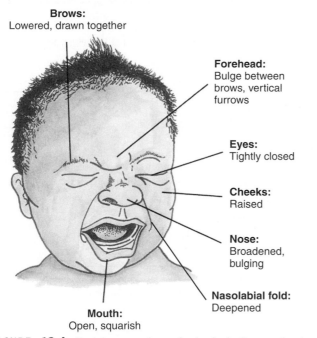

Brows:
Lowered, drawn together

Forehead:
Bulge between brows, vertical furrows

Eyes:
Tightly closed

Cheeks:
Raised

Nose:
Broadened, bulging

Nasolabial fold:
Deepened

Mouth:
Open, squarish

FIGURE **12-4.** Facial expression of physical distress is the most consistent behavioral indicator of pain in infants. (From Hockenberry MJ, Wilson D, Winkelstein ML et al: *Wong's nursing care of infants and children,* ed 7, St. Louis, 2003, Mosby.)

metabolism and clearance, they are safe at smaller doses by continuous infusion.[28,96] By 3 to 6 months of age, infants metabolize and clear opioids at rates similar to older children, and opioid use is no more dangerous in pediatrics than it is in adults.[28] No current research or practice standards endorse the withholding of pain medication before examination and diagnosis.[40] Although myths continue to affect practice, research now clearly demonstrates that pathophysiologic findings do not substantiate these myths. Opioid administration in neonates, infants, and children is safe.

Pediatric Pain Assessment

Anticipating and predicting painful experiences require the use of developmentally appropriate assessments and are paramount to successful pain management in pediatrics.[2] Because pain is a unique, individualized experience, the ED nurse must believe his or her patient's report and take into consideration age, race, gender, culture, cognition, emotions, and past experiences, all of which cannot be captured by any single assessment tool.[6] Although the clinical standard for pain assessment in children is self-report, this standard is limited to verbal, cognitively appropriate children. Figure 12-4 illustrates facial changes that may be observed in the infant in pain. Unidimensional tools such as the Oucher Scale, the visual analog scale, the color analog scale, the FACES Pain Rating Scale (Figure 12-5), and the Poker Chip Tool, have all been validated in ages 3 and above.* A numeric scale (Figure 12-6) may be used with children 5 years of age or above. Multidimensional tools such as FLACC (Table 12-5) and the Premature Infant Pain Profile (PIPP) rely on behavioral and physiologic observations and have been validated multiculturally in nonverbal as well as cognitively impaired infants and children.[6,65]

Pediatric Pain Interventions

Appropriate initial and ongoing assessment directly contributes to successful pain management. Optimal pediatric pain management should employ both nonpharmacologic and pharmacologic interventions whenever feasible. This process should always begin with preparing the child and family for the procedure. Table 12-4 identifies age-specific interventions to be used concurrently for procedural pain.

---

*References 10, 11, 35, 62, 63, 119.

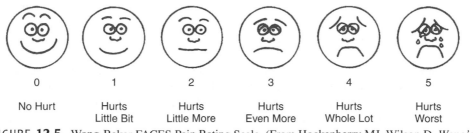

0	1	2	3	4	5
No Hurt	Hurts Little Bit	Hurts Little More	Hurts Even More	Hurts Whole Lot	Hurts Worst

FIGURE **12-5.** Wong-Baker FACES Pain Rating Scale. (From Hockenberry MJ, Wilson D. *Wong's nursing care of infants and children,* ed 8, St. Louis, 2007, Mosby.)

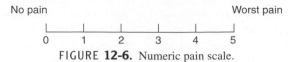

FIGURE **12-6.** Numeric pain scale.

Table 12-5. **FLACC (FACE, LEGS, ACTIVITY, CRY, AND CONSOLABILITY): 3 MONTHS TO 7 YEARS**

Categories	Scoring		
	0	1	2
Face	No particular expression or smile	Occasional grimace or frown; withdrawn, disinterested	Frequent to constant frown, clenched jaw, quivering chin
Legs	Normal position or relaxed	Uneasy, restless, tense	Kicking or legs drawn up
Activity	Lying quietly, normal position, moves easily	Squirming, shifting back and forth, tense	Arched, rigid, or jerking
Cry	No cry (awake or asleep)	Moans or whimpers, occasional complaint	Crying steadily screams or sobs; frequent complaints
Consolability	Content, relaxed	Reassured by occasional touching, hugging, or being talked to; distractable	Difficult to console or comfort

Each of the 5 categories is scored from 0 to 2, resulting in a total score between 0 and 10. Prior to scoring, awake children are observed for 2 minutes, asleep for 5 minutes.

From Markel S, Voepel-Lewis T, Shayevitz J et al: The FLACC: a behavioral scale for scoring postoperative pain in young children, *Pediatr Nurs* 23:293, 1997. © 2002, The Regents of the University of Michigan. Used with permission.

Table 12-6. **PEDIATRIC PROCEDURAL SEDATION RECOMMENDATIONS**

Drug Name	Standard Dose	Maximum Dose
Midazolam	0.05-0.1 mg/kg IV over 2-3 min	Child <5 yr: 6 mg IV/IM Child >6 yr: 10 mg IV/IM
Ketamine	1-1.5 mg/kg IV or IM (slow titration)	Rate of administration should not exceed 0.5 mg/kg/min
Propofol	1-1.5 mg/kg IV (slow titration)	3-3.5 mg/kg
Chloral hydrate	Low dose 25-50 mg/kg PO (may repeat in 30 min) High dose 60-80 mg/kg PO (peaks 30-90 min)	Infant: 1 g Child: 2-2.5 mg/kg

Data from Mace S: Pain management and procedural sedation in pediatric patients. In Mace S, Ducharme J, Murphy M, editors: *Pain management and sedation,* New York, 2006, McGraw-Hill; Custer JW, Rau RE, Johns Hopkins Hospital, Children's Medical and Surgical Center: *The Harriet Lane handbook: a manual for pediatric house officers,* ed 18, Philadelphia, 2009, Mosby.
IM, Intramuscular; *IV,* intravenous; *PO,* by mouth.

Lidocaine, EMLA cream (eutectic mixture of lidocaine and prilocaine), and LMX4 when combined with distraction techniques have been shown to be effective and safe in managing pain associated with vascular access, injections, lumbar puncture, and minor surgical procedures.[19,53] The S-Caine Patch (lidocaine and tetracaine) and buffered lidocaine are effective in diminishing pain associated with vascular access when combined with distraction and music therapy in older children.[88] Vapocoolants have a rapid onset and in combination with distraction are efficient methods of reducing the pain associated with injections and immunizations.[66] Sucrose, along with swaddling, breast-feeding, maternal positioning, and touching have been shown to be as effective in reducing pain associated with heel sticks, vascular access, injections, and urethral catheterization as other therapies for infants up to 3 months of age.[29,98] TAC (tetracaine, adrenaline, and cocaine) and LET (lidocaine, epinephrine, and tetracaine) are topical anesthetics that provide initial pain relief to open wounds requiring irrigation and suturing.[6] These agents should be applied to open wounds for approximately 15 to 20 minutes or until blanching around the edges occurs and before the use of local anesthetic blocks and suturing or irrigation to minimize the pain associated with these procedures. These agents should not be applied to fingertips, toes, or penis or any area with decreased circulation. More complex or lengthy procedures (e.g., diagnostic imaging, fracture reduction, and laceration repair) often cannot be successfully performed with distraction and topical anesthetics alone. Table 12-6 lists common anesthetic and sedative-hypnotic agents and dosages used for procedural sedation.[56]

Table 12-7. PEDIATRIC PHARMACOLOGIC RECOMMENDATIONS FOR MILD TO MODERATE PAIN

Medication	Route	Dose
Acetaminophen	PO	10-15 mg/kg q 4 hr (75 mg/kg/day max)
	PR	First dose 20-40 mg/kg, then same as PO
Ibuprofen	PO	4-10 mg/kg q 6 hr
Ketorolac (age >2 yr)	IV	0.5 mg/kg to max 15 mg single dose
	IM	1 mg/kg to max 30 mg single dose

Data from Bauman BH, McManus JG Jr: Pediatric pain management in the emergency department, *Emerg Med Clin North Am* 23(2):393, 2005.
IM, Intramuscular; *IV,* intravenous; *PO,* by mouth; *PR,* by rectum.

Table 12-8. PEDIATRIC PHARMACOLOGIC RECOMMENDATIONS FOR MODERATE TO SEVERE PAIN

Medication	Route	Dose for Child <50 kg	Dose for Child >50 kg
Codeine	PO	0.5-1 mg/kg q 3-4 hr	30-60 mg q 3-4 hr
Oxycodone	PO	0.1-0.2 mg/kg q 3-4 hr	5-10 mg q 3-4 hr
Hydrocodone	PO	0.05-0.2 mg/kg q 4-6 hr	5-10 mg q 4-6 hr
Morphine	IV/subcutaneous	0.1 mg/kg q 2-4 hr	5-8 mg q 2-4 hr
Fentanyl	IV/subcutaneous	0.5-1 mcg/kg q 1-2 hr	25-50 mcg q 1-2 hr
Hydromorphone	IV/subcutaneous	0.02 mg/kg q 2-4 hr	1 mg q 2-4 hr

Data from Bauman BH, McManus JG Jr: Pediatric pain management in the emergency department, *Emerg Med Clin North Am* 23(2):393, 2005.
IV, Intravenous; *PO,* by mouth.

Nonopioids, including acetaminophen and NSAIDs such as ibuprofen and ketorolac, provide excellent relief for mild to moderate pain (Table 12-7). Oral opioids such as codeine, oxycodone, and hydrocodone are often required to manage moderate to severe pain.[42] Morphine and fentanyl are excellent choices for treating severe pain.[6,42] Table 12-8 suggests routes and doses for these agents.[6] Children and infants are at the same risk for respiratory depression and apnea as adults. These risks can be greatly diminished by careful dose and rate selection and appropriate ongoing assessment and monitoring.[56]

In addition to the variety of pharmacologic interventions, nonpharmacologic interventions should be combined with pharmacologic interventions to help optimize pain relief for all pediatric patients with pain in the ED setting. Table 12-4 suggests possible age-specific, nonpharmacologic techniques.

SUMMARY

From a greater understanding of pain pathophysiology specific to adults and children, to validated multidimensional assessment tools, to cutting-edge pharmacologic and non-pharmacologic interventions, the opportunity for today's emergency nurse to provide safe and effective pain relief to both adult and pediatric patients is enormous. Emergency nurses can lead a culture change and optimize excellent pain management for all of our patients. This can be facilitated by increasing and promoting education specific to pain, using current research to guide practice, serving as a patient advocate, and always maintaining an active voice.

REFERENCES

1. American Academy of Pain Medicine, American Pain Society and American Society for Addiction Medicine *Definitions related to the use of opioids for the treatment of pain: consensus document from the American Academy of Pain Medicine, the American Pain Society, and the American Society of Addiction Medicine,* 2001.
2. American Academy of Pediatrics, Committee on Psychological Aspects of Child and Family Health: The assessment and management of acute pain in infants, children, and adolescents, *Pediatrics* 108(3):793, 2001.
3. American College of Emergency Physicians: *Pain management in the emergency departments.* Retrieved September 22, 2007, from http://www.acep.org/practres.aspx?id=29596.
4. American Pain Society: *Principles of analgesic use in the treatment of acute pain and cancer pain,* ed 5, Glenview, Ill, 2003, The Society.
5. Arendts G, Fry M: Factors associated with delay to opiate analgesia in emergency departments, *J Pain* 7(9):682, 2006.
6. Bauman BH, McManus JG Jr.: Pediatric pain management in the emergency department, *Emerg Med Clin North Am* 23(2):393, 2005.
7. Baumann BM, Holmes JH, Chansky ME et al: Pain assessments and the provision of analgesia: the effects of a templated chart, *Acad Emerg Med* 14(1):47, 2007.
8. Benjamin L, Dampier C, Jacox A et al: *Guideline for the management of acute pain in sickle-cell disease, quick reference guide for emergency department clinicians,* Glenview, Ill, 2001, American Pain Society.

9. Berry P, Covington E, Dahl J et al: *Pain: current understanding of assessment, management, and treatments*, Glenview, Ill, 2006, American Pain Society.

10. Beyer JE, Denyes MJ, Villarruel AM: The creation, validation, and continuing development of the Oucher: a measure of pain intensity in children, *J Pediatr Nurs* 7(5):335, 1992.

11. Bieri D, Reeve RA, Champion GD et al: The Faces Pain Scale for the self-assessment of the severity of pain experienced by children: development, initial validation, and preliminary investigation for ratio scale properties, *Pain* 41(2):139, 1990.

12. Bijur PE, Latimer CT, Gallagher EJ: Validation of a verbally administered numerical rating scale of acute pain for use in the emergency department, *Acad Emerg Med* 10(4):390, 2003.

13. Birnbaum A, Esses D, Bijur PE et al: Randomized double-blind placebo-controlled trial of two intravenous morphine dosages (0.10 mg/kg and 0.15 mg/kg) in emergency department patients with moderate to severe acute pain, *Ann Emerg Med* 49(4):445, 2007.

14. Blumstein HA, Moore D: Visual analog pain scores do not define desire for analgesia in patients with acute pain, *Acad Emerg Med* 10(3):211, 2003.

15. Boyd RJ, Stuart P: The efficacy of structured assessment and analgesia provision in the paediatric emergency department, *Emerg Med J* 22(1):30, 2005.

16. Brice M: Care plans for patients with frequent ED visits for such chief complaints as back pain, migraine, and abdominal pain, *J Emerg Nurs* 30(2):150, 2004.

17. Campbell P, Dennie M, Dougherty K et al: Implementation of an ED protocol for pain management at triage at a busy level I trauma center, *J Emerg Nurs* 30(5):431, 2004.

18. Cantees K, Yealy D: Pain management in the trauma patient. In Peitzman A, Rhodes M, Schwab C et al, editors: *The trauma manual*, Philadelphia, 1998, Lippincott-Raven.

19. Carraccio C, Feinberg P, Hart LS et al: Lidocaine for lumbar punctures: a help not a hindrance, *Arch Pediatr Adolesc Med* 150(10):1044, 1996.

20. Chang AK, Bijur PE, Meyer RH et al: Safety and efficacy of hydromorphone as an analgesic alternative to morphine in acute pain: a randomized clinical trial, *Ann Emerg Med* 48(2):164, 2006.

21. Chao A, Huang CH, Pryor JP et al: Analgesic use in intubated patients during acute resuscitation, *J Trauma* 60(3):579, 2006.

22. Coman M, Kelly A: Safety of a nurse-managed, titrated analgesia protocol for the management of severe pain in the emergency department, *Emerg Med* 11(3):128, 1999.

23. Corbett AD, Henderson G, McKnight AT et al: 75 years of opioid research: the exciting but vain quest for the Holy Grail, *Br J Pharmacol* 147(1 suppl):S153, 2006.

24. Cordell WH, Keene KK, Giles BK et al: The high prevalence of pain in emergency medical care, *Am J Emerg Med* 20(3):165, 2002.

25. Cutshall A, Fenske L, Kelly R et al: Creation of a healing enhancement program at an academic medical center, *Complement Ther Clin Prac* 13(4):217-223, 2007.

26. Ducharme J, Matheson K: What is the best topical anesthetic for nasogastric insertion? A comparison of lidocaine gel, lidocaine spray, and atomized cocaine, *J Emerg Nurs* 29(5):427, 2003.

27. Dunajcik L: Chronic nonmalignant pain. In McCaffery M, Passero C, editors: *Pain clinical manual*, ed 2, St. Louis, 1999, Mosby.

28. Emergency Nurses Association: *Emergency nursing pediatric course*, Des Plaines, Ill, 2004, The Association.

29. Evans JC, McCartney EM, Lawhon G et al: Longitudinal comparison of preterm pain responses to repeated heelsticks, *Pediatr Nurs* 31(3):216, 2005.

30. Fink WA Jr: The pathophysiology of acute pain, *Emerg Med Clin North Am* 23(2):277, 2005.

31. Fosnocht DE, Heaps ND, Swanson ER: Patient expectations for pain relief in the ED, *Am J Emerg Med* 22(4):286, 2004.

32. Fosnocht DE, Swanson ER: Use of a triage pain protocol in the ED, *Am J Emerg Med* 25(7):791, 2007.

33. Fosnocht DE, Swanson ER, Bossart P: Patient expectations for pain medication delivery, *Am J Emerg Med* 19(5):399, 2001.

34. Franck LS: A pain in the act: musings on the meaning for critical care nurses of the pain management standards of the Joint Commission on Accreditation of Healthcare Organizations, *Crit Care Nurse* 21(3):8, 2001.

35. Franck LS, Greenberg CS, Stevens B: Pain assessment in infants and children, *Pediatr Clin North Am* 47(3):487, 2000.

36. Fry M, Ryan J, Alexander N: A prospective study of nurse initiated panadeine forte: expanding pain management in the ED, *Accid Emerg Nurs* 12(3):136, 2004.

37. Garbez RO, Chan GK, Neighbor M et al: Pain after discharge: a pilot study of factors associated with pain management and functional status, *J Emerg Nurs* 32(4):288, 2006.

38. Gerik SM: Pain management in children: developmental considerations and mind-body therapies, *South Med J* 98(3):295, 2005.

39. Gilboy N, Tanabe P, Travers D et al: *Emergency Severity Index, version 4: implementation handbook*, Rockville, Md, 2005, Agency for Healthcare Research and Quality.

40. Gradin M, Eriksson M, Holmqvist G et al: Pain reduction at venipuncture in newborns: oral glucose compared with local anesthetic cream, *Pediatrics* 110(6):1053, 2002.

41. Green D, Kelly A, Priestley S et al: *Pain management package WH: Emergency Departments of Western Health, Australia, 2003-2006.*

42. Hatfield L, Messner E, Lingg K: Evidence-based strategies for the pharmacological management of pediatric pain during minor procedures in the emergency department, *Top Emerg Med* 28(2):129, 2006.

43. Heins JK, Heins A, Grammas M et al: Disparities in analgesia and opioid prescribing practices for patients with musculoskeletal pain in the emergency department, *J Emerg Nurs* 32(3):219, 2006.

44. Holdgate A, Pollock T: Systematic review of the relative efficacy of non-steroidal anti-inflammatory drugs and opioids in the treatment of acute renal colic, *BMJ* 328(7453):1401, 2004.

45. Howard RF: Current status of pain management in children, *JAMA* 290(18):2464, 2003.

46. Huether S, Defriez C: Pain, temperature regulation, sleep and sensory function. In McCance K, Huether S, editors. *Pathophysiology: the biologic basis for disease in adults and children*, ed 5, St. Louis, 2006, Mosby.

47. Hwang U, Richardson LD, Sonuyi TO et al: The effect of emergency department crowding on the management of pain in older adults with hip fracture, *J Am Geriatr Soc* 54(2):270, 2006.

48. International Association for the Study of Pain: *ISAP pain terminology*, September 6, 2007, http://www.isap-pain.org/terms-p.html#Pain.

49. Jacox A, Carr D, Chapman C et al: *Acute pain management: operative or medical procedures and trauma*, Clinical practice guideline No. 1, ACHPR publication No. 92-0032, Rockville, Md, 1992, U.S. Department of Health and Human Services, Agency for Health Care Policy and Research.

50. Joranson DE, Ryan KM, Gilson AM et al: Trends in medical use and abuse of opioid analgesics, *JAMA* 283(13):1710, 2000.

51. Kelly AM: A process approach to improving pain management in the emergency department: development and evaluation, *J Accid Emerg Med* 17(3):185, 2000.

52. Kharasch S, Saxe G, Zuckerman B: Pain treatment: opportunities and challenges, *Arch Pediatr Adolesc Med* 157(11):1054, 2003.

53. Kleiber C, Sorenson M, Whiteside K et al: Topical anesthetics for intravenous insertion in children: a randomized equivalency study, *Pediatrics* 110(4):758, 2002.

54. Knopp RK, Dries D: Analgesia in acute abdominal pain: what's next?, *Ann Emerg Med* 48(2):161, 2006.

55. Lee WW, Burelbach AE, Fosnocht D: Hispanic and non-Hispanic white patient pain management expectations, *Am J Emerg Med* 19(7):549, 2001.

56. Mace S: Pain management and procedural sedation in pediatric patients. In Mace S, Durcharme J, Murphy M, editors: *Pain management and sedation*, New York, 2006, McGraw-Hill.

57. Mahadevan M, Graff L: Prospective randomized study of analgesic use for ED patients with right lower quadrant abdominal pain, *Am J Emerg Med* 18(7):753, 2000.

58. Max M, RP, Edwards W et al: *Principles of analgesic use in the treatment of acute pain and cancer pain*, Glenview, Ill, 1999, American Pain Society.

59. Maxwell K, Streetly A, Bevan D: Experiences of hospital care and treatment seeking for pain from sickle cell disease: qualitative study, *BMJ* 318(7198):1585, 1999.

60. McCaffery M, Passero C: Assessment: underlying complexities, misconceptions, and practical tools, In McCaffery M, Passero C, editors: *Pain: clinical manual*, ed 2, St. Louis, 1999, Mosby.

61. McCaig L, Nawar E. *National Hospital Ambulatory Medical Care Survey: 2004 emergency department summary—advance data from vital and health statistics*, Hyattsville, Md, 2006, National Center for Health Statistics.

62. McCormack HM, Horne DJ, Sheather S: Clinical applications of visual analogue scales: a critical review, *Psychol Med* 18(4):1007, 1988.

63. McGrath PA, Seifert CE, Speechley KN et al: A new analogue scale for assessing children's pain: an initial validation study, *Pain* 64(3):435, 1996.

64. Melzack R: From the gate to the neuromatrix, *Pain* (6 suppl) S121, 1999.

65. Merkel S, Voepel-Lewis T, Malviya S: Pain assessment in infants and young children: the FLACC scale, *Am J Nurs* 102(10):55, 2002.

66. Meunier-Sham J, Ryan K: Reducing pediatric pain during ED procedures with a nurse-driven protocol: an urban pediatric emergency department's experience, *J Emerg Nurs* 29(2):127, 2003.

67. Montgomery R, Fink R: Pain management. In Oman K, Koziol-McLain J, editors: *Emergency nursing secrets*, ed 2, St. Louis, 2007, Mosby.

68. Musselman E, Owens I: *Pain protocol for university ED: Indiana University Emergency Department*, Indianapolis, 2006, Clarian Health Partners.

69. Neighbor ML, Honner S, Kohn MA: Factors affecting emergency department opioid administration to severely injured patients, *Acad Emerg Med* 11(12):1290, 2004.

70. Nelson BP, Cohen D, Lander O et al: Mandated pain scales improve frequency of ED analgesic administration, *Am J Emerg Med* 22(7):582, 2004.

71. Overton-Brown P, Higgins J, Bridge P: What does the triage nurse do? *Emerg Nurse* 8(10):30, 2001.

72. Pack-Mabien A, Labbe E, Herbert D et al: Nurses' attitudes and practices in sickle cell pain management, *Appl Nurs Res* 14(4):187, 2001.

73. Philpott S, Mason J, Aisiku I: Patient satisfaction in the emergency department management of acute sickle cell pain, *Acad Emerg Med* 12(5 suppl):1, 2005.

74. Platt A, Eckman JR, Beasley J et al: Treating sickle cell pain: an update from the Georgia comprehensive sickle cell center, *J Emerg Nurs* 28(4):297, 2002.

75. Platt OS, Thorington BD, Brambilla DJ et al: Pain in sickle cell disease: rates and risk factors, *N Engl J Med* 325(1):11, 1991.

76. Prevost S: Relieving pain and providing comfort. In Martin P, Fontaine D, Hudack C et al, editors: *Critical care nursing: a holistic approach*, ed 8, Philadelphia, 2005, Williams & Wilkins.

77. Probst BD, Lyons E, Leonard D et al: Factors affecting emergency department assessment and management of pain in children, *Pediatr Emerg Care* 21(5):298, 2005.

78. Puntillo K, Neighbor M, O'Neil N et al: Accuracy of emergency nurses in assessment of patients' pain, *Pain Manag Nurs* 4(4):171, 2003.

79. Raftery KA, Smith-Coggins R, Chen AH: Gender-associated differences in emergency department pain management, *Ann Emerg Med* 26(4):414, 1995.

80. Ranji SR, Goldman LE, Simel DL et al: Do opiates affect the clinical evaluation of patients with acute abdominal pain? *JAMA* 296(14):1764, 2006.

81. Ritsema TS, Kelen GD, Pronovost PJ et al: The national trend in quality of emergency department pain management for long bone fractures, *Acad Emerg Med* 14(2):163, 2007.

82. Rockett IR, Putnam SL, Jia H et al: Assessing substance abuse treatment need: a statewide hospital emergency department study, *Ann Emerg Med* 41(6):802, 2003.

83. Rupp T, Delaney KA: Inadequate analgesia in emergency medicine, *Ann Emerg Med* 43(4):494, 2004.

84. Schaffler R: Pain management, In Hoyt S, Selfridge-Thomas J, editors. *Emergency nursing core curriculum*, ed 6, St. Louis, 2007, Mosby.

85. Seguin D: A nurse-initiated pain management advanced triage protocol for ED patients with an extremity injury at a level I trauma center, *J Emerg Nurs* 30(4):330, 2004.

86. Serpell M: Pharmacological treatment of chronic pain, *Anaesth Intensive Care Med* 6(2):39, 2005.

87. Serpell M: Anatomy, physiology and pharmacology, *Surgery* 24(10):350, 2006.

88. Sethna NF, Verghese ST, Hannallah RS et al: A randomized controlled trial to evaluate S-Caine Patch for reducing pain associated with vascular access in children, *Anesthesiology* 102(2):403, 2005.

89. Shapiro BS, Benjamin LJ, Payne R et al: Sickle cell-related pain: perceptions of medical practitioners, *J Pain Symptom Manage* 14(3):168, 1997.

90. Siderias J, Guadio F, Singer AJ: Comparison of topical anesthetics and lubricants prior to urethral catheterization in males: a randomized controlled trial, *Acad Emerg Med* 11(6):703, 2004.

91. Silen W: *Cope's early diagnosis of the acute abdomen,* ed 17, New York, 1987, Oxford University Press.

92. Silen W: *Cope's early diagnosis of the acute abdomen,* ed 20, New York, 2000, Oxford University Press.

93. Silka PA, Roth MM, Moreno G et al: Pain scores improve analgesic administration patterns for trauma patients in the emergency department, *Acad Emerg Med* 11(3):264, 2004.

94. Singer AJ, Konia N: Comparison of topical anesthetics and vasoconstrictors vs lubricants prior to nasogastric intubation: a randomized, controlled trial, *Acad Emerg Med* 6(3):184, 1999.

95. Singer AJ, Stark MJ: Pretreatment of lacerations with lidocaine, epinephrine, and tetracaine at triage: a randomized double-blind trial, *Acad Emerg Med* 7(7):751, 2000.

96. Siwiec J, Porzucek I, Gadzinowski J et al: Effect of short term morphine infusion on Premature Infant Pain Profile (PIPP) and hemodynamics, *Pediatr Res* 45(5):69A, 1999.

97. Stalnikowicz R, Mahamid R, Kaspi S et al: Undertreatment of acute pain in the emergency department: a challenge, *Int J Qual Health Care* 17(2):173, 2005.

98. Stevens B, Yamada J, Beyene J et al: Consistent management of repeated procedural pain with sucrose in preterm neonates: is it effective and safe for repeated use over time? *Clin J Pain* 21(6):543, 2005.

99. Suresh S: Chronic and cancer pain management, *Curr Opin Anaesthesiol* 17(3):253, 2004.

100. Taddio A, Goldbach M, Ipp M et al: Effect of neonatal circumcision on pain responses during vaccination in boys, *Lancet* 345(8945):291, 1995.

101. Taddio A, Shennan AT, Stevens B et al: Safety of lidocaine-prilocaine cream in the treatment of preterm neonates, *J Pediatr* 127(6):1002, 1995.

102. Tanabe P, Buschmann M: A prospective study of ED pain management practices and the patient's perspective, *J Emerg Nurs* 25(3):171, 1999.

103. Tanabe P, Buschmann M: Emergency nurses' knowledge of pain management principles, *J Emerg Nurs* 26(4):299, 2000.

104. Tanabe P, Ferket K, Thomas R et al: The effect of standard care, ibuprofen, and distraction on pain relief and patient satisfaction in children with musculoskeletal trauma, *J Emerg Nurs* 28(2):118, 2002.

105. Tanabe P, Myers R, Zosel A et al: Emergency department management of acute pain episodes in sickle cell disease, *Acad Emerg Med* 14(5):419, 2007.

106. Tanabe P, Steinmann R, Anderson J et al: Factors affecting pain scores during female urethral catheterization, *Acad Emerg Med* 11(6):699, 2004.

107. Tanabe P, Thomas R, Paice J et al: The effect of standard care, ibuprofen, and music on pain relief and patient satisfaction in adults with musculoskeletal trauma, *J Emerg Nurs* 27(2):124, 2001.

108. Tcherny-Lessenot S, Karwowski-Soulie F, Lamarche-Vadel A et al: Management and relief of pain in an emergency department from the adult patients' perspective, *J Pain Symptom Manage* 25(6):539, 2003.

109. Thomas SH, Silen W, Cheema F et al: Effects of morphine analgesia on diagnostic accuracy in emergency department patients with abdominal pain: a prospective, randomized, trial, *J Am Coll Surg* 196(1):18, 2003.

110. Todd KH, Deaton C, D'Adamo AP et al: Ethnicity and analgesic practice, *Ann Emerg Med* 35(1):11, 2000.

111. Todd KH, Ducharme J, Choiniere M et al: Pain in the emergency department: results of the pain and emergency medicine initiative (PEMI) multicenter study, *J Pain* 8(6):460, 2007.

112. Todd KH, Green C, Bonham VL Jr et al: Sickle cell disease related pain: crisis and conflict, *J Pain* 7(7):453, 2006.

113. U.S. Food and Drug Administration: *FDA public health advisory: FDA announces important changes and additional warnings for COX-2 selective and non-selective non-steroidal anti-inflammatory drugs (NSAIDS)*. Retrieved September 22, 2007, from http://www.fda.gov/Cder/drug/advisory/COX2.htm.
114. Waldrop RD, Mandry C: Health professional perceptions of opioid dependence among patients with pain, *Am J Emerg Med* 13(5):529, 1995.
115. Weisman SJ, Bernstein B, Schechter NL: Consequences of inadequate analgesia during painful procedures in children, *Arch Pediatr Adolesc Med* 152(2):147, 1998.
116. Weissman DE, Haddox JD: Opioid pseudoaddiction: an iatrogenic syndrome, *Pain* 36(3):363, 1989.
117. Wilsey B, Fishman S, Rose JS et al: Pain management in the ED, *Am J Emerg Med* 22(1):51, 2004.
118. Wolfe TR, Fosnocht DE, Linscott MS: Atomized lidocaine as topical anesthesia for nasogastric tube placement: a randomized, double-blind, placebo-controlled trial, *Ann Emerg Med* 35(5):421, 2000.
119. Wong DL, Baker CM: Pain in children: comparison of assessment scales, *Pediatr Nurs* 14(1):9, 1988.
120. Yee AM, Puntillo K, Miaskowski C et al: What patients with abdominal pain expect about pain relief in the emergency department, *J Emerg Nurs* 32(4):281, 2006.

CHAPTER 13

Family Presence During Resuscitation

Jennifer Kingsnorth-Hinrichs

Patient- and family-centered care is an essential aspect of emergency nursing. Nursing manages care from a holistic approach.[10,22,23] Emergency nursing has recognized the role of the family at the bedside during emergency care and simple procedures. The benefits of a patient- and family-centered care delivery model support family presence during resuscitation as an essential part of providing quality care to patients and families.

Family presence during resuscitation is the essence of family support, allowing family members to benefit from being together during crisis. The family has the opportunity to offer each other and the patient support, alleviate the sense of helplessness, work through the reality of a situation, and potentially be able to share the final moments of a loved one's life. Family presence during resuscitation is not offered in all emergency departments. Emergency nurses must recognize the benefits of family presence during resuscitation and advocate for the option of family presence as the gold standard in all emergency departments.

This chapter will provide an overview of the evidence in support of family presence and outline the benefits of family presence for patient and families, as well as health care professionals. Information on how to implement family presence, education for health care professionals, and the barriers the emergency nurse may encounter during implementation will also be provided in this chapter.

EVIDENCE

In 1982 Foote Hospital in Jackson, Michigan, experienced two events in which family members refused to leave the bedside during the resuscitation of their loved one. Foote Hospital, like most hospitals, had a policy of "no family presence" during resuscitation and took this opportunity to examine their practice. Findings revealed that 72% of families surveyed would prefer to be in the resuscitation room and 71% of staff supported the practice of family presence. In addition, the hospital's Advanced Cardiac Life Support Committee found no difference in resuscitation events regardless of family presence.[11,18] These findings launched a substantial base of research outlining the benefits of family presence during resuscitation.

Following Foote Hospital's lead, other researchers conducted surveys to examine the attitudes of family members toward family presence during resuscitation. Meyers et al[27] conducted a retrospective study on the beliefs of family members (N = 25) who had experienced the death of a loved one in the emergency department. Although none of the families surveyed was present in the resuscitation room, 80% reported they would have chosen to be present and 96% stated families should have the choice. A year later Boie et al[8] surveyed parents' (N = 400) attitudes toward family presence during resuscitation and invasive procedures. Overall, 81% wanted to be present if the child was conscious.[8]

The percentage dropped to 71% if the child was unconscious. If the child was likely to die, 83% of parents wished to be present.

The second phase of research reported the positive effects of family presence on family members. Overwhelmingly studies have proven that families want the option to be present and will choose to be so if family presence is facilitated.[3,6,11,24,25] Foote Hospital surveyed family members who were offered the option of family presence during resuscitation. The majority of families, 94%, stated that after experiencing family presence, they would choose to be present again.[6,29] In these studies, families stated that having knowledge of the care their loved one was receiving, as well as the ability to have the opportunity to provide comfort, assisted with attaining closure.

Multiple studies have demonstrated that family presence has been instrumental in meeting the emotional needs of families.[*] Engaging families in an active role, encouraging the family to touch, talk, support, and soothe the patient, allows the family members to become empowered in the care of their loved one. Studies including perspectives from both families and health care providers conclude that family presence is helpful to the patient, family, and staff.[†]

Post resuscitation evaluation of the effects of family presence has found no traumatic memories for family members.[10,28] Holzhauser et al[20] did find a significant relationship between families who were present during resuscitation and the belief that their presence was beneficial to the surviving patient. In the same study 96% of family members present in the resuscitation room believed that their presence assisted in accepting the outcome of their loved one's illness or injury.[20]

Despite the overwhelming evidence of the benefits of family presence for the patient and family, some health care providers express concern that the resuscitation is too traumatic for family members.[9,11,18,28,34] Robinson et al[34] conducted a study to examine the psychological effect of witnessing the resuscitation of a loved one. Findings included no reported fear of the events in the resuscitation room. Families also stated contentment with the decision to remain present and that grief was eased by sharing the last moments of life with their loved one. Grief scores of the families remaining present were lower than the control group families who did not have the option of family presence.[34]

Studies have been conducted to evaluate the incidents in which family members have interrupted care, have been asked to leave the room, or felt faint/ill. O'Connell et al[31] found that 4% (N = 197) of families were asked to leave the resuscitation room after they had chosen to be present. Reasons for leaving included enhanced provider comfort during intubation (1%), concern about possible child abuse (less than 1%), providing a brief break for emotionally overwhelmed family members or family members displaying inappropriate

behavior (1%), and providing support to an inconsolable family member (1%).[31] Merlevede et al[26] reported that families who left the resuscitation room on their own indicated that they left because of fear of disturbing the treatment of the patient and indicated a sense of remorse.

The patient experience in family presence is limited due to the number of precipitous deaths that occur with cardiovascular resuscitation. Current data reveal a survival rate of less than 17% for in-hospital cardiac and/or pulmonary arrest patients.[32] This limitation elicited a hypothetical survey by Benjamin et al[7] to discern if people wanted to have their loved ones present during resuscitation. This study found that 72% (N = 200) reported that having family present in the room was positive. Other random studies conducted to gather information on the needs of the patients found that over half of those surveyed preferred to have family members present[16,25] and most individuals thought their preferences for family presence should be determined at admission.[16]

Eichhorn et al[12] studied actual patient response to family presence 2 months after the resuscitation event. Findings provided overwhelming support for the benefits the patient felt in having family members present, which outweighed any risk for their family member. Myers et al[28] reported patient themes paralleled those of family members. Patients stated they received comfort in knowing the family member was present and could comfort them and be an advocate for their care. Patients stated they had a right to family presence, indicating that having a family member present assisted in making them a real person to the health care provider.

Numerous "what-if-we-tried-it" surveys of health care workers have been conducted. More than 4,000 nurses, physicians, residents, and other health care providers at medical meetings and professional organizations have been surveyed about hypothetical family presence events. The main themes that have emerged include the following: less than half of the providers favor family presence; nurses (greater than 90%) are more likely to support family presence during resuscitation than physicians (greater than 75%); providers are more likely to support family presence during simple procedures versus resuscitation; an increase in support of family presence exists if there is an identified support person; health care providers who have experienced family presence during resuscitation are more supportive of the practice (63% to 86%); and experienced physicians are more comfortable than those early in their practice.[24,28,30,39]

Benefits to the health care provider have also been reported from actual family presence events. Providers have found that family presence during resuscitation provides the health care worker an opportunity to increase communication with the family,[31] thus enhancing education in real time as interventions unfold. Families are able to obtain a grasp of the situation as they watch the events in the room and the intensity and speed with which the health care providers deliver care, giving the family a sense that everything was done to save the life of their loved one.[11,24,28] Despite the outcome of the resuscitation, health care providers find that families are able to make better decisions and have a better

---

Box 13-1	ORGANIZATIONS THAT SUPPORT FAMILY PRESENCE

Agency for Healthcare Research and Quality (AHRQ)
Ambulatory Pediatrics Association (APA)
American Academy of Pediatrics (AAP)
American College of Emergency Physicians (ACEP)
American College of Surgeons (ACS)
American Heart Association (AHA)
American Pediatric Surgical Association
American Trauma Society (ATS)
Association of Professional Chaplains
Child Life Council
Emergency Nurses Association (ENA)
Maternal and Child Health Bureau
National Association of Children's Hospitals and Related Institutions (NACHRI)
National Association of Emergency Medical Technicians (NAEMT)
National Association of Pediatric Nurse Practitioners (NAPNAP)
National Association of Social Workers
Society for Academic Emergency Medicine (SAEM)
U.S. Department of Health and Human Services

---

understanding of the care that was provided. Litigation against health care providers decreases.[31] There is also support in the literature that family involvement in the resuscitation room affirms the patient's humanity.[28,34] It allows a sense of closure for families of patients who do not survive, allowing them the opportunity to say good-bye.

ORGANIZATIONAL SUPPORT

A significant number of national organizations support family presence during resuscitation. In 1993 the Emergency Nurses Association (ENA) became the first major organization to endorse family presence during resuscitation. Since that time ENA[14] has published interdisciplinary guidelines and educational resources for implementation of family presence during invasive procedures and resuscitation. Since 1993 there have been numerous published guidelines, recommendations, and endorsements of family presence for health care providers. In 2006, 18 national organizations convened to publish the *Report of the National Consensus Conference on Family Presence*.[20] Organizations represented can be found in Box 13-1.

Family presence guidelines have been included in several professional training curricula. ENA has included family presence in the Emergency Nursing Pediatric Course[13] and the Trauma Nursing Core Course.[15] The American Heart Association (AHA) has included information on the option of offering family presence during resuscitation since the *2000 Guidelines for Cardiopulmonary Resuscitation and Emergency Cardiovascular Care* in the Advanced Cardiac Life Support course.[2] The AHA in conjunction with the American

Academy of Pediatrics (AAP) in the Pediatric Advanced Life Support course and the Pediatric Emergency Assessment Resuscitation and Stabilization course,[35] and the AAP and the American College of Emergency Physicians (ACEP) in the Advanced Pediatric Life Support course present the option of offering family presence during resuscitation.

Consistent themes among national professional health care organizations include the following: the patient- and family-centered care philosophy should be instituted with all families; all families should be offered the option of family presence during procedures and resuscitations; an interdisciplinary approach to family presence should be integrated, including use of a designated and trained family presence facilitator (FPF) to guide the family through the experience; structured family presence guidelines, policies, or procedures should be developed before implementation of family presence; provider education should be completed for all staff involved in the resuscitation measures; and additional research is needed.[2]

IMPLEMENTATION

Positive implementation of family presence during resuscitation starts with a person or a group of people who have a commitment to support families during crisis. These champions are knowledgeable about the literature and support family presence during resuscitation and the benefits it can offer. This knowledge assists champions in their ability to influence key stakeholders to develop a well-represented task force that comprises frontline staff and key leadership staff. The task force composition should be interdisciplinary, including but not limited to nursing, social work, physicians, respiratory care, pastoral care, and other disciplines as appropriate. Inclusion of the family will help ensure that the program is designed to meet the needs of the patient and family, ensure that family support resources are identified, and foster greater patient and family satisfaction.

Institutional Assessment

Once a task force or working group is established, an institutional and departmental assessment should be conducted to evaluate factors that will influence the success of the program. This assessment identifies the support for family presence during resuscitation, as well as the barriers and resistance to it. A complete organizational/departmental assessment can be found in the ENA guideline *Presenting the Option for Family Presence*.[13] Important factors in the institutional assessment, along with examples of questions the institution must answer, can be found in Box 13-2.

Assessment results demonstrate an institution's current attitude in respect to the patient- and family-centered care model. These results can dictate an institution's need for guideline development for the family presence experience. Important elements of the guideline should include role delineation of the health care providers and staff; a method to provide psychosocial-spiritual support to families; determining the definition of family; limitation in the number and/or age of family members in the resuscitation room; an assessment of families before, during, and after resuscitation; and a procedure for terminating family presence if necessary.

Family Limitations

Each individual institution must agree on the definition of family within the guideline. Does your institution adhere to the patient- and family-centered care definition, which states a family member is any person who plays a significant role in the family? Or does your institution believe that a family member is a blood relative or legal guardian? Ensuring that all staff understand institutional beliefs will alleviate confusion as to who should be offered the option of family presence.

How many family members should be allowed in the resuscitation room is another pressing question that needs to be addressed in the institutional guideline. To answer this question, an institution must be realistic about the abilities of the FPF to ensure that each person is screened and can continually be assessed for any behavioral cues indicating inability to cope with the situation. Institutions must also look at physical space in the resuscitation room. It is important to recognize that there may be circumstances in which this element of the guideline will have to be evaluated.

The task force must answer the question as to age limit of the family members in the resuscitation room. Does your institution have an existing policy that defines the age of visitors? Are there appropriate resources available for a child to debrief after taking part in a resuscitation event? Again, this is an element in which case-by-case decisions are made.

Roles and Responsibilities

Patient care roles in the resuscitation room should not be affected because family members are in attendance. Nurses, physicians, respiratory therapists, and other health care personnel should continue to provide critical hands-on care to the patient as clinically dictated. Surveys of health care providers illustrate that the quality of care did not change when families were in the room.[19]

The addition of the role of the FPF is a key factor to the success of a program for family presence during resuscitation. The FPF provides direct support to the family. The FPF is responsible for screening the family before entering the resuscitation room, ensuring the resuscitation team is agreeable to family presence, and ensuring that all staff members are aware that family is present. The FPF prepares the family for the sights and sounds within the resuscitation room—preparing the family for what they are about to witness. Only after this is complete does the FPF enter the resuscitation room with the family.

In the resuscitation room the FPF is responsible for providing continued support to the family. The FPF is able to help the family determine where to stand to be close to the patient without interrupting patient care. The FPF explains medical jargon that is overheard, explains procedures that

---

Box 13-2	**ORGANIZATIONAL ASSESSMENT** [42]

ORGANIZATIONAL STRUCTURES AND AUTHORITY

- What is the organizational hierarchy—formal or informal?
- Who is the legitimate authority versus who is truly in power?
- Who is a potential champion in the management structure?
- Mission and Vision of Organization/Department
- Are the mission, vision, and values of the organization consistent with the patient- and family-centered care model?
- Are the mission and vision reflected in management practices? Clinical practices?

CURRENT PRACTICES

- What is the current visitation policy? Are family members visitors?
- Is family participation in care reflected in policy and procedure?
- Are patients and/or families invited to take part in clinical initiatives?
- Are family needs assessed during critical situations? If so, by whom?
- Are patients asked on admission if they prefer to have family presence during critical events? If so, how is this communicated to staff and integrated into the plan of care?

STAFF/PATIENT/FAMILY ATTITUDES AND BELIEFS

- Do the majority of staff support family presence?
- What barriers to family presence have been identified?
- What are the staff concerns related to family presence?

HUMAN AND FISCAL RESOURCES

- Who/what roles are involved in the care of a patient during a resuscitation situation?
- Is family support and/or patient information provided in the same manner 24 hours a day, seven days a week?
- How much time will champions devote to the project? Will other duties be reassigned?
- Is funding available to support staffing needs?

PHYSICAL PLANT LIMITATIONS

- Is there a private waiting room for families in crisis?
- Can treatment areas be set up differently to accommodate family members at the bedside?

RISK MANAGEMENT CONCERNS

- Are there risk management concerns related to family presence?
- If a problem occurs when a family is present, are there any additional procedures related to reporting and follow-up of the incident?

FOLLOW-UP SERVICES

- Is there a bereavement follow-up in process?
- Are staff provided an opportunity for a break following a death or resuscitation event?
- Do staff and management know how to contact the Employee Assistance Program?

---

are occurring, and facilitates answers to questions the family may have. He or she must continually assess the family response to the actions and behaviors within the resuscitation room and intervene if the family becomes overwhelmed.

The FPF must be able to remove a family member if he or she becomes distressed to a point at which care could be compromised. It is essential that the FPF recognize escalation of behavior so removal or intervention to deescalate can occur. This is an essential component to ensuring patient care is not interrupted.

Social work staff and nursing staff are clear choices to fulfill the needs of this role. Pastoral care staff or child life therapists have also been successful, although knowledge of medical jargon can be a challenge requiring education. In order to consistently provide family presence during resuscitation, the team must be cognizant of the resources within an institution and develop a plan that will work at that institution.

Support After Resuscitation

Because only 17% of all patients requiring cardiac resuscitation survive, each facility should have a process in place that assists families after the death of a loved one. The FPF may be able to further assist the family by explaining "next steps," including what they will see and hear and what they can expect when they reenter the room to see their loved one's body. The recommendations should incorporate providing support for the family as they view the body, as well as the importance of time alone for the family. Recommendations should also include letting the family know when it is okay to leave. The support person needs to make sure to provide the family with information on the disposition of the body, including a contact person and phone numbers.[15]

Bereavement follow-up services should be established to support families after a loss. A bereavement program provides for periodic contact with families. A variety of approaches can be used to implement such a program. If not already established, a follow-up process should be included as part of the program for family presence during resuscitation.

Evaluation

It is important to validate the family presence experience through formal evaluation of the guidelines implemented. This evaluation should include representation from the interdisciplinary team, the patient (if appropriate), and the family. This evaluation should include the implementation process outlined in the guidelines, the outcome of the event, and the behavior of the family before, during, and after the resuscitation event.

It is recommended that institutions with a fully implemented family presence program maintain a database of family presence events. Database information that could be collected for a family presence registry is found in Box 13-3.

EDUCATION

Education on family presence during resuscitation must be provided for all disciplines that have the potential to be involved in resuscitation efforts. The level of education will

---

Box 13-3   ELEMENTS FOR FAMILY PRESENCE DATABASE

- Family behavior upon initial screen
- Determination to offer the family presence option
- Families decision to be or not to be present
- Family behavior and coping within the resuscitation room
- Family presence facilitator availability to remain with the family
- Who were the family members in the room? How many family members were in the room?
- Was the family asked to leave the room at any time? Why? Who made the request?
- Outcome of resuscitation and determination of next level of psychosocial-spiritual care

---

depend on the discipline, the department, the level of involvement in the resuscitation, and the level of acceptance. Education should include the following elements:
- The institutional guideline
- Role of the FPF or support person
- Evaluation of the experience
- Advocating for family presence during resuscitation

Advocating for the concept of family presence may be an easy task or a more difficult task, depending on the current attitudes of staff. Early adopters are easy, so education should be targeted to the late adopters, or the staff that need proof the concept will work. Promoting the concept should include literature on the benefits of family presence during resuscitation, including family attitudes; staff attitudes before and after implementation of family presence; and impact on the grieving process. Do not be afraid to address potential barriers to family presence. Many health care providers are concerned about increases in litigation, traumatic ramifications to the family, and interruption of patient care. Use the literature to address the falsity of these barriers. Illustrate the means by which the institutional guideline will ensure that negative outcomes will not occur. Examples of statistics that have a powerful effect on staff include the following:
- Of surveyed families, 98% would choose to be present during resuscitation.[27]
- Greater than 75% of physicians trained in family presence lend support.[24,28,30,38]
- Greater than 90% of nurses trained in family presence lend support.[24,28,30,38]
- Of families present during resuscitation, 94% would choose to do it again.[6,11,28]
- Less than 4% of families are asked to leave the resuscitation room.[24]
- No increase in litigation has been shown.[19,31]

Education on the guidelines will vary depending on the guidelines adopted by individual institutions. All staff with resuscitation roles must be educated about the elements of the guideline and the impact the guideline has upon their roles. It is imperative to the success of the family presence program that all disciplines (physicians [emergency medicine; surgery; anesthesia], nurses, and ancillary staff) have an understanding of the guideline for family presence during resuscitation. Each staff member must be able to verbalize the method by which families will be offered the family presence option. All staff should be aware of the roles and responsibilities of the FPF, including the initial and ongoing assessment of the family and preparing and supporting the family for the resuscitation event. Staff should also understand that the FPF does not provide direct patient care. Staff interested in assuming the role of the FPF should have additional education related to the specific functions of the role. FPFs need to be educated on initial screening of the family, identifying families that meet criteria as outlined in the guideline, and how to present the option of being present during resuscitation. Identification of behavioral signs and physical symptoms of family members requires education. Highlight behaviors, such as hysteria and/or combative behaviors, that deter the FPF from offering family presence. Some cultures are expected to "act out" differently than others, yet this is often interpreted as escalation. Including techniques of de-escalation can be useful, because families may appear emotionally uncontrollable initially, but through interaction with the FPF can eventually regain composure in order to enter the resuscitation room. It must be recognized that different staff roles have expertise in these areas and should be consulted to assist with education. For example, social services staff are skilled at de-escalation and assessment of the family. Case studies of family behavior during crisis, as well as role-playing, are examples of educational techniques that may be used to ensure the practice and competency of FPF staff.

In addition to preparation of the family for the family presence experience, the FPF must have knowledge of medical jargon that may be heard in the resuscitation room, procedures that may be performed, and space available for families to stand. Nurses serving in the FPF role will need little education in the verbiage of resuscitation; however, social workers and chaplains may need extensive review in understanding the events in the resuscitation environment. To determine educational needs, invite a variety of social workers and chaplains into resuscitation rooms to audit the event, noting procedures, verbiage, and equipment that may be unfamiliar. Education can be tailored to the findings of the audit. Institutions may also want to supply the FPF with pocket cards or other resources to use as a quick reference.

Documentation and evaluation of family presence in the resuscitation room by the FPF should be outlined in their education. It is imperative that the documentation reflect the family behavior throughout the family presence experience, starting at the first encounter and ending with the termination of the resuscitation event. Documentation should include the patient outcome of the resuscitation and the next level of care. Documentation of the events will assist in evaluation of the family presence experience. This documentation may also provide a history of family behavior during crisis, lending itself to future family presence options.

SUMMARY

The benefits of family presence extend to the patient, family, and health care provider. As described in the literature, families experience a sense of control when they have the knowledge that appropriate treatment was given to their loved one. It is through family presence that families have the opportunity to support their loved one and have the opportunity to spend the final moments of life with a loved one.

Patients' benefits from family presence parallel family benefits. Patients surviving resuscitation events report that they felt supported by their family member's presence. They felt as if someone in the room actually cared for them and helped the health care team see them as a real person. The benefits to the patient are more difficult to prove because of the limitation of sample size due to death. There remains opportunity for further research on the effects of family presence on both adult and pediatric patients following a resuscitation event. The health care provider benefits in having the satisfaction that the needs of the patient and family were met. Acceptance of family presence across the health care continuum will better meet the needs of the patient and family.

REFERENCES

1. American Heart Association: Guidelines 2000 for cardiopulmonary resuscitation and emergency cardiovascular care, *Circulation* 102(8 suppl):I-1, 2000.
2. American Heart Association: American Heart Association guidelines for cardiopulmonary resuscitation and emergency cardiovascular care, *Circulation* 112(24 suppl):IVI, 2005.
3. Barratt F, Wallis D: Relatives in the resuscitation room: their point of view, *J Accid Emerg Med* 15:109, 1998.
4. Bauchner H, Vinci R, Bak S et al: Parents and procedures: a randomized control trial, *Pediatrics* 98:861, 1996.
5. Bauchner H, Waring C, Vinci R: Parental presence during procedures in an emergency room: results from 50 observations, *Pediatrics* 87:544, 1991.
6. Belanger J, Reed S: A rural community hospital's experience with family-witnessed resuscitation, *J Emerg Nurs* 23(3):238, 1997.
7. Benjamin M, Holder J, Carr M: Personal preferences regarding family members' presence during resuscitation, *Acad Emerg Med* 11:750, 2004.
8. Boie ET, Moore GP, Brummett C et al: Do parents want to be present during invasive procedures performed on their children in the emergency department? A survey of 400 parents, *Ann Emerg Med* 34(1):70, 1999.
9. Chalk A: Should relatives be present in the resuscitation room? *Accid Emerg Nurs* 3(2):58, 1995.
10. Craven R: The effects of illness on family function, *Nurs Forum* 11(2):186, 1972.
11. Doyle CJ, Hank P, Burney RE et al: Family participation during resuscitation: an option, *Ann Emerg Med* 16(6):673, 1987.

12. Eichhorn DJ, Meyers TA, Guzzetta CE et al: During invasive procedures and resuscitation: hearing the voice of the patient, *Am J Nurs* 101(5):48, 2001.
13. Emergency Nurses Association: *Emergency nursing pediatric course (ENPC)*, ed 3, Des Plaines, Ill, 2004, The Association.
14. Emergency Nurses Association: *Presenting the option for family presence*, ed 3, Des Plaines, Ill, 2007, The Association.
15. Emergency Nurses Association: *Trauma nursing core course (TNCC)*, ed 6, Des Plaines, Ill, 2007, The Association.
16. Grice AS, Picton P, Deakin CD: Study examining attitudes of staff, patients and relatives to witnessed resuscitation in adult intensive care units, *Br J Anaesth* 91(6):802, 2003.
17. Hampe SO: Needs of the grieving spouse in the hospital setting, *Nurs Res* 24(2):113, 1975.
18. Hanson C, Strawser D: Family presence during cardiopulmonary resuscitation: Foote Hospital emergency department's nine-year perspective, *J Emerg Nurs* 18(2):104, 1992.
19. Helmer S, Smith S, Dort J et al: Family presence during trauma resuscitation: a survey of AAST and ENA members, *J Trauma* 48(6):1015, 2000.
20. Henderson DP, Knapp J: Report of the National Consensus Conference on Family Presence, *J Emergency Nursing* 32:23, 2006.
21. Holzhauser K, Finucane J, De Vries S: Family presence during resuscitation: a randomized controlled trial of the impact of family presence, *Austr Emerg Nurs J* 8:139, 2006.
22. Institute for Family-Centered Care: Family-centered care: questions and answers, *Adv Fam Centered Care* 5(1):5, 1999.
23. Johnson B: Changing roles of parents in health care, *Child Health Care* 19:234, 1990.
24. Mangurten JA, Scott SH, Guzzetta CE et al: Effects of family presence during resuscitation and invasive procedures in a pediatric emergency department, *J Emerg Nurs* 32(3):225, 2006.
25. Mazer M, Cox L, Capon A: The public's attitude and perception concerning witnessed cardiopulmonary resuscitation, *Crit Care Med* 34(12):2925, 2006.
26. Merlevede E, Spooren D, Henderick H et al: Perception, needs and mourning reactions of bereaved relatives confronted with a sudden unexpected death, *Resuscitation* 61:341, 2004.
27. Meyers TA, Eichhorn DJ, Guzzetta CE: Do families want to be present during CPR? A retrospective survey, *J Emerg Nurs* 24(5):400, 1998.
28. Meyers TA, Eichhorn DJ, Guzzetta CE et al: Family presence during invasive procedures and resuscitation, *Am J Nurs* 100(2):32, 2000.
29. Morse JM, Pooler C: Patient-family-nurse interactions in the trauma-resuscitation room, *Am J Crit Care* 11:240, 2002.
30. Nibert AT: Teaching clinical ethics using a case study: family presence during cardiopulmonary resuscitation, *Crit Care Nurse* 25(1):38, 2005.
31. O'Connell KJ, Farah MM, Spandorfer P et al: Family presence during pediatric trauma team activation: an assessment of a structured program, *Pediatrics* 120(3):e565, 2007.
32. Peberdy MA, Kaye W, Ornato JP et al: Cardiopulmonary resuscitation of adults in the hospital: a report of 14,720 cardiac arrest from the National Registry of Cardiopulmonary Resuscitation, *Resuscitation* 58(3):297, 2003.
33. Powers KS, Rubenstein JS: Family presence during invasive procedures in the pediatric intensive care unit, *Arch Pediatr Adolesc Med* 153:955, 1999.
34. Robinson SM, Mackenzie-Ross S, Campbell-Hewson GL et al: Psychological effect of witnessed resuscitation on bereaved relative, *Lancet* 352(9128):614, 1998.
35. Sacchetti A, Lichenstein R, Carraccio CA et al: Family member presence during pediatric emergency department procedures, *Pediatr Emerg Care* 12(4):268, 1996.
36. Sacchetti A, Paston C, Carraccio C: Family members do not disrupt care when present during invasive procedures, *Acad Emerg Med* 12:477, 2005.
37. Shapira M, Tamir A: Presence of family member during upper endoscopy, *J Clin Gastroenterol* 22:272, 1996.
38. Timmermans S: High touch in high tech: the presence of relatives and friends during resuscitative efforts, *Sch Inq Nurs Pract* 11(2):153, 1997.
39. Wolfram RW, Turner ED: Effects of parental presence during children's venipuncture, *Acad Emerg Med* 3(1):58, 1996.

CHAPTER 14

Organ and Tissue Donation

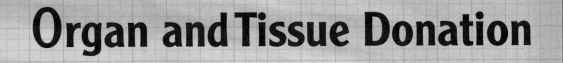

Nancy Bonalumi

Every hour another person in the United States dies because of the lack of an organ to provide a lifesaving transplant. In 2006 more than 97,000 people were on the organ donor waiting list in the United States, but less than 29,000 transplants were performed that year.[7] The number of adult and pediatric candidates for transplantation has increased significantly over the past decade, with adult candidates increasing by 19% and pediatric candidates by 16%.[1] The lack of organs is the result of a lack of organ donors. In 2005 there were 13,091 individuals under the age of 70 who met the criteria for cardiac and brain death and were eligible to be organ donors. Of these, only 58%, or 7,593, became actual donors, providing just over 23,000 organs. Living donors, primarily of kidneys, contributed about 6,800 more organs.[13]

Everyone who is near death or dies in the hospital should be considered a potential candidate for organ donation. There are very few absolute exclusion criteria (e.g., human immunodeficiency virus [HIV], cancer, systemic infection) and no firm upper or lower age limits. In a 2005 survey 95% of respondents indicated they support or strongly support organ donation, and almost 53% had granted permission for donation of organs by either signing a donor card or indicating it on a driver's license.[1] Nearly all respondents (97%) indicated they would donate a loved one's organs if they knew their wishes. Sixty-two percent of survey participants stated they would be a living donor for a family member. Yet, despite the increased public awareness and expressed willingness to support organ donation, the number of people waiting for transplants outgrows potential donors by more than three to one.[5]

Barriers to donation include failure of hospitals to identify potential donors and notify an organ procurement organization (OPO), failure to discuss donation with families, use of requestors who are not knowledgeable about the donation process, and cultural barriers between potential donor families and the medical staff who are discussing donation. Increased focus on identifying potential donors and improving the consent process is needed in all hospitals so that families wanting to donate have that opportunity. Any request for donation must be delivered in the most culturally sensitive and efficacious manner.[1]

In the emergency department (ED) setting it is imperative to determine the potential for donation from patients who have died or whose death is imminent. Emergency nurses have a unique and vital role to play in supporting the decision-making and organ procurement process. The emergency nurses' presence with patients and families during critical moments provides an opportunity to disseminate information, ascertain the patient's or family's wishes, and ensure that those wishes are followed. The emergency nurse should contact the local OPO to ensure that trained designated requestors approach families about donation. Several studies have shown that consent rates are higher when a neutral designated requestor asks for consent. If the ED staff are involved in the request process, families may get the impression that the people caring for their loved one may not be providing appropriate lifesaving care if they are anticipating organ donation.

OVERVIEW AND HISTORY

The first reported medical transplant occurred in the third century. However, significant advances in medical transplantation began early in the twentieth century with the first successful transplant of a cornea (Table 14-1).

Improved surgical techniques and a sequence of three events resulted in transplants becoming a viable option to save and meaningfully extend lives. The first event was the development in the late 1960s of the first set of neurologic criteria for determining death. These criteria allowed persons to be declared dead upon the cessation of all brain activity. The second event, occurring shortly after Dr. Christian Barnard's successful transplant of a heart in November 1967, was the adoption of the first Uniform Anatomical Gift Act in 1968. The most significant contribution of the act was to create a right to donate organs, eyes, and tissue, allowing individuals to donate their or their loved one's organs or tissues. The Uniform Anatomical Gift Act was revised in 1987 and again in 2006 to address changes in circumstances and in practice. The last event was the development of immunosuppressive drugs that prevented organ recipients from rejecting transplanted organs. This permitted many more successful organ transplants, thus contributing to the rapid growth in the demand for organs.[13]

Table 14-1. MILESTONES IN ORGAN AND TISSUE TRANSPLANTATION

Date	Event
1682	Meekran attempted to replace a portion of a soldier's cranium with the skull bone from a dog.
1800	Corneal graft surgery was performed by Wolfe.
1860s	Grahm developed and used a wooden hoop dialyzer to treat renal failure patients.
1881	Skin grafting was tried as a temporary means for treating a severe burn.
1893	Williams attempted transplanting a sheep's pancreas into a human.
1902	Ullman attempted transplanting kidneys in a goat model.
1940s	Sir Peter Medawar treated skin grafts with cold refrigeration; he also worked on immune response and rejection phenomenon.
1940s	Kolft designed the dialysis machine that is the basis for machines used today.
1954	Merrill and colleagues implemented dialysis therapy.
1954	Murray and Harrison performed the first kidney transplantation between living identical twins.
1963	Starzl performed the first liver transplantation.
1963	Hardy performed the first lung transplantation.
1967	Lillehei performed the first kidney and pancreas transplantation.
1967	Barnard performed the first heart transplantation.
1968	Uniform Anatomical Gift Act of 1968 was adopted as law in all 50 states. The law allows the individual to decide to become an organ or tissue donor and introduces the option of donor cards that identify the person's wishes.
1968	*Harvard Criteria for Determination of Brain Death* was published.
1981	Shumway performed the first heart-lung transplantation.
1984	Organ Transplant Act (PL 98-507) was passed.
1986	Report of Organ Transplantation Task Force was published, which led to the development of the United Network for Organ Sharing (UNOS), a private, nonprofit agency that serves as a clearinghouse for organs and tissues.
1986	The United States was divided into 11 UNOS regions with a single organ procurement organization (OPO) designated for each region. Figure 14-1 shows these regions.
1987	Consolidated Omnibus Reconciliation Act of 1986 (PL 99-272) was revised so that hospitals receiving Medicare funding must meet standards for education of patients and staff.
Late 1980s	Uniform Anatomical Gift Act was passed on a state-by-state basis.
1996	Congress authorized mailing organ and tissue donation information with income tax refunds (sent to approximately 70 million households).
1997	National Organ and Tissue Donation Initiative was launched by the U.S. Department of Health and Human Services to increase the number of organs and tissues available for donation. The final rule for organ, tissue, and eye donation for hospitals to participate in Medicare and Medicaid was published.
1998	Final rule for donation took effect, which requires each hospital to contact their OPO in a timely manner about those whose death is imminent or those who die in the hospital. Provisions limit discussion of donation to OPO staff or trained hospital staff.
2002	Up-to-the-minute data on the number of people waiting for organ transplants in the United States became available online through the Organ Procurement and Transplantation Network (OPTN).
2003	Secretary of the U.S. Department of Health and Human Services, Tommy G. Thompson, designated April as National Donate Life Month.

To address the nation's critical organ donation shortage and improve the organ matching and placement process, the U.S. Congress passed the National Organ Transplant Act in 1984. This act established the Organ Procurement and Transplantation Network (OPTN) (http://www.optn.org) to maintain a national registry for organ matching and seeks to ensure the success and efficiency of the U.S. organ transplant system. OPTN responsibilities include facilitating the organ matching and placement process through the use of the computer system and a fully staffed Organ Center operating 24 hours a day; developing consensus-based policies and procedures for organ recovery, distribution (allocation), and transportation; collecting and managing scientific data about organ donation and transplantation; maintaining a secure Web-based computer system containing the nation's organ transplant waiting list and recipient/donor organ characteristics; and providing professional and public education about donation and transplantation and the critical need for donation. Under federal law, all U.S. transplant centers and OPOs must be members of the OPTN to receive any funds through Medicare.[7]

In response to the need for donors, the U.S. Department of Health and Human Services launched the National Organ and Tissue Donation Initiative in December 1997, which required hospitals to work collaboratively with OPOs and mandated hospitals to contact their local OPO in a timely manner about individuals whose death is imminent or who die in the hospital. Only OPO staff or trained hospital staff referred to as designated requestors should approach families about organ donation. A designated requestor is defined in the rule as an individual who has completed a course offered or approved by the OPO.[4]

ORGAN DONATION BEST PRACTICES

The Health Resources and Services Administration launched the Organ Donation Breakthrough Collaborative in 2003 to identify and promote organ donations. The goal is to develop best practices in organ donation so they can be shared by all OPOs and hospitals.[1]

Organizational Structure

Hospitals need to have a strong culture of accountability, with hospital leadership across many levels (administrators, physicians, nurses, etc) participating in organ donation initiatives. A collaborative and integrated relationship between hospitals, local OPOs, transplant centers, and medical examiners' offices is desired. Benchmarking donation rates against local and national levels is encouraged.[1]

Early Referral

Initial identification of potential donors often occurs in the ED setting. Notification of brain death to the local OPO is mandated by the Centers for Medicare and Medicaid Services and is a standard of The Joint Commission. Developing "triggers," such as a low Glasgow Coma Scale score, may assist ED providers with identifying patients at risk for progression to brain death. Early notification of a potential donor gives the local OPO representative adequate time to determine the suitability of the donor and to prepare the family for the request to donate a loved one's organs or tissue.[1]

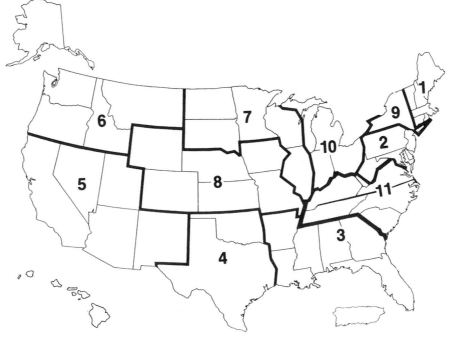

FIGURE **14-1.** United Network of Organ Sharing regional map.

Table 14-2. **COMPARISON OF STANDARD AND PRESUMPTIVE PHILOSOPHICAL APPROACHES TO REQUESTS FOR ORGAN DONATION**

Standard	Presumptive
Requestors act as grief counselors	Requestors are part of the medical team that specializes in organ donation
Requestors view themselves as advocates of the families of potential donors	Requestors view themselves as advocates for both donors and recipients
Requestors use value-neutral language: I'm here to provide you with information about organ donation	Requestors use value-positive language: I'm here to provide you with the opportunity to donate your loved one's organs
The approach is passive: Did you ever discuss organ donation with your loved one?	The approach is active: The overwhelming majority of people in the United States support organ donation and transplantation
Requestors raise the possibility of donation: We will support you in whatever choice you make	Requestors are affirmative about donation: Most people, if given the chance to save a life, will do it
The request for consent is non-presumptive: If you decide to donate…	The request to donate is presumptive: When you decide to donate…

From Zink S, Wertlieb S: A study of the presumptive approach to consent for organ donation, *Crit Care Nurse* 26(2):129, 2006.

Cultural Competence

Information must be provided to families in a culturally sensitive manner. One noted success has been to train requestors who mirror the community population, which reduces cultural and language barriers. Historically, nonwhites donate at a significantly lower rate, but when a requestor of similar ethnic or racial background addresses the family, the donation rate among these groups has increased.[9]

Presumptive Consent

Over the past decade, organ donation rates have been stagnant. Many states have required families to give consent even if the patient has indicated organ donation wishes. Other states assume expressed wishes such as a driver's license designation is consent, and families are not given an opportunity to override that consent. Refusal by families to consent to donation is a major barrier to organ donation. The presumptive approach is based on two philosophical assumptions: (1) most Americans will save a life if the opportunity presents, and (2) organ donation is the right thing to do. This approach is characterized by a shift in the language used by a requestor when addressing the family of a potential donor (Table 14-2).

Historically, requestors use a "value-neutral" approach in which organ donation is described in an unbiased manner. Consent is achieved by overcoming all the objections a family has to the organ donation concept. Presumptivity assumes the person consenting to donation has a desire to help others and to save lives. The benefits of donation are emphasized, and the clinical aspects of donation, which often generate a visceral response in the family, are avoided. Using the presumptive approach, consent to donate is indicated by the family by small affirmations during the course of the conversation. The traditional request for consent often has led to a negative reply simply because the family is unable to make one more decision in an overwhelmingly stressful time. Removing the forcefulness and finality of a traditional request alleviates the pressure on the family. Ongoing research on this method of obtaining consent will determine if this method is successful in increasing the rate of organ donation.[14]

In-House Coordinators

A demonstrated increase in potential donor referrals and actual organ donation has been noted when a local OPO assigns an in-house coordinator to large trauma centers. The role of the in-house coordinator is to be a member of the acute care team and to represent the local OPO. Being on site improves communications, increases the use of standards and audits as tools to improve performance, and allows the coordinator to serve as a liaison between clinical teams, local OPOs, and donor families.[10]

OTHER STRATEGIES TO INCREASE ORGAN DONATION
Living Donor Donation

Although most organ and tissue donations occur after the donor has died, some organs and tissues can be donated while the donor is alive. The first successful transplant in the United States was made possible by a living donor and took place in 1954. A man donated a kidney to his identical twin brother. As a result of the growing need for organs for transplantation, living donations have increased as an alternative to deceased donation, with about 6,000 living donations taking place each year. Most living donations happen among family members or between close friends. Some living donations take place between people unknown to each other.[5] Single kidney donation is the most frequent living donor procedure. Living individuals can donate one of their two kidneys, and the remaining kidney provides the donor with the necessary function needed to remove waste from his or her body. A living donor can donate one of two lobes of his or her liver. This is possible because liver cells in the remaining lobe of the liver grow or regenerate until the liver is almost back to its original size. This regrowth of the liver occurs in a short time in both the liver donor and the liver recipient. It is also possible for living donors to donate a lung or part of a lung, part of the pancreas, or part of the intestines. Although these organs do not regenerate, both the donated portion of the organ and the portion remaining with the donor are fully functioning.[5]

Each potential living donor is evaluated to determine his or her suitability to donate. The evaluation includes both the possible psychologic response and physical response to the donation process. This is done to ensure that no adverse outcome, physical, psychologic, or emotional, will occur before, during, or following the donation. Generally, living donors should be physically fit, in good health, between the ages of 18 and 60, and not have a current or past history of diabetes, cancer, high blood pressure, kidney disease, or heart disease. The decision to be a living donor must be weighed carefully as to the benefits versus the risks for both the donor and the recipient. Often the recipient has very little risk because the transplant will be lifesaving. However, the healthy donor does face the risk of an unnecessary major surgical procedure and recovery. Living donors may also face other risks. A small percentage of donors have had problems with maintaining life, disability, or medical insurance coverage at the same level and rate once donation has occurred. Living donors may also have financial concerns because of possible delays in returning to work due to unforeseen medical problems.[5]

Donation After Cardiac Death

Approximately three out of every four organs that are transplanted are recovered from deceased donors. The most rapid increase in organ recovery from deceased donors is in the category of donation after "cardiac death." This is defined as death declared on the basis of cardiopulmonary criteria (irreversible cessation of circulatory and respiratory function) rather than the neurologic criteria used to declare "brain death" (irreversible loss of all functions of the entire brain).[5]

The process of obtaining organs from donors after cardiac death was common until the 1960s with the development of brain-death criteria. At that time organ procurement and preservation techniques were primitive, and the physiologic functions of organs from brain-dead, heart-beating donors were superior.[1] Given the critical shortage of organs and improved preservation techniques, organ recovery from non-heart-beating donors has reemerged and is known as donation after cardiac death.[1] According to one estimate, at least 22,000 people who die each year of cardiac arrest outside of a hospital could be potential organ donors.[11]

The Organ Procurement and Transplantation Network/ United Network for Organ Sharing (OPTN/UNOS) has developed rules for donation after cardiac death.[6] According to these rules, the process begins with the selection of a suitable candidate and the consent of the legal next of kin before the withdrawal of care and retrieval of organs. Life-sustaining measures are withdrawn under controlled circumstances in the surgical setting. Once the donor is pronounced dead, the organs are then recovered. To avoid obvious conflicts of interest, neither the surgeon nor others involved in the organ procurement can participate in the end-of-life care or declaration of death.[13]

In January 2007 The Joint Commission implemented its first accreditation standard for donation after cardiac arrest. According to this standard, hospitals with the necessary resources must develop donation policies in conjunction with their local OPO that address opportunities for recovery of organs from patients after asystole.[8]

THE DONATION PROCESS

When a patient dies, the local OPO representative determines if the patient is a potential organ or tissue donor. Four key steps must be completed before the retrieval of organs or tissue:

1. Determination and declaration of death
2. Medical examiner's approval (as required by state law)
3. Notification of the local OPO
4. Consent from the next of kin

Determination of Death

Traditionally death was believed to occur when a person's heart stopped beating. As technology evolved, a patient could be maintained on mechanical support devices. Consequently, determination of death by brain-death criteria became a recognized practice. A patient must be declared dead for the donation process to begin. The 1981 Uniform Determination of Death Act defines brain death in the following manner: an individual who has sustained either (1) irreversible cessation of circulatory or respiratory functions or (2) irreversible cessation of all functions of the entire brain, including the brain stem. A determination of death must be made in accordance with accepted medical standards. After death has been determined, it must be documented in the patient's medical record, including the time of death. If the local OPO has not evaluated the patient for suitability as a donor, then required notification is undertaken at this time, before a designated requestor discusses donation with the family.

Eligibility Criteria

Medical criteria that may prevent donation of organs and some tissues from a patient include presence of a documented septicemia, communicable disease such as hepatitis, or possibility that the patient is at high risk for HIV. It is also important to note that those with metastatic cancer are eligible for tissue donation. Almost any person with most forms of cancer, including cancers that have metastasized, is eligible to donate corneas for transplantation or research. Again, the key is to contact the local OPO to determine suitability for donation before discussing donation with the family.

Medical Examiner's Approval

The medical examiner must be notified when a donation takes place under certain circumstances, including the following:
1. Homicide
2. Suicide
3. Accidental death
4. Death within 24 hours of admission
5. Patient is admitted in comalike state and dies
6. Death of a person 18 years of age or less
(Medical examiner regulations vary slightly from state to state.)

Each state has specific criteria. Before these criteria are included in a donation policy, the hospital should contact the state medical examiner for more information. Notation of communication with the medical examiner should be included in the patient's medical record.

Obtaining Consent for Donation

According to the Emergency Nurses Association position statement entitled *Role of the Emergency Nurse in Organ and Tissue Donation,*[3] emergency nurses are often the first to interact with and provide support to families of potential donors as they perform all possible measures to save a patient's life. They are able to "set the stage" for donation consent from family members by establishing and maintaining trust with the families before the declaration of brain death or asystolic arrest.[12] Supporting the family or next of kin in the donation process is one of the more difficult yet potentially rewarding responsibilities that emergency nurses assume in their professional careers. Assisting a family through the donation process offers the family a measure of comfort and consolation. The comfort is not necessarily experienced at the time of the death, but later when the death has been realized. Knowing that their loved one has been able to help another often helps families cope with the loss and continue their lives.

The best person to support the family through donation is a professional who has developed rapport with the family. The person designated to carry out this responsibility should be familiar with the donation process and comfortable with his or her own feelings about death and the donation of tissues and organs. Emergency nurses are in an ideal position to support the family during the process of donation. They have been working with the family and patient throughout the admission and have in most situations developed the greatest rapport with the family.

Physicians, emergency nurses, social workers, and pastoral care providers are all examples of team members that contribute to the donation process. The local OPO representative, designated requestor, and family supporter are key roles in the process. Each hospital, in collaboration with the local OPO, will determine who fills these roles. The person who approaches the family about donation and who provides information about donation to the family must be a trained designated requestor or local OPO representative. The emergency nurse may participate as a supporter or

designated requestor in the process, dependent upon training and hospital protocols. Emergency nurses in supporter roles may need less intense training than individuals in requestor roles. Each institution may have an established protocol for offering donation to a family, and this protocol should be given consideration before proceeding.

Some institutions may have a program in collaboration with the local OPO to train staff members as designated requestors. These requestors, along with the local OPO staff, are the only people who can approach families about their options for donation. The emergency nurse caring for the patient who has just died may not be familiar with the process of donation. The requestor can be a great resource and can assist with the process. The nurse can also talk to the local OPO for support in this matter; a coordinator from the agency can obtain consent from the family in person or over the telephone. Telephone consent requires two witnesses on the phone to confirm donation. An ED education program can be requested concerning the donation process. As discussed earlier, a presumptive approach to requesting organ donation is gaining interest and may lead to increased response rates from potential donor families.

The Impact of Family Presence During Resuscitation on Organ Donation

Many EDs across the United States are offering the option of family presence during resuscitation and invasive procedures. Family presence is most commonly defined as "the presence of family in the patient care area, in a location that affords visual or physical contact with the patient during invasive procedures or resuscitation events."[3] Studies have found that family members who remained with relatives during cardiopulmonary resuscitation (CPR) and invasive procedures reported that the experience removed doubt about what was happening and reinforced that everything possible was done. Family members who do not choose the option to be present during CPR attempts may be more likely to suffer psychologic difficulties during bereavement compared with those who witness unsuccessful resuscitations.[2] The option to be present during a resuscitation should be given to families when the patient's clinical condition indicates the patient may not survive.

Notification of Death

Before the family is made aware of the opportunity to donate organs or tissue, they must be told the patient has died. The family must be comfortable with the knowledge that everything possible was done to prevent death and that all available treatments were implemented. The family's sense of devastation may be extreme; members are grieving and unlikely to believe that death has occurred. Discussion of anything immediately following the discussion of death may be impossible. The family needs time to grieve and to grasp what has happened before they are asked to consider another critical decision.

Patients who survive a critical event may be admitted to a critical care setting where a series of tests are administered to determine that the criteria for brain death have been met. When death is to be declared by brain-death criteria, the family has more time to adjust to the fact that death has occurred. Helping the family understand that death has occurred is difficult. Information must be provided for the family by the primary physician in terms they can understand and must be educationally reinforced by the primary nurse and other available health care professionals.

When the patient in the ED is declared dead by the criterion of cardiac asystole, death is physically more obvious to the family. Grasping the reality of the event is poignant. Death as a result of cardiac arrest is recognized as a tangible end point. Family members have less time to consider possible options or treatments and to adjust to their loss. Donation after cardiac death is an option that should be offered to families in this circumstance.

Emotions can be labile. The family may be in shock, engulfed by many different emotions and feelings. Family members may have had little to do with this particular family member recently or they may feel responsible for the death. Families often ask themselves what could have been done to prevent death or how this death might have been made easier. Before the option of donation is broached, family members should be given time to gain control of their thoughts and adjust, if possible, to the reality that a family member has died and is not going to return.

Family Assessment and Support

If family members are in the ED, they must be provided a private room or location that is comfortable, quiet, and allows those present an opportunity to share feelings of loss and grief. Realizing that the family member is dead is the greatest hurdle the family must overcome. Viewing the body of the person who has just died can be a critical step in this process. A support person such as a chaplain or social worker should be available if the family chooses to view the deceased. Being culturally competent in the beliefs and practices of various religious, racial, and ethnic groups surrounding death is crucial to successfully caring for the family of the deceased.

Assessment of what the family knows or what they have been told is of great importance before offering the option of donation. Until the family can accept that death has occurred, donation should not be discussed. The family must hear the words *death* and *dead* when references are made to the status of its family member. A common error in health care is to refer to the death euphemistically. For example, the nurse may say that the patient "has just expired," "passed on," "will no longer be with us," that "there is no hope," or "it is over." Saying the word *dead* when talking to the family is straightforward and prevents misinterpretation. Because of shock and denial, the family may not comprehend the impact of the message that there is "no hope" for their loved one. This understanding is critical in the case of the family of a patient considered dead by brain-death criteria.

Other goals when assessing the family should include assessment of the family's cultural and religious background and its impact on donation. A decision not to offer donation because of religious and cultural biases based on assumptions about the family's last name and background has no place in the process. The choice belongs to the family.

If a family says no to donation, that response is perfectly reasonable. Donation is not an option for every family or every person. Whatever the decision about donation, it is the right one for that family or person and should be accepted. The emergency nurse's role is to give the family the choice of donation along with the right information about donation and to support the family's decision.

Family Education

The family needs information about donation to decide what is right for the family and what the family member would have wished. Detailed, understandable information is essential. The family should not be coerced into a decision about donation and its benefits, even if using a presumptive approach to consent.

The family needs to know that if they grant permission for donation, the donation will be carried out promptly. A slight chance exists of changes in physical appearance related to incisions required for different donations. The family should know that this causes no disfigurement that would prevent an open casket or alter funeral arrangements. Although it is important to address the topic of disfigurement, it is also very important to discuss the benefits of organ donation as discussed in the section on presumptive consent.

Because there are so few absolute exclusion criteria today, the screening questions families must answer are minimal. Tissue and organ retrieval occur after permission is given by the family and when recovery teams can be arranged to recover the tissue.

Procurement of internal organs and some tissue takes place in an operating suite. Multitissue, multiorgan procurement procedure is usually completed in 4 to 5 hours. The local OPO provides technical staff to recover the eyes, valves, and skin. If the family made special funeral arrangements, they should inform the emergency nurse or donation coordinator of those plans. Eyes may be recovered in the morgue.

A donation coordinator from the local OPO is available for support during any donation process. For most donations of internal organs, the coordinator comes to the hospital to evaluate the patient and meet the family, obtains consent from the family, and coordinates the donation procurement process. In the case of tissue donation only, the coordinator is less likely to be at the hospital but is available for consultation and ensures that necessary support is available. The coordinator works with the emergency nurse, other contact staff at the hospital, and the respective procurement teams.

THE PROCUREMENT PROCESS

Tissue and organ donors are managed differently. The potential organ donor declared brain dead still has a beating heart. Patients who are donors after cardiac death or who are tissue donors have been declared dead and have a non-beating heart. Management of the tissue or organ donor is discussed in the sections below. These patients must be managed carefully to ensure viable tissues and/or organs for transplant. Tissues and organs that can be transplanted are listed in Box 14-1.

Tissue Procurement

Tissue procurement is less complex than internal organ procurement. The coordinator from the procurement agency arranges for arrival of recovery teams and works with nursing staff in the operating suite to set up surgery times and conditions convenient for all parties involved.

Maximum time allowed for recovery of tissue after asystole is approximately 10 hours for bone, 6 to 10 hours for heart valves, and 24 hours for corneas and skin. These time limits may vary, depending on the procurement agency and availability of refrigeration. The preferred time of recovery is that time closest to asystole.

After death the eye donor should be maintained in a refrigerated room if available, with the head elevated at 20 degrees and the eyes taped closed with paper tape. Artificial tears may be instilled in each eye before taping, but this is not mandatory. Cool compresses can be placed over the eyes to prevent swelling and ease the procurement process. Recovery of eyes is a clean procedure using sterile technique and requires only 20 to 30 minutes. The eye tissue is packed in preservative solution; the container is placed on ice and dispatched to the respective eye recovery center for processing. Corneas are generally transplanted within 24 to 48 hours.

For recovery of heart valves, the entire heart is removed from the donor. The valves are dissected from the heart, their integrity examined, and the entire heart examined for pathologic conditions. Serologic examinations are performed,

and after a brief quarantine, usually 40 days, valves are released for homograft transplant according to size and need. The donor has a single incision on the chest that does not prevent an open casket if the family so wishes.

If the process of skin recovery is available in the region, this procedure can also take place in the morgue. A clean room and sterile technique are required. A dermatome is used to recover skin from the buttocks, thighs, back, and abdomen. A split-thickness graft, removed from the top surface of the body, is barely visible unless the donor has a dark tan or is of high pigment. After skin is recovered, it is treated with antibiotics, prepared surgically for grafting, and stored at 70° F. The recovered skin is used for temporary grafts in severely burned patients to provide protection from infection, fluid shifts, and other complications of burns.

Solid-Organ Procurement

Recovery of solid organs for transplant may be complex and requires cooperation of team members representing many different disciplines. Hemodynamic maintenance of the donor is necessary before the procedure. The donation coordinator supports the family and works with the nursing staff to manage the donor until time of the procurement.

After the patient has been accepted as a donor and all organs to be recovered have been assigned to receiving patients, recovery teams convene. The donor is transported to the operating room fully supported by mechanical means and is hemodynamically maintained in the operating room according to goals outlined previously. The donor is maintained throughout the organ dissection and mobilization of the respective tissues until organs and tissues are freed for immediate removal and preservation. Organs are removed from the donor, examined individually in a sterile back basin, flushed with preservative solution, and packed in a sterile container for transport or immediate transplant (in the case of the heart, heart and lung, and single lung). For kidneys, approximately 24 hours may elapse before transplantation takes place. For the pancreas and liver, time to transplant ranges from 6 to 20 hours. Tissue typing is primarily carried out between kidney donor and recipient and in some cases between heart, heart and lung, and single-lung donor and recipient.

FINANCIAL CONSIDERATIONS

The donor's family does not pay for any costs associated with patient management or donation from the time the patient has brain death criteria established through organ procurement. The recipient, third-party insurance, Medicare, or Medicaid pays all costs related to the donation. All charges related to the donation process should be removed from the deceased donor's bill. The local OPO coordinator should inform the family of this during the discussion about consent.

Box 14-1	TRANSPLANTABLE ORGANS AND TISSUES
Tissue	**Organ**
Cornea	Liver
Bone	Kidney
Pancreatic islet cell	Heart
Bone marrow	Pancreas
Ligaments	Intestines
Tendons	
Heart valves	
Skin	
Veins	
Middle ear	

The average cost of transplantation in 2005 ranged from $210,000 for a single kidney to over $800,000 for multiorgan transplants such as liver-pancreas-intestine. Health insurance may cover some or most of these costs, but insurance policies vary widely. Medicare and Medicaid are publicly funded health insurance programs that can help eligible people pay for the costs of transplantation.[14]

SUMMARY

The emergency nurse has significant responsibility related to tissue and organ donation. By contacting the local OPO, emergency nurses provide the family with the opportunity to donate tissue and/or organs when a patient meets the criteria for brain death or dies in the ED. The Emergency Nurses Association position statement *Role of the Emergency Nurse in Organ and Tissue Donation*[3] (http://www.ena.org/about/position) provides additional evidence to support the role of emergency nurses in organ and tissue donation. It is important that emergency nurses be knowledgeable about identification of potential donors, life support of potential donors, and accessing resource personnel from state or local transplant teams. It is within the role of the emergency nurse to facilitate, coordinate, and intervene with families of potential organ donors.

For too long the concept of donation has been associated solely with trauma victims: patients maintained and declared dead by brain-death criteria in the critical care setting. Almost any person who dies can be a donor of some tissue or organ for transplantation. This is an integral part of the emergency nursing care for patients and families in crisis.

REFERENCES

1. Bratton SL, Kolovos NS, Roach ES et al: Pediatric organ transplant needs, *Arch Pediatr Adolesc Med* 160:468, 2006.
2. Clark AP, Aldridge MD, Guzzetta CE et al: Family presence during cardiopulmonary resuscitation, *Crit Care Nurs Clin North Am* 17:23, 2005.
3. Emergency Nurses Association: *Role of the emergency nurse in organ and tissue donation*, 2004. Retrieved August 28, 2007, from http://www.ena.org/about/position.
4. *National Organ and Tissue Donation Initiative*, Washington, DC, 2007, U.S. Department of Health and Human Services. Retrieved August 15, 2007, from http://www.hhs.gov/news/press/1999pres/990519.html.
5. *Organ and tissue donation from living donors*, Washington, DC, 2007, U.S. Department of Health and Human Services. Retrieved August 20, 2007, from http://www.organdonor.gov/transplantation/donation.htm.
6. *Organ donation: opportunities for action*, Washington, DC, 2006, Institute of Medicine. Retrieved August 19, 2007, from http://nap.edu.
7. Organ Procurement and Transplantation Network: *Data*, Richmond, Va, 2007, United Network for Organ Sharing. Retrieved August 14, 2007, from http://www.optn.org/data.
8. Organ Procurement and Transplantation Network: *OPTN/UNOS board addresses protocols for donation after cardiac death, standards for transplant physicians and surgeons*, Richmond, Va, 2007, United Network for Organ Sharing. Retrieved August 28, 2007, from http://www.optn.org/news/newsDetail.asp?id=829.
9. Pietz CA, Mayes T, Naclerio A et al: Pediatric organ transplantation and the Hispanic population: approaching families and obtaining their consent, *Transplant Proc* 36:1237, 2004.
10. Shafer TJ, Ehrle RN, Davis KD: Increasing organ recovery from a level 1 trauma center, *Prog Transplant* 14:250, 2004.
11. Steinbrook R: Organ donation after cardiac death, *N Engl J Med* 357(3):209, 2007.
12. The Joint Commission: *Revised standard regarding procurement and donation of organs and other tissues*, Oak Brook, Ill, 2007. Retrieved August 27, 2007, from http://www.jointcommission.org/Library/ThisMonth/tm_05_07.htm.
13. The National Conference of Commissioners on *Uniform State Laws: Uniform Anatomical Gift Act*, Chicago, 2006. Retrieved August 14, 2007, from http://www.anatomicalgiftact.org.
14. Zink S, Wertlieb S: A study of the presumptive approach to consent for organ donation, *Crit Care Nurse* 26(2):129, 2006.

CHAPTER 15

Palliative and End-of-Life Care in the Emergency Department

OVERVIEW OF PALLIATIVE AND END-OF-LIFE CARE

Palliative care is a comprehensive and specialized way to approach patients and families who face life-threatening or severe advanced illness and focuses on alleviating physical, psychologic, emotional, and spiritual suffering and promoting quality of life.[8] Palliative care emphasizes communication, advanced care planning, and symptom management using a multidisciplinary approach.[16,23] Multidisciplinary palliative care teams include professionals from nursing, medicine, chaplaincy, social services, and psychology and lay volunteers. Palliative care can coexist with disease-modifying interventions and starts with the initial diagnosis of illness or injury continuing through the time of the patient's death and beyond to the survivors in the form of bereavement care. Palliative care is patient and family centered and respects personal, cultural, and spiritual values, wishes, and goals of the patient and family. End of life is a phase in the palliative care trajectory that usually focuses on the care of the person who is imminently dying. Fewer life-sustaining treatments are employed or recommended during the end-of-life phase.

In the emergency department (ED), suffering and death are common. According to the Centers for Disease Control and Prevention, approximately 317,000 persons died in U.S. EDs in 2003.[20] In addition, the ED is a fast-paced, high-stress,

and high-anxiety department where staff make decisions regarding patient care with suboptimal levels of information.[4] The ED is a place of transition where patients receive initial diagnostics and stabilizing treatment and then are transferred out or discharged from the ED. This may give a false impression that the sole focus of the ED is on diagnosis and initial curative treatment, when in fact palliative care is provided to patients to help relieve pain, anxiety, and other distressing symptoms and emotions of patients and families.

Many patients who come to the ED may need palliative care. Patients who present usually have a chief complaint of a symptom such as pain, dyspnea, or nausea. Common presentations of patients who need advanced palliative or end-of-life care include patients with advanced stages of illness such as congestive heart failure, chronic obstructive pulmonary disease (COPD), dementia, and severe trauma. Other patient populations that can benefit from end-of-life care are the family of a sudden infant death syndrome (SIDS) patient or the family of a woman who has miscarried.

We live in a rescue-oriented culture where cardiopulmonary resuscitation and other advanced procedures are routinely employed. However, some patients may not need these aggressive, heroic measures; rather, they may need care-and-comfort measures, especially at the end of life. It is important for the emergency nurse to recognize that some interventions they have at their disposal such as intubation and chest compressions may not be appropriate for patients near the end of life, and careful exploration regarding life goals and expectations for care will help determine what interventions may be appropriate for each situation.

Emergency nurses play a pivotal role in helping formulate an appropriate plan of care that takes into consideration the patient's and family's beliefs and desires while providing only those interventions that are beneficial and appropriate. The Emergency Nurses Association (ENA) has developed a position statement to help emergency nurses provide optimal end-of-life care.[10] Last, it is important to ask the patient, if possible, who is considered to be family. Determining who is considered family allows the nurse to understand who should receive information, be allowed in the treatment area, be consulted to can help make care decisions.[14]

PALLIATIVE CARE PRINCIPLES IN THE EMERGENCY DEPARTMENT

There are many definitions of palliative care. However, common among the various definitions are that palliative care is multidisciplinary, patient and family centered, and includes symptom management; emotional and psychologic care; social care; spiritual/existential care; communication and advanced care planning; and bereavement care for the survivors.[11,16,22,27] Core palliative and end-of-life principles of symptom management, emotional, psychologic, social, and spiritual care will be covered.

Symptom Management

Commons symptoms at the end of life are listed in Box 15-1. It is important for emergency nurses to assess for these symptoms and intervene to reduce their severity. Although all of these symptoms are important, in this chapter the focus will be on the common symptoms seen in the ED such as pain, dyspnea, nausea/vomiting, and constipation.[21]

Nurses must assess and reassess for the presence or improvement of symptoms before and after any intervention. Importantly, many interventions can be viewed as both palliative and therapeutic. For example, if a patient with end-stage congestive heart failure (CHF) comes to the ED with a chief complaint of dyspnea, the nurse may administer furosemide (Lasix) as a palliative treatment to relieve the dyspnea from pulmonary edema. Furosemide is considered more palliative than therapeutic for end-stage CHF and pulmonary edema. Another example is if a patient with end-stage cancer comes to the ED with severe fatigue and dyspnea secondary to anemia, packed red blood cell (PRBC) units may be administered in an attempt to relieve the fatigue and dyspnea. In this example the blood administration is viewed as palliative more than disease modifying because the anemia is a chronic condition that will not be reversed.

Box 15-1	COMMON SYMPTOMS AT THE END OF LIFE
Pulmonary	Dyspnea
	Cough
	Head/nasal congestion
	"Death rattle"
	Respiratory distress/respiratory depression
Neurologic/ Functional	Pain
	Spinal cord compression
	Weakness
	Fatigue
	Immobility
	Insomnia
	Confusion/dementia/delirium
	Memory changes
Gastrointestinal	Nausea/vomiting
	Dysphagia
	Anorexia
	Weight loss
	Unpleasant taste
	Ascites
	Constipation/obstipation/bowel obstruction
	Diarrhea
	Incontinence of bowel
	Hiccups
Urinary	Incontinence of bladder
	Bladder spasms
	Changes in function or control
Integumentary	Decubitus
	Mucositis
	Candidiasis
	Pruritus
	Edema
	Hemorrhage
	Infection (e.g., herpes zoster)
	Diaphoresis
Psychiatric	Depression
	Anxiety
Other	Fever

Modified from Ferrell BR: *HOPE: Home Care Outreach for Palliative Care Education Project,* Duarte, Calif, 1998, City of Hope.

Pain

Pain is defined as an unpleasant sensory and emotional experience associated with actual or potential tissue damage or described in terms of such damage.[12] This definition reflects the multidimensional aspects of pain and takes into consideration the physiologic, emotional and social effects of this symptom. Another commonly cited definition of pain is "pain is whatever the person says it is, experienced whenever they say they are experiencing it."[19] It is important to recognize that pain is a subjective symptom, and self-report is a valid measure of pain. However, in patients who are not able to communicate their pain due to an altered level of consciousness, language barriers, aphasia, or other factors, the patients are considered to be in pain until it is proven otherwise. Because families may spend a significant time with the patient and understand the baseline comfort level, the patient's family may be able to determine if the patient is in pain. The family should be asked by the nurse if they perceive that the patient is in pain or has any other symptom.

A common issue for emergency nurses is understanding the unique characteristics and differences between acute and chronic pain. Commonly patients who have severe acute pain present with behaviors such as yelling, writhing, grimacing, and other visible signs of discomfort. However, patients who have chronic pain (i.e., pain that lasts for weeks to months beyond acute tissue injury) may lack these visible signs of discomfort, yet they experience pain nonetheless. Acute and chronic pain differ significantly, and emergency nurses should continue to believe patients who verbalize they are in pain, regardless of the outward behaviors. It is important to note that patients may be experiencing severe pain and may be able to sleep. This phenomenon can be attributed to exhaustion and is contrary to the commonly held perceptions that pain will stop sleep. Chapter 12 explains pain pathophysiology, assessment, and management in more detail.

Patients who present with adverse side effects of opioids such as oversedation and respiratory depression (respiratory rate less than 8 breaths/min) should receive very small doses of naloxone (Narcan) to reverse the side effects without reversing the analgesic effects. Abruptly reversing both the analgesic and side effects, using naloxone, may precipitate abstinence syndrome, which can cause a range of symptoms, including anxiety, myalgias, tachycardia, hypertension, pulmonary edema, and cardiopulmonary collapse. One method of administering naloxone in patients to reverse the side effects without reversing the analgesia is as follows[7]:

1. Stop opioid administration.
2. Dilute 0.4 mg naloxone (one ampule) with normal saline to a total volume of 10 mL (1 mL = 0.04 mg).
3. Remind the patient to breathe; though narcotized, patients report hearing concerned staff and being unable to open their eyes or respond. Reminders to "take a deep breath" are often followed.
4. Administer 1 mL intravenously (IV) (0.04 mg) every 1 minute until the patient is responsive. A typical response is noted after 2 to 4 mL with deeper breathing and greater level of arousal. Gradual naloxone administration should prevent acute opioid withdrawal.
5. If the patient does not respond to a total of 0.8 mg naloxone (2 ampules), consider other causes of sedation and respiratory depression (e.g., benzodiazepines, stroke).
6. The duration of action of naloxone is considerably shorter than the duration of action of most short-acting opioids. A repeat dose of naloxone, or even a continuous naloxone infusion, may be needed.
7. Wait until there is sustained improvement in consciousness before restarting opioids at a lower dose.

Box 15-2	MODIFIED BORG SCALE	
Scale	**Severity**	
0	No breathlessness* at all	
0.5	Very, very slight (just noticeable)	
1	Very slight	
2	Slight breathlessness	
3	Moderate	
4	Somewhat severe	
5	Severe breathlessness	
6		
7	Very severe breathlessness	
8		
9	Very, very severe (almost maximum)	
10	Maximum	

From Borg G: Psychophysical bases of perceived exertion, *Med Sci Sports Exerc* 14(5):377, 1982.
*The term *breathlessness* was added for clarification of the scale.

Remember, patients may have a respiratory rate of 8 breaths/min while sleeping.

Dyspnea

Dyspnea is defined as a sense of breathlessness or shortness of breath and can be extremely distressing and frightening for both the patient and those who witness it. Many diseases cause dyspnea, including lung diseases such as COPD, pneumonia, and pulmonary embolisms; heart diseases such as congestive heart failure; end-stage renal disease; anxiety; metabolic disorders; anemia; and financial, legal, family, or spiritual issues. Initial management of dyspnea is to focus on the underlying causes and intervene with any disease-modifying treatments as appropriate. However, in some cases, the underlying cause of dyspnea may not be identified. It is important to recognize that dyspnea is a subjective symptom and the treatments need to be tailored to the amount of subjective dyspnea the patient experiences. Objective data such as oxygen saturation (SaO_2) may not correlate with the amount of dyspnea a patient is experiencing.

Assessment of dyspnea can include using a numeric rating scale such as the modified Borg scale. The modified Borg scale is a scale ranging from 0 to 10 and has been validated for use in the ED (Box 15-2). Trending the modified Borg scores will let the nurse know whether the interventions are effective in treating the dyspnea.

There are three pharmacologic approaches used commonly for dyspnea: oxygen, opioids, and anxiolytics. Although opioids and anxiolytics have side effects that include possible respiratory depression and sedation, these medications can be administered with careful titration and monitoring to avoid the adverse side effects. In addition, nonpharmacologic interventions such as positioning the patient, distraction, guided imagery, and the use of a fan to move air across the face have been shown to be effective in managing dyspnea.

Nausea and Vomiting

There are many causes of nausea and vomiting, and these symptoms are frequently seen in the ED. Nausea and vomiting can be effectively managed if the correct medications are chosen based on an accurate assessment of the underlying pathophysiology.

Two organ systems are particularly important in nausea and vomiting: the brain and the gastrointestinal (GI) tract.[8] In the brain the chemoreceptor trigger zone at the base of the fourth ventricle, the cortex, and the vestibular apparatus are areas involved in stimulating nausea and vomiting. In the GI tract the gastric and small intestine linings have chemoreceptors that are responsible for nausea and vomiting.

If stimulated, the neurotransmitters serotonin, dopamine, acetylcholine, and histamine can cause nausea and vomiting. These four neurotransmitters are found in the chemoreceptor trigger zone; however, in the vestibular apparatus, acetylcholine and histamine are predominant. In the GI tract, serotonin is the major neurotransmitter responsible for nausea and vomiting. The cortex is more complex and is not associated with specific neurotransmitters. Knowing the physiology of nausea and vomiting will help the emergency nurse understand which antiemetic might be most helpful in managing the nausea and vomiting.

Dopamine-mediated nausea is the most common form of nausea. Dopamine antagonists are classified into two categories: phenothiazines and butyrophenone neuroleptics. The phenothiazines include medications such as prochlorperazine (Compazine), promethazine (Phenergan), metoclopramide (Reglan), and trimethobenzamide (Tigan). The butyrophenone neuroleptics include haloperidol (Haldol) and droperidol (Inapsine). Both the phenothiazines and butyrophenone neuroleptics have the potential to cause drowsiness and extrapyramidal side effects.

Serotonin antagonists are commonly used in the ED. Often these medications are very effective, especially with chemotherapy-induced nausea, nausea from GI distension, or with nausea that is refractory to other therapies. They are expensive and should be stopped if a short trial does not control the nausea. Medications in this drug category include ondansetron (Zofran) and granisetron (Kytril).

Histamine antagonists may also be used in nausea that may be due to medications such as opioids or chemotherapeutic agents. The histamine antagonists may also have anticholinergic properties as well. Medications in this category include diphenhydramine (Benadryl), meclizine (Antivert), or hydroxyzine (Vistaril or Atarax).

Anticholinergic agents are effective if the nausea is caused by a disturbance in the vestibular apparatus. Medications in this class may be combined with other classes of antiemetics. An example of an anticholinergic medication is scopolamine.

Adjunctive agents that may also be used in combination with the above medications include dexamethasone, tetrahydrocannabinol (THC), and lorazepam (Ativan). The mechanisms of action are unclear but have been proven to be effective in clinical trials.

Constipation

Constipation can be a very painful and distressing symptom with many causes. With opioid use, many symptoms decrease with long-term use except for constipation. Therefore a bowel regimen should be in place for all patients receiving opioids. Prevention of constipation is the best strategy in managing constipation.

The most helpful class of medications for constipation is the stimulant laxatives. Stimulant laxatives increase the peristaltic activity of the GI tract. Agents in this class include prune juice, senna preparations, and bisacodyl. Osmotic laxatives draw water into the bowel lumen, thereby increasing the stool volume and the moisture content in the stool. Medications in this class include milk of magnesia, magnesium citrate, and lactulose. Detergent laxatives, also known as stool softeners, increase the water content in the stool and facilitate the dissolution of fat in water, increasing the stool volume. Medications in this class include sodium docusate and a Phospho-soda enema. Lubricant stimulants lubricate the stool and irritate the bowel, thus increasing the peristaltic activity. Glycerin suppositories and mineral oil are two examples of lubricant stimulants. Last, large-volume enemas such as warm water or soapsuds enemas may be used to distend the colon and increase peristalsis.

Emotional, Psychologic, Social, and Spiritual Care

Emergency nurses are experts at delivering aggressive, heroic measures to patients in distress. However, another aspect of good emergency nursing practice is taking care of the patient's and family's emotional, psychologic, social, and spiritual needs. Patients and families come to the ED in crisis, and their coping skills are challenged. Patients and families may exhibit taxing behaviors because they have distressing symptoms and feel out of control. In addition, patients' existential distress may amplify their symptom experience.

Simple interventions that emergency nurses may employ to address these concerns are to communicate clearly and often to the patient and family about the plan of care and what to expect during their stay in the ED and to encourage them to seek support from trusted members of their social network, such as calling their chaplain, family, or friends. Anticipating their needs may help avert an escalation of distress. Family presence during resuscitation is an important method of providing care to survivors and is another way to provide family-centered care (see Chapter 13). It is important to address the family's and patient's common inability to retain information related to their stress level. The need for repetition of information is essential. Families often report not receiving information, when in fact it was communicated. They may have received the information at a time when they were unable to process and respond.

COMMUNICATION ISSUES IN PALLIATIVE AND END-OF-LIFE CARE

Emergency nurses witness suffering and death frequently in the ED. Caring for patients in distress may become routine, and staff may become desensitized to the suffering around them.[25] This desensitization can have a profound impact on the nurse's ability to communicate effectively and respectfully with patients, families, and colleagues. At the same time, patients and families are often unfamiliar with death and dying. They come to the ED in crisis with unexpected injuries or illnesses, chronic disease exacerbations, or perhaps with terminal illnesses, seeking symptom management and lifesaving or life-prolonging treatment.[4] The patients and families are in crisis and seek help and answers from emergency clinicians.

To avoid feeling unprepared to handle these situations, it is important that the emergency clinician work with other disciplines such as social services, chaplaincy services, and trained volunteers to role-play these scenarios and to create policies and procedures surrounding issues such as death notification, bereavement services, follow-up contact, and written information about what to do following a death.[13,17]

The following areas of communication are essential in delivering quality end-of-life care: deciding on a plan of care and death notification/delivering serious news.

Deciding on a Plan of Care

There are seven trajectories to approaching death in the ED: (1) dead on arrival; (2) prehospital resuscitation with subsequent death in the ED; (3) prehospital resuscitation with survival to admission; (4) terminally ill and comes to the ED; (5) frail and hovering near death; (6) alive and interacting on arrival, but arrests in the ED; and (7) potentially preventable death by omission or commission.[5,8] Although emergency clinicians are skilled at resuscitation, there are dying trajectories that require different care interventions than resuscitative measures. Some dying trajectories benefit from aggressive symptom management and humanistic care, whereas others call for more aggressive heroic interventions such as chest compressions, defibrillation, and intubation.

Recognition of poor prognoses and framing beneficial interventions as best for the patient will determine the plan of care.[6] Although resuscitative measures are the standard of care, they may not be appropriate for all patients near the end of life. Taking the time to discuss with the survivors and surrogate decision makers which interventions are appropriate to the situation may help establish the best treatment goals. Fear of liability may be a concern of emergency clinicians.[3,4] However, expanding the definition of a "success" from the traditional concept of the patient being resuscitated back with a pulse to aggressive palliative care management will ease clinicians' feelings of abandoning the patient.[3]

Death Notification/Delivering Serious News

Notifying survivors about sudden and unexpected deaths or giving serious news can be stressful for clinicians.[13] Death notification can be in person, over the telephone, or may include assistance from other agencies such as police departments. Dr. Kenneth Iserson[13] has written an excellent resource to improve death notification. Dr. Iserson strongly recommends developing policies and procedures related to death notification. Death notification can be divided into four stages: prepare, inform, support, and afterwards (PISA). An introductory review of PISA follows.

In the prepare stage, there are four activities to prepare to give serious news: anticipate, identify, notify, and organize. Nurses should anticipate the needs of bereaved survivors, such as arranging a quiet room to include comfortable places to sit, tissues, a telephone for the survivors to notify others, a "panic button" to summon help if needed, and members of other disciplines that will be helpful such as a chaplain or a child-life specialist. Nurses should also have a list of agencies that survivors may need to contact such as the medical examiner/coroner's office, funeral homes, and bereavement services.

The health care team should also positively identify the individual who has died and identify the name and relationship of the person who will be notified. The health care team should have the complete information about the circumstances surrounding the death and any details that may be comforting to the survivors. Notification of the death to the key survivors should be done by the most experienced individual with support from other staff members. Sit at the same level as the survivors. If multiple fatalities occurred in one incident, attempt to notify all the primary survivors at the same time. Notification of the primary care provider is important as well.

Organization of the health care team allows for smoother communication with difficult news. If there is more than one victim, assign one staff member to each group of survivors. Escort the survivors to a more comfortable and quiet room. Be sure that all clinicians are wearing identification badges and are presentable and do not have blood or other body fluids on their clothing when giving the serious news. Accurately identify which family is in which room, if multiple casualties were involved. If a staff member such as a social worker or chaplain has already interacted with the family, be sure to have that staff member present when giving the serious news. Before you enter the room, give yourself a moment to think about what you are going to say and perhaps practice with another staff member if you feel uncomfortable. Be sure to let the health care team know that you are going to give serious news and are not to be interrupted.

In the inform stage, two activities are central: introductions and delivering the news. Before the serious news is given, identify the persons in the room and ask them to explain their relationship to the patient. Introduce yourself and the other health care team members with you and their role in the patient's care. Always refer to the patient by his or her name, and avoid terms such as "the victim," "the decedent," or "our patient."

When giving the news, first ask the survivors what they know about the events to get an understanding about what is known and not known. Then briefly describe the prehospital and hospital events that led up to the serious condition or death, including any resuscitative efforts. Use clear, nontechnical language, and avoid jargon. If the survivor asks you if the person is dead, he or she is giving you two pieces of information: (1) the survivor is ready for the news, and (2) he or she may be ready to cope with the answer that the person is dead.

The hardest part about death notification is using a "D" word—"dead," "died," or "death." Avoid using euphemisms such as "passed away," "no longer with us," "did not make it," "gone," or other confusing term. Using these ambiguous terms can create confusion for the survivors, and they may not understand the very important point that the patient is dead. If the survivors do not seem to understand, use another "D" word. After giving the serious or bad news, pause for a couple of moments to let the news sink in and for the survivors to react. Be prepared for any type of reaction to the news, including, but not limited to, disbelief, denial, anger, guilt, or exacerbation of a medical condition.

In the support stage the activities by the health care team are designed to support the survivors who are grieving. Not all survivors may need these activities in this stage; however, the emergency nurse should be prepared to provide support based on his or her assessment of the survivors. Reassure the survivors that everything that could be done was done and that any cultural or religious customs will be honored to the best of the health care team's ability. Ensure that information is collected in a respectful manner—it is not possible to honor cultural or religious customs unless the team is aware of them. Spiritual care is often an excellent resource for this process. Emergency nurses should also assuage the family's guilt and mental anguish. Often survivors question their role and sometimes blame themselves for not seeking help sooner. Relieve this guilt by reassuring them that the event was not their fault, unless it is very obvious that this is not true.

Reassure the survivors that the patient did not suffer. Useful phrases such as "most people with a bad head injury never have a memory of the accident" or "[the patient's name] was not conscious, and we do not believe that he [or she] was in pain."

In pediatric death, challenge any unrealistic expectations parents may have about their roles. Remind the parents that there was no way to protect their child from this death, unless this is not the case. Also, in pediatric deaths nurses should help the parents and other family members realize that they are grieving for not only the child but also the hopes, dreams, and expectations they had for the child.

Assist the survivors by being available to answer questions, and provide comfort measures such as water, tissues, calling other family members, listening to their stories and concerns, facilitating cultural or spiritual rituals, and allowing the survivors time to view the patient. In addition,

protecting the families and survivors from the media or graphic footage is important to providing privacy in this distressing time.

Last in the support stage, emergency nurses should provide a written list of local contacts for funeral arrangements, medical examiner/coroner's office, and support groups such as SIDS, murder victims, older adult survivors, and pediatric death. Conclude the encounter with the survivors by asking if they have any other questions and providing them a contact phone number at the hospital if they have any additional questions. Advise the survivors that everything that they need to do in the hospital is complete and that they may leave whenever they feel ready. Accompany the survivors to the exit or to their transportation to provide them support.

BIOETHICAL CONSIDERATIONS

There are several ethical and legal issues that are specific to end-of-life care. Many of these issues are governed by local, state, or national laws and regulations. However, it is important to note that we should not confuse that which is legal with what is the most ethical thing to do. Common bioethical considerations in the ED include advance directives, organ and tissue donation, postmortem procedures, autopsy, withholding or withdrawing life-sustaining measures, the principle of double effect, assisted suicide, and euthanasia.

Advance Directives

Since the landmark court case of Karen Ann Quinlan more than 30 years ago, patients have been encouraged to express their thoughts and feelings on end-of-life decisions with an advance directive. Because of this court case the Patient Self-Determination Act was passed in 1991 to alleviate this fear. This act states that at the time of a patient's admission to the hospital, patients (or parents or guardians of children) must be presented with information about advance directives and their rights in making medical care decisions. These wishes then become a part of the patient's permanent record. Many people fear being kept alive by medical technology beyond what they feel is a meaningful existence. No one should have the power to overrule the decisions of the individual, particularly when it comes to choosing the manner of death. The advance directive should be a guide to the individual's wishes and is based on the concept that the patient is competent and has a right to refuse treatment. These documents become effective only when the patient loses decision-making capacity. Decision-making capacity can be summarized as follows[8]:

- Ability to understand:
  - Does the patient have the ability to understand the basic information needed to make a decision?
- Ability to evaluate:
  - Can the patient reason and weigh the consequences of the decision?
  - Does the patient make a decision?
  - Is the decision reasonably consistent over time?

- Ability to communicate:
  - Can the patient communicate the decision?

But what if there is no advance directive? Medical ethicists have been trying to answer that question despite considerable legal uncertainty in this area.

Advance directives come in three forms: living will, durable power of attorney for health care, and do not resuscitate (DNR)/do not attempt resuscitation (DNAR)/allow natural death (AND). A living will is a legal document in which an individual can direct treatment modalities against extraordinary measures in the event of irreversible coma and terminal illness. The legality of this document varies from state to state and from country to country; however, it does not ensure a patient's right to die regardless of geographic location. The durable power of attorney for health care designates a surrogate decision maker when a patient is unable to make decisions. The patient can specify limits or parameters for the type of medical treatment that must be followed by the designated surrogate.

The DNR/DNAR/AND is an order that should be documented on the chart. A witness may be required in some areas. The DNR order addresses what lifesaving measures should be initiated, specifying limits such as cardiopulmonary resuscitation only, medications only, or no defibrillation. Despite the presence of a DNR order, every effort is made in these situations to ease pain and make the patient comfortable. Advance directives vary from state to state, so health care professionals must be familiar with stipulations in their respective states. Allow natural death recognizes that death is a natural course of illness and that no interventions will be attempted to alter the course of the disease.

In most states, prehospital DNR orders are recognized as valid in the ED.[8] A pitfall in emergency nursing and medicine is the failure to determine if a DNR order or an advance directive exists or to ignore these documents. It is important to have discussions after reading these documents to determine what the goals of care are for the patient and proxy decision maker in order to provide the care that is consistent with their wishes.

Society has obviously done its part by passing this act, forcing health care providers to confront questions that the individual may shy away from and may not want to address with patients. Despite written evidence of the patient's wishes, it is still difficult for many caregivers to let go. Most health care providers are as uncomfortable with the idea of death as the families. Health care professionals have been trained to preserve life, not to practice death care. Establishing a good patient-family–health care provider relationship in the ED may be difficult in a crisis situation. Unfortunately, it may be difficult if not impossible to identify the patient's wishes in the ED. Living wills, advance directives, and other documents may not be immediately available in the ED. Families in crisis may not be able to make a decision. It is critical for the emergency nurse to maintain ongoing contact with the patient and family throughout a crisis event. Families may find it easier to ask for information and advice from the nurse. Making yourself available to assist families with these difficult issues as they arise is a vital nursing function.

Organ and Tissue Donation

Federal law (Public Law 99-5-9; Section 9318) and Medicare regulations require that hospitals give the surviving family members the chance to authorize donation of their family member's tissues and organs.[3] Initiating the conversation about organ and tissue procurement can be difficult. However, some families have asked to donate organs or tissues. An important aspect surrounding organ or tissue procurement is respecting the family's grieving process and giving them all the information that they need to make a decision with which they will be comfortable. Organs and tissues can be procured after cardiac death or brain death. The following guidelines are helpful in working with families and organ/tissue procurement organizations[15]:

1. First, follow your hospital's protocol for organ procurement. Your hospital's protocol will identify who is to serve as a liaison between the family and the transplant program staff.
2. Recent guidelines by the Centers for Medicare and Medicaid Services (CMS) require that hospitals inform their organ procurement office of all deaths that occur and that trained staff discuss organ donation and obtain consent.
3. Arrange for the regional transplant program personnel to provide annual updates on organ donation. Doing so will ensure that staff members have current information on caring for the potential donor and updated information on legislation in your state.
4. Respect each staff member's individual beliefs. Identify which staff members believe in organ donation, and work with them to enhance the skills needed to speak with families and provide care to the donor. We all know that some staff members are "good" in certain situations, such as starting IVs, so find out who is "good" with organ donation.
5. Be knowledgeable about state and federal regulations; post guidelines in a conspicuous place. These regulations are variable from state to state and country to country. Nurses should ensure that they are familiar with their organization's protocol, as well as regional directives and/ or resources that may assist them.

Postmortem Procedures

The practicing of certain skills such as endotracheal intubation, cricothyrotomy, central line placement, and other procedures on the newly deceased patient is a sensitive topic. There is a balance between the need for health care providers to master these skills to be prepared for future situations that call for these high-risk, low-frequency skills and the respect for the patient and the wishes of the survivors. The ENA and the American College of Emergency Physicians (ACEP) have developed position statements that clearly define their positions.[1,9] ENA's position is as follows:

- ENA agrees with the need to teach and practice many of these skills. The critical, life-threatening nature of the situations requiring these procedures demands competence and confidence on the part of the provider.
- ENA believes that criteria must be met by those individuals who wish to practice these procedures:
  - The individual must have a legitimate need to master this skill.
  - The practitioner should be prepared, through a structured learning process, to maximize the educational experience.
- ENA believes that consent must be obtained from the family for the performance of invasive procedures. The method of obtaining this consent may vary, depending upon the needs of the institution, and could take the following forms:
  - An addition to the initial admission form.
  - An addition to the consent for autopsy or donation.
  - A separate form.
  - Public disclosure.
  - A provision in living wills.

Autopsy

The decision to perform an autopsy is usually made by the medical examiner or coroner's office in the county in which the patient died. EDs should develop policies and procedures delineating when to contact the medical examiner or coroner. Regulations vary from state to state and even within states. ED clinicians should consult with their local medical examiner, coroner, and other agencies to determine the local regulations, preferences, and procedures.

Several factors are taken in account to determine if an autopsy is warranted.[15] The first factor is the cause of death. Any death associated with a known or suspected criminal activity is cause for an autopsy. Second, autopsies are performed to determine the cause of any sudden, traumatic, or unexpected death. Last, family members may request an autopsy. In the last case, the autopsy may be performed by any pathologist rather than the medical examiner.

Withholding or Withdrawing Life-Sustaining Measures

Withholding or withdrawing treatments is challenging to emergency clinicians because we are trained and commonly are called upon to institute resuscitation interventions. However, morally and legally, withholding or withdrawing treatments is justified and has strong roots in the common law that reflects the American regard for self-determination and is supported by the ethical principles of autonomy, beneficence, and nonmaleficence.[18] Patients and surrogate decision makers may be allowed to refuse or withdraw a treatment at any time according to hospitals' patients' bill of rights. Refer to your hospital's policy on the patients' bill of rights.

Withholding treatment is considered morally equivalent to withdrawing treatment—the end result is that the patient is without the treatment; however, it is more difficult for emergency clinicians to withhold a treatment than it is to withdraw a treatment.

Principle of Double Effect

The ethical principle of double effect distinguishes between the intended and unintended consequences of a particular action. In certain cases an action has two effects: one good and one bad.[26] In a situation where there is no alternative but to cause harm in trying to fulfill one's duty to bring about good for a patient, the action is still permissible.[24]

The principle of double effect is most commonly applied when pain medication is being administered to a dying patient. Opioids are used to relieve pain and other symptoms of suffering. The relief of suffering is the good effect. However, opioids also have the potential adverse or bad effect of causing respiratory and cardiovascular depression, which may, if left untreated, lead to death. If the nurse's intention is to relieve pain and suffering, yet the nurse incidentally foresees that the patient may die, it is morally and legally permissible to administer the opioid if the intention is to relieve suffering. If the primary intention is to have the patient die, then it is not morally or legally permissible to administer the opioid. In end-of-life cases, it is important to note that the patient will eventually die as a result of the natural disease progression, regardless of the opioid administration. The main issue is whether the nurse will allow the suffering to continue until the patient dies or the nurse will attempt to relieve the suffering. It is good nursing practice to relieve the suffering of patients.

Assisted Suicide and Euthanasia

Distinguishing between the two concepts of assisted suicide and euthanasia is important both ethically and legally. Assisted suicide is defined as the act of providing the means to commit suicide knowing that the recipient plans to use the means to end his or her life. Provider-assisted suicide specifically refers to a provider making available medications or other interventions with the understanding that a patient plans to use them to commit suicide and subsequently does so.[23] Euthanasia is defined as someone other than the patient committing an act with the intent to end the person's life. Euthanasia is further divided into (1) voluntary euthanasia, in which an action is taken by another to end the patient's life at the patient's request; and (2) nonvoluntary euthanasia, in which an action is taken by another to end the person's life without the patient's knowledge or consent.[23]

Oregon is the only state with laws that sanction assisted suicide. Worldwide, the Netherlands represents a positive working model of euthanasia with creation of specific criteria and guidelines for performing euthanasia. Euthanasia is also legal in Australia and Colombia.

Because of these moral choices, palliative care and subsequent management of a patient's dying process is often the responsibility of nurses. Ethicists, physicians, and nurses play an active role in the decision making that precedes withdrawal of life support. Ethicists concern themselves with the ethics of the decision-making process, the definition of death, and even considerations about giving pain medications that may be thought to shorten the patient's life. Numerous professional organizations have issued guidelines to assist in this decision-making process and give us an avenue to explore with patients and their families when death becomes imminent. But after the decision is made and goals to a good death are obtained, the ethicists leave and care of the dying patient is left up to the nurse. A clear understanding of the goals must be specified for this dying patient so that a "good death" can be achieved. Many times the major and only goal is comfort care with family support.

CARE FOR THE CAREGIVER

Some deaths will affect individuals on a significant level, perhaps because the death of the patient may remind us of a death of someone close to us. Death of children, fetal demise, a mass casualty, death of someone the clinician knows, or a particularly horrific, traumatic death can have a profound impact on the clinician. It is important for the clinician to recognize that a death was meaningful in order to manage the stress of the event. Colleagues must be supportive and discover ways to support each other rather than dismissing the impact the death has on a clinician.

There are many strategies that can be used to cope with the event. Some strategies can be used immediately after the incident; other strategies are more long term. Examples of strategies include asking to be relieved from care responsibilities and taking a break, if possible; asking for reassignment to another part of the ED, if possible; finding a colleague or friend with whom you can discuss the event— consider speaking with your manager about stress debriefing; self-reflection—taking a moment to reflect on how you feel after exposure to the event. What do you think? How do you behave? Pay attention to any physical symptoms and to thoughts and feelings; use self-monitoring—assess your responses to traumatic situations, and compare them with your normal responses. Minimize the impact of negative thoughts; focus on what you did right. Include therapies that follow basic health principles such as incorporating physical exercise, meditation, humor, music, relaxation (e.g., acupressure, reflexology, therapeutic massage), guided imagery, proper nutrition, and getting adequate rest.[2]

It is important to recognize symptoms and signs of compassion fatigue (burnout) and posttraumatic stress. Working in the ED is hard work with many demands on clinicians' time, resources, and physical and emotional abilities. Recognition of symptoms and signs of traumatic stress is important in maintaining a healthy home and work life. Dealing with death on a constant basis can take its toll on our well-being. Therefore it is imperative to monitor ourselves and each other. Symptoms of compassion fatigue and posttraumatic stress may include increase in the number of sick

days, indecision, difficulty with problem solving, isolation or withdrawal, behavioral outbursts, denial and shock, fixation on a single detail, immobilization, feeling of extreme serenity, emotionally numbing responses, and intrusive responses.[2] Signs of burnout or posttraumatic stress may include tachycardia, increased respiratory rate, or elevated blood pressure.[2]

SUMMARY

Palliative and end-of-life care are cornerstones of good emergency nursing care and supplement other therapies that nurses initiate in the ED. Technologic advances that have brought about improved health care and greater choices in medical services have also resulted in questions concerning not how, but when, to make use of these choices and improvements. People still want to die with dignity, and we as health care providers should enable them to do just that. The manner in which these issues are handled will influence not only the medical outcome but also the quality of patient and family care.

REFERENCES

1. American College of Emergency Physicians: *Ethical issues in emergency department care at the end of life*, 2007. Retrieved December 4, 2007, from http://www. acep.org/practres.aspx?id=29440.
2. Badger JM: Understanding secondary traumatic stress, *Am J Nurs* 101(7):26, 2001.
3. Campbell M, Zalenski R: The emergency department, In Ferrell BR, Coyle N, editors: *Textbook of palliative care*, ed 2, New York, 2006, Oxford University Press.
4. Chan GK: End-of-life care models and emergency department care, *Acad Emerg Med* 11(1):79, 2004.
5. Chan GK: *Trajectories of approaching death in the emergency department*. Paper presented at the third Mediterranean Emergency Medicine Congress, Nice, France, September 1-5, 2005.
6. Chan GK: End-of-life issues in the emergency department. In Hoyt KS, Selfridge-Thomas J, editors: *Emergency nursing core curriculum*, St. Louis, 2007, Saunders.
7. Dunwoody CJ, Arnold R: *Fast fact and concept #039: using naloxone*, 2007. Retrieved December 4, 2007, from http://www.eperc.mcw.edu/fastFact/ff_39.htm.
8. Emanuel L, Quest T, editors: *Education in palliative and end-of-life care for emergency medicine*, Chicago, 2007, The EPEC Project.
9. Emergency Nurses Association: *The use of the newly deceased patient for procedural practice*, 2002. Retrieved August 2, 2006, from http://www.ena.org/about/position/PDFs/Use-of-NewlyDeceased.PDF.
10. Emergency Nurses Association: *End-of-life care in the emergency department* [position statement], 2005, The Association. Retrieved August 2, 2006 from http://www.ena.org/about/position/endoflife.asp.

11. Field MJ, Cassel CK: *Approaching death: improving care at the end of life*, Washington, DC, 1997, Institute of Medicine.

12. International Association for the Study of Pain: IASP *pain terminology*, 2007. Retrieved December 8, 2007, from http://www.iasp-pain.org/AM/Template.cfm?Section=General_Resource_Links&Template=/CM/HT-MLDisplay.cfm&ContentID=3058#Pain.

13. Iserson KV: The gravest words: sudden-death notifications and emergency care, *Ann Emerg Med* 36(1):75, 2000.

14. Kamienski MC: Family-centered care in the ED, *Am J Nurs* 104(1):59, 2004.

15. Kelly CT: Death and dying in the emergency department, In Oman KS, Koziol-McLain J, Scheetz LJ, editors: *Emergency nursing secrets*, Philadelphia, 2001, Hanley & Belfus.

16. Lasts Acts: *Means to a better end: a report on dying in America today*, 2002. Retrieved March 1, 2009 from http://www.wjf.org/files/publications/other/meansbetterend.pdf.

17. Li SP, Chan CW, Lee DT: Helpfulness of nursing actions to suddenly bereaved family members in an accident and emergency setting in Hong Kong, *J Adv Nurs* 40(2):170, 2002.

18. Luce JM, Alpers A: End-of-life care: what do the American courts say? *Crit Care Med* 29(2 suppl):N40, 2001.

19. McCaffery M, Pasero C: *Pain: clinical manual*, ed 2, St. Louis, 1999, Mosby.

20. McCaig LF, Burt CW: *National Hospital Ambulatory Medical Care Survey: 2003 emergency department summary—advance data from vital and health statistics*, No. 358, Hyattsville, Md, 2005, National Center for Health Statistics.

21. McClain K, Perkins P: Terminally ill patients in the emergency department: a practical overview of end-of-life issues, *J Emerg Nurs* 28(6):515, 2002.

22. National Consensus Project for Quality Palliative Care: *Clinical practice guidelines for quality palliative care*, 2004, National Consensus Project. Retrieved October 16, 2004, from http://www.nationalconsensusproject.org/Guidelines_Download.asp.

23. Puntillo KA, Benner P, Drought T et al: End-of-life issues in intensive care units: a national random survey of nurses' knowledge and beliefs, *Am J Crit Care* 10(4):216, 2001.

24. Sulmasy DP: Commentary: double effect—intention is the solution, not the problem, *J Law Med Ethics* 28(1):26, 2000.

25. Walters DT, Tupin JP: Family grief in the emergency department, *Emerg Med Clin North Am* 9:189, 1991.

26. Williams G: The principle of double effect and terminal sedation, *Med Law Rev* 9(1):41, 2001.

27. World Health Organization: *Cancer pain relief and palliative care*, Geneva, Switzerland, 1990, World Health Organization.

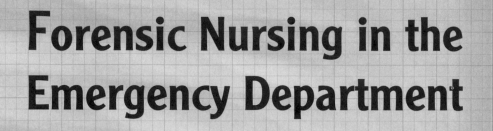

CHAPTER 16

Forensic Nursing in the Emergency Department

Daniel J. Sheridan, Katherine R. Nash, and Heidi Bresee

FORENSIC NURSING DEFINED

Every day in emergency departments (EDs) worldwide, skilled nurses provide care to patients presenting with injuries sustained by trauma and violence. These injuries occur from a wide variety of mechanisms, including motor vehicle crashes, missile injuries, burns, interpersonal violence, mass disasters, and bioterrorist acts. Most of these patients survive; some do not. ED nurses are uniquely positioned to identify, evaluate, and medically treat these patients and to preserve and collect any potential forensic evidence that may be on or with the patient.

When an ED nurse provides care to victims of violent events, that ED nurse is providing forensic nursing care. Based on writings by Lynch,[17-19,21] the person most often credited for coining the phrase "forensic nursing," the International Association of Forensic Nurses (IAFN) defines forensic nursing as follows:

> The application of nursing science to public or legal proceedings; the application of the forensic aspects of health care combined with the bio-psycho-social education of the registered nurse in the scientific investigation on and treatment of trauma and/or death of victims and perpetrators of abuse, violence, criminal activity and traumatic accidents.[10]

More succinctly, forensically trained nurses provide care to patients whose reasons for being in the ED have the likelihood of ending up in a civil or criminal proceeding and/or a legal hearing or arbitration.

In addition, experienced ED nurses may choose to offer their skills to a legal process by being expert witnesses or content expert consultants. This area of forensic nursing is called legal nurse consulting. A growing number of experienced nurses are being trained and hired to be death scene investigators, yet another forensic nursing subspecialty.

HISTORY OF FORENSIC NURSING

Lynch[20] tracks the origins of forensic nursing to the early 1980s and links it to the development of improvements in the science of clinical forensic medicine. However, the origins of forensic nursing began at least 10 years earlier with the development of the rape victim advocate (RVA) movement and the creation of the first sexual assault forensic evidence kits. The first three victim assistance programs in the United States began in 1972, of which two were rape crisis centers.[37]

In 1974 Burgess and Holmstrom,[3] a nurse researcher and sociologist, respectively, coined the phrase "rape trauma syndrome." They developed an intervention and treatment schema involving crisis intervention counseling that is still routinely taught in sexual assault nurse examiner (SANE) training programs.

The first three nurse-run SANE programs were developed in the late 1970s in Memphis, Tennessee,[33] Minneapolis,

Minnesota,[14] and Amarillo, Texas.[1] Today, there are over 530 SANE programs (mostly ED-based) in hospitals throughout America, Canada, and other countries around the world.

Drake[6] and Parker and Schumacher[24] were the first to conduct nurse-based research in domestic violence that guided future intervention studies. Campbell[5] began to look at domestic homicide and misogyny (hatred of women) and developed a tool, the Danger Assessment (DA), that could be administered by nurses to help identify women at risk for being killed by an intimate partner. In 1986, Hadley in Minneapolis and Sheridan in Chicago created the first ED-based family violence intervention programs.[31]

A growing number of SANE programs are expanding their forensic nursing services to include assessment and documentation of intimate partner violence; elder and vulnerable person abuse and neglect; and assaults, shootings, and knifings not related to family violence. For any hospital-based violence intervention program to succeed, it must have a multiprofessional component.[30] Within the hospital, ED nurses who work within a violence intervention program must develop collaborative relationships with such professionals as physicians, physician assistants, nurse practitioners, social workers, mental health professionals, and chaplains. Externally, ED nurses need to develop referral, networking, and consultative relationships with adult and child protective service agencies, law enforcement personnel, local prosecutors, and the state's attorney general's office.

ROLES AND RESPONSIBILITIES OF THE EMERGENCY DEPARTMENT NURSE WITH FORENSIC TRAINING
Reporting Suspected Abuse/Neglect

All states within the United States, including the District of Columbia, have statutes mandating health professionals to report suspected child maltreatment, and most states have statutes mandating health professionals to report abuse/neglect of elder or vulnerable adults. Fewer states have statutes that require mandatory notification of authorities of intimate partner violence or crime victims in general. ED nurses, mental health professionals, social workers, and medical examiners are examples of mandatory reporters. ED nurses need to know the mandatory reporting requirements for where they work and must have readily available the appropriate hotline or reporting numbers.

Physical, emotional, and educational neglect are types of maltreatment or neglect, as are refusal of health care, delay in medical care, abandonment, expulsion from home, inadequate supervision, inadequate nutrition or clothing, permitted chronic truancy, inattention to special education needs, exposure of the child or vulnerable individual to domestic violence, permitted drug or alcohol abuse, and refusal or delay in obtaining psychiatric care. It is essential for the

ED nurse caring for patients experiencing these forms of maltreatment or neglect to make the appropriate referrals to child or adult protective services.

Once the ED nurse has identified a case of potential abuse or neglect, he or she must involve other members of the multidisciplinary team to assist in conducting a thorough assessment and to plan post-ED case management. Acquiring and documenting a comprehensive history is a critical step in the assessment of abuse/neglect. Patients should be interviewed separately, and if the person(s) accompanying the patient attempts to block the patient's privacy, the ED nurse must intercede on the patient's behalf.

Documentation as Evidence

Thorough nursing documentation is part of excellent patient care, but one cannot understate its importance and value as forensic evidence. Nursing documentation should provide an accurate and forensically useful picture of what the trained ED nurse hears, sees, and smells when assessing the patient. Because wounds heal and histories of events may change over time, most ED nurses have a single opportunity to provide investigators and jury members an objective and detailed account of the patient's experience, sometimes minutes after a traumatic event.

ED nurses should maintain consistent organization in their writing to prevent the likelihood of forgetting any one section. One example of organizing style is the classic **SOAP** format: **S**ubjective history, **O**bjective data, **A**ssessment with diagnosis, and **P**lan for further testing or follow-up. All handwritten documentation should be legible to laypeople.

When documenting the patient's history, one should provide sufficient and forensically useful detail, using direct quotations from the patient whenever possible.[29] Patient statements recorded in the medical record may be admissible in court as exceptions to hearsay. Nursing documentation of a patient's history may be admissible under the medical exception to hearsay as long as it is relevant to the treatment of the patient's physical or psychologic condition.[29]

Another exception to hearsay is an "excited utterance," which is a spontaneous statement made under duress. An example of excited utterance is when a trauma patient being wheeled into the ED by paramedics yells, "My husband shot me! He said he's going to kill our kids. You've got to find my kids before he does." Such spontaneous utterances should also be documented even if the patient is cognitively impaired from alcohol, drugs, medications, dementia, or psychologic conditions. The ED nurse should document the history of any injuries and pre-ED treatments. Any delay in treatment should also be noted. If a caregiver is responsible for the patient's care, the ED nurse should document his or her explanation of any injuries or delays in medical treatment.

When documenting a patient's report of events, one should be careful not to sanitize statements or "medicalize" terms. If a patient's spouse threatened him or her, document the entire threat in quotation marks. Document verbatim what the trauma patient says, such as "My husband said, 'If I can't have you, you fu%$ing bitch, no one is going to have you.' Then he shot me and laughed when I begged him to call 911." Not only will that documented statement be valuable and powerful in court, it is also very significant for nurses and medical providers in planning interventions to address the patient's psychologic response to being shot.

A 5-year-old child may not describe his genitalia using the medical or adult term *penis*. Instead the nurse should use the patient's term, clarifying with the patient its location. For example, a child may report, "He touched my pee-pee [penis]."

ED nurses must remain objective in their documentation, limiting bias and subjectivity. If a patient presents to the ED reporting chest pain, the ED triage nurse would never consider writing "alleged chest pain" as the chief complaint. Similarly, the ED nurse should never document in the medical record "alleged sexual assault, alleged child abuse, or alleged domestic violence." The use of the word "alleged" or documenting that the patient "claims" he or she was assaulted is pejorative (biased) and sends a message that the ED nurse does not believe the patient. Replace the words "alleged" and "claimed" with "reported" or "suspected."

Another example of judgmental and biased documentation frequently found in medical records is the use of the word "refused," such as "The patient refused medication." To be more objective in one's charting, replace the word "refused" with "declined" or use the words "said," "stated," or "reports." For example, "Patient declined medications" or "Patient said she does not want to make a police report." ED nurses should not document their feelings and emotions.

Collecting Evidence in the Emergency Department

Because ED nurses are often the first individuals to come into contact with victims of violence, they have the important responsibility of recognizing, collecting, and preserving key forensic evidence. Ultimately, the first priority for these patients is their medical stability. However, nurses often overlook crucial forensic evidence that can be forever lost as they cut off the patient's clothing and clean/dress their wounds. Later in this chapter there will be a discussion of simple procedures that can be used to maximize evidence collected by a forensically trained ED nurse while not inhibiting lifesaving medical treatments.

Emergency Nurses Association Position Statement

The Emergency Nurses Association (ENA)[7] identifies forensics as a part of conscientious emergency nursing practice. The comprehensive nature of ED nurses' care of forensic patients lends itself to the inclusion of evidence collection procedures in daily practice. Even though nursing schools do not traditionally teach evidence collection and associated documentation, the ENA position statement *Forensic Evidence Collection* outlines the importance of ED nurses' having the knowledge and skills in collecting evidence and documenting appropriately using both written and

---

Box 16-1	**EMERGENCY NURSES ASSOCIATION POSITION STATEMENT ON FORENSIC EVIDENCE COLLECTION**

- ENA believes that it is the emergency nurse's role not only to provide physical and emotional care to patients, but also to help preserve the evidence collected in the emergency department.
- ENA supports collaboration with emergency physicians, social service, and law enforcement personnel to develop guidelines for forensic evidence collection and documentation in the emergency care setting.
- ENA encourages emergency nurses to become familiar with the concepts and skills of evidence collection, photographic and written documentation, as well as testifying in legal proceedings.

From Emergency Nurses Association: *Position statement: forensic evidence collection.* Retrieved June 1, 2008, from http://www.ena.org/position/pdfs/forensicevidence.pdf. *ENA,* Emergency Nurses Association.

---

photographic techniques (Box 16-1). A multidisciplinary approach should also be used by an ED to create its own evidence collection procedures. Finally, the ENA also emphasizes the importance of maintaining chain of custody, where appropriate.

What Is Evidence?

Forensic evidence is defined as anything presented in court to support or refute a theory or statement.[21] Evidence may be presented by the prosecution (criminal case), plaintiffs (civil case), or defendants. Evidence may be tangible, such as a medical record, DNA, clothing, bullets, and photographs, or intangible, such as the patient's reported history, excited utterances, and odors. Trace evidence involves small, minute quantities of physical material that has transferred from one location to another due to contact.[4] Such evidence is not always easily visible to the naked eye. Therefore everything that arrives with the patient will need to be preserved for closer scrutiny in the crime laboratory, as will be subsequently discussed.

Gloves should be worn at all times when collecting or handling potential evidence to prevent contamination. According to Locard's principle of exchange, when two objects come into contact, a mutual exchange of evidentiary material occurs.[4] ED nurses need to be aware of this principle and protect evidence as described in the following sections.

Identifying/Collecting/Preserving Physical Evidence

In a criminal case the person ultimately responsible for physical evidence in the legal system is the police officer. Sometimes the police are not yet involved at the time the patient is receiving care. Without ED nurses' first recognizing, preserving, and collecting physical evidence, its potential value may be lost forever. The police may have difficulty in effectively investigating the criminal matter. This can result in an inability to prosecute or the prosecution of the wrong person. Ultimately, the person responsible for the violence and suffering may go unpunished, capable of causing more harm.

SEMEN AS EVIDENCE. A 2006 study found that forensic evidence collection from body sites in children and adolescent victims of rape were unlikely to generate semen more than 24 hours after the incident.[36] Items of clothing and linens proved to have a greater yield of DNA, highlighting the significant role the ED nurse can play in collecting and securing potential evidence.

However, semen can be found in adult sexual assault patients many days after the reported assault. In a growing number of jurisdictions, the cutoff time for collection of DNA evidence in adolescents and adults has been extended from 72 hours to 120 hours (5 days) to 168 hours (one week).[35] Ensuring the evidence is in a locked or secured environment is essential to proving chain of custody. An example of a secure environment for evidence storage would be a locked closet with numerous shelves, each dedicated to one patient. Another example would be a locked multidrawer metal file cabinet that has had air holes drilled for ventilation. Access to the keys to evidence lockers needs to be restricted. Evidence should be released to law enforcement with proper documentation included to establish each person involved in the chain of custody.

CLOTHES. Clothing can tell an important story of the violent event. Consideration must be taken to properly collect clothing that may include DNA, patterned injuries such as bullet holes, or other valuable evidence that can prove crucial in abuse cases. For example, gunpowder residue can help experts determine the firearm distance, whereas blood or other body fluids may identify the individuals involved. Shoes can also be linked to footprints at the crime scene or display imprints from the brake pedal before a vehicle collision.

When a trauma patient comes through the door of an ED, one of the first steps in assessing and treating the patient is to remove all the patient's clothing. Typically this is done by cutting them off using shears and throwing the clothes on the floor in a pile. Do not cut through damaged areas of the clothing (e.g., a bullet hole) because this can distort their appearance. Clothes placed directly on the floor easily become contaminated. Instead, ED nurses can simply place two clean hospital sheets on the floor, one on top of the other, before the trauma patient's arrival. As the articles of clothing are removed from the patient, they can be quickly laid on top of the two sheets. Each piece of clothing should be kept separate to prevent cross-contamination. If the patient can undress himself or herself, have the patient do so while standing over two hospital sheets. The top sheet will catch any debris or trace evidence that falls off the patient while undressing. In both situations, collect the top sheet that has come in contact with the clothes or patient. Also, collect the sheet from the

emergency medical services (EMS) stretcher and/or hospital stretcher if possible.

With gloved hands, place each piece of clothing or sheet in an individual clean paper bag; do not use plastic. Paper bags are air permeable and facilitate drying of contents. If the clothes are moist, they should be allowed to air dry as much as possible before packaging. Moisture leads to bacterial or mold growth, resulting in denaturizing of proteins and DNA material.[4] Plastic bags allow moisture condensation, resulting in similar biologic degradation of evidence. The paper bags should be sealed with tape because staples can damage the contents or injure the handler. The ED nurse should date and initial over the tape, which makes it easy to determine if someone has opened the bag. Finally, document what articles of clothing were collected, and provide a brief description of each item (e.g., collected: brown shorts with stain noted to left leg, white short-sleeve shirt with defect noted to chest with surrounding stain).

STAINS OR OTHER DEBRIS. Suspicious stains on the patient's skin can be swabbed with a sterile cotton-tipped applicator moistened with sterile water. Swabs should be obtained of the exterior of gunshot wounds before surgery or cleaning. Stains on deceased individuals should not be swabbed unless permission is obtained from the local medical examiner or coroner. If the stain is dry, moisten the swab with sterile water. The swab must then be air dried before packaging it in a clean envelope or box. A simple method of air drying is to invert a Styrofoam cup and poke the end of the applicator through the bottom or side of the cup. This holds the applicator while it dries and limits cross contamination. Once the applicator is placed in the envelope, the envelope should be sealed with tape. Licking the envelope can result in cross contamination and risk for disease exposure. The collector should write on the envelope the appearance and location of the stain, and initial over the tape.

In the case of firearm injuries, special consideration should be taken with the patient's hands. The ED nurse should not clean the hands in an attempt to remove dried blood or other debris. Paper bags should be applied until the victim's hands can be tested for gunpowder residue.

Other debris, such as hair, soil, leaves, or paint can also be collected. Take a sheet of clean white paper and fold it into thirds vertically, and then horizontally. Open the paper and in the center place the collected debris using a swab or rubber-tipped forceps. Refold the paper, and place it in a clean envelope, sealing and labeling it as described above. To collect minute debris (e.g., glitter), one can also use the sticky side of a piece of transparent tape. Once the debris is collected, place the tape on a glass slide, which one can obtain from the hospital laboratory. Wrap the slide in white paper, then seal and label it.

PROJECTILES. Bullets, BBs, and other projectiles are sometimes removed during surgery or injury treatment. They may contain trace evidence, and ballistic markings may link them back to their weapon of origin. Metal projectiles should never be handled using forceps without rubber tips because the projectiles may be scratched, making it more difficult to forensically evaluate them. Each projectile should be placed in an *individual* small rigid container (e.g., urine cup) along with sterile gauze to minimize movement. Holes should be placed in the lid to allow air to circulate.[8] Firearms should always be secured by police.

The ED nurse should never label bullet wounds as entrance or exit wounds in the documented assessment.[26,30] The belief that entrance wounds are always smaller than exit wounds is a generality, and even forensic pathologists can struggle to differentiate entrance from exit wounds.[16] For example, if a bullet enters the body after ricocheting off a structure, it may strike the body in a tumbling rotation creating a large entrance wound. It may then strike a large bone in the body, splintering the bullet. Most of the bullet splinters may stay in the body, but a small splinter may then exit the body, creating a much smaller hole.

NEEDLES AND KNIVES. Tremendous care should always be taken when collecting or handling sharp objects. They need to be secured in a way that will preserve trace evidence without injuring the collector or other personnel handling the evidence. These objects hold important value in their trace evidence. Needles may contain toxic substances, and a knife blade may contain fingerprints. They should not be handled using forceps without rubber tips for the same reason as projectiles. They should be carefully packaged in appropriate cardboard boxes or tubes. Needles can be placed in glass tubes or gauze-filled specimen containers with air holes to allow ventilation.

Emergency Department Forensic Evidence Recovery Kit

To ease the incorporation of evidence collection into a busy ED, nurses should be trained to use a patient evidence recovery kit (PERK).[15] These inexpensive kits can be created to house all necessary materials for quick and easy access (Table 16-1). Within the kit there are supplies to collect and preserve clothing, swabs, debris, projectiles, and other physical evidence, as well as a procedure manual outlining the steps.

Maintaining Chain of Custody

Without authenticity, forensic evidence is of limited value.[9] In order to be accepted at court, physical evidence must be accompanied by documentation that demonstrates the item's location and responsible party at any given time. If chain of custody is not maintained or documented, an entire case may be lost. Each time the evidence changes hands (e.g., nurse to police) a receipt is generated and signed by both parties. Such a paper trail demonstrates a continuous chain in the custody of the evidence, with each custodian being a link in the chain.[27] Chain of custody forms can be obtained from a local police department. If a form is not readily available, document the transfer of evidence in the nurses' notes with both parties' signatures.[9]

Table 16-1. CONTENTS OF A PATIENT EVIDENCE RECOVERY KIT	
Item	**Number**
Evidence collection procedures	
Large white envelopes	5
White paper	10
Sterile cotton-tipped applicators	10
Sterile urine specimen cups	3
Sterile gauze (4 × 4 inches)	3
Large paper bags	5
Small paper bags	5
Glass slides	3
Various size cardboard boxes	3
Transparent tape	1
Rubber-tipped forceps (clean)	1
Permanent marker	1
Digital camera	
Chain of custody forms	

While in possession of the evidence, the ED must provide a safe and secure location for it to be stored. The number of individuals with access and adequate air circulation must be considered. An excellent and inexpensive example is a four-drawer file cabinet with holes drilled in the sides. Each drawer can be used for a different patient. The key to the cabinet needs to be accessible to the nursing staff but secured and monitored. An ideal solution is to house the key in an electronic medication dispensing machine (e.g., Pyxis). Such a machine has restricted access and provides a log of those who have accessed a specific drawer. Finally, a sign-in and sign-out sheet should be attached to the file drawer as an additional paper trail.

Use of Body Maps and Photographs

To accurately document the location of injuries or physical evidence, an ED nurse should include a body diagram/map (Figure 16-1) *and* photographs in addition to the written nursing note. The body diagram should show clearly the location, type of injury or evidence collected, and a brief description. Photographs should never replace body diagrams, because they may be lost or poorly representative.

Different camera technologies available for ED nurses include 35-mm cameras and digital cameras. For many years, 35-mm film was the forensic gold standard, but with its cost and delay in development, it has fallen out of favor with most forensic programs. Polaroid forensic cameras are no longer being sold, and film for these Polaroid cameras is no longer being manufactured. Therefore EDs that are still using Polaroid cameras need to invest in a new camera documentation system.

Many forensic sexual assault intervention programs use digital cameras. Photographs with this technology are instantaneous, can be retaken if not adequate, and replicated and enlarged for court. Digital photographic images must be

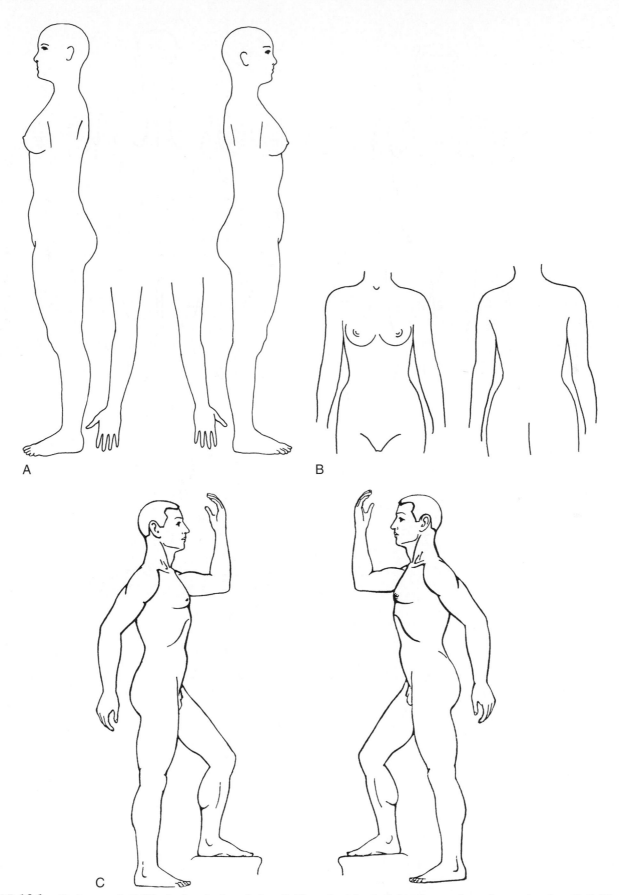

FIGURE 16-1.   Body map. **A,** Full body, female, lateral view. **B,** Thoracic abdominal, female, anterior and posterior view. **C,** Full body, male, lateral view.

Continued

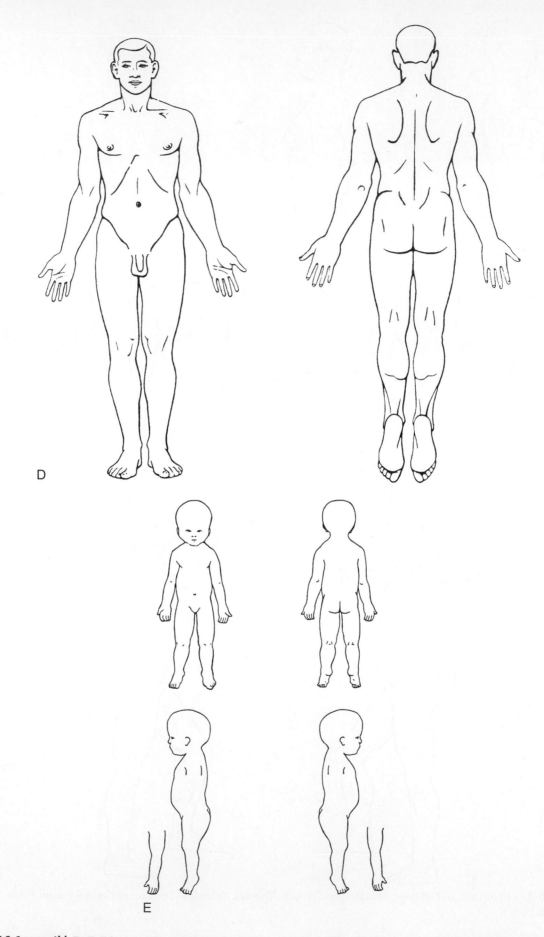

FIGURE **16-1—cont'd D,** Full body, male, anterior and posterior view. **E,** Infant, ventral, dorsal, and left and right lateral view.

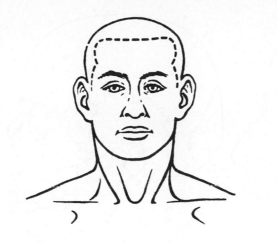
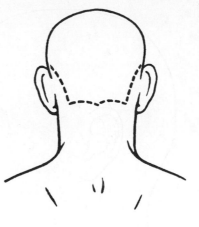

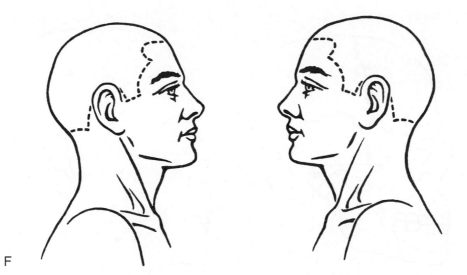

F

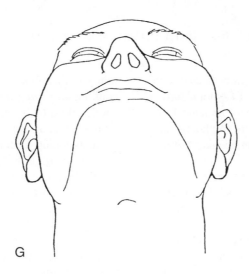

G

FIGURE **16-1—cont'd F,** Head and face diagrams. **G,** Submental view.

Continued

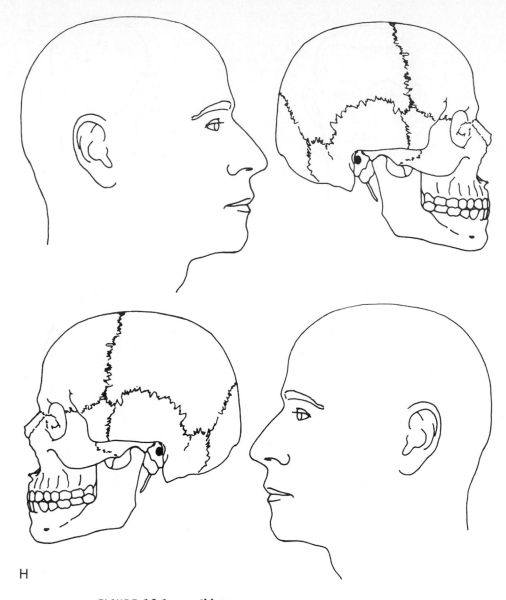

FIGURE **16-1—cont'd H,** Head and skull, lateral view.

stored securely on a computer, uploaded into an electronic medical record or burned onto a disc. The ED should have a well-developed policy and procedure for photographic documentation of injuries that includes "consent to photograph" forms and identifies when photographs can be taken without signed consent.

Whenever possible, the ED nurse should take the photographs and not delegate that role to a social worker or advocate. ED nurses are qualified to testify as to what injuries are present in the photographs, whereas social workers and advocates are not qualified to testify about wounds. Although digital images can be more readily altered or manipulated than film images, the ED nurse can testify to the photographs' unaltered nature and that the images are true and accurate representations of what the nurse assessed and treated in the ED.

When photographing an injury, start with a frontal identification shot of the patient about 6 feet away. Include the injury in this photograph if possible. Then the nurse should continue to photograph an injury by cutting the distance by about a third (4 feet away), finishing with a close-up image (about 2 feet away). By following this "rule of thirds," one prevents taking a photograph of an injury without orientation to its location.[28] Close-up photographs of the injury should be taken with and without a scale to help establish size. A scale may be a ruler or any item of a standard size (e.g., penny).

Lighting can affect the color of injuries, so the ED nurse should use a variety of sources. For example, fluorescent light, frequent in hospital settings, gives bruises a yellow or greenish color in photographs.[25] Finally, great care should be used in labeling the photographs with the patient's name, date, and case or medical record number. To limit confusion, one disc or roll of film should be used for each individual patient. If multiple patients are seen using the same digital memory or film, photograph the patient's identifying

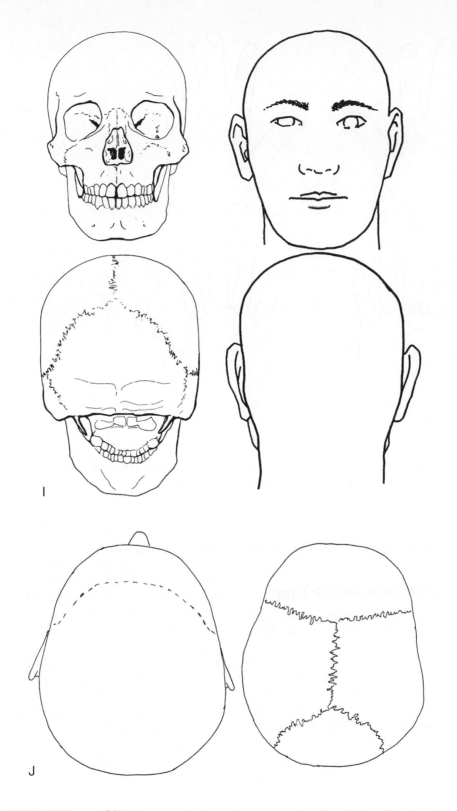

FIGURE **16-1—cont'd I,** Head and skull, anterior and posterior view. **J,** Top of head and skull.

Continued

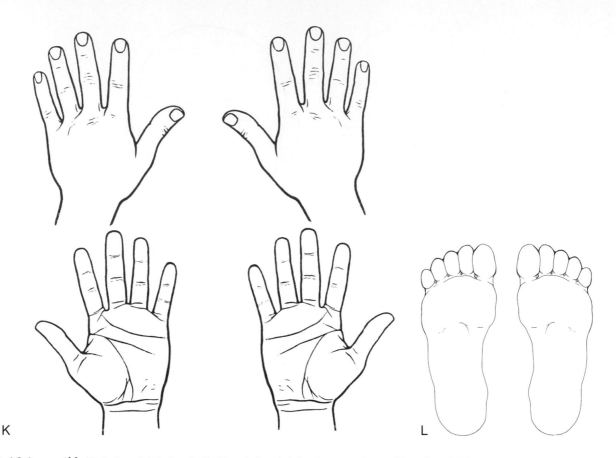

FIGURE **16-1—cont'd K,** Left and right hands. **L,** Feet, left and right plantar surfaces. (From Lynch VA: *Forensic nursing,* St. Louis, 2006, Mosby. Courtesy of the Metropolitan Dade County Medical Examiner Department, Dade County, Florida.)

information before photographing his or her injuries and again at the conclusion.

Correct Use of Common Medical Forensic Terms

It is critically important that ED nurses use correct medical forensic terminology when describing wounds. There are several terms commonly misused by ED personnel. For example, the terms *bruise* and *ecchymosis* are not synonymous; neither are the terms *laceration* and *cut.*[28-30]

Bruises are caused by blunt or compressive forces that damage blood vessels, resulting in bleeding either under the skin or in another organ. Ecchymotic lesions are usually caused by slow, hemorrhagic leakage of blood into the skin related to aging, medications, or underlying medical or hematologic conditions. Not every wound that is open and bleeding is a laceration. Lacerations are caused by the tearing or splitting of the skin or other organ by blunt or shearing forces. Cuts or incisions are caused by the cutting of the skin or other organ by a sharp object such as a knife or scalpel.[28-30]

The age of a bruise cannot be accurately estimated solely by looking at its color.[23] Bruise color charts still found in nursing textbooks were never developed using evidence-based research. In fact, the available research demonstrates that when clinicians attempt to date bruises by either looking directly at the contusion or a picture of the bruise, the clinicians' estimation of the age of the bruise is no more accurate than chance.[2,12,22] If the patient is a good historian, the ED nurse could document that the estimated age of the bruise is consistent with the history provided.

Traumatized patients often present with patterned injuries, which show on the skin the shape or outline of the object(s) used to inflict the injury. An example of a patterned injury is a triangular burn, with the shape, size, and appearance consistent with an iron. Documenting in the ED record the presence of patterned injuries can be invaluable in court.

Many victims of interpersonal violence or sexual assault experience reported strangulation. In abuse cases there are basically two types of strangulation, ligature and manual.[30] Ligature strangulation takes place whenever a cordlike object is wrapped around the neck and tightened. Common ligatures include ropes, electrical wires, telephone cords, clothing, and torn sheets. If a person has very long hair, it can be used as a ligature. Ligature strangulation usually leaves a ligature mark that is often a combination of a compression bruise mixed with an abrasion.

In manual strangulation the assailant uses some part of his or her body to compress the neck of the patient. Hands and headlocks are quite common. Visible injuries to the neck after strangulation can be rare,[34] even though the risk for death from strangulation is high. Although bruising or fingernail scratch marks may be absent on the neck, the ED nurse needs to assess whether the patient has any point tenderness. In addition, the ED nurse needs to ask the patient if there is any subjective change in the patient's voice quality or pain on swallowing.

Any form of strangulation can result in ruptured capillaries in and around the eyes and face called petechiae. However, strangulation does not always produce petechiae, and petechiae around the eyes and face can be caused by other mechanisms such as severe vomiting and strenuous activities such as childbirth.

Patients who have been strangled to unconsciousness or near unconsciousness may experience loss of bladder or bowel control.[32,34] The patient may be too embarrassed to share this finding. The ED nurse needs to be comfortable sharing with the patient that incontinence is common when strangled and it would be okay to share that with the nurse.

Patients who have survived strangulation, even in the absence of visible physical findings, need to be hospitalized with close supervision and 24-hour pulse oximetry monitoring, and they need to be in a setting where they can be promptly intubated if respiratory complications develop.[11,34]

SUMMARY

All EDs, large or small, rural, suburban, and urban, treat patients who have been victimized by violent acts (i.e., motor vehicle crashes, gunshot and stab wounds, physical assault, sexual assault, and neglect). Although there are a growing number of formal nursing educational programs that prepare nurses to be forensic specialists,[31] most of the forensic care of these patients will be provided by the ED nurse. The care provided needs to adhere to several well-published criteria of care. The ED nurse must do the following:
1. Be nonjudgmental
2. Document thorough, unbiased histories in the nursing record
3. Document physical findings on body maps and via photographs
4. Involve supporting disciplines when developing safety and discharge planning
5. Meet mandatory reporting requirements
6. Be ready and willing to testify to the ED nursing care

REFERENCES

1. Antognoli-Toland P: Comprehensive program for examination of sexual assault victims by nurses: a hospital-based program in Texas, *J Emerg Nurs* 11(3):132, 1985.
2. Bariciak ED, Plint AC, Gaboury I et al: Dating of bruises in children: an assessment of physician accuracy, *Pediatrics* 112(4):804, 2003.
3. Burgess AW, Holmstrom LL: Rape trauma syndrome, *Am J Psychiatry* 131(9):981, 1974.
4. Cabelus NB, Spangler K: Evidence collection and documentation. In Hammer RM, Moynihan B, Pagliaro EM: *Forensic nursing: a handbook for practice*, Sudbury, Mass, 2006, Jones & Bartlett.
5. Campbell JC: Misogyny and homicide of women, *Adv Nurs Sci* 8(4):67, 1981.
6. Drake VK: Battered women: a healthcare problem in disguise, *Image* 14:40, 1982.
7. Emergency Nurses Association: *Position statement: forensic evidence collection*. Retrieved June 1, 2008, from http://www.ena.org/about/position/pdfs/forensicevidence.pdf.
8. Fulton DR, Assid P: Evidence collection in the emergency department. In Lynch VA, Duval JB, editors: *Forensic nursing*, St. Louis, 2006, Mosby.
9. Hoyt CA: Evidence recognition and collection in the clinical setting, *Crit Care Nurs Q* 22(1):19, 1999.
10. International Association of Forensic Nurses: *What is forensic nursing?* 2006. Retrieved July 16, 2008, from http://www.iafn.org/displaycommon.cfm?an=1&subarticlenbr=137.
11. Kuriloff DB, Pincus RL: Delayed airway obstruction and neck abscess following manual strangulation injury, *Ann Otol Rhinol Laryngol* 98:824, 1989.
12. Langlois NEI, Gresham GA: The ageing of bruises: a review and study of the colour changes with time, *Forensic Sci Int* 50:227, 1991.
13. Ledray L, Chaignot MJ: Services to sexual assault victims in Hennepin County, *Eval Change,* special issue:131, 1980.
14. Ledray LE: Sexual assault nurse clinician: an emerging area of nursing expertise. In Andrist LC, editor: *Clinical issues in perinatal and women's health nursing*, vol 4, Philadelphia, 1993, Lippincott.
15. Lenehan G: Forensic nursing: an ED forensic kit, *J Emerg Nurs* 21:440, 1995.
16. Lew E, Dolinak D, Matshes E: Firearm injuries. In Dolinak D, Matshes E, Lew E, editors: *Forensic pathology: principles and practice*, Boston, 2005, Academic Press.
17. Lynch VA: *Clinical forensic nursing: a descriptive study in role development,* unpublished master's thesis, Arlington, 1990, University of Texas Health Science Center at Arlington.
18. Lynch VA: Forensic aspects of health care: new roles, new responsibilities, *J Psychosoc Nurs* 31(11):5, 1993.
19. Lynch VA: Forensic nursing: what's new? *J Psychosoc Nurs* 33(9):1, 1995.
20. Lynch VA: Forensic nursing science. In Hammer RM, Moynihan B, Pagliaro EM, editors: *Forensic nursing: a handbook for practice*, Sudbury, Mass, 2006, Jones & Bartlett.
21. Lynch VA: The specialty of forensic nursing. In Lynch VA, Duval JB, editors: *Forensic nursing*, St. Louis, 2006, Mosby.

22. Mosqueda L, Burnight K, Liao S: The life cycle of bruises in older adults, *J Am Geriatr Soc* 53(8):1339, 2005.
23. Nash KR, Sheridan DJ: Can one accurately date a bruise: the state of the science, *J Forensic Nurs*, 2009 (in press).
24. Parker B, Schumacher DM: The battered wife syndrome and violence in the nuclear family of origin: a controlled pilot study, *Am J Public Health* 67:760, 1977.
25. Pasqualone GA: Forensic photography. In Lynch VA, Duval JB, editors: *Forensic nursing*, St. Louis, 2006, Mosby.
26. Randall T: Clinician's forensic interpretations of fatal gunshot wounds often miss the mark, *JAMA* 269(16): 2058, 1993.
27. Saferstein R: Evidence collection and preservation. In Lynch VA, Duval JB, editors: *Forensic nursing*, St. Louis, 2006, Mosby.
28. Sheridan DJ: Forensic identification and documentation of patients experiencing intimate partner violence, *Clin Fam Pract* 5(1):113, 2003.
29. Sheridan DJ: Treating survivors of intimate partner abuse: forensic identification and documentation. In Olshaker JS, Jackson MC, Smock WS: *Forensic emergency medicine*, ed 2, Philadelphia, 2007, Lippincott Williams & Wilkins.
30. Sheridan DJ, Nash KR, Hawkins SL et al: Forensic implications of intimate partner abuse. In Hammer RM, Moynihan B, Pagliaro EM: *Forensic nursing: a handbook for practice*, Sudbury, Mass, 2006, Jones & Bartlett.
31. Sheridan DJ, Taylor WK: Developing hospital-based domestic violence programs, protocols, polices and procedures, *AWHONNS Clin Issues Perinat Womens Health Nurs* 4(3):471, 1993.
32. Smith DJ, Mills T, Taliaferro EH: Frequency and relationship of reported symptomology in victims of intimate partner violence: the effect of multiple strangulation attacks, *J Emerg Med* 21(3):323, 2001.
33. Speck P, Aiken M: 20 years of community nursing service, *Tenn Nurse* 58(2):5, 1995.
34. Strack GB, McClane GE, Hawley D: A review of 300 attempted strangulation cases. I, Criminal legal issues, *J Emerg Med* 21(3):303, 2001.
35. U.S. Department of Justice Office on Violence Against Women: *A national protocol for sexual assault medical forensic examinations: adults/adolescents*. NCJ 206554, Washington, DC, 2004, U.S. Department of Justice, 2004, http://www.safeta.org/associations/8563/files/National%20Protocol.pdf.
36. Young K, Jones J, Worthington T et al: Forensic laboratory evidence in sexually abused children and adolescents, *Arch Pediatr Adolesc Med* 160:585, 2006.
37. Young M, Stein J: *The history of the crime victim's movement in the United States: a component of the Office for Victims of Crime oral history project*, 2004, Justice Solutions, National Association of Crime Victim Compensation Boards, National Association of VOCA Assistance Administrators, and the National Organization for Victim Assistance, http://www.ojp.usdoj.gov/ovc/ncvrw/2005/pg4c.html.

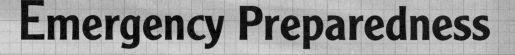

CHAPTER 17

Emergency Preparedness

Kathy S. Robinson

Disasters—natural and manmade events that dramatically affect life and property to catastrophic proportions—are fortunately rare, largely unpredictable, and yet inevitable. Historic events such as the attack on the World Trade Center in 2001 and Hurricane Katrina in 2005 reinforce the need for a national coordinated emergency response. Emergency responders, including nurses, are compelled by a sense of duty as the magnitude of any disaster unfolds and graphic images of human suffering are replayed over various media outlets. However, responding to human need is not as simple as grabbing a few supplies and jumping on the next bus to help. In 1995 a nurse was killed by falling debris in Oklahoma City in the aftermath of the explosion at the Alfred P. Murrah Building, illustrating the need for protective equipment and proper training. Hundreds of rescue and medical personnel who showed up via public transportation and private vehicles had to be turned away in the Gulf Coast region following Hurricane Katrina. Although professional skills were needed in specific locations, local officials did not have the means to feed or shelter unexpected personnel, verify professional credentials, or spare the resources to identify and coordinate proper work assignments in the midst of the actual event. Stockpiles of unrequested, unused supplies still sit in southern warehouses today. One of the greatest lessons learned during such events is that advance planning and preparation about the roles, responsibilities, and resource management strategies are essential to matching personnel, equipment, and supplies with the people and communities that need them most. Many mistakenly view the federal government (and in particular, the Federal Emergency Management Agency [FEMA]) in a lead and primary role in this regard. In reality, local emergency managers make intrastate and interstate requests for assistance long before a federal disaster response is activated by the governor of an affected state. These activations typically occur when local and state resources are exhausted or insufficient to meet the demands of the incident. FEMA is just one of many federal departments or agencies that may be called upon to assist rescue and recovery efforts.

The Homeland Security Act of 2002 refers to domestic incident management from an "all-hazards" perspective, in other words, any potential hazard that threatens a jurisdiction within our country's borders. The terms *emergency preparedness* and *domestic preparedness* are frequently used interchangeably. Under the initial U.S. Department of Homeland Security (DHS) reorganization in 2003, the Emergency Preparedness and Response Directorate contained most of the pre-DHS FEMA functions and staff, which were geared mostly toward natural disasters such as hurricanes and floods. The focus of this chapter addresses preparedness and response from an emergency management perspective, so the term *emergency preparedness* has been retained even though the more contemporary term is *domestic preparedness*.

Table 17-1. MAJOR FEDERAL LEGISLATIVE MILESTONES

Year	Milestone or Legislative Action	Key Elements
1803	Congressional Act	One of the first federal actions to provide local financial assistance (Portsmouth, NH, devastated by fire)
1934	Flood Control Act	Authorized U.S. Army Corps of Engineers to design and build flood control projects
1950	Civil Defense Act	Created shelter, evacuation, and training programs that state and local governments would implement
1950s	Ad hoc legislation	Provided disaster assistance funds following a series of hurricanes
1968	National Flood Insurance Act	Created the National Flood Insurance Program (NFIP)
1974	Disaster Relief Act	Coordinated federal response and recovery efforts through the NFIP
1979	Executive order by President Carter	Federal Emergency Management Agency (FEMA) created
1988	Robert T. Stafford Disaster Relief and Emergency Assistance Act	Amended Disaster Relief Act—constituted statutory authority for most federal disaster response activities, encourages hazard mitigation measures to reduce losses from disasters, authorized creation of the Federal Response Plan, required all states to prepare their own Emergency Operations Plans
1994	Stafford Act amended	Incorporated most of the former Civil Defense Act of 1950
1995	Nunn-Lugar Act	Core purpose was to reduce the nuclear threat to the United States domestically and abroad; it became the first federal legislation reflecting the government's concern for domestic disaster management resulting from terrorism
1996	Emergency Management Assistance Compact	Provided form and structure to interstate mutual aid
2001	Patriot Act	Significantly increased the surveillance and investigative powers of law enforcement agencies in the United States
2002	Homeland Security Act	Established Department of Homeland Security and refocused the country on terrorism
2002	Public Health Security and Bioterrorism Preparedness and Response Act	Related to public health preparedness and improvements, controls on biologic agents, protecting food, drug, and drinking water supplies; created state bioterrorism preparedness block grant program
2006	Pandemic and All-Hazards Preparedness Act	Transferred the National Bioterrorism Hospital Preparedness Program (NBHPP) from the Health Resources and Services Administration (HRSA) to the assistant secretary for preparedness and response (ASPR); ASPR is the principal advisor to the secretary of health and human services on public health and medical preparedness and response

Emergency nurses routinely plan, assess, adapt, and respond, and they can easily transition to unpredictable and chaotic environments while caring for patients. To serve as active participants in a disaster response, emergency nurses should gain additional skills and knowledge through an understanding of the Incident Command System (ICS) and of the various disciplines of emergency management—mitigation, preparedness, response, recovery, and communications[5]—before a disaster occurs.

EVOLUTION OF EMERGENCY MANAGEMENT

As a function of public health and safety, emergency management is an essential role of the government. During the Cold War era, the principal disaster risk in the United States was believed to be a nuclear attack by the Soviet Union. Individuals and communities were encouraged to build bomb shelters, and every community had a civil defense director (usually retired military personnel). Preceded by a string of natural disasters in the 1960s, a national focus on emergency management in the 1970s resulted in the formation of FEMA during the Carter administration. In the 1970s new categories of catastrophes also became evident—those caused by human error or malfeasance and involving chemicals or other toxic agents.[10] A new type of disaster without precedent was revealed in 1978 when toxic waste, buried in the Love Canal some 30 years earlier, was identified as the source of an alarming rate of cancer and birth defects in local residents. President Carter used emergency authority granted in disaster relief legislation to relocate families from the affected area.[2]

Several federal legislative milestones have been identified over the last decade making federal assistance available at the local level (Table 17-1). One of the most significant pieces of emergency management legislation was enacted by Congress in 1988. The key provision of the Robert T. Stafford Disaster Relief and Emergency Assistance Act included authorization (statutory authority) for most federal disaster response activities. The Stafford Act also encouraged hazard mitigation measures to reduce losses from disasters, authorized creation of the Federal Response Plan, and required all states to prepare their own Emergency Operations Plans. The Federal Response Plan, a landmark federal document when it was released in 1992, identified and organized Emergency

Support Functions (ESFs) as a mechanism for grouping activities most frequently used to provide federal support, both for declared disasters and emergencies under the Stafford Act and for non–Stafford Act incidents. ESF #8, the Public Health and Medical Services Annex,[3] was revised in 2007 and is categorized into the following core functional areas:

- Assessment of public health/medical needs
- Health surveillance
- Medical care personnel
- Health/medical/veterinary equipment and supplies
- Patient evacuation
- Patient care
- Safety and security of drugs, biologics, and medical devices
- Safety of blood and blood products
- Food safety and security
- Agriculture safety and security
- Worker safety and health
- All-hazard public health and medical consultation
- Technical assistance and support
- Behavioral health care
- Public health and medical information
- Vector control
- Potable water/wastewater and solid waste disposal
- Fatality management
- Veterinary medical support
- Human services coordination

Before Hurricane Katrina in 2005, Hurricane Andrew, which ravaged the state of Florida in 1992, was the most expensive disaster in United States history. At the time, Florida was ill-prepared to handle a disaster the magnitude of Hurricane Andrew. The state was not capable of providing adequate assessments of its damage and was unprepared to make appropriate requests for assistance. As a result, the Southern Regional Emergency Management Assistance Compact (SREMAC) was created through the Southern Governors Association. This compact "allowed states to assist each other with some certainty of the expectations and responsibilities involved, which in turn increased the likelihood of their doing so at considerably reduced risk of suit or of great expense. It also allowed states to provide assistance to one another either in advance of FEMA aid where it was forthcoming, or in place of FEMA aid where it was not."[1] Using SREMAC as a model, the U.S. Congress ratified the Emergency Management Assistance Compact (EMAC) as Public Law 104-321 on October 19, 1996, and today 50 states, the District of Columbia, Puerto Rico, and the U.S. Virgin Islands have enacted legislation to become members of EMAC.

In the months following the 2001 attack on the World Trade Center, President George W. Bush created the Homeland Security Council within the executive branch of the federal government and began issuing a series of executive orders commonly known as "Homeland Security Presidential Directives" or HSPDs, which record and communicate presidential decisions about the homeland security policies of the United States. Among them, in February 2003 President Bush issued Homeland Security Presidential Directive (HSPD)-5, *Management of Domestic Incidents,*[6] which directs the secretary of homeland security to develop and administer a National Incident Management System (NIMS). The system is intended to provide a nationwide template to enable federal, state, local, and tribal governments to work effectively together to manage a range of domestic incidents. Under NIMS, the president leads the federal government's response effort to ensure that the necessary coordinating structures, leadership, and resources are applied quickly and efficiently to large-scale catastrophic incidents. Under the NIMS structure, the secretary of homeland security is the principal federal official for domestic incident management. HSPD-5 requires all federal departments and agencies to adopt NIMS and to implement it across all programs. The directive also requires federal departments and agencies to mandate compliance with NIMS as a condition for federal preparedness assistance (i.e., grants, contracts, and other activities). As a result, NIMS became an essential component of the United States health care system through the National Bioterrorism Hospital Preparedness Program. Originally administered by the Health Resources and Services Administration (HRSA), the National Bioterrorism Hospital Preparedness program is now located in the United States Department of Health and Human Services (DHHS) under the assistant secretary for preparedness and response (ASPR). The focus of the program has become all-hazards preparedness and not solely bioterrorism. NIMS also identifies the basic principles of ICS.

Overview of ICS and NIIMS

According to FEMA, one of the most important "best practices" incorporated into NIMS is ICS, a standard, on-scene, all-hazards incident management system already in use by firefighters, hazardous materials teams, rescuers, and emergency medical teams. ICS has been established by NIMS as the standardized incident organizational structure for the management of all incidents.

The concept of ICS was developed more than 30 years ago, in the aftermath of a devastating wildfire in California. During 13 days in 1970, 16 people died, 700 structures were destroyed, and over one-half million acres burned. The cost and loss associated with these fires totaled $18 million per day. Although all of the responding agencies cooperated to the best of their ability, numerous problems with communication and coordination hampered their effectiveness. As a result, Congress mandated that the U.S. Forest Service design a system to effectively coordinate interagency actions and to allocate resources that would be applicable to multiple-fire situations. This system became known as Firefighting Resources of California Organized for Potential Emergencies (FIRESCOPE). FIRESCOPE ICS is primarily a command and control system delineating job responsibilities and organizational structure for the purpose of managing day-to-day operations for all types of emergency incidents.

By 1980, FIRESCOPE ICS training was under development. Recognizing that, in addition to the local users for whom it was designed, the FIRESCOPE training could satisfy the needs of other state and federal agencies, the National Wildfire Coordinating Group (NWCG) conducted an analysis of FIRESCOPE ICS for possible national application. Also during the 1970s the NWCG was chartered to coordinate fire management programs of the participating federal and state agencies.

By 1981, ICS was widely used throughout southern California by the major fire agencies. It was quickly recognized that ICS could help public safety responders provide effective and coordinated incident management for a wide range of situations: floods, hazardous materials incidents, earthquakes, and aircraft crashes. This system was flexible enough to manage catastrophic incidents involving thousands of emergency response and management personnel. By introducing relatively minor terminology and organizational and procedural modifications to FIRESCOPE ICS, ICS became adaptable to an all-hazards environment.

In 1982, all FIRESCOPE ICS documentation was revised and adopted as the National Interagency Incident Management System (NIIMS). In the years since FIRESCOPE and NIIMS were blended, the FIRESCOPE agencies and the NWCG have worked together to update and maintain the Incident Command System Operational System Description (ICS 120-1). This document would later serve as the basis for the NIMS ICS, created by HSPD-5 in 2003 and implemented by DHS in 2004. In December 2008, FEMA published a revision to NIMS, superseding the March 2004 version. It expands on the original version released in 2004 by clarifying existing NIMS concepts, better incorporating preparedness and planning, and improving the overall readability of the document. The revised document also differentiates between the purposes of NIMS and the National Response Framework (NRF) by identifying how NIMS provides the action template for the management of incidents, whereas the NRF provides the policy structure and mechanisms for national-level policy for incident management. The basic tenets of NIMS remain the same. There have been several improvements to the revised NIMS document that will aid in readability and usefulness of preparing, preventing, and responding to incidents, including a reordering of the key components to emphasize the role of preparedness and to mirror the progression of an incident. Additional information is available at http://www.fema.gov/emergency/nims/.

ICS Requirements for Hospitals and Practitioners

NIMS requires that all federal, state, local, tribal, private sector, and nongovernmental personnel with a direct role in emergency management and response must be NIMS and ICS trained.[4] This includes all emergency services–related disciplines such as emergency medical services (EMS), hospitals, public health, fire service, law enforcement, public works/utilities, skilled support personnel, and other emergency management response, support, and volunteer personnel. FEMA does not review or endorse commercial or proprietary courses. Currently the only approved training courses that meet NIMS competencies are provided through FEMA's Emergency Management Institute (EMI) and through approved local and state providers. EMI serves as the national focal point for the development and delivery of emergency management training. Courses are available online, and registration is free. It is anticipated that emergency nurses who wish to participate in disaster response under NIMS will be required to have this training in the future. Additional information is available at http://www.training. fema.gov/EMIWeb/. Emergency nurse managers involved or interested in hospital preparedness are encouraged to consider FEMA Independent Study Courses IC 100 and 200 HC for hospitals and health care systems. The Hospital Incident Command System (HICS, formerly HEICS) is an important foundation for the more than 6,000 hospitals in the United States in their efforts to prepare for and respond to various types of disasters. All HICS materials posted at www.emsa. ca.gov/dms2/dms2.asp are NIMS compliant and meet the requirements for hospital training when attended through EMI or an approved local or state provider. All hospitals were required to be fully compliant with NIMS activities delineated by FEMA[9] as of September 30, 2008, for hospitals to remain eligible for federal preparedness and response grants, contracts, or cooperative agreement funds.

Credentialing of Emergency Responders

Three principal efforts among FEMA's HSPD-5 initiatives are directed at supporting NIMS' policies to improve mutual aid processes. These include establishment of common performance standards for training emergency responders, use of common definitions for typical response resources (National Mutual Aid and Resource Management Initiative or "Resource Typing"), and implementing a national system for credentialing emergency responders that can be used to easily support mutual aid through the verification of the identity and qualifications of emergency response personnel. The credentialing system, currently referred to as the National Emergency Responder Credentialing System (NERCS) can help prevent unauthorized (i.e., self-dispatched or unqualified) personnel access to an incident site. Most homeland security experts agree that once the system is fully operational, access to a disaster scene will be restricted to those with a documented mission assignment and authorization to provide assistance through interstate mutual aid agreements.

National Bioterrorism Hospital Preparedness legislation in 2002 mandated that a state-based national system be implemented to meet the needs of hospital workforce emergency surge capacity. The Emergency System for Advance Registration of Health Professional Volunteers (ESAR-VHP) was developed and is currently operational in several states. The system comprises four levels based on the types of credentials required of a given health profession and what can be verified. Information about ESAR-VHP is available at http://www.hrsa.gov/esarvhp/.

DOMESTIC PREPAREDNESS AUTHORITY AND PLANNING AT THE FEDERAL LEVEL

Many federal agencies share roles and responsibilities with regard to domestic preparedness, requiring them to work in a collaborative manner. Under the Public Health Security and Bioterrorism Preparedness and Response Act of 2002, Congress outlines the need for DHHS to focus on public health emergencies and hospital needs in an effort to expand the physical capacity of our nation's hospitals and other health care facilities. Under the Federal Response Plan, DHHS is clearly responsible for ESF #8 (public health and medical services), as discussed earlier in this chapter. However, the Homeland Security Act of 2002 empowers the DHS to ensure the effectiveness of "emergency response providers" and incorporate all incident management disciplines into a unified structure under the national response plan. Although the primary responsibility for ESF #8 is assigned to DHHS, DHS retains primary responsibility for emergency response providers

defined in the act as "emergency response, emergency medical (including hospital emergency facilities), and related personnel, agencies, and authorities who are deployed from state-to-state using EMAC or other agreements for mutual aid."

The multiplicity of federal documents in the last decade reveals the complexity of creating a national system that adequately addresses domestic preparedness. The Federal Response Plan created in 1992 was replaced by the National Response Plan in 2004, which was amended in 2005 (Table 17-2). The National Response Framework (NRF) was developed by the DHS to replace all previous documents. DHS hails the 2008 framework as "flexible, scalable, and adaptable" and shifts many previously viewed federal responsibilities to state and local authorities. Online details of the NRF can be found in the NRF Resource Center at http://www.fema.gov/emergency/nrf/. It calls for separate operational and strategic plans to be developed around 15 national planning scenarios that are intended as a reference to help identify the critical tasks and capabilities that would be required in a coordinated national effort to manage major events (Box 17-1).

Table 17-2. CHRONOLOGY OF FEDERAL PREPAREDNESS DOCUMENTS

Year	Title	Description/Online Location
1992	Federal Response Plan	Guide for all-hazards approach to domestic incidents. Organizes Emergency Support Functions (ESFs) into categories reflecting various disciplines. The ESFs provide the structure for coordinating federal interagency support for a federal response to an incident. They are mechanisms for grouping functions most frequently used to provide federal support to states and federal-to-federal support, both for declared disasters and emergencies under the Stafford Act and for non–Stafford Act incidents (unavailable online)
2002	National Strategy for Homeland Security	Intended to mobilize and organize our nation to secure the U.S. homeland from terrorist attacks (http://www.whitehouse.gov/infocus/homeland/nshs/2007/index.html)
2004	National Incident Management System (NIMS)	Integrates emergency preparedness and response into national framework for incident management. Incident Command Structures are based on three organizational systems: incident command, multiagency coordination, public information (http://www.fema.gov/emergency/nims/nims_doc.shtm)
2004	National Response Plan	Uses the National Incident Management System (NIMS) to establish standardized training, organization, and communications procedures for multijurisdictional interaction and clearly identifies authority and leadership responsibilities (http://www.dhs.gov/nrp)
2005	National Response Plan amended	Updates reflect organizational changes within Department of Homeland Security (http://www.dhs.gov/nrp)
2005	National Preparedness Goal	Proposes to strengthen the preparedness of the United States to prevent, protect against, respond to, and recover from terrorist attacks, major disasters, and other emergencies
2005	National Strategy for Pandemic Influenza	Guides nation's preparedness and response to an influenza pandemic (http://www.pandemicflu.gov)
2006	National Strategy for Pandemic Influenza: Implementation Plan	Establishes 300+ actions for federal departments and agencies. Sets expectations for state and local governments and other nonfederal entities in response to an influenza pandemic (http://www.pandemicflu.gov)
2006	Pandemic Influenza Preparedness, Response, and Recovery Guide for Critical Infrastructure and Key Resources	Provides contingency planning process for a pandemic. Also provides business planners with sector-specific and common pandemic information planning variables keyed to escalating disaster phases (http://www.pandemicflu.gov)

(Continued)

Table 17-2. CHRONOLOGY OF FEDERAL PREPAREDNESS DOCUMENTS—CONT'D

Year	Title	Description/Online Location
2007	Community Strategy for Pandemic Influenza Mitigation	Designed to provide community guidance to reduce contact between people during a pandemic (www.pandemicflu.gov)
2007	National Preparedness Guidelines	Finalizes development of the national goal and its related preparedness tools. Encourages the development of capabilities that directly support and enable implementation of the concepts presented in NIMS and National Response Plan (http://www.fema.gov/pdf/government/npg.pdf)
2008	National Response Framework	Presents an overview of key response principles, roles, and structures that guide the national response (http://www.fema.gov/emergency/nrf/)
2008	National Incident Management System (NIMS) revised	Clarifies existing NIMS concepts, better incorporates preparedness and planning, improves the overall readability of the document, and reorders the key components to emphasize the role of preparedness and to mirror the progression of an incident. Complete description of revisions provided at (http://www.fema.gov/pdf/emergency/nims/NIMSWhatsNew.pdf)
2008	National Incident Management System (NIMS) Voluntary Standards for the Credentialing of Personnel Draft published in *Federal Register* for public comment	In development. Does not mandate a federal technical standard but asks state and local agencies to voluntarily adopt interoperable identification credentials. The Guidelines offer advice on registration and enrollment, eligibility, and risk assessments, issuance, verification and use, expiration and revocation, and redress and waiver. The Federal Docket is available at (http://www.regulations.gov/fdmspublic/component/main?main=DocketDetail&d=FEMA-2008-0015)

Box 17-1   NATIONAL PLANNING SCENARIOS

Nuclear Detonation: 10-kiloton Improvised Nuclear Device	Natural Disaster: Major Earthquake
Biological Attack: Aerosol Anthrax	Natural Disaster: Major Hurricane
Biological Disease Outbreak: Pandemic Influenza	Radiological Attack: Radiological Dispersal Device
Biological Attack: Plague	Explosives Attack: Bombing Using Improvised Explosive Device
Chemical Attack: Blister Agent	Biological Attack: Food Contamination
Chemical Attack: Toxic Industrial Chemicals	Biological Attack: Foreign Animal Disease
Chemical Attack: Nerve Agent	Cyber Attack
Chemical Attack: Chlorine Tank Explosion	

Data from the Homeland Security Counsel: The national planning scenarios. Washington, DC, 2006, The Author.

A companion to the National Preparedness Guidelines, the Targeted Capabilities List[11] (TCL), published by DHS in 2007, is a national-level, generic model of operationally ready capabilities defining all-hazards preparedness. Using the National Strategy for Homeland Security,[8] various federal statutes, presidential directives, and related doctrine, the TCL provides an all-hazards taxonomy showing the alignment of all homeland security activities toward mission achievement (Figure 17-1). This illustrative approach effectively communicates the national concept for all providers in responding to our nation's disasters. A basic understanding of these tenets can assist emergency nurses in making competent decisions, identifying resources, and functioning within legal parameters while serving a disaster response.

HOMELAND SECURITY MISSION AREAS: PREVENT-PROTECT-RESPOND-RECOVER

Whether part of a hospital staff, disaster medical assistance team (DMAT), or other community group organizing to assist during a disaster, emergency nurses can play leadership roles in personal and community domestic preparedness. Using the Homeland Security All-Hazards Taxonomy, as well as a full range of publications available from national organizations and federal agencies on disaster preparedness as a guide, Tables 17-3 to 17-6 are intended to stimulate thinking and create awareness of the types of activities that emergency nurses can perform on a personal and professional basis through the four mission stages related to homeland security:

1. Prevent
2. Protect
3. Respond
4. Recover

Originally intended to guide federal strategies in regard to terrorist attacks, these mission areas remain pertinent in the nation's response to all natural and manmade hazards. (Tables 17-3 to 17-6 are not intended to provide comprehensive planning recommendations or substitute for consultation or collaboration with local planning authorities).

Text continued on p.197.

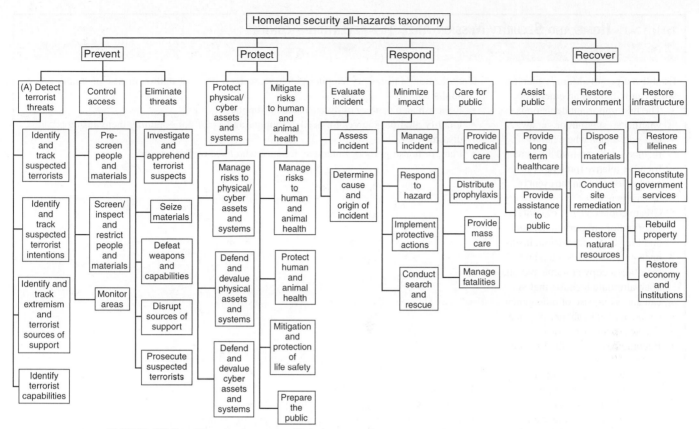

FIGURE **17-1.** Homeland security all-hazards taxonomy. (From U.S. Department of Homeland Security: *Targeted capabilities list, a companion to the national preparedness guidelines.* 2007.)

Table 17-3. **HOMELAND SECURITY MISSION AREA 1: PREVENTION**	
Personal	**Professional**
Learn what type of disasters can occur in your area and how to prepare for them	Participate in hospital planning efforts intended to help mitigate the effect of the disaster • Identify departmental lead and support in planning, training, and meeting activities to maintain preparedness expertise • Establish surveillance and detection plans to help identify unusual clusters of cases • Monitor CDC and public safety Web sites for current information and warnings • Reevaluate and drill hospital evacuation plans • Work with community leaders to establish medical surge plans • Work with hospital administration, community, and law enforcement leaders on ways to identify essential personnel for access through roadblocks, checkpoints, and hospital entrances during a disaster • Consider mutual aid agreements with community and public safety groups that can help transport stranded personnel and/or equipment during a disaster • Establish mutual aid agreements with EMS agencies for priority patient transport services during a disaster • Consider the use of alternate care sites in conjunction with public health, emergency management, and EMS authorities • Establish alternate staffing plans when employees cannot get to work or are confined to work • Identify a special area on the hospital's Web site to communicate with employees during a disaster, and educate them about going there for information; consider the hospital's Web site as a means to request resources and supplies along with drop-off information • Include local media venues when establishing an overall communications plan • Establish security plans for facility, equipment, vehicles, and personnel • Reevaluate mutual aid agreements • Evaluate the hospital's ability to provide interoperable communications • Consider the feasibility of a hospital-based emergency operations center, and identify responders, roles, and responsibilities

(Continued)

Table 17-3.   HOMELAND SECURITY MISSION AREA 1: PREVENTION—CONT'D

Personal	Professional
Establish a personal/family plan for what you will do in an emergency • The first important decision is whether to stay put or get away • Consider a plan where family members call or e-mail the same friend or relative (preferably in another location) in the event of an emergency • Create copies or lists of contact information, important account and financial information, insurance policies, cards, etc., and maintain a copy at home and one at an alternate location that you can access in case of emergency • Create a plan to shelter in place • Create a plan to get away • Become familiar with alternate routes • Plan how to take care of your pets	Identification of necessary supplies purchase, storage, and distribution in case of supply chain disruption • Establish an inventory of disaster-related supplies • Identify multiple sources for needed supplies and a plan for obtaining them during a disaster • Plan for housing, food, water, etc. for staff who must remain at work
Get a kit of emergency supplies (minimum 3-day supply) • Battery-powered radio with extra batteries • Water • Nonperishable food • Necessary medications • First-aid kit • Antibacterial hand products • Filter masks • Plastic sheeting and duct tape • Garbage bags and plastic ties for personal sanitation • Warm clothes and sleeping bag for each member of the family	Reevaluate infection control plans • Model exceptional infection control practices • Educate staff on known or potentially emerging threats • Encourage co-workers to maintain recommended vaccinations • Plan to offer medical countermeasures to personnel and their families
Learn about what to expect following a disaster in terms of immediate services, and help educate friends and family members about the need to prepare	Include public health authorities, law enforcement community, 911, and EMS in hospital planning efforts, and establish phone trees to communicate with own personnel before, during, and after a major event

CDC, Centers for Disease Control and Prevention; EMS, emergency medical services.

Table 17-4.   HOMELAND SECURITY MISSION AREA 2: PROTECTION

Personal	Professional
Report suspicious persons, packages, or vehicles to the proper authorities	Organize • Decision guidance for PPE • Consider patient flow, use of alternate care facilities • Consider medicolegal implications when equipment and supplies become scarce, and collaborate with hospital ethics committees to preestablish equipment use protocols • Establish fatality management plan with public health and local medical examiner to deal with large numbers of fatalities • Consider plans to identify alternate security personnel if hospital security and local law enforcement become unable to respond

Table 17-4. HOMELAND SECURITY MISSION AREA 2: PROTECTION—CONT'D

Personal	Professional
Find out about the disaster plans at your workplace, your children's school or day care center, and other places where your family spends time	Training needs • Ensure clinical educators are current and informed on a range of emergency preparedness topics and ready to provide "just in time" training in the event of a disaster
Make sure to maintain cash on hand (ATMs and banking services may become unavailable)	Equipment • Become familiar with national resources such as the Interagency Board or *Concept of Operations for the Acute Care Center* to assist in determining local stockpiles (see http://www.iab.gov/Documents.aspx and http://www.nnemmrs.org/surg) • Check with national specialty organizations for sample checklists and equipment lists to support advance planning needs
Conduct fire and emergency evacuation drills at home	Exercise • Review national exercises (such as TOPOFF) and real-time "after action reports" to establish best practice suggestions that might be used to support local needs • Test local response plans through drills and exercises to identify strengths and weakness of the plan and to reinforce roles and responsibilities among all levels of responders • Conduct "lockdown" exercises to identify departmental vulnerabilities in advance of an MCI
Replace stored water and stored food every 6 months	Evaluate • Review outcomes of local exercises, and identify strengths and weaknesses to share with participants • Identify community partners that may have been overlooked in planning and exercise opportunities, and invite them to future meetings
If you are considering volunteer opportunities for future deployment: 1. Get involved with a response team now (such as a DMAT, Medical Reserve Corps, or hospital response team) 2. Discuss deployment expectations with your employer in advance to ensure support; do not expect that you can simply take leave when a need arises because needs may exist or increase at your own facility during a disaster 3. Obtain expected and necessary training 4. Check with local health department, and maintain proper vaccinations and immunizations for health care workers (such as Tdap, hepatitis, and influenza) 5. Participate in drills with your team 6. Check with your state health department or SBN for rules and regulations that pertain to interstate licensing requirements to ensure proper credentialing	Improve • Address weaknesses, and work to eliminate them • Conduct regional conferences to educate personnel on "lessons learned" at all levels • Revise protocols, policies, and plans as needed • Repeat exercise

ATM, Automated teller machine; *DMAT,* disaster medical assistance team; *MCI,* mass casualty incident; *PPE,* personal protective equipment; *SBN,* state board of nursing; *TOPOFF,* Top Officials (preparedness exercise).

Table 17-5. HOMELAND SECURITY MISSION AREA 3: RESPONSE

Personal	Professional
Remain calm and patient, and put your plans into action	Gain situational awareness • Estimate number of victims • Estimate severity of injuries • Anticipate personnel and equipment needs • Coordinate activities and requests with health and public safety officials

(Continued)

Table 17-5. HOMELAND SECURITY MISSION AREA 3: RESPONSE—CONT'D

Personal	Professional
Give first aid, and get help for seriously injured people Listen to your battery-powered radio for news and instructions	• Assess situation, and report to chain of command • Initiate hospital EOC Activate resources • Hospital disaster plans • Local and regional disaster plans • Security plan • Establish triage and decontamination areas as needed • Establish private family waiting area outside the ED, and assign support personnel to facilitate information • Alter traffic patterns around hospital entrances, and restrict access to the ED to essential equipment and personnel
Check for damage in your home • Use flashlights. Do not light matches or turn on electrical switches if you suspect damage • Sniff for gas leaks, starting at the water heater. If you smell gas or suspect a leak, turn off the main gas valve, open windows, and get everyone outside quickly • Shut off any other damaged utilities • Clean up spilled medicines, bleaches, gasoline, and other flammable liquids immediately Remember to … • Confine or secure your pets • Call your family contact—do not use the telephone again unless it is a life-threatening emergency • Check on your neighbors, especially elderly or disabled persons • Make sure you have an adequate water supply in case service is cut off • Stay away from downed power lines	Coordinate response • Provide point of contact to support incident commander and facilitate exchange of information • Ensure real-time supply monitoring • Patient tracking systems • Hospital resource tracking systems • Establish a fatality/missing person information telephone number to report unidentified fatalities, incorporating this information into a national patient tracking system Demobilize • Maintain ongoing awareness of personnel needs • Rotate staff to prevent burnout • Provide comfort stations, hydration and nourishment, restroom facilities, and private areas for debriefing • Arrange for on-site grief counselors to support victims, families, and staff • Replenish equipment and supplies between patient surges

ED, Emergency department; *EOC,* emergency operations center.

Table 17-6. HOMELAND SECURITY MISSION AREA 4: RECOVER

Personal	Professional
Maintain an evacuation box large enough to carry the following: • A small amount of traveler's checks or cash and a few rolls of quarters • Negatives for irreplaceable personal photographs, protected in plastic sleeves • A list of emergency contacts that includes doctors, financial advisors, clergy, reputable repair contractors, and family members who live outside your area • Copies of important prescriptions for medicines and eyeglasses and copies of children's immunization records • Health, dental, or prescription insurance cards or information • Copies of your automobile, flood, renter's, or homeowner's insurance policies (or at least policy numbers) and a list of insurance company telephone numbers • Copies of other important financial and family records (or at least a list of their locations) • Backup of computerized financial records • A list of bank account, loan, credit card, driver's license, investment account (brokerage and mutual funds), and Social Security numbers • Safe deposit box key	Identify needs and resources • If forced to evacuate, ensure safety and security of premises before reentry • Gain awareness of impact on staff (both personal and professional) • Acknowledge staff accomplishments • Anticipate workforce leaves of absence, and plan to adjust schedules as necessary • Physical inspection of facilities • Reevaluate critical infrastructure (i.e., intact physical space, disruption to utilities and lines, sanitation) • Inventory supplies, and reestablish supply chain • Identify status of ancillary services, and communicate availability to staff

Table 17-6. HOMELAND SECURITY MISSION AREA 4: RECOVER—CONT'D	
Personal	**Professional**
Consult American Red Cross and other Web sites for recovery guides	Promote community restoration • Address mental health needs • Public relations strategies to identify available resources (ensure consistent messages throughout hospitals and health care systems) • Consider temporary expansion of services to address surge of primary care needs • Monitor CDC and public information Web sites for any postevent instructions • Attend postincident community briefings

CDC, Centers for Disease Control and Prevention.

SUMMARY

Emergency preparedness is every citizen's responsibility and perhaps a greater responsibility for those working in health professions. Emergency nurses interested in deployment opportunities during disasters must receive proper ICS and disaster-related safety training and participate in state credentialing programs *in advance* of a disaster. Some hospitals and health systems have established and equipped medical teams who could provide emergency response during a disaster. The state public health office, the state emergency preparedness office (usually located within the health department,) the state Emergency Management Agency, or the state hospital association may have more information in this regard. Most jurisdictions will not accept self-deployed responders during a disaster because of the challenges created by on-site logistics, credentialing, and liability. Individual responders are generally not requested; however, individuals who organize and train together as a team (such as a local or state ENA chapter, Community Emergency Response Team [CERT], or Medical Reserve Corps) could be eligible for funding and grants and could be requested and deployed through the EMAC process to support a mutual aid response. Opportunities for individuals may also exist through the National Disaster Medical System.[7] Most important, emergency preparedness begins at home. Personal preparedness assists us with being ready to support ourselves and our families when affected and to respond as health care professionals when needed.

REFERENCES

1. Bullock J: *The emergency management assistance compact: creating a network of management in times of emergency,* 1996. Retrieved August 30, 2007, from http://www.clearhq.org/Bullock.htm.
2. EPA, *New York State announce temporary relocation of Love Canal residents* (press release), 1980. Retrieved August 7, 2007, from http://www.epa.gov/history/topics/lovecanal/03.htm.
3. *Federal response framework ESF #8—public health and medical services annex,* 2007, U.S. Department of Homeland Security. Retrieved September 22, 2007, from http://www.fema.gov/emergency/nrf/.
4. *FY07NIMS training guidelines,* 2007, Federal Emergency Management Agency. Retrieved September 22, 2007, from http://www.fema.gov/pdf/emergency/nims/TrainingGdlMatrix.pdf.
5. Haddow GD, Bullock JA: *Introduction to emergency management,* ed 4, Burlington, Mass, 2007, Elsevier Butterworth-Heinemann.
6. *Homeland security presidential directive/HSPD-5,* 2003, The White House. Retrieved August 21, 2007, from http://www.whitehouse.gov/news/releases/2003/02/20030228-9.html.
7. *National disaster medical system,* 2007, U.S. Department of Health and Human Services. Retrieved August 21, 2007, from http://www.hhs.gov/aspr/opeo/ndms/index.html.
8. *National strategy for homeland security,* Washington, DC, 2002, U.S. Department of Homeland Security. Retrieved August 21, 2007, from http://www.dhs.gov/xabout/history/publication_0005.shtm.
9. NIMS implementation activities for hospitals and healthcare systems, 2006, Federal Emergency Management Agency. Retrieved February 19, 2008, from http://www.fema.gov/pdf/emergency/nims/imp_hos.pdf.
10. Rubin CB, editor: *Emergency management: the American experience 1900-2005,* Fairfax, Va, 2007, Public Entity Risk Institute, .
11. *Targeted capabilities list,* 2007, Washington, DC, U.S. Department of Homeland Security.

CHAPTER 18

Nuclear, Biologic, and Chemical Agents of Mass Destruction

Knox Andress

WEAPONS OF MASS DESTRUCTION: THE THREAT

Emergency nursing requires preparation for many types of disasters and mass casualty incidents (MCIs), including those caused by nuclear, biologic, or chemical (NBC) agents, collectively referred to as potential weapons of mass destruction (WMD). The United States Code, Title 50, defines WMD as "any weapon or device that is intended or has the capacity to cause death or serious bodily injury to a significant number of people through the release, dissemination, or impact of (a) toxic or poisonous chemicals or their precursors; (b) a disease organism; or (c) radiation or radioactivity." WMD are used or stockpiled by both terrorists (domestic and foreign) and military agencies because their primary purpose is to kill, injure, sicken, threaten, or strike fear in a target population. Because of the potential for such a widespread psychologic effect, WMD have also been termed weapons of mass effect (WME).[45] This chapter outlines the characteristics and medical response considerations for NBC agents of mass destruction.

Who Threatens

Both domestic and foreign terrorist threats could involve NBC agents. These threats include lone individuals, political and special-interest groups, nonaligned groups, doomsday or religious cults, and insurgents.[8] Domestic terrorists are those from the United States. They may be individuals such as Ted Kaczynski (i.e., the "Unabomber"); Timothy McVeigh, who was convicted of the Murrah Federal Building bombing; or Eric Rudolph (Olympic Park Bomber). Domestic terrorists may also belong to hate-associated organizations such as the Ku Klux Klan (KKK); ecology "special interest" groups like the Earth Liberation Front (ELF), which was responsible for multiple acts of arson to vehicles and buildings; religious cults such as the Aum Shinrikyo, which was responsible for the sarin gas attacks in Japan; and/or followers of the Bhagwan Shree Rajneesh, who were responsible for sickening hundreds of residents in (the city of) The Dalles, Oregon. Foreign terrorists may belong to organizations such as al Qaeda, Hamas, and/or may be state sponsored.[10] Terrorists seek to injure, kill, cause destruction, and instill fear for their personal or political agenda. The use or threatened use of WMD agents is a federal crime with the FBI having jurisdictional authority.

Why Nuclear, Biologic, and Chemical Agents

NBC agents are practical tools for terrorism. NBC weapons require only small quantities of an agent or pathogen to achieve a high impact. NBC agents are easy to conceal and transport and can be hard to detect. Many of these small, potent agents do not have a characteristic odor or other obvious physical characteristics. NBC components are widely available within the community, are readily made, and are relatively inexpensive. Bioweapons have been cited as "the poor man's atomic bomb" because of their potentially high impact and relatively low cost.[36] Materials can be found in local factories, hardware stores, industrial settings, school laboratories, universities, and hospitals.

Mass Casualty Differences

There are differences between the mass casualties arising from a natural disaster and those resulting from terrorism involving NBC components. MCIs occur every day, resulting in injured persons presenting to the emergency department (ED). MCIs may result from manmade events such as a transportation crash or from natural events such as an earthquake, hurricane, tornado, or epidemic. Natural disasters are not premeditated, whereas terrorism is a planned and perpetrated event. Terrorism or threats of terrorism are federal crimes and require collaboration with multiple organizations, which includes following chain of custody when collecting the victim's personal belongings. Responders need to be aware of possible secondary terrorism devices intended for the rescuers.[5] There is a greater potential for death and destruction with NBC agents. Many natural disasters come with some sort of warning beforehand; however, there is usually little to no preparation for an act of terrorism. MCIs involving NBC agents, whether accidental (e.g., Chernobyl, Russia) or intentional (e.g., Tokyo, Japan) will result in reactions of anxiety and increased fear of possible exposure or contamination. Persons with exacerbations of preexisting psychogenic illnesses may also present to the ED.[24] Hospital and emergency medical services (EMS) systems could easily become overwhelmed.

NUCLEAR-RADIOLOGIC THREATS

Most people are exposed to some level of environmental radiation every day. Ionizing radiation sources are used in commercial food sterilization processors, smoke detectors, medical therapy devices, radiopharmaceuticals, and radiography devices to name a few. A nuclear threat may be the result of an accident or malfunction, or it may involve a terrorist's use of a radioactive source either alone, in combination with an explosive, or in a nuclear detonation. A nuclear detonation is considered the least likely threat-scenario because of its complexity and the security processes in place; however, it may create the greatest destructive impact.[39] The nuclear detonations at Hiroshima and Nagasaki, Japan, during World War II were some of the first accounts of overt nuclear-radiologic threats against man. Current nuclear threats are considered to come from nations such as North Korea and Iran and from both domestic and foreign terrorist elements.

Types of Nuclear-Radiologic Devices

Potential radiologic and nuclear threats include the following:

- *Radiologic exposure device (RED):* A radioactive source is placed where numerous individuals can be unknowingly irradiated. An RED could be placed in a common public location, or radioactive material could be placed in food or drink, causing internal irradiation as experienced by the Soviet dissident Alexander Litvinenko.[25]
- *Radiologic dispersal device or RDD (dirty bomb):* A radioactive source is combined with/in a traditional explosive device. The bomb explodes and spreads radioactive particulate and aerosolized radiation sources. Geographic areas and people within the plume incur varying levels of contamination. Injuries can arise from explosion burns, blast, radioactive contaminates, contaminate inhalation, and shrapnel injuries.
- *Nuclear installation or reactor:* Intentional (sabotage) or unintentional (cracks or meltdown) damage to a reactor can release high levels of radiation via contaminated steam and smoke.
- *Improvised nuclear device:* A fabricated or crude nuclear bomb that could result in a 10- to 20-kiloton blast similar to the explosion that destroyed Nagasaki, Japan. Fissile materials could be acquired by terrorists to create this WMD.[27,41]
- *Thermonuclear weapon:* A weapons-grade, atomic or hydrogen bomb. This device creates energy from atomic fission or fusion. The effects of a 1-kiloton blast (equivalent to 1,000 tons of TNT) over 1 minute would be as follows:
  - Blast range of approximately 400 yards
  - Thermal radiation burns approximately 400 yards out
  - High rates of radioactive fallout up to ½ mile from blast
  - Gamma and neutron radiation up to ½ mile from blast
  - Electromagnetic pulse (EMP) that would destroy or damage computer microchips and circuits (an aerial burst would increase the effects of an EMP)

All of these nuclear threats have the potential to release ionizing radiation in the form of alpha, beta, and gamma rays; neutrons; and x-rays in either a particulate matter or "wavelike" form.

Radiation Basics

Radiation is energy emitted from a source and is a constant occurrence in our natural environment. We are surrounded by low-level, background radiation coming from the soil, sun, and certain products within our living space and workplace.[26] There are two principal radiation forms, nonionizing and ionizing, and it is the ionizing radiation that poses the potential health risks addressed here. Ionizing radiation has enough energy that it can break chemical bonds of impacted atoms, creating energized, or ionized particles. There are two forms of ionizing radiation: waves (electromagnetic) and particles. Types of ionizing radiation include alpha, beta, gamma, neutron, and x-rays. Under the correct conditions and amounts, the ionized particles can interact with living cells, creating free radicals that cause chemical changes within those cells. Biologic damage can occur to cellular DNA bonds, proteins, and membranes and can be expressed later as tissue alterations, mutations, tumors, or cancers.

Types of Radiation

Ionizing radiation may be emitted directly in the forms of alpha or beta particles along with gamma and or x-rays. Neutrons are indirectly ionizing particles because they do not carry an electrical charge

- Alpha particle radiation is composed of two neutrons and two protons, is very energetic, and highly ionizing. Alpha is the least penetrating, traveling several centimeters in air, and particles can be blocked by a sheet of paper, clothing, or by the outer layer of dead human skin. There is a minimal external-exposure threat, but inhalation or absorption/internalization can be a serious hazard.
- Beta radiation is emitted from the nucleus. It is a smaller particle than alpha and penetrates moderately, moving up to a few meters in air and a few millimeters through tissue. Beta particles can be blocked with glass, wood, or plastic. Beta particles and energy can cause skin injury known as "beta burns" over time.
- Gamma rays and x-rays are high-energy, wavelike forms of radiation that can penetrate deeply and are difficult to shield. Gamma rays travel farther and require special shielding such as appropriate amounts of lead or concrete.
- Neutrons are highly penetrating and energetic particles emitted from the nucleus. Neutrons, like gamma rays and x-rays, require special shielding.[37]

Dose

To understand exposure one must study or measure the dose of radiation. Radiation measurement factors include the activity (A), absorbed dose (D), and the dose-equivalent (H). Activity is a measurement of ionized particles discharged and is measured in a unit called a curie (Ci). More curies present means more radioactivity. The time it takes for a quantity of radioactive material to decay by half of its original amount is its "half-life." A Geiger counter is used to detect and measure radioactive decay. Absorbed dose (D), or rad, is energy deposited in the tissue per unit mass of irradiated tissue. The rad is the U.S. standard unit of measurement, whereas the International System (SI) of units for the absorbed dose is the gray (Gy). Dose-equivalent (H) is measured in rems, comprises the absorbed dose (D), and is weighted for the effectiveness of causing biologic damage.[26] The Sievert is the SI unit used to measure dose-equivalent. Dose-equivalant assists by providing a common scale for all types of radiation tissue damage

Everyone receives natural, background radiation exposure from his or her living and working environment. The annual natural background radiation dose a person receives

from sun, soil, building materials, etc., is approximately 300 millirem (300 mrem). Airline passengers flying from Los Angeles to New York might receive 2.5 mrem of cosmic radiation, whereas an unprotected ED nurse potentially receives 5 mrem during a portable chest x-ray examination. Other typical patient radiation doses include the following: bone scan, 400 mrem; abdominal computerized tomography (CT) scan, 760 mrem; barium enema, 870 mrem; and cardiac catheterization, 45,000 mrem. The goal is to keep radiation exposure and contamination levels as low as reasonably achievable (ALARA).

The hospital radiation safety officer or health physicist can assist with calculating dose exposures and monitoring the effectiveness of decontamination actions.

Protection Principles: Time, Distance, Shielding

Principles for protection from the effects of ionizing radiation include factors of time, distance, and attenuation or shielding. Limiting time spent near a radioactive source limits dosage and possible effects. Remain as far away from a source as possible. The intensity of ionizing radiation is minimized by the inverse of the distance squared (i.e., the greater the distance, the less of a dose received). Radiation attenuation or shielding with proper materials can reduce radiation exposure and dose received. Proper shielding materials are a factor of the type of radiation emitted, with alpha particles being blocked by clothing or paper and beta particles by a thicker plastic or wood material, which can impede absorption. Gamma rays, neutrons, and x-rays require substantially more shielding with appropriate amounts of lead (aprons or lead-lined rooms), concrete (radiation bunkers), or earth (berms).

Exposure, Contamination, and Incorporation

Radiation injury begins after external or internal exposure (contamination) or irradiation occurring from exposure to a penetrating radioactive source. The body's incorporation or uptake of radioactive contaminants results in systemic injury. Contamination occurs after internal or external exposure to radioactive materials by inhalation, ingestion, or when deposited on the body or clothing. Patients considered potentially contaminated should be surveyed and appropriately decontaminated.

External irradiation exposure does not make the victim radioactive or pose a threat to caregivers. A person contaminated with radioactive isotopes should be medically stabilized, appropriately decontaminated, and referred for further treatment and evaluation.[9]

Internal contamination results when radioactive contaminants are blast embedded, inhaled, or ingested. This might occur to victims near a detonated RDD when radioactive fragments and bomb particulates become imbedded or nuclear material is aerosolized and inhaled. Incorporation begins when the cells and tissues of the body's radiosensitive system cells, such as bone marrow stem cells, gastrointestinal (GI) villi, liver cells, and thyroid cells, begin uptake of the radioactive contamination.[37]

Acute Radiation Syndrome

The acute illness arising from a significant and penetrating, partial- or whole-body irradiation is referred to as acute radiation syndrome (ARS). Ionizing radiation affects the most radiosensitive cells first, which include those involving hematopoiesis, digestion, and the central nervous system (CNS).[3] ARS is subdivided into three syndromes that are based on the body's affected system and includes potential cutaneous radiation injury.

Body Systems Affected

The order of syndrome appearance is based on cell radiosensitivity and the absorbed dose. Syndromes include the hematopoietic syndrome, the GI syndrome, CNS or neurovascular syndrome, and cutaneous radiation injuries.

HEMATOPOIETIC SYNDROME. Bone marrow stem cells and accessory cells are most notably radiosensitive, and their irradiation results in increasingly rapid cellular death and alterations in blood component formation. The destruction of bone marrow stem cells and similar systems results in lymphopenia, pancytopenia, sepsis, and hemorrhage. Radiation doses resulting in a hematopoietic syndrome may be seen in an exposure of 0.3 to 0.7 Gy (30 to 70 rads).[19] The rate of decline in absolute lymphocytes over a 2-day period is used to help predict radiation level exposure.

GASTROINTESTINAL SYNDROME. Destruction of microvilli and GI tract lining occurs with absorbed doses of 6 to 10 Gy (600 to 1000 rads). Mucosal lining breakdown and sloughing of the intestinal wall results in diarrhea, severe nausea, vomiting, abdominal pain, and subsequent systemic effects that could include fever, GI bleeding, dehydration, and anemia. The LD_{100}, or lethal dose for 100% of the population, is approximately 10 Gy (1000 rads).

CENTRAL NERVOUS SYSTEM SYNDROME. CNS syndrome is equated with an expectant or fatal outcome. CNS syndrome may be noted after absorbed doses of 20 to 50 Gy (2000 to 5000 rads) and is indicated by nervousness, confusion, altered level of consciousness, convulsions, and death. Symptoms can begin minutes after exposure to this intense irradiation.

CUTANEOUS RADIATION INJURY. Radiation injury to the skin and tissues can occur with doses as low as 2 Gy (200 rads). Because minimal energy is required, injury can occur without other ARS symptoms. An example would be the beta burns resulting from beta radiation. Dermal and underlying tissue damage increases as dose is increased. Radiation burn injuries can present over weeks or months and are staged and graded. Symptoms can include itching, tingling, edema, erythema, ulcerations, and the injuries may result in dry or moist desquamation and necrosis. Pain management and infection control are important for care.

Acute Radiation Syndrome Stages

ARS symptoms are also classified into a sequence of four phases or stages. Stage development is dependent on cell radiosensitivity and dose and type of radiation received. The four stages of ARS are prodromal, latent, manifest illness, and recovery or death. The prodromal or nausea-vomiting-diarrhea stage is dose dependent. It usually begins minutes to days after exposure, and symptoms may last for days The latent phase occurs hours to weeks after the prodromal stage and is marked as a period when the patient feels and may look healthy. In the manifest illness stage symptoms due to the particular syndrome appear and may last from hours to months. The recovery or death stage lasts from days to years, again depending on the syndrome.[19]

Diagnosis and Treatment

ARS follows a predictable course of illness after substantial irradiation. Complete blood count (CBC) analysis can be correlated to exposure level. ARS should be evaluated with serial CBC analysis with a focus on lymphocyte count every 2 to 3 hours for the first 8 to 12 hours after exposure, and then every 4 to 6 hours for the subsequent 2 to 3 days.[33] Dosimetry for exposure dose levels can also be quantified via genetic assay with dicentric chromosome analysis considered the "gold standard." Record all symptoms, including nausea, vomiting, diarrhea, skin erythema, and any blistering, as well as their time of onset. The onset time of vomiting has been correlated to prognosis and exposure level. Treatment considerations will be largely supportive based on ARS symptoms, including antiemetics and fluids. Other possible treatments include stem cell replacement, cytokines, and if internalized or incorporated, cathartics, chelators, and binding agents, some of which may be implemented in the ED.

Planning

- Stabilize the patient first. Ensure airway, breathing, and circulation.
- If contamination is suspected, decontaminate appropriately and survey for effectiveness.
- An exposure without contamination does not need decontamination.
- Treat any traumas, burns, or other injury symptoms. Provide supportive care.
- Notify public health and law enforcement.
- Obtain laboratory specimens, including serial CBC, human leukocyte antigen (HLA), and serum amylase. Other specimens collected might include swab samples from body orifices and urine specimens if contamination or a substantial dose was internalized. Consider dicentric chromosomal assay.
- Consult specialists, including the hospital radiation safety officer, health physicist, Radiation Emergency Assistance Center Training Site (REAC/TS), and/or the Armed Forces Radiobiology Research Institute (AFRRI).[24]

BIOLOGIC AGENTS

Biologic pathogens have been researched, weaponized, and employed by armies against their opponents for hundreds of centuries. Pathogens were used in the Middle Ages, during the French and Indian War, by Germany in World War I, and Japan in World War II. In 1984 The Dalles, Oregon, was the scene for the first known biologic attack in the United States. There the Rajneeshee, a religious cult, attempted to gain control of the local county government by spraying salmonella on salad bars and throughout public venues before a county election. Over 500 persons became ill.[46] The September 2001 anthrax attacks on various U.S. news media offices and two U.S. Senate offices resulted in 22 infections including 5 deaths. Today both domestic and foreign terrorists have developed and deployed bioweapons. Countries with offensive biologic weapons programs have included South Africa, United States, Soviet Union, Great Britain, Iraq, Syria, North Korea, and Iran. The signing of the 1972 Biological Weapons Convention Treaty by a majority of nations, including the United States, ended offensive biologic weapons development for the signing countries. Although also signing, the Soviet Union reportedly continued clandestine research, development, and production of genetically altered "super pathogens" well into the 1990s. Production activities were curtailed and facilities closed after defecting Soviet microbiologists revealed ongoing bioweapons activities and facility locations.[2]

Biologic Threats: Bacteria, Viruses, and Toxins

Biologic threat agents include bacteria, viruses, and toxins. Bacteria are single-celled microorganisms that may form spores and produce a tissue inflammatory reaction. Viruses are the simplest pathogen, consisting of protein-coated RNA or DNA. Viruses require a host cell and can cause a variety of cell-specific diseases. Viral diseases may end in vascular damage and multiple system organ failure. Toxins are nature's poisons and are more deadly than comparable amounts of any manmade chemical agent.[49] Toxins or their precursors may be found in the outside garden (ricin) or may exist in the kitchen pantry (botulinum).

The infection methods or delivery routes include inhalation, ingestion, injection, and dermal contact. Examples include inhalation of respiratory droplets infected with a virus such as smallpox, ingestion of salmonella, or dermal contact with anthrax spores. Many biologic agents are contagious from person to person.

The Centers for Disease Control and Prevention (CDC) has categorized certain bacterial, viral, and toxin biologic threats into Category A, B, and C diseases or agents. Categorization factors include ease of dissemination; transmissibility; potential for high morbidity and mortality; potential for social disruption; surveillance needs, and ease of production among others. The CDC Category A agents are anthrax, botulism, plague, smallpox, tularemia, and viral hemorrhagic fevers (VHFs), including Ebola, Marburg, Lassa, and Machupo.[13] All suspected biologic agent cases should result in notification of the infection control practitioner, appropriate hospital personnel, and public health officials.

Epidemiology: The Clues

A biologic attack or infectious outbreak will be insidious, but there will be clues. Clues include infections unusual for a geographic region; increased deaths among the immunocompromised; multiple, similar outbreaks of disease; multiple, drug-resistant pathogens; increased or many sick and dying animals; physical evidence; or agent delivery device. Disease surveillance factors during triage and medical history might include travel history, infectious contacts, activities over the previous 3 to 5 days, and employment history.[49] The hospital infection control practitioner along with local and state public health officials should be notified for any suspected Category A patient.

CDC Category A Bacteria

ANTHRAX. *Bacillus anthracis* is a rod-shaped, grampositive, spore-forming bacteria endemic within certain agricultural regions and livestock populations and may cause woolsorter's disease from handling contaminated hides or fluids. Spore inoculation may result in cutaneous anthrax; spore ingestion may result in GI anthrax; whereas spore inhalation may result in respiratory or inhalational anthrax. Infection results in bacterial migration to regional lymph nodes, producing an edema-factor toxin or a lethal-factor toxin.[30] Inhalational anthrax is the most lethal variation and may result in mediastinitis, as opposed to pneumonia, as evidenced by a widened mediastinum on chest x-ray films.

Manifestations. Cutaneous anthrax results in itching skin and papular lesions that become vesicular and ulcerative. Ulcerative areas may develop moderate to severe edema. The lesions develop a black eschar within 1 to 2 weeks. There is a slight possibility that cutaneous anthrax could be transmitted by contact with another person.

Gastrointestinal anthrax arises from spore germination within the upper or lower intestinal tract. Upper GI tract involvement results in edema, lymphadenopathy, and sepsis. Lower GI tract involvement includes symptoms of bloody diarrhea, ascites, abdominal pain, and sepsis associated with a partially necrotic lower intestine.

Inhalational anthrax victims may initially feel like the seasonal flu victim. Those infected may experience a 2- to 6-day incubation period followed by a dry cough, myalgias, fatigue, and fever. Victims may experience a short period of improvement followed by a sudden onset of high fever, respiratory distress, shock, and death possibly with 24 to 36 hours. Patients may develop a mediastinitis, and approximately 50% will have hemorrhagic meningitis.

Treatments. Standard precautions are needed when caring for anthrax or potentially anthrax-exposed patients.[5] Avoid any contact with wound drainage. Anthrax victims will require specimen cultures and then antibiotics. Treatments approved by the Food and Drug Administration (FDA) include ciprofloxacin, levofloxacin, doxycycline, and penicillin. Other care includes supplemental oxygen, managing respiratory compromise, and supportive care. A vaccination regimen involving six courses is available to the Department of Defense, whereas a new civilian anthrax vaccination protocol is being developed by the CDC.

Planning.

- Hospitals, including EDs, should have a protocol and/or plan to deal with potentially contaminated mail and "white powder" events.
- Report suspected cases to the infection control practitioner and public health officials.
- Use standard precautions, and avoid wound drainage contact.

PLAGUE. Plague, or *Yersinia pestis*, is a non–spore-forming, gram-negative bacillus responsible for pandemics in AD 541 and 1346, the latter known as the "Black Death" or "great pestilence." Found in certain rodents, including some rats, ground squirrels, and prairie dogs, *Y. pestis* is endemic to the western United States and every continent except Australia. *Y. pestis* is transmitted to humans by bites from fleas that have been feeding and living on infected rodents, including rats and mice.[35]

This disease has several variations, including bubonic, septicemic, and pneumonic plague. The bubonic version is transmitted to the human's regional lymph nodes, causing adenitis or bubos (large, painful, inflamed lymph nodes), hence its name—bubonic plague. *Y. pestis* can progress from a bubonic to septicemic plague; however, neither is contagious person to person. A few individuals may develop a secondary pneumonic plague, which is highly contagious and spread via respiratory droplets.[18] Pneumonic plague probably represents the most significant biowarfare or terrorism threat. Techniques to aerosolize and induce pneumonic plague were developed in the later years of U.S. and Soviet Union biowarfare production. The World Health Organization (WHO) reported that if 50 kg of *Y. pestis* were released over a city of 5 million inhabitants, approximately 150,000 would develop pneumonic plague and 36,000 would die. Other contagious inhabitants would flee the city, and the infection would spread.[11]

Manifestations. Bubonic plague symptoms, including chills, fever, weakness, and the development of painful bubos, begin 2 to 8 days after a bite from an infected flea. Bubos tend to form in the axilla, groin, or cervical region, and their pain restricts movement of the affected areas.[38] Untreated, the disease will progress into a fatal septicemic or possible pneumonic plague.

Pneumonic plague symptoms should start with a 1- to 6-day incubation period followed by high fever, myalgias, chills, headache, chest pain, and cough with bloody sputum. If untreated, dyspnea, cyanosis, and shock may result in death. Other complications for pneumonic and septicemic plague may include acral gangrene, which can affect the fingers, toes, earlobes, nose, and/or penis.

The diagnosis of plague is made by history, Gram stain and cultures of lymph node aspirates, and sputum and CSF samples. Bipolar, "safety-pin" staining may be present with a Wright, Giemsa, or Wayson stain.[5]

Treatment. Patients with confirmed bubonic plague require standard precautions. Those patients being ruled out for bubonic versus pneumonic plague or diagnosed probable

pneumonic plague require strict respiratory droplet precautions. Antibiotics are required as soon as possible after culture specimens are collected. Antibiotic therapy considerations for active disease and postexposure prophylaxis include streptomycin, gentamicin, doxycycline, ciprofloxacin, and chloramphenicol.[35]

Planning

- The hospital laboratory/microbiology should be notified when plague is suspected.
- Report suspected cases to the infection control practitioner and public health officials.
- Cohort patients if large numbers of suspected pneumonic plague victims make isolation impractical.

TULAREMIA. Tularemia, caused by the bacterium *Francisella tularensis*, is a potentially fatal illness that occurs naturally in the United States, North America, and Eurasia. It is commonly called "rabbit fever" because it is found in small animals, especially rodents, rabbits, squirrels, and hares. Tularemia is one of the most pathogenic diseases known, requiring as few as 10 organisms via inoculation or inhalation to cause infection.[49] It has been studied as a potential bioweapon for years. The Japanese investigated *F. tularensis* as a weapon in Manchurian research units between 1932 and 1945. Russia, the United States, and other countries have previously experimented and stockpiled *F. tularensis* as an offensive weapon. By 1973 the United States had destroyed its offensive arsenal.[23] Because of its ease of infection, dissemination, and capacity to cause illness and death, *F. tularensis* is considered a dangerous potential biologic weapon. Although human tularemia infections may occur with ingestion, contact, or aerosol inhalation, it is not transmissible person to person.

Manifestations. Infection takes place through bacilli contact with mucous membranes, GI tract, and the lungs. Symptoms of tularemia appear 3 to 5 days after exposure but can take up to 14 days. Like other flulike illnesses, symptoms can include sudden fever, chills, headaches, sore throat, dry cough, diarrhea, muscle aches, and progressive weakness.[15] Manifestations can include pleuritic chest pain, shortness of breath with pneumonias, hemoptysis, hilar lymphadenopathy, and sepsis.

Treatment. Standard precautions are warranted for suspected tularemia patients. Diagnosis will be made by sputum Gram stain and blood cultures. Designated national reference laboratories can aid in rapid diagnostic testing and identification. Immediate antimicrobial treatments, with streptomycin as drug of choice or gentamicin, are usually indicated for adults and children. A tularemia vaccine is available as an investigational new drug (IND) and under review by the FDA.

Planning

- After an aerosol delivery expect multiple victim presentations with similar symptoms.
- Report suspected cases to the infection control practitioner and public health officials.
- Implement standard precautions for suspected tularemia patients.

CDC Category A Viruses

SMALLPOX. Smallpox is caused by one of two species of poxvirus, variola minor or variola major. Variola major, hereafter called smallpox, is a highly virulent and contagious disease that spreads person to person by aerosols or droplet nuclei via cough, sneeze, and direct contact. It results in a fever, characteristic rash, and death rate of 30%. Smallpox had been a significant cause of illness and death in developing countries until the 1970s, when the last outbreak occurred in Somalia in 1977.[17] By 1980 WHO certified the eradication of smallpox among the world's populations. The only specimens known to exist are in the CDC Laboratory in Atlanta, Georgia, and the Vector Laboratory in Moscow, Russia.

Smallpox has been a consistent choice for biologic warfare using contagious pathogens. Variola was probably first employed as a weapon between 1754 and 1767, during the French and Indian War, when British soldiers distributed infected blankets to the American Indians.[49] The Indian death rate from this contagious disease was approximately 50%. In 1796 Edward Jenner's cowpox vaccination prevented the spread of smallpox. Dr. Ken Alibek, a microbiologist and former director of the Soviet biologic weapons program, reported Soviet efforts to further weaponize smallpox in a variety of munitions. This included developing industrial quantities of genetically altered smallpox and other pathogens that would be more virulent and resistant to possible drug therapies.[2]

Manifestations. Smallpox inoculation occurs via face-to-face encounter or contact with infected body fluids, contaminated objects, and bedding. The incubation period ranges from 7 to 17 days, after which the virus spreads to lymph nodes and multiplies. The first symptoms include high fever and may include malaise, headache, body aches, and sometimes nausea and vomiting. During the next 2 to 4 days, the most contagious phase, a rash develops on the tongue and in the mouth. The rash then spreads to the face, arms, legs, and distally to the hands and feet. Fever may fall. The rash evolves into fluid-filled, painful bumps that later thicken and develop a characteristic central depression or umbilicus. Fever rises, and the bumps turn into sharply raised pustules that crust over and scab. The person is considered contagious until the scabs fall off.[34]

Treatment. Smallpox is very contagious. Evaluation and care should be in a negative pressure environment using strict airborne and contact infection control precautions. Diagnosis is made by clinical presentation, positive tissue cultures, and/or positive virus identified with electron microscopy. Smallpox treatment is supportive. Antivirals and immune globulin may aid treatment, though vaccination remains the most effective prevention tool.

Planning

- Any case of smallpox indicates bioterrorism and is considered a federal crime; therefore criminal investigation should be anticipated.
- Identify a response team within the ED whose members are protected by recent smallpox vaccination.
- Report suspected cases to the infection control practitioner and public health officials.

VIRAL HEMORRHAGIC FEVERS. VHF refers to an illness characterized by fever and bleeding disorders caused by one of four virus families. VHF illnesses are caused by distinct families of RNA viruses that cause high fevers, vascular abnormalities, sepsis, hemorrhaging, and multisystem organ failure. The four VHF virus families are Filoviridae (Marburg and Ebola), Arenaviridae (Lassa fever), Flaviviridae (yellow fever), and Bunyaviridae (Rift Valley fever).[42] These pathogens are endemic to parts of Africa, Central and South America, and the Middle East, with infections usually transmitted during insect bites or contact with infected body fluids. Other diseases that belong to this group include hantaviruses, Crimean-Congo fever, and others. Several countries have investigated weaponizing VHFs because of contagiousness along with high morbidity and mortality rates.[32] The VHFs are limited in treatment and vaccine options.

Manifestations. VHF symptoms include fever, myalgias, rash, weakness, hypotension, prostration, jaundice, and bleeding complications, including conjunctival injection, petechiae, disseminated intravascular coagulation, and shock. Laboratory findings will likely indicate thrombocytopenia and may indicate renal or liver failure.

Treatment. Most VHF viruses are very contagious. Patients should be placed in a private room with with standard, droplet and contact precautions. Airborne precautions including negative pressure might also be chosen for patients with respiratory involvement or those undergoing pulmonary procedures or treatments that stimulate coughing.[49] Most VHFs do not have a vaccine; however, yellow fever is the exception. Arenaviruses, bunyaviruses, and those VHFs of unknown causes may be effectively treated with ribavirin.[14] The majority of VHF treatment will be supportive, including intravenous fluids, hemodynamic monitoring, ventilation, dialysis, and antibiotics for secondary infections. Needle punctures and anticoagulant therapies are contraindicated.

Planning

- Additional barriers might be necessary to prevent contact with large amounts of body fluids and/or secretions.
- Fever and hemorrhaging from any site is characteristic for VHF.
- Report suspected cases to the infection control practitioner and public health officials.

CDC Category A Toxin

Toxins are harmful substances naturally produced by living organisms and can be more toxic per unit measure than any manmade chemical or synthetic poison. Toxins tend not to cause illness via contact (except trichothecene mycotoxins [T2 mycotoxins]) or spread person to person.[29] Toxins are usually ingested, but their aerosol versions can be inhaled. Examples of toxins include botulinum, the most potent neurotoxin; ricin, a deadly cytotoxin; staphylococcal enterotoxin B (SEB), which causes incapacitating gastroenteritis; and the T2 mycotoxins, the only dermally active toxin. Of these, botulinum is the only CDC Category A toxin.[12]

BOTULINUM. *Clostridium botulinum* is the spore-forming, anaerobe bacillus that produces botulinum toxin and is the most poisonous substance by weight known.[47] Botulism is a neuroparalytic disease occurring naturally in three forms: foodborne, infant botulism, and wound botulism. Inhalational botulism would be an unnatural occurrence and a result of a biologic attack. Properly manufactured, dispersed, and inhaled, a single gram of botulinum would kill more than 1 million people. Botulism has been an agent for bioterrorism and bioweapons development for years. During the 1930s, the Japanese Unit 731 fed botulinum cultures to prisoners in biologic warfare experiments. Countries that have developed and stockpiled, or are thought to be developing, botulism weapons include the United States, Soviet Union, Iraq, Iran, North Korea, and Syria. As an agent of bioterrorism, the doomsday cult Aum Shinrikyo unsuccessfully attempted aerosolized botulism attacks on multiple Japanese locations between 1990 and 1995.[4]

Manifestations. Signs and symptoms begin 6 hours to 2 weeks after exposure and are the same for all forms of botulism, including inhalational. Disease symptoms depend on the rate and amount of toxin absorbed. Neurologic symptoms include symmetrical, descending flaccid paralysis with bulbar palsies including ptosis, blurred vision, diplopia, dysphagia, and dysphonia.[5] Patients may appear comatose, requiring months of mechanical ventilation before recovery. Clinical diagnosis is made by bulbar palsy with descending paralysis. Positive *C. botulinum* specimen cultures and mouse neutralization assay can confirm diagnosis.

Treatment. Standard precautions are appropriate when caring for botulism victims. Therapy for botulism includes early use of type-specific botulinum antitoxin after rapid diagnosis. Supportive care may include extended mechanical ventilation and enteral or parenteral tube feeding.

Planning
- Report suspected cases to the infection control practitioner and public health officials.
- The ED or hospital encountering botulism should consider foodborne substances, including home-canned products and potential contaminated illegal drug use.
- There is no person-to-person spread of botulism.

CHEMICAL AGENTS

Chemical agents can be used as weapons of mass destruction and have been deployed by various nations' military and by terrorists. Many chemical components of a terrorism attack are readily available in the community. These threats can be found in local hardware stores, schools, laboratories, and in tankers transiting community highways and railroads. Depending on their primary effect, most chemical agents can be classified as nerve agents, vesicants, blood agents, or pulmonary/choking agents. Chemical agent response will require coordination with EMS, poison control and planning for effective decontamination and appropriate personal protective equipment use by hospital first receivers and decon team.

Some of the first uses of chemical weapons included toxic smoke directed by Spartan allies in 423 BC; the use of poisons in hollow, explosive mortar shells during the 15th and 16th centuries and the deployment of chlorine gas in World War I.[48] Chemical weapons used during recent military engagements have included mustard agents, phosgene, cyanide, and probably sarin. Many nations, including the United States and Soviet Union, signed the 1972 Biological Weapons Convention Treaty indicating they would eliminate biologic and chemical weapons, but intelligence sources have indicated continued offensive chemical weapons operations by some signatory nations.

Nerve Agents

Nerve agents were developed specifically for warfare. As the most toxic of chemicals, they are likened to very powerful organophosphates. These agents are acetylcholinesterase (AChE) inhibitors, disrupting and blocking the effects of the enzyme acetylcholinesterase. The result is accumulated acetylcholine at the receptor sites, causing repeated stimulation of the nerve. Nerve agents were discovered while a German scientist was trying to develop an insecticide during the late 1930s and have been called "bug poison for people."[16] Since that time nerve agents such as tabun (GA), sarin (GB), soman (GD), cyclosarin (GF), and VX have been developed and stockpiled by various countries for military deployment. The G (German) agents are volatile and soluble in water. VX is not nearly as volatile or soluble. VX is persistent in the environment with an oilylike nature and therefore presents a greater contact hazard.

The United States began destruction of its stockpiles of nerve agents with the signing of the 1972 Biological Weapons Convention Treaty.[31] In 1988 Iraqi military reportedly bombed a Kurdish community of 80,000 with a cocktail of chemical agents, including sarin, soman, mustard gas, and other agents. Although nerve agents have been historically developed and controlled by the military, they have also been used by terrorists. A "low-potency" sarin was made and released by the doomsday cult Aum Shinrikyo in Matsumoto, Japan, and on Tokyo, Japan, subways in 1995. The Tokyo subway release killed 12 people and sent over 5000 to area hospitals seeking evaluation and treatment.[40,51]

Manifestations

Nerve agents disrupt nerve impulse transmission and result in overstimulation of nerves, producing nicotinic effects (skeletal muscle twitching, cramping, weakness, flaccid paralysis, tachycardia, and high blood pressure) and muscarinic effects (pinpoint pupils; miosis; hypersecretion by salivary, lacrimal, sweat, and bronchial glands; nausea, vomiting, and diarrhea). CNS effects can include behavioral changes, irritability, seizures, and apnea. Mild/moderate exposure symptoms may include localized sweating, fasciculations, nausea, vomiting, weakness, and dyspnea. Severe exposure symptoms include unconsciousness, seizures, convulsions, apnea, and flaccid paralysis.[1,9] Exposure is toxic in all amounts with little difference between a lethal and survivable dose. Exposure can occur through inhalation, dermal/eye contact, ingestion, or injection. Exposure signs and symptoms are remembered with the mnemonic SLUDGEM:

S   Salivation and increased secretions
L   Lacrimation
U   Urinary incontinence
D   Defecation, incontinence
G   Gastrointestinal distress
E   Emesis
M   Miosis

Treatment

Decontamination and antidote delivery for the nerve agent exposure are critical. Following exposure, clothing should be removed and the patient properly decontaminated as quickly as possible. Up to 75% to 90% of the chemical contamination can be stopped by removing the victim's clothing. Respiratory support, including supplemental oxygen, suctioning of secretions, and possible intubation, may be necessary. Diazepam may be necessary for seizure activity.

Nerve agent antidotes include atropine and pralidoxime chloride (2-PAM Cl). The United States military has developed Mark 1 antidote kits that comprise two autoinjectors: one autoinjector delivers 2 mg atropine in 0.7 mL diluent IM, and the other contains 600 mg of 2-PAM Cl in 2 mL diluent. Emergency department management includes administration of the antidotes with dosage based on age and degree (mild, moderate, or severe) of symptom presentation. The antidotes are given until the symptoms begin to subside; therefore large doses may be required. Seizures are treated with diazepam.[21]

Planning

* Nerve agents are extremely toxic and can cause death within minutes to hours after exposure.
* Patients presenting to the ED are a potential threat from vapor off-gassing or contaminant contact.
* First receivers need to be adequately protected and trained for the chemical casualty decontamination response.
* Report suspected cases to the infection control practitioner, public health officials, and law enforcement.

Vesicants

The vesicants, or blister agents, are manmade chemicals that cause vesicles or skin blisters with potential systemic effects and include sulfur, three variations of nitrogen mustard (H1, H2, and H3), lewisite, and phosgene oxime. Vesicants have been used in warfare since World War I, during the 1980s Iran-Iraq war, and reportedly by Iraq against the Kurds in 1988.[44] Vesicants can cause dermal burns and represent a contact and inhalation threat. The mustard gases are named because of their distinctive garlicky or mustard odor. Sulfur mustard is a terrorist threat because it is inexpensive and can be dispersed as a droplet or vapor. Mustards are oily, stable, persist in the environment, and attack the skin, mucous membranes, lungs, and blood-forming organs.[22] Mustard exposure

is not immediately painful on contact and has a latent reaction period, whereas lewisite produces immediate pain and discomfort. The mustard agents and phosgene oxime do not have an antidote, but lewisite does—British antilewisite (BAL).

Manifestations

Exposure to vesicants will most likely occur via contact or inhalation, but ingestion of contaminated food or water is possible. Symptoms can include eye tearing and conjunctivitis, eyelid swelling, blepharospasms, itching, redness, ophthalmic injury, burning and blisters especially in warm, moist areas (axilla, groin, etc.). Other symptoms include throat and mucous membrane burning, hoarseness, shortness of breath, cough, abdominal pain, emesis, and diarrhea. Inhalation of a vesicant can lead to systemic effects, pulmonary edema, and death. Substantial mustard gas exposures can induce bone marrow stem cell suppression, leucopenia, and subsequent decreased immunity.[20,48]

Treatment

Treatment for exposure to vesicants is mostly supportive but begins with immediate decontamination because injury begins within 2 minutes of exposure. Eye exposures receive copious irrigations, topical mydriatics, and antibiotics. Bronchodilators may be helpful. Supportive care objectives are to relieve symptoms, promote healing, and prevent secondary infection and may take months.

Planning

* Sulfur mustard victims may complain of a mustard, garlic, or onion odor. Ocular exposures may produce a sensation of grittiness in the eyes.
* Antibiotic therapy should be guided by laboratory and culture sensitivity findings.
* Report suspected cases to the infection control practitioner and public health officials.

Blood Agents: Cyanides

Blood agent is an antiquated term for a chemical category that includes mostly cyanides, powerful chemicals that kill quickly by interfering with the blood's ability to transport oxygen to tissues. Although not an ideal weapon for war, due to its rapid evaporation and dispersion, hydrogen cyanide (HCN) was used as a weapon by France in World War I, allegedly by Japan in World War II, and by the Iraqi government in the 1980s against the Kurds. Cyanide (as Zyklon B) was used as an agent of genocide during World War II to kill gas chamber victims in concentration camps.

In recent history, various individuals and groups have used cyanide as an agent in murder and mass suicide. The range of settings and modes of delivery illustrate the versatility and ease of use of cyanide in intentional poisonings. Some of these recent events include the following:

* In July 2004 a 19-year-old from Maryland was sentenced to life in prison after being convicted of poisoning his best friend's soda with cyanide.

- In 1982 seven Chicagoans were killed after ingesting cyanide-laced Extra Strength Tylenol capsules.
- In 1978 in Jonestown, Guyana, 913 followers of Rev. Jim Jones committed suicide with cyanide-laced Kool-Aid.

Because cyanide possesses many of the characteristics of an "ideal" terrorist weapon, the CDC and the Department of Homeland Security consider it to be among the most likely agents of chemical terrorism.

- Cyanide is used in many industries and is transported throughout the country via rail and highway and is therefore plentiful, readily available, and can be easily accessed by terrorists via theft or hijacking attempts.
- Unlike many biologic or nuclear weapons, cyanide does not require special scientific or technical knowledge to use.
- Because of its rapidly lethal mechanism of action, cyanide is capable of causing mass incapacitation and casualties, as well as mass confusion and panic created by the difficulty in identifying the source.
- Cyanide requires large quantities of a specific resource (antidote) to combat—a major public health readiness obstacle in most countries.

Exposure to cyanide can occur through several methods. Because it is absorbable into the body through inhalation, contact, or ingestion, the ease of dispersal is of grave concern. Most often discussed is the release of hydrogen cyanide gas into an enclosed space such as an office building, subway, or stadium. But cyanide salts also could be introduced into pharmaceuticals or the food and water supply. Terrorists are likely to initiate an explosion and fire as a secondary component of the act of terrorism. The resulting fire and burning contents including plastics could become a source of cyanide exposure, especially if in an enclosed area such as a tunnel.[6]

Manifestations

Cyanide effectively blocks aerobic metabolism and energy production, resulting in cellular hypoxia and cellular death. No amount of supplemental oxygen can overcome the deficit in affected cells, and anaerobic metabolism causes high levels of lactic acid to accumulate. At moderate to high exposure concentrations, cyanide can kill very quickly—within minutes to hours, depending on the route of exposure. A cellular asphyxiate, cyanides can cause severe respiratory distress and death. However, if recognized and diagnosed in a timely manner, cyanide poisoning can be effectively treated.

Cyanide is reported to have a smell like bitter almonds; however, 60% of the population is genetically unable to detect this odor. Symptoms of exposure include anxiety, tachypnea, agitation, vertigo, weakness, nausea, confusion, lethargy, convulsions, bradypnea, apnea, cardiac dysrhythmias, and death.

Occasionally, excessive venous saturation may result in a rose-colored or cherry-red skin.[48] Other effects may include headache and significant eye, nose, and throat irritation. Elevated plasma lactate levels are also useful as a surrogate marker for elevated cyanide levels.[6,28]

Treatment

Exposure treatment includes immediate movement into a well-ventilated area or into fresh air and supplemental oxygen. Cyanide gas is lighter than air, making decontamination by immediate clothing removal in a clean air environment very effective. Several therapeutic treatments exist for acute cyanide poisoning: an antidote kit including sodium nitrite, sodium thiosulfate, amyl nitrite components and more recently, hydroxocobalamin, which counteract the effects of cyanide; buffer agents such as sodium bicarbonate to counteract the effects of severe metabolic acidosis that accumulates in the bloodstream following HCN exposure; sympathomimetics such as epinephrine to augment coronary and cerebral blood flow during the low flow states associated with HCN poisoning; anticonvulsants such as diazepam, lorazepam, midazolam, and phenobarbital for the treatment of repeated or prolonged generalized seizures.

Planning

- Victims may report smelling bitter almonds, or caregivers might smell bitter almonds on patient's breath.
- Victims may appear with rose-colored or cherry-red skin.
- Report suspected cases to law enforcement and public health officials.
- Provide antidote kit(s) for EMS units.

Pulmonary and Choking Agents

Used as weapons during World War I, pulmonary and choking agents are found in great quantities within the community and are transported daily on highways and railways. These agents include chlorine, phosgene, ammonia, and those chemicals that cause stress to the respiratory tract and irritate and damage lung tissue. Inhalation of pulmonary or choking agents can create noncardiac pulmonary edema, leading to asphyxiation.[43] When these chemicals come in contact with moisture, they begin forming acids or alkalis, causing inflammation, irritation, burns, or delayed tissue injury. Although primarily an inhalation threat, these chemical exposures may also occur via skin contact, ingestion, or ocular exposure.

Manifestations

Patients may take on the smell of the product to which they were exposed. Patients may report an acrid, pungent odor with chlorine exposure or the scent of new-mown hay, which is a characteristic odor of phosgene.[50] Exposure to these agents can result in eye irritation, conjunctivitis, coughing, wheezing, chest tightness, headaches, nausea, choking sensation, dyspnea, cyanosis, respiratory distress, and symptoms of pulmonary edema, including copious frothy sputum. Moderate to significant exposures to some agents, including phosgene, may result in a relatively asymptomatic or latent period that may last for hours. The latent period is usually followed by dyspnea, hypoxia, and pulmonary edema brought about by simple exertion.

There are no diagnostic laboratory findings or tests for pulmonary or choking agent exposure.

Treatment

Care is supportive. There are no antidotes for the choking/pulmonary agents. Actions include removal from the agent source and thorough decontamination. Medical therapies may include airway maintenance, including possible intubation; respiratory support with supplemental oxygen and possible mechanical ventilation; and administration of inhaled bronchodilators. Dermal exposures should be decontaminated with large volumes of tap water. Ocular exposures should receive large volumes of saline irrigation and thorough evaluation. Patients should be in a high Fowler's position to promote chest excursion and respiratory ease.[51] Patients exposed to phosgene should also be forced to rest and not be allowed to exert themselves because of the potential latent period effects.

Planning

- First receivers need to be adequately protected and trained for the chemical casualty decontamination response.
- Decontaminate with copious amounts of water, paying particular attention to warm, moist areas, including axilla and groin.
- Report suspected cases to the infection control practitioner and public health officials.
- Plan for victim forced rest after exposure.

SUMMARY

Emergency nursing requires knowledge and preparation for many kinds of MCIs. Terrorism and disasters involving NBC agents are a documented source of MCI victims throughout history. NBC agents are relatively inexpensive, widely available, and offer a potential for high impact and terror by causing dramatic death and illness. The increase in domestic and foreign terrorism, along with geopolitical instability in many countries, indicates the potential for more NBC events. Effective emergency nurse response planning begins with potential threat awareness and appropriate medical treatments. This chapter has briefly summarized NBC medical effects and response planning for emergency nurses.

REFERENCES

1. Agency for Toxic Substances and Disease Registry: *Nerve agents tabun (GA) CAS 77-81-6, sarin (GB) CAS 107-44-8, soman (GD) CAS 96-64-0, and VX CAS 5078269-9.* Retrieved January 1, 2008 from http://www.atsdr.cdc.gov/tfacts166.pdf.
2. Alibek K: *Biohazard,* New York City, 1999, Random House.
3. Armed Forces Radiobiological Research Institute: *Medical management of radiological casualties: handbook,* Bethesda, Md, 1999, The Institute.
4. Arnon S, Schechter R, Inglesby T et al: Botulinum toxin as a biological weapon: medical and public health management, *JAMA* 285:1059, 2001.
5. Bartlett J, Greenburg M: *PDR guide to terrorist response,* Montvale, NJ, 2005, Thompson PDR.
6. Baskin ST, Brewer TG: *Medical aspects of chemical and biological warfare,* Washington, DC, 1997, Office of the Surgeon General, Department of Army.
7. Borio L, Inglesby T, Peters C et al: Hemorrhagic fever viruses as biological weapons: medical and public health management; *JAMA* 287:2397, 2002.
8. Bowman S: Weapons of mass destruction: the terrorist threat, *CRS Report for Congress.* Retrieved March 7, 2002, from http://www.fas.org/irp/crs/RL31831.pdf.
9. Buchberg J, Miller K: *Hospital responses to radiation casualties.* Retrieved 2004, from Health Physics Society. Retrieved January 1, 2008 from http://www.medicalphysics.org/apps/medicalphysicsedit/HPS04CH25.pdf.
10. Burgess M: *A brief history of terrorism,* Center for Defense Information. Retrieved July 2, 2003, from http://www.cdi.org/program/issue/document.cfm?DocumentID=1381&IssueID=138&StartRow=1&ListRows=10&append URL=&Orderby=DateLastUpdated&ProgramID=39 &issueID=138.
11. Center for Biosecurity, University of Pittsburgh Medical Center: *Yersinia pestis (plague).* Retrieved October 2007, http://www.upmc-biosecurity.org/website/focus/agents_diseases/fact_sheets/plague.html.
12. Centers for Disease Control and Prevention: *Bioterrorism agents.* Retrieved January 1, 2008 http://www.bt.cdc.gov/agent/agentlist_category.asp
13. Centers for Disease Control and Prevention: *Bioterrorism agents/diseases.* Retrieved January 11, 2009, from http://www.bt.cdc.gov/Agent/agentlist.asp.
14. Centers for Disease Control and Prevention: Interim Guidance for Managing Patients with Suspected Viral Hemorrhagic Fever in U.S. Hospitals. Retrieved January 10, 2009, from http://www.cdc.gov/ncidod/dhqp/bp_vhf_interimGuidance.html
15. Centers for Disease Control and Prevention: *Key facts about tularemia.* Retrieved October 2003, from http://www.bt.cdc.gov/agent/tularmia.
16. Centers for Disease Control and Prevention: *Chemical emergencies: facts about sarin.* Retrieved May 2004, from http://www.bt.cdc.gov/agent/sarin/basics/facts.asp.
17. Centers for Disease Control and Prevention: *Smallpox fact sheet.* Retrieved August 2004, from http://www.cdc.gov/smallpox.
18. Centers for Disease Control and Prevention: *Plague fact sheet.* Retrieved January 2005, from http://www.bt.cdc.gov/agent/plague/factsheet.asp.

19. Centers for Disease Control and Prevention: *Acute radiation syndrome: a fact sheet for physicians.* Retrieved March 2005, from http://www.bt.cdc.gov/radiation/arsphysicianfactsheet.asp.

20. Chemical casualty treatment. In *Jane's chem-bio handbook,* ed. 6, Alexandria, Va, 2000, Jane's Information Group.

21. *Chemical terrorism—primary care preparedness—mustards,* 2003, Institute for BioSecurity, St. Louis University School of Public Health. Retrieved January 1, 2008 from http://www.bioterrorism.slu.edu/bt/products/ahec_chem/scripts/Mustard.pdf.

22. Dennis D, Inglesby T, Henderson D et al: Tularemia as a biological weapon: medical and public health management, *JAMA* 285:2763, 2001.

23. Department of Homeland Security Working Group on Radiological Dispersal Device (RDD) Preparedness, Medical Preparedness and Response Sub-Group. Retrieved May 1, 2003, from http://www1.va.gov/emshg/docs/Radiologic_Medical_Countermeasures_051403.pdf.

24. DiGiovanni C: Domestic terrorism with chemical or biological agents: psychiatric aspects, *Am J Psychiatry* 156(10):1500, 1999.

25. *Doctors seek poisoning clues during autopsy,* December 2, 2006, CNN. Retrieved January 1, 2008 from http://edition.cnn.com/2006/WORLD/europe/12/02/uk.spy.autopsy/index.html.

26. Eckhardt R: "Ionizing radiation: it's everywhere," *Los Alamos Science,* pp. 23-27. Retrieved November 25, 1995, from http://library.lanl.gov/cgi-bin/getfile?23-01.pdf.

27. Ferguson C, Potter W: *Improvised nuclear devices and nuclear terrorism,* 2005, The Weapons of Mass Destruction Commission, No. 2. Retrieved January 1, 2008 http://www.wmdcommission.org/files/No2.pdf.

28. Flomenbaum NE et al: *Goldfrank's toxicologic emergencies,* New York, 2006, McGraw-Hill.

29. Franz D: Defense against toxin weapons. In *Textbook of military medicine, medical aspects of chemical and biological warfare,* Office of the Surgeon General, Department of the Army, Washington, D.C., 1997, Borden Institute.

30. Friedlander A: Anthrax. In *Textbook of military medicine, medical aspects of chemical and biological warfare,* Office of the Surgeon General, Department of the Army, Borden Institute, Washington, D.C., 1997.

31. Geldblat J: The biological weapons convention—an overview, International Review of the Red Cross, No. 318, pp. 251-265, 1997. Retrieved January 1, 2008 from http://www.icrc.org/Web/Eng/siteeng0.nsf/html/57JNPA

32. Grace C: *Viral hemorrhagic fevers,* (March 2003) University of Vermont College of Medicine. Retrieved January 1, 2008 from http://www.fahc.org/Healthcare_Providers/Healthcare_Providers_Contribution/Bioterrorism_Curriculum/Email_1_March_3_20.pdf.

33. *Guidance for radiation accident management: managing radiation emergencies,* Radiation Emergency Assistance Center/Training Site. Retrieved January 1, 2008 from http://orise.orau.gov/reacts/guide/syndrome.htm.

34. Henderson D, Inglesby T, Bartlett J et al: Smallpox as a biological weapon: medical and public health management, *JAMA* 281:2127, 1999.

35. Inglesby T, Dennis D, Henderson D et al: Plague as a biological weapon: medical and public health management, *JAMA* 283:2281, 2000.

36. Lyell L: Chemical and biological weapons: the poor man's bomb. Retrieved October 4, 1996, from North Atlantic Assembly, http://www.fas.org/irp/threat/cbw/BIOWEAPONS_FULL_TEXT2.pdf.

37. McCann D: Radiation poisoning: current concepts in the acute radiation syndrome, *Am J Clin Med* 3(3):13, 2006.

38. McGovern T, Friedlander A: Plague. In *Textbook of military medicine,* part 1, Falls Church, Va, 1997, Office of the Surgeon General.

39. *Medical management of radiological casualties: handbook,* Bethesda, Md. Retrieved January 1, 2008, from Armed Forces Radiobiology Research Institute.

40. Olson K: Aum Shinrikyo: once and future threat? *Emerg Infect Dis* 5(4):513, 1999.

41. *Radiological and nuclear terrorism: medical response to mass casualties,* 2006, Centers for Disease Control and Prevention. Retrieved January 1, 2008 from http://www.bt.cdc.gov/radiation/masscasualties/training.asp.

42. San Francisco Department of Public Health: *Infectious disease emergencies: viral hemorrhagic fevers.* Retrieved August 2005, from http://www.sfcdcp.org/UserFiles/File/PDF/vhf.pdf.

43. Sidell F, Patrick W, Dashiell T: Pulmonary agent effect. In *Jane's chem-bio handbook,* ed 6, Alexandria, Va, 2000, Jane's Information Group.

44. Sidell F, Urbanetti J, Smith W et al: Vesicants. In *Textbook of military medicine, medical aspects of chemical and biological warfare,* Office of the Surgeon General, Department of the Army, Borden Institute Washington, DC, 1997.

45. Thomas L, Cohon J, Augustine N, et al: Preventing the entry of weapons of mass effect into the United States, January 10, 2006, Homeland Security Advisory Council, Weapons of Mass Effect Task Force. Retrieved January 1, 2008 from http://www.dhs.gov/xlibrary/assets/hsac_wme-report_20060110. pdf.

46. Tucker J: Historical trends related to bioterrorism: an empirical analysis, *Emerg Infect Dis* 5(4):6, 1999. Retrieved October 20, 2007, from http://www.cdc.gov/ncidod/eid/vol5no4/tucker/htm.

47. *U.S. Army medical management of biological casualties handbook,* ed 5, US Army Medical Research, Institute of Infectious Diseases, Fort Detrick, Frederick, Md, August 2004.

48. U.S. Army Medical Research Institute of Chemical Defense: *Medical management of chemical casualties handbook,* ed 3, Chemical Casualty Care Division, USAMRICD, Aberdeen Proving Ground, Md, July 2000.

49. *U.S. Army Medical Research Institute of Infectious Diseases Handbook,* ed 5, US Army Medical Research, Institute of Infectious Diseases, Fort Detrick, Frederick, Md, August 2004.

50. Urbanetti J: Toxic inhalational injury. In *Textbook of military medicine: medical aspects of chemical and biological warfare,* Office of the Surgeon General, Department of the Army, Borden Institute, Washington, D.C., 1997.

51. Yasufumi A, Arnold J: Terrorism in Japan, *Prehosp Disaster Med* 18(2):106, 2003.

SUGGESTED READINGS

Axtman K: The terror threat at home often overlooked, *Christian Science Monitor,* December 29, 2003. Retrieved January 1, 2008 from http://www.csmonitor.com/2003/1229/p02s01-usju.html.

Alibek, K; *Biohazard.* Random House, New York, 1999.

Centers for Disease Control and Prevention: *Interim guidelines for hospital response to mass casualties from a radiological incident.* Retrieved December 2003, from http://www.bt.cdc.gov/radiation/pdf/MassCasualtiesGuidelines.pdf.

Centers for Disease Control and Prevention: *Chemical emergencies: vesicant/blister agent poisoning.* Retrieved February 2005, from http://emergency.cdc.gov/agent/vesicants/tsd.asp.

Centers for Disease Control and Prevention: *Glossary of radiological terms.* Retrieved January 10, 2009, from http://www.bt.cdc.gov/radiation/glossary.asp#primer

Eisenman D, Stein B, Tanielian T, et al: Terrorism's psychogenic effects and their implications for primary care policy, research and education, *J Gen Intern Med* 20: 772-775, 2005.

Fact sheet: terrorism and cyanide, 2007, Cyanide Poisoning Treatment Coalition. Retrieved January 5, 2008, from http://www.cyanidepoisoning.org/pages/terrorism.asp.

Keim M: Terrorism involving cyanide: the prospect of improving preparedness in the prehospital setting, *Prehosp Disaster Med* 21(2):S56, 2006.

Lung damaging agents. In *Treatment of chemical agent casualties and conventional military chemical injuries,* Field Manual 8-285, Washington, DC, December 1995, Department of the Army, Navy, Air Force and Commandant Marine Corps. Retrieved January 1, 2008 from http://www.globalsecurity.org/wmd/library/policy/army/fm/8-285/ch5.pdf.

Miller J, Engelberg S, Broad W, *Germs: biological weapons and America's secret war,* Simon & Schuster, 2001, New York.

Occupational Health and Safety Administration: Best practices for hospital-based first receivers of victims from mass casualty incidents involving the release of hazardous substances. Retrieved January 2005, from http://www.osha.gov/dts/osta/bestpractices/firstreceivers_hospital.pdf

CHAPTER 19

Management of the Critical Care Patient in the Emergency Department

Carol Rhoades, Reneé Semonin Holleran, Lori Carpenter, and Colin Grissom

CRITICAL CARE IN THE EMERGENCY DEPARTMENT

Critical care patients remaining for extended periods of time in the emergency department (ED) have become increasingly more common over the past decades.[26] Multiple reasons for "boarding" of critical care patients in the ED have been identified. Some of these are a lack of inpatient critical care beds, the ongoing nursing shortage, and increasing ED visits despite a decrease in EDs. Ultimately, when hospital beds are full, patients cannot be transferred from the critical care units to floor beds, which results in critical care patients boarding in the ED. Other reasons that account for the increase in boarding of critical care patients in the ED are a lack of policies and procedures to facilitate patient movement from the ED to a critical care unit, lack of administrative support to improve patient flow, and lack of regionalization of health care resources to admit patients.[13]

Inpatient care of the critically ill or injured patient results in different needs than the typical initial stabilization provided in the ED. Additional education, equipment, and resources are needed to ensure safe and competent critical care. Two recent studies demonstrated that hospital mortality rates increased as the length of time waiting for an inpatient critical care bed increased once an admission order to a critical care unit was received.[12,14]

Management of the critically ill or injured patient necessitates that the ED have skilled critical care clinicians and equipment and an area where patients can be closely monitored. Many EDs are not designed to provide this type of care and do not have the appropriate equipment for invasive monitoring. Observation units have been created in EDs to alleviate some of the pressure related to limited inpatient beds. However, there are times when these units and other areas of the ED may be used to manage critical care patients. There are many unpredictable critical conditions that can occur in patients admitted to an ED observation unit, including dyspnea, shock, cardiac arrest, and death. The focus of this chapter is to discuss the common clinical conditions and interventions needed when emergency nurses care for the critically ill or injured patient boarding in the ED. Included in this chapter is the management of the artificially ventilated patient, selected invasive lines, and sepsis.

MECHANICAL VENTILATION

Mechanical ventilation of a critically ill or injured patient can be challenging in the ED. Ventilator settings, alarms, patient positioning, and oral care are just a few of the issues that need to be addressed.

Box 19-1	DEFINITIONS FOR MECHANICAL VENTILATION

- *Acute lung injury (ALI):* A severe form of ARDS characterized by acute hypoxemic respiratory failure, diffuse bilateral pulmonary infiltrates on chest x-ray film, pulmonary wedge pressure <18 mm Hg and PaO_2/FIO_2 ratio of <300.
- *Acute respiratory distress syndrome (ARDS):* The same definition as ALI except the PaO_2/FIO_2 ratio is <200.
- *Barotrauma:* Damage to the lung tissue due to high airway pressures. Alveolar rupture may lead to pneumothorax, pulmonary interstitial edema, and pneumomediastinum.
- *FIO_2:* Fraction of inspired oxygen ranges from 0.21 (21%) to 1.0 (100%). The normal ambient air FIO_2 is 0.21.
- *Functional residual capacity (FRC):* The volume of air remaining in the lungs at the end of normal expiration.
- *Ideal body weight (IBW):* The expected weight of a person based on sex and height.
  Males: IBW = 50 kg + 2.3 kg for each inch over 5 feet.
  Females: IBW = 45.5 kg + 2.3 kg for each inch over 5 feet.
- *I:E ratio:* The ratio of inspiratory time to expiratory time. Under normal conditions the expiratory phase is passive and is twice as long as the active inspiratory phase (1:2).
- *Inspiratory flow:* The rate at which a breath is delivered on a ventilator. It is measured in liters per minute. The higher the flow, the faster the breath is delivered.
- *Inspiratory time (T_i):* The time over which a tidal volume is delivered or a pressure maintained (depending on mode). Set as I:E ratio or inspiratory flow.
- *Mean airway pressure:* The average pressure to which the lungs are exposed over one inspiratory/expiratory cycle.
- *Minute ventilation (V_E):* The volume of air that moves in and out of the lungs in 1 minute. It is the product of the tidal volume and respiratory rate. V_E = Vt × rate.
- *Peak inspiratory pressure (PIP):* The measurement in the lungs at the peak of inspiration as measured on the ventilator manometer.
- *PEEP:* Positive end-expiratory pressure. A therapy used in mechanical ventilation to provide airway pressure at the end of expiration to increase the volume of gas remaining in the lungs at the end of expiration (FRC). Ideally it will increase the surface area of the alveoli to decrease the shunting of blood through the lungs and improve gas exchange.
- *Plateau pressure:* A constant pressure value that is maintained during the inspiratory phase of ventilation. It is measured by pressing the pause or hold button during mechanical inspiration.
- *Sensitivity:* A measure of the amount of negative pressure that must be generated by a patient to trigger a mechanical ventilator into the inspiratory phase.
- *Tidal volume (Vt):* The volume of air inspired or expired in a single breath during regular respiration.
- *Volutrauma:* The volume-related overdistention injury of alveoli inflicted by mechanical ventilation.
- *V/Q:* Ventilation to perfusion ratio. Normal is 0.8. A high V/Q is indicative of dead space ventilation, and a low V/Q is indicative of shunt ventilation.
- *VR:* Ventilatory rate. Also referred to as frequency (f).

Indications for Intubation and Mechanical Ventilation

Intubation is indicated in a variety of clinical situations but generally falls into one of three main categories: failure to maintain a patent airway, inadequate oxygenation, or ineffective ventilation.

Failure, or Anticipated Failure, to Protect or Maintain a Patent Airway

The following groups of patients are at a higher risk for airway issues:

- Obtunded or comatose patients with loss of gag reflex: traumatic brain injury (TBI), overdose, anoxia, cerebral vascular accident, cerebral aneurysm, etc.
- Patients with a partial or complete obstruction: edema due to inhalation injury, neck trauma, epiglottitis, laryngeal edema, bronchospasm, foreign object aspiration, burns
- Patients receiving some pharmacologic therapy: benzodiazepine therapy for status epilepticus, sedation/paralysis for TBI to control increased intracranial pressures or to obtain diagnostic imaging in combative patients

Inadequate Oxygenation

A shunt occurs when alveoli are perfused but not ventilated, as in pneumonia, acute respiratory distress syndrome (ARDS), acute lung injury (ALI), pulmonary hemorrhage or pulmonary contusion, and atelectasis. Dead space ventilation results when alveoli are ventilated but not perfused, as in pulmonary embolus, hypotension, and low cardiac output states such as cardiogenic shock.

Diffusion abnormality is caused by the obstruction or restriction of gas exchange across the capillary-alveolar membrane, as in pulmonary edema or pulmonary fibrosis. Inadequate oxygenation can also occur because of an inability of the cells to extract oxygen, such as in sepsis, carbon monoxide poisoning, or cyanide poisoning.

Inadequate Ventilation

Inadequate ventilation may result from neurologic causes such as spinal cord injury, traumatic brain injury, overdose, and Guillain-Barré syndrome. Muscular abnormalities that result from myopathies and myasthenia gravis will contribute to the failure to ventilate. Finally, anatomic causes such as pleural effusions, hemothorax, pneumothorax, flail chest, and abdominal hypertension may impair ventilation.

Definitions

There are important definitions related to mechanical ventilation that emergency nurses should be familiar with. Box 19-1 contains a summary of these.

Classification of Mechanical Ventilators

There are two types of ventilators: positive pressure and negative pressure. It is highly unlikely that negative pressure ventilation (e.g., iron lung, cuirass) would ever be used in the

ED setting. There are two types of positive pressure ventilation that will be used in the ED. The ventilator type is named for the parameter that terminates the inspiratory cycle of the ventilator: volume-controlled and pressure-controlled.

Volume-Controlled, Pressure Variable

This is the most common mode of ventilation. The tidal volume (Vt) is preset and delivered during the inspiratory phase of the ventilator cycle. Depending on the compliance and resistance of the lung, the pressure required to deliver the set tidal volume will vary. The advantage of this mode is that the patient receives guaranteed minute ventilation volumes. The disadvantage is the potential for lung injury when high pressures are required to deliver the set tidal volume in patients with low lung compliance.

Modes include controlled mandatory (or controlled) ventilation, assist-control (AC) ventilation, and synchronized intermittent mandatory ventilation (SIMV).

Pressure-Controlled, Volume Variable

In this mode of ventilation, the inspiratory pressure is preset and the ventilator will deliver a breath until that pressure is reached. The tidal volume delivered to reach that pressure will vary depending on the compliance and resistance of the lung. The advantage of this mode is that it limits the distending pressure of the lung. The mean airway pressure can be manipulated by prolonging the inspiratory time, thus reducing the potential for high peak or plateau pressures. The disadvantage is that the minute ventilation volume is not guaranteed and requires more attentive monitoring to prevent hypoventilation or hyperventilation.

Modes of Ventilation

Modes include pressure control and pressure support ventilation.

Controlled Mandatory Ventilation (CMV)

Method: Delivers a set respiratory rate at a set tidal volume, overriding any respiratory effort by the patient. This may cause physical discomfort for the patient and is usually used if the patient is unconscious or has received a neuromuscular blocking agent.

Set parameters: Fraction of inspired oxygen (FIO_2), Vt, ventilatory rate (VR), positive end-expiratory pressure (PEEP), ratio of inspiratory to expiratory time (I:E) or inspiratory time (T_i).

Variable parameters: Peak inspiratory pressure (PIP).

Assist-Control Ventilation

Method: The ventilator will deliver a set number of respirations at a set tidal volume. Sensitivity is set at a level to recognize the patient's respiratory effort with delivery of an additional full tidal volume with each spontaneous respiratory effort. The sensitivity can be adjusted so that it takes a specific amount of respiratory effort to recognize the respiratory effort.

The patient receives a breath whenever he or she wants one without having to work hard for it. Patients can hyperventilate in this mode, and minute ventilation should be monitored and the patient adequately sedated if indicated.

Set parameters: FIO_2, Vt, VR, flow, PEEP, sensitivity.

Variable parameters: PIP.

Synchronized Intermittent Mandatory Ventilation

Method: A set tidal volume at a set rate is delivered every minute. This type of ventilation allows the patient to breathe spontaneously but does not provide a spontaneous breath with additional tidal volume support. Sensitivity is set to ensure that the ventilator synchronizes the tidal volume breaths with the spontaneous breaths. A similar mode, intermittent mandatory ventilation (IMV), does not synchronize with the patient's spontaneous breaths.

Patients with ALI or ARDS will have a difficult time generating sufficient effort to open the demand valve and breathe through the endotracheal tube without ventilatory assistance.

SIMV can be used in combination with pressure support to allow a spontaneous breath attempt to trigger the ventilator to give a pressure-limited breath.

Set parameters: FIO_2, Vt, VR, I:E or Ti, PEEP, sensitivity.

Variable parameters: PIP, sensitivity.

Pressure Controlled Ventilation (PCV)

Method: There is no guaranteed minute ventilation with this mode; therefore close monitoring to prevent hypoventilation and hypoxia is required. If the VR is set too fast, auto-PEEP can develop (see discussion of complications). Sensitivity is set to recognize the patient's respiratory effort, and a full preset pressure is delivered with each ventilatory attempt (as opposed to assist-control, where volume is the set parameter). The sensitivity can be adjusted to require a specific amount of effort to occur for the patient's respiratory effort to be recognized.

Mean airway pressure is increased by prolonging the inspiration time. In some patients, increasing the mean airway pressure without increasing PIP may require prolonging the inspiratory time to improve the oxygen benefit.

Set parameters: FIO_2, VR, PIP, PEEP, Ti or I:E

Variable parameters: Vt, flow.

Pressure Support Ventilation (PSV)

Method: Provides inspiratory support to a spontaneously breathing patient. The patient determines the rate and with each spontaneous effort triggers the ventilator to deliver a flow to the preset pressure limit. The pressure is maintained throughout inspiration.

This is often used for ventilator weaning purposes by gradually decreasing the pressure support provided.

Set parameters: FIO_2, PIP, sensitivity, PEEP.

Variable parameters: VR, Vt, Ti.

Continuous Positive Airway Pressure (CPAP)

Method: No volume or pressure breaths are provided. The patient breathes spontaneously at his or her own rate and own tidal volume while the ventilator maintains a constant pressure throughout the respiratory cycle. This mode is used primarily to assess the patient's ability to ventilate and oxygenate before extubation. It is also used in patients who have no oxygenation or ventilation abnormalities but only need airway protection, as in patients who are alert and awake but have laryngeal edema or airway compression. This mode should be used with caution in patients who have the potential to decompensate neurologically or hemodynamically.

Set parameters: PEEP, FiO_2.

Variable parameters: VR, Vt.

Preventing Injury From Mechanical Ventilation

A variety of strategies have been developed to reduce ventilator-associated injuries usually caused by high plateau pressures and high inspiratory pressures. The strategy most likely to be encountered in the ED is permissive hypercapnea.

Permissive Hypercapnea

Permissive hypercapnea is a lung protective strategy that decreases alveolar ventilation to prevent lung injury due to high volumes and high pressures. It involves the use of low tidal volumes (4 to 6 mL/kg ideal body weight [IBW]) and pressure-limited ventilation. The arterial carbon dioxide pressure ($PaCO_2$) is allowed to rise gradually, and the pH is allowed to drop to between 7.2 and 7.25. Acidosis at this level is generally well tolerated.[20] Permissive hypercapnea is not appropriate for patients with head injuries or severe metabolic acidosis.

Inverse-Ratio Ventilation (IRV)

The normal I:E ratio is reversed so that the inspiratory phase is longer than the expiratory phase. (2:1 to 4:1). It is usually done in the pressure control mode (PC/IRV).

The longer inspiratory time lowers the peak inspiratory pressure and plateau pressure while increasing the mean airway pressure. This prevents the potentially damaging effects of cyclical opening and closing of alveoli by maintaining a constant pressure and improving oxygenation.

This form of ventilation is extremely uncomfortable and almost always requires chemical paralysis and sedation.

Other Advanced Ventilatory Strategies

Further studies are needed to determine improved patient outcomes in the following modes.

HIGH-FREQUENCY OSCILLATORY VENTILATION. High-frequency oscillatory ventilation (HFOV) is characterized by high respiratory rates, generally between 180 and 360 breaths/min, with very low tidal volumes of 1 to 3 mL/kg. In HFOV the pressure oscillates, maintaining a constant distending pressure. Gas is pushed into the lungs during inspiration and pulled out during expiration. It is used in patients who have hypoxia refractory to normal mechanical ventilation. High-frequency ventilators for the adult population are not readily available.

AIRWAY PRESSURE-RELEASE VENTILATION (BILEVEL). Airway pressure-release ventilation (APRV) is a time-cycled, pressure-limited form of ventilation that maintains a constant positive airway pressure (similar to plateau pressure) and has a regular, brief, intermittent release of airway pressure allowing for removal of carbon dioxide. This method allows the patient to breathe spontaneously so chemical paralysis is not required.

Depending on the brand of ventilator, a modified version of APRV provides pressure support during the spontaneous respiratory effort.

Tidal volume is variable, requiring close attention to the patient's minute ventilation to prevent hypercapnea or hypocapnia.

Selecting Ventilator Settings

Ventilator mode and settings are determined by physician preference, clinical assessment, and degree of alteration in oxygenation and/or ventilation. Under the guidance of the physician, the respiratory therapist is the most skilled and knowledgeable person to set up and monitor ventilator parameters. The emergency nurse should be familiar with the concepts and therapies used and participate in collaborative discussions on the goal of ventilatory support.

Tidal Volume (Using Volume-Controlled Ventilation)

A Vt that is too high places the patient at risk for overinflation injury. Patients with acute lung injury or ARDS should be started on a Vt of 6 mL/kg IBW. In a randomized controlled study, the ARDS Network compared patient outcomes when using 6 mL/kg IBW versus the traditional 12 mL/kg IBW. Plateau pressure was maintained at less than 30 cm H_2O, and Vt in the low-volume group was dropped as low as 4 mL/kg if necessary to meet this limitation. The low-volume group had a 22% relative reduction in mortality.[1] A Vt of 8 mL/kg IBW is appropriate for patients with chronic obstructive pulmonary disease (COPD) and asthma so that fewer breaths are given at a higher Vt to allow for a longer exhalation time.

A Vt of 8 to 9 mL/kg should be adequate for people with normal lungs. Patients with neuromuscular disease may benefit from a slightly higher Vt to prevent atelectasis.

Pressure (Using Pressure-Controlled Ventilation)

Pressure will need to be adjusted as compliance changes (i.e., increase pressure support with decreased compliance, and decrease with increased compliance). Start with a pressure support of 20 cm H_2O, and adjust to a tidal volume of 6 to 8 mL/kg.

Rate

Respiratory rates that are set too fast place the patient at risk for inadequate expiratory time. When initially selecting the rate, consider the minute ventilation and the tidal volume.

The desired minute ventilation is usually 5 to 10 L/min. The initial rate will generally range from 8 to 18 breaths/min depending on the tidal volume selected and the degree of acidosis. Draw a specimen for arterial blood gas (ABG) analysis 20 minutes after changing ventilator settings. Further adjustments of the rate depend on the clinical goal and patient response. The goal may be based on a $PaCO_2$ range (as in traumatic brain injury) or a pH range (as in passive hypercarbia). In summary, increased rate equals increased pH and decreased $PaCO_2$, whereas decreased rate equals decreased pH and increased $PaCO_2$.

FiO_2

If the patient's arterial oxygen pressure (PaO_2) is unknown, start with a FiO_2 of 60% to 100%. The percentage of oxygen can be weaned down while monitoring oxygen saturation levels and arterial blood gases. The FiO_2 and PEEP should be managed to maintain the PaO_2 in the middle of the normal range for the given altitude. Patients with head injuries or heart problems should have a PaO_2 at the upper end of normal. ARDS and ALI patients can tolerate a PaO_2 in the lower end of the range so that lower FiO_2 and PEEP can be used, thereby lessening the chance of oxygen toxicity. Prolonged periods with a FiO_2 greater than 0.6 (60%) are associated with lung injury; however, it should be used, if necessary, to prevent hypoxemia.

PEEP

PEEP exerts pressure in the patient's airway, above atmospheric level, to prevent alveolar collapse by increasing the functional residual capacity (FRC). PEEP can be used in any mode of ventilation. Most patients should receive 5 cm H_2O of PEEP to prevent atelectasis. Use PEEP with extreme caution (usually only 3 cm H_2O) in COPD and asthma patients to prevent further air trapping. PEEP is used in conjunction with FiO_2 to improve oxygenation. Higher levels of PEEP are helpful to decrease FiO_2 to less than 0.6 (60%). PEEP greater than 10 cm H_2O can cause decreased venous return and hypotension. The hemodynamic effects of PEEP should be monitored closely.

I:E Ratio

The normal inspiratory/expiratory ratio is 1:2 or 1:3. Patients with obstructive airway disease, such as asthma or COPD, should have longer expiratory times of 1:4 or longer to prevent air trapping and alveolar overdistention. In this patient population, increasing the rate, which shortens the expiratory time in an attempt to lower the $PaCO_2$, may actually increase $PaCO_2$ and worsen the clinical condition.[42]

Sensitivity

The sensitivity is set to recognize the patient's spontaneous respiratory effort. It is usually set at −1 to −2 cm H_2O. A setting that is too high will cause increased patient effort, and a setting that is too low may cause overtriggering of the ventilator and hyperventilation.

PIP

The PIP alarm should be set at 10 to 15 cm H_2O higher than baseline. This will alert staff to decreased lung compliance or conditions that do not allow full exhalation. Lung compliance will often decrease with fluid resuscitation and capillary leak associated with the inflammatory response. This will increase the peak inspiratory pressure.

Management of the Patient on Mechanical Ventilation

Chapter 30 contains information about specific treatment of patients with pulmonary disease and ABG analysis. FiO_2 and PEEP are the settings used to improve oxygenation (PaO_2). It is often a delicate balance of increasing the PEEP to achieve a FiO_2 below 0.6 while maintaining the mean arterial blood pressure above 65 mm Hg. Vt and VR are the settings used to adjust $PaCO_2$. The emergency nurse needs to continuously monitor the patient's heart rate, electrocardiogram (ECG) pattern, and pulse oximetry readings. End-tidal CO_2 monitoring ($EtCO_2$) is a useful adjunct in the assessment of ongoing endotracheal tube placement in the trachea. It is of limited value in correlating to $PaCO_2$ in hemodynamically unstable patients or in patients with ventilation/perfusion (V/Q) mismatch. A self-inflating resuscitation bag should be kept at the patient's bedside at all times in the event of mechanical failure. Suction equipment should be readily available. Endotracheal tube depth should be noted on the patient's chart and assessed whenever the patient is moved or becomes agitated, air bubbles are noted in the airway, low or high PIP alarms are activated, vocal sounds are heard, or when there is any question of tube displacement. Be aware of and document the patient's baseline FiO_2, mode of ventilation, PIP, PEEP/pressure support and tidal volume; documentation of these should occur every 2 hours while receiving mechanical ventilation. Assess the patient for any changes. Goals of oxygenation and ventilation should be clear. If no adjustment parameters are given, the ED nurse should notify the physician when any value falls outside the desired range.

Ventilator Management

Ventilator alarms should be on at all times and set to the maximum volume. Immediately evaluate the cause of any ventilator alarm. Table 19-1 contains a summary of how to troubleshoot ventilator alarms.

Monitor for signs and symptoms of barotrauma (see complications discussed later in the chapter).

Disconnect the patient from the ventilator and ventilate with a self-inflating resuscitation bag if there is any question as to whether the patient is being adequately ventilated. Be sure that the resuscitation bag has good oxygen flow, and use a PEEP valve if the patient is PEEP dependent (requires PEEP to adequately oxygenate). If it is necessary to sedate and administer a neuromuscular blocking agent to maintain adequate oxygenation, adjust the respiratory rate to the

Table 19-1. TROUBLESHOOTING VENTILATOR ALARMS

Initial assessment:
- *Airway:* Is the endotracheal tube still in? Check ETT insertion depth, check end-tidal CO_2, check breath sounds.
- *Breathing:* Check breath sounds, look for chest excursion, check pulse oximetry, check patient color.
- *Circulation:* Check the pulse, ECG, and blood pressure.

Alarm	Possible Causes	Management
Apnea	Insufficient spontaneous breathing by a patient in the CPAP or pressure support mode	• Switch ventilator mode to one that provides a set rate
High airway pressure	ETT obstruction: sputum, kink, biting Increased compliance or resistance: circumferential burns, bronchospasm, lung collapse, pneumothorax, endobronchial intubation, worsening of lung process Anxiety/fear/pain/fighting ventilator	• Suction the airway • Treat cause of resistance • Adjust mode or settings • Rule out hypoxia before treating agitation • Chest radiography analysis • Change ventilator mode to one that is better tolerated and/or provide sedation/analgesia
Low airway pressure	Ventilator disconnect Leak in ventilator system Cuff leak Inadvertent extubation	• Ensure that all connections are intact and tight • Troubleshoot ETT cuff • Bag-mask device if ETT was dislodged
Oxygen pressure low	Oxygen cylinder is empty Cylinder valve is closed Unit not connected to the wall terminal	• Check wall and cylinder connections • Bag-mask ventilation until resolved

CPAP, Continuous positive airway pressure; *ETT,* endotracheal tube.
* Remove patient from the ventilator, and manually bag with a resuscitation bag if there is any compromise.

patient's premedication minute ventilation and repeat an ABG analysis.

Complications of Mechanical Ventilation

There are multiple complications that may occur with mechanical ventilation. The following is a discussion of some that the emergency nurse may come across in the ED.

HYPOTENSION. Positive pressure ventilation increases intrathoracic pressure and subsequently decreases venous return and cardiac output. In patients with marginal or low volume status, the decrease in venous return will cause hypotension. The greater the positive pressure applied, the more profound the hypotensive response. This is most apparent when the PEEP is greater than 10 cm H_2O. Hemodynamic status should be monitored closely with any increase in PEEP and immediately after intubation. Optimizing fluid status will lessen the degree of hypotension.

VOLUTRAUMA. Volutrauma is the overdistention injury of alveoli inflicted by mechanical ventilation. It is most closely associated with high PIP. It is thought that this damage degrades surfactant, disrupts epithelial and endothelial cell barriers, and increases cytokine levels and inflammatory cells in the lung.[16,55] Lung-protective ventilatory strategies should be used in all patients with ALI or ARDS.

BAROTRAUMA. Barotrauma is the damage caused to lung tissue because of high airway pressures and rupture of alveoli. This may lead to a pneumothorax, tension pneumothorax, subcutaneous emphysema, or pneumomediastinum. Symptoms include hypotension, tachycardia, decrease in arterial oxygen saturation (SaO_2), decrease in central venous oxygen

saturation/mixed venous oxygen saturation ($ScvO_2/SvO_2$), decrease in cardiac output, decreased breath sounds, unequal chest excursion, and deviated trachea. Large tidal volumes should be avoided and PIP and plateau pressures monitored carefully.

AUTO-PEEP. Auto-PEEP, also called intrinsic PEEP, occurs when a ventilator breath is not completely exhaled before the next delivered inspiratory breath (stacking breaths). This occurs most frequently in patients with asthma or COPD who require longer exhalation times. High tidal volumes along with high respiratory rates will also cause auto-PEEP. The resultant increasing pressures will cause barotrauma, volutrauma, hypotension, and death. Assessing for auto-PEEP includes monitoring the PIP and the respiratory waveforms on the ventilator for increasing baselines. If auto-PEEP is identified, the patient should be disconnected from the ventilator and allowed to completely exhale.

OXYGEN TOXICITY. A FiO_2 of greater than 0.5 for a long duration may cause the production of oxygen free radicals that damage pulmonary epithelium; inactivate surfactant; and form intraalveolar edema, interstitial thickening, and pulmonary fibrosis.[55] The extent of injury is related to the level of FiO_2 and the duration of exposure. Using PEEP in conjunction with FiO_2, if tolerated hemodynamically, will facilitate weaning the FiO_2 to less than 0.5. With severe ARDS/ALI it may not be possible to lower FiO_2 below 50%. However, treatment of hypoxemia and hypotension takes precedence over the possibility of oxygen toxicity.

INFECTION. Ventilator-associated pneumonia (VAP) is a serious and potentially life-threatening consequence of intubation and is defined as a nosocomial pneumonia that develops after 48 hours of intubation and mechanical ventilatory support.[44] VAP is the most common and fatal nosocomial infection of critical care, affecting between 9% and 27% of intubated patients.[46] VAP doubles the risk for dying, prolongs the duration of ventilation, and increases the length of stay in the critical care unit, total hospital length of stay, and cost of hospitalization.[44,46] VAP may be prevented by using the following measures:

- Rigorous hand washing
- Sterile suction technique
- Avoiding the routine use of saline lavage
- Aseptic airway technique
- Bronchial hygiene
- Regular oral care
- Elevating the head of the bed 30 degrees

Summary

To provide safe and competent mechanical ventilation the emergency nurse needs to be familiar with the functioning and management of ventilators. Mechanical ventilation can support critically ill or injured patients, but when inappropriately managed, can cause unnecessary harm.

INVASIVE MONITORING

Every year the number of critically ill patients presenting to the ED increases, and so does their length of stay in the ED. The focus on early diagnosis and therapy for myocardial infarction, stroke, sepsis, and other time-dependent emergencies has called upon ED personnel to initiate monitoring and therapy that has traditionally fallen to the critical care units. Familiarity with the principles and management of hemodynamic monitoring, as well as its limitations, is essential to accurately interpreting the data obtained. The goal of hemodynamic monitoring is to initiate and guide therapy in patients at risk for tissue hypoperfusion and subsequent organ dysfunction.

General Monitoring Principles

Several general principles can be applied when preparing for and monitoring patients with invasive lines:

- A catheter is inserted into the desired location (blood vessel or brain) for direct measurement. The catheter is connected to the transducer via monitoring tubing.
- The monitoring tubing that connects the catheter to the transducer is stiff, low-compliance tubing that prevents distortion of the signal from the blood vessel or brain to the transducer.
- The transducer system (unless using fiberoptic) is fluid filled and maintained with a flush solution. The solution is usually normal saline, with or without heparin added depending on hospital protocol, and is flushed before connection to the catheter. The transducer senses the pressure signal from the blood vessel or brain, converts it to an electrical waveform, and displays it on the monitor.

- Air should be removed from the flush solution and drip chamber when the bag is spiked. This will prevent air from entering the system should the fluid level become low or the bag turned on its side.
- The flush bag is pressurized to 300 mm Hg to overcome the pressure of the system and prevent backflow of blood.
- The transducer system allows very low infusion rates into the catheter to prevent clotting (2 to 3 mL/hr). The tubing should be disabled (clamped) when connected to intracranial monitoring systems. A fast-flush on the transducer allows for bypass of the restricted flow of fluid for initial priming of the system and for clearing of blood from the system.
- The tubing should be checked and cleared of all air bubbles, including stopcock ports. Air bubbles distort the waveform and can result in inaccurate measurements.
- Open-ended (vented) stopcock caps used for zeroing should be replaced with dead-end covers. This prevents serious blood loss should the stopcock become inadvertently turned to the open position. It also helps maintain sterility.
- Connections should be tight and placed where they can be visualized regularly. Loose connections can result in serious blood loss or infection.
- Set the monitor to the appropriate scale for the pressure being measured. Generally this is a scale of 0 to 20 mm Hg or 0 to 40 mm Hg for central venous pressures (CVP) and pulmonary artery pressures (PAP), 0 to 100 mm Hg for arterial pressure readings, and 0 to 50 mm Hg for intracranial pressure monitoring.
- The transducer should be properly aligned with the reference point when zeroing. For CVP, pulmonary artery (PA) catheters, and arterial pressures this is the phlebostatic axis located at the level of the fourth intercostal space and the midway point between the anteroposterior chest walls. Transducers used for intracranial pressure monitoring are usually placed at the level of the lateral or fourth ventricle—the tragus of the ear is a good reference point. Transducers placed above the reference point will result in a falsely elevated pressure, and transducers below the reference point will result in a false low value.
- Patency of the line should be checked regularly and whenever the waveform appears dampened.
- Coagulation status should be reviewed, considered, and reversed, if necessary, before insertion of any invasive line.

Arterial Blood Pressure Monitoring

Direct arterial blood pressure monitoring is accomplished with the insertion of a catheter into an artery. Although generally inserted into the radial artery, the brachial, femoral, and dorsalis pedis arteries can also be cannulated. The catheter is attached to a fluid-filled transducer system that converts the pressure to an electrical waveform and displays it on the monitor for concurrent continuous readings. The arterial waveform is pulsatile and depicts the systolic and diastolic phases of the cardiac cycle. The dicrotic notch on the waveform separates the systolic and diastolic phases (Figure 19-1).

The arterial pressure is determined by the cardiac output and the systemic vascular resistance (volume of blood flow versus resistance of the vessels). The relationship between pressure, flow, and volume is very complex; however, hypotension generally represents a failure of compensatory mechanisms after large-scale circulatory changes.[51] The sympathetic stress response will maintain a normal blood pressure despite declining blood volume and flow until it becomes exhausted. Blood pressure measurements are a useful screening tool and are helpful with trend assessment, but as a solitary measurement, they are of limited physiologic significance.[51]

The mean arterial pressure (MAP) represents the perfusion pressure. Diastole is longer than systole, so the MAP is not calculated by averaging the two numbers. Most monitoring systems do the math for you. The calculation is as follows:

$$\frac{\text{Systolic blood pressure [SBP]} + (2 \times \text{Diastolic blood pressure [DBP]})}{3}$$

An Allen's test is traditionally performed before radial artery cannulation. This procedure assesses for collateral blood flow to the hand by the ulnar artery in the event that the radial artery becomes occluded or damaged. The process involves having the patient clench his or her hand in a fist while the clinician applies direct pressure simultaneously to the radial and ulnar arteries, occluding flow. Ask the

patient to open his or her fist, and release pressure on the ulnar artery. If collateral flow is intact, the hand will turn pink within 7 seconds. If color does not return for greater than 15 seconds, another site should be selected.

Indications for Arterial Monitoring

Arterial lines are indicated for the following:

- Close monitoring of patients who are, or have the potential to be, hemodynamically unstable.
- Frequent blood gas analysis.
- Guiding titration of vasoactive medications. Small changes in an infusion dose of vasoactive medications may result in a large swing in blood pressure. Direct arterial blood pressure monitoring will detect potentially harmful changes immediately so that dosage adjustments can be quickly managed.
- Monitoring MAP for cerebral perfusion pressures (CPP) in patients with neurologic injury.
- Intraaortic balloon pump therapy.

Complications of Arterial Monitoring

Complications of arterial lines are not common. They include ischemic tissue necrosis due to occlusion of blood flow to the insertion site, infection, thrombus formation, vasospasm, embolism, hematoma, and pseudoaneurysm. Assessment of blood flow distal to the insertion site should be performed at least every 2 hours.

CVP Monitoring

Central venous catheters are traditionally placed in the superior vena cava via the internal jugular, external jugular, or subclavian vein or into the inferior vena cava via the femoral vein. The femoral site should be avoided for pressure monitoring purposes because the reliability at that distance from the right atrium is questionable. Recent studies suggest that the use of ultrasound-guided central line insertion reduces complications and improves the success of insertion, particularly with less experienced operators.[33,37] Readings may be measured intermittently when fluids are being infused through the port, or they may be read continuously via the same fluid-filled transducer system as used in the arterial line. Multiport catheters, such as triple-lumen catheters, are particularly helpful when vasoactive medications are being infused or when continuous CVP monitoring and simultaneous port utilization is desired. The CVP is reflective of right atrial pressures caused by stretch of the muscle fibers in the heart chambers. It can represent intravascular volume status if that "stretch" is caused by blood volume in the right atria and ventricle. However, CVP values are also influenced by venous wall and right ventricle compliance, which can rapidly accommodate a wide variation in blood volume. Although there is no direct correlation of CVP to blood volume, it does provide valuable data regarding the tolerance of volume loads. Patients with fluid overload, stress, cardiac failure, and chronic renal failure are sensitive to fluid volume loads. If a titrated fluid bolus is administered and results in a large and

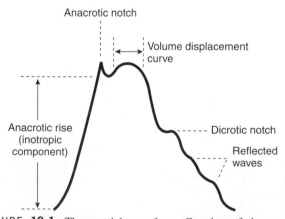

FIGURE 19-1. The arterial waveform. Creation of the arterial pressure wave and acceleration of blood flow correlate with the inotropic upstrike. The rounded shoulder represents blood volume displacement and distention of the arterial walls. Normally the peak of both the inotropic and volume displacement phases are equal in amplitude. The descending limb represents diastolic runoff of blood; the dicrotic notch separates systole from diastole. Additional humps on the downslope relate to pulse waves reflected from the periphery. (From Davoric GO: *Handbook of hemodynamic monitoring,* ed 2, Philadelphia, 2004, Saunders.)

sustained increase in CVP, then cardiac capacitance is limited. Likewise, hypovolemic and septic patients do not tolerate delayed or inadequate fluid resuscitation. In both cases, careful titration of fluids is required.[51] Central venous pressure readings are most helpful during the early stages of illness or injury when volume changes are acute. Causes of elevated CVP include increased intravascular volume, increased intrathoracic pressure, impaired right ventricular function, cardiac tamponade, pulmonary hypertension, chronic left ventricular function, or increased intraabdominal pressures. Causes of decreased CVP include hypovolemia, sudden blood or fluid loss, venodilation, or reduced intrathoracic pressures. Because CVP can be affected by position and intrathoracic pressure, readings should be taken in the supine position and read at the end of expiration at the established zero reference point (phlebostatic axis). Normal values are 2 to 6 mm Hg but are variable from patient to patient. (Water manometer systems measure in centimeters of water, instead of mercury. Normal is 3 to 11 cm H_2O.) Accuracy is best produced when monitoring trends rather than a single CVP measurement. Changes in CVP readings should be noted during and after fluid challenges and with the initiation and titrating of vasoactive agents. CVP is a useful adjunct to clinical assessment and should be evaluated along with the clinical presentation.

Indications for the Insertion of a CVP Monitor

CVP is useful in guiding fluid resuscitation after trauma, surgery, sepsis, or other emergency conditions with suspected blood volume deficit or excess. It is especially useful when using early goal-directed therapy guidelines for sepsis in which end points in fluid resuscitation are tied to specific measurements. Infusing vasoactive medications through a central line greatly reduces the risk for irritation to peripheral veins and potential infiltration and necrosis of surrounding tissue.

The guidelines for sepsis management also recommend monitoring $ScvO_2$. Monitoring $ScvO_2$ involves drawing a blood sample from the central venous catheter and sending it for ABG analysis, or using an inline bedside monitor

specifically developed for this purpose. $ScvO_2$ gives a generalized interpretation of the balance between oxygen supply and demand. Although the debate continues regarding the correlation of $ScvO_2$ and SvO_2 during the early stages of sepsis, there is good evidence that a low $ScvO_2$ during the early stages of shock is directly correlated with increased morbidity and mortality; correcting this imbalance leads to better outcomes.[30,45,57] Under normal conditions a hemoglobin molecule becomes almost 100% saturated with oxygen as it passes through the lungs. The tissues extract approximately 25% of the oxygen from the hemoglobin molecule, and it returns to the heart with approximately 75% saturation. If saturation falls below 75%, this may be reflective of either an inadequate supply of oxygen (i.e., low cardiac output, decreased hemoglobin, and low arterial saturations) or an increase in metabolic demand. Therapy to improve increased oxygen consumption includes volume, inotropes, and blood transfusions.

Complications Related to CVP Monitoring

Complications are generally associated with line insertion and include pneumothorax, hemothorax, or artery puncture. Patients with indwelling catheters are at higher risk for infection.

PA Pressure Monitoring

The PA catheter can be inserted into the internal jugular, subclavian, femoral, brachial, or basilic vein. The PA catheter is usually inserted through an introducer catheter.

There are several types of PA catheters, depending on clinical indication. Catheters can provide SvO_2 measurement, transvenous pacing, and continuous cardiac output monitoring, and some have extra infusion ports. The most common catheter used is a quad-lumen catheter with a lumen containing a thermistor for measuring cardiac output. The right atrial pressure is measured through the proximal port of the catheter; the pulmonary artery systolic and diastolic pressures and pulmonary wedge pressures are measured through the distal port. Figure 19-2 depicts a Swan-Ganz catheter.

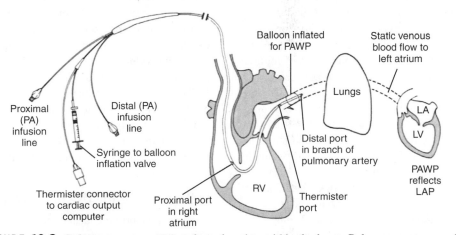

FIGURE **19-2.** Pulmonary artery (*PA*) catheter location within the heart. Pulmonary artery wedge pressure (*PAWP*) is an indirect measure of left arterial and left ventricular end-diastolic pressure. *LAP,* Left arterial pressure; *RV,* right ventricle; *LA,* left atrium; *LV,* left ventricle. (From Kersten LD: *Comprehensive respiratory nursing,* Philadelphia, 1989, WB Saunders.)

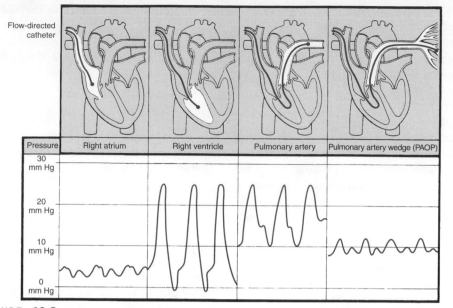

FIGURE 19-3. Bedside hemodynamic monitoring via flow-directed, balloon-tipped catheter capable of thermodilution cardiac output determination. *PAOP,* Pulmonary artery occlusion pressure. (From Urden LD, Stacy KM, Lough ME: *Thelan's critical care nursing: diagnosis and management,* ed 5, St. Louis, 2008, Mosby.)

Insertion is guided by monitoring waveforms as the catheter tip passes through the right atrium, right ventricle, and pulmonary artery (Figure 19-3). Once the catheter tip is in the pulmonary artery, the balloon is inflated and the catheter is advanced until it lodges in a smaller branch of the pulmonary artery. This is the pulmonary wedge pressure (PWP), also called pulmonary artery wedge (PAW) or pulmonary capillary wedge pressure (PCWP).

When the balloon is inflated, blood flow stops and the catheter tip senses pressures indirectly from the left atrium, which is reflective of left ventricular end-diastolic pressures (LVEDP) or the "filling pressure." Pressures are reflective of stretch of the muscle fibers caused by fluid in the left ventricle and thus allow for assessment of fluid status. However, as with CVP pressure measurements, stretch is not caused solely by volume changes, but is influenced by the compliance of the ventricles and the vascular system. Positive end-expiratory pressure, pericardial tamponade, rigid chest wall, increased intraabdominal pressures, and cardiac function all reflect pressure, not volume, of the cardiopulmonary structures and will affect accuracy of the interpretation of volume status.[49] If the ventricle is stiff, small changes in volume may result in large changes in pressure measurements. A more compliant ventricle will accommodate an increase in volume with less stretch and therefore lower pressure measurement. Factors that decrease ventricle compliance (stiffness) include ischemia, left ventricular hypertrophy, restrictive cardiomyopathies, and shock states. Factors that increase ventricular compliance include afterload reduction (antihypertensive, intraaortic balloon pump therapy, etc.) cardiomyopathies (nonrestrictive), and the resolution of ischemia.

The PWP, although not a direct indicator of blood volume, will provide some indication of capacitance for additional fluids. If pressure initially increases after a fluid bolus and then settles within the normal range, it is probably safe to administer more fluid. However, if the PWP climbs to a higher level and remains high after 30 to 60 minutes, the capacity for additional fluids is limited.[51] Mitral valve stenosis yields elevated PWPs that do not correlate with LVEDP. In patients without pulmonary disease, the pulmonary artery diastolic pressure (PAD) can also be used to estimate the LVEDP instead of the PWP. When conditions permit and a correlation has been established in the patient, the PAD pressure is often used to decrease the frequency of balloon inflation and the associated risks, or when the balloon is not functional. Pulmonary artery and wedge pressures are affected by intrathoracic pressures and should be read at end-expiration. The appearance of the location of end-expiration on the PA waveform tracing will depend on whether or not the patient is on positive pressure ventilation. Misreading of end-expiration may result in a large discrepancy of documented and actual values. Treatment based on erroneous values can prove harmful to the patient.

The exact effect of PEEP on PWP is not fully clear. However, patients should not be removed from PEEP to take a reading. Not only does this have the potential to cause hypoxia that may be difficult to reverse, but it will also cause an increase in venous return and the value will be of questionable significance.

Indications for the Use of PA Catheters

PA catheters provide access to direct measurements for a variety of cardiac parameters that can assist in the evaluation of patients with confusing clinical presentation or with rapid hemodynamic changes. Table 19-2 discusses cardiac parameters.

Table 19-2. CARDIAC PARAMETERS

Parameter	Abbreviation	Calculation	Measurement	Normal Values	Evaluation
Cardiac output	CO	HR × SV	The amount of blood ejected from the ventricle in a minute	4-8 L/min	Pump effectiveness and ventricular function
Cardiac index	CI	CO/BSA		2.4-4.0 L/min	Cardiac output by body weight
Mean arterial pressure	MAP	$\dfrac{SBP + (DBP \times 2)}{3}$	The average pressure throughout the vascular system during systole and diastole	70-105 mm Hg	Indicates adequacy of coronary and tissue perfusion
Central venous pressure	CVP	Direct pressure reading	Indirect measurement of the right atrium filling pressures.	2-6 mm Hg	Right ventricular function and volume assessment
Right atrial pressure	RA	Direct pressure reading	Filling pressure of the right atrium	2-6 mm Hg	Right ventricular function
Pulmonary artery pressures (systole/diastole)	PAP PAS PAD	Direct pressure reading	Pressures in the pulmonary artery during systole and diastole	15-25 mm Hg 0-5 mm Hg	PAS: Reflects RV pressure during systole PAD: Reflects the diastolic pressure in the pulmonary vasculature
Pulmonary wedge pressure	PWP	Direct pressure reading	Amount of myocardial fiber stretch at the end of diastole	6-12 mm Hg	Preload. The volume in the ventricle at the end of diastole. Used in fluid assessment.
Systemic vascular resistance	SVR	$\dfrac{(MAP - RA) \times 80}{CO}$	Resistance, impedance, or pressure that the ventricle must overcome to eject blood volume	800-1200 dynes/sec/cm^2	Afterload. Resistance against the left ventricle.
Stroke volume	SV	$\dfrac{CO}{HR} \times 1000\ mL/L$	The amount of blood ejected from the left ventricle with each contraction	60-100 mL/beat	Influenced by preload (PWP), afterload (SVR), and contractility
Stroke volume index	SVI	$\dfrac{SV}{BSA}$		33-47 mL/beat/m^2	Stroke volume by body weight
Pulmonary vascular resistance	PVR	$\dfrac{(MAP - PWP) \times 80}{CO}$	Resistance, impedance, or pressure that the right ventricle must overcome to eject blood volume into the pulmonary system	<250 dynes/sec/cm^2	Resistance against the right ventricle.

BSA, Body surface area; *DBP,* diastolic blood pressure; *HR,* heart rate; *RV,* right ventricle; *SBP,* systolic blood pressure.

The cardiac parameters and oxygen transport measurements are used to monitor patients with acute myocardial infarction, shock, trauma, or other critical illnesses in which the fluid and circulatory status is not clear.[51] In addition to its prognostic value, the PA catheter helps guide pharmacologic and fluid therapy. PA catheters take time and skill to place correctly and potentially pose serious complications. Clinicians should weigh the risk versus benefit for each individual patient before inserting a catheter in the ED and should not proceed if it cannot be safely inserted or monitored.

Complications Related to PA Catheters

In addition to the complications listed for central line access, the following complications have also been reported:

- *Balloon rupture:* Related to overinflation of the balloon and may cause air embolism and embolic balloon fragments. The balloon should be inflated slowly and should not exceed manufacturer's inflation values. If no resistance is felt when inflating the balloon, or if blood is returned through the balloon port, efforts should be discontinued and the physician notified.
- *Knotting:* Loops in the catheter usually caused by repeated withdrawal and advancement. This is problematic not only in obtaining readings, but in catheter removal as well. It may require surgical removal.
- *Pulmonary artery perforation:* Rupture may occur (1) during insertion, (2) with undetected prolonged wedging of the balloon, (3) because of shearing forces of cardiac pulsation, or (4) when catheter tip is located at a distal artery bifurcation

when the balloon is inflated.[59] Perforation often presents with massive hemoptysis and can be fatal. To minimize this occurrence, do the following: (1) perform constant monitoring of pressure waveforms to detect inadvertent wedge; (2) inflate balloon slowly, and stop as soon as PWP tracing is obtained; (3) keep inflation time to a minimum; (4) use only air, not fluid, to inflate the balloon; (5) avoid high-pressure flush; and (6) never flush when the catheter is in wedge.

- *Thrombus or embolus:* Most catheters are heparin bonded to prevent thrombus formation. High-pressure system flushes can release any thrombi formation on the catheter and should be avoided.

- *Arrhythmias:* Every patient should have continuous ECG monitoring both during insertion and while the catheter is in place. Premature ventricular contractions (PVCs) frequently occur when the catheter is in the right ventricle. The PA pressure waveform should be monitored continuously and consulted for right ventricular pressure (RV) waveform whenever increased ectopy is noted. If hospital policy permits, the nurse should pull the catheter back until the right atrial pressure (RA) waveform is obtained and then notify the physician.

- *Valvular damage:* Never withdraw the catheter with the balloon inflated.

Intracranial Pressure Monitoring

Intracranial pressure (ICP) is a measurement of the relationship between the contents of the brain: cerebrospinal fluid (CSF) (10%), blood (10%), and brain tissue (80%). The Monro-Kellie doctrine hypothesizes that when the volume of one brain component increases there is a corresponding and compensatory decrease in one of the other brain components. Under normal conditions, compliance between the three components maintains an ICP between 0 and 15 mm Hg. Once the compensatory mechanisms within the rigid confines of the brain reach capacity, the ICP will increase. At its limits, small changes in one of the components will result in a significant increase in the ICP (Figure 19-4).

There is an inverse correlation with the magnitude and the duration of increased ICP and morbidity and mortality. Guidelines for treatment thresholds vary, but generally for adults it is 20 to 25 mm Hg, for children from 1 to 5 years it is 15 mm Hg, and for infants it is 10 mm Hg.[2,34,36-38] The body's autoregulatory system maintains a constant cerebral blood flow within a MAP range of 50 to 150 mm Hg. The MAP is the main driving force of blood supply to the brain. The MAP is met with resistance from the opposing force of the ICP. The difference between the two is the cerebral perfusion pressure (CPP):

$$MAP - ICP = CPP$$

Severe increases in ICP will reduce the CPP and the cerebral blood flow (CBF). CPP that is too low causes ischemia, and CPP that is too high causes elevated ICP. The average CPP is 80 to 100 mm Hg; if it falls below 50 mm Hg, hypoperfusion and ischemia occur. CPP should be maintained at 60 to 70 mm Hg unless ordered otherwise.[10]

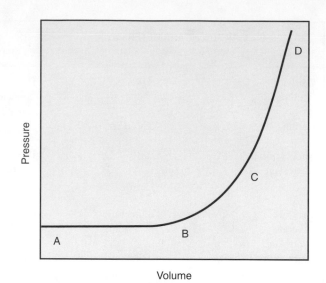

FIGURE **19-4.** Pressure-volume curve. From point *A* to point *B*, intracranial pressure remains constant with the addition of volume and brain compliance is high. At point *B* brain compliance begins to change and intracranial pressure (ICP) rises slightly. From point *B* to point *C*, compliance is low and ICP rises with increases in intracranial volume. From point *C* to point *D*, small increases in volume cause significant ICP elevations. (From McQuillan KA, Thurman PA: Traumatic brain injuries. In McQuillan KA, Makic Flynn MB, Whalen E et al, editors: *Trauma nursing: from resuscitation through rehabilitation,* ed 4, St. Louis, 2009, Saunders.)

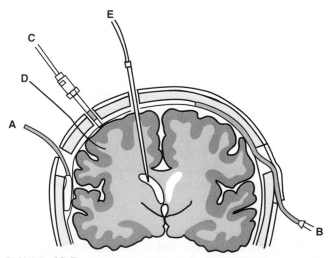

FIGURE **19-5.** Coronal section of the brain showing potential sites for placement of intracranial pressure monitoring devices. *A,* Epidural; *B,* subdural; *C,* subarachnoid; *D,* intraparenchymal; *E,* intraventricular. (From McNair ND: Intracranial pressure monitoring. In Clochesy JM, Breu C, Cardkin S at al, editors: *Critical care nursing,* ed 2, Philadelphia, 1996, Saunders.)

An ICP monitoring device is necessary to calculate the CPP. Multiple modalities for measuring cerebral blood flow, oxygenation, temperature, and pressures are available.

ICP measurements can be obtained via intraventricular catheter, subdural, epidural, subarachnoid, or intraparenchymal transducers (Figure 19-5). Table 19-3 contains a description of ICP monitoring devices.

Table 19-3. ICP MONITORING DEVICES

Device	Description	Transducer Options	Advantage	Disadvantage
Ventriculostomy catheter	A catheter is inserted into the lateral ventricle	Fiberoptic External strain gauge Internal strain gauge	Most accurate measurement of ICP Allows drainage and sampling of CSF Can be rezeroed externally	Can be difficult to place Highest risk for infection May get occluded Accidental excess CSF drainage
Subdural probe or catheter	A probe or catheter is placed into the subdural space	Fiberoptic External strain gauge Internal strain gauge	Easy to insert	Does not allow CSF drainage Poor accuracy
Epidural sensor	A sensor is placed in the epidural space	Fiberoptic External strain gauge	Easy to insert	Does not allow CSF drainage Indirect pressure measurement Poor accuracy
Intraparenchymal probe	A probe is placed into the brain parenchyma	Fiberoptic Internal strain gauge	Easy to insert Good accuracy	Does not allow CSF drainage Poor accuracy
Subarachnoid screw	The tip of hollow bolt is placed into the subarachnoid space	Fiberoptic External strain gauge	Easy to insert	Does not allow CSF drainage Poor accuracy

CSF, Cerebrospinal fluid; *ICP,* intracranial pressure.

The reference point for zeroing the transducer is the foramen of Monro, which corresponds externally with the external auditory meatus (tragus of the ear). Transducer systems can be external strain gauge (fluid filled) or fiberoptic. Fiberoptic transducers are zeroed before insertion and do not require further rezeroing or leveling after insertion. The cables are fragile, and care must be taken not to bend or twist the probe. The zero can drift slowly over time. Fluid-filled catheters require regular rezeroing, so any zero-drift can be corrected. Leveling with the zero reference point (external auditory meatus) must be consistent and adjusted with change in patient position. Although the ventriculostomy catheter is considered the most accurate of ICP monitoring devices, cerebral edema and collapsed ventricles often make placement difficult. This is the only device that allows for the drainage of CSF for ICP control or sampling of CSF for laboratory assessment. Accuracy of CPP calculations requires that the arterial catheter (for MAP) and the ICP zero reference points be the same.[49] The foramen of Monro should be used as the reference point for both monitors. The ICP waveform is similar to arterial waveforms in that it is a pulsatile waveform. Normal ICP waveforms have three distinctive waves that become altered in pathologic conditions: P1 or percussion wave, P2 or tidal wave, and P3, known as the dicrotic wave (Figure 19-6). The P1 wave has higher amplitude than the P2 wave, except when cerebral compliance becomes compromised and autoregulation is impaired.[34] A P2 wave equal to or greater than the P1 wave is indicative of an increase or impending increase in ICP.

Dampened waveforms call for assessment of the monitoring system for leaks or obstruction.

Indications for the Use of ICP Monitoring

Evidenced-based traumatic brain injury (TBI) guidelines call for the placement of an ICP monitoring device for patients with severe traumatic brain injury (Glasgow Coma Scale score

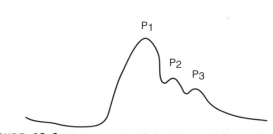

FIGURE **19-6.** Components of the intracranial pressure wave. From McQuillan KA, Thurman PA: Traumatic brain injuries. In McQuillan KA, Makic Flynn MB, Whalen E et al, editors: *Trauma nursing: from resuscitation through rehabilitation,* ed 4, St. Louis, 2009, Saunders/Elsevier.)

of less than 8) with abnormal computed tomography (CT) scan or with a normal CT scan and two or more high-risk indicators. High-risk indicators include (1) age greater than 40 years, (2) posturing motor response, and (3) systolic blood pressure less than 90 mm Hg.[10] ICP monitoring is also used, though less frequently, with management of subarachnoid hemorrhage and stroke.

See Chapter 33 for specific therapies.

Complications Related to the Use of ICP Monitors

Infection: Infection is a complication related to the use of ICP monitors. Ventriculostomy catheters have a higher incidence of infection than other devices. Strict aseptic technique should be maintained on insertion and when manipulating or accessing the device. A sterile occlusive dressing should be applied and maintained.

Ventricular collapse, herniation, or hemorrhage: When draining CSF from a ventriculostomy catheter, only small amounts should be removed at a time (2 to 3 mL). Drainage systems can be set up to monitor continuously or to drain when a predetermined ICP is reached (using the gravity principle). Changing the level of the head without changing the level of the drainage system can cause CSF to drain beyond what is desired or to not drain at all when ICP is elevated. If CSF is drained too rapidly, brain tissue can shift into the space evacuated by the CSF, causing stretching and tearing of vessels, resulting in hemorrhage or herniation. In traumatic-brain-injured patients, the problem is not with overdrainage of CSF but collapse of the ventricles. This may cause loss of waveform and pressure reading but does not damage the brain or neurologic function.[56] In the ED setting it is safest to keep the system on the monitor mode with the alarm on, and drain CSF when the ICP reaches the treatment threshold unless otherwise ordered by the physician.

Fluid entering system: Fluid-filled transducer lines should be connected to a plain pressure tubing without a flush system. When the only transducer system that is available contains a flush system, it must be disabled and clamped. The line should be well marked, indicating that it is an ICP line, to prevent accidental infusion of fluid into the brain.

CSF leakage or air entering the system: Make sure all connections are tightened. When using a fluid-filled transducer system, ensure that it has been cleared of air and bubbles. Remove air when spiking the bag, and fill the drip chamber with fluid. Bubbles will interfere with the transmission of pressure and will give inaccurate ICP measurements.

Occlusion: Occlusion may arise from blood or brain in the system and will demonstrate as a dampened waveform. Notify the physician when unable to drain CSF from a ventriculostomy catheter. Do not directly flush the catheter unless specific guidelines and training have been established. The tubing (not the catheter) can be flushed.

Fiberoptic catheters are fragile and can break easily, which would require replacement. Handle the catheter gently, and protect from external damage. Ensure the connections are tight so that the catheter does not dislodge.

Summary

Invasive monitoring can provide important information about the patient's condition and response to selected treatments. However, the emergency nurse must be familiar with the indications for the use of invasive monitoring, how to use the equipment, and how to recognize and manage complications related to their use in the ED.

SEPSIS

Severe sepsis and septic shock continue to have a mortality rate of 30% to 50% despite an improved understanding of pathogenesis and advances in technology. In the United States there are an estimated 751,000 cases of severe sepsis annually with approximately 215,000 deaths, eclipsing the death rate attributed to myocardial infarction. Sepsis is the

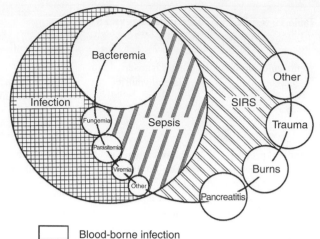

Blood-borne infection

FIGURE 19-7. Interrelationships between systemic inflammatory response syndrome (SIRS), sepsis, and infection. (From Bone RC, Balk RA, Cerra FB et al: Definitions for sepsis and organ failure and guidelines for the use of innovative therapies in sepsis, *Chest* 101:1644, 1992.)

leading cause of death in the critical care unit and the tenth leading cause of death in the United States.[3] Because the incidence of severe sepsis increases markedly with age, the number of cases will continue to rise as the population ages. The incidence of sepsis is also increased in patients who are immunocompromised, critically ill, have indwelling catheters, and are very young.

Definitions

In 1991 a consensus conference between the American College of Chest Physicians (ACCP) and the Society of Critical Care Medicine (SCCM) was assembled to clarify the definition of sepsis along the continuum of inflammatory response.[7,9,18] Before this time, terminology was poorly defined and inconsistently applied. It was the intent of this group that using universal terminology to describe the inflammatory response would improve collecting reliable epidemiologic data and outcome research. Consensus conference definitions include the following:

- *Infection:* The inflammatory response by a host to the invasion of a microorganism.
- *Bacteremia:* The presence of bacteria in the bloodstream.
- *SIRS:* Systemic inflammatory response syndrome is a nonspecific systemic response to a variety of insults. The causative factor is not necessarily specific to infection and can include inflammatory responses to trauma, pancreatitis, shock, burns, ischemia, or surgery. Figure 19-7 demonstrates the interrelationships between SIRS, sepsis, and infection. To meet the criteria for SIRS, two or more of the criteria in Box 19-2 must be met.
- *Sepsis:* The systemic inflammatory response specifically attributed to an infection or a presumed infection. Two or more of the criteria for SIRS (see Box 19-2) are present, and there is reasonable clinical evidence that an infection is present. Blood cultures do not need to be positive.

Box 19-2	SIRS MANIFESTATIONS

- Temperature <96.8° F (36° C) or >100.4° F (38° C)
- Heart rate >90 beats/min
- Respiratory rate >20 breaths/min (or $PaCO_2$ <32 mm Hg)
- Abnormal WBC counts
  - >12,000/mm^3
  - <4000/mm^3
  - >10% bands

SIRS, Systemic inflammatory response syndrome; *WBC*, white blood cell.

- *Severe sepsis:* The presence or presumed presence of an infection, as well as single or multiple organ dysfunction, hypoperfusion, or hypotension. Hypoperfusion may present as lactic acidosis, oliguria, and/or acute change in mental status.
- *Septic shock:* A subset of severe sepsis marked by hypotension that does not respond to adequate volume resuscitation. Hypotension is defined as SBP less than 90 mm Hg, MAP less than 60 mm Hg, or a decrease in SBP by greater than 40 mm Hg from baseline. Blood pressures that are normal but require vasopressor support to maintain are included in the septic shock definition.
- *Multiple organ dysfunction syndrome (MODS):* The potentially reversible dysfunction of at least two organs requiring medical intervention to maintain body equilibrium. Table 19-4 provides system presentation of organ ischemia and dysfunction.

Recent randomized, controlled studies have approached the treatment of sepsis in an aggressive and time-dependent manner similar to acute myocardial infarction and stroke.[45] Success in reducing mortality in these studies prompted a group of international experts representing critical care and infectious disease to develop evidence-based guidelines for the management of sepsis and septic shock, with a heavy focus on early diagnosis and treatment in the initial hours of presentation.[15] The Surviving Sepsis Campaign is a collaborative effort by the Society of Critical Care Medicine, the European Society of Intensive Care Medicine, and the International Sepsis Forum to improve awareness and treatment of sepsis and to decrease mortality rate by 25% by 2009. These guidelines were initially presented in 2004 and include 45 recommendations for the resuscitation and management of septic patients.

Pathophysiology

Sepsis is the result of a series of complex events of cellular, humoral, and inflammatory interactions within a host that is manifested by systemic inflammation and coagulation.[39] Initially a localized response to a pathogen results in cellular activation of monocytes to stimulate the release of proinflammatory cytokines such as interleukin-1, interleukin-6, and tumor necrosis factor. These cytokines

Table 19-4.	EFFECTS OF ORGAN ISCHEMIA
System	**Presentation**
CNS	Acute change in mental status
	Confusion
	Comatose
Respiratory	Hypoxia/hypoxemia
	Ventilation/perfusion mismatch
	Adult respiratory distress syndrome (ARDS)
	Acute lung injury (ALI)
Cardiovascular	Decreased ejection fraction
	Biventricular dilation
Renal	Oliguria
	Anuria
	Elevated creatinine level
	Acute renal failure
Metabolic/Endocrine	Hyperglycemia
	Lactic acidosis
	Adrenal insufficiency
	Hypothyroidism
	Catabolic
Hepatic	Elevated liver enzyme levels
	Hyperbilirubinemia

CNS, Central nervous system.

produce compounds that cause local vasodilatation and the release of cytotoxic chemicals to fight and destroy the pathogen.[22] In normal circumstances this proinflammatory response is balanced with antiinflammatory cytokines to promote wound healing and maintain homeostasis. However, in sepsis the initial proinflammatory response spins out of control, causing damage to the endothelium and release of the cytotoxic material into the bloodstream.[15] Further damage to the endothelium leads to extravasation of cellular fluid, interstitial edema, decreased intravascular volume, and relative hypovolemia. The mass production of nitric oxide by cytokines and tumor necrosis factor causes systemic vasodilatation and hypotension. As a result, oxygen supply to tissues does not keep up with oxygen demand, and global tissue hypoxia and shock ensue. This marks the transition into severe sepsis and septic shock.[11,53] In addition, damage to the endothelium causes stimulation of the coagulation and complement cascades, causing microcirculatory coagulation, platelet aggregation, and thrombus formation.[29]

Diagnosis

Because the mortality of sepsis increases exponentially as it progresses to septic shock and organ dysfunction, early identification and treatment of severe sepsis is essential. However, the identification of severe sepsis is not clear-cut because many of the symptoms identified in the early stages of sepsis are common in a wide variety of conditions in addition to inflammatory response. Thus diagnosis of sepsis is often determined through a combination of detailed history and assessment that lead to a high degree of suspicion. Vital signs in the early stages of sepsis do not adequately reveal the level of global hypoperfusion, even though damage that will affect morbidity and mortality is well under way.[43] The combination of history, symptoms associated with SIRS, and laboratory values suggestive of infection or hypoperfusion, such as elevated serum lactate, should indicate the need for immediate resuscitation.

Laboratory findings on presentation to the ED vary depending on the stage of sepsis. Early findings will be reflective of SIRS, including abnormal white blood count and/or an increase in immature cells. As the inflammatory response advances, signs of hypovolemia may be evident, presenting as hemoconcentration with elevation of hematocrit and hemoglobin. Hypoperfusion of organs and tissues may present as hypoxemia, metabolic acidosis, elevated lactate, elevated liver enzymes, and hyperbilirubinemia. As the coagulation cascade is stimulated, thrombocytopenia, prolonged thrombin time, and low fibrinogen levels develop.

Imaging studies to identify the source of sepsis should be obtained as quickly as possible. The stability of the patient and risks of transport and placement in confined areas should be considered and risks weighed thoughtfully.

Emergency Department Management

The landmark study by Rivers et al compared standard therapy with early goal-directed therapy (EGDT) in the treatment of patients who presented to the ED with sepsis and serum lactate levels greater than 4 mmol/L or refractory hypotension related to infection.[24,35,41,45] In this study the patients were treated for 6 hours in the ED before transfer to the intensive care unit (ICU), at which point the study was discontinued. The treatment goal involved implementing a systematic process using set hemodynamic parameters to guide treatment and reverse global hypoperfusion without causing further stress on myocardial function. The in-hospital mortality rates in standard therapy and EGDT therapy were 46.5% and 30.5%, respectively. The EGDT group also had significantly shorter hospital lengths of stay, lower organ dysfunction scores, and a twofold decrease in acute respiratory failure, hypotension, and sudden episodes of cardiopulmonary complications, such as cardiac arrest. Subsequent studies have validated the results of this study.[28,40,54]

Likewise, it appears that the timing of initiating therapy is of equal importance. Similar studies involving patients admitted to the ICU in later phases of sepsis and septic shock did not demonstrate any benefit to patient outcome, and in some cases increased mortality.[17,19]

With this evidence, the Surviving Sepsis Campaign was developed, and the distribution of guidelines for the resuscitation and management of severe sepsis and septic shock patients was initiated. Some of the guidelines are supported by consensus expert opinion only, but others are evidence based and supported by clinical research (such as EGDT).[39] Although the principles are based on solid clinical practice, not all of the guidelines will meet every patient scenario. It is important for clinicians to use their judgment in applying the guidelines as the individual circumstance dictates. Whether intensive care is brought to the ED or the patient is delivered to the ICU, it is clear that treatment should be implemented without delay.

Initial Priorities

The priorities of treating severe sepsis and septic shock in the ED are (1) patient stabilization, (2) early identification of sepsis, (3) early hemodynamic stabilization and support, (4) source identification, and (5) prompt administration of appropriate antibiotics. The principles of airway-breathing-circulation should always take the highest priority. Patients may present in an advanced stage of septic shock with altered mental status and inability to protect their airway. Patients who are chronically ill, elderly, or debilitated may have limited respiratory reserve. These patients may require intubation if oxygenation, ventilation, or airway cannot be maintained. Continuous monitoring of heart rate, blood pressure, urine output, and oxygen saturation should be initiated and maintained throughout resuscitation.

FLUID RESUSCITATION. Fluid resuscitation should begin as soon as sepsis or septic shock is recognized. An elevated serum lactate level is a useful indicator of hypoperfusion and is often present even when blood pressure is normal.[8,11,50] Clinicians should not wait for hypotension before initiating fluid resuscitation if signs of hypoperfusion are present. The debate on colloids versus crystalloids continues. A multicenter double-blind study of almost 7000 heterogeneous intensive care patients randomized to resuscitation fluids of either 4% albumin or normal saline showed no significant difference in primary outcomes after 28 days.[47] Whatever fluid is selected, the goal of therapy is to achieve a CVP of 8 to 12 mm Hg. When using crystalloids, start with 20 mL/kg administered rapidly, and repeat as necessary, monitoring the patient's response carefully. It is not unusual for patients to require a large volume of fluid (5 to 10 L) during the resuscitation phase; this is dependent on the degree of vasodilatation and hypovolemia.

BLOOD PRESSURE CONTROL. Blood pressure monitoring is optimized with the use of an arterial catheter that should be placed as soon as time and resources permit. A MAP of 65 mm Hg or greater is the goal during resuscitation. It is preferable to first attempt to reverse hypotension with volume resuscitation; however, it may be necessary to initiate vasopressors in conjunction with volume resuscitation to sustain life. Fluid resuscitation to restore an adequate intravascular volume is the priority. The use of vasopressors without adequate volume resuscitation is harmful. Norepinephrine and dopamine are favored over phenylephrine and epinephrine.[5] Some studies support the use of norepinephrine as the preferential vasopressor to support MAP in septic shock, although dopamine may have some benefit. Norepinephrine is a more potent vasoconstrictor than dopamine and may be superior over dopamine in reversing hypotension. Alternately, dopamine has inotropic qualities that may make it a better choice in patients with compromised cardiac function, but excessive tachycardia may result. There is good evidence that low-dose dopamine does not protect kidneys or improve any of the patient outcome indicators. Low-dose dopamine should not be used in treating severe sepsis or septic shock.[48]

The SCCM guidelines recommend that vasopressin be used only when the blood pressure is not responsive to well-established vasopressors. Vasopressin has been shown to decrease hepatosplanchnic flow as well as cardiac output. If this agent is used as an additional vasopressor for treatment of septic shock, then the dose should be constant at 0.04 units/min.[21]

OXYGEN DELIVERY AND CONSUMPTION. Low $ScvO_2$ or SvO_2 and an elevated serum lactate level are indicators that oxygen delivery is not meeting cellular demand. If the $ScvO_2$ remains less than 70% after hypovolemia and hypotension are reversed, clinicians should consider reversing the deficit. This can be accomplished by transfusion of packed red blood cells if hematocrit is less than 30% and/or initiation of a dobutamine infusion to improve cardiac contractility. Dobutamine should always be used in conjunction with vasopressors in patients with hypotension. Attempts to achieve supranormal levels of oxygen delivery have proven potentially harmful and are not recommended.[19] If dobutamine is not tolerated due to tachycardia or hypotension, clinicians may consider reducing oxygen demand and consumption through intubation, sedation, and paralysis.

ANTIMICROBIAL THERAPY. The early initiation of appropriate antibiotic therapy is associated with improved morbidity and mortality.[23,31] The Kumar study showed that for every hour of delay in initiating appropriate antimicrobial therapy in patients with persistent hypotension, survival would decrease by 7.6%. Survival was 77.2% for patients who were started on effective antibiotics in the first 30 minutes of hypotension, whereas survival of patients who were not started on antibiotics for 6 hours was only 42.0%. Administration of antibiotics early in the ED treatment period should be a priority because it likely will lead to an improvement in patient outcome. The Surviving Sepsis Campaign guidelines call for the initiation of antimicrobial therapy within the first hour after severe sepsis is diagnosed.[15] Cultures should be obtained before antibiotic administration, but treatment should not be delayed if they cannot be obtained.

RECOMBINANT HUMAN ACTIVATED PROTEIN C. Protein C plays an important role in the inflammatory response as an antiinflammatory, anticoagulant, and profibrinolytic, offsetting some of the proinflammatory pathophysiologic processes in sepsis.[25] Protein C levels are low in sepsis. The Recombinant Human Activated Protein C Worldwide Evaluation in Severe Sepsis (PROWESS) trial investigated the effect of the administration of recombinant activated protein C (rhAPC; drotrecogin alpha [activated]) on patients with sepsis-induced organ dysfunction.[6] The rhAPC group showed a 6.1% absolute decrease in mortality and a relative risk reduction of 19.4% over a 28-day period. Because rhAPC has anticoagulant properties, it is associated with increased risk for bleeding, most notably in the pediatric population. The use of drotrecogin alpha (activated) is currently recommended for adult patients at high risk for death despite optimized treatment using the principles of EGDT, and where no contraindications exist. Contraindications are primarily associated with patients at higher risk for bleeding such as recent surgery, hemorrhagic stroke, traumatic brain injury, and high-risk trauma. Outcome benefit may be tied to the timing of rhAPC administration, and studies have suggested that administration should be initiated within 24 to 48 hours.[6,27,58]

HYDROCORTISONE. Patients who are refractory to fluid resuscitation and require high-dose vasopressor therapy may have relative adrenal insufficiency. The lack of adrenal reserve is associated with worse outcome.[32,52] Fluid-resuscitated, hemodynamically unstable patients on vasoactive agents should have an adrenocorticotropic hormone stimulation test or a baseline cortisol level drawn and then be started on low-dose hydrocortisone (50 mg).[4]

Assessment, Management, and Evaluation of the Patient With Sepsis in the Emergency Department

The assessment, management, and evaluation of the patient with sepsis in the ED require a focused team approach. The following is a summary of that care.

ASSESSMENT
1. Airway, breathing, circulation, disability, and exposure (ABCDE) assessment and implementation of critical interventions
2. Obtain history of present illness to localize potential origin of infection
   a. *Head:* ear, sinus, or throat pain; swollen lymph glands; nasal drainage
   b. *Neck:* pain, stiffness
   c. *Chest:* shortness of breath, cough, pleuritic pain, pulmonary secretions, congestion
   d. *Abdomen:* nausea, vomiting, diarrhea, abdominal pain (generalized or localized), loss of appetite
   e. *Renal/pelvic/genital:* vaginal or urethral drainage; flank, back, or pelvic pain; urinary frequency, hematuria, oliguria, or dysuria; bladder fullness; cloudy urine
   f. *Extremities:* obvious deformities, open fractures, cellulitis
   g. *Soft tissue:* erythema, pain beyond borders of erythema, localized edema, bullae, blebs
   h. *General:* headache, malaise, chills, body aches, weakness, dizziness, altered level of consciousness
   i. *Past medical and surgical history:* Immunocompromising conditions, prosthetic devices, recent exposures to communicable diseases
3. Physical assessment: signs of infection, SIRS, sepsis
   a. *Fever:* core temperature greater than 101.4° F (38° C)
   b. *Hypothermia:* core temperature less than 96.8° F (36° C)
   c. *Tachypnea:* respiratory rate greater than 20 breaths/min
   d. Altered mental status
   e. Significant peripheral edema
   f. *Hypotension:* SBP less than 90 mm Hg, mean arterial pressure less than 70 mm Hg, SBP decrease of more than 40 mm Hg from patient's baseline

g. Absent bowel sounds

h. Delayed capillary refill

i. *Physical examination indicating localized infection:* crackles, rhonchi, or dullness to percussion on chest examination; abdominal distention, localized tenderness, rebound tenderness or guarding; erythema, crepitus, edema, tenderness; any purulent drainage; meningismus; petechial or purpuric rash

4. Diagnostic assessment associated with SIRS and sepsis

a. Hyperglycemia (greater than 120 mg/dL) not associated with diabetes

b. White blood cell (WBC) count greater than 12,000/mm^3, WBC count less than 4,000/mm^3, WBC count normal, but with greater than 10% bands

c. Plasma C-reactive protein greater than 2 standard deviations (SD) above the normal value

d. *Arterial hypoxemia:* PaO$_2$ less than 60 mm Hg

e. *Oliguria:* urine output less than 0.5 mL/kg/hr for more than 2 hours

f. *Elevated creatinine:* greater than 0.5 mg/dL

g. *Thrombocytopenia:* platelet count less than 100,000/mm

h. *Coagulation abnormalities:* international normalized ratio (INR) greater than 1.5 baseline or greater than 4.0

i. *Hyperbilirubinemia:* total bilirubin greater than 4 mg/dL

j. *Hyperlactatemia:* greater than 2 mmol/L

MANAGEMENT. The management of a patient who is septic should be based on the following:

a. Maintain/establish airway, breathing, and circulation.

b. *Obtain cultures:* Thirty to fifty percent of patients presenting with symptoms of severe sepsis have positive blood cultures. Cultures from all sources, including blood, urine, wounds, secretions, CSF, etc., should be drawn before initiation of antimicrobial therapy. At least two sets of cultures are recommended. In addition to at least one percutaneous site, blood cultures should be drawn simultaneously from any vascular device that has been in place greater than 48 hours. This may aid in the determination of the source of infection.

c. *Administer antibiotics:* Antibiotics should be administered within 3 hours of patient admission to the ED. Antibiotic selection should be sufficiently broad to cover all likely pathogens. Although the concern for antibiotic-resistant organisms is noted, the marginal physiologic reserve of patients in severe sepsis and septic shock warrants the use of broad-spectrum antibiotics until the pathogen and antibiotic susceptibilities are identified.

d. Administer fluid bolus with crystalloid or colloid solution if the patient is hypotensive or serum lactate is greater than 4 mmol/L.

   • Rapid bolus with crystalloid solution starting with at least 20 mL/kg over 15 to 30 minutes.

   • Insert an indwelling urinary catheter.

   • Assess blood pressure, heart rate, urine output, and arterial oxygen saturation during the course of each fluid bolus.

   • Repeat boluses as necessary until heart rate is less than 110 beats/min, MAP is greater than 70 mm Hg, or the patient is fluid compromised (e.g., pulmonary edema).

   • If using EGDT, administer fluid until CVP is 8 to 12 mm Hg.

e. *Treat ongoing hypotension as ordered:* Blood pressure goals and treatments are best monitored by the placement of an arterial catheter and continuous, ongoing measurements. Assist with placement if ordered, and monitor circulation distal to catheter site. If the patient is unresponsive to fluid resuscitation (patient remains hypotensive with CVP 8 to 12 mm Hg or at least 40 mL/kg has been given), vasopressor therapy should be initiated as directed by the physician. The preferred route of infusion of vasoactive drugs is through a central line as soon as it is available. Titrate the vasopressor carefully. Care should be taken not to overshoot treatment goals and cause unnecessary hypertension, especially in patients with preexisting cardiac disease. This can add strain to the workload of the heart and worsen cardiac output and cellular perfusion. Range of accepted MAP is 65 to 85 mm Hg.

f. *Assess oxygen delivery:* If using the EGDT guidelines and a central venous catheter is in place, assess the ScvO$_2$ (or SvO$_2$ if a pulmonary catheter has been placed). The goal ScvO$_2$ is greater than 70% and is manipulated using fluid resuscitation, dobutamine, and red blood cell transfusion (if Hct less than 30%).

Start dobutamine at 2.5 to 5 mcg/kg/min, and titrate to 20 mcg/kg/min to reach the goal of ScvO$_2$ of 70%. Monitor the blood pressure closely on initiation and titration of dobutamine. Vasopressors should be infused simultaneously to adjust for hypotension. Discontinue dobutamine if hypotension is persistent or if heart rate becomes excessively high.

ONGOING EVALUATION. Continuously monitor and record heart rate, blood pressure, urine output, and if available ScvO$_2$ and CVP. Monitor mental status. Reevaluate lactate levels intermittently throughout resuscitation to guide adequacy of resuscitation. If infusing vasoactive agents through a peripheral line, assess skin around insertion site for signs of infiltration and tissue damage. Adjust titration of vasopressor agents to maintain MAP between 65 and 85 mm Hg. Prepare the patient for transport to radiology for imaging for further diagnosis when deemed sufficiently stable.

Prepare and transport the patient to the critical care unit for further care and evaluation.

SUMMARY

The basis of early goal-directed therapy is the prompt identification of systemic hypoperfusion, indicating the potential for progression of sepsis to severe sepsis. Initiation of therapy should be considered time dependent and instituted without delay. The source of infection should be investigated, cultures drawn, and appropriate antibiotics administered as soon as possible. The treatment of sepsis and septic shock is both time dependant and labor intensive. It is only with the collaboration of the emergency and critical care departments that the impact on patient care can be fully realized. The role of the emergency nurse is essential to the success of implementation of sepsis guidelines. It is the bedside nurse who will initiate therapy, evaluate response, and identify obstructions with implementing strategies.

REFERENCES

1. Acute Respiratory Distress Syndrome Network: Ventilating with lower tidal volumes as compared with traditional tidal volumes for acute lung injury and the acute respiratory distress syndrome, *N Engl J Med* 342:1301, 2000.
2. Addelson P, Kochanek P: Head injury in children, *Child Neuro* 12:2, 1999.
3. Angus DC, Linde-Zwirble WT, Lidicker J et al: Epidemiology of severe sepsis in the United States: analysis of incidence, outcome, and associated costs of care, *Crit Care Med* 29:1303, 2001.
4. Annane D, Sebille V, Dharpentier C et al: Effect of treatment with low doses of hydrocortisone and fludrocortisone on mortality in patients with septic shock, *JAMA* 288:862, 2002.
5. Beale RJ, Hollenberg SM, Vincent JL et al: Vasopressor and inotropic support in septic shock: an evidence-based review, *Crit Care Med* 32(11 suppl):S455, 2004.
6. Bernard GR, Vincent JL, Laterre PF et al: Efficacy and safety of recombinant human activated protein C for severe sepsis, *N Engl J Med* 344:699, 2001.
7. Bone RC, Balk RA, Cerra FB et al: Definitions for sepsis and organ failure and guidelines for the use of innovative therapies in sepsis, *Chest* 101:1644, 1992.
8. Broder G, Weil M: Excess lactate: an index of reversibility of shock in human patients, *Science* 143:1457, 1964.
9. Brun-Buisson C, Doyon F, Carlet J et al: Incidence, risk factors, and outcome of severe sepsis and septic shock in adults: a multicenter prospective study in intensive care units—French ICU Group for Severe Sepsis, *JAMA* 274:968, 1995.
10. Bullock R, Chestnut RM, Clifton G et al: *Guidelines for the management of severe head injury*, New York, 2000, Brain Trauma Foundation.
11. Cady L, Weil M, Afifi A et al: Quantitation of severity of critical illness with special reference to blood lactate, *Crit Care Med* 1:75, 1973.
12. Chalfin D, Trzeciak S, Likourezos A et al: Impact of delayed transfer of critically ill patients from the emergency department to the intensive care unit, *Crit Care Med* 35:1, 2007.
13. Clark K, Normile L: Delays in implementing admission orders for critical care patients associated with length of stay in emergency departments in six mid-Atlantic states, *J Emerg Nurs* 28:489, 2002.
14. Clark K, Normile L: Influence of time-to-interventions for emergency department critical care patients on hospital mortality, *J Emerg Nurs* 33:6, 2007.
15. Dellinger RP, Carlet JM, Masur H et al: Surviving Sepsis Campaign guidelines for management of severe sepsis and septic shock, *Crit Care Med* 32(3):858, 2004.
16. Dreyfuss D, Saumon G: Ventilator-induced lung injury: lessons from experimental studies, *Am J Respir Crit Care Med* 157:294, 1998.
17. Gattinoni L, Brazzi L, Pelosi P et al: A trial of goal-oriented hemodynamic therapy in critically ill patients: SvO2 Collaborative Group, *N Engl J Med* 333:1025, 1995.
18. Gupta S, Jonas M: Sepsis, septic shock and multiple organ failure, *Anesth Intensive Care Med* 7(5):143, 2005.
19. Hayes MA, Timmins AC, Yau EH et al: Elevation of systemic oxygen delivery in the treatment of critically ill patients, *N Engl J Med* 330:1717, 1994.
20. Hirvela ER: Advances in the management of acute respiratory distress syndrome: protective ventilation, *Arch Surg* 135:126, 2000.
21. Holmes CL, Walley KR, Chittock DR et al: The effects of vasopressin on hemodynamics and renal function in severe septic shock: a case series, *Intensive Care Med* 27:1416, 2001.
22. Hotchkiss RS, Karl IE: The pathophysiology and treatment of sepsis, *N Engl J Med* 348:138, 2003.
23. Houck P, Bratzler D, Nsa W et al: Timing of antibiotic administration and outcomes for Medicare patients hospitalized with community-acquired pneumonia, *Arch Intern Med* 164:637, 2005.
24. Huang DT, Gilles C, Dremsizov TT et al: Implementation of early goal-directed therapy for severe sepsis and septic shock: a decision analysis, *Crit Care Med* 35(9):2090, 2007.
25. Huges M: Recombinant human activated protein C, *Int J Antimicrob Agents* 28:90, 2006.
26. Institute of Medicine: *The future of emergency care in the United State health system,* Report brief, June 2006, National Academy of Science, Washington, D.C.
27. Johnston J, Pulgar S, Ball D et al: The impact of timely drotrecogin alfa (activated) administration on hospital mortality and resource use, *Crit Care Med* 31:A73, 2003.
28. Jones AE, Foct A, Horton JM et al: Prospective external validation of the clinical effectiveness of an emergency department-based early goal-directed therapy protocol for severe sepsis and septic shock, *Chest* 132(2):425, 2007.
29. Karemova A, Pinsky DJ: The endothelial response to oxygen deprivation: biology and clinical implications, *Intensive Care Med* 27:19, 2001.
30. Krafft P, Steltzer H, Hiesmayr M et al: Mixed venous oxygen saturation in critically ill septic shock patients: the role of defined events, *Chest* 103:900, 1993.

31. Kumar A, Roberts D, Wood K et al: Duration of hypotension before initiation of effective antimicrobial therapy is the critical determinant of survival in human septic shock, *Crit Care Med* 34(6):1589, 2006.

32. Lamberts S, Bruining H, de Jong F: Corticosteroid therapy in severe illness, *N Engl J Med* 337:1285, 1997.

33. Leung J: Real-time ultrasonographically-guided internal jugular vein catheterization in the emergency department increases success rates and reduces complications: a randomized, prospective study, *Ann Emerg Med* 48:540, 2006.

34. March K: Application of technology in the treatment of traumatic brain injury, *Crit Care Nurs Q* 23(3):26, 2000.

35. Martin GS, Mannino DM, Eaton S et al: The epidemiology of sepsis in the United States from 1979 through 2000, *N Engl J Med* 348(16):1546, 2003.

36. McQuillan KA: The neurologic system: system wide elements, In Alspach J, editor: *Core curriculum for critical care nursing*, ed 6, St. Louis, 2006, Saunders/Elsevier.

37. Mey U, Glasmacher A, Hahn C et al: Evaluation of an ultrasound-guided technique for central venous access via the internal jugular vein in 493 patients, *Support Care Cancer* 11(3):148, 2003.

38. Meyer P, Legros C, Orliaguet G: Critical care management of neurotrauma in children: new trends and perspectives, *Childs Nerv Syst* 15:732, 1999.

39. Nguyen HB, Rivers EP, Abrahamian FM et al: Severe sepsis and septic shock: review of the literature and emergency department management guidelines, *Ann Emerg Med* 48:28, 2006.

40. Nguyen HG, Corbett SW, Stille R et al: Implementation of a bundle of quality indicators for the early management of severe sepsis and septic shock is associated with decreased mortality, *Crit Care Med* 35(4):1005, 2007.

41. Otero RM, Nguyen HB, Huang DT et al: Early goal-directed therapy in severe sepsis and septic shock revisited: concepts, controversies, and contemporary findings,, *Chest* 130(5):1579, 2006.

42. Phipps P, Garrard C: The pulmonary physician in critical care: acute asthma in the intensive care unit, *Thorax* 58:81, 2003.

43. Rady MY, Rivers EP, Nowak RM: Resuscitation of the critically ill in the ED: responses of blood pressure, heart rate, shock index, central venous oxygen saturation, and lactate, *Am J Emerg Med* 14:218, 1996.

44. Rello J, Ollendorf DA, Oster G et al: Epidemiology and outcomes of ventilator-associated pneumonia in a large US database, *Chest* 122:2115, 2002.

45. Rivers E, Nguyen B, Havstad S et al: Early goal-directed therapy in the treatment of severe sepsis and septic shock, *N Engl J Med* 345:1368, 2001.

46. Safdar N, Dezfulian C, Collard HR et al: Clinical and economic consequences of ventilator-associated pneumonia: a systematic review, *Crit Care Med* 33:2184, 2005.

47. The SAFE Study Investigators: Finfer S, Bellomo R, Boyce N et al: A comparison of albumin and saline for fluid resuscitation in the intensive care unit, *N Engl J Med* 350:2247, 2004.

48. Sakr Y, Reinhart K, Vincent JL et al: Does dopamine administration in shock influence outcome? Results of the sepsis occurrence in acutely ill patients (SOAP) study, *Crit Care Med* 34(3):589, 2006.

49. Schulman C. End point of resuscitation: choosing the right parameters to monitor, *Dimens Crit Care Nurs* 21(1):2, 2002.

50. Shapiro N, Howell M, Talmor D et al: Serum lactate as a predictor of mortality in emergency department patients with infection, *Ann Emerg Med* 45:524, 2005.

51. Shoemaker W, Parsa M: Invasive and noninvasive monitoring. In Grenvik A, Ayres A, Holbrrok P et al, editors: *Textbook of critical care*, ed 4, Philadelphia, 2000, Saunders.

52. Soni A, Pepper G, Wywinski P et al: Adrenal insufficiency occurring during septic shock: incidence, outcome, and relationship to peripheral cytokine levels, *Ann J Med* 98:266, 1995.

53. Symeonides S, Balk RA: Nitric oxide in the pathogenesis of sepsis, *Infect Dis Clin North Am* 13(2):449, 1999.

54. Trzeckak S, Delinger RP, Abate NL et al: Translating research to clinical practice: a 1-year experience with implementing early goal-directed therapy for septic shock in the emergency department, *Chest* 129:225, 2006.

55. Udobi K, Childs E, Touijer K: Acute respiratory distress syndrome, *Am Fam Physician* 67(2):315, 2003.

56. University of Southern California Neurosurgery: *Ventriculostomies*. Retrieved October 1, 2007, from http://uscneurosurgery.com/infonet/5036/ventriculostomy%20new.htm#indications.

57. Varpula M, Tallgren M, Saukkonen K et al: Hemodynamic variables related to outcome in septic shock, *Intensive Care Med* 31:1066, 2005.

58. Vincent J, Benard G, Beale R et al: Drotrecogin alfa (activated) treatment in severe sepsis from the global open-label trial ENHANCE: further evidence for survival and safety and implications for early treatment, *Crit Care Med* 33:2266, 2005.

59. Voyce SJ, McCaffree DR: Pulmonary artery catheters, In Irwin R, Rippe J, editors: *Intensive care medicine*, ed 5, Philadelphia, 2003, Lippincott Williams & Wilkins.

UNIT IV

MAJOR TRAUMA EMERGENCIES

CHAPTER 20

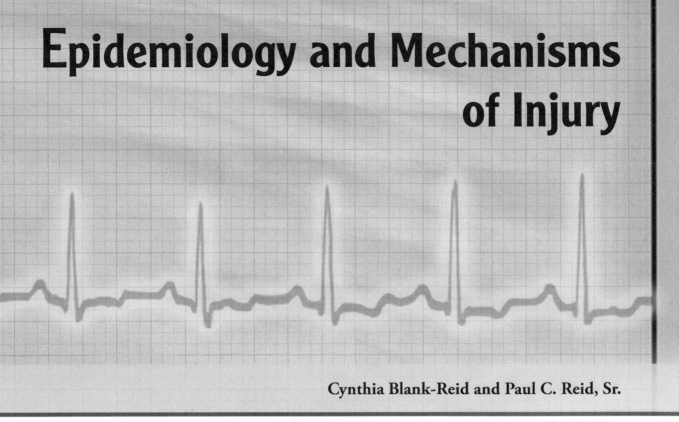

Epidemiology and Mechanisms of Injury

Cynthia Blank-Reid and Paul C. Reid, Sr.

Epidemiology and mechanism of injury (MOI) are separate and distinct disciplines, yet they are closely intertwined in the trauma literature. Epidemiology is the branch of medicine that studies the causes, distribution, and control of disease in populations.[2] It defines the scope of injuries in terms of their incidence and identifies associated factors and determinants of specific types of injury. An understanding of MOI, the study of how energy is transferred from the environment to the individual, equips health care providers with the knowledge to anticipate injuries, diagnosis, treatments, and complications of traumatic injury. Common patterns of injury are observed with specific mechanisms, and this knowledge can assist with the rapid detection of suspected injuries. Unless death occurs immediately, the outcome of an injured person depends not only on injury severity, but also on the speed and appropriateness of treatment.

Knowledge of both epidemiology and MOI helps shape health care by allowing providers to deliver evidence-based care and understand the populations who are at risk for particular injuries and those who need to be targeted for specific prevention programs. It also provides the ability to evaluate the effectiveness of these programs over time. Nurses who care for trauma patients clearly recognize the need for prevention and control strategies to curb mortality and morbidity. Perception of trauma as preventable events rather than acts of random unexpectedness ("accidents") is essential for

the success of prevention programs. Throughout this chapter the terms *trauma* and *injury* are used interchangeably.

EPIDEMIOLOGY

The epidemiology of trauma is particularly important because of the implications for social and public policy, legislation, and injury prevention programs. Understanding the scope of any problem is central to successful planning and implementation of legal, environmental, and educational remedies. Data elements such as incidence, prevalence, age, sex, race or ethnicity, geographic distribution, and morbidity or mortality are the sources of epidemiologic surveillance and serve to quantify aggregates.

Trauma is a disease that remains a leading cause of death for Americans of all ages regardless of gender, race, or economic status. Millions of Americans are injured each year and survive.[4] Whether the injury is fatal or nonfatal, the patient and his or her family, friends, and employers will all have to face adjustments in their lives. Refer to Table 20-1, the Centers for Disease Control and Prevention's (CDC's) 10 leading causes of death by age-group.

Trauma is the leading cause of death for children over 1 year and adults under 45 years of age. Trauma is also the main cause for loss of work years because it predominately affects a younger population who are in their prime working years. The great social, personal, and economic

Table 20-1. **TEN LEADING CAUSES OF DEATH BY AGE-GROUP IN THE UNITED STATES FOR 2005, ALL RACES, BOTH SEXES**

Rank	<1	1-4	5-9	10-14	15-24	25-34	35-44	45-54	55-64	65+	All Ages
					Age-Groups						
1	Congenital Anomalies 5,552	Unintentional Injury 1,664	Unintentional Injury 1,072	Unintentional Injury 1,343	Unintentional Injury 15,753	Unintentional Injury 13,997	Unintentional Injury 16,919	Malignant Neoplasms 50,405	Malignant Neoplasms 99,240	Heart Disease 530,926	Heart Disease 652,091
2	Short Gestation 4,714	Congenital Anomalies 522	Malignant Neoplasms 485	Malignant Neoplasms 515	Homicide 5,466	Suicide 4,990	Malignant Neoplasms 14,566	Heart Disease 38,103	Heart Disease 65,208	Malignant Neoplasms 388,322	Malignant Neoplasms 559,312
3	SIDS 2,230	Malignant Neoplasms 377	Congenital Anomalies 196	Suicide 270	Suicide 4,212	Homicide 4,752	Heart Disease 12,688	Unintentional Injury 18,339	Chronic Low. Respiratory Disease 12,747	Cerebro-vascular 123,881	Cerebro-vascular 143,579
4	Maternal Pregnancy Comp. 1,776	Homicide 375	Homicide 121	Homicide 220	Malignant Neoplasms 1,717	Malignant Neoplasms 3,601	Suicide 6,550	Liver Disease 7,517	Diabetes Mellitus 11,301	Chronic Low. Respiratory Disease 112,716	Chronic Low. Respiratory Disease 130,933
5	Placenta Cord Membranes 1,110	Heart Disease 151	Heart Disease 106	Congenital Anomalies 200	Heart Disease 1,119	Heart Disease 3,249	HIV 4,363	Suicide 6,991	Unintentional Injury 10,853	Alzheimer's Disease 70,858	Unintentional Injury 117,809
6	Unintentional Injury 1,083	Influenza & Pneumonia 110	Cerebro-vascular 52	Heart Disease 146	Congenital Anomalies 504	HIV 1,318	Homicide 3,109	Cerebro-vascular 6,381	Cerebro-vascular 10,028	Influenza & Pneumonia 55,453	Diabetes Mellitus 75,119
7	Respiratory Distress 860	Septicemia 85	Influenza & Pneumonia 51	Chronic Low. Respiratory Disease 55	Diabetes Mellitus 202	Diabetes Mellitus 617	Liver Disease 2,688	Diabetes Mellitus 5,691	Liver Disease 7,126	Diabetes Mellitus 55,222	Alzheimer's Disease 71,599
8	Bacterial Sepsis 834	Cerebro-vascular 62	Chronic Low. Respiratory Disease 49	Influenza & Pneumonia 55	Cerebro-vascular 196	Cerebro-vascular 546	Cerebro-vascular 2,260	HIV 4,516	Suicide 4,210	Unintentional Injury 36,729	Influenza & Pneumonia 63,001
9	Neonatal Hemorrhage 665	Perinatal Period 58	Benign Neoplasms 40	Septicemia 45	Complicated Pregnancy 183	Congenital Anomalies 436	Diabetes Mellitus 2,045	Chronic Low. Respiratory Disease 3,977	Nephritis 4,141	Nephritis 36,416	Nephritis 43,901
10	Necrotizing Enterocolitis 546	Chronic Low. Respiratory Disease 56	Septicemia 36	Cerebro-vascular 43	Influenza & Pneumonia 172	Influenza & Pneumonia 354	Influenza & Pneumonia 934	Viral Hepatitis 2,314	Septicemia 3,912	Septicemia 26,243	Septicemia 34,136

WISQARS Produced By: Office of Statistics and Programming, National Center for Injury Prevention and Control, Centers for Disease Control and Prevention.
Data Source: National Center for Health Statistics (NCHS), National Vital Statistics System.
From Centers for Disease Control and Prevention, National Center for Injury Prevention and Control: *Web-based Injury Statistics Query and Reporting System (WISQARS)*, 2005, http://www.cdc.gov/ncipc/wisqars.
HIV, Human immunodeficiency virus; *SIDS*, sudden infant death syndrome.

costs associated with traumatic injuries makes trauma a major public health problem in the United States.

Trauma in the United States

Age

For children under 1 year old, the leading cause of a fatal injury is unintentional suffocation due to choking or strangulation. Motor vehicle crashes (MVCs) are a leading cause of death throughout childhood; the incidence is particularly high in 1- to 3-year-olds, who are too frequently unrestrained passengers.

The high rate of injury for individuals 15 to 24 years of age may be caused by experimentation with drugs and alcohol in combination with poor judgment and risk-taking behaviors. The risk for MVC is higher among 16- to 19-year-olds than any other age-group. Drivers in this age-group are four times more likely than older drivers to crash, based on number of miles driven.[18] Teens are at risk because of the following:

- *Inexperience:* They often fail to recognize or underestimate the dangers in hazardous situations. They are more likely to speed, run red lights, make illegal turns, ride with an intoxicated driver, and drive after using alcohol or drugs.[19]
- *Low rates of seat belt usage:* Compared with other age-groups, teens have the lowest rate of seat belt usage.[5] Among teen drivers who were killed in crashes after drinking and driving, 74% were not wearing seat belts.[5]
- *Alcohol and driving:* Studies show that 25% of teenage drivers who died in an MVC had a blood alcohol concentration (BAC) of 0.08% or higher, which is above the legal BAC limit for adult drivers.[8,27]

The 65 and older age-group is the fastest growing segment of the U.S. population. As the U.S. population grows older, more and more people become vulnerable and are dependent on others to meet their most basic needs. Individuals more than 75 years of age have the highest death rate from injuries, which is attributed to multiple factors, including their frailer state of health and preexisting medical conditions. Age has been shown to be independently associated with increased mortality after trauma. Falls continue to be the most common cause of nonfatal and fatal injuries in adults ages 65 and older.[5] Drivers who are 65 and older have the highest death rate per mile driven except for teenage drivers. Older drivers drive less, but they are more likely to crash and die in the collision.[10,13] Estimates indicate that more than 40 million older adults will be licensed drivers in 2020.[4,22] In addition, age is a major factor in determining the risk for a cervical spine injury in auto-pedestrian injuries. Those over the age of 65 years are 12 to 14 times more likely to sustain a cervical spine injury than pediatric patients.[32]

Of the 11 million people age 65 years and older who are hospitalized annually, a significant percentage (52%) of injury-related admissions are due to fractures.[4,22] Of interest is that medical costs for the geriatric population are 2.5 times

greater than for younger patients with similar injuries; this is due to longer lengths of stay, higher incidence of complications, and more intensive care unit days.[22,23]

Gender

Gender, along with age variances, is related to the incidence and type of injury incurred. Males are 2.5 times more likely to be injured than females. This statistic is significant because of their participation in more hazardous activities and greater risk taking. This fact continues throughout the life span, as rates for motor vehicle (MV)–related injuries are twice as high for older men than women.[5] The pedestrian fatality rate is also more than twice as high for men as for women.[5]

Race

Injury and death rates vary with race and income. The reasons for these variations are multifactorial and not completely understood. However, knowledge of the differences observed has been used to target prevention programs toward specific populations or geographic areas. For African Americans and whites, no matter what the MOI, the higher the income, the lower the death rate. The number of MVCs decreases in a depressed economy, whereas homicides and suicides increase. The highest homicide rate occurs in the African American population, the highest suicide rate is seen in whites and Native Americans and the lowest death rate occurs in Asian Americans.

African Americans have a pedestrian death rate that is 1.7 times that of whites.[5] African American men age 65 and older have one of the highest MV-related death rates when sorted by age, sex, and race.[5] Homicide is the leading cause of death for African Americans age 10 to 24 years of age.[5] The drowning rate for 5- to 14-year-old African Americans is 3.2 times higher than that of whites.[3,11]

Asian-Pacific and Native American women age 65 years and older have the highest death rates when sorted by age, sex, and race.[5] Homicide is the second leading cause of death for Asian-Pacific Islanders for those age 10 to 24 years.[5]

Hispanics have a mortality rate 1.8 times higher than non-Hispanics if they are a pedestrian who has been injured.[5] Homicide is the second leading cause of death for Hispanics among people age 10 to 24 years.[5]

Native Americans 19 years or age and younger are at greater risk for preventable injury-related deaths than are all other children and youth in the United States. They have twice the average rate of traumatic deaths than their counterparts in any other racial group. Injuries and violence account for 75% of all deaths among Native Americans in this age-group. MVCs are the leading cause of fatality followed by homicide, drowning, and fires.[4] The rates for pedestrian deaths in auto-pedestrian injuries are three times higher for Native Americans and Alaska Natives than whites.[5] The drowning rate overall for Native Americans and Alaska Natives is 1.8 times higher than that for whites; in children age 5 to 14 years the drowning rate is 2.6 times higher.[3,11] Native American men age 20 years and older are (1) twice as

Box 20-1	ESSENTIAL CONCEPTS FOR MECHANISMS OF INJURY
Acceleration	Increase in velocity or speed of a moving object.
Acceleration-deceleration	Increase in velocity or speed of object followed by decrease in velocity or speed.
Axial loading	Injury occurs when force is applied upward and downward with no posterior or lateral bending of the neck.
Cavitation	Creation of temporary cavity as tissues are stretched and compressed.
Compression	Squeezing inward pressure.
Compressive strength	Ability to resist squeezing forces or inward pressure.
Deceleration	Decrease in velocity or speed of a moving object.
Distraction	Separation of spinal column with resulting cord transection, seen in legal hangings.
Elasticity	Ability to resume original shape and size after being stretched.
Force	Physical factor that changes motion of body at rest or already in motion.
High velocity	Missiles that compress and accelerate tissue away from the bullet, causing a cavity around the bullet and the entire tract.
Inertial resistance	Ability of body to resist movement.
Injury	Trauma or damage to some part of the body.
Kinematics	Process of looking at an accident and determining what injuries might result.
Kinetic energy	Energy that results from motion.
Low velocity	Missiles that localize injury to a small radius from center of the tract with little disruptive effect.
Muzzle blast	Cloud of hot gas and burning powder at the muzzle of a gun.
Shearing	Two oppositely directed parallel forces.
Stress	Internal resistance to deformation, or internal force generated from application load.
Tensile strength	Amount of tension tissue can withstand and ability to resist stretching forces.
Tumbling	Forward rotation around the center; somersault action of the missile can create massive injury.
Yaw	Deviation of bullet nose in longitudinal axis from straight line of flight.

likely to die from an MVC, (2) nearly twice as likely to die from fire and burn injuries, and (3) five times more likely to drown than their counterparts in other races. They are also four times more likely to commit suicide and three times more likely to be murdered.[9]

Firearm-Related Injuries

The CDC began tracking firearm injuries in the early 1960s. Firearm violence and firearm-related deaths have been increasing at a steady rate for over 40 years.[5] Firearm injury disproportionately affects young people, resulting in lives cut short or forever affected as a result of their use. Firearms (especially handguns) are effective lethal weapons with the capability to escalate often-impulsive acts of interpersonal violence or suicidal thoughts into death. The United States has wrestled with firearms and the consequences of their use and misuse for years. Compared with other industrialized countries, the firearm death rate in the United States is eight times the average rate of its economic counterparts.[21] Among all industrialized countries, more men are killed by firearms than women; however, women in the United States die at a much higher rate from firearm injuries then their counterparts in other high-income countries.[21]

Alcohol

Alcohol plays a significant role in all types of trauma, including MVCs, family violence, suicides, homicides, and altercations. Alcohol alters judgment and coordination, so it frequently contributes to injury-producing events.

An alcohol-related MVC kills someone every 31 minutes and nonfatally injures someone every 2 minutes.[8,26] The CDC's research has found that about 68% of the children killed in alcohol-related crashes were riding in cars driven by drivers who had been drinking.[5] One study demonstrated that child passenger restraint use decreased as the BAC of the child's driver increased.[29]

Geography and Chronology

Geographic differences exist in injury mortality. Physical environment or geographic area also characterizes injury rates. Homicides and suicides occur more often in urban areas, whereas unintentional injuries are more numerous in rural areas. Injury and death rates are greater on weekends with the peak on Saturday. More injuries are seen in July—probably as a result of summer recreational activities.

MECHANISM OF INJURY

Trauma is now recognized as a disease process with MOI as part of its etiology. Strong assessment skills are essential for health care providers because treatment of trauma patients is contingent on identifying all injuries. Unfortunately, even when the clinician has strong assessment skills some injuries go undetected if the "index of suspicion" is not sufficient. Understanding MOI and maintaining a high index of suspicion enable caregivers to predict and locate occult injuries more quickly and save time initiating essential treatment. Injury should be considered present until definitively ruled out in the hospital setting.

Human beings are exposed to potential injury in multiple forms during the course of a normal day. Injury, defined as trauma or damage to a part of the body, occurs when an uncontrolled or acute source of energy makes contact with the body and the body cannot tolerate exposure to it. Energy originates from numerous sources, including kinetic (motion or mechanical), chemical, electrical, thermal, and radiation. Absence of heat and oxygen causes injuries such as frostbite, drowning, or suffocation. Kinetic energy is defined as energy that results from motion.[14,22,24] The majority of traumatic injuries are caused by absorption of kinetic energy. Box 20-1 defines essential concepts for understanding mechanisms of injury.

Severity of trauma depends on the wounding agent. There are three major classifications of traumatic disease: blunt injury, penetrating injury, and thermal injury. Energy transfer can result in any one of these individual categories or in any combination of these wounding forces.

Kinematics

Kinematics is the process of looking at an event and determining what injuries are likely to occur given the forces and motion involved. Physics is the foundation on which kinematics is based. Understanding essential laws of physics is the first step toward understanding kinematics.

Newton's First Law of Motion

Newton's first law of motion states that a body at rest remains at rest and a body in motion remains in motion unless acted on by an outside force. Pedestrians struck by a vehicle, blast injury patients, and people with gunshot wounds (GSW) are examples of stationary objects set in motion by energy forces. Moving objects interrupted or acted on to stop their motion are illustrated by people falling from a height, vehicles hitting a tree, or vehicles braking to a sudden stop.[14,24]

Law of Conservation of Energy

The law of conservation of energy states that energy is neither created nor destroyed but changes form. As a car decelerates slowly, the energy of motion (acceleration) is converted to friction heat in braking (thermal energy).[14,24]

Newton's Second Law

Newton's second law states that force equals mass multiplied by acceleration or deceleration.[14]

Kinetic Energy

Kinetic energy (KE) equals one half the mass (M) multiplied by the velocity squared (V^2).[14] This law is evidenced in firearm injuries—the mass (the bullet) is small, but because of the velocity (speed) with which the bullet is propelled, substantial energy is transferred to the body.

Patient Assessment

Initially trauma patients may not appear seriously injured because of strong compensatory mechanisms that maintain adequate vital signs. All members of a trauma team must anticipate injuries by recognizing potential patterns of injury related to the energy and force of the trauma. Assessment, resuscitation, and stabilization efforts based on this knowledge enable health care providers to evaluate hidden or internal injuries based on these predicted patterns. Health care providers should correlate reported mechanisms to actual or potential injuries. Patients, family, and friends may have reasons to fabricate, falsify, or deny the actual event. Consequently, injuries identified in the examination may not correspond to the reported mechanism. Eliciting a careful history of the injury during initial assessment is vital. Accurate information, especially about MOI, can reduce morbidity and mortality in many circumstances.

When assessing a trauma patient, the emergency nurse should identify mechanisms associated with major force or energy transfer (e.g., pedestrian hit by vehicle traveling faster than 20 mph, falls from more than 20 feet, MVC with major vehicular damage, speed change of more than 20 mph, vehicle rollover, ejected occupant, death of occupant). Some injuries are significant because of potential complications, such as two or more long bone fractures; flail chest; penetrating trauma to the head, neck, chest, abdomen, or groin; and any combination of these patterns with burns over the head, face, or airway.[14,22] Patients with significant injuries require close monitoring for complications or changes in hemodynamic stability.

Certain questions elicit valuable information regarding the MOI and are helpful in assessing potential injuries. When a MV is involved, asking the following questions is important:

- What type of vehicle was the patient driving (large or small)?
- What was the estimated speed at the time of the crash?
- Were seat belts or restraint devices used? Were the devices applied appropriately? Were air bags installed, and did they deploy?
- Where was the patient in the vehicle (driver, front passenger, or rear-seat passenger)? If ejected, how far was the patient thrown or found from the vehicle?
- How much damage was done to the vehicle? Where was the majority of damage? Was there intrusion into the passenger space? How much?
- Was there any steering wheel deformity?

If the patient was involved in a fall, the following questions should be asked:

- What was the approximate height of the fall?
- Were any objects struck during the fall?
- What was the surface where the patient landed?
- In what position was the patient found after the fall?

With penetrating injury the following questions should be asked:

- What was the wounding agent (e.g., knife, gun, arrow, ice pick)?
- What was the size and length of the agent?

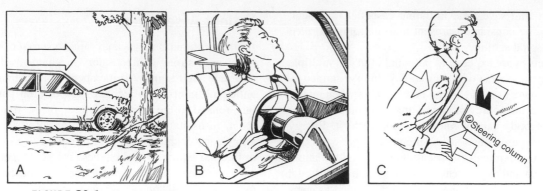

FIGURE 20-1. The three collisions of a motor vehicle collision. **A,** Auto hits tree. **B,** Body hits steering wheel, causing broken ribs. **C,** Heart strikes chest wall, causing blunt cardiac injury.

- If a firearm was used, what was the caliber? What was the distance between the fired weapon and the patient?

Patients with penetrating trauma must be assessed for other types of trauma such as falls or assaults. Patients may be exposed to more than one wounding force.

A detailed history is not always possible and is often impractical. Valuable information can be obtained from family members, prehospital personnel, police, firefighters, bystanders, or eyewitnesses; however, these resources are often overlooked or are unavailable in a hectic emergency department (ED). Management of life-threatening injuries must take priority over obtaining a detailed history; however, every effort should be made to obtain as much historical data as possible.

After airway/cervical spine protection, breathing, circulation, and neurologic function have been assessed and supported, a rapid head-to-toe assessment should be performed. Patients with penetrating trauma are generally easier to assess than those with blunt trauma because injuries are usually focused in one area. Surface trauma may or may not be present with blunt injuries; therefore assessment tends to be more difficult. During the secondary survey, injuries can be found by systematically examining the patient who is completely undressed. Maintaining a high index of suspicion for probable injuries based on certain MOIs and performing a detailed physical assessment will minimize the risk for missed injuries.

Blunt Injury

Blunt trauma is characterized as an injury with no opening in the skin or communication to the outside environment. Definitive diagnosis of blunt trauma is challenging. The extent of injuries is not always obvious; however, these injuries may indeed be life-threatening. Depending on the tissue injured and properties associated with this tissue, certain diagnostic studies are more helpful than others. Air-filled organs, such as lungs and bowel, are subject to blast and compressive injuries. Crush injuries to solid organs (e.g., liver and spleen) may present with minimal external signs of injury, but because energy associated with blunt trauma is transmitted in all directions, organs and tissues can rupture or break if pressure is not released.[14,22]

Examples of blunt force events include MVCs, falls, contact sports, and assaults. Direct impact causes the greatest injury. Injuries result when energy is released on impact with the body. Various body tissues respond differently; tissue may move and displace with impact or rupture from the force.

Forces commonly associated with blunt trauma include acceleration, deceleration, shearing, and compression forces. Acceleration injuries occur when velocity (speed) is transferred to a stationary or slower-moving object; deceleration injuries occur when velocity or forward momentum is abruptly stopped. Shearing injuries occur when two oppositely directed parallel forces are applied to tissue. Compression injuries occur with a squeezing inward pressure applied to tissues. An example of these forces is seen with blunt injury to the thoracic aorta. Rapid deceleration causes the aorta to bend and stretch. Shearing damage occurs when stretching forces exceed vessel elasticity. Shearing damage causes the aorta to dissect, rupture, tear, or form an aneurysm.[28]

MOTOR VEHICLE COLLISIONS. Before a collision the occupant and vehicle are moving at the same speed. At the time of collision the vehicle and the occupant decelerate to a speed of zero, but at different rates. Deceleration forces are transferred to the body in three points of collision (Figure 20-1).[14,22] The first collision occurs when the vehicle strikes another object. As the vehicle stops, the driver or occupant continues to move forward. The second collision occurs when the driver or occupant strikes the steering column, windshield, restraint system, or another structure in the car. The body stops; however, internal organs continue to move until they collide with another organ, cavity wall or structure or they are restrained suddenly by vasculature, muscles, ligaments, or fascia—the third collision point. A fourth collision may occur when unsecured objects in the vehicle collide with the occupant (e.g., unrestrained passengers, bottled drinks, sports equipment). Different damage occurs with each collision; therefore each collision point must be considered separately to avoid missed injuries.

One way to estimate injuries in a MVC is to look at the vehicle. Because this is not possible in the ED, the emergency

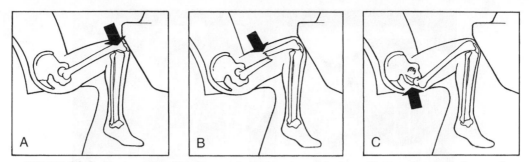

FIGURE **20-2.** Down and under pathway. **A,** Dislocation of the knee. **B,** Fracture of the femur. **C,** Dislocation from the acetabulum.

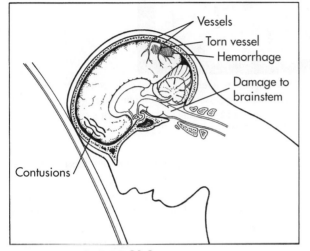

FIGURE **20-3.** Brain injury.

nurse should ask prehospital providers about vehicular damage—interior and exterior. Some prehospital personnel take instant photographs (i.e., digital), allowing hospital providers to see vehicular damage firsthand. The picture can then become a permanent part of the medical record.

Frontal Impact. Frontal impact occurs when the front of a vehicle impacts another object (e.g., another vehicle, tree, bridge abutment). The first collision results in damage to the front end. The more severe the damage and the faster that the vehicle was traveling, the greater the probability for severe injury due to the amount of energy transferred.

Multiple injuries may occur when a person comes to a sudden stop. The use of restraints does reduce the energy absorbed by the body, minimize direct contact with nonyielding interior structures, and prevent ejection from the vehicle. Interior structures, such as the windshield, steering wheel, dashboard, or instrument panel, injure the occupants when direct contact is made. After the vehicle stops, occupants in the front seat continue to move down and under, or up and over, the dashboard.

Down and Under. One path an occupant may travel after a frontal impact is down and under. The occupant continues forward movement downward into the steering column or dashboard. The person's knees impact the dashboard; however, the upper legs absorb most of the energy. This mechanism may cause patellar dislocations, midshaft femur

fractures, and posterior dislocations or fractures of the acetabulum or femoral head (Figure 20-2). When one of these injuries is identified, the patient should be carefully evaluated for the other associated injuries.

Up and Over. Continued forward motion from a frontal collision can carry the body up and over, so the head, chest, and/or abdomen strike the steering column, dashboard, or windshield. Head injuries, such as contusions and scalp lacerations, skull fractures, facial fractures, cerebral hemorrhage, or cerebral contusions can occur.

The brain does not stretch easily, so if one part of the brain moves in one direction, the rest follows. The skull stops suddenly after striking the steering wheel, windshield, or another stationary object, but the brain continues to move forward and strikes the inside of the skull.[14,22] This area of the brain is compressed and may sustain ecchymosis, edema, or contusion. This type of injury is called a "coup injury," and it occurs when the damaged area forms directly at the site of contact. As this injury is occurring, the other side of the brain continues to move forward and may be disrupted and shear away from tissue and vascular attachments (Figure 20-3). A contrecoup injury occurs on the side opposite the direct contact because of the movement of the brain within the skull (recoil or "bounce-back"). This impact can cause two separate injuries, shear injury and compression injury, to the same organ, the brain.

When the head collides with an object, injury to the cervical spine can also occur. The spiderweb effect of a broken windshield suggests the possibility for cervical spine injury. If prehospital providers report a spiderweb effect, caregivers must maintain a high index of suspicion for a spinal injury.

Chest injuries occur when the thorax is compressed against the steering column. Injuries include fractured ribs and sternum, anterior flail chest, blunt cardiac injury, and pulmonary contusion. Thoracic vertebral injuries occur as energy travels up or down the thoracic spine; however, these injuries are less common because the thoracic vertebrae are so well protected.

Compression injuries to the abdomen may result in ruptured hollow organs (e.g., the stomach or intestines) that spill their contents into the abdominal cavity, whereas fractured or lacerated solid organs (e.g., the liver and spleen) are associated with significant blood loss. Organs in the abdominal

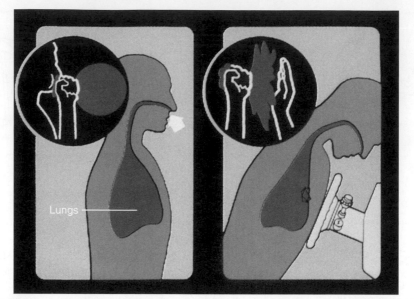

FIGURE **20-4.** Compression of lung against closed glottis by impact on anterior or lateral chest wall produces effect like that of compressing a paper bag when opening is closed tightly by hands: the paper bag ruptures, and so does the lung. (From National Association of Emergency Medical Technicians: *PHTLS: prehospital trauma life support,* ed 6, St. Louis, 2007, Mosby.)

cavity are attached to the abdominal wall by the mesentery, ligaments, and vasculature. As organs continue their forward motion, attachments can be torn or lacerated.

The steering column is often referred to as a modern-day battering ram and can be the most lethal part of a vehicle.[14,22] When steering wheel deformity is reported, the index of suspicion for neck, face, thoracic, or abdominal injuries should increase significantly. Injuries caused by this collision may or may not be readily visible. Lacerations of the chin and mouth, contusion and ecchymosis of the neck, traumatic tattooing of the chest and abdomen, and bruising of the chest and abdomen may be obvious or subtle. Internal occult injuries may be secondary to compression forces, shearing forces, and displacement of kinetic energy.[14,22]

Certain organs are more susceptible to shear injuries because of ligamentous attachments (e.g., liver, spleen, bowel, kidneys, and aortic arch). Compression forces commonly injure the lungs, diaphragm, heart, and bladder. Respiratory distress in trauma patients may be caused by injuries such as a pneumothorax, flail chest, and pulmonary contusion. A diaphragmatic hernia or a ruptured diaphragm can also cause respiratory distress and is characterized by bowel sounds in the chest. If a trauma patient has a contused chest wall, a blunt cardiac injury should be considered.

In frontal and lateral impacts a mechanism sometimes called the "paper bag effect" leads to pneumothorax. The driver or occupant sees the collision about to happen, inhales deeply, and holds his or her breath. The glottis closes and seals the lungs. As the chest impacts, the lungs burst like paper bags (Figure 20-4).

Frontal impacts are also characterized by extremity injuries. Fractures of the lower extremities, ankles, and feet occur when the occupant extends the feet or are secondary to vehicle intrusion into the passenger compartment. An unrestrained back-seat passenger doubles the risk for injury to front-seat occupants during frontal impact.

Rear Impact. Rear-impact collisions occur when a stationary object or a slower-moving object is struck from behind. Initial impact accelerates the slower-moving or stationary object and may force the vehicle into a frontal collision. When the vehicle suddenly decelerates, hyperextension of the neck may occur, especially when headrests are not properly positioned. Neck ligaments may be strained or torn. If the vehicle strikes another object or is slowed by the driver applying the brake, rapid forward deceleration occurs. The crash then involves two points of impact, rear and frontal, which increases the chance for occupant injuries. Injuries common to each mechanism must be assessed.

Lateral or Side Impact. When a vehicle is struck on either side ("T-boned"), most injuries are dependent on vehicle deformity because the vehicle either remains in place or moves away from the point of impact. If the vehicle remains in place, energy is transferred or changed to vehicle damage rather than the energy of motion. Trauma to the occupants can be more severe because of intrusion into the interior compartment. The greater the intrusion, the more significant the injury can be. More than 10 to 12 inches of intrusion is considered significant.

With side-impact or lateral collisions, occupants generally receive most injuries on the same side of their body as the vehicle impact. A second collision may occur between occupants if another passenger is in the vehicle. The head and shoulder of one occupant may impact the other occupant's head and shoulder. When a patient has an injury on the side opposite impact, caregivers should assess both occupants for associated injuries.

Figure 20-5 illustrates injuries from a side-impact collision. Flail chest, pulmonary contusion, and rib fractures are

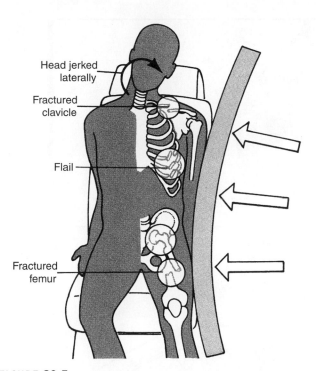

FIGURE **20-5.** Potential injury sites in lateral-impact collision. Injury is still possible in lateral crash with air bag inflation; however, injuries are usually fewer with air bag inflation than without. (From Neff JA, Kidd PS: *Trauma nursing: the art and science,* St. Louis, 1993, Mosby.)

possible chest injuries. Numerous musculoskeletal injuries can occur. Energy from an impact can pin the occupant's arm against the car, causing injury to the chest wall and clavicle or force the femoral head through the pelvis, causing a pelvic or acetabulum fracture.[14,22] Strain on the lateral neck can cause spinal fractures or ligament tears. Side impacts can cause spine fractures, with associated neurologic deficit, more often than rear collisions. Other injuries may include a splenic injury when impact is on the driver's side and liver injury when the impact is on the passenger side.

Rotational Impact. Rotational impact occurs when the corner of one vehicle strikes another stationary vehicle, a vehicle traveling in the opposite direction, or a slower vehicle. The point of impact on the second car stops forward motion, and then the rest of the vehicle rotates until all energy is transformed. As the car is hit, the occupant's forward motion continues until it impacts with the side of the car as the vehicle begins rotating. Injuries that occur in rotational impacts are a combination of those seen in frontal and lateral impacts.

Vehicle Rollover. Vehicular rollover is when a vehicle flips over, regardless of whether the motion is end over end, or side over side. In rollovers, injuries are sometimes difficult to predict. Occupants frequently have injuries in the same body areas where damage occurs to the vehicle. Just as the vehicle impacts at different angles, several times, so does the occupant's body and internal organs. In the rollover mechanism, the chance for axial loading injuries is increased.

Ejection. Ejection is when an occupant is thrown from the vehicle. Occupants who are ejected sustain injuries at the

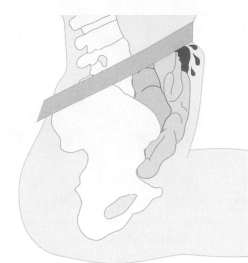

FIGURE **20-6.** A seat belt that is positioned above the rim of the pelvis allows the abdominal organs to be trapped between the moving posterior wall and the belt. Injuries to the pancreas and other retroperitoneal organs, as well as blowout ruptures of the small intestine and colon, result. (From McSwain N, Paturas J: *The basic EMT: comprehensive prehospital patient care,* ed 2, St. Louis, 2003, Mosby.)

point of impact and when energy is transferred to the entire body; spinal fractures and severe traumatic brain injuries occur at a higher rate in ejections. Occupants who are ejected have a much greater chance of dying than occupants who remain in the vehicle, and those at greatest risk are unrestrained occupants.[4]

Restraint Systems. The first mandatory child restraint use law was enacted in Tennessee in 1978, and now all 50 states and the District of Columbia have child restraint laws. The first mandatory seat belt law was enacted in New York State in 1984, and since that time every state and the District of Columbia have also enacted seat belt laws. Restraint systems are designed to prevent injuries and decrease their severity by allowing occupants to decelerate at the same rate as the vehicle rather than being thrown against interior structures or being ejected from the vehicle. Restraints also keep occupants from striking each other within the compartment. Worn properly, safety restraints reduce fatalities and the severity of injuries.

The most effective restraint system is the three-point restraint, which is a shoulder harness and lap belt. Three-point restraints decrease severity of the "second" collision, reducing facial, head, and abdominal injuries and long-bone fractures.[14,24] The National Highway Traffic Safety Agency (NHTSA) has reported that lap and shoulder safety belts "reduce the risk of fatal injury to front-seat passenger car occupants by 45% and the risk of moderate-to-critical injury by 50%." More people are now using occupant protection.[25,26]

Injuries caused by a shoulder-lap belt fastened loosely or worn above the anterior iliac crest (Figure 20-6) include compression to abdominal organs such as the pancreas, liver, and spleen; possible rupture of the diaphragm with herniation of abdominal organs; and anterior compression fractures of the

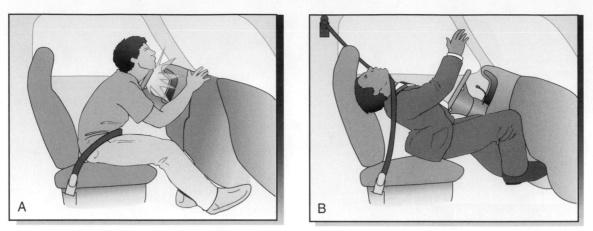

FIGURE 20-7. **A,** Without the diagonal strap the forward motion of the upper body can cause severe injuries to the face, head, and neck. **B,** When worn alone, the diagonal strap retards forward motion but produces an excessive force on the neck. Neck injuries as severe as decapitation have been reported. (From McSwain N, Paturas J: *The basic EMT: comprehensive prehospital patient care,* ed 2, St. Louis, 2003, Mosby.)

| Box 20-2 | INJURIES WITH APPROPRIATE RESTRAINT SYSTEMS |

SPINAL

Cervical vertebral fractures from flexion forces
Neck sprains secondary to hyperextension
Lumbar vertebral fractures secondary to flexion-distraction forces

THORACIC

Soft tissue injuries of the chest wall associated with belt placement
Sternal fractures with or without blunt cardiac injury
Fewer than three rib fractures if restrained; more than four if unrestrained
Trauma to breast in females

ABDOMINAL

Soft tissue injuries (contusions, abrasions, ecchymosis)
Seat belt friction burns or abrasion where seat belt rests
Injuries to small bowel secondary to crushing and deceleration
Ruptured aorta secondary to longitudinal stretching of the vessel
Injuries to the liver, pancreas, gallbladder, and duodenum secondary to crushing forces

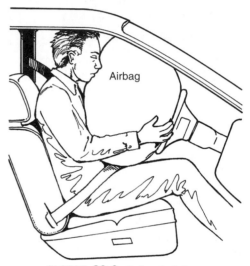

FIGURE 20-8. Inflated air bag.

lumbar spine. Diaphragmatic rupture occurs from increased intraabdominal pressure from the misplaced lap belt. Figure 20-7 illustrates the consequences of incorrect use of lap belts and shoulder straps. Lap belts worn alone allow injuries to the face, head, neck, and chest, whereas shoulder belts worn without a lap belt can cause severe neck injuries.

Properly used restraints transfer energy from the impact to the restraint system instead of to the occupant. Injuries received when seat belts are used properly are generally not life-threatening, or the chance of sustaining a life-threatening injury is greatly reduced. Box 20-2 describes injuries that occur even with proper seat belt use.

Air Bags. Air bags were designed to protect front-seat occupants in frontal deceleration collisions by inflating from the center of the steering column or the dashboard or both at impact (Figure 20-8), cushioning the head and chest, and then rapidly deflating. Since 1998 all new passenger cars have been equipped with driver and front-seat passenger air bags. Some newer vehicles also have side-impact air bags. Injuries reported from air bag deployment include facial trauma, such as tattooing, ecchymosis, and corneal abrasions. Abrasions and ecchymosis from air bag deployment are seen on forearms. Air bags, however, are not considered primary restraint systems but are "supplemental" to lap and shoulder belts. An ongoing Special Crash Investigation Program sponsored by NHTSA provides data associated with adult passengers, drivers, and children who sustain fatal or serious injuries in "minor or moderate severity air bag deployment crashes."[25]

Drivers and passengers should sit at least 10 inches away from the steering column/dashboard and tilt the seat rearward for vehicles with air bags. Serious injuries have been reported in small drivers who adjust the seat closer to the

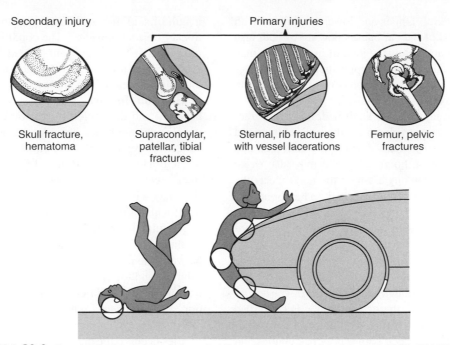

Secondary injury   Primary injuries

Skull fracture, hematoma

Supracondylar, patellar, tibial fractures

Sternal, rib fractures with vessel lacerations

Femur, pelvic fractures

FIGURE 20-9. Potential primary injury sites of child pedestrian. (Modified from Neff JA, Kidd PS: *Trauma nursing: the art and science,* St. Louis, 1993, Mosby.)

steering wheel. Infants and children placed in the front seat have been seriously injured or killed by inflating air bags. The NHTSA Web site (http://www.nhtsa.dot.gov) has a section that discusses the most updated information on rules and regulations governing on and off switches for air bags. The following points regarding driving in a car equipped with air bags are recommended by NHTSA[25]:

- Children 12 years and younger should ride in the back seat of cars.
- Never use a rear-facing child-restraint seat in a seat with an air bag.
- Always wear a lap and shoulder belt even in vehicles equipped with air bags.
- When driving a car equipped with an air bag, sit at least 10 inches away from the steering wheel and tilt the seat rearward.
- There are some situations authorized by NHTSA that permit air bag deactivation if the vehicle is not equipped with an air bag off switch.

MVC Preventive Measures. Because MVCs account for more than half the injuries associated with blunt trauma, preventive measures are an ongoing concern. Research has shown that the number of MVCs can be reduced by highway design changes, enforcement of speed limits, and improvements in vehicle design. Safety changes made in highway design include separating opposing streams of traffic, installing breakaway barriers and nonskid road surfaces, and removing obstacles from the roadside. Enforcing the speed limit also reduces injuries from MVCs because speed is a determining factor in the severity of injuries. The greater the speed or velocity, the more energy dissipated and the more severe the injury. The size and design of vehicles also affect injury. Small cars are associated with more injuries and deaths than

larger cars. Changes in interior design can decrease injuries seen in occupants. Examples of this include incorporation of side air bags and additional padding on dashboards.

FARM EQUIPMENT. The majority of fatalities associated with tractors are crushing injuries when the tractor overturns.[6] When tractors turn over, it is generally to the side; however, they can overturn to the rear. Rear overturns do not allow the driver to jump free or be thrown clear. Other mechanisms of injury include thermal burns from ignited fuel or hot engine parts and chemical burns from diesel fuel, hydraulic fluid, gasoline, or battery acid.

PEDESTRIAN INJURIES. When a vehicle strikes a pedestrian, injuries can be predicted based on the person's age or size. Children and adults have different patterns of injuries because of their size differences and orientation to the vehicle.

In children, frontal impacts usually occur because children tend to freeze and face the approaching vehicle. The femur or chest of the child impacts the bumper or hood depending on the child's height. The child is then thrown backward with his or her upper back or head impacting the ground or pavement, where contralateral skull injuries occur. Very small children are rarely thrown clear of the vehicle because of their low center of gravity, size, and weight. A child may be knocked down and under the vehicle, then run over or dragged. Multisystem trauma should be suspected in any child hit by a car. A combination of injuries referred to as Waddell's triad often occurs when a child is struck by a car (Figure 20-9). Waddell's triad is characterized by injuries to the chest, head, and femurs.

Adults struck by a vehicle sustain injuries to the lower extremities along with head, chest, and abdominal injuries. Adults try to protect themselves by turning sideways, so the impact is usually lateral. Upper and lower leg impact with the bumper and hood of the car causes bowing of both legs with fractures above and below the joint of impact. This may also cause ligament damage to the opposite knee from associated strain. Figure 20-10 shows points of impact when an adult is struck by a vehicle.

Another common injury in an adult pedestrian is a fractured pelvis. As the patient folds over, the upper femur and pelvis strike the front of the hood while the abdomen and chest strike the top of the hood. The head may also strike the hood of the car, or the angle where the hood meets the windshield. The patient then rolls off the hood and onto the pavement or into the windshield. The victim may be able to protect the face and head with the arms during this forward motion. If the victim is thrown any distance, he or she can be run over by a second vehicle. Tire mark impressions may be found on the clothing or skin of victims who are run over.

SCHOOL BUSES. Although the incidence of crashes involving school buses is low, the general public is concerned that safety restraints are not standard equipment. Understanding the epidemiology associated with school bus injuries and deaths is an example of how a problem must be identified before implementing those strategies that will have the most effect on prevention of such injuries. The majority of deaths involving school buses are not to bus occupants. Data indicate that promoting safety around school buses being used for transport of children is one of the necessary prevention strategies.[28] NHTSA has a free school bus safety program for teaching children how to be cautious and vigilant around school buses.

MOTORCYCLE CRASHES. Injuries occurring from motorcycle crashes (MCCs) depend on the amount and type of kinetic energy and part of the body impacted. Head, neck, and extremity injuries occur more frequently with MCC because of the lack of protection afforded the riders. Clues to the amount of force sustained during a collision include the length of skid marks, deformity of the motorcycle, and stationary objects impacted. The condition of an MCC rider is often similar to an occupant ejected from a vehicle (Figure 20-11). There are four types of motorcycle impacts with predictable injuries, which are listed below.

Head-on Impact. The motorcycle impacts an object head-on, and the cycle flips forward so the rider strikes or travels over the handlebars. As the rider strikes the handlebars, abdominal and chest injuries and shearing fractures of the tibia can occur. Bilateral femur fractures occur if the rider's feet are trapped by the foot pegs at the time of impact. A helmet will provide limited protection to the rider's head, but it will not protect the neck.

Angular Impact. The cycle is struck at an angle and falls on the rider so that one side of the rider's body is crushed between the motorcycle and the ground or the object struck. Injuries tend to occur to the lower extremities, such as open fractures of the tibia or fibula, crushed legs, ankle dislocation, and soft tissue injuries.

Ejection. When a rider is ejected from the motorcycle, injuries occur to the body part that is hit at the time of impact and the point of impact when the body lands. Energy from the impact is absorbed by the rest of the body. Ejection from a motorcycle has a high potential for severe injuries.

Laying the Bike Down. This maneuver is used by professional riders to separate themselves from their bikes when they see an impending collision. This maneuver slows down the rider as the bike is turned sideways, and the rider drags the inner leg. The most common injuries seen with laying the bike down are minor fractures, abrasions, and crush injuries to lower legs. Figure 20-12 shows road burns that occurred in a rider who was not wearing protective clothing.

ALL-TERRAIN VEHICLES. All-terrain vehicles (ATVs) have two basic designs: three-wheeled or four-wheeled. Four-wheeled ATVs offer easier handling and more stability than

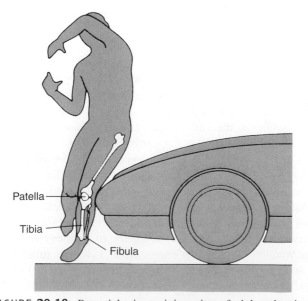

FIGURE **20-10.** Potential primary injury sites of adult pedestrian. (From Neff JA, Kidd PS: *Trauma nursing: the art and science,* St. Louis, 1993, Mosby.)

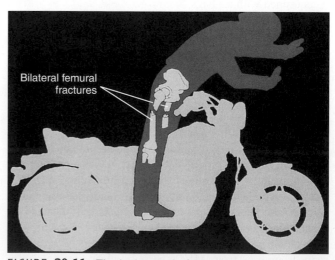

FIGURE **20-11.** The body travels forward and over the motorcycle, impacting the thighs and femurs into the handlebars. The driver can also be ejected. (From National Association of Emergency Medical Technicians: *Prehospital trauma life support,* ed 6, St. Louis, 2007, Mosby.)

three-wheeled, which when turned sharply are prone to roll-over because of a higher center of gravity. Some states have enacted laws defining the minimum operator age and requiring helmets for all riders.

The most common MOIs associated with ATVs are rollovers, rider falling off, and the vehicle hitting a stationary object and causing forward deceleration of the rider. Injuries depend on which part of the rider's anatomy is struck and the mechanism involved. Head, spine, and chest injuries involving the ribs, sternum, and clavicles have been reported.

SNOWMOBILES. Snowmobiles are used for work and play. Injuries commonly seen are similar to those associated with ATVs. The snowmobile has a low center of gravity and low clearance. Crush injuries are frequently seen because it turns over more easily and is heavier than most ATVs. Significant neck injuries can occur if the rider runs into an unseen wire fence or rope. Patterns of injury depend on the mechanism and the part of the body affected. Hypothermia is a significant risk if the rider is not adequately clothed for the weather or is not found immediately after the injuring event.

WATERCRAFT. Watercraft or boating injuries can occur from colliding with another boat or an obstruction in the water. Occupants of boats are not provided with restraint systems, and the boats are not built to absorb the energy associated with impacts as motor vehicles are. There is also the potential for drowning or hypothermia when occupants are ejected into the water. Other injuries may be similar to those seen in people ejected from a vehicle. It is always advised for occupants of watercraft to use Coast Guard–approved personal floatation devices.

In recent years, personal watercraft (PWC), such as waverunners and jet skis, have become popular recreational vehicles. The injury rate is about 8.5 times higher with PWCs than with motorboats.[11] Different styles allow the driver to sit, stand, or kneel while operating the watercraft, with some

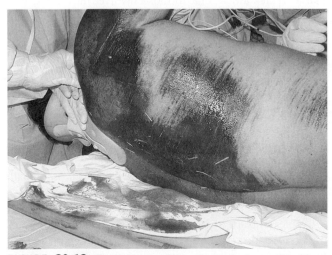

FIGURE **20-12.** Road burns after a motorcycle crash without protective clothing. (From McSwain N, Paturas J: *The basic EMT: comprehensive prehospital patient care,* ed 2, St. Louis, 2003, Mosby.)

PWCs large enough to carry two to three passengers. A high speed can be obtained quickly with most PWCs, so collisions can occur with other watercraft or objects in the water. The potential for injury is very similar to the injury patterns seen with ATVs. Rectal, vaginal, and perineal trauma may occur when passengers or drivers hit the water (buttocks first) or seat at high speeds. Drowning and hypothermia are additional complications associated with PWC accidents.

BICYCLE CRASHES. Several mechanisms for bicycle collisions exist; the most common are collisions with a MV or pedestrian and falling off the bicycle. Most deaths related to bicycles are the result of a collision with a MV. A rider usually loses control and falls off because of hazardous ground surfaces, performing stunts, speeding, or generalized lack of skill.

Bicycle crashes have common patterns of injuries. The spokes of a bicycle wheel can fracture the feet when feet are caught in the wheel. These injuries may cause the person to be thrown and sustain other injuries. Properly installed wheel guards decrease spoke-related injuries.

When a rider is thrown over the handlebars as a bike impacts an object and tips forward, the rider without a helmet may suffer injuries similar to someone ejected from a MV (e.g., head, neck, abdomen, and chest injuries). If the rider impacts the middle bar or seat, straddle injuries such as vaginal tears, scrotal injuries, and perineal contusions occur. Riders can also sustain serious abdominal injuries from coming into contact with the bicycle handlebars. These injuries can range from pancreatic, liver, and spleen tears to stomach injuries to bowel perforations.

Bicycle-mounted child seats are another cause of injuries with bicycle use. The child may fall from the seat, the seat can detach from the bicycle, the bike can tip over, or the child's extremity may be caught in wheel spokes. Head and facial injuries are common and often severe. Child seats mounted on bicycles do not provide protection to the child's head and face, and the child is not developmentally ready for self-protection; therefore helmets should be worn by all children in bicycle-mounted seats.

Injuries can occur to bicycle riders from rear-view mirrors that extend from trucks or vans. Significant head, neck, and facial injuries and severe deep lacerations to the head and neck can occur and can be fatal.

FALLS. Vertical deceleration is the wounding force associated with falls. Severity and types of injuries seen depend on the height of the fall, area of the body impacted, and the landing surface. Falls are more likely to result in severe injury when the distance is three times greater than the victim's height; however, any fall greater than the person's standing height has the potential for significant injury. Different patterns of injuries are seen with different types of falls. Small children tend to land on the head because it is the largest/heaviest part of their body. Certain injuries occur when a person falls from a height and lands feet first. A trio of injuries, called the Don Juan syndrome, includes bilateral calcaneus fractures, compression fractures of the vertebrae (usually thoracolumbar), and bilateral Colles fractures.

Table 20-2. SPORTS-RELATED INJURIES	
Sport	**Potential Injuries**
Boxing	Cumulative brain damage, ocular injuries, lacerations, nasal fractures, hand fractures
Gymnastics	Spinal cord injuries, extremity fractures, sprains, strains
Football	Spinal cord injuries, head injuries, knee strains, fractures, lacerations
Skiing	Head injuries, lower extremity fractures, and exposure to elements
Ice hockey	Facial fractures, soft tissue injuries, lacerations
Running	Lower extremity injuries, strains, sprains
Baseball	Head injuries, ocular injuries, fractures, lacerations, sprains, strains
Basketball	Lower extremity sprains, strains, fractures, lacerations, contusions
Horseback riding	Head injuries, bite wounds, crush wounds
Inline skates	Wrist fractures, head injuries, lower extremity fractures
Bungee jumping	Major impact-related injuries, intraocular hemorrhages, spinal cord injuries, peroneal nerve injuries, soft tissue injuries

Data from Centers for Disease Control and Prevention: *Preventing injuries in America: public health in action,* 2004. Retrieved July 17, 2007, from http://www.cdc.gov.

Energy transfer initially causes bilateral calcaneus fractures, then displaces upward and causes other injuries, including femur fractures, hip dislocations or fractures, vertebral compression fractures, and basilar skull fractures. Wrist fractures occur from acute flexion as the person falls forward onto his or her outstretched arms. Deceleration forces of this nature can also cause secondary renal injuries.

If a person lands on other areas of the body, injuries occur at those impact points and to the rest of the body. If impact is on the wrist, energy is transferred upward through the elbow and shoulder, whereas impact on the knee transfers energy upward to the hip. Another point of impact may be the head, as seen in diving injuries. With this impact, injuries occur because the weight and force of the torso, pelvis, and legs bear down on the head and cervical spine. This type of injury is known as a compression injury or axial loading injury. Vertebral bodies are compressed and wedged, producing vertebral fragments that can penetrate the spinal cord.[30]

Falls affect older adults in a significant way. It is estimated that one of three adults ages 65 and older fall per year, and 50% of those hospitalized are at risk for death within a year's time of the fall.[5,14,22,30] Falls that result in fractures of the hip in adults ages 65 and over have some particular characteristics: (1) 84% of them occur at home, (2) 76% occur indoors, (3) 76% occur while the victim is standing, (4) 72% fall in a sideways direction, (5) 47% occur when the victim is moving forward, (6) very few falls (10%) are related to wet or slippery surfaces, and (7) 13% of falls occur as a result of some manifestation of another medical condition such as dizziness, seizures, or sudden paralysis. Research has been replicated that demonstrates that extrinsic factors such as objects in the environment (e.g., furniture, cords, loose mats) are associated with only 25% of falls and that intrinsic factors such as balance and gait are more frequently associated with falls that result in fractures.[1,14,24,31] Factors that increase the probability of falls in older adults include deterioration in health, physical changes associated with aging (i.e., loss of visual acuity), use of prosthetic devices (e.g., canes, walkers), and environmental hazards (e.g., slippery surfaces, stairs, poor lighting, unexpected objects in walkways).

To lessen the chances of falls, floor surfaces should be covered with nonslip materials and handgrips provided on both sides of walkways. Handgrips are especially helpful in bathrooms. Floors and stairs can be covered with resilient materials that lessen the chance of injury if a fall occurs. Improved lighting in hallways and on stairs helps older adults avoid tripping. Lighting should be concentrated on landings, where falls are most likely to occur. Lighting should provide uniform levels so that older adults do not have to make rapid visual adjustments to variable light intensity.

SPORTS- AND RECREATION-RELATED INJURIES. Injuries associated with sports are generally caused by compressive forces or sudden deceleration as well as by twisting, hyperflexion, and hyperextension. Factors that contribute to injuring events include lack of protective equipment, lack of conditioning, and inadequate training of the participant. Mechanisms associated with recreational sports and sportslike activities are similar to those involved in MVCs, motorcycle collisions, and bicycle crashes. Potential mechanisms associated with individual sports are numerous; however, the general principles are the same as with falls and MVCs.

- What energy or forces impacted the victim?
- What parts of the body are affected by the energy or force?
- What are the obvious injuries?
- What injuries are associated with the involved energy or force?

Damaged equipment, such as broken snow skis or football, lacrosse, or bicycle helmets, can help establish impact sites. Table 20-2 describes injuries associated with various sports.

Adolescents 10 to 14 years of age have the highest rates of sports- and recreation-related injury.[15] An estimated 1.6 to 3.8 million sports- and recreation-related traumatic brain injuries occur in the United States every year.[22,24] Collegiate and high school football players who have at least one concussion are at an increased risk for another concussion.[16]

MOTORIZED AND NONMOTORIZED SCOOTERS.
The new lightweight aluminum nonmotorized scooters hit the commercial market in the year 2000; an older version was sold in the years 1998 and 1999. The majority of those injured on scooters are children younger than 15 years of age and male. Injuries from using scooters include fractures or dislocations, lacerations, contusions and abrasions, and strains and sprains. Injuries are predominately to the arms and hands, the head and face, and to the leg and foot. The CDC has made the following recommendations for scooter use[25]:

- Scooter riders should wear helmets that meet Consumer Product Safety Commission standards.
- Scooter riders should wear knee and elbow pads.
- Scooters should be used on "smooth, paved surfaces without traffic."
- Scooters should not be used on "water, sand, gravel, or dirt."
- Scooter riding should be avoided at night.
- Supervision should be provided for young children using scooters.

Penetrating Trauma

Penetrating injuries are caused by foreign objects in motion that penetrate the body. Energy created by the foreign object dissipates into surrounding tissues. Evaluation and assessment of penetrating trauma depends on the wounding agent, how the energy dissipates, distance from the patient to weapon, and the characteristics of the tissues struck. Examples of penetrating trauma include GSWs, stab wounds, and impalements. The tissue penetrated and underlying structures damaged determine severity of the injury. Patients sustaining penetrating trauma may also suffer blunt injuries, for instance, falling down a flight of stairs after being shot.

Ultimately, the extent of damage will be governed by an interaction of three factors: (1) the character of the wounding instrument (e.g., knife, gun, bomb fragment), (2) its velocity at the time of impact, and (3) the characteristics of the tissue through which it passes.

STAB WOUNDS. Stab wounds are considered low-velocity injuries and therefore low energy transfer. Damage is the result of the sharp cutting edge of the wounding agent; minimal secondary trauma occurs. A narrow, pointed object (e.g., an ice pick) will cause a microscopic crush injury, which will be confined to the path of the instrument's apex. If the instrument is tapered and flat (e.g., a dagger), there will also be fraying and crushing in the tissues as they are stretched to accommodate the wide edge of the blade close to the shaft. If a blunter instrument is used (e.g., an axe), there will be a greater area of crushed tissue and the force applied to achieve the same degree of penetration will also include blunt injury.

For patients with penetrating trauma from a stab wound, knowing the position of the attacker and the patient, the type of weapon used, and gender of the attacker can identify the projected path of the weapon. Women tend to stab downward, whereas men tend to stab upward.

Damage from a stab wound depends on the location of the penetrating object. Tissue damage is generally isolated

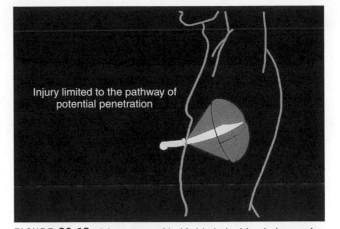

FIGURE 20-13. Movement of knife blade inside victim produces damage, limited to path of penetration. (Modified from Prehospital Trauma Life Support Committee of the National Association of Emergency Medical Technicians in Cooperation With the Committee on Trauma of the American College of Surgeons: *PHTLS: basic and advanced prehospital life support,* ed 4, St. Louis, 1999, Mosby.)

to the area of penetration (Figure 20-13); however, a single wound can penetrate several body cavities, causing lethal injuries. For example, the weapon can enter the thoracic and abdominal cavities with just one penetration. Chest wounds at the level of the nipple or below can involve the abdominal cavity and underlying organs.

More than one wound may exist. It is also important to remember that small wounds can hide extensive internal damage caused by weapon movement. Internal damage is directly proportional to the length of the wounding object and to the density of tissue affected.

IMPALEMENTS. Impalements are generally low-velocity injuries that occur from falls, MVCs, or secondary to a flying or falling object. Impaled objects should be stabilized and removed only when the patient is in a controlled environment such as an operating room where surgical support and intervention is immediately available.

GUNSHOT WOUNDS. Handguns, shotguns, and rifles are responsible for most firearm injuries. Ballistics is the science of the study of the motion of projectiles. A penetrating wound occurs when the missile remains in the body and there is only an entrance wound; a perforating wound occurs when the missile passes out of the body and thus creates an entrance and an exit wound (Figure 20-14). The size of the entrance wound will vary directly with the size (caliber) of the missile. The size and shape of the wound are also subject to the missile's flight pattern at the time of impact (yaw). (Figure 20-15 demonstrates these movements). Also affecting the size and shape of the wound is the shape of the projectile (i.e., a smooth bullet or a jagged shell fragment). Once the missile is inside the body, the degree of damage is a result of the interaction between the body itself and the projectile and depends upon the consistency of the tissues being traversed by the missile and the characteristics of the weapon that launched it.

Missile velocity determines tissue deformation and extent of cavitation.[14] Velocity is generally described as low or high. Low-velocity missiles travel at speeds below 2500 ft/sec and have little disruptive effect on tissues. Injuries are localized at the center of the tract with a small radius of distribution. The temporary cavity is two to three times the diameter of the missile.[14,22] Low-velocity missiles push tissues aside along the path. Side arms such as pistols and submachine guns fall into this type of category.

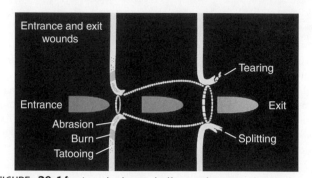

FIGURE **20-14.** A spinning missile produces a 1- to 2-mm abraded edge along wound if it enters straight. If it enters at an angle, abraded side is on bottom of missile, with more skin contact, and covers a much wider area. Difference in entrance and exit wounds is also depicted. Exit wounds are generally longer and more explosive. (Modified from Prehospital Trauma Life Support Committee of the National Association of Emergency Medical Technicians in Cooperation With the Committee on Trauma of the American College of Surgeons: *PHTLS: basic and advanced prehospital life support,* ed 4, St. Louis, 1999, Mosby.)

High-velocity missiles (HVMs) travel at speeds above 2500 ft/sec and cause more serious injuries because of high cavitation and energy transfer.[14] High-velocity missiles create a cavity around the bullet and the bullet tract by compressing and displacing tissue. As kinetic energy is transferred from the bullet to the tissue, the cavity enlarges. A tract temporarily displaces tissue laterally and forward as the missile moves forward. Behind or following the missile, negative pressure contaminates the wound by pulling in foreign material. These cavities can be 30 to 40 times the diameter of the bullet. Figure 20-16 describes the cavitational differences between low-velocity and high-velocity bullets. High-velocity wounds often require debridement because of extensive tissue disruption. An example of this type of missile would be one fired from a modern-day rifle. Entrance and exit wounds

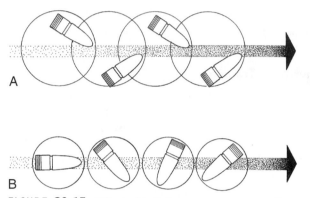

FIGURE **20-15.** Effect of bullet movement on wounding potential. **A,** Yawing. **B,** Tumbling.

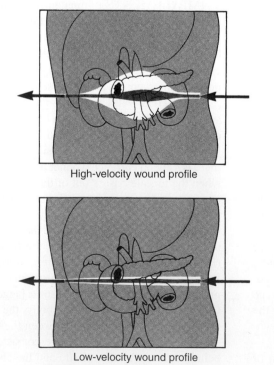

High-velocity wound profile

Low-velocity wound profile

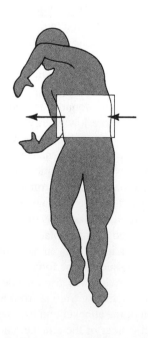

FIGURE **20-16.** Potential injury path of high- and low-velocity bullets. (From Neff JA, Kidd PS: *Trauma nursing: the art and science,* St. Louis, 1993, Mosby.)

with high-velocity missiles differ with types of tissues and body areas hit.[22] Exit wounds may be larger when the missile travels through smaller structures such as an extremity because all energy has not dissipated by the time the bullet exits; cavitation and missile movement is still occurring. Exit wounds tend to be small in dense tissue because cavitation is complete and most energy is dissipated. If the bullet fragments while traveling through the tissues, no exit wound is found. Because entrance and exit wounds may have differing characteristics in differing circumstances, documentation should include only a description of the wound and not identification as either an entrance or exit wound.

Deformation of the bullet is another important factor when assessing GSWs. Energy production increases when missiles change shape on impact. Types of bullets that produce greater kinetic energy include soft-nosed, flat-nosed, and hollow-point bullets that mushroom on impact. Refer to Table 20-3 for the characteristics of bullets by shape.

Another feature of GSWs is the muzzle blast seen with close-range wounds or when the gun is pressed against the skin. Immediately on firing, a cloud of burning powder and hot gas is released from the muzzle. If a muzzle blast is evident, tattooing from burning particles, abrasions, and burn marks at the entrance wound are seen.

Blast Injuries

Blasts are not as common in the United States as in some other countries; however, the potential for hazardous explosions at chemical plants, oil refineries, shipyards, and other industrial settings does exist. Terrorist activity has increased the concern for explosions in urban areas. Explosions can occur anywhere because of the large amount of volatile materials carried by rail or truck. Blasts occur when explosives are detonated and changed to gases. As the gas expands, an equal volume of air is displaced and travels after the blast wave. Disruption of tissue, evisceration, and traumatic amputation can occur from this mass movement of air. When the explosive casing ruptures, the casing fragments become high-velocity projectiles.[14,24]

The greater density of water allows a blast wave to travel more rapidly and farther in water than air. Consequently, injuries associated with underwater blasts are usually more severe. Closed-area explosions cause more damage than open-area ones because of the potential inhalation of smoke and toxic gases.

Blast injuries occur in three phases or impact points. Figure 20-17 diagrams how injuries occur from an explosive

Table 20-3. CLASSIFICATION OF BULLETS BY SHAPE	
Shape	**Composition**
Pointed nose Round nose	Certain kinds are called "soft points" and on impact will flatten and "mushroom" back on themselves, increasing the amount of damage.
Hollow-Pointed nose	Made with a depression at the tip of their noses and deform on impact. It is thought that by becoming deformed, these bullets will increase the amount of damage.
Flat nose	One type is "Dum-Dum" bullets which were developed by the British in 1897 at their garrison in Dum Dum, India. The Hague Convention outlawed them for military use.

Reprinted from Emergency Nurses Association: *Trauma nursing core course: provider manual, ed 6,* Des Plaines, Ill, 2007, The Association.

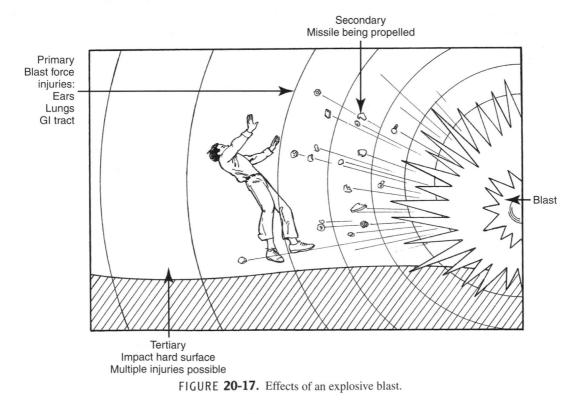

FIGURE **20-17.** Effects of an explosive blast.

blast, and Table 20-4 describes common injuries. As explosives change to an expanding mass of heated gas, primary injuries occur because of concussive effects of the pressure wave. Concussion injuries are frequently overlooked because they are not obvious and may occur without external signs of trauma; however, these injuries are usually the most severe. Injuries associated with this mechanism include brain and spinal cord injuries, rupture of air-containing organs, and tearing of membranes and small vessels. The associated heat wave can also cause burns on areas of the body facing the explosion.

Fragments of glass, rocks, or metal debris become high-velocity projectiles and can cause secondary injuries: impalements, fractures, traumatic amputations, burns, and soft tissue injuries such as contusions, abrasions, and lacerations.

The third point of impact occurs when the victim is thrown through the air and becomes a missile. Tertiary injuries associated with this mechanism are similar to those seen when people are ejected from vehicles or fall from heights, and these injuries generally occur at the point of impact. Structural collapse during the blast can lead to crush injuries.

Specific Mechanisms of Injury

BURNS. Deaths from fires and burns are the fifth most common cause of unintentional injury deaths in the United States.[7] Data reveal that on average in the United States someone dies in a fire every 2 hours and someone is injured as a result of fire every 29 minutes. Cooking is the primary cause of residential fires. Smoking is the leading cause of fire-related deaths. Alcohol contributes to about 40% of residential fire deaths.[7] Those at greatest risk for fire-related deaths and sustaining burns are the following:

- Children ages 4 and younger
- Adults ages 65 and older
- The poorest Americans
- African Americans and Native Americans

- Those living in rural areas
- Those living in manufactured homes or substandard housing.

Although the number of fatalities and injuries caused by residential fires has declined gradually over the past several decades, many residential fire–related deaths remain preventable and continue to pose a significant public health problem. Fortunately, the incidence of serious burns and subsequent hospitalizations has decreased by 50% over the last two decades. Unfortunately, burn injury is the third leading cause of death for all children and the second leading cause of death for those between 1 and 4 years.[7] Annually there are approximately 1.25 million burn injuries, causing 51,000 hospitalizations and death for approximately 10% of those patients.[7] Those under age 5 and over age 65 are the most susceptible to scald burns from hot liquids; these injuries may lead to hospitalization but rarely lead to death.[7] Those older than age 65 sustain the majority (75%) of burns from clothing ignition resulting from cigarette smoking or use of stoves and space heaters.[1]

Contact with electrical current leading to electrical burns causes approximately 1000 deaths per year, and another 80 deaths per year are due to lightning. It has been estimated that care for a burn victim in a hospital may cost between $36,000 and $117,000. Death of a person in a fire costs between $250,000 and $1.5 million when lost years of estimated productivity are considered in the calculation.[1,7]

SUBMERSION INJURIES. Submersion (drowning and near-drowning) results in injury secondary to oxygen deprivation. Blunt trauma is frequently associated with these events due to the increased use of watercraft and the reality that the individuals involved have either fallen into the water or they were involved in an untoward chain of events, a reason why they could not be rescued or rescue themselves. Males account for 80% of drownings in the United States.[5,31] Alcohol is involved in about 25% to 50% of adolescent and adult deaths associated with water recreation.[17] Alcohol influences balance,

Table 20-4.	MECHANISMS OF BLAST INJURIES		
Mechanism	**Causation**	**Primary Organs Affected**
Primary	Initial blast or air wave. It is important to try and determine what type of blast occurred (steam, chemical, gas, electrical, etc.) so that pre-hospital providers can be safe and secondary complications can be avoided with the patients.	Affects primarily air-filled organs: Tympanic membranes—rupture and permanent deafness can occur Lungs—pneumothorax, alveolar rupture, air embolus GI—intestinal and stomach contusions and rupture CNS—concussion syndrome, various types of focal and diffuse cerebral hemorrhage, cerebral air embolism
Secondary	Flying debris, which act as projectiles	Injuries will vary depending on the size of the projectiles and what and where they hit
Tertiary	The distance an individual's body travels from the blast and where it has impacted	Injuries are similar to those in an individual who has been ejected from a MVC or fallen from a great height
Miscellaneous	Inhalation of dust or toxic gases, thermal burns, radiation, etc.	Lungs, skin, eyes

Reprinted from Emergency Nurses Association: *Trauma nursing core course: provider manual,* ed 6, Des Plaines, Ill, 2007, The Association.
CNS, Central nervous system; *GI,* gastrointestinal; *MVC,* motor vehicle crash.

coordination, and judgment, and its effects are heightened by sun exposure and heat.[30] Up to 70% of boating-related deaths were the result of drowning; 86% of people who drowned were not wearing personal flotation devices.[5,31] Most drownings occur at sites without lifeguards.[5,31]

For every child 14 years and younger who drowns, three will receive ED care for nonfatal submersion injuries. Nonfatal incidents can cause brain damage that results in long-term disability ranging from memory problems and learning disabilities to persistent vegetative state. Children under the age of 1 year most often drown in bathtubs or toilets.[5] The overall age-adjusted drowning rate for African Americans is 1.4 times higher than for whites.[11]

VIOLENCE-RELATED INJURIES. Violence-related injures are defined as those that result from the intentional use of physical force or power against oneself, another person or a group or community. This definition encompasses injuries that result from acts of interpersonal violence such as homicide, child maltreatment, youth violence, intimate partner violence, and other types of assaults. It also includes acts of self-directed violence such as suicide, suicide attempts, and self-mutilation. Violence adversely affects the health and welfare of all Americans through premature death, disability, medical costs, and lost productivity. Medical costs and productivity losses due to interpersonal and self-directed violence in the United States are significant and difficult to quantify.[12] See Chapters 48 to 50 for further discussion of child abuse and neglect, intimate partner violence, and elder abuse and neglect.

SCHOOL VIOLENCE. Although the number of incidents has decreased steadily since 1992, the number of multiple-victim incidents has increased. Most incidents were homicides involving firearms.[5] More than 50% of school-associated violent deaths occurred at the beginning or end of the school day or during lunch. School-associated homicide rates are highest near the start of each school semester; suicide rates are generally higher in the spring semester.[5] Male students are more likely to be involved in a physical fight than female students (41% versus 25%).[5]

SUICIDE/SELF-INFLICTED VIOLENCE. Like other forms of violence, suicide is another category that is underreported. Each year in the United States more people commit suicide than die from homicide. CDC data indicate that 87 people take their own life every day.[5] Although females attempt suicide more often than males, males are four times as likely to die from suicide. Suicide is the third leading cause of death among young people ages 15 to 24 years.[20] Suicide rates are highest among those ages 65 and older. Data indicate that Americans over age 65 average one suicide every 90 minutes, with men constituting 85% of these suicides.[5] Standard definitions for suicide do not exist, and the definitions used in federal and state legislation vary drastically. These inconsistencies contribute to confusion and a lack of consensus about the magnitude of the problem. Although there are numerous methods for suicide (e.g., toxicological overdose, hanging, asphyxiation), 56% of suicides are committed with a firearm.[20]

Overall, poisoning (66%) and cuttings/piercings (18%) are the most common forms of self-inflicted injuries. Males are six times more likely to sustain a firearm injury, whereas self-inflicted poisonings were 60% higher for females than males.[12]

PREVENTION

Traumatic injuries have physical, emotional, and financial consequences that can affect the lives of individuals, families, and society. Some injuries can result in temporary or permanent disability or death. Because of this, injury prevention programs were developed in the hopes of stopping the injury from ever occurring.

The Haddon Injury Matrix is the most widely used epidemiologic model of injury prevention.[5] This model describes a two-dimensional approach to injury and its causes. The first dimension encompasses the three factors of injury: host or human factors, the agent or vector of energy transfer, and the physical and social environment. The second dimension in this model is the phase of injury. The preevent phase is amenable to primary prevention strategies designed to stop the injuring event from occurring by acting on its cause (e.g., installing pool fences, divided highways). The injury event phase is amenable to secondary prevention strategies that attempt to prevent an injury or reduce the seriousness of an injury when an event actually occurs (e.g., wearing safety restraints, bicycle helmets). The post–injury event phase is amenable to tertiary prevention strategies that attempt to reduce the seriousness of an injury after the event has occurred by providing adequate care (e.g., trained prehospital and ED staff). Injury prevention programs can be constructed that target specific factors or phases of injury or both. Table 20-5 describes possible injury prevention strategies to reduce falls in older adults using the Haddon Matrix. In general most injury control strategies can be classified according to three *E*'s: engineering and technologic interventions, enforcement and legislative interventions, and education and behavioral interventions. For example, a program designed to prevent falls in older adults may include engineering/technologic innovations such as specially designed padded underwear, enforcement/legislation interventions such as regulations related to restraint use, and education/behavioral interventions such as the CDC's *Check for Safety: A Home Fall Prevention Checklist for Older Adults.*

The Emergency Nurses Association (ENA) offers a wide variety of injury prevention programs and materials through the Injury Prevention Institute; programs include alcohol prevention education, bike and helmet safety, child passenger safety, gun safety, and healthy aging. An example of an injury prevention strategy adopted at the state level is the gradual phasing in of licensing of young drivers so that they drive mainly in the daylight, have no other teenagers in the car, and need to be with an experienced driver. Additional examples of injury programs are the ThinkFirst diving program, and the National Rifle Association's Eddie the Eagle gun safety program for children.

Table 20-5. THE HADDON INJURY MATRIX TO PLAN PREVENTION STRATEGIES			
Phases	Human Factors	Vehicle or Vector Factors	Environmental Factors
Preevent	Reduce use of sedatives	Correct defects in safety equipment (e.g., walkers, wheelchairs)	Use of safety bars, handrails, side rails on beds
Event	Consider reduction in severity of preexisting medical conditions (e.g., vertigo, imbalance)	Cover exposed skin areas with protective barriers to reduce severity of injury (e.g., elbow and knee pads)	Reduction of clutter in the patient's environment
Postevent	Consider if patient is on anticoagulants or other medications and their effects on subsequent bleeding or physiologic response to shock and trauma	Have patients avoid areas where they could become trapped after a fall and where access to help is minimal	Implementation of comprehensive emergency response protocols and systems

Not all injury prevention programs are successful. The key is to implement an evaluation system that measures the impact of the program. Some may view the prevention of one death or one injury as a success, but when scarce resources are available in public health, the impact of expense must be justified. It is difficult to determine the effect of some programs; for example, a red ribbon tied around one's side-mounted mirror or educational programs for teens and drunk-driving prevention.

Access to the Internet provides innumerable resources for prevention programs through federal, state and local nonprofit and private organizations, companies, and foundations. The key to preventing many unintentional injury deaths and disabling injuries among children is effective supervision, yet this behavioral component of injury prevention lacks conceptual and methodologic clarity.[5]

SUMMARY

Treatment of trauma patients depends on identifying all injuries and rapidly intervening to correct those that are life threatening. Consideration of mechanisms of injury is essential to identifying patients with possible underlying injuries who require further evaluation and treatment.

REFERENCES

1. Adelmen AA, Daly MP: *Twenty common problems in geriatrics*, New York, 2001, McGraw-Hill.
2. *American Heritage dictionary*, ed 3, Boston, 1992, Houghton Mifflin.
3. Brenner RA, Triumble AC, Smith GS et al: Where children drown, United States, 1995, *Pediatrics* 108(1):85, 2001.
4. Centers for Disease Control and Prevention: *Preventing injuries in America: introduction*, 2004. Retrieved July 17, 2007, from http://www.cdc.gov.
5. Centers for Disease Control and Prevention: *Preventing injuries in America: public health in action*, 2004. Retrieved July 17, 2007, from http://www.cdc.gov.
6. Centers for Disease Control and Prevention: *Agriculture fact sheet*, 2007. Retrieved July 17, 2007, from http://www.cdc.gov/ncipc/factsheets/agriculture.htm.
7. Centers for Disease Control and Prevention: *Fire deaths and injuries: fact sheet*, 2007. Retrieved July 17, 2007, from http://www.cdc.gov/ncipc/factsheets/fire.htm.
8. Centers for Disease Control and Prevention: *Impaired driving: fact sheet*, 2007. Retrieved July 17, 2007, from http://www.cdc.gov/ncipc/factsheets/driving.htm.
9. Centers for Disease Control and Prevention: *Injuries among Native Americans: fact sheet,* 2007. Retrieved July 17, 2007, from http://www.cdc.gov/ncipc/factsheets/nativeamericans.htm.
10. Centers for Disease Control and Prevention: *Older adult drivers: fact sheet*, 2007. Retrieved July 17, 2007, from http://www.cdc.gov/ncipc/factsheets/older.htm.
11. Centers for Disease Control and Prevention: *Water-related injuries: fact sheet*, 2007. Retrieved July 17, 2007, from http://www.cdc.gov/nipc/factsheets/drown.htm.
12. Corso PS, Mercy JA, Simon TR et al: Medical costs and productivity losses due to interpersonal and self-directed violence in the United States, *Am J Prev Med* 32(6):474, 2007.
13. Delliner AM, Langlois JA, Li G: Fatal crashes among older drivers: decomposition of rates into contributing factors, *Am J Epidemiol* 155(3):234, 2002.
14. Emergency Nurses Association: *Trauma nursing core course: provider manual*, ed 6, Des Plaines, Ill, 2007, The Association.
15. Gotsch K, Annest JL, Holmgreen P et al: Non-fatal sports and recreational-related injuries treated in emergency departments—United States, July 2000-June 2001, *MMWR Morb Mortal Wkly Rep* 51(33):736, 2002.
16. Guskiewicz KM, Weaver N, Padua DA et al: Epidemiology of concussion in collegiate and high school football players, *Am J Sports Med* 28(5):643, 2000.
17. Howland J, Mangione T, Hingson R et al: Alcohol as a risk factor for drowning and other aquatic injuries. In Watson RR, editor: *Alcohol and accidents,* Drug and alcohol abuse reviews, vol 7, Totowa, NJ, 1995, Humana Press.

18. Insurance Institute for Highway Safety: *Fatality facts: teenagers 2002,* Arlington, Va, 2004, The Institute.

19. Jonah BA, Dawson NE: Youth and risk: age differences in risky driving, risk perception, and risk utility, *Alcohol, Drugs and Driving* 3:13, 1987.

20. Kochanek KD, Murphy SL, Anderson RN et al: Deaths: leading causes for 2002, *Natl Vital Stat Rep* 53(5): 1, 2004.

21. Krug EG, Powell KE, Dahlberg LL: Firearm-related deaths in the United States and 35 other high-and upper middle-income countries, *Int J Epidemiol* 27:214, 1998.

22. Mattox KL, Feliciano DV, Moore EE, editors: *Trauma,* ed 6, New York, 2008, McGraw-Hill.

23. McQuillan K, Whalen E, Makic MBF, editors: *Trauma nursing: from resuscitation through rehabilitation,* ed 4, Philadelphia, 2008, Elsevier.

24. McSwain NE, Frame S, Salomone JP, editors: *Pre-hospital trauma life support (PHTLS),* St. Louis, 2003, Mosby.

25. National Highway Traffic Safety Administration, U.S. Department of Transportation: *Traffic safety facts 2003,* Washington, DC, 2004, The Administration.

26. National Highway Traffic Safety Administration, U.S. Department of Transportation: *Traffic safety facts 2003 data: pedestrians,* Washington, DC, 2004, The Administration.

27. National Highway Traffic Safety Administration, U.S. Department of Transportation: *Traffic safety facts 2003 data: young drivers,* Washington, DC, 2004, The Administration.

28. Porter RS: Blunt trauma. In Bledsoe BE, Porter RS, Cherry RA, editors: *Paramedic care: principles and practice,* Upper Saddle River, NJ, 2001, Prentice-Hall.

29. Shults RA: Child passenger deaths involving drinking and drivers—United States, 1997-2002 [published erratum appears in *Morb Mortal Wkly Rep* 53(5):109, 2004], *Morb Mortal Wkly Rep* 53(4):77, 2004.

30. Stevens JA, Dellinger AM: Motor vehicle and fall related deaths among older Americans 1990-1998: sex, race and ethnic disparities, *Inj Prev* 8:272, 2002.

31. U.S. Coast Guard, Department of Homeland Security: *Boating statistics 2005.* Retrieved July 3, 2007, from http://www.uscgboating.org/statistics/accident_stats. htm.

32. Yanar H, Demetriades D, Hatzizacharia P et al: Pedestrians injured by automobiles: risk factors for cervical spine injuries, *J Am Coll Surg* 205(6):794, 2007.

CHAPTER 21

Head Trauma

Beth Broering

Traumatic brain injury (TBI), a leading cause of death and permanent disability, is a major public health problem both in the United States and internationally. Over 2 million persons in the United States sustain a brain injury each year, more than 8 times the number of people diagnosed with breast cancer and 34 times the number of people diagnosed with human immunodeficiency virus/acquired immunodeficiency syndrome.[10,18,22] There are an estimated 50,000 deaths, over 200,000 hospitalizations, and more than 1 million emergency department (ED) visits.[18] TBI has resulted in more than 5 million persons in the United States living with permanent disabilities, many requiring lifelong assistance with activities of daily living.[18] According to the Centers for Disease Control and Prevention (CDC), the estimated direct and indirect costs of TBI were more than 60 billion dollars in 2000, with the average lifetime cost per survivor of TBI requiring hospitalization being $111,578 and the average cost per fatality being $454,717.[10,18,30]

Mechanisms of injury include blunt, penetrating, and blast forces that disrupt the vascular and neuronal structures inside the cranial vault, leading to a complex cascade of cellular and biochemical processes. A small percentage of patients with severe TBI will have concomitant fracture of the cervical spine. Falls are a common mechanism of injury in all ages but particularly in the pediatric population and those over 65 years of age. Persons of all ages sustain head injuries from motor vehicle crashes; however, those 15 to 24 years of age are at greatest risk. Other motorized vehicles (e.g., all-terrain vehicles, motorcycles, dirt bikes) have become an increasing cause of TBI in children and young adults.[5,9,21] Along with mechanisms, the forces of energy are important to understand. Brain injuries can result from acceleration, deceleration, rotational, or deformation forces. Table 21-1 provides an overview of the common energy forces associated with TBI.

Penetrating injuries occur most commonly from firearms but can also result from any sharp object that penetrates the scalp and skull. The extent of damage to brain tissue is determined by the point of entry, depth and angle of entry, and force of entry. Although all types of penetrating injuries are potentially lethal, gunshot wounds have the highest associated mortality rate. Blast injuries, the most common cause of TBI for military troops deployed to war zones, can occur in any type of explosion. Blast injury is often a combination of both blunt and penetrating forces. The impact of the blast waves moving through the victim's body causes shearing of neuronal structures, while flying debris might produce penetrating injuries.

It is important for the emergency nurse to have an understanding of the mechanisms of injury and forces involved to ensure appropriate management and minimize the potential for secondary brain injury, complications, and missed injuries.

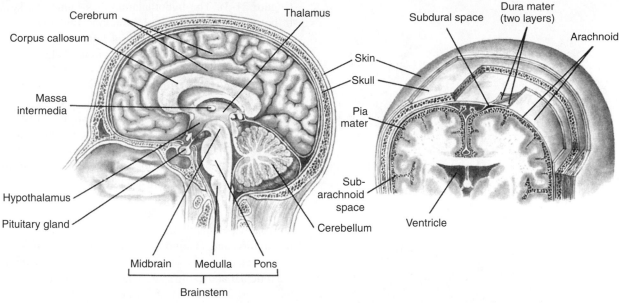

FIGURE **21-1.** Brain structures. (From Thompson JM, McFarland G, Hirsch J et al: *Mosby's clinical nursing,* ed 5, St. Louis, 2002, Mosby.)

This chapter begins with a brief review of anatomy and physiology. It also provides an overview of assessment techniques focusing primarily on adult patients with TBI. Current management options for TBI are also discussed. For a more complete discussion on pediatric injuries, refer to Chapter 28.

ANATOMY AND PHYSIOLOGY
Anatomy

The hair, scalp, skull, meninges, and cerebrospinal fluid (CSF) protect the brain from injury (Figure 21-1). Five layers of tissue form the scalp: skin, subcutaneous tissue, galea aponeurotica, ligaments, and periosteum. The cranium, composed of the frontal, parietal, temporal, and occipital bones, joins with the facial bones to form the cranial vault, a rigid, nonexpandable cavity that can hold a volume of approximately 1700 mL. Bones of the cranium consist of three layers (Figure 21-2). The outer and inner tables are composed of hard cortical or compact bone. The diploë or middle layer is made up of soft cancellous bone. The structure of the cranial bones provides significant protection to the brain parenchyma. The skull is divided into the supratentorial and the infratentorial space. The cerebral hemispheres and the diencephalon are contained in the supratentorial space. The infratentorial space contains the cerebellum and the brainstem. Other bony structures of importance are depressions at the base of the skull called the anterior, middle, and posterior fossae. The frontal lobe is located in the anterior fossa. The deeper middle fossa contains the parietal, temporal, and occipital lobes. The posterior fossa is the largest and deepest and supports the brainstem and cerebellum.

Three layers of meninges surround the brain and provide additional protection. The outermost meninx is the dura mater (meaning "tough mother"), which consists of two

Table 21-1.	**ENERGY FORCES ASSOCIATED WITH TRAUMATIC BRAIN INJURY**	
Type of Force	**Description**	**Result**
Acceleration forces	When the head is struck by a moving object	Skull fractures Contusions Hematomas
Deceleration forces	When the head is moving and strikes a stationary object (e.g., head hits the steering wheel of a car, ejected occupant hits head on the ground)	Skull fractures Contusions Coup-contrecoup injuries Hematomas
Acceleration-deceleration forces	Combination of injuries due to rapid changes in the velocity of the brain	Coup-contrecoup injuries Diffuse axonal injuries Hematomas
Rotational forces	Side-to-side and twisting movement of brain tissue	Diffuse axonal injuries
Deformation forces	Direct blows or compression of the skull with resultant change in shape of the skull	Severity and extent of injury often determined by the velocity of blow or the length of compression

layers of tough fibrous tissue. The inner layer of the dura mater produces prominent folds that subdivide the interior of the cranial cavity. The largest of these folds forms the falx cerebri, which separates the brain into the right and left cerebral hemispheres. The next-largest fold is the tentorium cerebelli, which divides the posterior cranial fossa into the superior

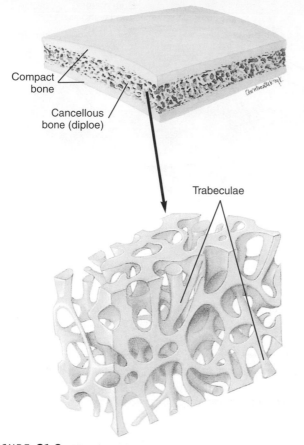

Compact bone

Cancellous bone (diploe)

Trabeculae

FIGURE 21-2. The three layers of "skull bone": outer layer of compact bone surrounding cancellous bone. Note the fine structure of compact and cancellous bone. (From Thibodeau GA, Patton KT: *Anatomy and physiology,* ed 6, St. Louis, 2007, Mosby.)

(supratentorial) and inferior (infratentorial) compartments. Potential spaces located above the dura mater (epidural) and below the dura mater (subdural) are at risk for hematoma formation because the middle meningeal artery lies in the epidural space, and veins are located within the subdural space. The middle meningeal layer is the arachnoid (spider-like) mater, a fine, elastic layer. Below the arachnoid mater, the subarachnoid space is a relatively large space that is normally filled with CSF and contains arachnoid villi, fingerlike projections that form channels for CSF absorption. Adhering to the surface of the brain is the pia mater (meaning "tender mother").

The cerebrum consists of two hemispheres separated by a longitudinal fissure. Each lobe of the cerebrum is responsible for specific functions. The frontal lobe coordinates voluntary motor movements and controls judgment, affect, and personality. Hearing, behavior, emotions, and dominant-hemisphere speech are controlled by the temporal lobe. Sensory interpretation occurs in the parietal lobe, whereas the occipital lobe is responsible for vision.

The cerebral hemispheres are connected with the midbrain by the diencephalon. The thalamus, hypothalamus, subthalamus, and epithalamus are located within the diencephalon

(Figure 21-3). The hypothalamus has numerous key roles in hormonal regulation and metabolic functions, including temperature regulation; release of hormones from the pituitary gland and adrenal cortex; emotional behaviors such as fear, rage, and pleasure; and activation of the sympathetic and parasympathetic functions of the autonomic nervous system.

The cerebellum is located in the posterior fossa adjacent to the brainstem and separated from the cerebrum by the tentorium cerebelli. Primary functions of the cerebellum are integration of motor function, maintenance of equilibrium, and maintenance of muscle tone.

The brainstem consists of the midbrain, pons, and medulla (see Figure 21-3). Although each structure has important pathway functions, the medulla contains the cardiac, respiratory, and vasomotor centers. The reticular formation, also located in the brainstem, is the central component of the reticular activating system and is responsible for arousal, the lowest level of consciousness, which is interpreted as wakefulness. Along with the primary cardiorespiratory centers, the brainstem contains many ascending and descending pathways that carry impulses between the spinal cord and the brain. In addition, all cranial nerves (CNs) with the exception of CN I and CN II originate in the brainstem. Table 21-2 describes the function of each CN.

The anatomic structure of the capillaries of the brain, the tight junctions between endothelial cells, and the surrounding neuroglia form the blood-brain barrier. The blood-brain barrier acts as a protective mechanism restricting the free movement of substances from the blood vessels into the interstitial spaces and CSF. The blood-brain barrier, although mainly protective in nature, can hinder the effectiveness of some drugs. In brain injury, the breakdown of the blood-brain barrier may potentiate cerebral edema.

Physiology

In the adult patient the skull is a closed box containing three volumes: the brain (80%), CSF (10%), and blood (10%). Intracranial pressure (ICP) is a dynamic state that reflects the pressure in the supratentorial space as exerted by the total of the three volumes, which under normal conditions is maintained in constant balance through multiple homeostatic mechanisms. Normal ICP is less than 10 mm Hg with an upper limit of approximately 15 mm Hg. If one or more of the volumes of the cranial contents increases, ICP will rise and, if not immediately corrected, will compromise cerebral blood flow. The Monro-Kellie hypothesis describes the concept of reciprocal changes in volume as a means of compensation and maintaining ICP. As one of the volumes increases, there must be reciprocal decreases in the other two volumes or ICP will rise. CSF is initially displaced out of the cranial compartment into the spinal subarachnoid space, and production of CSF is reduced. Once CSF is maximally displaced, there is vasoconstriction and compression of the cerebral venous system. Sustained ICP greater than 20 mm Hg represents intracranial hypertension. If ICP continues to

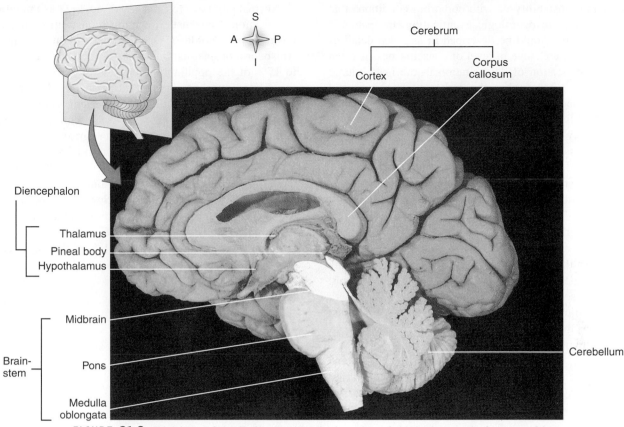

S
A ✦ P
I

Cerebrum
Cortex
Corpus callosum

Diencephalon

Thalamus
Pineal body
Hypothalamus

Midbrain

Brain-stem

Pons

Medulla oblongata

Cerebellum

FIGURE **21-3.** Divisions of the brain. A midsagittal section of the brain reveals features of its major divisions. (From Thibodeau GA, Patton KT: *Anatomy and physiology,* ed 6, St. Louis, 2007, Mosby.)

rise, arterial blood flow is compromised. These compensatory mechanisms have a finite ability to reduce volume and maintain ICP. As the intracranial volume increases beyond the compensatory threshold, there are sharp increases in ICP (Figure 21-4). Failure to reduce ICP may cause ischemia and necrosis of brain tissue.

The brain requires a constant supply of oxygen and nutrients, primarily glucose, to maintain function. It receives 15% of the cardiac output and consumes approximately 20% of the body's oxygen supply. Cerebral blood flow is maintained through highly sensitive and complex mechanisms of autoregulation. Cerebral autoregulation is the ability of the brain to maintain a constant blood flow over a wide range of metabolic demands and systemic mean arterial pressures (normally 50 to 150 mm Hg).[3,8,9,23,26] This is accomplished through vasoconstriction or vasodilation of the cerebral blood vessels. For example, if metabolic demands rise, the cerebral vessels will vasodilate to increase cerebral blood flow, oxygen, and glucose delivery. Cerebral blood flow also remains relatively constant with changes in systemic pressure. The cerebral vessels vasoconstrict when systemic pressure is high and vasodilate as systemic pressures begin to fall. Cerebral autoregulation can be impaired or lost, either locally or globally, after brain injury. When cerebral autoregulation is disrupted, cerebral blood flow becomes dependent on the systemic blood pressure.

Cerebral perfusion pressure (CPP) is the pressure gradient across the brain or the pressure difference between the arterial blood entering the brain and the venous blood exiting. Adequate delivery of oxygen and nutrients requires adequate CPP (i.e., CPP ≥50 mm Hg).[2,6,13,23] CPP plays an important role in regulating cerebral blood flow. As CPP falls, the cerebral vessels will vasodilate to maintain cerebral blood flow. If CPP drops too low, the cerebral vessels collapse, and cerebral blood flow will actually fall, resulting in ischemia and neuronal cell death. CPP is calculated by subtracting the ICP from the systemic mean arterial pressure (MAP) (Box 21-1).

PATIENT ASSESSMENT

After ensuring adequate control of airway, breathing, and circulation (ABCs), the emergency nurse should perform a neurologic assessment. The goals of the neurologic assessment in brain-injured patients include detection of life-threatening injuries and establishing a baseline assessment that can be used as a comparison in subsequent examinations. A complete neurologic assessment, including mental status, level of consciousness or Glasgow Coma Scale (GCS) score, pupillary size and reactivity, CN assessment, reflexes, and motor symmetry and strength, can be performed in the awake and hemodynamically stable patient. In a patient with hemodynamic instability or with comorbid conditions that prevent a complete neurologic examination, the patient's neurologic status should be described in as much detail as possible. A subtle change in level of consciousness is often the earliest indication of deterioration in the head-injured patient. Box 21-2 describes the early and late signs and symptoms of increased ICP.

Table 21-3 lists the components of the GCS, an objective, and universally accepted measure of a patient's neurologic status.[27] Assessment of level of consciousness should be directed toward acquiring the highest-level or best response with the least stimulus. Completing the GCS allows assignment of numeric values to clinical changes. Interpretation of the GCS must be correlated with other clinical assessment findings. Other physiologic conditions such as hypotension, hypoxia, alcohol intoxication, or substance abuse may falsely lower the initial GCS. Eye and facial trauma may make assessment of eye opening inaccurate or difficult. Motor response may be difficult to assess in patients with spinal cord injuries. In addition, the emergency nurse must also consider the accuracy of response in the non–English-speaking patient. However, in the acute resuscitation a GCS score of 8 or less represents coma, and the nurse must assume the patient has sustained a severe head injury until further clinical and diagnostic studies can be completed.

Normal pupillary response to direct light examination is constriction. Consensual reaction (constriction of the opposite pupil) should occur with direct light examination. Anisocoria or unequal pupils are a normal finding in 15% to 17% of the population, so assessment of reactivity in the dilated pupil is critical. Sluggish pupillary response may be the first indication of increasing cerebral edema and rising ICP. An oval pupil is also commonly seen in patients with increasing ICP.[2] With aggressive intervention the oval pupil will often return to normal size, shape, and reactivity as ICP is reduced. If ICP cannot be controlled, the pupil will become dilated and nonreactive. CN III exits the brainstem and lies at the junction of the midbrain and the tentorial notch. Any increase in downward pressure at the tentorial notch compresses the third CN, resulting in unilateral pupil dilation (Figure 21-5). Bilateral fixed and dilated pupils are indicative of impending transtentorial herniation.

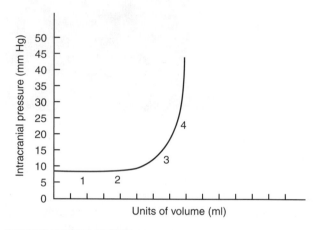

STAGES ON THE CURVE

Stage 1: There is a high compliance and low elastance. The brain is in total compensation, with accommodation and autoregulation intact. An increase in volume does not increase ICP.

Stage 2: The compliance is lower and elastance is increasing. An increase in volume places the patient at risk of increased ICP.

Stage 3: There is high elastance and low compliance. Any small addition of volume causes a great increase in pressure. There is a loss of autoregulation, and there may be symptoms indicating increased ICP, such as systolic hypertension with an increasing pulse pressure, bradycardia, and slowing of respiratory rate (Cushing's triad). With the loss of autoregulation and the rise in the systolic blood pressure as a result of the Cushing response, decompensation occurs. The ICP passively mimics the blood pressure.

Stage 4: Finally, when the patient is in stage 4, the ICP rises to terminal levels with little increase in volume. Herniation occurs as the brain tissue shifts from the compartment of greater pressure to the compartment of lesser pressure.

FIGURE **21-4.** Intracranial volume-pressure curve. *ICP,* Intracranial pressure. (Modified from Lewis SM, Heitkemper MM, Dirksen RF, editors. *Medical-surgical nursing: assessment and management of clinical problems,* ed 7, St. Louis, 2007, Mosby.)

Table 21-2. CRANIAL NERVES AND THEIR FUNCTIONS

Cranial Nerve	Function	Physiologic Effects
I. Olfactory	Sensory	Smell
II. Optic	Sensory	Vision
III. Oculomotor	Motor	Extraocular movement of eyes, raises eyelid, constricts pupils
IV. Trochlear	Motor	Allows eye to move down and inward
V. Trigeminal	Motor and sensory	Facial sensation, mastication, and corneal reflex
VI. Abducens	Motor	Allows eye to move outward
VII. Facial	Motor and sensory	Movement of facial muscles, closes eyes, secretes saliva and tears
VIII. Vestibulo-cochlear	Sensory	Hearing and equilibrium
IX. Glossopharyn-geal	Motor and sensory	Gag reflex, swallowing, and phonation
X. Vagus	Motor and sensory	Voluntary muscles for swallowing, involuntary to visceral muscles (heart, lungs)
XI. Spinal accessory	Motor	Turns head, shrugs shoulders
XII. Hypoglossal	Motor	Tongue movement for swallowing

The oculomotor (CN III), trochlear (CN IV), and abducens (CN VI) nerves control extraocular eye movements. In the conscious patient, extraocular movements should be assessed. Conjugate gaze is movement of both eyes simultaneously in the same direction. This indicates the brainstem and cerebral cortex are functioning. Disconjugate gaze is when one eye is deviated from the normal midposition with the patient at rest. Ask the patient to follow a finger through the six directions of gaze. If any of the three CNs are injured, there will be paralysis or paresis of the extraocular muscles, leading to a disconjugate gaze. Ptosis (drooping eyelid) may also be observed with injury to the oculomotor nerve. Patients may also complain of diplopia as the eyes move through the different positions. Injuries can be unilateral or bilateral; therefore it is important to assess each eye separately and observe for consensual and/or conjugate response.

With severe brain injury it is important to evaluate the integrity of brainstem function. The oculocephalic (doll's eye) reflex tests the integrity of pontine centers.[2,6] A doll's eye examination is performed only in an unconscious patient after the cervical spine has been cleared. To perform the doll's eye examination, briskly rotate the patient's head

---

BOX 21-1 CEREBRAL PERFUSION PRESSURE

MAP − ICP = CPP
Example: Mean arterial pressure = 90 mm Hg
Intracranial pressure = 15 mm Hg
90 mm Hg − 15 mm Hg = 75 mm Hg

CPP, Cerebral perfusion pressure; *ICP*, intracranial pressure; *MAP*, mean arterial pressure.

Box 21-2 SIGNS AND SYMPTOMS OF INCREASED INTRACRANIAL PRESSURE

EARLY

Level of conscious deteriorates: Patient may become, restless, more confused, agitated or combative
Headache
Nausea/vomiting
Slowed or slurred speech
Blurred vision or diplopia
Pupillary changes: Delayed/sluggish reactivity to light, pupil becomes ovoid, unilateral change in pupil size or shape
Decreased strength and sensation

LATE

Progressive decline in level of consciousness to coma
Projectile vomiting (without nausea)
Speech significantly impaired, may only groan
Impaired brainstem reflexes (corneal, gag)
Motor posturing
Unilateral or bilateral pupil that enlarges and becomes fixed
Irregular respirations
Cushing's response
Cardiac dysrhythmias
Abnormal reflexes (Babinski's)

Table 21-3. GLASGOW COMA SCALE

Response	Score	Significance
EYE OPENING		
Spontaneously	4	Reticular activating system is intact; patient may not be aware
To verbal command	3	Opens eyes when told to do so
To pain	2	Opens eyes in response to pain
None	1	Does not open eyes to any stimuli
VERBAL STIMULI		
Oriented, converses	5	Relatively intact CNS, aware of self and environment
Disoriented, converses	4	Well articulated, organized, but disoriented
Inappropriate words	3	Random, exclamatory words
Incomprehensible	2	Moaning, no recognizable words
No response	1	No response or intubated
MOTOR RESPONSE		
Obeys verbal commands	6	Readily moves limbs when told to
Localizes to painful stimuli	5	Moves limb in an effort to remove painful stimuli
Withdrawal	4	Pulls away from pain in flexion
Abnormal flexion	3	Decorticate rigidity
Extension	2	Decerebrate rigidity
No response	1	Hypotonia, flaccid: suggests loss of medullary function or concomitant spinal cord injury

From Geegaard WG, Birow MH: Head. In Marx J, Hockberger R, Walls R: *Rosen's emergency medicine: concepts and clinical practice*, ed 6. St. Louis, 2006, Mosby. Modified from Teasdale G, Jennett B: Assessment of coma and impaired consciousness: a practical scale, *Lancet* 2(7872):81, 1974.
CNS, Central nervous system.

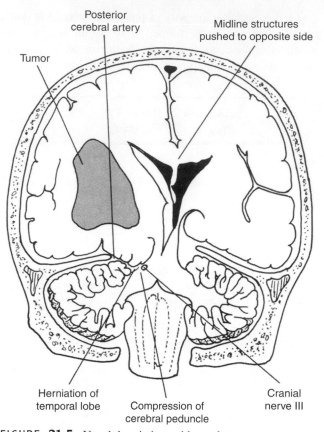

FIGURE **21-5.** Uncal herniation with oculomotor nerve compression. (From Barker E: *Neuroscience nursing: a spectrum of care,* ed 3, St. Louis, 2008, Mosby.)

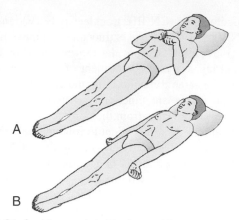

FIGURE **21-6.** Abnormal. **A,** Flexion. and **B,** Extension. (Modified from Urden LD, Stacy KM, Lough ME: *Thelan's critical care nursing: diagnosis and management,* ed 5, St. Louis, 2006, Mosby.)

to the right and then to the left while holding the eyelids open and watching the eye movements. If the reflex is present (brainstem is intact), the patient's eyes deviate away from the direction the head is rotated. Loss of brainstem integrity is presumed when eyes remain midline with rotation of the head or move in a disconjugate manner. The oculovestibular response (cold calorics) also assesses the integrity of the brainstem and is only evaluated in the unconscious patient. The head should be flexed to approximately 30 degrees, and 20 to 50 mL of cold saline is injected into the external auditory canal. Rapid nystagmus-like deviation of the eyes toward the irrigated ear is the normal response. No movement, disconjugate movement, or asymmetric movement indicates interruption in the functional connection between the medulla and midbrain. Severe dizziness and vomiting occur with this test in a conscious patient, so the ice water test is contraindicated in semiconscious or conscious patients. Another contraindication is tympanic membrane rupture.

A patient's motor examination includes assessment for strength and symmetry when possible. Bilateral extremities should be assessed at the same time for comparison and to identify subtle abnormalities or differences. Refer to Chapter 22 for a more detailed description of the motor examination. A central noxious stimulus should be used to elicit a motor response in the uncooperative or unconscious patient. Central stimulation (e.g., trapezius pinch or sternal rub)

produces an overall body response. Peripheral stimulation (e.g., nail bed pressure) is also important to assess to differentiate between a spinal cord injury and brain or brainstem injury. Voluntary purposeful movement should be distinguished from abnormal posturing. Abnormal motor responses include inequality in movement and strength from side to side and posturing. Posturing may be spontaneous or elicited by verbal or painful stimuli. Abnormal flexion posturing (previously called decorticate posturing) is rigid flexion with arms flexed toward the core and lower extremities extended. This type of posturing is associated with lesions above the midbrain. Abnormal extension posturing (previously called decerebrate posturing) is rigid extension of the arms with wrist flexion and rigid extension of lower extremities and is associated with an insult to the brainstem. Figure 21-6 illustrates abnormal flexion and extension posturing. Lateralization occurs when patients with TBI present with unilateral abnormal motor posturing. In a patient with hemiparesis contralateral to a fixed and dilated pupil, herniation should be suspected.[2,6]

A detailed CN examination may be delayed until the secondary or focused survey but should be completed in all patients who are awake and can cooperate. In the severely injured patient the examination may be limited to pupillary responses (CN III), and corneal (CN V and VII) and gag reflexes (CN X).

Assessment of vital signs is an integral part of every initial assessment of a trauma patient. In the patient with brain injury, because of the significant influence the brain and brainstem have on cardiac and respiratory functions, changes in heart rate, blood pressure, and ventilatory rate may be indicators of neurologic deterioration. After major trauma and brain injury the body frequently is in a hyperdynamic state. As ICP rises, the body's compensatory response is to increase systemic pressure in an attempt to maintain CPP. Hypertension is a common manifestation of severe brain injury. Increased heart rate and cardiac output are also part of the body's compensatory response. There are a variety of cardiac dysrhythmias associated with traumatic brain injuries. Bundle branch blocks and atrial fibrillation may be seen with contusions, atrial and ventricular ectopy with subdural hematomas, and ST and T-wave changes with severe brain injuries.[7] Along with ventilatory rate, the pattern of breathing, work of breathing, and auscultation of breath sounds should be assessed. Respiratory pattern changes are common after severe brain injury and can assist in determining the level of brainstem dysfunction (Table 21-4).[2,8]

Temperature changes not only are common in brain injury but also may contribute to secondary injury if the temperature is not controlled. Hypothermia is frequently a result of environmental exposure and the infusion of cold or room temperature intravenous fluids and blood products. Hypothermia is defined as a core temperature of less than 95° F (35° C). Hyperthermia may be seen with hypothalamic damage. Hyperthermia (core temperature >100.4° F [38° C]) increases the cerebral metabolic rate and oxygen requirements. In order to compensate, cerebral blood flow must increase, which results in increased ICP. In the acute resuscitation, one must also consider preexisting infection as a source of the hyperthermia if environmental factors have been eliminated. If cooling measures are necessary, shivering must be avoided because it further increases the metabolic demands.

With severe brain injury and progressive or uncontrolled intracranial hypertension, the body exhibits a syndrome of vital sign changes called the Cushing's reflex or Cushing's response. The presence of the Cushing's response is a late finding and indicates that ICP has reached life-threatening levels. These changes include hypertension, widening pulse pressure, and bradycardia and are related to pressure on the medullary areas of the brainstem.[2] The systolic pressure increases in an attempt to overcome the compression of the cerebral arteries and diminished flow to the brain (from ICP). Blood pressure that is decreased with brain injuries indicates a poor prognosis.

PATIENT MANAGEMENT

Management of a brain-injured patient begins in the prehospital setting. Patients with severe brain injury likely benefit from early intubation and targeted ventilation.[31] In addition, it is important to ensure that these patients are transported to trauma centers with neurosurgical and neurocritical care capabilities as early as possible to reduce morbidity and mortality.[14] Communication with prehospital providers during transport allows ED and trauma personnel to be adequately prepared to receive and resuscitate the patient. Once the patient is admitted into the ED, initial stabilization of the brain-injured patient is directed toward maintenance of oxygenation, ventilation, restoration of circulating blood volume, and maintenance of systemic blood pressure to ensure adequate cerebral perfusion. Patients with a GCS less than 8 are considered to have a significant brain injury and require endotracheal intubation to protect their airway, to minimize the risk for aspiration, and to ensure adequate ventilation. Because hypoxia has a significant contribution to the morbidity and mortality of the brain-injured patient, oxygen

saturations should be maintained above 90% and PaO_2 levels greater than 60 mm Hg.[13] Circulatory management is directed at maintaining systolic blood pressure at greater than 90 mm Hg to ensure adequate CPP. Isotonic crystalloids are the fluids of choice in the initial resuscitation along with blood products based on estimated prehospital and ongoing blood loss. Hypotonic solutions should be avoided in the brain-injured patient because they can potentiate cerebral edema. Although a lower hemoglobin and hematocrit level is often considered acceptable in the trauma patient, in the brain-injured patient, it is essential to maximize oxygen-carrying capacity and oxygen delivery.[13]

Once the patient is initially stabilized, diagnostic studies to evaluate the type, location, and extent of the brain injury are completed. Table 21-5 discusses some of the diagnostic studies with regard to purpose and advantages. Currently the primary radiographic study for the evaluation of brain injury in the ED phase of care is the computed tomography (CT) scan. Skull radiographs are no longer indicated because CT scanning has become much more efficient, as well as sensitive, for both skull fractures and intracranial lesions.[15] More recently, helical CT with multidetector technology allows for extremely rapid imaging and much higher quality images along with the ability to do three-dimensional reconstruction.[15] Other studies include cerebral angiography and magnetic resonance imaging (MRI). Cerebral angiography is useful when there is suspicion of cerebral vascular abnormality (aneurysm). MRI is beneficial to further delineate the extent of diffuse axonal injury and brainstem injury; however, this is less commonly indicated as part of the acute evaluation. All patients with significant brain injury and alterations in level of consciousness must also be evaluated for cervical spine injury through spine radiographs or CT imaging.

After initial stabilization of the patient, the emergency nurse should consider other interventions that promote optimal neurologic recovery. In the remainder of this section, the emphasis will be directed toward the patient with a severe brain injury incorporating the Guidelines for the Management of Severe Traumatic Brain Injury published by the Brain Trauma Foundation and the American Association of Neurological Surgeons Joint Section on Neurotrauma and Critical Care.[13] Management of patients with mild traumatic brain injuries will be discussed in the section on specific injuries. In addition, an integral component of caring for brain-injured patients is inclusion of the family or significant other in the plan of care. Brain injuries can be overwhelming for the family; psychosocial support and education regarding the injury cannot be overemphasized and should begin in the ED phase of care.

Hyperventilation

Traditionally hyperventilation was used as a means of reducing ICP by vasoconstriction of cerebral vessels, which decreased cerebral blood flow and ultimately cerebral volume. However, now cerebral blood flow studies illustrate

Table 21-4. PATTERNS OF BREATHING

Breathing Pattern	Description	Location of Injury
HEMISPHERIC BREATHING PATTERNS		
Normal	After a period of hyperventilation that lowers the arterial carbon dioxide pressure ($Paco_2$), the individual continues to breathe regularly but with a reduced depth.	Response of the nervous system to an external stressor—not associated with injury to the CNS.
Posthyperventilation apnea (PHVA)	Respirations stop after hyperventilation has lowered the PCO_2 level below normal. Rhythmic breathing returns when the PCO_2 level returns to normal. (Usually an intact cerebral cortex will trigger breathing within 10 seconds, regardless of PCO_2.)	Associated with diffuse bilateral metabolic or structural disease of the cerebrum.
Cheyne-Stokes respirations (CSR)	The breathing pattern has a smooth increase (crescendo) in the rate and depth of breathing (hyperpnea), which peaks and is followed by a gradual smooth decrease (decrescendo) in the rate and depth of breathing to the point of apnea when the cycle repeats itself. The hyperpneic phase lasts longer than the apneic phase (represents an amplitude change).	Bilateral dysfunction of the deep cerebral or diencephalic structures, seen with supratentorial injury and metabolically induced coma states unrelated to neurologic dysfunction, also may be seen in CHF.
BRAINSTEM BREATHING PATTERNS		
Central reflex hyperpnea (Central neurogenic hyperventilation [CNH])	A sustained deep, rapid, but regular pattern (hyperpnea) occurs, with a decreased $Paco_2$ and a corresponding increase in pH and increased Po_2.	May result from CNS damage or disease that involves the midbrain and upper pons; seen after increased intracranial pressure and blunt level trauma.
Apneusis	A prolonged inspiratory cramp (a pause at full inspiration) occurs. A common variant of this is a brief end-inspiratory pause of 2 or 3 seconds often alternating with an end-expiratory pause.	Indicates damage to the respiratory control mechanism located at the pontine level; most commonly associated with pontine infarction but documented with hypoglycemia, anoxia, and meningitis.
Cluster breathing	A cluster of breaths has a disordered sequence with irregular pauses between breaths.	Dysfunction in the lower pontine and high medullary areas.
Ataxic breathing	Completely irregular breathing occurs, with random shallow and deep breaths and irregular pauses. Often the rate is slow.	Originates from a primary dysfunction of the lower pons or upper medulla.
Gasping breathing pattern (agonal gasps)	A pattern of deep "all-or-none" breaths is accompanied by a slow respiratory rate.	Indicative of a failing medullary respiratory center.

From Boss BJ: Concepts of neurologic dysfunction. In McCance KL, Huether SE: *Pathophysiology: the biologic basis for disease in adults and children*, ed 5, St. Louis, 2006, Mosby.
CHF, Congestive heart failure; *CNS*, central nervous system.

Table 21-5. DIAGNOSTIC EVALUATION FOR HEAD INJURY

Diagnostic Examination	Purpose	Comments
Cervical spine radiographs	Visualization of all seven cervical vertebrae to rule out injury	Tomograms or CT scans of the cervical spine may be necessary to rule out injury.
CT scan	Detect intracranial injuries—bleeds, hematomas, cerebral edema	Patients may require sedation to obtain adequate CT scan.

CT, Computed tomography.

there is a substantial reduction in cerebral blood flow within the first few hours of injury.[13,25] Numerous studies have now concluded that hyperventilation can actually be more detrimental to the severely injured brain by causing further ischemia.[1,13,25,29,31] Hyperventilation reduces cerebral blood flow without consistently decreasing ICP. In addition, autoregulation may be interrupted, further compromising blood flow to the injured area. In the acute resuscitation with evidence of significant neurologic deterioration or when ICP is refractory to other measures, hyperventilation may be used as a temporizing measure; however, the PCO_2 should be maintained at greater than or equal to 30 mm Hg.[13] Prophylactic hyperventilation should be avoided.

Table 21-6. COMPARISON OF INTRACRANIAL PRESSURE MONITORS

Type	Site	Advantages	Disadvantages
Subarachnoid bolt or screw	Subarachnoid space	Can be used with small or collapsed ventricles; does not penetrate brain parenchyma; low infection rates; low cost; ease and safety of insertion that can be performed quickly	Does not allow CSF drainage or withdrawal; becomes occluded; may have dampened waveform to give unreliable readings after a few days; blood or brain tissue may herniate into bolt; less accurate at higher ICP elevations
Intraventricular catheter (IVC) or ventriculostomy	Ventricles	Ventricular site provides more accuracy; CSF cultures can be collected; allows CSF to be withdrawn to control ICP; contrast materials can be injected for radiologic studies	Risk for hemorrhage due to invasiveness; increased risk for infection; risk for CSF leak at site; artifacts may cause dampening of recordings; more difficult to insert, especially for collapsed, small or displaced ventricles
Epidural or subdural sensor	Epidural or subdural space	Ease of insertion; least invasive; recommended in case of meningitis and CNS infection; less risk for infection; does not require recalibration	Slower response time; fragile; can become wedged against skull; affected by heat or febrile patient; expensive; diaphragm can rupture; less accurate; unable to sample or drain CSF
Intraparenchymal	Brain parenchyma	Quick insertion, accurate, reliable approach when ventricular access is not an option	Unable to drain CSF; may become clogged

From Barker E: *Neuroscience nursing: a spectrum of care,* ed 3, St. Louis, 2008, Mosby.
CSF, Cerebrospinal fluid; *ICP,* intracranial pressure.

Hyperosmolar Therapy

Hyperosmolar therapy is aimed at reducing ICP through several mechanisms: plasma expansion and reduced blood viscosity, improved cerebral blood flow with a concomitant decrease in cerebral blood volume, and finally by creating an osmotic gradient that pulls water from cerebral tissue into the vascular space.[4,6,13,32] Mannitol has been widely used as a method to control ICP. Along with its osmotic properties, mannitol has neuroprotective properties, including free radical scavenging. Mannitol should be administered at doses of 0.25 to 1 g/kg. Mannitol should only be administered in bolus doses, and the Guidelines for Severe Traumatic Brain Injury do not support the use of continuous infusions.[13] More recently, hypertonic saline in various strengths (3%, 7.5%, and 10%) has been used and studied as an additional hyperosmolar agent for the management of increased ICP. The principal effect of hypertonic saline on ICP is through the osmotic gradient created in the brain and subsequent reduction of water content. Along with an osmotic change, hypertonic saline has been shown to alter hemodynamics, including increased MAP and vasoregulatory and immunologic effects.[17] Some reported advantages of hypertonic saline over mannitol include a longer duration of therapeutic modification and immunomodulation.[4,17] Currently there are no recommended doses or concentrations of hypertonic saline in adults. Use of 3% saline as a continuous infusion is recommended in children with severe brain injury.[13]

ICP Monitoring, ICP and CPP Management

Recommended indications for invasive management of intracranial hypertension include abnormal admission CT scan with GCS ≤8. Indications in the presence of normal CT scan are two or more of the following: age greater than 40 years, abnormal motor posturing, or systolic blood pressure less than 90 mm Hg. ICP monitoring aids in the detection of intracranial mass lesions, limits unnecessary use of adjunctive therapies to control ICP, facilitates drainage of CSF (through ventricular catheters), and helps guide therapy and predict outcome.[13] The ultimate goal of ICP monitoring is to optimize ICP and cerebral perfusion. There are several types of monitoring systems available. Table 21-6 describes the most common types of monitoring methods along with advantages and disadvantages. Studies have shown that ventricular catheters with an external strain gauge are the most accurate means of monitoring ICP. Many facilities use a fiberoptic monitor and external strain gauge device simultaneously to ensure accurate ICP monitoring (Figure 21-7).

Management of elevated ICP includes measures that ensure adequate cerebral blood flow. Scientific evidence has clearly established that maintaining ICP below 20 mm Hg improves outcomes. Treatment should be initiated when ICP is greater than 20 mm Hg for more than 5 minutes. Sedation with benzodiazepines and opioid analgesia are first-line agents to assist in minimizing the noxious effects of endotracheal intubation and other stimuli, pain from other traumatic injuries, and the control of ICP.[3,13] Common benzodiazepines include midazolam (Versed) and lorazepam (Ativan). Midazolam (Versed) has the advantage of being short acting with small intermittent dosing. Propofol has become widely used due to its rapid onset and short duration of action, allowing for repeat neurologic assessments in the brain-injured patient who requires sedation. Propofol may have additional beneficial properties of maintaining or improving cerebral autoregulation.[16] High-dose propofol is not recommended

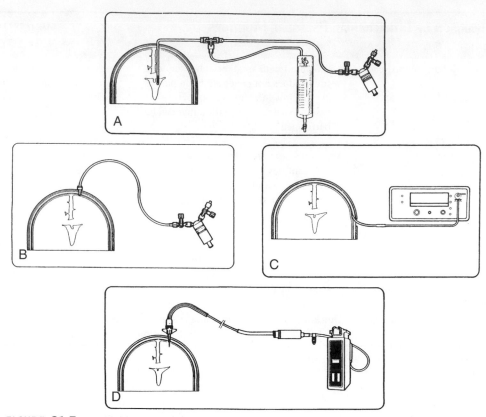

FIGURE **21-7.** **A,** Ventricular pressure monitoring system. **B,** Subarachnoid pressure monitoring system. **C,** Epidural pressure monitoring system. **D,** Intraparenchymal pressure monitoring system. (From Thelan LA et al: *Critical care nursing: diagnosis and management,* ed 5, St. Louis, 1998, Mosby.)

due to the risk for propofol infusion syndrome and increased mortality.[13]

In conjunction with management of intracranial hypertension, cerebral perfusion must be maximized. Current recommendations are to maintain cerebral perfusion between 50 mm Hg and 70 mm Hg.[13] Augmented CPP has demonstrated enhanced cerebral blood flow and may help to maintain the autoregulatory mechanisms in the injured brain. CPP management is directed at keeping patients normovolemic and avoiding excessive hypotonic fluids. Vasopressors are widely used to augment systemic blood pressure and MAP and thus improve CPP. There have been no clinical studies to compare the various vasopressors; however, phenylephrine (Neo-Synephrine), norepinephrine (Levophed), and vasopressin are the most frequently used agents. Along with fluids and pressures, maintaining a hematocrit level at 30% to 35% with administration of blood products improves oxygen delivery. Maintaining CPP at higher than 70 mm Hg with fluids and pressors is associated with increased risk for acute respiratory distress syndrome (ARDS).[13] Paralytic agents can also be used in conjunction with sedatives and analgesics to reduce skeletal muscle activity, metabolic rate, and oxygen consumption. Short-acting paralytic agents are frequently part of institutional rapid sequence intubation protocols. Both short- and long-acting paralytics may be beneficial in the ED management

of the brain-injured patient to facilitate diagnostic studies and help reduce the noxious stimuli associated with the acute resuscitation.

In the last decade, technology that allows for continuous monitoring of brain tissue oxygenation and temperature (PbtO$_2$) in conjunction with ICP has become available. The monitor is placed in the white matter of the brain 2 to 3 cm below the dura. Normal white matter brain tissue oxygen is approximately 25 to 30 mm Hg.[1,13,20,33] Low values of PbtO$_2$ are associated with a poorer outcome. In conjunction with traditional ICP and CPP management, using the PbtO$_2$ levels to guide therapy may improve outcomes of patients with severe brain injury. A full discussion of this technology is beyond the scope of this text.

Additional Treatment Modalities

Early seizure activity should be treated with appropriate anticonvulsants. Prophylactic use of anticonvulsants is not recommended for prevention of late postinjury seizure activity. Barbiturate therapy may be considered for patients with refractory intracranial hypertension. Hemodynamic stability should be confirmed before induction of barbiturate coma. No evidence exists to support routine use of glucocorticoids in brain injury. Follow-up of patients who received steroids after brain injury reveals no difference in outcomes. If cervical spine injury has been ruled out and the patient is hemodynamically stable, elevate the head of the bed 30 to 45 degrees, which may decrease ICP. Maintaining the head in neutral alignment also facilitates venous drainage.

SPECIFIC INJURIES

Brain injuries can be classified by their mechanism (blunt or penetrating), by severity (mild, moderate, or severe), or by the type of injury (fracture, focal brain injury, diffuse brain injury). Patients with mild brain injuries have an initial GCS of 14 to 15. Frequently these patients are evaluated and treated in the ED and may be discharged home after a short period of observation. Moderate brain injures are classified as those patients with initial GCS of 9 to13. Moderate brain injuries are associated with structural damage (e.g., contusions) and have a high potential for deterioration because of increasing cerebral edema and ICP. They require frequent neurologic assessments and a high index of suspicion for potential deterioration (Box 21-3).[6] Severe brain injuries are those patients who have initial GCS of 8 or less. These injuries are often associated with significant structural damage, they have a high mortality rate, and patients who survive frequently have long-term or permanent cognitive and physical disabilities. Aggressive management to ensure adequate oxygenation and prevention of hypotension is essential in these patients to prevent secondary brain injury.

Focal Injuries

Scalp Lacerations

The scalp protects the brain from injury by acting as a cushion to reduce energy transmission to underlying structures. Excessive force applied to the scalp often causes a laceration. The scalp has an extensive vascular supply with poor vasoconstrictive properties, causing lacerations to bleed profusely. Bleeding can be controlled with direct pressure to the affected area followed by wound repair and tetanus prophylaxis as indicated. Staples or clips may also be used for rapid closure.

Skull Fractures

Skull fractures occur when energy applied to the skull causes bony deformation. Clinical presentation of skull fractures is directly correlated to type of fracture, area involved, and damage to underlying structures. A linear skull fracture is nondisplaced and associated with minimal neurologic deficit (Figure 21-8). Supportive care is usually all that is required for optimal neurologic recovery.

When energy displaces the outer table of bone below the inner table of the adjoining skull, a depressed skull fracture occurs (Figure 21-9). Surgical elevation is required when depressed bone fragments become lodged in brain tissue. Open depressed skull fractures are surgically elevated and repaired as soon as possible because of increased risk for infection.

Box 21-3	RISK STRATIFICATION IN PATIENTS WITH MINOR HEAD TRAUMA

HIGH RISK

Focal neurologic findings
Asymmetric pupils
Skull fracture on clinical examination
Multiple trauma
Serious, painful, distracting injuries
External signs of trauma above the clavicles
Initial Glasgow Coma Scale score of 14 or 15
Loss of consciousness
Posttraumatic confusion/anemia
Progressively worsening headache
Vomiting
Posttraumatic seizure
History of bleeding disorder/anticoagulation
Recent ingestion of intoxicants
Unreliable/unknown history of injury
Previous neurologic diagnosis
Previous epilepsy
Suspected child abuse
Age >60 yr, <2 yr

MEDIUM RISK

Initial Glasgow Coma Scale score of 15
Brief loss of consciousness
Posttraumatic amnesia
Vomiting
Headache
Intoxication

LOW RISK

Currently asymptomatic
No other injuries
No focality on examination
Normal pupils
No change in consciousness
Intact orientation/memory
Initial Glasgow Coma Scale score of 15
Accurate history
Trivial mechanism
Injury >24 hr ago
No or mild headache
No vomiting
No preexisting high-risk factors

From Geegaard WG, Birow MH: Head. In Marx J, Hockberger R, Walls R: *Rosen's emergency medicine: concepts and clinical practice,* ed 6. St. Louis, 2006, Mosby.

A basilar skull fracture develops when enough force is exerted on the base of the skull to cause deformity. The base of the skull includes any bony area where the skull ends and is not limited to the posterior aspect of the skull. A basilar skull fracture may be visualized on a radiograph; however, this is not always true. Approximately 25% of basilar skull fractures are not seen on radiographs; therefore diagnosis is usually made on the basis of clinical findings. Basilar skull fractures that overlay the middle meningeal artery may cause

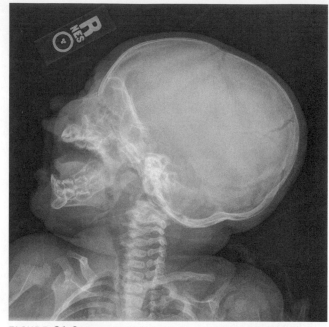

FIGURE **21-8.** Linear skull fractures in a 1-month-old child who was a victim of child abuse.

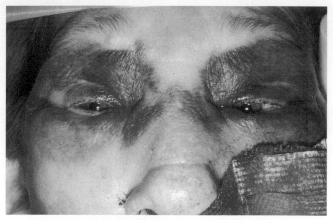

FIGURE **21-10.** Raccoon eyes.

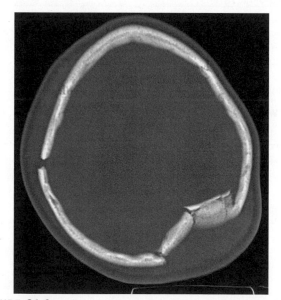

FIGURE **21-9.** Severely depressed skull fracture in a patient after a fall.

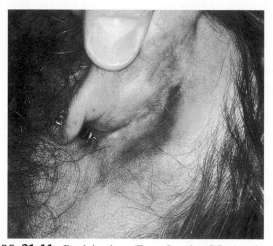

FIGURE **21-11.** Battle's sign. (From London PS: *A color atlas of diagnosis after recent injury,* London, 1990, Wolfe Medical Publications.)

a subgaleal hematoma. Disruption of the middle meningeal artery is the cause of more than 75% of epidural hematomas. A basilar skull fracture may also cause intracerebral bleeding.

Neurologic changes that occur with a basilar skull fracture range from mild changes in mentation to combativeness and severe agitation. Combative behavior is often considered a hallmark of a basilar skull fracture. Clinical manifestations of a basilar skull fracture include periorbital ecchymoses (raccoon eyes) (Figure 21-10) from intraorbital bleeding, Battle's sign (ecchymosis over the mastoid

process) (Figure 21-11) 12 to 24 hours after initial injury, hemotympanum (blood behind the tympanic membrane caused by a fracture of the temporal bone), and CSF leak from the nose or ear caused by temporal bone fracture. If the tympanic membrane is intact, fluid drains through the eustachian tube and appears as CSF rhinorrhea. However, absence of visible CSF does not eliminate the possibility of a basilar skull fracture. If a CSF leak is considered, test the fluid draining from the nose on filter paper. Formation of two distinct rings is called the "halo" or "ring" sign and indicates presence of CSF. Clear fluid should be tested for glucose, a normal finding in CSF.

Diagnostic interventions include CT scanning. Additional interventions focus on protecting the patient from injury, preventing infection, and using nasal drip pads as needed for rhinorrhea. Nasal packing is not recommended. Frequent neurologic assessment with ongoing reassessment is essential for early identification of deterioration in neurologic function.

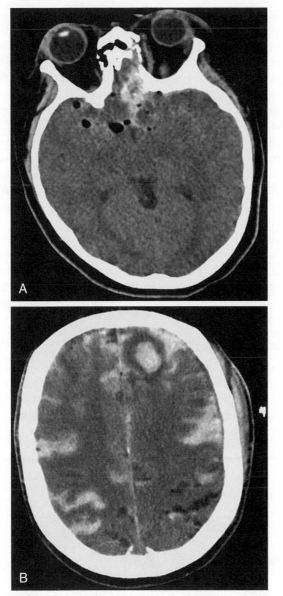

FIGURE **21-12.** **A,** Right temporal contusion in a patient after motor vehicle collision. **B,** Large left hemorrhagic contusion in a man who hit a deer. He also has a large amount of subarachnoid hemorrhage.

Contusion

Cerebral contusion is a bruise on the surface of the brain that occurs from movement of the brain within the cranial vault (Figure 21-12, *A* and *B*). When an acceleration-deceleration injury occurs, two contusions may result, one at the initial site of impact (coup) and one on the opposite side of the impact (contrecoup). The clinical presentation varies with size and location of the contusion. Commonly occurring symptoms include altered level of consciousness, nausea, vomiting, visual disturbances, weakness, and speech difficulty. Interventions focus on preservation of neurologic function, control of pain, and adequate hydration. Patients with cerebral contusions require admission and serial neurologic assessments. Contusions often increase in size over the first

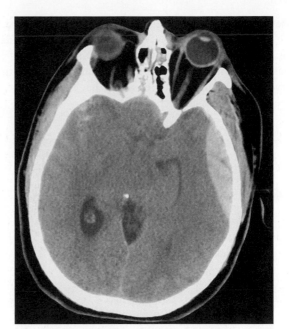

FIGURE **21-13.** Epidural hematoma.

12 to 24 hours, causing deterioration in neurologic status due to increased ICP. In patients with very large contusions at initial presentation, some neurosurgeons may elect to surgically evacuate the contusion and leave the bone flap off to allow for swelling of the brain.

Epidural Hematoma

Epidural hematoma is bleeding between the skull and dura mater (Figure 21-13), usually resulting from a direct blow to the head. A skull fracture and injury to the middle meningeal artery may also be present. A torn middle meningeal artery with arterial bleeding leads to a rapidly forming hematoma, with associated morbidity and mortality of more than 50%. Approximately half of the patients with an epidural hematoma have no evidence of skull fracture. Signs and symptoms include a brief period of unconsciousness followed by a lucid period, then another loss of consciousness. This brief lucid period is considered a hallmark of an epidural hematoma; however, it does not occur in all patients. If alert, the patient with an epidural hematoma complains of severe headache and may exhibit hemiparesis and a dilated pupil on the side of injury. Large epidural hematomas require emergent surgical evacuation; however, small hematomas may be managed conservatively with serial neurologic examinations and repeat diagnostic imaging, particularly in a patient who has minimal neurologic deficits on initial presentation to the ED.

Subdural Hematoma

Subdural hematomas occur more frequently than other intracranial injuries and have the highest morbidity and mortality of all hematomas. Bleeding into the subdural space between the dura mater and the arachnoid leads to subdural hematoma (Figure 21-14). A subdural hematoma may be acute, subacute, or chronic. When acute, the hematoma usually results from dissipation of energy that ruptures bridging veins in the subdural space. Clinical features are loss of consciousness; hemiparesis; and fixed, dilated pupils. Surgical intervention within 4 hours of injury has the best potential for neurologic recovery.

Subacute subdural hematomas develop 48 hours to 2 weeks after injury. The clinical presentation is progressive decline in level of consciousness as the hematoma slowly expands. The brain compensates as a result of slow blood collection over time, so decline in neurologic function occurs gradually. After the subdural is drained, the patient improves quickly with little or no lasting neurologic deficit.

Chronic subdural hematomas, seen more frequently in older adults, progress slowly. Blood collects over weeks to months; by the time a person is examined, the causative mechanism may have been forgotten. Chronic subdural hematomas are initially tolerated by older adults because of brain atrophy associated with aging. As the brain decreases in size, the space within the cranial vault increases. A hematoma collects over time without obvious changes in neurologic status until its size is sufficient to produce a mass effect. Treatment of a chronic subdural consists of burr holes and a subdural drain. Patients become more alert after the subdural is drained.

Other Focal Injuries

Intraventricular hemorrhage (Figure 21-15) and intracerebral clots (Figure 21-16) are types of focal injuries. Management depends on the size of the clot and source of bleeding. Surgical evacuation may be necessary in concert with medical management of increased ICP.

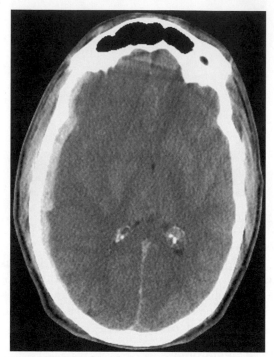

FIGURE **21-14.** Subdural hematoma.

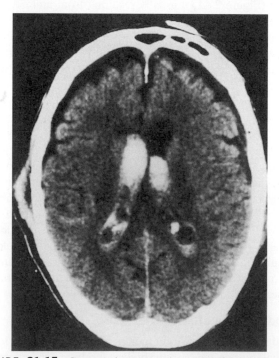

FIGURE **21-15.** Computed tomography scan of head showing intraventricular hemorrhage secondary to motor vehicle collision. (From Parrillo JE, Bone RC: *Critical care medicine: principles of diagnosis and management,* St. Louis, 1995, Mosby.)

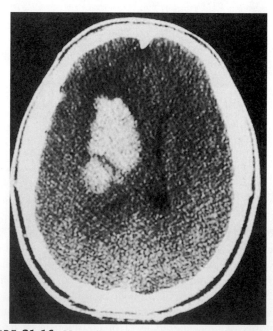

FIGURE **21-16.** Nonenhanced computed tomography scan showing large right hemispheric clot in 26-year-old male patient who sustained closed-head injury from a motor vehicle collision. Note mass effect on right lateral ventricle. (From Parrillo JE, Bone RC: *Critical care medicine: principles of diagnosis and management,* St. Louis, 1995, Mosby.)

Diffuse Brain Injuries

Mild Traumatic Brain Injury (Concussion)

Previously called concussion, mild traumatic brain injury (MTBI) can occur as a result of a direct blow to the head or from an acceleration or deceleration injury in which the brain collides with the inside of the skull. Previously, MTBI was defined as a loss of consciousness without defined changes on initial diagnostic imaging. It is now known that there is some degree of neurochemical as well as axonal disruption associated with MTBI, and this is the basis for the persistence of symptoms known as post-concussive syndrome. An MTBI may be associated with cognitive, physical, emotional, and sleep disturbances (Table 21-7). Acutely, it is typically associated with a loss of consciousness followed by transient neurologic changes such as nausea, vomiting, temporary amnesia, headache, and possible brief loss of vision.

Care for the patient with an MTBI includes observation, especially with prolonged loss of consciousness (greater than 2 to 3 minutes). With protracted nausea and vomiting, hospital admission may be considered to avoid dehydration. Nonnarcotic analgesia may be administered for headache. Narcotics affect the level of consciousness and interfere with ongoing patient assessment. Patients with an MTBI may be discharged with a responsible adult who will observe the patient overnight for possible complications, such as confusion, difficulty walking, altered level of consciousness, projectile vomiting, and unequal pupils. Discharge teaching includes instructions on how to assess neurologic status in the home and when to contact the primary care provider. Because MTBI is associated with some degree of structural changes, many experts in the field are now recommending periods of "brain rest" along with physical rest after a brain injury.[11,12,24,28] Patients should not return to sports, work, school, or engage in high-risk activities until all symptoms of the brain injury are gone. It is also recommended that there is a gradual return to work and school. With the increasing awareness and emphasis on MTBI in sports, in 2007 the CDC published several booklets for parents, athletes, coaches, and physicians on the diagnosis and management of MTBI.

Headache, memory loss, concentration difficulties, and difficulty with activities of daily living are characteristic of postconcussion syndrome. Clinical manifestations of this syndrome may persist for weeks or months and occasionally permanently after the patient's initial injury. Interventions include supportive treatment and recognition that this is a true physiologic consequence of what was perceived as a minor head injury.

Diffuse Axonal Injury

The phrase "diffuse axonal injury" (DAI) illustrates the major pathophysiologic event associated with the most severe form of TBI. This injury is almost always the result of blunt trauma that causes shearing and disruption of neuronal structures, predominantly white matter. Prognosis for diffuse axonal injuries depends on the degree of injury (mild, moderate, or severe) and severity of damage from any secondary injury. The terms *mild, moderate,* and *severe* reflect the clinical presentation of diffuse axonal injury and should not be confused with the grading system indicating the actual underlying pathophysiology of DAI.

Mild DAI is characterized by loss of consciousness for 6 to 24 hours. Initially the patient may exhibit abnormal flexion or extension posturing but improves rapidly within 24 hours. Return to baseline neurologic status may occur over days, but periods of amnesia may be present.

Moderate DAI is a coma lasting longer than 24 hours, possibly extending over a period of days. Brainstem dysfunction (abnormal flexion or extension posturing) is evident almost immediately and may continue until the patient begins to wake. Patients with moderate DAI usually recover but rarely return to full preinjury neurologic function.

Severe DAI is characterized by brainstem impairment that does not resolve. Victims of severe DAI remain comatose for days to weeks. Autonomic dysfunction may also be present. Overall prognosis for severe diffuse axonal injury is extremely poor. Early CT scans may be unremarkable; however, serial examinations reveal areas of edema and

Table 21-7. SIGNS AND SYMPTOMS ASSOCIATED WITH MILD TRAUMATIC BRAIN INJURY

Physical	Cognitive	Emotional	Sleep
• Headache	• Feeling mentally "foggy"	• Irritability	• Drowsiness
• Nausea	• Feeling slowed down	• Sadness	• Sleeping less than usual
• Vomiting	• Difficulty concentrating	• More emotional	• Sleeping more than usual
• Balance problems	• Difficulty remembering	• Nervousness	• Trouble falling asleep
• Dizziness	• Forgetful of recent information or conversations		
• Visual problems	• Confused about recent events		
• Fatigue	• Answers questions slowly		
• Sensitivity to light	• Repeats questions		
• Sensitivity to noise			
• Numbness/Tingling			
• Dazed or stunned			

From *Heads up: facts for physicians about mild traumatic brain injury,* Atlanta, 2007, Centers for Disease Control and Prevention.

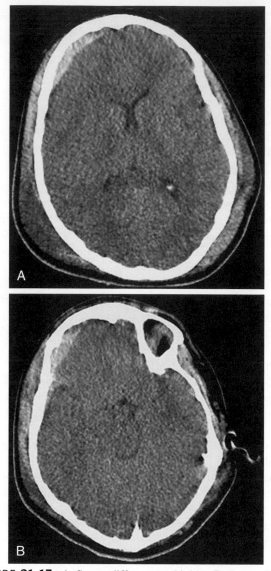

FIGURE **21-17. A,** Severe diffuse axonal injury. **B,** Severe diffuse axonal injury with right subdural hematoma.

microvascular hemorrhage (Figure 21-17). Treatment for all degrees of DAI includes general supportive care, prevention of further brain injury, and support for the family.

SUMMARY

Despite advances in our understanding of the pathophysiologic changes of brain injury and advances in diagnostic technology and monitoring capabilities, TBI remains a major cause of death and long-term disability. Management of the severely injured patient in the acute resuscitation should focus on aggressive airway and ventilatory management to ensure adequate oxygenation along with restoring intravascular volume, preventing hypotension, and ensuring adequate cerebral perfusion. Maximizing outcomes for the severely brain-injured patient requires a collaborative multidisciplinary team from the time of injury throughout the continuum of care. Although there has been much research

on managing severe brain injuries, the emergency nurse will care for many more patients with mild and moderate brain injuries. It is essential that emergency care providers recognize the patient at risk for deterioration and ensure repeated neurologic assessments. Finally, there must be additional emphasis placed on patient education and the public's understanding of MTBI.

REFERENCES

1. Adamides AA, Winter CD, Lewis PM et al: Current controversies in the management of patients with severe traumatic brain injury, *ANZ J Surg* 76(3):163, 2006.
2. Barker E: The adult neurologic assessment. In Barker E: *Neuroscience nursing: a spectrum of care*, ed 3, St. Louis, 2008, Mosby.
3. Barker E: Intracranial pressure and monitoring. In Barker E: *Neuroscience nursing: a spectrum of care*, ed 3, St. Louis, 2008, Mosby.
4. Bayir H, Clark RS, Kochanek PM: Promising strategies to minimize secondary brain injury after head trauma, *Crit Care Med* 31(1):S112, 2003.
5. Bazarian JJ, Garcia M: All-terrain vehicle–related traumatic brain injuries in the US, *Acad Emerg Med* 11(5): 514, 2004.
6. Biros MH, Heegard W: Head trauma. In Marx JA, Hockberger RS, Walls RM: *Rosen's emergency medicine: concepts and clinical practice*, ed 5, St. Louis, 2002, Mosby.
7. Blank-Reid C, McClelland RN, Santora TA: Neurotrauma: traumatic brain injury. In Barker E: *Neuroscience nursing: a spectrum of care*, ed 3, St. Louis, 2008, Mosby.
8. Boss BJ, Wilkerson RR: Concepts of neurologic dysfunction. In McCance KL, Huether SE: *Pathophysiology: the biologic basis for disease in adults and children*, ed 5, St. Louis, 2006, Mosby.
9. Brandenburg MA, Archer P, Mallonee S: All-terrain vehicle–related central nervous system injuries in Oklahoma, *J Okla State Med Assoc* 98(5):194, 2005.
10. Brener I, Harman JS, Kelleher KJ et al: Medical costs of mild to moderate traumatic brain injury in children, *J Head Trauma Rehabil* 19(5):405, 2004.
11. Centers for Disease Control and Prevention: *Heads up: facts for physicians about mild traumatic brain injury*, 2007, Centers for Disease Control and Prevention.
12. Concussion (mild traumatic brain injury) and the team physician: a consensus statement, *Med Sci Sports Exerc* 37(11):2012, 2005.
13. Guidelines for the management of severe traumatic brain injury, ed 3, *J Neurotrauma* 24(suppl 1):561, 2007.
14. Hartl R, Gerber LM, Iacono L et al: Direct transport within an organized state trauma system reduces mortality in patients with severe traumatic brain injury, *J Trauma* 60(6):1250, 2006.
15. Iaia A, Barker E: Neurodiagnostic studies. In Barker E: *Neuroscience nursing: a spectrum of care*, ed 3, St. Louis, 2008, Mosby.

16. Johnston AJ, Steiner LA, Chatfield DA et al: Effects of propofol on cerebral oxygenation and metabolism after head injury, *Br J Anaesth* 91(6):781, 2003.

17. Knapp JM: Hyperosmolar therapy in the treatment of severe head injury in children: mannitol and hypertonic saline, *AACN Clin Issues* 16(2):199, 2005.

18. Langlois JA, Rutlan-Brown W, Thomas KE: *Traumatic brain injury in the United States: emergency department visits, hospitalizations, and deaths*, 2004, Centers for Disease Control and Prevention.

19. Littlejohns LR, Bader MK: Guidelines for the management of severe head injury: clinical application and changes in practice, *Crit Care Nurse* 21(6):48, 2001.

20. Littlejohns LR, Bader MK: Prevention of secondary brain injury: targeting technology, *AACN Clin Issues* 16(4):501, 2005.

21. Miller B, Baig I, Hayes J et al: Injury outcomes in children following automobile, motorcycle, and all-terrain vehicle accidents: an institutional review, *J Neurosurg* 10(5):S182, 2006.

22. Nolan S: Traumatic brain injury: a review, *Crit Care Nurs Q* 28(2):188, 2005.

23. Roth P, Farls K: Pathophysiology of traumatic brain injury, *Crit Care Nurs Q* 23(3):14, 2000.

24. Ruff R: Two decades of advances in understanding mild traumatic brain injury, *J Head Trauma Rehabil* 20(1):5, 2005.

25. Stocchetti N, Maas AIR, Chieregato A et al: Hyperventilation in head injury, *Chest* 127(5):1812, 2005.

26. Sugerman RA: Structure and function of the neurologic system. In McCance KL, Huether SE: *Pathophysiology: the biologic basis for disease in adults and children*, ed 5, St. Louis, 2006, Mosby.

27. Teasdale G, Jennett B: Assessment of coma and impaired consciousness: a practical scale, *Lancet* 2(7872):81, 1974.

28. Terrell TR: Concussion in athletes, *South Med J* 97(9): 837, 2004.

29. Thomas SH, Orf J, Wedel SK et al: Hyperventilation in traumatic brain injury patients: inconsistency between consensus guidelines and clinical practice, *J Trauma* 52(1):47, 2002.

30. Thompson K, Antony A, Holtzman A: The costs of traumatic brain injury, *NC Med J* 62(6):376, 2001.

31. Warner KJ, Cushieri J, Copass MK et al: The impact of prehospital ventilation on outcome after severe traumatic brain injury, *J Trauma* 62(6):1330, 2007.

32. White H, Cook D, Venkatesh B: The use of hypertonic saline for treating intracranial hypertension after traumatic brain injury, *Anesth Analg* 102(6):1836, 2006.

33. Zauner A, Daughtery WP, Bullock MR et al: Brain oxygenation and energy metabolism. I. Biological function and pathophysiology, *Neurosurgery* 59(2): 289, 2002.

CHAPTER 22

Spinal Trauma

Jennifer Wilbeck

Trauma to the spinal column and the spinal cord can result in devastating and life-threatening injuries. Each year approximately 11,000 acute spinal cord injuries occur in the United States. The vast majority of those injured are males under age 38 years. Males have remained the gender most commonly injured for decades; however, the average age at injury has steadily increased over the past three decades as the same trend has been observed in the general United States population. The estimated cost for care ranges from $218,500 to more than $741,400 during the first year after the patient's injury. Lifetime costs vary based on age of the patient and site of the injury. High cord injuries in young patients cost just under $3,000,000 per year. Although prehospital care, medical, surgical, and technologic advances have contributed to an increased life span for those who have suffered a spinal cord injury, the life expectancy of these patients remains lower than for patients with no spinal injury.[21]

Spinal trauma can occur as a result of both blunt and penetrating trauma. The most common mechanism of injury is a motor vehicle crash, accounting for nearly half of acute spinal cord injuries.[21] Motor vehicle crashes cause spinal cord injuries through rollovers, occupant ejection, and collisions with pedestrians. Spinal trauma also commonly results from falls, acts of violence (including penetrating wounds from guns or knives), and sports injuries. In older adults, falls are the leading cause of trauma.[2] Although the number of spinal injuries due to falls is continually rising, the number of injuries resulting from violence has trended down since the mid-1990s.[16] Increased participation in extreme sports and outdoor activities such as in-line skating, snowboarding, and bicycling have also contributed additional sources for spinal cord injuries.

In the past, many people with spinal cord injuries died from respiratory complications such as aspiration and pneumonia.[34] Establishment of spinal cord injury care systems has decreased complications from spinal cord injuries and improved survival of those injured. Spinal cord patients need to be transferred to the appropriate definitive care facility as soon as possible to decrease complications and costs that may occur related to the injury.

Care of the patient with spinal trauma begins in the prehospital environment with rapid identification of actual injury or potential for injury based on the mechanism of injury, immediately followed by appropriate spinal protection interventions. Recent studies indicate that patients with head injuries are at higher risk for also having cervical spine injuries, particularly if the patient is unconscious or has a focal neurologic deficit.[11,14] On arrival in the emergency department (ED), the patient should be fully evaluated to rule out concomitant life-threatening injuries such as tension pneumothorax or intraabdominal bleeding while spine protection is continued.

Emergency care of the patient with spine trauma requires an organized, multidisciplinary approach. Patient survival

272

Table 22-1. Examples of Spinal Tracts and Their Functions

Spinal Tract	Function
Dorsal column (ascending)	Proprioception, pressure, and vibration
Lateral spinothalamic tract (ascending)	Pain and temperature
Anterior spinothalamic tract (ascending)	Light touch, pressure, and itch sensation
Spinocerebellar tract (ascending)	Proprioception to the cerebellum
Pyramidal tracts (descending)	Voluntary control of skeletal muscle
Extrapyramidal tracts (descending)	Automatic control of skeletal muscle

Data from Seeley R, Stephens T, Tate P: *Anatomy and physiology*, ed 6, Boston, 2003, McGraw-Hill.

and quality of life after the acute injury depend on the emergency care a patient receives. This chapter discusses anatomy and physiology of spine trauma, mechanisms of injury, patient assessment and initial interventions, specific injuries, and current research related to management of acute spine injury.

ANATOMY AND PHYSIOLOGY
Vertebral Column

The vertebral column serves as bony support for the head and trunk and provides protection for the spinal cord. A total of 7 cervical vertebrae, 12 thoracic vertebrae, 5 lumbar vertebrae, 1 sacral vertebra (composed of 5 fused vertebrae), and 1 coccygeal vertebra (composed of 4 fused vertebrae) constitute the vertebral column. Each vertebra is composed of a body, a vertebral arch, and a vertebral foramen. The arch of the vertebra is composed of two pedicles, two laminae, four articular processes (facets), two transverse processes, and the spinous process, which can be felt when palpating the posterior spine.[27,33]

The cervical vertebrae are the most frequently injured vertebrae because they are the most mobile part of the spine and because they are so small and delicate.[27] The rib cage provides stability to the vertebrae from T-1 to T-10 and keeps this portion of the spine relatively immobile. Because the thoracic vertebrae are so strong, fractures and/or dislocations at this level should increase suspicion for spinal cord injury.[19] The lumbar vertebrae are the largest and strongest in the vertebral column.[27,33]

Ligaments attach to the transverse and spinous processes to connect the vertebral bodies and provide support and stability to the vertebral column. They also limit the spinal column from excessive flexion and extension. Between the vertebral bodies are discs that act as shock absorbers and articulating surfaces for the adjacent vertebral bodies.[33,35]

Spinal Column

The spinal cord extends from the brain, through the foramen magnum, and down the vertebral column to the level of L2. This mass of nerve tissue regulates body movement and function through transmission of nerve impulses. The diameter of the spinal cord is largest in the cervical and lumbar regions and tapers in the lower thoracic area. In adults it terminates in a cone-shaped structure, known as the conus medullaris, at the L1 or L2 level. Spinal nerve roots that exit below the conus medullaris are referred to as the cauda equina.[5,27,31]

The primary function of the spinal cord is to regulate bodily function and movement by transmitting nerve impulses between the brain and the body. Cross-sectional views of the spinal cord reveal a butterfly-shaped core composed of gray matter, surrounded on the outer edges by white matter. The gray matter contains nerve cell bodies and is divided into three distinct regions, each with specific characteristics: the posterior (dorsal), intermediolateral (lateral), and anterior (ventral) horns. The posterior, or dorsal, horn contains sensory interneurons and axons whose cell bodies are located in the dorsal root ganglion. The intermediolateral, or lateral, horn contains cell bodies with autonomic nervous system function. The anterior, or ventral, horn contains somatic motor neurons that leave the spinal cord via the spinal nerves.[27,31]

The white matter of the spinal cord consists of multiple ascending and descending pathways (referred to collectively as "spinal tracts"), which are individually named based on their origins and terminations. These tracts run parallel to the spinal cord's vertical axis and transmit action potentials to and from the brain to other parts of the spinal cord. Table 22-1 lists some of these specific tracts and describes their functions.[27,31]

Spinal Nerves

The spinal cord has 31 pairs of spinal nerves that exit the spinal cord bilaterally and provide pathways for involuntary responses to specific stimuli. There are 8 cervical nerves, 12 thoracic nerves, 5 lumbar nerves, 5 sacral nerves, and 1 coccygeal nerve. The spinal nerves innervate voluntary striated muscle and are responsible for the majority of the communication between the spinal cord and the rest of the body. Each of these nerves has a posterior root that transmits sensory impulses from the periphery into the spinal cord and an anterior root that transmits motor impulses from the spinal cord out to the periphery. Table 22-2 lists the spinal nerve muscle innervations and their corresponding expected patient response. The dorsal root of these nerves innervates a distinct region of the body surface known as a dermatome.[27,33] Assessment of the 28 dermatomes provides information about function to sensory areas of the spinal cord. Figure 22-1 illustrates the sensory dermatomes.

Vascular Supply

The vascular supply for the spinal cord comes from branches of the vertebral arteries and the aorta. The anterior and posterior spinal arteries branch off the vertebral artery at the cranial base and descend parallel to the spinal cord.[31] Because spinal cord arteries cannot develop collateral blood supply, injuries to these arteries can be devastating.

PATIENT ASSESSMENT

The emergency nurse should perform primary and secondary assessments of injured patients while simultaneously performing interventions to stabilize the airway, breathing, and circulation. All patients with multisystem injuries or significant mechanisms of injury must be suspected of having a spinal injury and should be completely immobilized.

Table 22-2.	SPINAL NERVE MUSCLE INNERVATION AND PATIENT RESPONSE	
Nerve Level	**Muscles Innervated**	**Patient Response**
C4	Diaphragm	Ventilation
C5	Deltoid	Shrug shoulders
	Biceps	Flex elbows
	Brachioradialis	
C6	Wrist extensor	Extend wrist
	Extensor carpi radialis longus	
C7	Triceps	Extend elbow
	Extensor digitorum communis	Extend fingers
	Flexor carpi radialis	
C8	Flexor digitorum profundus	Flex fingers
T1	Hand intrinsic muscles	Spread fingers
T2 to T12	Intercostals	Vital capacity
L1	Abdominal	Abdominal reflexes
L2	Iliopsoas	Hip flexion
L3	Quadriceps	Knee extension
L4	Tibialis anterior	Ankle dorsiflexion
L5	Extension hallucis longus	Ankle eversion
S1	Gastrocnemius	Ankle plantar flexion
		Big toe extension
S2 to S5	Perineal sphincter	Sphincter control

Spinal protection involves manual immobilization of the patient's head until a rigid cervical collar, lateral head support such as head blocks or rolled sheets, and backboard have been applied. The entire spine should be immobilized using a backboard with straps across the chest, abdomen, and knees.[11,14,18]

Once the initial assessment and resuscitation have been completed, the patient should be removed from the backboard as soon as safely possible. Patients who have sustained spinal trauma, particularly those with sensory losses, are at great risk for developing skin breakdown, putting the patient at increased risk for additional injury and infection.[14,20]

After the patient's critical needs have been met, the emergency nurse may then perform a more focused assessment related to spinal injury. The initial assessment includes obtaining mechanism of injury and other history, as well as performing a focused examination of the spine and spinal cord.

Mechanisms of Injury

Mechanisms of spine injury include blunt and penetrating forces. The vertebrae, spinal cord, and nerve roots may be injured as a result of fractures, dislocations, or subluxation. The cord may also be injured through direct penetration by a bullet, knife, or other sharp object, or by adjacent injuries resulting in localized edema that compresses the spinal cord. Six basic types of movement can injure the spinal cord. These are illustrated in Figure 22-2 and summarized in Table 22-3.

The following mechanisms have been identified as being commonly associated with cervical spine injuries: fall from a height greater than or equal to 3 feet or five stairs; axial loading; motor vehicle collision at a high rate of speed with rollover or ejection; collision involving a motorized recreational vehicle; and bicycle collisions.[30] In addition, spinal injuries should be suspected if a fall results in fractures of the heels[7] or if an unrestrained (no seat belt) patient presents with facial injuries.

History

In addition to the mechanism of injury, the following pieces of history may indicate a potential spinal cord injury: history of significant trauma and altered mental status from intoxication; history of seizure activity since the incident; any complaint of neck pain or altered sensation in the upper extremities; complaint of neck tenderness; history of loss of consciousness; injuries to the head or face. When obtaining the history, the emergency nurse should ask the patient about neck pain and changes in sensation or movement since the time of injury. Any history of incontinence before arrival in the ED is important to identify because it may signal a spinal cord injury.[11,18,30]

If the patient is unconscious, prehospital history may be the only source of information available concerning the patient's condition and behaviors immediately after the incident; thus the emergency nurse should obtain as much information from prehospital personnel as possible. Patients who are unconscious or have any altered mental status and those with distracting injuries are at a higher risk for missed cervical spine injury because their injuries are more easily overlooked and they are unable to report any indicative symptoms.[14,30]

Inspection

The emergency nurse should observe the patient for obvious signs of spinal injury, including deformity of the vertebral column, cervical edema, and ballistic wounds in the neck, chest, or abdomen. Abrasions or contusions at the level of the lap or shoulder belt in restrained patients can indicate spinal injuries at those levels.[14]

The patient's ventilatory pattern and effort may also indicate a cord injury. Injuries to the spinal cord between C3 and C5 can result in progressive respiratory insufficiency secondary to significant respiratory muscle dysfunction when diaphragmatic innervation by the phrenic nerve is altered. Injuries to the cord below C5 lead to decreased intercostal and abdominal muscle function, in turn altering the normal mechanics of ventilation and increasing the work of breathing.[5,18,34]

The patient's ability to move and perceive pain during procedures such as arterial punctures or intravenous catheter insertion is another important observation. The patient should be able to wiggle his or her toes and fingers and to lift arms and legs. The inability to do so indicates some type of spinal injury. Continued penile erection (priapism) can occur with loss of sympathetic nervous system control and may indicate a cervical spine injury.[19]

Leakage of cerebral spinal fluid (CSF) from the nose or ears may also be noted. Confirm the presence of CSF using the halo test (as discussed in Chapter 21). Due to the high incidence of simultaneous closed head injuries and cervical spine injuries, patients with CSF leaks raise even higher suspicion for serious spinal trauma.

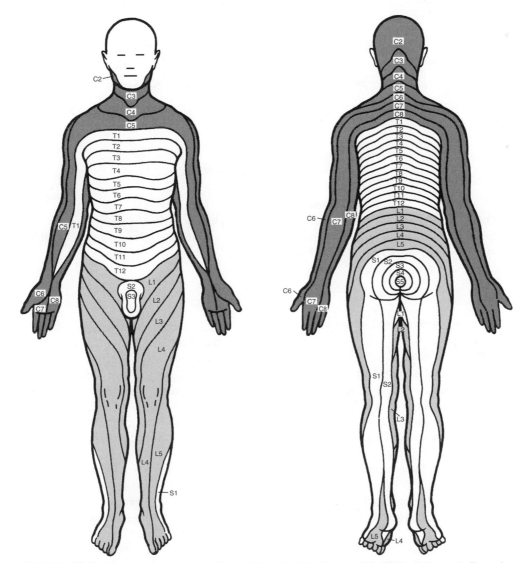

FIGURE **22-1.** Sensory dermatomes. (From Marx JA, Hockberger RS, Walls RM, et al: Rosen's *emergency medicine: concepts and clinical practice,* ed 6, St. Louis, 2006, Mosby.)

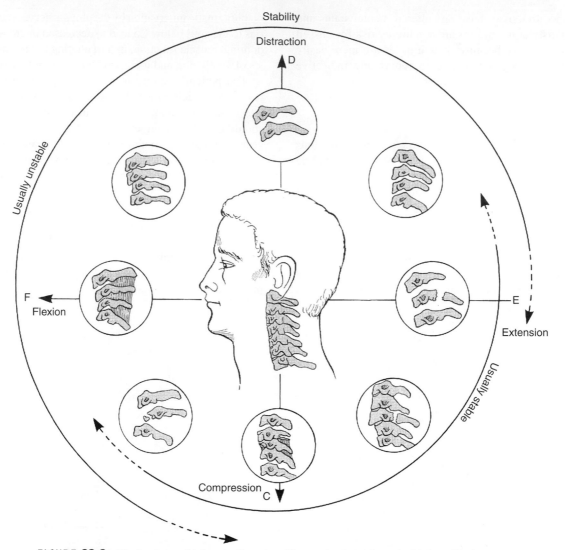

FIGURE **22-2.** Mechanisms of injury to the spine. The mechanism of cervical injury (flexion versus extension) determines the type of cervical spine fracture or dislocation. (From Moore EE, editor: *Early care of the injured patient,* ed 3, Philadelphia, 1990, Decker.)

Palpation

Injuries above the T4 level usually disrupt the sympathetic nervous system, causing vasodilation below the level of the injury. If the patient is diaphoretic, sweat is present above rather than below the level of the injury. In addition, a patient with a spinal cord injury becomes poikilothermic, assuming the temperature of his or her surroundings, because of loss of sympathetic tone. This can leave the patient at great risk for becoming hypothermic.[5]

Pulse rate and quality should be palpated. In neurogenic shock the pulse is slow and strong, whereas in hypovolemic shock it is rapid and weak.[5]

Strength and symmetry of movement in all four extremities should be evaluated (see Table 22-2). A quick motor evaluation should include flexion and extension of the arms,

flexion and extension of the legs, flexion of the foot, extension of the toes, and sphincter tone.

Sensory status may be assessed by evaluation of dermatomes. The patient should be able to distinguish between sharp and dull sensations using a safety pin or cotton swab. Testing should begin at the level of no reported sensation and proceed upward to identify the level at which feeling returns.

The presence of sacral or perineal sensations should also be assessed.[14] If sacral sensations are present in patients with other focal deficits (termed "sacral sparing"), an incomplete spinal cord injury should be suspected.

Finally, the patient's entire spinal column should be gently palpated for pain, tenderness, crepitus, and step-off deformity. Palpation requires that the patient be logrolled by at least three team members to maintain spinal alignment.[14]

Table 22-3. CATEGORIES OF MOVEMENT THAT MAY RESULT IN SPINAL CORD INJURY

Category	Mechanism of Injury
Hyperextension	The head is forced back, and the vertebrae of the cervical region are placed in an overextended position.
Hyperflexion	The head is forced forward, and the cervical vertebrae are placed in an overflexion position.
Axial loading	A severe blow to the top of the head causes a blunt downward force on the vertebrae and the spinal column.
Compression	Forces from above and below compress the vertebrae.
Lateral bend	The head and neck are bent to one side, beyond the normal range of motion.
Overrotation and distraction	The head turns to one side, and the cervical vertebrae are forced beyond normal limits.

Table 22-4. REFLEXES TESTED IN SPINAL TRAUMA

Reflex	Spinal Cord Level
Biceps	C5-C6
Brachioradialis	C5-C6
Triceps	C6-C7
Superficial abdominal (above umbilicus)	T8-T10
Superficial abdominal (below umbilicus)	T10-T12
Knee jerk	L2-L4
Ankle	S1
Anal wink	S2-S4
Plantar response	L5-S1

Data from: Bickley L: *Bates' guide to physical examination and history taking*, ed 9, Philadelphia, 2007, Lippincott Williams & Wilkins.

If the cervical collar is removed for this procedure, manual stabilization must be maintained.

Reflex Testing

The emergency nurse may perform an assessment of the patient's reflexes. Reflexes are summarized in Table 22-4.

Radiographic Evaluation

Radiographic evaluation of the injured patient is performed to assess alignment, identify fractures or ligamentous injuries, and identify spinal cord compression by bone or soft tissues. Commonly a three-view x-ray film series of the cervical spine is obtained, and all seven cervical vertebrae, including the C7-T1 junction, must be visualized to rule out cervical spine injuries.[11,23] When all of the cervical vertebrae cannot be visualized, a swimmer's view (open-mouth series) may be used to evaluate integrity of the odontoid body and C1 and C2 vertebrae. In addition to cervical films, patients with a history of a fall or significant chest and abdominal trauma should also have thoracic and lumbosacral spine films obtained. Patients with an altered mental status require complete spinal radiographic evaluation.[30]

Increasing availability of computed tomography (CT) and magnetic resonance imaging (MRI) has affected the evaluation of patients with suspected spinal trauma. CT scanning provides extremely sensitive detection of cervical spine skeletal injuries and is often used when C7 to T1 cannot be visualized on plain films.[18,23] It has also been suggested that CT be used as the primary imaging modality of the cervical spine in geriatric patients.[2] MRI is less sensitive to bony injuries and is therefore often used in conjunction with CT scans to evaluate suspected spinal injuries. Ligamentous and intervertebral disc injuries, spinal cord and surrounding vascular integrity, as well as the surrounding soft tissue, are best evaluated by MRI.[9,23] In addition, MRI is superior to CT in evaluating spinal cord injury without radiographic abnormality (SCIWORA).[9]

STABILIZATION

Initial stabilization of a patient with spinal trauma begins with recognition and treatment of life-threatening injuries such as airway and vascular compromise. The airway is evaluated while maintaining cervical spine control. Therapeutic interventions are directed at ensuring an adequate airway, maintaining ventilations, supporting adequate circulation, and preventing further injury.

Airway Management

The patient with cervical spine trauma is at risk for hypoxia, respiratory arrest, and aspiration. Spinal cord injuries may compromise muscles of respiration, and localized edema can cause airway obstruction, particularly in penetrating neck trauma. Initial clearing of the airway may safely be done with a controlled chin lift or jaw thrust. Advanced airway management such as endotracheal intubation should be considered early, especially in patients with injuries at the C5 level or above. Any airway maneuvers require that the cervical spine remain adequately protected. The emergency care team must also initiate interventions to minimize postinjury edema.[11,14,34]

Cervical Spine Protection

Although there is a lack of clinical research and considerable debate addressing cervical spine protection procedures, the standard at this time remains to err on the side of caution and continue using cervical spine stabilization

---

Box 22-1   **SPINAL PROTECTION PROCEDURE**

Cervical spine stabilization should be performed as a team. Generally, four people should work together. Note that some patients (such as those with a compromised airway, neck deformities, or penetrating injuries) may not be able to tolerate lying flat. Massive neck swelling that may result from a penetrating injury may prohibit the use of a cervical collar. Towel rolls and tape may be a safer method of securing such patients to the board and allowing for evaluation of the patient's injury.

1. Leader is positioned at the head of the patient with hands on each side of the patient's head. Manual in-line stabilization is maintained throughout the entire procedure by placing the leader's hands on the patient with fingers along the mandible.
2. Assess the patient's motor and sensory level by asking the patient to wiggle his or her toes and fingers. Touch the patient's arms and legs to determine sensory response.
3. One assistant applies and secures an appropriately fitting cervical collar. Follow the directions for sizing that comes with each collar. An ill-fitting collar can cause pain, occlude the patient's airway, or fail to give appropriate immobilization.
4. Straighten the patient's arms and legs, and position team members so that they are both on the same side of the patient at the shoulders and hips.
5. On the leader's count, the patient is rolled on the backboard as a unit.
6. Straps should be placed so that the patient is secured to the backboard at the shoulders, hips, and proximal to the knees.
7. The patient's head should be further immobilized with head blocks or towel rolls. Tape or straps should not be placed across the chin.
8. Manual in-line stabilization is maintained until the head and neck are immobilized.
9. The patient's motor and sensory function should be reassessed after the patient is immobilized.

Modified from Emergency Nurses Association: *Trauma nursing core course provider manual,* ed 6, Des Plaines, Ill, 2007, The Association; Bailes J, Petschauer M, Guskiewicz K et al: Management of cervical spine injuries in athletes, *J Athl Train* 42:126, 2007.

Box 22-2   **HELMET REMOVAL PROCEDURE**

Various helmets are available for those sports in which head protection is recommended. Motorcycling, bicycling, in-line skating, kayaking, ice hockey, football, and auto racing are just a few. The careful removal of this gear is imperative for protection of the cervical spine. In order to accomplish safe helmet removal, baseline understanding of various helmet types is needed.

(NOTE: Never attempt to remove a helmet alone; airway protection can be achieved with most helmets in place, and the potential for complicating an injury with a difficult removal is great.)

1. One person should apply in-line stabilization by placing his/her hands on each side of the helmet with fingers on the patient's mandible. (This person is in control of the head and neck.)
2. The second person then cuts or removes the helmet straps. After doing so, the second person places the thumb of one hand at the angle of the mandible, wrapping the remaining fingers along the other side of the mandible. Using the other hand, pressure is applied to the occipital region of the patient's head. Doing so shifts the responsibility of in-line stabilization to the second person.
3. The person at the top may now remove the helmet. When doing so, the helmet must be stretched laterally to clear the ears. If the helmet includes full facial coverage, glasses must be removed first and the helmet may need to be tilted backward and raised to clear the nose. The second person maintains in-line stabilization throughout this process.
4. Following helmet removal, the person at the top places his/her hands on either side of the patient's head with his/her palms over the patient's ears. In-line stabilization is continued in this position until the patient is secured on a backboard and any cervical immobilization devices are in place.

Modified from American College of Surgeons: Helmet removal from injured patients. Retrieved October 7, 2007, from http://www.facs.org/trauma/publications/helmet.pdf.

---

devices in all patients with potential for cervical spine injury.[6] The emergency nurse must ensure that spinal protection devices are appropriately applied to prevent further neurologic injury in patients with an unstable spinal injury.[11,18] Box 22-1 summarizes this procedure. The equipment required to protect the cervical spine includes a rigid cervical collar, lateral head immobilizer, and full backboard with straps.

A rigid cervical collar is applied to decrease head and neck movement. When applying a cervical collar, the emergency nurse should follow manufacturer's directions for size selection and application. Cervical collar application should occur only after the patient's head has been placed in a neutral in-line position, and in-line stabilization should be maintained throughout application. Rigid cervical collars should not obstruct the patient's mouth or airway or interfere with ventilations.

Placing the patient on a backboard does not completely protect the spine. The head must be stabilized laterally with a commercial head immobilizer, towel rolls and tape, or by taping the patient's head to the backboard. Tape or straps should never obstruct the patient's airway. The patient should be secured to the backboard at the chest, abdomen, and knees before the head is secured.

If the patient has a helmet in place, it should be removed before application of the cervical collar and before the patient is placed on the backboard. Box 22-2 and Figure 22-3 illustrate this procedure.

Circulation Management

Patients with spinal trauma may experience hypotension as a result of neurogenic or hypovolemic shock. Injuries to the spinal cord at the level of T6 or above may cause loss of sympathetic vasomotor tone, leading to hypotension and bradycardia. This shock state (known as neurogenic shock) prevents a compensatory increase in the heart rate in response to

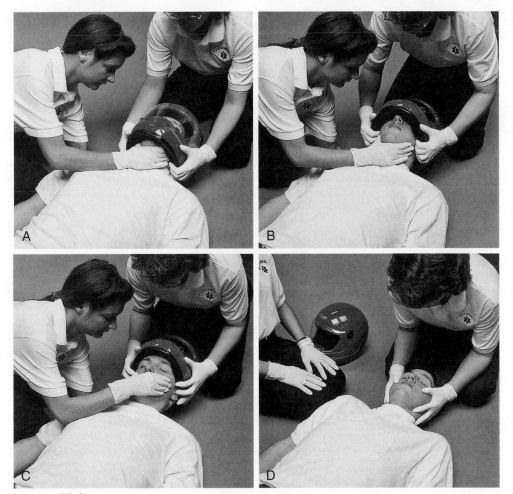

FIGURE **22-3.** Helmet removal. **A,** The helmet and the head are immobilized in an in-line position. The patient's mandible is grasped by placing the thumb at the angle of the mandible on one side and two fingers at the angle on the other side. The other hand is placed under the neck at the base of the skull, producing in-line immobilization of the patient's head. **B,** The side of the helmet is carefully spread away from the patient's head and ears. **C,** The helmet is then rotated to clear the nose and removed from the patient's head in a straight line. **D,** After removal of the helmet, in-line immobilization is applied as is a rigid cervical collar. (From Sanders M: *Mosby's paramedic textbook,* ed 2, St. Louis, 2000, Mosby.)

hypotension.[5] Injuries that could lead to hypovolemic shock (e.g., tension pneumothorax, hemothorax, or intraabdominal bleeding) should be ruled out.

If the cause of the patient's hypotension is not clear, intravenous crystalloid solutions should be used to correct hypovolemia. Vasoactive medications may be considered once fluid deficits have been corrected. If the hypotension is due to neurogenic shock rather than hypovolemia, maintenance of circulation will not be restored with crystalloids but will require judicious use of vasopressors.[8,18]

Pharmacologic Management

If the patient arrives in the ED soon after an injury, high-dose methylprednisolone (MP) may be administered. The effects of some biochemical responses have reportedly been reduced when MP is administered within 8 hours of injury.

The primary benefits reported were limited edema to the spinal cord, reduction in ischemia, and prevention of cellular death. Although administration of MP remains the current standard of care for spinal cord injury, recent research has begun to question its effectiveness. Newer studies have indicated that patients who receive high-dose MP are at greater risk for wound infections, pneumonia, decubitus ulcer formation, and urinary tract infections. If given, standard dosing is an initial bolus of 30 mg/kg over 15 minutes followed 45 minutes later by a continuous infusion of 5.4 mg/kg/hr for 23 hours.[8,13,15]

Additional Interventions

The patient with an acute spinal cord injury needs a urinary catheter to facilitate bladder emptying and to monitor urinary output during resuscitation. A gastric tube should be inserted to protect the patient from gastric distention and subsequent aspiration that can result from decreased peristalsis.[18,34]

The emergency nurse must recognize that the patient with a spinal cord injury has lost the ability to control body temperature. The patient should be kept warm and protected from unnecessary exposure. Increasing the room temperature, applying warm blankets, or using a commercial warmer are interventions to keep the patient normothermic. Intravenous fluids should also be warmed before administration, particularly if large amounts are infused.[26] These interventions are even more crucial in geriatric patients with spinal cord injuries because older patients have a lower basal metabolic rate and are more prone to problems maintaining body temperature in the absence of injury.[2]

Finally, because patients with spinal injuries may lose the sensations of pain and pressure, skin care is crucial. Prolonged immobilization leads to ischemic pressure ulcers. To reduce the occurrence of this complication, the backboard should be removed as soon as safely possible.[11,18,20] Padding bony prominences and placing a clean, dry sheet under the patient will further protect the patient's skin.

Cervical Tongs and Skeletal Fixation

Unstable cervical fractures may initially be stabilized in the ED with application of cervical tongs or halo devices to provide consistent traction and minimize cord compression, although doing so does carry a risk for increasing neurologic deficits.[18] Two types of tongs are currently used: MRI-compatible Gardner-Wells tongs and Crutchfield tongs.[10,18] Halo fixation devices provide the most rigid immobilization of all cervical orthotic devices and may be used for stabilization of C1, C2, and odontoid fractures, as well as single-column cervical spine injuries and cervical fractures in patients with ankylosing spondylosis.[14,25] Halo traction devices are contraindicated when the patient has an unstable skull fracture or traumatized skin at pin insertion sites.

When cervical traction is applied in the ED, the emergency nurse may assist with this procedure. The procedure should be explained to the patient, and if the patient's condition warrants, sedation should be administered to decrease anxiety and ensure patient comfort. Following application of tongs, ensure that any weights are hanging freely at all times. If a halo is used, necessary tools (including a wrench) for emergent removal should be taped to the halo vest. Cervical films should be obtained following application of tongs or halo device.[18]

PSYCHOSOCIAL CARE

Spinal trauma elicits a tremendous amount of anxiety and fear from both the patient and the family. The major concern of many patients and families is whether the patient will be able to move, walk, or "be the same" again. Unfortunately, this cannot be answered fully in the ED. The emergency nurse's discussions with the patient and family should be based on honesty. All questions should be answered, and all procedures should be explained. The family should be allowed to see the patient as soon as possible and remain there. Being truthful from the beginning and focusing care on prevention of further injury are important emergency nursing interventions.

SPECIFIC SPINAL CORD INJURIES

Spinal cord trauma encompasses both primary and secondary injuries. The initial impact from blunt or penetrating forces results in the primary injury. Examples of primary injuries include vertebral fractures or dislocations, torn ligaments, and spinal cord transections. Figure 22-4 identifies common fractures of the vertebral column. Secondary injuries to the spinal cord may develop within minutes of the initial injury. Microscopic hemorrhages and edema lead to spinal cord hypoperfusion (often complicated by hypotension in shock states), hypoxia, and endogenous biochemical responses. Secondary injuries extend the initial injury, increase morbidity, and limit future recovery, so the emergency nurse must be alert to these and provide interventions to minimize their development.[5,11,22]

Injuries of the vertebral column may occur with or without associated spinal cord injury. Although they are the most devastating, not all spinal cord injuries involve transection (or severing) of the spinal cord. Contusions, lacerations, vascular damage, hemorrhage, and transection are all possible injuries to the spinal cord. When they do occur, spinal cord transections may be complete or incomplete. Complete spinal cord transections lead to loss of all motor and sensory function below the level of an injury and account for almost 50% of all spinal cord injuries.[12] Patients with incomplete spinal cord transections will have partial preservation of some motor and/or sensory tracts.

Complications related to spinal cord injury are based on the location of the injury. An injury to the cervical spine puts the patient at risk for pulmonary and ventilatory problems. A low-thoracic spine injury causes loss of abdominal muscle functions, decreased respiratory reserves, and gastric distension.[34] Injury to the lumbosacral area of the spinal cord may cause loss of temperature regulation and bowel and bladder function. Injuries to the spinal cord at any level may lead to muscle flaccidity and the loss of reflexes below the level of injury. Due to decreased mobility from spinal injuries, all spinal cord injury patients are at risk for developing deep venous thrombosis, decubitus ulcers, and pulmonary emboli.[18,34]

Spinal and Neurogenic Shock

When a complete spinal cord injury occurs, all motor and sensory functions cease below the level of injury. Spinal shock is characterized by loss of reflexes and motor and sensory function below the level of the injury. The onset is usually immediate, and the intensity and duration are determined by the level of injury. Patients with spinal shock exhibit flaccid paralysis, areflexia, and bowel or bladder dysfunction. In addition, spinal shock disrupts the patient's ability to thermoregulate the body, causing the patient to assume the temperature of the surrounding air.[5]

Neurogenic shock, a form of distributive shock, may also be seen with injuries above the T6 level. Temporary disruption of the sympathetic nervous system causes bradycardia and hypotension.[5,18] Neurogenic shock leads to further spinal

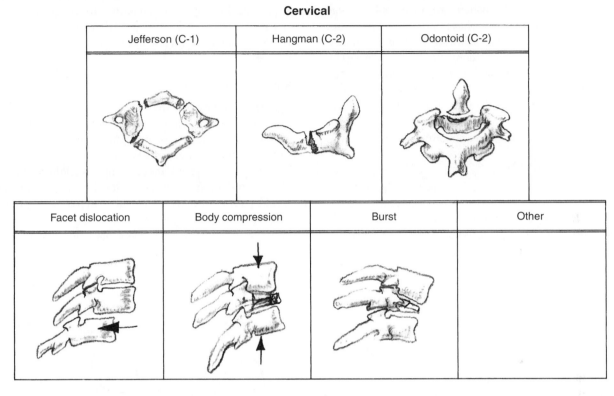

FIGURE 22-4. Common vertebral column fractures. (Modified from *Orthopaedic knowledge: update–I,* Chicago, 1984, American Academy of Orthopaedic Surgeons.)

cord hypoperfusion and must be recognized and treated early to prevent further damage to the spinal cord.

Incomplete Spinal Cord Injury

There are many types of incomplete cord injuries, and they are classified according to the affected spinal tracts. Regardless of the specific type of injury, patients with incomplete spinal cord injuries have asymmetric reflexes and flaccid paralysis, with some preserved sensations below the level of their injury. The specific types of incomplete cord syndromes are based on these characteristics and include central cord syndrome, anterior cord syndrome, posterior cord syndrome, Brown-Séquard syndrome, and nerve root injuries.[5] Confirmation of an incomplete lesion is based on evaluation of sensory and motor functions as defined by the American Spinal Injury Association.

Central Cord Syndrome

Central cord syndrome (Figure 22-5) is caused by hyperextension and results in swelling to the central portion of the spinal cord. This syndrome causes greater loss of function in the upper extremities than in the lower extremities.[5,12] Bowel and bladder function typically are maintained.

Anterior Cord Syndrome

Anterior cord syndrome (Figure 22-6) usually results from disruption of the anterior spinal artery, which supplies the motor and sensory pathways in the anterior portion of the spinal cord. The patient has a loss of motor function and pain and temperature sensations below the level of the injury. Vibratory sense, touch, pressure, and proprioception remain intact because the posterior column is preserved.[3,5,12]

Posterior Cord Syndrome

Posterior cord syndrome is rare and results from hyperextension injuries that damage the dorsal column of the spinal cord. Light touch and proprioception are impaired but not completely lost.[3,5]

Brown-Séquard Syndrome

Brown-Séquard syndrome is an uncommon injury resulting from hemisection of the cord (Figure 22-7). The most common cause is a penetrating injury such as a gunshot, knife, or missile-fragment penetration. Brown-Séquard syndrome is characterized by ipsilateral (same side) paresis or hemiplegia and loss of motor function, touch, pressure, vibratory sense, and proprioception. Contralateral (opposite side) losses include decreased sensation to pain and temperature changes.[5,12]

Nerve Root Injuries

Injuries to nerve roots may also occur as a result of spinal cord trauma. Common injuries include conus medullaris and cauda equina syndromes, both of which result from nerve root compression, most often secondary to other vertebral fractures or disk herniation. Conus medullaris syndrome occurs with compression at the level of T12 and results in flaccid paralysis of the legs with variable sensory deficits below the level of injury. Cauda equina syndrome occurs with compression of the nerve roots below the L1 level of the cord. Patients with cauda equina syndrome present with

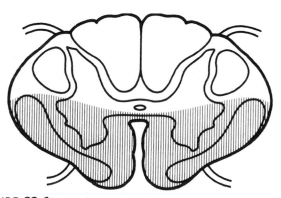

FIGURE 22-6. Anterior cord syndrome. (Modified from Rosen P, Barkin RM, Hockberger RS et al: *Emergency medicine: concepts and clinical practice,* ed 4, St. Louis, 1998, Mosby.)

Area of cord injury

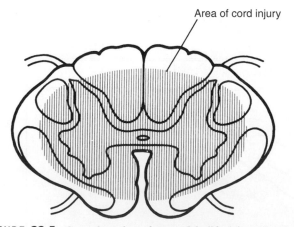

FIGURE 22-5. Central cord syndrome. (Modified from Rosen P, Barkin RM, Hockberger RS et al: *Emergency medicine: concepts and clinical practice,* ed 4, St. Louis, 1998, Mosby.)

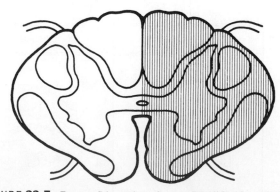

FIGURE 22-7. Brown-Séquard syndrome. (Modified from Rosen P, Barkin RM, Hockberger RS et al: *Emergency medicine: concepts and clinical practice,* ed 4, St. Louis, 1998, Mosby.)

a triad of symptoms, including saddle paresthesias, bowel or bladder dysfunction, and lower extremity weakness. In both syndromes the patient loses anal sphincter tone.[4,5,28]

Penetrating Injuries

Penetrating injuries to the spinal cord are usually the result of gunshot wounds and stab wounds and account for at least one fourth of all new spinal cord injuries. The emergency nurse should note the presence of any ballistic type of wounds or punctures. Because the exact path of penetrating objects is not known, visceral injuries must be suspected and ruled out. If the missile passes through the abdominal viscera into the spinal cord, the patient is at great risk for central nervous system infection and antibiotic prophylaxis is required. If the patient is brought to the ED with the wounding object in place, the emergency nurse should leave the object in place and stabilize it.[24,29] Bullets and wounding objects such as a knife are evidence and should be handled carefully to maintain integrity of the evidence.

Spinal Cord Injury Without Radiographic Abnormality

SCIWORA is a condition in which neurologic deficits are present in the absence of identified radiographic abnormalities on plain films or on CT. Although most often seen in the pediatric population, SCIWORA is not uncommon in middle-age or geriatric patients and accounts for up to 12% of spinal cord injuries.[32] In children, the condition is often attributed to anatomic differences allowing for ligamentous laxity in the cervical spine. In adults, disc prolapse and cervical spondylosis have also been noted as causes in addition to ligamentous injuries. As previously discussed, MRI has been found invaluable in diagnosing this condition.[17]

Autonomic Dysreflexia

Autonomic dysreflexia is a complication of spinal cord injury above the T6 level that can occur anytime following the resolution of spinal shock. This life-threatening emergency occurs when stimulation of the sympathetic nervous system leads to a massive, uncontrolled cardiovascular response. Multiple stimuli below the level of injury can trigger this response. Commonly a full bowel or bladder is responsible for triggering the response, but stimulation of the skin or cutaneous pain receptors may also cause an autonomic dysreflexia crisis. Signs and symptoms of autonomic dysreflexia include sudden severe headache, hypertension, nausea, bradycardia, and sweating above the level of injury with coolness below the level of injury. The patient may also complain of nasal stuffiness and appear quite anxious.[5]

Treatment of autonomic dysreflexia begins with identifying the cause of the sympathetic response. Once the cause of the dysreflexia is identified, such as a full bladder or constipation, the nurse can begin to rapidly intervene. If the bladder is full, inserting a urinary catheter or irrigating an existing one may relieve the symptoms. Medications to relieve constipation or urinary retention, as well as antihypertensive medications, may be administered.[5] When medications are used to lower a patient's blood pressure, the patient must be closely monitored to prevent a precipitous drop in blood pressure and to quickly identify any serious complications. After the emergency is resolved, the emergency nurse should work with the patient and family to develop interventions to prevent another occurrence.

SUMMARY

Spinal trauma is not as common as other types of injury, but its consequences are devastating. Its impact is extremely expensive and far-reaching across the population. Patients are generally young and require extensive physical and psychosocial care, often for the remainder of their lives. Emergency care of these patients involves resuscitation to decrease and prevent further injury to the spinal cord.

Current research focuses on preventing and treating the effects of secondary injuries that occur with spinal cord damage and regrowth of the damaged cells.[18] Techniques for regeneration of the injured spinal cord tissue through stem cell transplantation and gene therapy are also being studied.[15]

Regardless of advances in research and treatment, the most successful way to lessen the impact of spinal trauma is prevention. Use of seat belts, air bags, new car construction such as reinforced side compartments, helmets, and other safety devices are some methods currently used to prevent spinal injury. Teaching children, adolescents, and adults the consequences of risky behaviors and extreme sports may eventually help decrease the uncommon but devastating consequences of this injury.

REFERENCES

1. American College of Surgeons: Helmet removal from injured patients. Retrieved October 7, 2007, from http://www.facs.org/trauma/publications/helmet.pdf.
2. Aschkenasy M, Rothenhaus T: Trauma and falls in the elderly, *Emerg Med Clin North Am* 24:413, 2006.
3. Bailes J, Petschauer M, Guskiewicz K et al: Management of cervical spine injuries in athletes, *J Athl Train* 42:126, 2007.
4. Bickley L: *Bates' guide to physical examination and history taking*, ed 9, Philadelphia, 2007, Lippincott Williams & Wilkins.
5. Boss B: Alterations of neurologic function, In McCance K, Huether S, editors: *Pathophysiology: the biologic basis for disease in adults and children*, St. Louis, 2006, Mosby.
6. Bulger E, Maier R: Prehospital care of the injured: what's new? *Surg Clin North Am* 87:37, 2007.
7. Campbell J, editor: *Basic trauma life support for paramedics and other advanced providers*, Upper Saddle River, NJ, 2004, Pearson Education.
8. Chestnut R: Management of brain and spine injuries, *Crit Care Clin* 20:24, 2004.

9. Cohen W, Giauque A, Hallam D et al: Evidenced-based approach to use of MR imaging in acute spinal trauma, *Eur J Radiol* 48:49, 2003.

10. Congress of Neurological Surgeons: Initial closed reduction of cervical spine fracture-dislocation injuries, *Neurosurgery* 50(3 suppl):S44, 2002.

11. Crosby E: Airway management in adults after cervical spine trauma, *Anesthesiology* 104:1293, 2006.

12. Freeborn K: The importance of maintaining spinal precautions, *Crit Care Nurs Q* 28:195, 2005.

13. Gomes J, Stevens R, Lewin J et al: Glucocorticoid therapy in neurologic critical care, *Crit Care Med* 33(6):1214, 2005.

14. Harris M, Sethi R: The initial assessment and management of the multiple-trauma patient with an associated spine injury, *Spine* 31:S9, 2006.

15. Hurlbert R: Strategies of medical intervention in the management of acute spinal cord injury, *Spine* 31:S16, 2006.

16. Jackson A, Dijkers M, DeVivo M et al: A demographic profile of new traumatic spinal cord injuries: change and stability over 30 years, *Arch Phys Med Rehabil* 85:1740, 2004.

17. Kaji A, Hockberger R: Imaging of spinal cord injuries, *Emerg Med Clin North Am* 25:735, 2007.

18. Lee T, Green B: Advances in the management of acute spinal cord injury, *Orthop Clin of North Am* 33:311, 2002.

19. Morgan K, McCance K: Alterations of the reproductive system. In McCance K, Huether S, editors: *Pathophysiology: the biologic basis for disease in adults and children*, St. Louis, 2006, Mosby.

20. Morris C, McCoy E, Lavery G: Spinal immobilisation for unconscious patients with multiple injuries, *BMJ* 329:495, 2004.

21. National Spinal Cord Injury Statistical Center: *Spinal cord injury facts and figures at a glance*, 2006. Retrieved October 4, 2007, from http://www.spinalcord.uab.edu.

22. Okonkwo D, Stone J: Basic science of closed head injuries and spinal cord injuries, *Clin Sports Med* 22:467, 2003.

23. Platzer P, Jaindl M, Thalhammer G: Clearing the cervical spine in critically injured patients: a comprehensive c-spine protocol to avoid unnecessary delays in diagnosis, *Eur Spine J* 15:1801, 2006.

24. Potter B, Groth A, Kuklo T: Penetrating thoracolumbar spine injuries, *Curr Opin Orthop* 16:163, 2006.

25. Rechtine G: Nonoperative management and treatment of spinal injuries, *Spine* 31(11 suppl):S22, 2006.

26. Richards C, Mayberry J: Initial management of the trauma patient, *Crit Care Clin* 20:1, 2004.

27. Seeley R, Stephens T, Tate P: *Anatomy and physiology*, ed 6, Boston, 2003, McGraw-Hill.

28. Small S, Perron A, Brady W: Orthopedic pitfalls: cauda equine syndrome, *Am J Emerg Med* 23:159, 2005.

29. Steinmetz M, Krishnaney A, McCormick W et al: Penetrating spinal injuries, *Neurosurg Q* 14:217, 2004.

30. Stiell I, Wells G, Vandemheen K et al: The Canadian C-spine rule for radiography in alert and stable trauma patients, *JAMA* 286:1841, 2001.

31. Sugerman R: Structure and function of the neurologic system. In McCance K, Huether S, editors: *Pathophysiology: the biologic basis for disease in adults and children*, St. Louis, 2006, Mosby.

32. Tewari M, Gifti D, Singh P et al: Diagnosis and prognostication of adult spinal cord injury without radiographic abnormality using magnetic resonance imaging: analysis of 40 patients, *Surg Neurol* 63(3):204, 2005.

33. Tortora G, Grabowski S: *Principles of anatomy and physiology*, ed 8, New York, 1996, HarperCollins.

34. Urdaneta F, Layon A: Respiratory complications in patients with traumatic cervical spine injuries: case report and review of the literature, *J Clin Anesth* 15:398, 2003.

35. Waxman S, deGroot J: *Correlative neuroanatomy*, Norwalk, Conn, 1995, Appleton & Lange.

CHAPTER 23

Thoracic Trauma

Nancy J. Denke

Chest trauma is a significant source of morbidity and mortality, accounting for 20% to 25% of trauma-related deaths in adults. Two thirds of these deaths occur before the patient reaches the hospital because of major disruption of the airway, impaired breathing, or lethal alterations in circulation (injury to the heart and/or great vessels). The incidence has increased markedly over the last 100 years because of high-speed vehicular travel and interpersonal violence. In children, thoracic trauma commonly occurs as part of multisystem injury, with 90% of childhood thoracic traumas being blunt injuries.[13] Chest trauma can result from either penetrating or blunt trauma, causing a spectrum of injuries ranging from a simple rib fracture to severe vital organ injuries. Mechanism of injury, force, trajectory, type of weapon, angle of impact, proximity to the patient, secondary factors such as fire, and overall physical attributes of the patient determine degree and type of injury. The physical nature of the chest wall allows for considerable elastic recoil; therefore the severity of thoracic trauma may need to be assessed, focusing on the potential for underlying damage based on mechanism of injury, rather than on the initial appearance of the patient.

Blunt trauma to the chest is more common than penetrating injury, accounting for more than 90% of thoracic injuries.[9] Blunt trauma may be caused by motor vehicle incidents, falls, exploding tires, or any mechanism where the force of impact (particularly sudden deceleration, compression, or a direct blow) causes internal structural damage to the chest wall, parenchyma, pleura, diaphragm, heart, trachea, and/or great vessels. Penetrating injuries are a result of direct application of a mechanical (e.g., projectile) force to tissue or organs and the energy that is transferred from the object to the body tissues. The velocity of the penetrating projectile is the single most important factor that determines the severity of the wound.[9] Blunt and penetrating injuries may be sustained in all types of trauma; therefore anticipation is key to the prompt management of patients with chest trauma.

Thoracic injury and treatment have been described for centuries; however, it was not until the end of World War II that a chest tube connected to underwater seal drainage became standard treatment for many thoracic injuries. Endotracheal intubation, anesthesia, and chest x-ray examinations developed in the nineteenth and early twentieth centuries, and advances in the past 50 years, such as improved ventilatory assistance, antibiotics, blood gas analysis, and specialized nursing care, have increased survival in patients with thoracic injuries. Despite these advances, mortality rates for thoracic trauma remain second only to brain and spinal cord injuries.[19]

Thoracic trauma requires systematic assessment for potentially lethal injuries followed by rapid intervention to prevent unnecessary complications and death. Eighty-five percent of patients with thoracic trauma can be managed by simple lifesaving treatments that do not require surgical

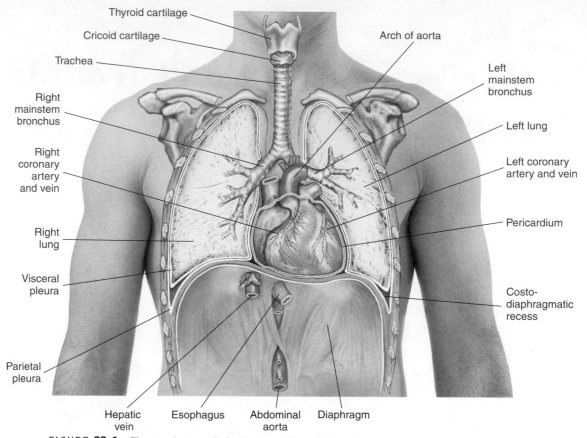

FIGURE 23-1. Chest and anatomic landmarks. (From Seidel HM, Ball JW, Dains JE et al: *Mosby's guide to physical examination,* ed 6, St. Louis, 2006, Mosby.)

interventions. This chapter discusses assessment and treatment of various thoracic injuries. Understanding the anatomy and physiology is essential.

ANATOMY AND PHYSIOLOGY

The thoracic cavity skeleton includes the sternum, ribs, costal cartilages, and thoracic vertebrae. The thorax is fairly mobile and expands easily to accommodate respiratory efforts. The ribs are elastic arches of bone that attach posteriorly to thoracic vertebrae and anteriorly to the sternum. Seven upper ribs are joined directly to costal cartilages, whereas ribs 8, 9, and 10 interface indirectly with the sternum through fusion of costal cartilage. Ribs 11 and 12 do not interface with the sternum. Beneath each rib lies a neurovascular bundle, containing an intercostal nerve, artery, and vein. The sternum has three parts: the manubrium, the body (corpus), and the xiphoid process (tip). The diaphragm forms the inferior border of the thorax, whereas the superior border is continuous with structures of the neck.

Internal thoracic structures are composed of organs and structures of the pulmonary, cardiovascular, and gastrointestinal systems (Figure 23-1). Pulmonary structures are located in the pleural space, whereas cardiovascular and gastrointestinal structures are located in the mediastinum, a cavity between the two pleural spaces.

Pulmonary System

Lungs are cone-shaped organs above the diaphragm that extend approximately 1½ inches above the clavicles. Each lung is located in a cavity lined with a serous membrane called the pleura. The visceral pleura covers the lungs, whereas the parietal pleura covers the rib cage, diaphragm, and pericardium. A potential space between these layers is the pleural cavity. Pleural cells secrete pleural fluid that separates the lungs but allows membranes to remain in contact and move without creating friction.

Normal breathing occurs through the processes of ventilation, which moves air in and out of the lungs, and respiration, which exchanges gases across alveolar-capillary membranes. During inspiration, phrenic nerve stimulation causes the diaphragm to contract and pull downward. As the diaphragm pulls downward, external intercostals pull the chest wall out, which enlarges the thoracic cavity. As lung capacity increases, intrathoracic pressure becomes negative (i.e., lower than atmospheric pressure). This negative intrathoracic pressure draws air into the lungs. During expiration this process is reversed as the diaphragm relaxes and moves up. Intercostal muscles compress the chest so that the lungs recoil passively. Intrathoracic pressure becomes more positive as lung capacity diminishes. Increasing positive intrathoracic pressure forces air out of the lungs.[9]

Cardiovascular System

The heart is located in the mediastinum positioned with the right ventricle anteriorly beneath the sternum. The pericardium, a three-layered sac that surrounds and protects the heart, is a fibrous envelope separated from the heart by the pericardial space, a potential space between the parietal pericardium and the visceral pericardium, or epicardium. The pericardium contains pericardial fluid (5 to 30 mL) that minimizes friction during cardiac contraction. The outer parietal pericardium is the fibrous pericardium, which attaches to the sternum, great vessels, and diaphragm to hold the heart in place. The heart itself is composed of three layers: the epicardium (the outermost layer of the heart), the myocardium (the middle, voluminous muscular layer), and the endocardium (the innermost layer of tissue that lines the chambers of the heart).

Four muscular chambers, two atria and two ventricles, contract rhythmically as they fill and empty with blood. The right atrium and ventricle receive deoxygenated blood from the body and pump the blood to the lungs for oxygenation. Oxygenated blood then enters the left side of the heart, which sends blood to the systemic circulation. The left heart is a high-pressure system; the right heart a low-pressure system. Valves separate chambers to prevent regurgitation of blood back into the atria and ventricles. Cardiac function and output depend on contractility, heart rate, preload (volume achieved during diastolic filling of the ventricles), and afterload (force or resistance against which the heart must pump to eject blood).

The thoracic aorta carries oxygenated blood to various tissues. Three anatomic parts of the aorta are recognized: ascending aorta, aortic arch, and descending aorta. The aortic arch is attached to the pulmonary artery by the ligamentum arteriosum. Near the ligamentum, a portion of the aorta branches off to form the left subclavian artery. At this point of the aorta, just distal to the ligamentum, the aorta is relatively immobile and is at increased risk for disruption. More than 85% of aortic injuries caused by acceleration or deceleration forces occur at this site.

Also in the mediastinum are the trachea, located posterior to the heart; the esophagus, posterior to the trachea; the phrenic nerve; and the diaphragm. Other thoracic cavity structures include the thymus gland in the anterior mediastinum behind the sternum and the subclavian and common carotid arteries.

PATIENT ASSESSMENT

The patient with obvious or suspected chest trauma must be promptly assessed because injury to thoracic structures may produce life-threatening alterations in ventilation and perfusion within minutes. Rapid assessment and intervention to support airway, breathing, and circulation (ABCs) are crucial. Protection of the cervical spine occurs simultaneously with assessment of airway patency. Assessment of rate, depth, and effort of breathing performed in conjunction

---

Box 23-1   INITIAL ASSESSMENT OF THORACIC TRAUMA

AIRWAY WITH CERVICAL SPINE PROTECTION

BREATHING

Spontaneous breathing
Rise and fall of the chest
Rate and pattern of breathing (such as shortness of breath, paradoxical chest wall movement, respiratory stridor)
Use of accessory muscles, diaphragmatic breathing, or both
Skin color (such as cyanosis)
Integrity of the soft tissues and bony structures of the chest wall (such as sucking chest wound, subcutaneous emphysema, upper abdominal injury)
Bilateral breath sounds
Tracheal deviation and jugular venous distention are considered late signs of airway compromise

CIRCULATION

Skin color, temperature, and moisture
Heart sounds
Vital signs
Blood pressure in upper extremities (equal or asymmetric)
Extremity pulses (equal, diminished, or absent)

ADDITIONAL CONSIDERATIONS

Pattern of abrasions or bruising
Wound size and location

---

with auscultation of breath sounds and inspection for symmetry and chest wall integrity is performed to identify overt and subtle injuries to the thorax. Supplemental oxygen is administered with a 100% nonrebreather mask or bag-mask device to maintain adequate oxygenation and ventilation. Life-saving interventions required during the initial patient assessment may include application of a three-sided occlusive dressing for an open pneumothorax or needle thoracentesis (decompression) for a tension pneumothorax. Assessment of circulation is performed with palpation of the central and peripheral pulses for quality, rate, skin color/temperature, and capillary refill. Obvious external bleeding is controlled with direct pressure. Internal bleeding is initially managed with replacement of intravascular volume; two large-bore intravenous lines should be established and warmed crystalloids (0.9% normal saline or lactated Ringer's) infused at a rapid rate. Boxes 23-1 and 23-2 highlight initial and secondary assessment of the patient with thoracic trauma. Therapeutic interventions are listed in Box 23-3.

The focused assessment sonography for trauma (FAST) examination has become an integral component of the initial assessment for patients with both blunt and penetrating trauma to the thorax and/or abdomen. It is a rapid noninvasive diagnostic study that can be performed at the bedside. (Table 23-1 describes strengths and limitations of the FAST examination.) The subxiphoid view obtained in this

---

Box 23-2	**SECONDARY ASSESSMENT OF THORACIC TRAUMA**

Assess pain.
Obtain patient history.
Identify mechanism of injury.
Determine time of the injury.
Determine what the patient remembers about the event.

Box 23-3	**THERAPEUTIC INTERVENTIONS FOR THORACIC TRAUMA**

Maintain patent airway.
Promote adequate ventilation.
Provide high-flow oxygen.
Assist ventilations.
Prepare for intubation.
Cover open chest wound.
Assist with chest tube insertion or needle thoracentesis (decompression).
Monitor bleeding from chest.
Prepare for autotransfusion.
Initiate two large-bore intravenous lines.
Facilitate essential imaging—ultrasonography, radiography, computed tomography.
Monitor cardiac rhythm continuously.
Monitor blood pressure, respiratory rate and effort, pulse oximetry, and level of consciousness every hour or more often if indicated by patient condition.
Document urine output and patient response to therapeutic interventions.
Facilitate surgical intervention.

Table 23-1. **STRENGTHS AND LIMITATIONS OF THE FAST EXAMINATION**

Strengths	Limitations
• Rapid (2-3 minutes) • Portable • Noninvasive • Can be done serially • Sensitive and specific for free fluid that is equal to a DPL or CT • Inexpensive	• Does not identify the source of bleeding or injuries that may not cause a hemoperitoneum • Limited in detecting <250 mL of peritoneal fluid • Poor diagnostic tool for identifying hollow viscus or retroperitoneal injury • Operator dependent • Obesity and subcutaneous air may interfere with the examination

CT, Computed tomography; *DPL*, diagnostic peritoneal lavage.

---

four-view study allows for the most rapid identification of pericardial injury. The interpretation is straight-forward: a positive subxiphoid examination is defined as "detection of pericardial fluid on the cardiac window."[23] The absence of fluid in the pericardial region represents a negative examination. The sensitivity of the FAST examination for detecting blood in the pericardial space has been reported at 96% to 100%.[10] Bedside ultrasonography is also being used to detect the accumulation of blood and air in the pleural space. Ultrasonography has been reported to have a higher sensitivity and specificity in detecting pneumothorax than chest radiography.[24]

SPECIFIC THORACIC INJURIES

Thoracic injuries include injuries of the chest wall, pulmonary system, cardiovascular system, and esophagus. Acuity is determined by the effect of the injury on ventilation and circulation.

Chest Wall Injuries

Rib Fractures

The exact incidence of rib fractures is unknown, but experts estimate a regional trauma center can expect 10% of all trauma admissions to have rib fractures. Fractures result from a direct or indirect blunt force or crush injury. Motor vehicle crashes (MVCs) and falls are the most common mechanisms of injury associated with rib fractures in the adult population. In the pediatric population, rib fractures are commonly the result of intentional injury in younger children, with recreational/athletic injuries being more common in the older pediatric population.

Rib fractures may occur in a single rib or multiple ribs and occur most often in the fourth through tenth ribs. These fractures are not considered life-threatening but can be associated with potentially life-threatening injuries to the underlying organs (most commonly the lungs). The patient often experiences pain/tenderness at the fracture site, so respirations are shallow (splinted) to avoid moving the chest wall. Fragments of fractured ribs can also act as penetrating objects, leading to the formation of a hemothorax or a pneumothorax. Subcutaneous emphysema or crepitus may also be present. Chest radiographs assist with diagnosis but are only 70% sensitive for detecting rib fractures. Fractures that separate the sternum from costal cartilage are not evident on a radiograph.

Fractures of the first and second ribs are rare due to the protection granted to them by the clavicle. Significant blunt force is required to fracture these ribs; therefore associated injuries to the underlying structures, the great vessels, and brachial plexus must be considered. Other injuries associated with upper rib fractures include injuries to the clavicles, scapulae, trachea, and lungs. Lower rib fractures (9 through 12) are associated with injuries to the spleen, liver, kidneys, or other abdominal contents, depending on location of the fracture(s).

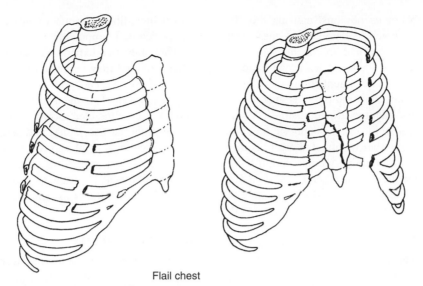

Flail chest

FIGURE **23-2.** Fracture of several adjacent ribs in two places with lateral flail or central flail segments. (From Marx J, Hockberger RS, Walls R: *Rosen's emergency medicine: concepts and clinical practice,* ed 6, St. Louis, 2006, Mosby.).

Treatment for most rib fractures is focused on the prevention of complications. Good pulmonary toilet, coughing, and deep breathing, in conjunction with use of an incentive spirometer and early mobilization, are recommended to prevent complications, including pneumonia or atelectasis. The use of binders or "strapping" is to be avoided in all patients. Patients with multiple rib fractures are usually admitted for observation. Those with severe injuries (eight or more fractured ribs, massive flail injury) may require internal fixation with plates and screws.

Pain management is essential because even one or two rib fractures can cause respiratory splinting, resulting in atelectasis and pneumonia. Oral, transdermal, or intravenous analgesia is available for many patients. Administration of an opioid in conjunction with a nonsteroidal antiinflammatory drug (NSAID) can provide some of the best analgesia; but the use of NSAIDs must be done with caution in older adults and should not be used until other injuries that may be associated with bleeding are ruled out. Monitoring the older adult patient for respiratory depression when giving opioids is also of utmost importance. Intercostal blocks provide complete analgesia allowing normal inspiration and coughing without the risks of respiratory depression. These blocks may be placed in the thoracic or high-lumbar positions, typically provide relief up to 12 hours, and can be repeated as needed. They are minimally invasive and provide a great deal of pain relief locally.

Older adult patients with rib fractures are at greater risk for complications because of diminished vital capacity that occurs with aging. Impaired ventilation worsens in all patients during the first few days after injury secondary to increasing chest wall edema and decreasing compliance. In an older adult patient with rib injury and diminished capacity, serial assessment is essential to prevent complications. Patients with decreased pulmonary function from asthma or chronic obstructive pulmonary disease also require careful ongoing assessment, in conjunction with good pulmonary toileting, because vital capacity in this population is also decreased.

Children have thin chest walls, and their bony thorax is more cartilaginous. Consequently, energy is easily transmitted to underlying thoracic structures without fracturing ribs. When rib fractures do occur in children, concurrent thoracic and abdominal injuries may be severe.[13]

Flail Chest

A flail chest is defined as fractures in two or more adjacent ribs in two or more places, or bilateral detachment of the sternum from costal cartilage (Figure 23-2). Mechanically a significant force diffused over a large area (i.e., the thorax) is usually required to create multiple anterior and posterior rib fractures.[4] Flail chest is usually associated with a fall, massive crush injury, or high-speed MVC. Flail chest commonly occurs in older adults secondary to their weakened structural components. A flail chest creates a free-floating, unstable segment that moves in opposition to normal chest wall movement. The flail segment moves in when the patient inspires and out with exhalation. The loss of coordinated chest wall movement results in hypoventilation of both lungs followed by atelectasis and eventually hypoxia. This injury is usually associated with an underlying pulmonary contusion that further compromises ventilation because of loss of pulmonary compliance, increased airway resistance, and decreased gas diffusion.

Diagnosis of flail chest is often made by direct observation—the affected area moves paradoxically from the rest of the chest. Muscular splinting of the chest immediately after injury may, however, mask a flail chest until hours later when intercostal muscles become fatigued and paradoxical movement becomes obvious, causing this diagnosis to be missed or delayed.[1,4] Paradoxical chest wall movement will not be demonstrated in the mechanically ventilated patient. Palpation of the chest wall may indicate abnormal motion and crepitus. The patient complains of pain and difficulty breathing. Plain chest radiographs may not be helpful because many times fractures are not visible. A computed tomography (CT) scan of the chest can provide significant information as to the number of ribs that are fractured and even early diagnosis of a pulmonary contusion; if there is any suspicion of involvement of the great vessels a CT angiography (CTA) should be performed. Blood gas analysis illustrates the severity of the hypoventilation caused by both the pulmonary contusion and the pain of the rib fractures and can be helpful as a baseline in assessing the need for mechanical ventilation. These values can also assist in the management of pain in these patients.[1]

Treatment consists of ensuring adequate oxygenation, judicious fluid administration, and pain management. Fluids are limited because of associated pulmonary contusion and potential development of acute respiratory distress syndrome (ARDS). Intubation and mechanical ventilation are not required for all patients, but patients should be monitored carefully for any change in respiratory status that indicates a need for more aggressive management (i.e., changes in respiratory rate, arterial oxygen tension, and work of breathing).[1] Patients who require mechanical ventilation are usually managed with continuous positive end-expiratory pressure (PEEP); continuous positive airway pressure (CPAP) may successfully be used for some patients. Patient-controlled analgesia (PCA) pumps, oral/transdermal/intravenous pain medications, intercostal blocks, and indwelling epidural catheters form the mainstay of current pain management. Surgical stabilization is rarely used.[4] Although surgical management of patients with severe flail chest is at present controversial, surgical stabilization has been indicated in specific clinical situations, such as when the patient fails to wean from the ventilator once a partial resolution of the pulmonary contusion is achieved, or in patients with deteriorating pulmonary function despite aggressive clearance of bronchial secretions and adequate analgesia.

Sternal Fracture

With the increased use of seat belts, shoulder restraints, and air bags in motor vehicles, there has been a decrease in the number of sternal fractures. Sternal fractures occur when tremendous force is applied to the chest, as with steering wheel impact, sporting injuries in which direct thoracic impact is sustained, or falls. Sternal fractures secondary to cardiac compressions during basic life support measures, or even stress fractures (as in weight lifters) do occur, but rarely. Occurrence is more common in the older adult population due to their inelastic/weakened bony thorax. The most common site of fracture is the junction of the manubrium and body of the sternum (angle of Louis, adjacent to the second intercostal space).[6] In addition to pain, a sternal fracture has significant potential for underlying cardiac and pulmonary injury, including pulmonary contusion, blunt cardiac injury, and pericardial tamponade.

The patient may experience dyspnea and localized pain with movement and may hypoventilate to avoid chest wall movement. Chest wall ecchymosis, sternal deformity, or crepitus may also occur. Treatment includes pain relief (as described above), a baseline electrocardiogram (ECG) to evaluate potential blunt cardiac injury, and serial patient examinations. If the fracture is displaced, operative reduction may be required. If cardiac symptoms are present, an echocardiogram may be obtained to evaluate myocardial performance. No surgical intervention is usually required. Patients are treated symptomatically.

Traumatic Asphyxia

Traumatic asphyxia results from a severe crush injury to the thorax caused by a strong crushing mechanism that remains in place for some time (e.g., being pinned under a heavy object). The pathophysiology involves two elements: a direct increase in thoracic and superior vena cava pressure from the crush injury combined with closure of the glottis, which further exacerbates the increase in central venous pressure.[11] Patients will present with cyanosis of the face and neck and subconjunctival and retinal hemorrhages. The face will appear to be moonlike because of the edema. There is some thought that the lower torso is protected because the inferior vena cava is compressed or obliterated during the "fear response" (Valsalva maneuver).[15] Neurologic symptoms such as loss of consciousness, seizure, or even blindness are generally transient.

Treatment is focused on supporting airway and ventilation and preventing secondary cerebral injury. If no cervical injury is suspected, the head of the bed should be elevated to 30 degrees to decrease the edema of the head. Serial neurologic examinations are required to monitor the patient. Outcomes are dependent on the degree of hypoxia and the extent of anoxic neurologic injury.[11]

Pulmonary Injuries

Laryngeal Injury

Fracture of the larynx is a rare, life-threatening injury. Common mechanisms of injury include striking the anterior neck on the steering wheel or dashboard, karate blows, and "clothesline" injuries when a snowmobiler or motorcycle rider hits a clothesline, wire, or tree limb with direct anterior neck impact. Females tend to have slimmer, longer necks, predisposing them to a higher susceptibility to laryngeal injury, in particular supraglottic injury; however, males (77% versus 33%) tend to present with the greater percentage of traumatic laryngeal injuries.[18] Laryngeal fractures are most commonly associated with intracranial injuries (13%), open neck injuries (9%), cervical spine fractures (8%), and esophageal injuries (3%).[18] Injury is suggested with a history of blunt trauma to the neck, even if the symptoms are subtle. The patient with laryngeal injury will likely present with one or more of the following symptoms: hoarseness, stridor, hematoma, ecchymosis, laryngeal tenderness, subcutaneous emphysema, crepitus, or loss of anatomic landmarks. The cornerstones of diagnostic evaluation in suspected laryngeal trauma are flexible laryngoscopy and CT scan[21]; angiography, esophagoscopy, or a Gastrografin swallow study should be considered for penetrating trauma to the area. Any patient with a laryngeal injury must be evaluated for a concomitant cervical injury, and patients with cervical injury need to be assessed for laryngeal injury.

In minor injuries to the larynx, close observation is essential for the first 24 to 48 hours. Keeping the head of the bed elevated 30 to 45 degrees in conjunction with the use of humidified air, keeping the patient NPO (nothing by mouth), and on voice rest will minimize edema and subcutaneous emphysema. Supplemental oxygen is not always needed. Histamine (H_2)-receptor antagonists and proton pump inhibitors can help reduce granulation tissue formation and tracheal stenosis; the efficacy of steroids is controversial. Intubation may worsen the preexisting injury (laceration or tracheal separation may occur during tube placement). Tracheostomy is indicated for the patient in respiratory distress and will be left in place for at least 5 days. Special consideration must be given to pediatric patients with laryngeal injuries and an unstable airway because local tracheotomy is not usually a viable option. It is suggested that these patients be managed in a manner similar to epiglottitis, using inhalation anesthesia with spontaneous respirations followed by rigid endoscopic intubation. Once the airway has been evaluated and secured in this manner, tracheotomy can be performed if needed.[21]

Penetrating trauma to the larynx is readily apparent and requires immediate surgical intervention. Associated injuries to the carotid artery or jugular vein may occur. Penetrating missile injuries have been associated with extensive tissue destruction related to the blast effect.[1] Injury to the cervical spine must also be considered in any patient with injury to the neck. Management of these injuries is similar to the above, but patients should be taken to the operating room as soon as possible for direct laryngoscopy, bronchoscopy, and esophagoscopy. Large mucosal injuries will require antibiotic use.

Tracheal Injury

Trauma to the trachea may be blunt or penetrating; mechanisms of injury are often the same as for laryngeal injuries. Blunt injuries can be subtle or acute. Noisy breathing may be the only indication of partial obstruction, whereas absent breathing suggests complete obstruction/disruption. If the patient has an altered level of consciousness, diagnosis is more difficult. Diagnostic evaluation includes bronchoscopy, CT scan, and laryngoscopy. Treatment includes operative interventions for severe blunt or penetrating injuries. Less acute injuries may be managed with intubation or tracheostomy.

Bronchial Injury

Major bronchial injuries are unusual and often overlooked.[1] Blunt trauma to the chest that causes bronchial injury has a high mortality because of delayed or missed diagnosis of the injury. Stab wounds or gunshot wounds of the bronchus are often identified during an operation performed for other reasons. Many patients die at the scene of the trauma, with most injuries occurring within 1 inch of the carina.[1] Signs and symptoms of bronchial injury include hemoptysis, subcutaneous emphysema, or tension pneumothorax with mediastinal shift. If air accumulates in the mediastinum, a crunching sound called Hamman's sign occurs. With bronchial disruption into both pleural spaces, bilateral tension pneumothoraces occur. The patient may present with dyspnea, tachycardia, and diminished or absent breath sounds. Persistent emphysema or air leak after chest tube insertion should increase the index of suspicion for this injury; bronchoscopy confirms the diagnosis. Treatment may be limited to airway support until inflammation and edema resolve; however, surgical intervention is required for patients with a significant tear.

Pneumothorax

Pneumothorax refers to accumulation of air in the pleural space resulting in partial or complete collapse of the lung as negative intrapleural pressure is lost (Figure 23-3). Pneumothorax may result from blunt or penetrating injuries. Laceration of lung tissue, often associated with rib fractures and subsequent air leak, is the most common cause of pneumothorax with blunt trauma.

A patient with a pneumothorax complains of chest pain and shortness of breath. Auscultation of the chest on the injured side demonstrates decreased or absent breath sounds; percussion demonstrates hyperresonance. Normal breath sounds can occur as a result of resonance within the thoracic cavity. Tachycardia and tachypnea are usually present. Chest radiography, chest CT, or ultrasonography is used to confirm the diagnosis of pneumothorax. The size of the pneumothorax is determined by the degree of lung collapse: small pneumothorax—15% or less occupation of the pleural cavity with air; moderate pneumothorax—15% to 60% occupation of the pleural cavity with air; large pneumothorax—60% or greater occupation of the pleural cavity with air.

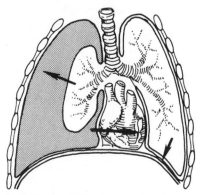

FIGURE 23-3. Closed pneumothorax. Simple pneumothorax is present in right lung with air in pleural cavity and collapse of right lung. (From Marx J, Hockberger RS, Walls R: *Rosen's emergency medicine: concepts and clinical practice,* ed 6, St. Louis, 2006, Mosby.)

Observation with serial chest x-ray examination may be the only treatment needed for a small, closed pneumothorax. Chest tube insertion is generally required for moderate to large pneumothoraces, patients who are symptomatic regardless of size of the pneumothorax, and patients requiring mechanical ventilation. The chest tube is most commonly placed in the fourth or fifth intercostal space, along the anterior axillary line. The chest tube may be attached to a Heimlich valve or a chest drainage system. A Heimlich valve will allow for complete evacuation of air that is not under tension. It does not require suction, allowing the patient to have greater mobility and less discomfort. More commonly the chest tube is connected to an underwater drainage system with suction to facilitate lung reexpansion.[1,22] Box 23-4 identifies essential components for chest drainage systems and discusses general nursing implications. Figure 23-4 illustrates a typical chest drainage system. A radiograph taken after insertion confirms tube placement. Oxygen administration, pain management, and serial chest radiographs to monitor lung reexpansion are standard treatment plans for all patients with a chest tube.

OPEN PNEUMOTHORAX. Open pneumothorax, or sucking chest wound, occurs when an opening in the chest is more than two thirds the diameter of the trachea. Air preferentially moves into the chest through the chest wall rather than through the trachea, escaping and collecting in the pleural space. This injury is usually the result of penetrating trauma to the chest wall; however, blunt trauma may also cause an open chest wound. An open chest wound causes loss of the negative intrathoracic pressure required for effective ventilation (Figure 23-5). Presenting symptoms may include chest pain, shortness of breath, hemoptysis, and occasionally hypotension. Breath sounds may be decreased or absent on the affected side, and a "sucking or hissing" sound may be heard with inspiration. Bubbles or froth often is observed

---

Box 23-4	CHEST DRAINAGE SYSTEMS—COMPONENTS AND MANAGEMENT[2,3]

FLUID COLLECTION CHAMBER

Fluid drains from the patient through a long tube to a collection chamber, marked for assessment of drainage.

WATER SEAL CHAMBER

Allows air to pass out, via bubbles, through the bottom of the chamber. Often calibrated for measuring intrathoracic pressure and may have float valve to protect patient from high negativity. With the water seal chamber, during spontaneous respirations, the water level should rise during inhalation and fall during exhalation. This oscillation is called tidaling and is one indicator of a patent pleural chest tube.

SUCTION CONTROL CHAMBER

Improves drainage and helps overcome the air leak. Keep suction control at −10 to −20 cm H_2O. Dry suction control systems provide many advantages: higher suction pressure levels can be achieved, set-up is easy, no continuous bubbling provides for quiet operation, and there is no fluid to evaporate, which would decrease the amount of suction applied to the patient. Instead of regulating the level of suction with a column of water, the dry suction units are controlled by a self-compensating regulator. Suction can be set at −10, −15, −20, −30, or −40 cm H_2O. The unit is preset at −20 cm H_2O when opened. Patient situations that may require higher suction pressures of −30 or −40 cm H_2O include a large air leak from the lung surface, empyema, a reduction in pulmonary compliance, or anticipated difficulty in expansion of the pulmonary tissue.

NURSING RESPONSIBILITIES

Secure all connections. Monitor catheters to prevent kinking. Monitor drainage output. Assess for air leaks. Maintain unit in upright position.

ASSESSING FOR AIR LEAKS

Look at the underwater seal. Leaks may originate with the patient or the drainage system. (Check the patient history. Would you expect a patient air leak?). For a patient receiving mechanical ventilation with positive end-expiratory pressure (PEEP), leaking causes continuous bubbling. Note the pattern of the bubbling. If it fluctuates with respirations (i.e., occurs on exhalation in a patient breathing spontaneously), the most likely source is the lung. Momentarily clamp chest tube at the dressing site with a toothless/padded clamp. Move the clamp incrementally toward the drainage unit—when you place the clamp between the source of the air leak and the water seal/air leak meter chamber, the bubbling will stop. If bubbling stops the first time you clamp, the air leak must be at the chest tube insertion site or the lung. If bubbling continues, leak is distal to the clamp. If bubbling stops before the end of the tubing, leak is in the tube, so tube must be replaced. If the unit is still bubbling when the very end of the tubing is clamped, the unit has the leak and should be changed. If the leak is at the insertion site, remove the chest tube dressing and inspect the site. Make sure the catheter eyelets have not pulled out beyond the chest wall. Replace the dressing. Notify physician of any new, increased, or unexpected air leaks that are not corrected by the above actions.

INDICATIONS OF PATENCY

Water level in the water seal should fluctuate with breathing, rising with inspiration and falling with expiration, and is an indicator of chest tube patency. If the patient is on mechanical ventilation, this pattern is reversed because breaths are delivered under positive pressure. Fluctuations stop when the lung is fully reexpanded or when the tube is kinked or compressed.

MILKING/STRIPPING THE TUBE

Vigorous milking or stripping can create dangerously high negative pressures, placing the patient at risk for mediastinal trauma. Use extreme caution, and follow your hospital policy.

TO CLAMP OR NOT TO CLAMP?

You should never clamp a chest tube during patient transport unless the chest drainage system becomes disrupted during patient movement, and then only if there is no air leak.

around the wound as air escapes through the bloodied wound. Immediate treatment consists of placing a sterile, nonporous, three-sided occlusive dressing over the injury. Taping three sides allows air to escape but prevents air from entering through the wound. After placement of this dressing, the patient should be carefully monitored for development of a tension pneumothorax. If symptoms suggesting a tension pneumothorax develop, the taped dressing must be removed immediately. A chest tube should be inserted to facilitate reexpansion of the lung. Definitive treatment of the open chest wound is operative closure. If the injury is caused by penetrating trauma with an impaled object, the object must be stabilized and left in place. NEVER REMOVE the object in the emergency department (ED).

TENSION PNEUMOTHORAX. Tension pneumothorax is a life-threatening condition that occurs when accumulation of air in one pleural space forces thoracic contents to the opposite side of the chest (Figure 23-6). Initial lung injury allows air into the pleural space with inspiration; however, air cannot escape with expiration. Air continues to accumulate and intrathoracic pressure increases, forcing thoracic contents away from the injured side. Eventually the lung on the opposite side, the heart, and great vessels are compressed as mediastinal shift occurs. Auscultation reveals decreased or absent breath sounds on the affected side and possibly decreased sounds on the unaffected side as that lung is compressed. If the patient is alert and able to speak, he or she may complain of chest pain, severe shortness of breath, and a feeling of impending doom. Compression of the heart causes cardiac dysrhythmias, decreases diastolic filling, and decreases cardiac output. Vena caval compression impairs venous return to the heart, which worsens diastolic filling and further decreases cardiac output. Neck vein distension occurs as venous return is impaired by compression of the heart; however, neck veins may remain flat if concurrent hypovolemia exists. The trachea eventually deviates to the unaffected side as mediastinal shift worsens.

Immediate needle decompression of the affected side is required. A 14- or 16-gauge catheter is inserted into the second intercostal space at the midclavicular line on the injured side. Hearing a rush of air upon needle insertion, with a rapid improvement in symptoms, confirms the diagnosis. Definitive therapy is chest tube insertion.

Hemothorax

A hemothorax is free blood in the pleural space (Figure 23-7) resulting from bleeding from lung parenchyma, heart and major vessel injury, or injury to internal mammary arteries. The most common cause is an injury to the intercostal arteries that results in bleeding into the pleural space. In addition to chest pain, shortness of breath, and decreased or absent

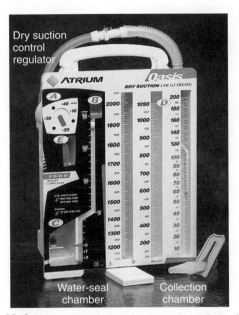

FIGURE 23-4. Chest tube drainage systems have three chambers: (1) collection chamber; (2) water-seal chamber, and (3) suction control chamber. Suction control chamber requires a connection to a wall suction source that is dialed up higher than the prescribed suction for the suction to work. (Courtesy Atrium Medical Corporation, Hudson, NH.)

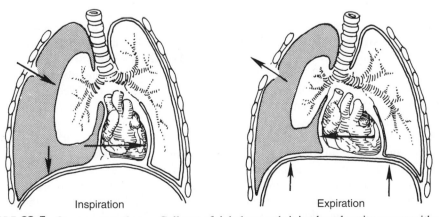

FIGURE 23-5. Open pneumothorax. Collapse of right lung and air in pleural cavity occurs with communication to outside through defect in chest wall. In sucking chest wound, lung volume is greater with expiration. (From Marx J, Hockberger RS, Walls R: *Rosen's emergency medicine: concepts and clinical practice,* ed 6, St. Louis, 2006, Mosby.)

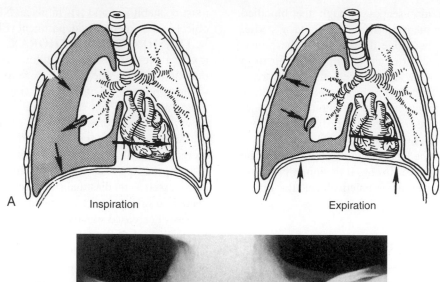

A   Inspiration   Expiration

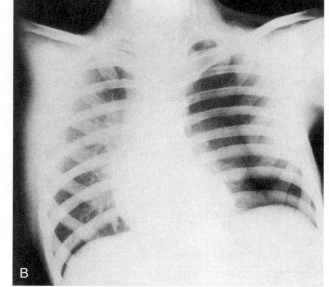

B

FIGURE **23-6.** **A,** Tension pneumothorax. Right pneumothorax under tension, total collapse of right lung, and shift of mediastinal structures to left. **B,** Radiograph of left tension pneumothorax with shift of mediastinal structures to right. Note subcutaneous emphysema in soft tissues of neck. (From Marx J, Hockberger RS, Walls J: *Rosen's emergency medicine: concepts and clinical practice,* ed 6, St. Louis, 2006, Mosby.)

breath sounds on the affected side, the patient has dullness on chest percussion. Signs and symptoms of hypovolemic shock and respiratory distress are often present. Treatment includes chest tube insertion (usually size 32 Fr or 36 Fr in an adult), high-flow oxygen by a nonrebreather mask, and large-bore intravenous lines for fluid replacement. Chest drainage should be carefully monitored to assess the need for autotransfusion and clots that occlude the tube. If blood return with chest tube insertion is 1000 mL or blood loss is 200 mL/hr for 3 to 4 hours, surgical intervention is indicated.[1] Persistent hypotension or massive air leak are additional indicators for surgery.[1] Patients with a hemothorax may also require insertion of a second chest tube to allow the lung to reexpand. FAST examination is used at some trauma centers in the initial evaluation of patients for hemothorax. Chest radiography may confirm the diagnosis, but an upright or decubitus film is often necessary; a CT scan may be used to identify and quantify the hemothorax.

AUTOTRANSFUSION. Autotransfusion, collecting and reinfusing the patient's own blood, is a valuable tool during resuscitation of select hypovolemic trauma victims. Blood shed into the thoracic cavity can be easily collected and infused. Significant intrathoracic blood loss (more than 350 mL) and wounds that are less than 4 to 6 hours old are potential indications for autotransfusion.[1,3] Autotransfusion is also useful when homologous blood is not available or the patient's religious convictions forbid homologous transfusion. Box 23-5 highlights specific advantages and disadvantages of autotransfusion. Autotransfusion is not appropriate when enteric contamination has occurred or is suspected (e.g., ruptured diaphragm), infection is present, patient has established coagulopathies or hepatic/renal insufficiency,

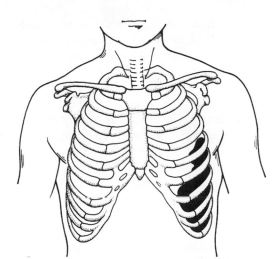

FIGURE **23-7.** Hemothorax. (From Danis DM, Blansfield JS, Gervasini AA: *Manual of clinical trauma care: the first hour,* ed 4, St. Louis, 2007, Mosby.)

or the blood has been in the autotransfuser for greater than 6 hours.

Autotransfusion requires a chest drainage unit and autotransfusion device and user competence with the process and collection device. An anticoagulant may be added before blood collection to prevent clotting during the collection phase and plugging of the blood filter and intravenous line during reinfusion. Citrate dextrose solution-A and citrate phosphate dextrose are the most common anticoagulants used; however, many trauma centers elect not to add an anticoagulant. Continuous monitoring of respiratory and cardiac status in conjunction with serial laboratory assessments must be performed.

Pulmonary Contusion

Pulmonary contusion is the most common, potentially lethal, chest injury seen in North America.[1] Almost 75% of patients with blunt chest trauma have an underlying pulmonary contusion, with mortality about 40%. Contusions occur when underlying lung parenchyma is damaged, causing edema and hemorrhage. Pulmonary laceration is usually not present. Concussive and compressive forces from blunt trauma are the most common cause of pulmonary contusion. Injury to lung parenchyma worsens progressively over time. Thoracic injuries associated with pulmonary contusion include rib fractures, flail chest, hemothorax, pneumothorax, and scapular fractures.[22]

Injury to the lung parenchyma causes ruptures and hemorrhages into pulmonary tissue, alveoli, and small airways. As a result, airways collapse, followed by loss of ventilation, pulmonary shunting, and hypoxemia. The subsequent inflammatory response impairs gas exchange and worsens the clinical picture. Diagnosis is based on the index of suspicion. Clinical evidence of dyspnea, hemoptysis, hypoxia, and possible chest wall abrasion or ecchymosis may be present. Fifty percent of patients with pulmonary contusion have no external physical findings. Auscultation rarely detects

abnormalities, but a baseline blood gas measurement may be helpful. The chest radiograph is usually not helpful during initial evaluation because the contused areas do not "blossom" until approximately 6 to 8 hours after injury unless the injury is severe. CT scan of the chest may be used to quantify the contusion because it is a more sensitive indicator of tissue injury.[4] Contusions change rapidly and usually improve within 72 hours and resolve within 3 to 5 days.

Treatment consists of placing the patient in semi-Fowler's position to facilitate lung reexpansion, suctioning, and chest physiotherapy. Intubation and mechanical ventilation may be required if the patient has severe hypoxia or the contusion affects more than 28% of the lungs, as quantified by a CT scan. In general, intubation and mechanical ventilation are more likely with larger contusions. Intubation may also be required if the patient exhibits signs of shock, has fractured eight or more ribs, is an older adult, or has underlying pulmonary disease; CPAP may be used on a trial basis in select patients. Fluids may be restricted when there is no evidence of hypovolemia.

Diaphragmatic Injury

Blunt or penetrating trauma may result in diaphragmatic injuries; 80% to 90% of blunt diaphragmatic ruptures result from MVCs. Lateral impact from an MVC is three times more likely than any other type of impact to cause a rupture.[23] The resulting large radial tears cause herniation of abdominal contents into the thorax. Penetrating trauma can cause small radial tears that may go unnoticed for several years, until the gradual herniation becomes apparent. Most injuries occur on the left side of the diaphragm; the reason for this is unclear, but the proximity of the right diaphragm to the liver may provide protection. When injuries do occur on the right, they may be difficult to identify because of the liver. Diaphragmatic injuries rarely occur alone. They are most commonly seen in conjunction with other blunt thoracic injuries, trauma to the liver or spleen and pelvic or long bone fractures. Three clinical phases of diaphragmatic injuries have been described: the acute phase, when the injury occurs; if not diagnosed early, the second, or latent, phase occurs. This phase is asymptomatic but may evolve into gradual herniation of abdominal contents. The diagnosis may be made later because of complications of herniation of abdominal contents into the pleural cavity. The third, or obstructive, phase is characterized by bowel or visceral herniation, incarceration, strangulation, and possible rupture of the stomach and colon. If herniation occurs, it can cause significant lung compression, leading to tension pneumothorax.[12]

The presence of dyspnea, abdominal or epigastric pain that radiates to the left shoulder (Kehr's sign), bowel sounds in the chest, and decreased breath sounds on the affected side suggest a possible ruptured diaphragm. The chest radiograph may demonstrate an elevated diaphragm, loss of the diaphragmatic shadow, irregularity of the diaphragm, or even a gastric tube noted to pass into the stomach and then curling into the chest. In the stable patient, the CT scan of the chest is the diagnostic tool of choice. If a diagnostic peritoneal lavage (DPL) is performed, lavage fluid may leak into the chest drainage system, if present. Treatment focuses on early identification (both in blunt and penetrating injuries) and prompt surgical repair to avoid morbidity and mortality form visceral herniation/strangulation and even cardiopulmonary compromise.

Cardiac and Great Vessel Injuries

Blunt Cardiac Injury

Formerly known as "cardiac contusion" or "cardiac concussion," blunt cardiac injury describes a spectrum of potential injuries to the heart resulting from blunt trauma to the anterior chest. Common mechanisms of injury include steering wheel impact during an MVC, falls, assaults, and direct blows from an object or large animal (e.g., kick from a horse). The myocardium may sustain a mild contusion or concussion injury or may have a severe injury that mimics acute myocardial infarction. An echocardiogram differentiates the extent of injury. A mild injury can cause cardiac dysrhythmias, yet the echocardiogram is normal. Extensive myocardial injury is characterized by 12-lead ECG changes, dysrhythmias, and some evidence of myocardial dysfunction on the echocardiogram.

The signs and symptoms of blunt cardiac injury are nonspecific. The spectrum of clinical presentations range from asymptomatic to cardiogenic shock, so many times the only information that you may have to suggest that the patient has blunt cardiac injury is the patient's history of blunt anterior chest trauma.[1,7] Some common presentations seen in this population are chest pain and skin abrasions or ecchymosis to the anterior chest. Chest pain associated with blunt cardiac injury mimics pain that occurs with ischemic chest pain. Unlike ischemic pain, however, pain with blunt cardiac injury does not respond to coronary vasodilators such as nitroglycerine.[7] Dysrhythmias associated with this injury include sinus tachycardia, atrial fibrillation/flutter, atrial and ventricular extrasystoles, and even ventricular tachycardia/fibrillation. The most common dysrhythmia is premature ventricular contractions, the incidence of which increases with age of the patient. Most of the lethal dysrhythmias and cardiac failures occur within 24 to 48 hours of the injury.

Serial ECGs and continuous cardiac monitoring are essential. A two-dimensional echocardiography (2-D Echo) is also recommended, although a transesophageal echocardiogram (TEE) is thought to be the more sensitive test. Echocardiograms are useful for differentiating cardiac dysfunction from other abnormalities such as pericardial tamponade, valve rupture, and pericardial effusion.[7] Diagnostic use of cardiac isoenzyme analysis has been largely abandoned because researchers have demonstrated lack of specificity and sensitivity for dysrhythmia development or injury with use of these enzyme values. Variable ECG findings occur in blunt cardiac injury. Specific findings include ST-segment and T-wave changes, prolonged QT interval, and right bundle branch block. Sequelae after injury include dysrhythmias, valve lesion and rupture, thromboembolic events, and heart failure. Treatment consists of cardiac monitoring of patients for at least 24 hours. Patients with abnormal ECGs or dysrhythmia should have a 2-D Echo. Patients with an abnormal echocardiogram should be treated symptomatically. Patients with normal serial ECGs or those who remain asymptomatic for 24 hours require no further treatment.

Penetrating Cardiac Injuries

Most penetrating cardiac injuries are caused by person-against-person violence or industrial incidents. Most victims of penetrating cardiac injuries arrive in the ED in cardiac arrest or with significant hypotension secondary to cardiac tamponade or hemorrhage. The right ventricle is the most frequently injured chamber because of its anterior position.[17] Other chambers injured are the left ventricle and right atrium. Gunshot wounds to the heart are significantly more lethal than stab wounds.[17] Penetrating injuries are associated with a high mortality (83%); only 20% to 25% of the victims reach the hospital alive.[1] Of those who arrive alive, only 20% are stable.[20] Patients who arrive with stable cardiac injuries have the best chance for survival with early diagnosis and treatment. Patients with injuries to the chest between the midclavicular lines, clavicles, and costal margins should be aggressively evaluated for cardiac involvement.[7]

Stabilization of the ABCs followed by echocardiography is recommended if the patient has cardiac activity. If the echocardiogram is negative, no further evaluation is indicated. Positive findings indicating tamponade suggest the need for a subxiphoid window. With positive subxiphoid exploration, cardiac surgery is indicated to repair the defect.[14,17,20] Use of the FAST examination has led to earlier diagnosis and definitive surgical intervention, with a specificity of 99.3% and sensitivity of 100% for identifying penetrating cardiac injury.[16]

Immediate thoracotomy in the ED may be indicated for selected patients presenting with penetrating chest trauma. The indications for this resuscitative procedure have been subject to considerable review. The best results are obtained in patients with a single penetrating injury to the anterior or precordial thoracic area and in patients who had a witnessed cardiac arrest in the ED. Holes in the myocardium, lungs, or great vessels can be temporarily plugged with the balloon of a urinary catheter, sutures, staples, clamps, or a finger while an operating room is readied. Box 23-6 describes considerations of the resuscitative thoracotomy.

Box 23-6	**RESUSCITATIVE THORACOTOMY**

CANDIDATES/INDICATIONS

Patient with penetrating chest trauma who arrives and deteriorates rapidly
Unresponsive hypotension (BP <70 mm Hg)
Rapid exsanguination from chest tube (>1500 mL)
Witnessed cardiac arrest in the department or just before arrival

CONTRAINDICATIONS

Blunt trauma with no witnessed cardiac activity or patient who arrests at the scene
Severe head injury

EQUIPMENT

No. 10 blade
Rib spreader
Metzenbaum scissors
Vascular clamps (long)
3-0 nonabsorbable suture (nylon, polypropylene) on round-bodied needles—multiple
Aortic clamp

TECHNIQUE

"Splash prep" chest with skin disinfectant
Incision made with a No. 10 blade from sternal border to midaxillary line fourth intercostal space
Insert retractor and open widely
Address the cause of arrest
Once you have done this, you can then clamp the descending aorta with the vascular clamp or with digital pressure.
Start internal compressions
Get patient to the OR for definitive care

RESULTS

Dismal in those that arrest before arrival and require CPR for a few minutes
Survival for blunt trauma patients who never exhibited any signs of life—0%
Survival for penetrating trauma patients without signs of life—0% to 5%

BP, Blood pressure; *CPR,* cardiopulmonary resuscitation; *OR,* operating room.

Cardiac Tamponade

Cardiac tamponade occurs when rapid accumulation of blood in the pericardial sac decreases ventricular filling. As the pericardial sac fills, blood presses on the ventricles, impairs ventricular filling and the heart's pumping ability, so cardiac output decreases. Figure 23-8 shows massive pericardial effusion with a "water bottle" appearance on chest radiograph.

Classic signs of cardiac tamponade are a complex of symptoms called Beck's triad: hypotension, muffled heart tones, and distended neck veins.[6] Hypotension is secondary to myocardial compression and decreased cardiac output as more blood accumulates in the pericardium. Muffled heart sounds are caused by the insulating ability of blood in the pericardium, whereas neck vein distension occurs because the heart cannot expand normally to accommodate blood return to the heart. Classic symptoms may not always be evident because of associated injuries such as hypovolemia. As the tamponade worsens, the patient exhibits air hunger, agitation, and deterioration in level of consciousness.

Knowing mechanisms of injury and location of the wounds is crucial for accurate assessment. Gunshot wounds and stab wounds to the chest are the most suggestive for this condition. Hemodynamically unstable patients with injuries to the chest should be immediately evaluated for tamponade using bedside sonography (e.g., FAST examination). In a stable patient, an echocardiogram and subxiphoid pericardial window are diagnostic tools of choice.

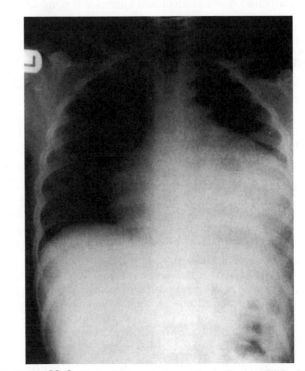

FIGURE 23-8. Pericardial effusion. (From Barkin RM: *Pediatric emergency medicine: concepts and clinical practice,* ed 2, St. Louis, 1997, Mosby.)

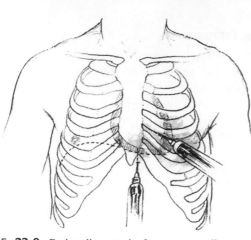

FIGURE 23-9. Pericardiocentesis for acute cardiac tamponade can be performed via a left subxiphoid or parasternal approach. The subxiphoid route is generally preferred for acute trauma. (From Davis JH et al: *Essentials of clinical surgery,* St. Louis, 1991, Mosby.)

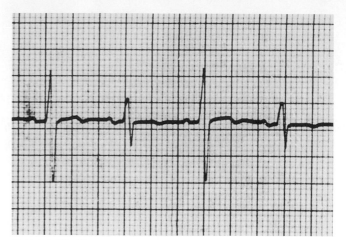

FIGURE 23-10. Lewis-lead electrocardiogram shows total electrical alternation of amplitude and configuration of P and QRS complexes. (From Sotolongo RP, Horton JD: Total electrical alternans in pericardial tamponade, *Am Heart J* 101:853, 1981.)

Pericardiocentesis (Figure 23-9) may be lifesaving for some patients with pericardial tamponade. It is a temporizing procedure performed to improve cardiac function while waiting for surgery. However, it is not the best diagnostic tool for most patients because of a significant false-positive rate and risks for secondary injuries such as coronary vessel laceration and dysrhythmia.[20] The ECG, chest radiograph, and central venous pressure readings are not reliable diagnostic tools because of inconsistent changes in assessment parameters for each.[20] Some patients exhibit an unusual rhythm known as electrical alternans (Figure 23-10). Early identification and prompt intervention are essential for patient survival.

Aortic Disruption

The majority of victims with aortic rupture caused by blunt trauma die at the scene of the injury; ascending aortic injuries are immediately fatal in most cases and descending aortic injuries carry an 85% fatality rate before arrival at the ED.[6] Aortic injury is commonly associated with horizontal or vertical acceleration or deceleration injuries such as high-speed MVCs and falls from a great height. A combination of shearing forces, compression of the aorta against the vertebral column, and an increase in intraluminal pressure inside the vessel at the time of the injuring event are responsible for disrupting aortic integrity.[8] The most common site of injury involves the area of the aorta just distal to the left subclavian artery adjacent to the ligamentum arteriosum (the site where the aorta is relatively fixed in place). The innominate artery at the aortic arch and the aortic valve are also common sites of injury.[17] Figure 23-11 demonstrates common sites of aortic disruption.

The patient may complain of chest pain or pain between the scapulae, often described as unrelenting and severe. Other symptoms include dyspnea and hemoptysis. A loud systolic murmur may be heard over the precordium if aortic valve integrity has been lost. Signs of hemorrhagic shock may be present. A discrepancy between blood pressure values in the right and left arms may occur, depending on the level of aortic injury. Acute coarctation syndrome can occur as sympathetic fibers in the aorta respond to the stretch stimulus from a torn intimal flap or hematoma. Blood pressure and pulse quality in the upper extremities are elevated, whereas pulses and blood pressure in the lower extremities are decreased or absent.[8]

The most common diagnostic test used to detect aortic disruption is a chest radiograph; the most common finding is mediastinal widening (Figure 23-12). A supine chest radiograph may not adequately demonstrate mediastinal widening. Other chest film findings include the presence of an "apical cap," a displaced esophagus (evidenced by visualization of a deviated orogastric/nasogastric tube), trachea deviated to the right, obliteration of the aortic knob, fracture of the first or second ribs, depression of the left mainstem bronchus, and massive left pleural effusion.[4,8,17] Radiographic findings are not specific or sensitive enough to pinpoint the injury; up to 28% of victims with aortic rupture have a normal chest radiograph.[17] The diagnostic standard for identification of aortic injury is the aortogram; however, this procedure is not without associated risks. Injection of radiopaque dye may worsen the tear in the aorta and cause complete disruption. Spiral chest CT may be used to provide aortic imaging. Another diagnostic option is TEE, used in some centers across the country, which visualizes the aorta from the posterior aspect via the esophagus.[5]

Definitive treatment for aortic disruption is immediate surgical repair. Management in the ED includes insertion of large-bore intravenous catheters and collection of blood for type and cross-match. Some patients require medical management with beta-blockers and antihypertensive agents when associated injuries preclude the safe induction of anesthesia.[8]

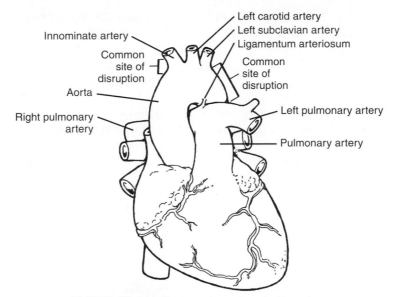

FIGURE **23-11.** Common sites of aortic disruption.

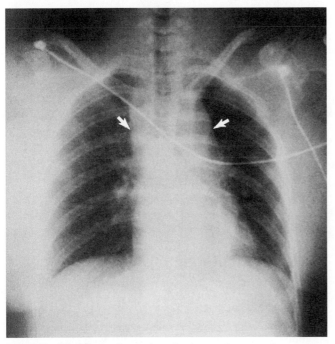

FIGURE **23-12.** Radiograph of chest. Arrows demonstrate widened mediastinum.

Esophageal Injury

Injury to the esophagus is rare and often lethal, almost universally the result of penetrating trauma. Instrumentation during invasive procedures such as endoscopy or intubation is the most common cause.[18] Caustic ingestions (acids or alkalis), crush injuries, and blast injuries also cause esophageal injury. Regardless of the mechanism, the final result is mediastinitis caused by contamination from saliva and gastric contents. The patient may experience pain to the neck, upper back, chest, or abdomen; dysphagia; dyspnea; subcutaneous emphysema of the neck and chest; Hamman's crunch, and

shock out of proportion to the apparent chest injury. Pneumothorax or hemothorax without rib fracture may be present. Chest tube drainage may contain particulate matter. Diagnosis is confirmed by contrast studies or esophagoscopy. Urgent surgical repair is indicated.

SUMMARY

Thoracic injuries are challenging, chaotic to manage, and potentially life-threatening due to compromises in breathing and circulation. Changes in diagnostic technology (e.g., FAST examinations and TEE) have made early identification of many of these serious injuries easier. With more research, management of chest injuries may change significantly. The patient with a thoracic injury requires rapid assessment and intervention. The emergency nurse must anticipate potentially lethal thoracic injuries and rapidly intervene.

REFERENCES

1. American College of Surgeons: Thoracic trauma. In *Advanced trauma life support for doctors (instructor course manual)*, ed 7, Chicago, 2004, The College.
2. Atrium Medical Corporation: *Chest drainage competency manual,* 2004. Retrieved June 14, 2008, from http://www.atriummed.com/PDF/CompetencyManual2004.pdf.
3. Baumann MH: What size chest tube? What drainage system is ideal? And other chest tube management questions, *Curr Opin Pulm Med* 9:276, 2003.
4. Bjerke HS: Flail chest, e-*Medicine,* 2006. Retrieved June 14, 2008, from http://www.emedicine.com/med/topic2813.
5. Cinnella G, Dambrosio M, Brienza N et al: Transesophageal echocardiography for diagnosis of traumatic aortic injury: an appraisal of the evidence, *J Trauma* 57(6):1246, 2004.

6. Emergency Nurses Association: Thoracic trauma. In *Trauma nursing core course provider manual*, ed 6, Des Plaines, Ill, 2007, The Association.

7. Ivatury RR: The injured heart. In Moore EE, Feliciano DV, Mattox KL, editors: *Trauma*, ed 5, New York, 2004, McGraw-Hill.

8. Khalil A, Tarik T, Porembka DT: Aortic pathology: aortic trauma, debris, dissection, and aneurysm, *Crit Care Med* 35(8 suppl):S292, 2007.

9. Khan AN: Thorax, trauma, *e-Medicine,* 2007. Retrieved June 14, 2008, from http://www.emedicine.com/radio/topic400.htm.

10. Kincaid EH, Meredith JW: Thoracic injuries: overview. In Flint L, Meredith JW, Schwab CW et al, editors: *Trauma: contemporary principles and therapy*, Philadelphia, 2008, Lippincott Williams & Wilkins.

11. Livingston DH, Hauser CJ: Trauma to the chest wall and lung. In Moore EE, Feliciano DV, Mattox KL, editors: *Trauma*, ed 5, New York, 2004, McGraw-Hill.

12. Matthews BD, Bui H, Harold KL et al: Laparoscopic repair of traumatic diaphragmatic injuries,, *Surg Endosc* 17(2):254, 2003.

13. Paidas CN: Thoracic trauma, *e-Medicine,* 2006. Retrieved June 14, 2008, from http://www.emedicine.com/ped/topic3001.htm.

14. Patel AN, Brennig C, Cotner J et al: Successful diagnosis of penetrating cardiac injury using surgeon-performed sonography, *Ann Thorac Surg* 76:2043, 2003.

15. Richards CE, Wallis DN: Asphyxiation: a review, *Trauma* 7(1):37, 2005.

16. Rozycki GS, Dente CJ: Surgeon-performed ultrasound in trauma and surgical critical care, In Moore EE, Feliciano DV, Mattox KL, editors: *Trauma*, ed 5, New York, 2004, McGraw-Hill.

17. Salim A: Mediastinal trauma, *Trauma* 3(1):33, 2001.

18. Schaefer SD: Laryngeal and esophageal trauma. In *Cummings otolaryngology*, ed 4, St. Louis, 2005, Mosby.

19. Sherwood SF, Harstook RL: Thoracic injuries. In McQuillan KA, Von Rueden KT, Harstook RL et al, editors: *Trauma nursing: from resuscitation through rehabilitation*, ed 3, Philadelphia, 2002, WB Saunders.

20. Suárez FJO, Mustelier JV, Arzola RC: Role of transesophageal echocardiography in assessment of penetrating heart trauma, *Internet J Cardiol* 4(2), 2007.

21. Thevasagayam MS: Laryngeal trauma: a systematic approach to management, *Trauma* 7(2):87, 2005.

22. Tribble RW, Nolan SP: Pneumothorax. In Cameron JL, editor: *Current surgical therapy*, ed 8, St. Louis, 2004, Mosby.

23. Welsford M: Diaphragmatic injuries, *e-Medicine*, 2007. Retrieved June 14, 2008, from http://www.emedicine.com/emerg/TOPIC136.HTM.

24. Zhang M, Liu ZH, Yang JX et al: Rapid detection of pneumothorax by ultrasonography with multiple trauma, *Crit Care* 10(4):R112, 2006. Retrieved June 14, 2008, from http://www.ccforum.com/content/10/4/R112.

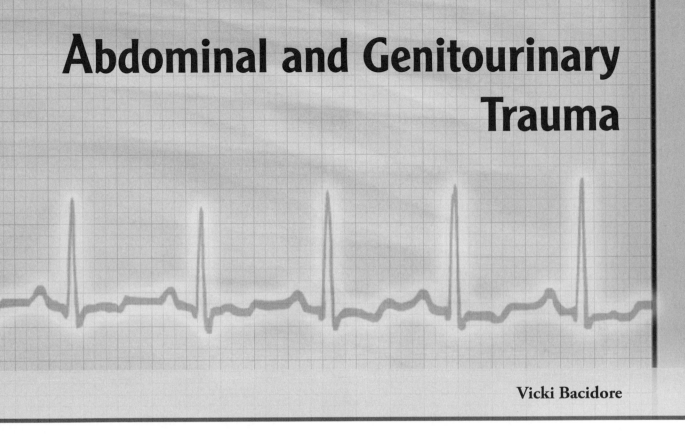

CHAPTER 24

Abdominal and Genitourinary Trauma

Vicki Bacidore

bdominal injuries are a significant source of morbidity and mortality, ranking third as a cause of traumatic death, preceded only by injuries to the head and chest. Although both penetrating and blunt injuries are common, blunt abdominal trauma is the leading cause of death and disability across all age-groups. One of the most frequent causes of preventable death is an abdominal injury that is unrecognized or missed by the emergency care provider.[13] The emergency nurse should initially manage patients with abdominal trauma in the same manner as all other trauma patients. Evaluation should begin with a rapid assessment and concurrent emergency management of any airway, breathing, circulation, and disability issues.

An understanding of the mechanism of injury and the forces involved in the wounding event allows the team to focus its assessment and raises the suspicion of specific organ involvement. Blunt injury occurs most often from motor vehicle crashes (MVCs). These injuries are often related to mechanisms of shearing, tearing, or direct-impact forces. Blunt abdominal trauma has a higher mortality rate than penetrating injuries because blunt injuries are more difficult to detect and are often associated with other concomitant injuries to the head, chest, and extremities. Multiple abdominal organ injuries are associated with higher mortality. Penetrating injuries are often caused by gunshots or stabbings but can be due to any sharp object. Stab injuries occur almost three times more often than gunshot injuries, are usually less destructive, and have a much lower mortality rate.[7] Penetrating trauma is more likely to involve vascular structures. Gunshot wounds can be deceiving because there is almost always some blast effect, and the dissipation of kinetic energy can damage structures that were not in direct contact with the bullet. Also, because of the force involved, the wound tract can close in on itself, making an accurate estimate of tissue damage difficult. See Chapter 20 for further discussion on blunt and penetrating trauma.

ANATOMY AND PHYSIOLOGY

Knowledge of the anatomic boundaries of the abdomen is important as one considers injury patterns, such as hollow-organ injury, vascular injury, solid organ injury, or injuries to the retroperitoneal area (Figure 24-1). The oval-shaped abdominal cavity extends from the dome-shaped diaphragm, a large muscle separating the thoracic cavity from the abdomen, to the pelvic brim. The pelvic brim stretches at an angle from the intervertebral disk between L5 and S1 to the pubic symphysis.

The abdomen is divided into three sections: the anterior abdomen, the flanks, and the posterior abdomen or back. The outer boundary of the abdominal cavity is the abdominal wall on the front of the body and the peritoneal surface on the back of the body. The abdomen extends upward

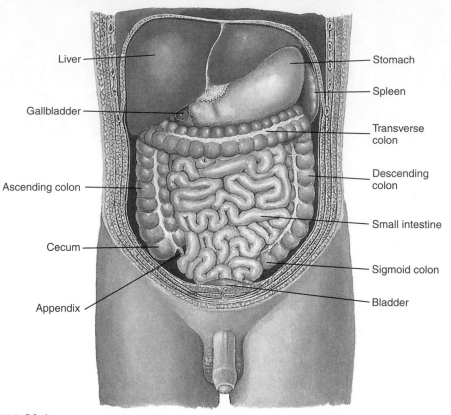

FIGURE **24-1.** Abdominal viscera. (From Seidel HM et al: *Mosby's guide to physical examination,* ed 6, St. Louis, 2006, Mosby.)

into the lower thorax at about the level of the nipples or the fourth intercostal space. The anterior part of the abdomen extends inferiorly to the inguinal ligaments and symphysis pubis, and laterally to the front of the axillary line. The flanks include the regions between the anterior and posterior axillary lines from the sixth intercostal space to the iliac crest. The back extends posteriorly between the posterior axillary lines, from the scapula to the iliac crests. The flanks and the back are protected by thick abdominal wall muscles that protect the region from low-velocity penetrating trauma.

Peritoneum

The peritoneum is a smooth, serous membrane that provides cover to the abdominal structures and allows the viscera to move within the abdomen without friction. The parietal peritoneum lines the abdominal wall, and the visceral peritoneum surrounds the organs of the abdomen. The mesenteries are double layers of the peritoneum; they surround, supply blood, and attach organs like the large and small bowel to the abdominal wall. Organs in the retroperitoneal space (e.g., kidneys, parts of the colon, duodenum, pancreas, aorta, and inferior vena cava) (Figure 24-2) are only partially covered by the peritoneum. In men the peritoneum is closed, but in women it is open where the ends of the fallopian tubes communicate with the peritoneum.

Solid Organs

The liver is a solid organ and is the largest organ in the abdomen. It is located in the right upper quadrant (RUQ) with extension into the midline and is extremely vascular. Circulation is through the hepatic artery and portal vein and represents about 30% of the total cardiac output. Aside from its metabolic functions, the liver releases bile to aid in fat emulsification and the absorption of fatty acids. It also filters and stores up to 500 mL of blood at any given time.

The spleen is also a large vascular organ located in the left upper quadrant (LUQ), beneath the diaphragm at the level of the ninth through eleventh ribs. The spleen is important in the body's immune function for its clearance of bacteria. It also filters and stores up to 200 mL of blood.

The gallbladder is a saclike organ located on the lower surface of the liver that acts as a reservoir for bile, one of the digestive enzymes produced by the liver. The liver continually secretes bile, and the gallbladder stores it until it is released through the cystic duct during the digestive process.

The kidneys are retroperitoneal organs that lie at the level of the twelfth thoracic vertebra to the third lumbar vertebra. The kidneys lie posterior to the stomach, spleen, colonic flexure, and small bowel. They are enclosed in a capsule of fatty tissue and a layer of renal fascia, which maintains their position. They are well protected by the vertebral bodies and the back muscles, as well as the abdominal viscera. They

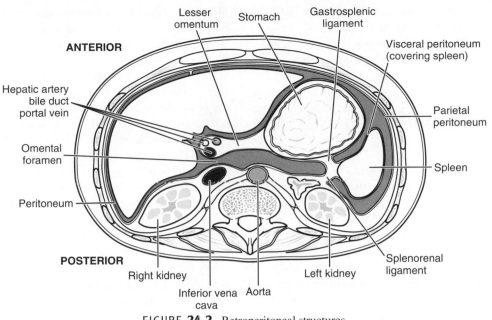

FIGURE **24-2.** Retroperitoneal structures.

are protected because of their deep location in the retroperitoneal space and by abdominal contents, muscles, and the vertebral spine. They filter blood and excrete body wastes in the form of urine.

The pancreas is located behind the stomach along the abdomen's posterior wall in the retroperitoneum. Its exocrine cells produce enzymes, electrolytes, and bicarbonate to assist in the digestion and absorption of nutrients. Its endocrine cells produce insulin, glucagon, and somatostatin, which are involved in carbohydrate metabolism.

Hollow Organs

The stomach is located in the LUQ between the liver and spleen at the level of the seventh and ninth ribs. Entry to the stomach is controlled by the lower esophageal sphincter (sometimes referred to as the cardiac sphincter), and exit is controlled by the pyloric sphincter. The stomach stores food, secretes acidic gastric secretions, mixes food with the secretions, and then propels the mixture into the duodenum.

The small bowel connects to the pyloric sphincter and fills most of the abdominal cavity because it is approximately 7 m long. It is composed of three sections: duodenum, jejunum, and ileum, and it is held in position by the adjacent viscera, the peritoneal membrane attachments to the posterior abdominal wall, and ligaments. It functions by releasing enzymes that aid in digestion and absorption.

The large bowel is about 1.5 m long; it connects with the ileum proximally and ends distally at the rectum. Its divisions consist of the ascending colon, transverse colon, descending colon, and the sigmoid colon. The primary functions of the large bowel are to absorb water and nutrients and store fecal matter until it can be eliminated.

The urinary bladder is an extraperitoneal organ that stores urine. When empty, it lies in the pelvic cavity, and when full, it can expand into the abdomen. Its blood supply is large and derived from branches of the iliac artery. The ureters are a pair of thick-walled, hollow tubes that carry urine from the kidneys to the urinary bladder. The female urethra is short and well protected by the symphysis pubis, whereas the male urethra is about 20 cm long and lies mostly outside of the body.

Reproductive Organs

The abdomen also contains organs of the reproductive system. The female reproductive system contains the uterus, a pear-shaped organ that allows implantation, growth, and nourishment of a fetus during pregnancy. The nongravid uterus is in the pelvis, and the gravid uterus is in the midline of the lower abdomen. The female ovaries, located in the pelvis, one on each side of the uterus, produce the precursors to mature eggs and produce hormones that regulate female reproductive function.

The male reproductive system contains the penis, the male external reproductive organ, as well as the testes. The penis has three vascular bodies (erectile tissue): the paired corpora cavernosa and the corpus spongiosum. A testis and epididymis lie in each scrotal compartment. Testicular blood supply is obtained via the spermatic cord and the testicular artery, the artery to the vas deferens, and the cremasteric artery. The scrotum is covered by a thin layer of skin and obtains its blood supply via the branches of the femoral and internal pudendal arteries.

Vascular Structures

The abdominal aorta lies left of the midline and bifurcates into the iliac arteries, which supply blood to the lower extremities. Three unpaired arteries originating from the abdominal aorta (the celiac trunk and the superior and inferior mesentery arteries) supply the abdominal organs. The celiac trunk branches into the hepatic, left gastric, and splenic arteries. The inferior vena cava is the major vein in the abdomen.

PATIENT ASSESSMENT
History

Because the patient with abdominal trauma may not exhibit any obvious injuries, it should be suspected based on the patient's chief complaint and mechanism of injury. Abdominal trauma should also be considered in a patient with multisystem trauma or history of injury with unexplained hypotension or tachycardia. Complaints of pain, rigidity, guarding, or spasms in the abdominal musculature are classic signs of intraabdominal injury. Peritoneal membranes may be irritated due to free blood, air, or gastric or intestinal contents within the peritoneal cavity. Irritation of the inferior surface of the diaphragm and phrenic nerve can cause referred pain to the left shoulder This finding, known as Kehr's sign, should alert the trauma nurse to a possible splenic injury. Patient history and assessment triggers that require further evaluation include the following[12]:

1. Presence of abdominal pain, tenderness, or distension
2. Mechanism of injury and prehospital details suggest potential for injury
3. Lower chest or pelvic injury
4. High-speed collisions or collisions in which there has been substantial deformity to the vehicle (particularly if the patient was unrestrained)
5. MVCs with fatalities or those in which there were others with substantial injuries
6. Unprotected injury (i.e., motorcycle crashes)
7. Inability to tolerate a delayed diagnosis (e.g., older adults, those with significant comorbid diseases)
8. Presence of distracting injuries (e.g., long-bone fractures)
9. Decreased level of consciousness/altered sensorium
10. Pain-masking drugs (e.g., ethanol, opiates)

Mechanisms of Injury

Understanding the mechanism of injury, the type of force applied, and the tissue density of the injured organ (solid, hollow) aids the trauma team by focusing the assessment and having a high index of suspicion regarding specific organ involvement. Blunt and penetrating abdominal trauma can cause extensive injury to the viscera, resulting in massive blood loss, spillage of intestinal contents into the peritoneal space, and peritonitis.

Blunt

Blunt trauma is the most common mechanism of injury seen in the United States; motor vehicle collisions are the leading mode of injury. This diffuse injury pattern puts all abdominal organs at risk for injury. The biomechanics of blunt injury involve a compression or crushing by direct energy transmission. If the compressive, shearing, or stretching forces exceed tissue tolerance limits, they are disrupted. This may result in injury to solid viscera (liver, spleen) or rupture of hollow viscera (gastrointestinal tract). Injury also can result from the movement of organs within the body. Some organs are rigidly fixed in place, whereas others are semifixed by ligaments, such as the mesenteric attachments of the intestines. During energy transfer, longitudinal shearing forces may cause rupture of these organs at their attachment points or where the blood vessels enter the organ. Examples of structures semifixed in place and therefore susceptible to injury include the mesentery and small bowel, particularly at the ligament of Treitz or at the junction of the distal small bowel and right colon. Falls from a height produce a unique pattern of injury. In this case, injury severity is a function of distance and the surface on which the victim lands. Intraabdominal injuries are uncommon from vertical falls; hollow visceral rupture is most frequent. Retroperitoneal injuries with significant blood loss, however, are common because force is transmitted up the axial skeleton.

Penetrating

Stab wounds directly injure tissue as the blade passes through the body. External examination of the wound may underestimate internal damage and cannot define the trajectory of the blade. Any stab wound in the lower chest, pelvis, flank, or back has caused abdominal injury until proven otherwise. Gunshot wounds injure in several ways. Bullets may injure organs directly, via secondary missiles such as bone or bullet fragments, or from energy transmitted from the bullet. Bullets designed to break apart once they enter a victim cause much more tissue destruction than a bullet that remains intact. Tissue disruptions presumed to be entrance and exit wounds can approximate the missile trajectory. Plain radiographs help to localize the foreign body, allowing prediction of organs at risk. Unfortunately, bullets may not travel in a straight line. Thus all structures in any proximity to the presumed trajectory must be considered injured.[12]

Motor Vehicle Crashes

In MVCs there are five typical patterns of impact: frontal, lateral, rear, rotational, and rollover. Each of these different mechanisms, with the exception of rear impact, has the potential to cause significant injury to the abdominal organs. In a rear-impact collision, the patient is less likely to have an abdominal injury if proper vehicular restraints are used. However, if restraints are improperly worn or not used at all, the potential for injury is great. Rollover impacts present the greatest potential to inflict lethal injuries. Unrestrained occupants may change direction several times with an increased risk for ejection from the vehicle. The occupants involved in a rollover may collide with each other, as well as with the vehicle interior, producing a wide range of potential injuries.

Inspection

Observe the lower chest for asymmetric chest wall movement, which may indicate lower rib fractures and liver, spleen or diaphragmatic injury. Look at the contour of the abdomen: distension may be due to massive bleeding, pneumoperitoneum, gastric dilation, or ileus produced by peritoneal irritation; a flat or concave abdomen may be indicative of a ruptured diaphragm with herniation of abdominal organs into the thoracic cavity. Assess for bruising, abrasions, or lacerations. Ecchymosis in the LUQ may indicate soft tissue injury or a splenic injury. Bruising or patterning over where the seat belt would be located or steering wheel–shaped contusions suggest a significant mechanism of injury, and other intraabdominal injuries should be suspected. Cullen's sign (i.e., periumbilical ecchymosis) may indicate intraperitoneal hemorrhage; however, this symptom usually takes several hours to develop. Flank bruising, Grey Turner's sign, may raise suspicion for retroperitoneal injury and bleeding. Old surgical scars should be noted because this may help narrow the search for organs that may be injured. Inspect for gunshot or stab wounds, and inspect the pelvic area for soft tissue bruising.

Percussion and Auscultation

Percussion has been used to detect the presence of free fluid in the abdomen. With the ready availability of more sensitive, noninvasive diagnostic techniques (e.g., ultrasonography and computed tomography [CT]), listening to percussion sounds to diagnose abdominal injury is outmoded.

All four quadrants of the abdomen should be auscultated for the presence and frequency of bowel sounds. The presence of bowel sounds is a reassuring indicator of peristalsis, but it is not reliable for ruling out visceral injuries. Up to 30% of patients have active bowel sounds in the presence of intraperitoneal bleeding or rupture of hollow viscera. Conversely, about 30% of patients who have absolutely no bowel sounds after careful listening for at least 5 minutes have no visceral damage.[15] An abdominal bruit may indicate underlying vascular disease or traumatic arteriovenous fistula. Auscultation of bowel sounds in the thoracic cavity, especially on the left side, may indicate the presence of a diaphragmatic injury.

Palpation

Beginning in an area where the patient has not complained of pain, palpate the abdomen for pain, rigidity, tenderness, and guarding in all four quadrants. To determine the presence of rebound tenderness, press on the abdomen and quickly release. Fullness and doughy consistency may indicate intraabdominal hemorrhage. Crepitus or instability of the lower thoracic cage indicates the potential for splenic or hepatic injuries associated with lower rib injuries. Pelvic instability indicates the potential for lower urinary tract injury, as well as pelvic and retroperitoneal hematoma.

Initial Stabilization

Initial stabilization of the patient with abdominal or genitourinary (GU) trauma follows the same sequence as for any patient with major trauma and begins by securing airway, breathing, and circulation. Two large-bore intravenous (IV) catheters should be secured for administration of crystalloids (e.g., lactated Ringer's solution or normal saline), blood products, and medications. Baseline laboratory studies are obtained, as well as a pregnancy test for any woman of childbearing age. Efforts should be made to limit hypothermia, including use of warm blankets and prewarmed fluids.

Medications
Analgesia

Pain relief is appropriate for most injuries. Morphine sulfate 2 to 5 mg or 0.1 mg/kg IV is commonly used. Fentanyl 50 to 100 mcg IV is an alternative agent. It has less histamine release than morphine and thus causes less hypotension; its shorter duration of action may be advantageous in trauma situations in which serial examinations are required. Avoid medications with antiplatelet activity potential such as nonsteroidal antiinflammatory drugs.

Antibiotics

Anaerobes and coliforms are the predominant organisms found in cases of intestinal perforation, and antibiotics active against these organisms should be given to decrease the incidence of intraabdominal sepsis.

Emergency Department Interventions
Urinary Catheter

A urinary catheter should be inserted to monitor urine output in all patients with major trauma. Before inserting a urinary catheter in patients with severe blunt trauma, a rectal examination needs to be performed to check the position of the prostate, look for any rectal blood, and check sphincter tone. If there is any suspicion of damage to the urethra as evidenced by blood at the urethral meatus, penile or perineal hematomas, a displaced prostate, or a severe anterior pelvic fracture, a retrograde urethrogram should be performed before a urinary catheter is inserted.[15]

Gastric Decompression

Early gastric decompression with a gastric tube is particularly important when there is a possibility of intraabdominal visceral damage or when the patient may have eaten or drunk recently. All trauma patients should be assumed to have full stomachs, even if they deny recent ingestion of food or liquids. The gastric tube may be a valuable diagnostic tool for revealing injury to the upper gastrointestinal tract; oral rather than nasal insertion of the tube is recommended in patients with concurrent head injury (i.e., basilar skull fracture) or midface injuries. Injured patients tend to swallow air, especially if they have any respiratory distress. Patients resuscitated with a bag-mask device can also have large amounts of air forced into their stomachs. The resulting distension of the stomach not only increases the chances of vomiting and aspirating, but also raises the diaphragm, increasing the resistance to ventilation.

Wound Care

Penetrating wounds should be covered with sterile dressings. In cases of traumatic eviscerations, the intraabdominal contents extrude through the abdominal wall and are exposed to the environment. To prevent further injury and to keep the exposed organs viable for surgical replacement, the extruded contents must be kept moist at all times with sterile saline–soaked dressings.[3] Eviscerated organs, especially the small bowel, should never be allowed to dry out. Never attempt to push the eviscerated contents back into the peritoneal cavity, which may further injure the tissue.[16]

Disposition

A trauma surgeon should be consulted for any patient suspected of having an abdominal or GU injury. The patient should be transferred to another facility if a trauma surgeon is unavailable. All patients with intraabdominal injuries require admission for emergent surgery or for observation. Stable and reliable patients with no identifiable injury can be discharged to home, as well as patients with stab wounds to the abdominal cavity that are found to be superficial after wound exploration. Discharged patients need to be provided with detailed instructions that describe signs of undiagnosed injury. Patients need to return if they experience increased abdominal pain or distension, nausea and/or vomiting, lightheadedness, syncope, or new or increased bleeding in urine or feces. All patients require close follow-up and repeat evaluation.

Diagnostic Evaluation

Diagnostic evaluation of a patient with abdominal trauma is based on the patient's hemodynamic stability. If the patient is or becomes hemodynamically unstable secondary to intraperitoneal injury, transfusion with fluids or blood is begun and the patient is prepared for surgery. If the patient's condition permits, major diagnostic tools, including radiology, CT, focused assessment sonography for trauma (FAST) examination, magnetic resonance imaging (MRI), angiography, diagnostic peritoneal lavage (DPL), and laparoscopy, may be used. Table 24-1 provides a comparison of DPL, FAST, and CT scans in blunt abdominal trauma.

Imaging

PLAIN FILMS. Plain films may reveal free intraperitoneal air, which is indicative of hollow-organ injury (e.g., bowel perforation); however, free air is more readily seen on CT than plain films.[16] Foreign bodies and missiles can also be identified. All penetrating wounds should be marked.

COMPUTED TOMOGRAPHY SCAN OF THE ABDOMEN AND PELVIS. A CT scan is noninvasive but requires a hemodynamically stable patient. It can reveal intraperitoneal injury, retroperitoneal injury, the source of intraabdominal hemorrhage, and occasionally, active bleeding. A CT scan can aid in evaluating the vertebral column and can be extended to visualize the thorax and pelvis. One advantage of the CT scan is the reduction of nontherapeutic laparotomies for self-limited injuries to the liver and spleen. Unfortunately, the CT scan is not accurate enough to detect injury to the pancreas, diaphragm, small bowel, and mesentery. Oral contrast is not routinely used at many trauma centers—the risk for aspiration is increased with administration of oral contrast, and the delay in imaging is potentially harmful. IV contrast is essential to increase the ability of CT scans to identify hemorrhage.

Table 24-1. COMPARISON OF DIAGNOSTIC TESTS

Procedure	Advantages	Disadvantages	Results
FAST (focused assessment sonography for trauma)	Noninvasive Provides rapid evaluation of hemoperitoneum	Operator dependent Hollow viscus injury rarely identified	As accurate as DPL Free fluid appears as black stripe Sensitivity/specificity of 85%-95%
CT (computerized tomography)	Provides most detailed images Useful in determining nonoperative management of solid injuries	Expensive Time consuming Use only on hemodynamically stable patients May miss injuries to diaphragm and gastrointestinal tract	High specificity
DPL (diagnostic peritoneal lavage)	Provides rapid evaluation of intraperitoneal blood Useful in unstable patients, patients with unreliable history, or inability to perform serial abdominal examinations	Invasive procedure Complications of bleeding, infection	Can have false-positive results leading to unnecessary laparotomy

From Hoyt KS, Selfridge-Thomas J, editors: *ENA's emergency nursing core curriculum,* ed 6, St. Louis, 2007, Saunders.

FOCUSED ASSESSMENT SONOGRAPHY FOR TRAUMA/ULTRASONOGRAPHY. FAST is a portable (bedside), rapid, accurate, and inexpensive diagnostic tool that is used to detect the presence of hemoperitoneum in patients primarily with blunt abdominal trauma. Four areas are examined: the hepatorenal fossa, the splenorenal fossa, the pericardial sac, and the pelvis (Figure 24-3). FAST is considered to be extremely sensitive, with the ability to detect as little as 100 mL of fluid. However, FAST is typically not considered positive until at least 200 to 500 mL of fluid is detected in the abdomen.[7] The disadvantage of FAST is its inability to diagnose hollow visceral and retroperitoneal injuries or intraperitoneal injuries not associated with hemoperitoneum. Ultrasonography can be used to rapidly outline kidney parenchyma and provide evidence of intraperitoneal fluid. It is operator dependent and is not accurate in distinguishing blood from other intraperitoneal fluids such as ascites. The FAST scan is being increasingly used in the initial assessment of trauma patients and has been incorporated into the recommendations for investigations of blunt trauma by the American College of Surgeons.[1]

MAGNETIC RESONANCE IMAGING. There is no rule for MRI in the diagnosis of abdominal trauma, and its use is typically reserved for spinal injuries and difficult-to-diagnose diaphragmatic injuries.

ANGIOGRAPHY. Angiography is typically reserved for the unstable patient with a pelvic fracture or splenic injury. It may also be used to further evaluate a patient in the setting of renal trauma when a vascular pedicle injury is suspected.

DIAGNOSTIC PERITONEAL LAVAGE. The evidence regarding the use of DPL versus the FAST examination is limited, and the most robust studies evaluate the use of DPL as a screening test before CT. Although the FAST examination has widespread use, DPL is still being used.[5] In blunt trauma, DPL is primarily indicated in the hemodynamically unstable patient who has multiple injuries. A DPL can discern solid and hollow visceral injury better than ultrasonography. A DPL can also be used in the diagnostic workup of a stab wound to the abdomen, lower chest, flank, or back to reveal intraperitoneal organ injury or an isolated diaphragmatic rupture. In blunt trauma and stab wounds to the anterior abdomen, flank, and back, a positive result consists of the following: aspiration of 10 mL or more of gross blood or red blood cells (RBCs) greater than 100,000/mm in the lavage fluid. [7] For lower chest stab wound and gunshot wounds, the cutoff for RBCs is 5000/mm.[7] Patients with equivocal findings should be observed for at least 24 hours. Many injuries will be to hollow viscera, and clinical manifestations should develop within that period. Elevated levels of peritoneal amylase may be indicative of small bowel or pancreatic injury. Other positive but less commonly documented DPL results include food fibers or the presence of fecal matter in the lavage fluid. As a precaution to minimize the risk for inadvertent injury to the stomach or bladder, a gastric tube and urinary catheter should be inserted before performing a DPL.

RETROGRADE URETHROGRAPHY. Retrograde urethrography is indicated for any suspected urethral injury. The procedure should be performed at a 30-degree oblique angle from the horizontal. The contrast is retrogradely injected into the urethra using a special catheter to occlude the urethral orifice to prevent reflux of contrast. Static images are then obtained. Dynamic images using fluoroscopy are preferred.

CYSTOGRAPHY. Cystography is indicated for any suspected bladder injury. A urinary catheter can be placed directly into the bladder, the urine drained, and the bladder refilled with contrast material. It is important to fully distend the bladder to avoid missing small injuries. Images are then obtained under retrograde urethrography.

ARTERIOGRAPHY. Arteriography is needed if the mechanism of injury suggests a renal artery injury, because it can provide detailed information regarding vascular injury.

INTRAVENOUS PYELOGRAPHY. Intravenous pyelography was formerly the only means to study the upper GU tract but today is less commonly used, being supplanted by CT.

Laboratory Studies

Initial hemoglobin and hematocrit levels do not reflect the amount of recent hemorrhage that may have occurred, but these values can serve as a baseline and are important if the patient will be going to surgery. In the absence of hypotension, a progressive decrease in hemoglobin and hematocrit levels can serve as a warning of continued bleeding, but this finding tends to be relatively late. Serum amylase levels must be interpreted in conjunction with other clinical findings; however, an increasing level or a persistently high amylase level is suggestive of pancreatic injury.[15]

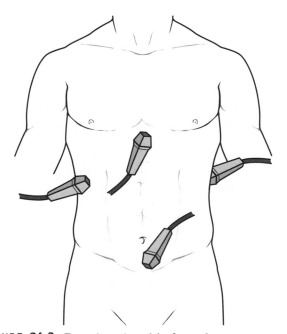

FIGURE 24-3. Four sites viewed in focused assessment sonography for trauma (FAST) examinations. (From Emergency Nurses Association: *Trauma nursing core course [TNCC]*, ed 6, Des Plaines, Ill, 2007, The Association.)

A urinalysis should be performed on any patient with suspected abdominal or pelvic damage as a guide to possible injury of the urinary tract and to detect diabetes mellitus or concomitant renal parenchymal disease. If the urine dipstick is positive for hemoglobin but has few or no red blood cells, one should suspect myoglobinuria. With minor microscopic hematuria, a detailed urologic workup is not generally indicated, but a repeat urinalysis is appropriate. Microscopic hematuria, heme-positive dipstick, and gross hematuria are the strongest indicators of GU injury. However, the degree of hematuria does not necessarily correlate with the degree of injury. Furthermore, blunt injury to the renovascular pedicle or penetrating ureteral injury may not produce gross or even microscopic hematuria. The best urine sample for the assessment of hematuria in the trauma patient is the first voided or catheterized specimen, because a later sample can often be diluted by diuresis.

A urine pregnancy test should be done in all women of reproductive age.[8]

SPECIFIC INJURIES
Abdominal Injuries
Spleen

Falls and MVCs commonly injure the spleen. However, less obvious injury patterns in activities such as sports (tackling in football or checking in lacrosse) can also cause injury. The spleen is one of the organs most often injured by blunt trauma. Its small size makes it a difficult target, so it is injured less often with penetrating trauma. Due to the spleen being encapsulated, injury may damage only the capsule or can actually fracture the spleen. Table 24-2 summarizes grading of splenic injury. Injury is suggested when the patient has sustained blunt trauma to the LUQ. The patient should be assessed for LUQ pain and tenderness, pain referred to the left shoulder (Kehr's sign), peritoneal irritation, and hypotension.

When assessing for bruising or pain in the LUQ, the presence of Kehr's sign suggests diaphragmatic irritation by peritoneal blood. Splenic injuries may cause significant hemodynamic instability. Shock and hypotension are present in as few as 30% of patients with splenic trauma.[11] Not all patients with splenic injury require surgery; those who are hemodynamically stable may be managed nonoperatively, focusing on serial abdominal examinations, vital signs, and laboratory values. Operative management is reserved for unstable patients, gunshot wounds, or injuries that violate all layers of the splenic capsule. The ultimate goal is to preserve the function of the spleen if possible. The CT scan is noninvasive and sensitive in stable patients. The FAST examination can be used for unstable patients.

Liver

The liver's size and anterior location make it an easy target for blunt and penetrating forces. The liver is one of the most commonly injured abdominal organs in blunt trauma. At any given time, 25% of circulating blood is in the liver, resulting in serious sequelae if injured. Overall mortality for liver injuries is

Grade	Category	Description
I	Hematoma	Subcapsular; involves less than 10% surface area; hematoma does not expand
	Laceration	Nonbleeding capsular tear; less than 1 cm deep
II	Hematoma	Subcapsular hematoma covering 10%-50% surface area
		Hematoma does not expand; intraparenchymal hematoma less than 2 cm wide
	Laceration	Capsular tear with active bleeding; intraparenchymal injury 1-3 cm deep
III	Hematoma	Subscapular hematoma involving more than 50% surface area or one that is expanding; intraparenchymal hematoma ≥5 cm or expanding; ruptured subscapular hematoma with active bleeding
	Laceration	More than 3 cm deep or involving intracellular vessels
IV	Hematoma	Ruptured intraparenchymal hematoma with active bleeding
	Laceration	Segmental laceration or one that involves hilar vessels
		Devascularization of more than 25% of spleen
V	Laceration	Shattered spleen
	Vascular	Hilar vascular injury; spleen is devascularized

Table 24-2. **SPLENIC INJURIES**

From Pearl WS, Todd KH: Ultrasonography for the initial evaluation of blunt abdominal trauma: a review in prospective trials, *Ann Emerg Med* 27:353, 1996.

10%. MVCs still account for the majority of hepatic injuries. Like the spleen, the liver is encapsulated, so injuries can affect only the capsule or fracture the liver itself. Table 24-3 summarizes graded liver injuries. Liver injuries are suggested when the patient has a direct blow to the RUQ from the eighth rib to the central abdomen. Clinical indications include RUQ pain and tenderness, bruising over the RUQ, or referred pain to the right shoulder. Hemodynamic instability is almost always present when the liver sustains major damage. The trauma team should consider acute hepatic injury if the patient remains hypotensive despite aggressive IV fluid resuscitation. The CT scan is noninvasive and sensitive in stable patients, and the FAST examination can be used for unstable patients. Surgical repair of liver injuries is determined by the extent of the injury and the patient's hemodynamic status. More than 50% of adults with liver injury are treated nonoperatively.

Stomach

The stomach is a hollow organ that can be easily displaced, so it is rarely injured with blunt trauma. Gastric and esophageal injuries occur more with multiorgan and multisystem

Grade	Category	Description
I	Hematoma	Nonexpanding subcapsular hematoma less than 10% of liver surface
	Laceration	Nonbleeding capsular tear less than 1 cm deep
II	Hematoma	Nonexpanding subcapsular hematoma covering 10% - 50% surface area; less than 2 cm deep
	Laceration	Less than 3 cm parenchymal penetration; less than 10 cm long
III	Hematoma	Subcapsular hematoma more than 50% of surface area or one that is expanding; ruptured subcapsular hematoma with active bleeding; intraparenchymal hematoma more than 2 cm wide
	Laceration	More than 3 cm deep
IV	Hematoma	Ruptured central hematoma
	Laceration	15%-25% hepatic lobe destroyed
V	Laceration	More than 75% hepatic lobe destroyed
	Vascular	Major hepatic veins injured
VI	Vascular	Avulsed liver

Table 24-3. LIVER INJURIES

From Pearl WS, Todd KH: Ultrasonography for the initial evaluation of blunt abdominal trauma: a review in prospective trials, *Ann Emerg Med* 27:353, 1996

injuries and are most commonly associated with penetrating trauma because of their size and anterior location.[13] Physical signs and symptoms associated with stomach injuries include LUQ pain and tenderness. Diagnosis is based on patient assessment, aspiration of blood via the gastric tube, and presence of free air on the abdominal radiograph. All patients with gastric injury require surgical exploration.

Large and Small Intestine

The intestines are hollow, highly vascular organs approximately 32 feet long that are fixed at various points in the peritoneal cavity. Their anterior location, relative lack of protection, vascularity, and fixed points of attachment make the intestines vulnerable to both blunt and penetrating injuries. Penetrating trauma, particularly stab wounds, can eviscerate the bowel or omentum. Management includes covering the evisceration with sterile saline–soaked pads, taking care not to pour saline onto pads that are in place on the wound. Wounds should then be covered with an occlusive dressing. Examine the back, because organs can eviscerate from penetrating injury to the posterior surface as well. Establish IV access, and prepare the patient for surgery. The intestines are frequently injured by inappropriately worn seat belts. Injury to the intestines usually causes rupture followed by spillage of chemical and bacterial contamination into the peritoneum. Initial signs and symptoms of intestinal injury include tenderness and rigidity. As time progresses and more peritoneal contamination occurs, the patient may develop

fever, elevated white blood cell count, abdominal distension, and hypoactive bowel sounds. Reassessments are important because peritoneal signs may be delayed and injuries can be missed on initial plain radiographs and CT scans.

Pancreas

The pancreas, a semisolid organ in the retroperitoneal space, is well protected by the liver and stomach, so it is more likely to be injured by penetrating trauma. Pancreatic injury from blunt trauma is more unusual but does occur; children sustain pancreatic injury in bicycle crashes when the handlebars are driven into the abdomen. Patients may present with epigastric or back pain. Cullen's sign is often associated with pancreatic injury and pancreatitis. The retroperitoneal location of the pancreas makes DPL an unreliable indicator of pancreatic injury. Elevated serum amylase level is also an unreliable indicator of pancreatic injury because up to 40% of all patients with pancreatic injury initially have a normal serum amylase level. Lipase is considered a better indicator of pancreatic injury. An assay for pancreatic fraction is proving more reliable; however, this test is not yet readily available. CT scan is noninvasive and sensitive to detect pancreatic injury. Endoscopic retrograde pancreatography has proven useful in identifying injury to the pancreatic duct. When surgery is required, every effort is made to preserve the pancreas because of its essential endocrine and exocrine functions. The majority of patients with pancreatic injury have other injuries, with associated hemorrhage being the major cause of death.

Diaphragm

Diaphragmatic rupture may be due to blunt or penetrating mechanisms. Rupture almost always occurs on the left side because the liver protects the right hemidiaphragm. Rupture should be suspected in all patients with thoracoabdominal injuries. In diaphragmatic rupture, abdominal organs herniate into the thoracic cavity, causing respiratory compromise secondary to lung compression. Bowel sounds may be auscultated in the chest cavity. Loss of negative pressure in the chest and inability of the diaphragm to function normally further compromise respiratory function. Cardiac output also decreases because of cardiac compression. Diagnosis is usually confirmed by a radiograph of the chest showing abdominal contents or the gastric tube in the left chest. CT scan or laparoscopy are more sensitive. These patients require immediate surgical repair. Mortality increases with delay in identification and treatment (see Chapter 23 for additional discussion).

Vascular Structures

Major vascular structures in the abdomen include the abdominal aorta, inferior vena cava, iliac artery, and hepatic veins. Vessels can be injured by blunt or penetrating mechanisms—injury of major abdominal vessels occurs in 5% to 10% of patients with blunt abdominal trauma. Disruption of vascular structures causes severe hemorrhage and death if damage is not repaired. Hemorrhagic shock from intraabdominal hemorrhage often leads to metabolic acidosis accompanied by coagulopathy and hypothermia—often referred to as the "lethal triad of trauma." Identification of injuries is often made in surgery, particularly in an unstable patient. A CT scan and arteriography may be used for the stable patient. Emergency management of patients with vascular injuries includes establishing IV access and providing rapid transport to the surgical suite.

Foreign Bodies

Abdominal injuries may result from foreign bodies in the stomach and rectum. This may be the result of ingestion, masturbation, autoeroticism, assault, confusion, or psychiatric illness. Body packing (i.e., drug-filled condoms or plastic bags swallowed or placed in the rectum) has been increasing over the past decade as drug smugglers attempt to bring opium, heroin, cocaine, amphetamines, or other drugs into various countries. Often these drugs will be wrapped in capsules, condoms, balloons, plastic bags, or latex glove fingers and swallowed or placed in the rectum, where they are prone to rupture. Not only may the patient suffer from the toxic effects of the drugs, but there have been some reports of gastrointestinal hemorrhage caused by prolonged pressure of the packets on the gastric mucosa. Body packing should be considered in patients who show signs of drug-induced toxic effects after a recent arrival from a city terminal.[6] Many patients do not acknowledge the presence of a foreign body during initial evaluation. Complaints are often vague and relate to pain or discomfort. Diagnosis is usually made using radiography. Removal of the foreign body may be done in the emergency department or may require surgical intervention, depending on the size, shape, and location of the foreign body.

Genitourinary Injuries

Most GU injuries occur from blunt force and are usually not immediately life-threatening. Red flags suggesting GU injury include the following[8]:

- Flank, abdominal, rib, back, or scrotal pain
- Inability to void spontaneously
- Hemodynamic instability
- Gross hematuria or blood at the urethral meatus or vaginal introitus
- Perineal ecchymosis
- High-riding prostate
- Pelvic fracture

In patients with GU trauma, symptoms are nonspecific and may be masked by or attributed to other injuries.

Renal Injuries

Renal injuries occur in up to 10% of patients with blunt abdominal trauma and account for more than 80% of all GU injuries.[10] The majority of renal injuries are due to blunt trauma forces as in MVCs. The patient should be assessed for abdominal pain and tenderness over the kidneys, denoting significant force transfer. There may be a large flank

Table 24-4.	**RENAL INJURY SCALE**
Grade	**Injury Description**
I	Contusion: Microscopic or gross hematuria; normal urologic studies
	Subscapular hematoma, nonexpanding, no laceration
II	Laceration of renal parenchyma <1 cm; no extravasation
	Perinephric hematoma, nonexpanding
III	Laceration of renal parenchyma >1 cm
	No urinary extravasation; no collecting system involvement
IV	Laceration involving collecting system
	Perinephric and paranephric extravasation
	Thrombosis of segmental renal artery
	Main renal artery or vein injury; hemorrhage controlled
V	Fractured kidney
	Thrombosis of main renal artery
	Avulsion of main renal artery or vein

Grades I and II are minor; Grades III, IV, and V are major.

From Dixon MD, McAninch JW: *American Urological Association update series, traumatic renal injuries, part 1: assessment and management,* Houston, 1991, The Association.

ecchymosis, palpable mass, or hematoma. Unfortunately, it is possible to have significant renal injury without any physical findings. Obtain a urinalysis, complete blood count, and chemistry panel to assess for hematuria, baseline hematocrit, and renal function. CT scan is the imaging study of choice because it can also reveal other abdominal injuries. Ultrasonography has a limited role but can reveal free fluid in the abdomen. Arteriography is most useful in showing injuries of the renal artery. Renal injuries can be graded from I to V depending upon the location (Table 24-4); grades I to III will usually not require operative management. Higher-grade lesions may require nephrectomy, especially in hemodynamically unstable patients.

Penetrating renal injury results in a higher renal loss than blunt injury. Evidence of penetrating trauma to the flank should be obvious on examination; however, gunshot trajectories with known entry points not involving the flank can still involve the kidney and should be managed by the trauma surgeon along with a urologist. Surgical exploration of the abdomen is required for most gunshot wounds regardless of the grade of the injury, with selective operative management for stab wounds.

Ureteral Injuries

The ureter is the least commonly injured part of the GU tract. The most common mechanism of ureteral injury is penetrating trauma. The patient should be assessed for this type of injury when there is an appropriate mechanism with or without abdominal pain. Penetrating injury can cause partial or complete ureteral transection. Hematuria may be detected on urinalysis, and a CT scan or arteriogram should be obtained.

Surgical repair is primarily done by direct reanastomosis or stenting and temporary diversion. Because of the high rate of missed ureteral injuries, the possibility should be considered in trauma patients with worsening abdominal pain, fever, leukocytosis, or an unexplained fluid collection that could represent a urinoma.[8]

Bladder Injuries

The likelihood of bladder injury varies by the severity of the mechanism and also by the degree of bladder distension at the time of the injuring event. The fuller the bladder is, the greater the opportunity for injury. Bladder injuries are usually associated with pelvic injuries from MVCs, falls from heights, and physical assaults to the lower abdomen. These mechanisms may cause a pelvic fracture to perforate the bladder. Signs and symptoms of bladder injuries are generally nonspecific but may present as gross hematuria, suprapubic pain and tenderness, difficulty voiding, bruising and ecchymosis around the bladder/thighs, and abdominal distension, guarding, or rebound tenderness. The presence of signs of peritoneal irritation may also indicate the possibility of an intraperitoneal bladder rupture. Urinalysis typically shows gross hematuria. Gunshot wounds to the bladder may result in microscopic hematuria. Rupture of the bladder can be seen on routine abdominal CT and more accurately with a CT cystogram. Intraperitoneal bladder rupture requires exploratory laparotomy and repair through a layered closure, whereas extraperitoneal injuries can be managed with bladder drainage alone. Urologic follow-up and antibiotics are needed to prevent long-term complications, including strictures, fistulas, infection, and delayed healing.

Urethral Injuries

Most urethral injuries occur as a result of blunt trauma and occur primarily in men because the male urethra is longer and found mostly outside the body, whereas the female urethra is shorter and more protected. Injuries are usually a result of high-energy impact or straddle mechanisms and should be considered with any pelvic fracture. For classification of male injuries, the urethra is divided into a posterior segment (prostatic and membranous) and anterior segment (bulbous and pendulous). Posterior-segment injuries are associated with pelvic ring fractures, whereas anterior injuries are the result of external blunt or straddle mechanisms. Evaluate the patient for blood at the urethral meatus (a contraindication to inserting a urinary catheter), a high-riding prostate, and pain, swelling, and ecchymosis in the penis or perineum. Gross hematuria is common. A retrograde urethrogram reveals extravasation of contrast anywhere along the course of the urethra, confirming the presence of disruption. If bladder filling is noted, then the lesion is considered partial, whereas no contrast ending up in the bladder is indicative of a complete tear. Minor injuries can be managed conservatively with passage of a catheter. Most injuries require suprapubic cystostomy and delayed repair of the urethral injury.

Foreign bodies of the urethra are usually the result of self-insertion; various medical case reports describe unusual and seemingly dangerous objects in the urethra. The objects identified have included nuts, bolts, pens, pencils, toothbrushes, pocket batteries, fishhooks, shards of glass, pistachio shells, and animal parts.[14] Patients may be too embarrassed to admit they inserted or applied any object and usually present when a complication or symptoms occur. The most common reason for consultation is dysuria. Other complaints are suprapubic or perineal pain, urethral discharge, hematuria, difficulty urinating, swelling, or abscess formation. Clinical diagnosis is based on history and should always be considered in patients with chronic urinary tract infections. Radiographic studies, including plain radiographs, are usually helpful for detecting radiopaque objects. Management is focused on removing the foreign body and treating complications. Foreign bodies below the urogenital diaphragm can usually be palpated and readily removed endoscopically. When they are above the urogenital diaphragm, greater manipulation is required; perineal urethrostomy or suprapubic cystostomy is performed.

Penile Injuries

Penile fracture typically occurs during vigorous sexual intercourse when the penis is misdirected against the partner's pubic bone or is self-inflicted by abrupt bending of the erect penis during masturbation. There is disruption of the tunica albuginea surrounding the corpora cavernosa. The patient may report a popping sound as the tunica tears, followed by pain, swelling, and rapid detumescence. On physical examination the penis is swollen and ecchymotic. The fracture line in the tunica is often palpable. There is associated urethral injury in up to one third of cases. Urinalysis will show microscopic and often gross hematuria. Retrograde urethrography should be performed to rule out a urethral injury, particularly in the presence of gross hematuria, inability to void, or blood at the urethral meatus. Early surgical treatment is essential to prevent complications such as deformity, impotence, erectile dysfunction, and urethral stenosis.

Penile amputation is a very rare occurrence and usually due to self-mutilation, violent assault, or a devastating complication of circumcision. Emergent urologic consultation is required for immediate reimplantation. Successful reimplantation has been accomplished up to 24 hours after amputation. The penis should be preserved in saline-soaked gauze, placed within a sterile plastic bag, and then placed on ice.[9]

Testicular Injuries

The testicles may be injured by a direct blow, MVCs, or sports-related activities. The right testicle, possibly because of its higher lying position, is more commonly injured than the left. Injuries include contusion, hematocele, rupture, dislocation, or traumatic torsion. Testicular injury can be difficult to distinguish on examination alone, and imaging is required to assess the extent of the damage. Findings can include significant pain, swelling, and ecchymosis in the scrotal area. An ultrasound study should include Doppler flow studies to assess arterial flow. Ice and adequate analgesia should be used while obtaining urologic consultation.

Do not delay consultation for imaging studies if the testicle appears ruptured. Complications of testicular trauma include testicular atrophy, infection, infarction, and infertility.

Straddle Injuries

Straddle injuries occur when a patient falls and takes the brunt of the fall on the perineum. These injuries commonly occur in young patients as they fall onto bicycle bars, motorcycles, and fences. On examination of the female patient a vulvovaginal laceration with extensive ecchymosis of the perineum may be evident. Straddle injuries are often accompanied by vulvar hematomas that can extend into the retroperitoneal space. Associated urethral injuries and rectal tears should be ruled out. Treatment for straddle injuries involves repair of the laceration with evacuation and drainage of hematomas. The most common complication of the immediate postoperative period is infection. Sexual dysfunction may also result.

SUMMARY

Abdominal trauma is very common but often missed because other injuries distract attention from the abdomen. The delay in the development of signs and symptoms further confounds the ability to identify problems. Moreover, the bulk of injuries are seen in young people, whose compensatory capacities are high. An objective evaluation of the abdomen is often necessary with ultrasonography followed by imaging studies dependent upon the patient's stability. Penetrating injuries, especially high-velocity gunshot wounds, carry an extremely high chance of internal injury, so virtually all of these patients will require laparotomy. Blunt injuries are harder to recognize and require a higher level of suspicion based on the mechanism of injury. The emergency nurse who understands anatomy and recognizes injury patterns and pathophysiologic consequences of injury as a basis for signs and symptoms will contribute significantly to the effective management of the patient with abdominal and genitourinary trauma.

REFERENCES

1. American College of Surgeons: Abdominal trauma. In *Advanced trauma life support program for doctors*, ed 7, Chicago, 2004, American College of Surgeons.
2. Campbell MR: Abdominal and urologic trauma, In Hoyt KS, Selfridge-Thomas J, editors: *ENA's emergency nursing core curriculum*, ed 6, St. Louis, 2007, Saunders.
3. Dickenson ET, Braslow B: Acute abdominal eviscerations, *J Emerg Med Serv* 31(1):70, 2006.
4. Emergency Nurses Association: *Trauma nursing core course (TNCC)*, ed 6, Des Plaines, Ill, 2007, The Association.
5. Griffen XL, Pullinger R: Are diagnostic peritoneal lavage or FAST safe screening investigations for hemodynamically stable patients after blunt abdominal trauma?: a review of the literature, *J Trauma* 62(3):779, 2007.
6. Hassanian-Moghaddam H, Abolmasoumi Z: Consequences of body packing of illicit drugs, *Arch Iran Med* 10(1):20, 2007.
7. Marx JA, Hockberger RS, Walls RM: *Rosen's emergency medicine: concepts and clinical practice*, ed 6, St. Louis, 2002, Mosby.
8. Roppolo L, Davis D, Kelly SP et al: *Emergency medicine handbook: critical concepts for clinical practice*, Philadelphia, 2007, Mosby.
9. Rosenstein D, McAninch JW: Urologic emergencies, *Med Clin North Am* 88:495, 2004.
10. Smith JK, Kenney PJ: Imaging of renal trauma, *Radiol Clin North Am* 41:1019, 2003.
11. Stone CK, Humphries RL: *Current emergency diagnosis and treatment*, New York, 2004, Lange Medical Books/McGraw-Hill.
12. Tintinalli JE, Kelen GD, Stapczynski JS: *Emergency medicine*, ed 6, New York, 2004, McGraw-Hill.
13. Todd SR: Critical concepts in abdominal injury, *Crit Care Clin* 20:119, 2004.
14. Van Ophoven A, DeKernion JB: Clinical management of foreign bodies of the genitourinary tract, *J Urol* 164(2):274, 2000.
15. Wilson RF: *Handbook of trauma: pitfalls and pearls*, Philadelphia, 1999, Lippincott Williams & Wilkins.
16. Yeug K, Chang M, Hsiao C et al: CT evaluation of gastrointestinal tract perforation, *Clin Imaging* 28(5):329, 2004.

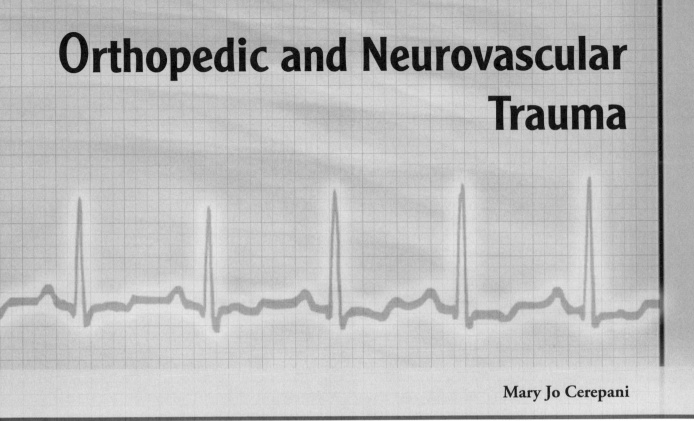

CHAPTER 25

Orthopedic and Neurovascular Trauma

Mary Jo Cerepani

Musculoskeletal injury is one of the most common types of trauma seen in the emergency department (ED) and is a significant cause of disability. Primary mechanisms for these injuries include motor vehicle crashes (MVCs), assaults, falls, sports and recreation, and injuries sustained at work or home. Bone, soft-tissue, and associated neurovascular injuries are rarely emergent unless accompanied by a life-threatening hemorrhage as in certain amputations and pelvic fractures. Fractures and soft-tissue injuries are primarily designated as urgent because of potential neurovascular injury with resultant limb disability and pain. Early intervention enhances preservation of limb and function. This chapter focuses on common orthopedic and neurovascular extremity injuries and appropriate therapeutic interventions. Related anatomy and physiology are briefly reviewed.

ANATOMY AND PHYSIOLOGY

The musculoskeletal system and related neurovascular structures consist of bones, joints, tendons, ligaments, muscles, vessels, and nerves. The skeletal system contains 206 bones, which provide support, strength, movement, and protection to the body and organs. Bones store a number of minerals, including calcium and phosphorus, and are involved in blood cell production. Bones are characterized by shape as long, short, flat, or irregular with the shape of a particular bone suited for a unique function or purpose. The skeleton is composed of two types of bones: cancellous and cortical. Cancellous (spongy) bone is found in the skull, vertebrae, pelvis, and long-bone ends. Cortical (dense) bone is found in the long bones. Bones are supplied by blood vessels, nerves, and lymphatic vessels that nourish bone tissue and allow the bone to repair injuries. The periosteum covers the bones and provides a point for attachment of muscle, as well as the blood supply for underlying bone tissue.

Bone is connected to other bone by stabilizing bands of elastic, fibrous connective tissue called ligaments. Nonelastic fibrous cords that connect muscle to bone are tendons. Dense connective tissue found between the ribs, in the nasal septum, ear, larynx, trachea, bronchi, between vertebrae, and on articulating surfaces is known as cartilage. Cartilage has a limited vascular supply, whereas bone tissue has abundant vascular structures.

Joints are classified as nonsynovial (immovable and slightly immovable) and synovial (freely movable). Synovial joints have two articulating surfaces covered with cartilage and are surrounded by a two-layered synovial membrane sac. The entire joint is encapsulated by dense, ligamentous material. Joints provide mobility and stability, flexion and extension, medial and lateral rotation, and abduction and adduction. Joint movement is enhanced by muscles and ligaments that overlie the joint.

Nerves and arteries lie in close proximity to bones and muscle groups, with arterioles distributed throughout the periosteum to provide nutrients. Nerves provide sensation and movement. The closeness of arteries and nerves to bone structures increases their risk for injury with trauma to soft tissue, muscles, bones, or joints.

PATIENT ASSESSMENT

Assessment of orthopedic trauma begins with assessment of the airway, breathing, and circulation (ABCs). Rapid assessment identifies major injuries of the head, cervical spine, chest, and abdomen and prioritizes essential interventions. After ensuring that no life-threatening injury has been left unattended, the nurse assesses and stabilizes any extremity injuries. Assessment of orthopedic injuries includes inspecting for edema, obvious deformity, presence of contusions, abrasions, lacerations, or puncture wounds and palpating for crepitus and point tenderness. A focused neurovascular evaluation is conducted for any injuries identified, noting the presence and/or absence of pain, pulses, paralysis, paraesthesia, pallor, temperature, and capillary refill.[6]

Before immobilization, open fractures should be stabilized and bleeding controlled. Open fractures with obvious bone protrusion or a deep laceration should be rinsed with sterile normal saline to remove gross contamination and covered with a dry sterile dressing.

Puncture wounds over a fracture site should not be irrigated because this can force bacteria deeper into the wound. Reduction of an open fracture should not be attempted in a prehospital setting because this may force contaminants into the wound, increasing risk for infection.

To control bleeding apply pressure directly to the injury site, edges of the wound, or an adjacent pressure point. Use of a tourniquet for hemorrhage control should be considered only as a last resort (life over limb) because of potential neurovascular compromise.

Immobilization

Immobilization should be accomplished as soon as possible to minimize further damage or complications secondary to bone fragments or neurovascular injury and to reduce pain in the injured limb. A splint should include the joints above and below the injury. Neurovascular status must be checked before and after immobilization. If neurovascular status is initially compromised, gradual traction may be used to promote return of neurologic or vascular function before splinting. If neurovascular status is compromised after splinting or traction, the splint should be removed and reapplied or the traction should be decreased. Angulation should be corrected only if it prevents immobilization or if neurovascular compromise is present. Splinting is best accomplished with an assistant to support the limb while a padded splint is placed and wrapped with a noncompressive bandage. Neurovascular status is rechecked after splinting.

Four basic types of splints exist, including soft splints such as pillows; hard splints such as padded board, cardboard, aluminum, plaster, fiberglass, or a ladder splint; inflatable air splints or vacuum splints; and traction splints, which reduce angulation and provide support.[5] Common splints that are used to immobilize the thumb/finger, wrist/forearm, elbow, and lower extremities are thumb spica, volar splint, boxer splint, sugar tong, and posterior splints (Figure 25-1).

Air splints were used extensively when first developed because they conformed well and provided visualization of the injured extremity. However, an air splint that is not open on the distal end does not allow for neurovascular checks without deflating or unzipping the splint (Figure 25-2). An air splint should be inflated only to the point where a finger can be slipped between the splint and the skin. Excessive pressure in the splint can compromise circulation. Air splints

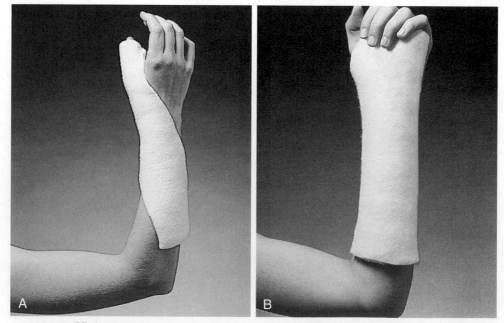

FIGURE **25-1.** Types of splints and their indications. **A,** Thumb spica splint. **B,** Volar splint.

also stick to the skin, cause irritation, and are difficult to remove in patients with excessive diaphoresis.

Several types of traction splints are available and are usually applied by prehospital providers. The Thomas ring splint, Sager splint, and Hare splint (Figure 25-3) are used for fractures of the midshaft of the femur or upper third of the tibia but should not be used for the hip, lower tibia or fibula, ankle, or a femur fracture with associated tibial-fibular fractures.

After immobilization the limb should be elevated and an ice pack applied to minimize swelling. Caution is advised because overzealous elevation may compromise arterial circulation and excessive, prolonged cold may damage tissues.

The patient should be completely disrobed and examined for anterior injuries and then logrolled to identify posterior injuries while maintaining adequate cervical spine protection. Rings should be removed if the injury involves the hand, arm, foot, or toes. Elevation and cooling measures should be maintained, and neurovascular status should be checked periodically.

Careful history should include circumstances of the injury (time and mechanism) and significant medical history, including acute and chronic alcohol use, medications, allergies, and tetanus immunization status. Time of last oral intake should be recorded, and the patient should be allowed nothing by mouth (NPO) if procedural sedation or surgical intervention is a possibility.

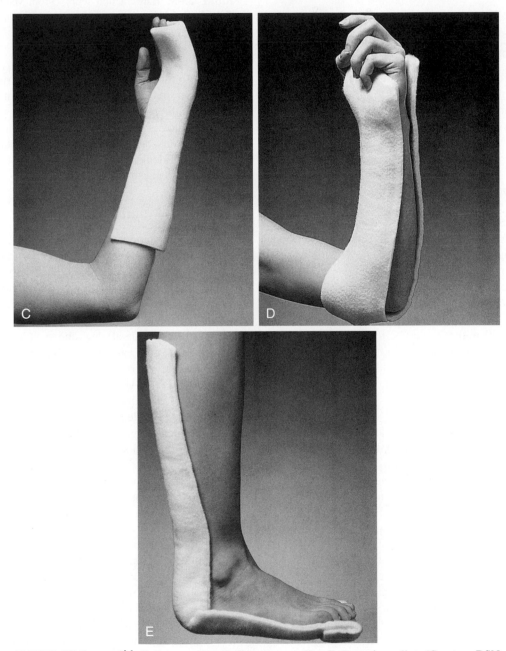

FIGURE **25-1—cont'd** **C,** Boxer splint. **D,** Sugar tong splint. **E,** Posterior splint. (Courtesy BSN Medical, Inc.)

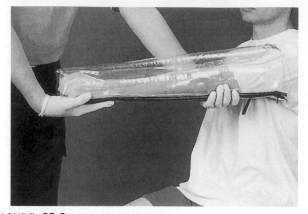

FIGURE **25-2.** Air splint. (From Stoy W: *Mosby's EMT: basic textbook,* ed 2, St. Louis, 2007, Mosby.)

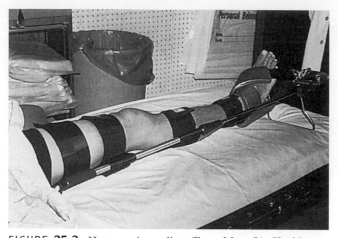

FIGURE **25-3.** Hare traction splint. (From Marx JA, Hockberger RS, Walls RM: *Rosen's emergency medicine: concepts and clinical practice,* ed 6, St. Louis, 2006, Mosby.)

SOFT TISSUE INJURIES

Soft-tissue injuries generally accompany orthopedic trauma and can involve skin, muscles, tendons, cartilage, ligaments, veins, arteries, and nerves; circulation and function can be compromised from soft-tissue injury. Common injuries to the skin include abrasions, avulsions, contusions, hematomas, lacerations, and puncture wounds.

Principles of nursing care are generally the same for various soft-tissue injuries. Inspection involves checking for wounds, swelling, hematomas, and bleeding, then assessing neurovascular status. A soft, bulky dressing is applied, and swelling can be minimized with elevation and cooling measures. Radiographs are used to rule out foreign bodies and fractures. Analgesia is administered as prescribed for isolated injuries, and antibiotics are administered for significant, contaminated wounds. Written discharge instructions discuss RICE: rest, ice (e.g., apply a covered ice bag to the injury for 20 minutes every 2 to 3 hours for 24 to 48 hours), compression, and elevation. (See Chapter 11 for more specific information.)

Fingertip Injuries

Fingertip injuries are frequently seen in the ED, with the most common type being a crush injury to the distal phalanx that occurs when a heavy object falls on the finger or the digit is caught in a door. Crush injuries can also be associated with a fracture. If a hematoma forms under the fingernail, it may cause a subungual hematoma (Figure 25-4), which requires nail trephination by penetrating the fingernail over the hematoma with a nail drill, scalpel, pencil cautery, or superheated paper clip to release blood under the nail and relieve pressure.[15]

Fingertip injuries caused by a high-pressure paint or grease gun have increased in recent years. This injury occurs when a person is cleaning the gun tip and a stream of paint or grease is released into the fingertip or hand under high pressure. A pressure greater than 7000 pounds per square inch has been associated with a high amputation rate.[9] Particular

attention to history and time of injury is crucial; the injury appears as a small pinhole in the fingertip but represents a serious, limb-threatening surgical emergency because material has been injected into the soft tissue of the involved limb. Treatment must not be delayed. Therapeutic intervention requires debridement of the paint- or grease-injected limb under general anesthesia.

Traumatic Amputations

Traumatic amputations occur among farm workers secondary to heavy farm machinery, in factory workers when a limb is caught by a heavy machine, and in motorcyclists when the motorcycle and driver collide with another vehicle. Other causes include snow blowers and lawn mowers. Body parts frequently amputated are digits (fingers, toes), distal half of the foot (transmetatarsal), leg (above, at, or below the knee), hand, forearm, arm, ears, nose, and penis.

Therapeutic interventions for amputations begin with stabilization of the ABCs, including administration of high-flow oxygen, initiation of two large-bore intravenous (IV) lines, control of bleeding, and rapid transportation to a facility for definitive care. If the body part is only partially amputated, the limb should be supported and splinted in a position of anatomic function. Figure 25-5 shows anatomic hand position. A completely amputated stump should be irrigated to remove gross contamination, dressed, and elevated. Antibiotics, a tetanus booster, and tetanus immune globulin, as indicated, should be initiated in the ED.

Whenever possible, the amputated part is preserved for reimplantation by wrapping it in saline-moistened gauze and placing it in a plastic bag or container. The sealed container is then placed on top of crushed ice and water. This cools the part without causing direct damage to tissue. If the amputated part is placed directly in water or on ice, cells can be damaged by water moving across the cellular membranes, including cellular freezing and death. Distilled water is not used because of its deleterious effect on tissue. Iodine should

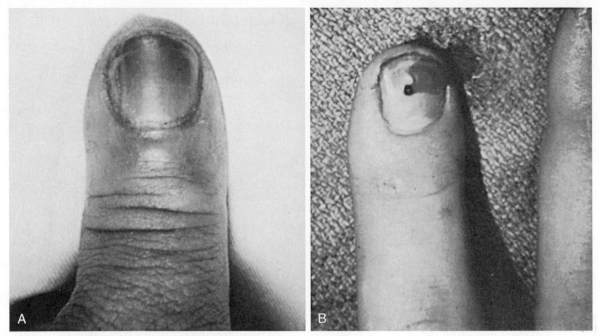

FIGURE **25-4. A,** Subungual hematoma. **B,** Subungual hematoma following trephination. (From Roberts JR, Hedges JR: *Clinical procedures in emergency medicine,* ed 4, Philadelphia, 2004, WB Saunders.)

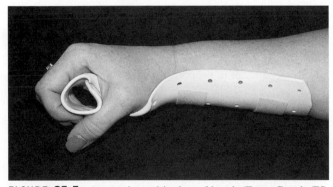

FIGURE **25-5.** Anatomic positioning of hand. (From Canale TS, Beaty JH: *Campbell's operative orthopaedics,* ed 11, St. Louis, 2007, Mosby.)

never be placed directly on the amputated part because of discoloration and its effects on tissue viability. Maintain the limb in correct anatomic position.

Reimplantation

After amputation, reimplantation may be possible. Limiting factors for successful reimplantation include availability of a reimplantation team, amount of damage to the attached and amputated parts, method of preservation of the amputated part, and time elapsed since the accident. Sharp, guillotine-like cuts have a better outcome than crush or avulsion type of injuries. Muscles can survive 12 hours of cold ischemia; bone, tendon, and skin can survive 24 hours; warm survival time is much less.[8] Predicted outcome of reimplantation is further determined by age, occupation, motivation, and general physical condition of the victim. Historically, upper extremity reimplantations are more successful than lower extremity reimplantations, and children typically have a better outcome with this type of reimplantation.

Impaling Injuries

Impaling injuries usually result from an industrial accident in which the victim falls onto a sharp, immobile object. Injuries with nails from a powered nail gun are also common. Nails used in these guns are coated with a special adhesive that can stick to tissue. Impaled objects should not be immediately removed; surgical removal may be required. Complications from this type of injury include infection and problems specific to the structures in which the object is impaled. Biologic substances such as wood carry an increased risk for infection.

Gunshot Wounds

Gunshot wounds usually result from hunting or acts of violence. Tissue damage depends on the type of weapon, size of ammunition used, distance from the weapon, and part of the body injured (Figure 25-6). Tissue, bones, organs, and vessels away from the bullet's unpredictable path may also be injured. Appearance of the entrance wound does not always reflect the amount of destruction beneath. An extremity injury may be associated with a truncal injury because of a projectile path through the chest into the arm or through the arm into the chest or because of multiple bullet wounds. (See Chapter 20 for further discussion of gunshot wounds.) Careful assessment, including neurovascular assessment of all limbs, is critical so that other wounds are

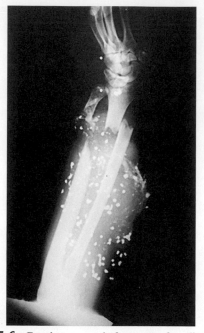

FIGURE 25-6. Gunshot wound fracture of radius and ulna with extensive soft-tissue damage. (From Frank ED, Long BW, Smith BJ: *Merrill's atlas of radiographic positioning and procedures,* ed 11, St. Louis, 2007, Mosby.)

not overlooked; immunization status needs to be verified. With gunshot wounds, evidence surrounding the wound site or powder burns on the hand should be carefully protected until the police can perform requisite testing. (See Chapter 16 for a detailed discussion of evidence collection and preservation.)

Tendon and Muscle Rupture

Tendon and muscle ruptures are generally related to sports or recreation; however, metabolic disease and age may be causative factors. Runners may experience a quadriceps tear, whereas a biceps tear can occur with minimal effort in middle-age or older individuals. Surgery may be required to restore function for complete tears. For an incomplete injury, treatment usually consists of rest and intermittent application of ice for 24 to 48 hours followed by heat.

An Achilles tendon rupture can occur in start-and-stop sports in which a person steps off abruptly on the forefoot with the knee forced in extension. The patient may also report hearing a loud crack or snap or sensation of something striking their posterior ankle. This causes sharp pain extending from the heel into the back of the leg, sudden inability to use the foot, and obvious deformity. A clinical tool to assist in the diagnosis is the Thompson test: the patient lies supine on the examination table with the feet hanging off the edge; the examiner squeezes each calf bilaterally and observes for plantar flexion. If a complete rupture has occurred, there is minimal or no foot movement (a positive Thompson's sign). A splint in plantar flexion should be applied and the patient prepared for surgery.[3]

Crush Injuries

Crush injuries frequently occur in industrial settings (e.g., arm caught in the wringer of an industrial washing machine, press, or conveyor; limbs or trunk caught between equipment). Injury may involve only the distal end of a digit or large areas of the body. Depending on the extent of damage, orthopedic, surgical, neurosurgical, or vascular-surgical intervention may be required.

Complications from crush injuries depend on the mechanism of injury and extent of tissue damage. With significant tissue necrosis, systemic crush syndrome can develop, characterized by myoglobinuria, extracellular fluid loss, acidosis, increased potassium, renal failure, shock, and cardiac disruption.[15]

Compartment Syndrome

Compartment syndrome occurs when swelling or compression-restriction causes pressure in the muscle compartment to rise to the point that microvascular circulation is interrupted. The resulting tissue ischemia threatens limb survival. Compartment syndrome is associated with severe soft-tissue injuries and fractures, casts, or a pneumatic antishock garment (PASG). Prolonged pressure directly on a limb, frostbite, or snakebite can also lead to compartment syndrome. It usually occurs in compartments of the lower leg and forearm (Figure 25-7). Symptoms develop 6 to 8 hours after injury but may be delayed 48 to 96 hours. Symptoms include deep, throbbing pain out of proportion to the original injury that is not relieved by narcotics, pain with passive flexion, decreased mobility of digits, paresthesia, coolness, pallor, and tenseness of overlying skin. Pulses may be absent, decreased, or palpable with compartment syndrome.

Irreversible tissue damage occurs within 4 to 6 hours of ischemia; therefore prompt physician notification is essential. The limb is positioned level with the heart, and neurovascular function is assessed hourly, or more often if indicated, to identify changes. Diagnosis is made by measuring compartment pressure with a syringe or catheter device (Figure 25-8). Pressures greater than 30 to 60 mm Hg usually require fasciotomy.[11] A high index of suspicion is necessary when caring for injured comatose patients who cannot verbalize increasing pain or paresthesia.[7]

Peripheral Nerve and Artery Injury

The most common causes of peripheral nerve and artery injuries are lacerations, penetrating wounds, fractures, and dislocations. Joints are well innervated and vascularized, so they are especially prone to nerve or artery damage. Familiarity with major nerves and arteries is necessary for assessment of tissue injuries.

Nerve injury may also occur from compression caused by prolonged PASG use or skeletal traction. Resolution of symptoms depends on the type of injury and length of time before compression is corrected. Partial nerve injury may

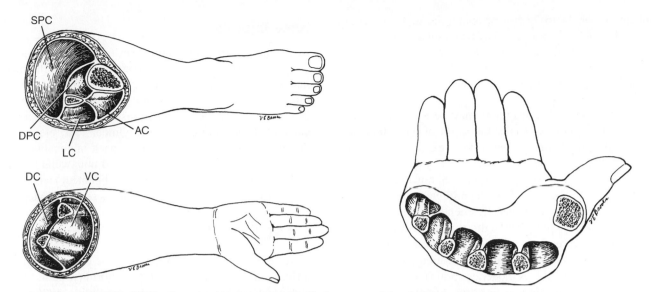

FIGURE **25-7.** Cross-section anatomy of calf, forearm, and hand showing fascial compartments (From Matsen FA III: *Compartmental syndromes,* New York, 1980, Grune & Stratton.)

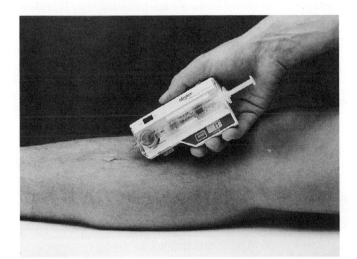

FIGURE **25-8.** The Stryker 295 intracompartmental pressure monitor. (Courtesy Stryker Surgical, Kalamazoo, Mich.)

be caused by a contusion that causes temporary paralysis and sensory deficit. Complete and total disruption of the nerve causes loss of all functions and usually requires surgical repair. Nerve evaluation and repair of an isolated injury may be done on an outpatient basis. Table 25-1 describes the assessment of common peripheral nerve injuries.

Axillary, brachial, radial, and ulnar arteries are the major arteries in the arms. Femoral, popliteal, anterior tibial, posterior tibial, and peroneal arteries are major arteries in the leg. High-impact and rapid-deceleration mechanisms are most likely to cause arterial injury. Assessment should evaluate pulse quality, skin color and temperature, capillary refill, bleeding, hematoma formation, and presence of bruits.

Arterial injuries may be difficult to discover; 10% to 15% of significant arterial disruptions can have detectable distal pulses.[12] A Doppler ultrasound should be used for pulses that

are difficult to palpate. Evaluation may require angiography; however, injury in association with an open fracture may be evaluated during surgery. Arterial injuries may not require repair if existing collateral circulation prevents ischemia. Complications of undiagnosed arterial disruptions include thrombosis, arteriovenous fistula, aneurysm, false aneurysm, and tissue ischemia with resultant limb dysfunction.[8]

Strains

A strain is a weakening or overstretching of a muscle at the point of attachment to the tendon. Strains may occur as a result of almost any type of movement, from twisting the ankle to wrenching forces caused by an MVC or violent muscle contraction. Strains are most often associated with athletic injuries.

A patient with a first-degree or mild strain complains of local pain, point tenderness, and slight muscle spasms. Therapeutic interventions include a compression bandage, intermittent elevation of the limb above heart level for 12 hours, application of a cold pack for the same period, and light weight bearing on the injured part.

With a second-degree strain the patient has local pain, point tenderness, swelling, discoloration, and inability to use the limb for prolonged periods. Therapeutic interventions include a compression bandage, elevation, and intermittent cold pack application for 24 hours; analgesia; and light weight bearing.

Severe strains (third-degree) cause complete disruption of the muscle or tendon. This disruption can cause a small avulsion fracture that can be seen on x-ray films. The patient complains of local pain, point tenderness, swelling, and discoloration. The patient often describes a "snapping noise" at the time of injury. Therapeutic interventions include a compression bandage or splints, elevation, and cold pack application for 24 to 72 hours; analgesia; and no weight bearing for 48 hours. Surgery may be required if a complete rupture occurs at the tendon-bone attachment site.

Sprains

Mechanism of injury for sprains may be the same as for strains, but a sprain is usually the result of more traumatic force. A sprain occurs when a joint exceeds its normal limit and damages ligaments. The patient may have a history of a popping or snapping sound. Sprains often occur in ankles, knees, and shoulders. In children, epiphyseal disruption is more common than ligamentous injury. A mild sprain (first-degree) produces slight pain and slight swelling. Therapeutic interventions include a compression bandage, elevation, intermittent cold pack application for 12 hours, and light weight bearing. A moderate sprain (second-degree) causes pain, point tenderness, swelling, and inability to use the limb for more than a brief period. Therapeutic interventions include compression bandage, elevation, intermittent cold pack application for 24 hours, and light weight bearing with crutches. A stirrup ankle brace is commonly applied to the ankle to prevent inversion and eversion of the ankle, but allow flexion and extension.

A severe sprain (third-degree) involves torn ligaments, which cause pain, point tenderness, swelling, discoloration, and inability to use the limb. Therapeutic interventions include a splint or cast, elevation, intermittent cold pack application for 48 hours, and light to no weight bearing with crutches (lower extremity injury).

Knee Injuries

Knee injuries are a common form of soft-tissue injury in which rotation or excess flexion strains or tears the medial meniscus, collateral ligament, or cruciate ligament. Symptoms include swelling, ecchymosis, effusion, pain, and tenderness. Therapeutic interventions include a compression bandage, knee immobilizer, or cylinder cast; elevation of the injured limb; intermittent cold pack application to the injured area for the first 24 hours; and non–weight bearing with crutch walking. If the injury is a ligament tear, surgical repair within 24 to 48 hours of injury is recommended.

FRACTURES

A fracture is a disruption or break in the bone. Patients may arrive in the ED with angulation, deformity, pain, regional and point tenderness, swelling, immobility, and/or crepitus. Other findings might include bony fragment protrusion, impaired neurovascular status, and occasionally shock.

Fractures are divided into two general categories: closed and open. With closed or simple fractures, the bone is broken but the skin is intact. Open or compound fractures are characterized by bone protrusion or puncture wounds in which the bone punctures the skin or a foreign object penetrates the skin and bone, causing a fracture. Table 25-2 describes etiology for various types of fractures with illustrations for each type in Figure 25-9.

Open fractures are considered contaminated and require prophylactic antibiotic therapy. These fractures are graded

Table 25-1. ASSESSMENT OF COMMON PERIPHERAL NERVE INJURIES

Nerve	Frequently Associated Injuries	Assessment Findings
Radial	Fracture of humerus, especially middle and distal thirds	Inability to extend thumb in "hitchhiker's sign"
Ulnar	Fracture of medial humeral epicondyle	Loss of pain perception in tip of little finger
Median	Elbow dislocation or wrist or forearm injury	Loss of pain perception in tip of index finger
Peroneal	Tibia or fibula fracture; dislocation of knee	Inability to extend great toe or foot; may also be associated with sciatic nerve injury
Sciatic and tibial	Infrequent with fractures or dislocations	Loss of pain perception in sole of foot

Table 25-2. CAUSES OF DIFFERENT TYPES OF FRACTURES

Type	Etiology
Transverse fracture	Sharp, direct blow
Oblique fracture	Twisting force
Spiral fracture	Twisting force while foot is firmly planted
Comminuted fracture	Severe direct trauma causes more than two fragments
Impacted fracture	Severe trauma, causes bone ends to jam together
Compression fracture	Severe force to top of head, sacrum, or os calcis (axial loading) forces vertebrae together
Greenstick fracture	Compression force; usually occurs in school-age children
Avulsion fracture	Forceful contraction of a muscle mass; causes a bone fragment to break away at the insertion point
Depressed fracture	Blunt trauma to a flat bone; usually associated with significant soft-tissue damage

by severity, then further categorized by wound size, amount of soft-tissue damage, injury to the periosteum, and vascular damage. Most open fractures require surgical debridement. A greater potential for shock exists with open fractures because of the potential for significant blood loss; closed injuries are more likely to tamponade and limit blood loss.[7] General nursing care includes fracture immobilization and establishing IV access for fluid replacement, antibiotics, analgesia, and anesthesia. Wound care includes irrigation with normal saline, covering with a dry sterile dressing, and verification of tetanus immunization status.

After evaluation of ABCs, specific limb injury assessment should be completed, followed by immobilization, elevation, and ice packs. Repeated neurovascular assessments are essential to identifying changes secondary to swelling. History should be obtained to determine mechanism of injury. The emergency nurse should also be alert for signs of abuse when the injury does not match the history. Understanding patterns of injury also facilitates assessment and identification of less obvious injuries.

When a limb suffers significant trauma, a fracture should be suspected until proven otherwise by radiologic studies. Radiography should include both anterior and lateral views because fractures may appear from only one angle.[4] Joints above and below the injury should be included in all radiographic evaluations.

Open fractures and certain closed fractures require surgical intervention. Ideally, patients with open fractures should have surgery within 8 hours of the injury.[5] The patient should be kept NPO and prepared for surgery. IV lines are inserted, and consent should be obtained before narcotics are administered. Prophylactic broad-spectrum antibiotics are given as soon as possible for open fractures and vascular injuries.

Fractures are associated with numerous complications. Jagged bone ends may lacerate vital organs, arteries, and nerves, causing hemorrhage and neurovascular compromise. Open fractures can result in serious infections that can lead to permanent limb dysfunction or limb loss. Long-term complications of fractures include nonunion, deformity, disability, avascular necrosis from decreased blood supply, and

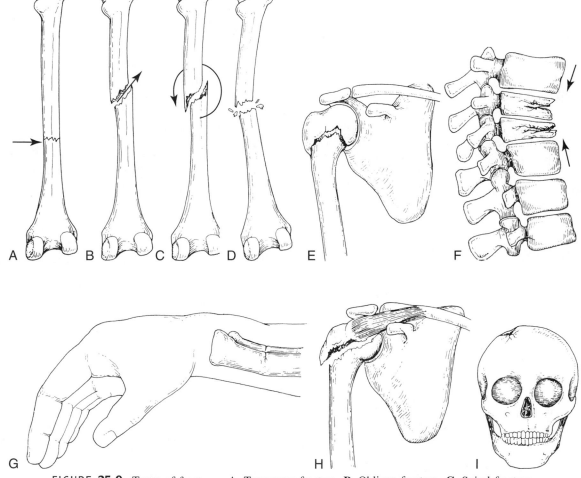

FIGURE 25-9. Types of fractures. **A,** Transverse fracture. **B,** Oblique fracture. **C,** Spiral fracture. **D,** Comminuted fracture. **E,** Impacted fracture. **F,** Compression fracture. **G,** Greenstick fracture. **H,** Avulsion fracture. **I,** Depressed fracture.

Volkmann's contracture (contracture in a group of muscles caused by ischemia) secondary to untreated compartment syndrome.[5]

Fat embolism is a relatively uncommon, but life-threatening, sequela of bone injury and usually presents 24 to 48 hours after injury. Seen most often with pelvic, femoral, or tibial fractures, this complication has a high mortality rate. A fracture causes release of fat particles into the bloodstream that embolize to end-organs, particularly the pulmonary vasculature. The patient suddenly develops tachycardia accompanied by elevated temperature, altered level of consciousness, tachypnea, cough, shortness of breath, cyanosis, petechiae over the upper half of the body—particularly in the axillae—and pulmonary edema leading to adult respiratory distress syndrome. Immediate therapeutic interventions include high-flow oxygen, support of ABCs, and possible administration of a corticosteroid.[7]

Fractures occur frequently among children 6 to 16 years old and older adults. Children's bones are softer and more porous and therefore more likely to have a partial or greenstick fracture.[14] Epiphyseal or growth plate (Salter-type) fractures may affect future bone growth because of early closure of the epiphyseal plate and resultant limb shortening (Figure 25-10). Angulation may occur with partial growth plate fractures because bone growth continues in the noninjured area. Epiphyseal fractures require close orthopedic follow-up for several months to monitor healing and identify growth abnormalities.[10] Another concern with pediatric fractures is bleeding. A child with a femur fracture can lose 300 to 1000 mL of blood, a significant amount given the child's body size and circulating blood volume.[1]

Older adult patients have brittle bones because of calcium loss associated with aging. This physiologic change combined with problems older adults have with balance increases the risk for falls and fractures. These patients may also have multiple medical problems that complicate recovery. Planning home care may be difficult for the older adult patient with a fracture who may be already challenged by normal activities of daily living. A cast and crutches cause greater loss of balance and impaired mobility.

Fracture Healing

Bone healing occurs over weeks or can take several months. Fracture healing is determined by the type of bone, type of fracture, degree of opposition, immobility, and general state of health.[7] Infection and decreased neurovascular supply hamper healing, as does chronic hypoxia. Conversely, exercise promotes bone healing. Alterations in healing are described as delayed, malunion (residual deformity), and nonunion (failure to unite).

Upper Torso Fractures

Bones in the upper torso that communicate with the upper extremities include the clavicle and scapula.

Clavicular Fracture

Fracture of the clavicle occurs in all age-groups but is particularly common in children and adolescents.[14] A fall on an arm or shoulder, such as contact injury when athletes run into each other or with direct frontal impact, is a frequently

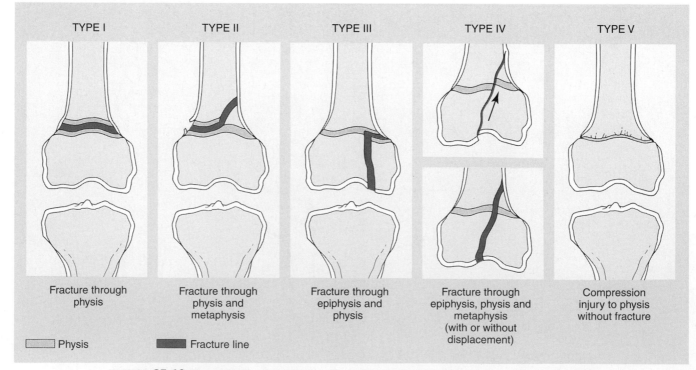

TYPE I	TYPE II	TYPE III	TYPE IV	TYPE V
Fracture through physis	Fracture through physis and metaphysis	Fracture through epiphysis and physis	Fracture through epiphysis, physis and metaphysis (with or without displacement)	Compression injury to physis without fracture

☐ Physis   ■ Fracture line

FIGURE 25-10. Salter-Harris classification. (From Zitelli BJ, Davis HW: *Atlas of pediatric physical diagnosis*, ed 4, St. Louis, 2002, Mosby.)

reported mechanism of injury. Eighty percent of fractures occur in the middle third of the clavicle. Patients complain of pain in the clavicular area with point tenderness, swelling, deformity, and crepitus found on assessment. The patient will not raise the affected arm and tilts the head toward the side of injury with the chin directed toward the opposite side. Neurovascular status of the arm should be assessed, including the axillary, median, ulnar, and radial nerve; distal pulses; and capillary refill. The arm should be supported and a sling or sling and swath applied; a figure-eight splint or clavicle strap may still be preferred for displaced fractures involving the middle third of the clavicle. The patient should be instructed to apply a cold pack intermittently to the injured area for 12 to 24 hours and to wear the sling or sling and swath at all times until there is no further pain with movement. A referral should be given for orthopedic follow-up. Complications include pneumothorax and hemothorax, particularly from the more serious frontal-impact injuries and brachial plexus injuries.

Scapular Fracture

Scapular fractures constitute 1% of all fractures, occurring primarily in young men.[15] This injury is usually caused by violent, direct trauma but may be seen with severe muscle contraction. Associated injuries include pulmonary contusions and rib fractures. Common mechanisms of injury include MVCs, falls, and crush injuries. Patients complain of point tenderness and pain during shoulder movement. Bone displacement and swelling over the injured area may be evident. Therapeutic interventions include assessment of neurovascular status of the affected arm, placement of a compression bandage over the scapula if bone is not displaced, sling and swath bandage or shoulder immobilizer for 1 to 2 weeks (Figure 25-11), and intermittent application of a cold pack for the first 24 hours. Complications include injuries to underlying ribs or viscera from the force required to cause the fracture.

Upper Extremity Fractures

Shoulder Fracture

A shoulder fracture is a fracture of the glenoid, humeral head, or humeral neck. Shoulder fractures occur frequently in older adult patients, resulting from a fall on an outstretched arm or direct trauma to the shoulder. When this same mechanism of injury occurs in a younger person, shoulder dislocation usually occurs. Fracture occurs in an older adult because of the weaker bone structure.

The patient arrives with pain in the shoulder area, point tenderness, immobility of the affected arm, gross swelling, and discoloration. The majority of injuries are impacted or nondisplaced fractures and require only a sling and swath or shoulder immobilizer. A Velpeau immobilizer (i.e., a sling with a strap attached to the elbow end that comes around the patient's back and attaches to the sling near the fingers) may also be used. A significantly displaced fracture may require open reduction or skeletal traction but is generally reduced with closed traction. This injury can complicate activities of daily living and requires extra planning for home care, particularly for an older adult patient living alone. Complications include neurovascular compromise (axillary nerve injury) and possible adhesive capsulitis or "frozen" (stiff) shoulder.

Upper Arm Fractures

Fractures of the upper arm (humeral shaft) are commonly seen in children and older adults (Figure 25-12). This type of fracture results from a fall on the arm, direct trauma, or

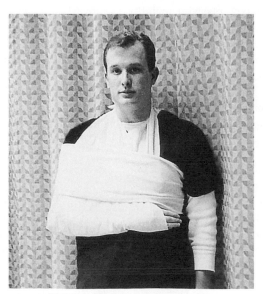

FIGURE **25-11.** Sling and swath.

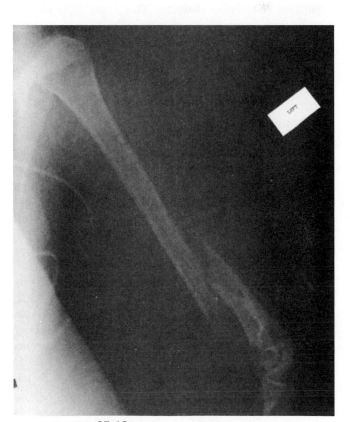

FIGURE **25-12.** Radiograph of humerus fracture.

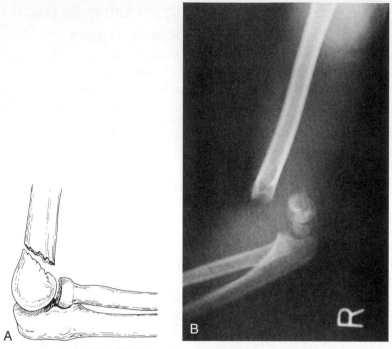

FIGURE **25-13.** **A,** Elbow fracture. **B,** Radiograph.

in association with dislocation of the shoulder and may also occur as a stress injury with lifting weights. The patient complains of point tenderness and significant discomfort. Swelling, inability or hesitancy to use the arm, severe deformity or angulation, and crepitus also occur. Therapeutic interventions include assessment for other injuries (e.g., chest trauma) and fracture management. The fracture is usually reduced by closed reduction with mild, steady, downward traction. Fractures of the proximal humerus are generally treated with a sling and swath; midshaft fractures are casted with a Y-shaped (sugar tong) splint applied from the axilla, around the elbow, and back to the shoulder (acromial process).[11] The patient should sit and lean forward during this procedure. The arm may be secured to the chest for additional stabilization. In addition to routine cast care instructions, the patient should be given instructions to exercise the wrist and fingers frequently. Radial nerve damage commonly accompanies fracture of the middle or distal portion of the humeral shaft.

Elbow Fractures

Elbow fractures (Figure 25-13) are seen most often in young children and athletes. These injuries occur with a fall on an extended arm or flexed elbow, such as a fall from a skateboard. Fractures of the elbow involve the distal humerus or head of the ulna or radius. Typically, supracondylar fractures of the humerus are extension injuries and are more likely to damage the brachial artery. Ulnar head fractures are generally the result of a direct blow and are usually comminuted.

Elbow fractures are associated with considerable swelling and potential neurovascular compromise. The arm should be splinted as found and a sling applied. Prompt initial neurovascular assessment should be followed by serial assessment every 30 to 60 minutes. If compromise is present, the arm may be flexed at a greater angle. When closed reduction is employed, the arm is casted and placed in a sling. Sling immobilization is usually sufficient for radial head fractures. Open reduction and fixation is required for comminuted or intraarticular fractures. Complications associated with elbow fractures include brachial artery laceration, nerve (median, radial, or ulnar) damage, and Volkmann's contracture.

Volkmann's contracture is due to ischemia of muscles and nerves from untreated compartment syndrome. The patient presents with inability to move his or her fingers, severe pain with manipulation, severe pain in forearm flexor muscles even after reduction, pulse deficit, swelling, extremity coolness, cyanosis, and decreased sensation. Temporary therapeutic intervention includes cast removal, extension of the forearm, and possible cold pack application. Prompt orthopedic consultation is essential for further therapeutic interventions. Nonintervention leads to atrophy and a clawlike deformity.

Forearm Fractures

Forearm fractures include fractures of the radius and ulna. Common in adults and children, forearm fractures usually result from a fall on an extended arm or a direct blow (Figure 25-14). The patient presents with pain, point tenderness, swelling, deformity, angulation, and occasionally shortening of the extremity. Therapeutic interventions include a splint to immobilize the fracture and a sling. Many fractures can be manipulated by closed reduction, then casted with the elbow

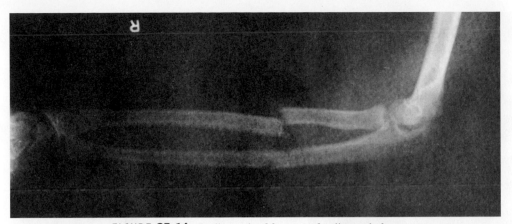

FIGURE **25-14.** Radiograph of fracture of radius and ulna.

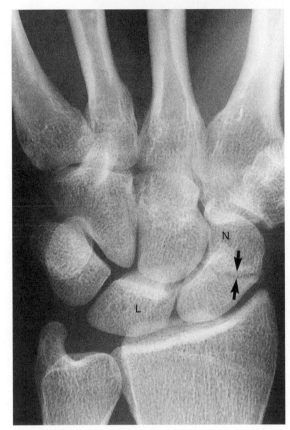

FIGURE **25-15.** Scaphoid fracture. (From Mettler FA: *Essentials of radiology,* ed 2, Philadelphia, 2005, WB Saunders.)

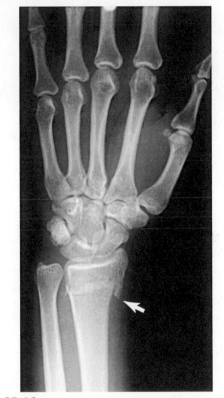

FIGURE **25-16.** Wrist fracture (radius). (From Ballinger PW: *Merrill's atlas of radiographic positions and radiologic procedures,* ed 8, St. Louis, 1995, Mosby.)

flexed 90 degrees. The shoulder and fingers should be free of the cast. If a sling is used, the entire arm and hand should be supported. The hand should not become dependent or droop at the wrist. Complications of forearm fractures include neurovascular compromise leading to Volkmann's contracture.

Wrist and Hand Fractures

CARPAL FRACTURES. The scaphoid is the carpal bone most prone to fracture (Figure 25-15). The patient complains of tenderness over the depression in the wrist on the thumb side of the hand (anatomic snuffbox). A specific navicular-view radiograph demonstrates scaphoid fractures best; however, fractures may not appear on radiographs for 2 to 4 weeks. If symptoms are present, a cast is placed regardless of negative radiographs. Complications include avascular necrosis or tissue death of the scaphoid from loss of blood supply.

WRIST FRACTURES. Fractures of the wrist include the distal radius, distal ulna, and carpal bones of the hand (Figure 25-16). The most common mechanism is a fall onto an extended arm and open hand, causing swelling and deformity. Fractures of the distal radius and ulna are the most

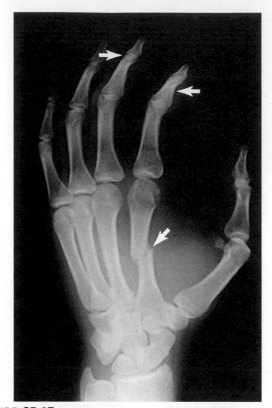

FIGURE **25-17.** Metacarpal fracture (From Frank ED, Long BW, Smith BJ: *Merrill's atlas of radiographic positioning and procedures,* ed 11, St. Louis, 2007, Mosby.)

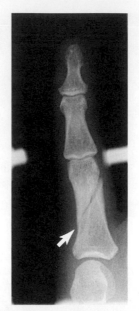

FIGURE **25-18.** Fractured fifth digit. (From Frank ED, Long BW, Smith BJ: *Merrill's atlas of radiographic positioning and procedures,* ed 11, St. Louis, 2007, Mosby.)

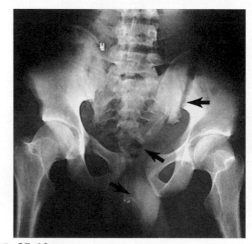

FIGURE **25-19.** Pelvis fracture. (From Frank ED, Long BW, Smith BJ: *Merrill's atlas of radiographic positioning and procedures,* ed 11, St. Louis, 2007, Mosby.)

common fracture, typically seen in older adults. A Colles' fracture may also occur in association with a calcaneus and vertebral fracture sustained in a fall from a height. Wrist fractures are generally manipulated with closed reduction and then casted. Some physicians may not prescribe a sling because it can hinder elevation; some prefer a hanging apparatus, such as an IV pole for the first 2 days of elevation, even for home care.

METACARPAL FRACTURES. Fractures of the metacarpals (Figure 25-17) are common athletic injuries, particularly during contact sports. Striking a person or wall with a closed fist causes a boxer's fracture, a midshaft fracture of the fifth metacarpal. Throwing a baseball may cause the distal attachment of the extensor tendon to tear loose along with a segment of bone, resulting in an avulsion fracture. Industrial crush injuries to the hand can also fracture metacarpals. If an open fracture occurs, a compression bandage is used to control bleeding.[2] Rings are removed before swelling increases and makes removal difficult. Metacarpal fractures are seldom displaced to any degree and are generally casted in the ED.

PHALANX FRACTURES. Fractured phalanges (fingers) are common in all age-groups (Figure 25-18). Symptoms are similar to those for carpal and metacarpal fractures with therapeutic interventions basically the same. Sometimes a phalanx fracture is associated with a hematoma beneath the fingernail (subungual hematoma), causing severe, throbbing pain. Therapeutic intervention for phalanx fractures is

usually splinting the finger. Occasionally, surgical reduction is necessary to realign fractured segments. Subungual hematoma is treated with nail trephination.

Pelvic Fractures

Pelvic fractures (Figure 25-19) occur most frequently in middle-aged and older adults and have a mortality rate of 8% to 13%. An estimated 65% of patients with pelvic fractures have sustained other concurrent injuries.[8] Mortality increases to 50% when the patient has an open pelvic fracture. Open fractures into the rectum or vagina constitute approximately 3% of pelvic injuries but have a 40% to 60% mortality.[9] Vehicular trauma, particularly in pedestrians, accounts for almost two thirds of pelvic fractures. Other

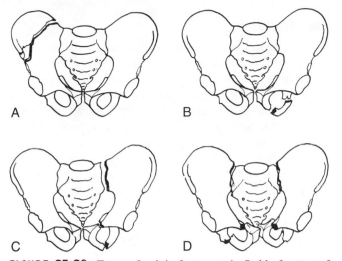

FIGURE **25-20.** Types of pelvic fractures. **A,** Stable fracture of the iliac, without disruption of the pelvic ring. **B,** Stable fracture of the ischial tuberosity. **C,** Unstable fracture of pubis symphysis involving the ischial tuberosity and pelvic ring. **D,** Unstable fracture involving the pubis symphysis and ischial tuberosity. (From Danis DM, Blansfield JS, Gervasini AA: *Handbook of clinical trauma care: the first hour,* ed 4, St. Louis, 2007, Mosby.)

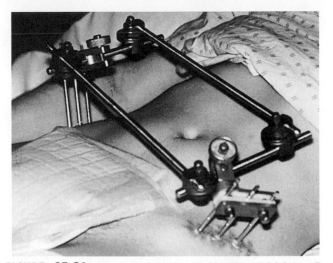

FIGURE **25-21.** External fixator: pelvis. (From Maher AB, Salmond SW, Pellino TA: *Orthopedic nursing,* ed 3, Philadelphia, 2002, WB Saunders.)

causes are direct trauma, falls from a height, sudden contraction of a muscle against a resistance, and even doing splits while waterskiing. Pelvic fractures are classified as stable or unstable, depending on disruption of the pelvic ring (Figure 25-20). A particularly unstable fracture results from vertical-shear force, which causes significant bone and tissue damage. Specific neurovascular structures at risk for injury with pelvic fractures include the iliac artery, venous plexus, and sciatic nerve. Large-volume blood loss from lacerated pelvic veins, arteries, or the fracture itself can occur as well as injury to the genitourinary system.[1]

Compression of the iliac wings causes tenderness over the pubis in the patient with a pelvic fracture. These patients can also have paraspinous muscle spasm, sacroiliac joint tenderness, paresis or hemiparesis, pelvic ecchymosis, and hematuria. Hemorrhagic shock resulting from associated blood loss should be suspected in the patient with tachycardia and hypotension.

Therapeutic interventions include high-flow oxygen, serial vital signs, and two large-bore IV lines for volume replacement titrated to blood pressure and pulse rate. The spine and legs are usually immobilized with a long spine board before the patient's arrival at the ED. After the long board is removed, the pelvis may be wrapped tightly with a sheet and secured with towel clips or a pelvic binder splint. This is done temporarily to assist in tamponading the bleeding from the pelvic fracture(s). Patients with pelvic fractures can bleed profusely because the pelvis is supplied with major arteries and a rich venous plexus, so a type and crossmatch for at least 4 to 5 units of blood should be done. Average blood loss for a closed fracture is 1500 to 3000 mL[13]; exsanguinating hemorrhage can occur with both closed and open fractures. A urinary catheter should be inserted cautiously

in the patient with pelvic trauma because of the potential for associated urethral injury. Never insert a urinary catheter when a patient has blood at the meatus or if there is penile deformity in a male patient.

Definitive interventions depend on the severity of the fracture. Less severe, non–weight-bearing injuries are treated with bed rest and traction. Unstable, weight-bearing fractures are treated with external fixation devices (Figure 25-21) or with open reduction using internal fixation devices. Hemorrhage from lacerated pelvic vessels may require an angiogram with embolization.

Complications from pelvic fractures include bladder trauma, genital trauma, lumbosacral trauma, ruptured internal organs, sepsis, shock, and death. Long-term complications include thrombophlebitis, fat embolism, chronic pain, and loss of function.

Hip Fractures

Hip fractures are common in older adults and are usually caused by falls or minor trauma (Figure 25-22). Conversely, major trauma accounts for most hip fractures in younger patients. Fractures can occur in the femoral head, femoral neck (intracapsular), and intertrochanteric region. Femoral head fractures are rare but generally are associated with a high-speed MVC. Symptoms associated with hip fractures include pain in the groin, hip, or knee; severe pain with leg movement; and immobility. Patients with greater trochanteric fractures can be ambulatory. Extracapsular trochanteric fractures are associated with pain in the lateral hip, shortening of the extremity, and a greater degree of external rotation.

Immediate therapeutic interventions include minimizing movement of the affected leg (e.g., splinting the hip to a long spine board or to the opposite leg). Monitoring serial vital signs is recommended because of the potential for blood loss. Early immobilization with Buck's traction or surgical intervention is often necessary. Complications of hip fracture include hypovolemia, shock, avascular necrosis with femoral head and neck fractures, and nonunion. These patients are generally at a greater risk for developing postoperative complications related to age and immobility.

Lower Extremity Fractures

Femoral Fracture

Femoral fractures (Figure 25-23) occur in all age-groups, usually secondary to major trauma. The patient has severe pain, inability to bear weight on the injured leg, deformity, swelling, and angulation. Severe muscle spasms cause significant pain and also cause the limb to shorten. Crepitus occurs over the fracture site as bone pieces move.

Initial therapeutic interventions include use of a traction splint (e.g., Hare, Sager, or Thomas) for immobilization. A long air splint with an enclosed foot or using the other leg as a splint is not recommended because these methods do not provide adequate stability. Associated injuries such as knee trauma are assessed. IV access is established, ideally in two sites, and vital signs are monitored frequently. Analgesia and volume replacement should be determined based on individual patient assessment. The patient should be prepared for traction, pin placement in the ED, or surgery.

The greatest complication of femoral fracture is shock secondary to hypovolemia. Average blood loss from a closed fracture is 1000 mL[13] and can exceed 3000 mL.[1] Severe muscle spasms can move bone ends, causing further soft-tissue injury, muscle damage, and pain. Neurovascular structures that can be damaged include the peroneal nerve, sciatic nerve, and popliteal artery.

Knee Fractures

Knee fractures may be supracondylar fractures of the femur or intraarticular fractures of the femur or tibia (Figure 25-24). This type of injury occurs in all age-groups and is usually the result of automobile, motorcycle, or automobile-pedestrian collisions that cause direct trauma to the knee. Patients complain of knee pain, inability to bend or straighten the knee (depending on position of the knee at the time of injury), swelling, and tenderness. Therapeutic interventions include a long leg splint or securing one leg to the other. Depending on extent of injury, the patient may require surgical repair. The knee will most likely be casted. The most common complication of knee fracture is neurovascular compromise of the peroneal or tibial nerve or the popliteal artery.

Patellar Fractures

Patellar fractures are seen in all age-groups (Figure 25-25) usually after direct trauma from a fall or impact with the dashboard. Indirect trauma such as a severe muscle pull can also cause fracture of the patella. The patient presents with knee pain and often has an obvious deformity of the patella. Open patellar fractures also occur. Therapeutic interventions include covering any open wound and applying a long leg splint. Radiographs of the affected limb should be obtained to determine extent of the fracture. Treatment for a nondisplaced patellar fracture is use of a long leg cylinder cast. If the fracture is displaced, reduction is attempted, with surgery if appropriate, to realign fractured parts. The patella

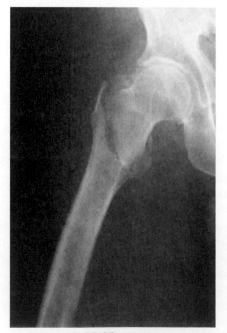

FIGURE **25-22.** Hip fracture.

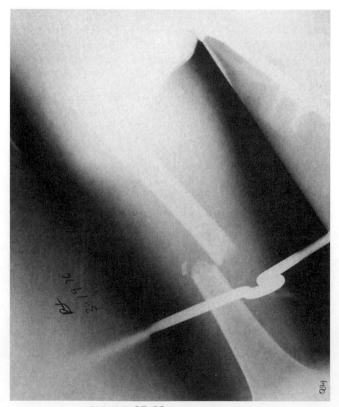

FIGURE **25-23.** Femur fracture.

is an important part of the knee that aids in leverage and protects the knee joint. Complete disruption of leg extension warrants surgery.

Tibial and Fibular Fractures

Tibial and fibular fractures are seen in all age-groups (Figure 25-26) secondary to direct trauma, indirect trauma, or rotational force. The patient has pain in the leg, point tenderness, swelling, deformity, and crepitus. Many tibial and fibular fractures are open. Open and closed tibial injuries should be splinted as they are found; realignment of an open fracture should not be attempted unless neurovascular compromise is present. Any open wounds should be covered with a dry sterile dressing. The patient with a stable, nondisplaced tibial fracture may be discharged in a long leg splint or cast. Open or closed reduction may be necessary when the fracture is unstable or displaced. Reduction of these fractures is followed by application of a splint or cast. Use of a cast or splint immediately after reduction is determined by the degree of edema and the potential for swelling to increase.

An isolated fibular fracture is unusual. A walking cast is usually applied because the fibula is not a weight-bearing bone. Complications of tibial and fibular fractures include blood loss up to 2 L, infection, soft-tissue damage, neurovascular compromise, compartment syndrome, and Volkmann's contracture.

Ankle Fractures

Fractures of the ankle involve the distal tibia, distal fibula, or talus and occur in all age-groups (Figure 25-27). Direct trauma, indirect trauma, or torsion can lead to open or closed ankle fractures. The patient complains of pain in the injured area, inability to bear weight on the extremity, point tenderness, swelling, and deformity. After closed reduction the patient is placed in a walking cast. Depending on the extent of injury, the patient may require open reduction and pinning. The most frequent complication is neurovascular compromise, particularly of the peroneal nerve.

Foot Fractures

TARSAL AND METATARSAL FRACTURES. Fractures of the tarsals and metatarsals (Figure 25-28) occur in all age-groups, usually from MVCs, athletic injuries, crush injuries, or direct trauma. Fifth metatarsal fractures can occur with inversion injuries of the foot. The patient complains of pain in the foot and hesitates to bear weight. Therapeutic intervention includes a compression dressing and soft splint. Minimally displaced fractures are treated with open-toed walking shoes or casts. With significant displacement, open reduction may be required. Crutches may be used to assist with weight bearing or non–weight bearing. Complications from this type of fracture are rare.

CALCANEUS FRACTURES. Fractures of the calcaneus are usually seen in young adults secondary to a fall in which the victim lands on his or her feet (Figure 25-29). The patient complains of pain in the heel, point tenderness, and swelling. Dislocation may also occur. Management includes reduction of the fracture when necessary and application of a below-the-knee, weight-bearing cast. Open reduction is occasionally necessary. Associated injuries seen with calcaneus fractures include lumbosacral compression fracture and Colles' fracture.

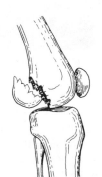

FIGURE **25-24.** Knee fracture.

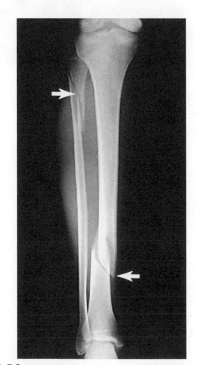

FIGURE **25-26.** Fracture of tibia and fibula. (From Frank ED, Long BW, Smith BJ: *Merrill's atlas of radiographic positioning and procedures,* ed 11, St. Louis, 2007, Mosby.)

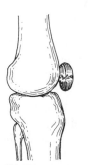

FIGURE **25-25.** Patella fracture.

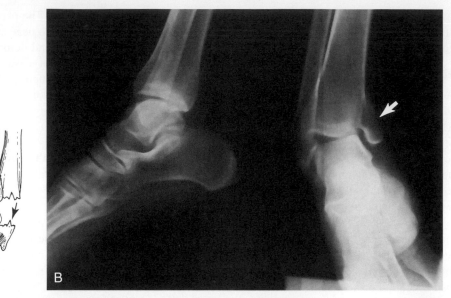

FIGURE **25-27.** **A,** Ankle fracture. **B,** Radiograph.

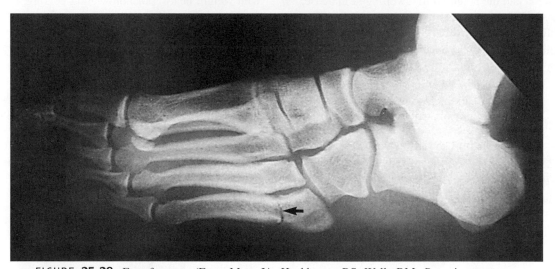

FIGURE **25-28.** Foot fracture. (From Marx JA, Hockberger RS, Walls RM: *Rosen's emergency medicine: concepts and clinical practice,* ed 6, St. Louis, 2006, Mosby.)

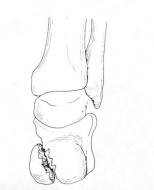

FIGURE **25-29.** Calcaneus fracture.

TOE (PHALANGEAL) FRACTURES. Fractures of the toes (Figure 25-30) occur in all age-groups secondary to kicking a hard object or running into an immovable object. The patient has pain in the toe, swelling, and discoloration. Felt or cotton is placed between the fractured toe and adjacent toe, then both toes are taped together (buddy taped) so the uninjured toe acts as a splint. The patient may bear weight as tolerated and is instructed to wear hard-soled shoes, such as wooden or hard-soled open-toed shoes, that do not put pressure on the toes. Complications are rare, but nail injury may occur.

DISLOCATIONS

Dislocations occur when a joint exceeds its normal range of motion so that joint surfaces are no longer intact. Partial (subluxation) or complete separation of both articulating surfaces can occur. Soft-tissue injuries within the joint capsule and surrounding ligaments; severe swelling; and nerve, vein, and artery damage may be observed with dislocations. Diagnosis can often be predicted before radiographs are taken by soliciting information about the mechanism of injury and noting clinical assessment findings.

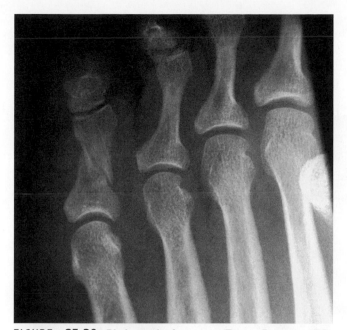

FIGURE **25-30.** Phalangeal fracture. (From Browner BD, Jupiter JB, Levine AM et al: *Skeletal trauma: basic science, management, and reconstruction,* ed 3, Philadelphia, 2003, WB Saunders.)

In general, dislocations produce severe pain, joint deformity, inability to move the joint, swelling, and point tenderness. Potential for vascular compromise also exists, so the distal pulse should be assessed carefully. Initial interventions include careful palpation of the joint and splinting the joint as it is found. Analgesia and sedation are given before reduction by the ED physician or orthopedist. Significant sedation (e.g., morphine, fentanyl, midazolam, methohexital, etomidate, propofol) may be required to reduce dislocations, so the patient requires careful monitoring. Nitrous oxide is used in some institutions. Complications related to dislocations include ischemia, aseptic necrosis, and recurrent dislocations.

Acromioclavicular Dislocation

Acromioclavicular separations (Figure 25-31) are commonly seen in athletes secondary to a fall or direct force on the point of the shoulder. The patient complains of great pain in the joint area and cannot raise the affected arm or bring the arm across the chest. Deformity, point or area tenderness, swelling, and hematoma over the injury site are also noted. The injury is classified in degrees of separation with third-degree injuries involving a complete separation of the joint. Treatment for first- and second-degree injuries involves reducing the separation, regaining anatomic alignment, and immobilizing the affected limb with a sling and swath. More involved third-degree injuries often require surgery for open reduction and wiring. The patient may experience painful range of motion after reduction.

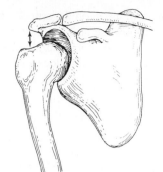

FIGURE **25-31.** Acromioclavicular separation.

Shoulder Dislocation

Dislocations of the shoulder usually occur in children and athletes. Two general categories are anterior and posterior dislocations.

Anterior shoulder dislocations occur as an athletic injury when the athlete falls on an extended arm that is abducted and externally rotated. The force pushes the head of the humerus in front of the shoulder joint (Figure 25-32). Posterior dislocations are rare and usually occur in patients with seizures when the arm is abducted and internally rotated. In all shoulder dislocations, the patient complains of severe pain in the shoulder area, inability to move the arm, and deformity. Deformity is sometimes difficult to see in posterior dislocation. An estimated 55% to 60% of shoulder dislocations seen in the ED are recurrent. The extremity is placed in the position of greatest comfort, then distal pulses are checked, followed by evaluation of skin temperature and moisture, and neurologic status. Radiographs are obtained before the joint is relocated unless neurovascular compromise has occurred. After the joint is relocated, it is immobilized with a sling and swath or shoulder immobilizer. Postreduction radiographs are obtained to confirm placement. The patient should be referred to an orthopedic surgeon. Complications from this type of injury are neurovascular compromise of the brachial plexus and axillary artery and associated fractures.

Elbow Dislocation

Dislocations of the elbow are seen most often in children, teenagers, and young adults. Elbow dislocation is a common athletic injury caused by a fall on an externally rotated arm or when a young child is jerked or lifted by a single arm (known as nursemaid's elbow). The patient complains of pain in the joint, which may feel "locked." Any movement can produce severe pain. Swelling, deformity, and displacement are also noted. The arm is immobilized in the position of greatest comfort. The joint is relocated, then immobilized after radiographs are obtained. The most common complication of this injury is neurovascular compromise to the median nerve or brachial artery.

Radial head subluxation (nursemaid's elbow) accounts for about 20% of upper extremity injuries in children and is seen in children ages 6 months to 5 years, most often in 1- to

3-year-olds. History of a pull on the arm or a fall is reported. The child refuses to use the arm but does not seem in pain or distress. The injury does not require radiographic studies if the dislocation can be easily relocated with good return of function; immobilization after reduction is not necessary.

Reduction of a nursemaid's elbow is accomplished by positioning the child with the elbow flexed 90 degrees, hypersupinating the wrist, and placing the thumb on the radial head. Upon hypersupination a click will be felt on the radial head, confirming the reduction was successful (Figure 25-33).

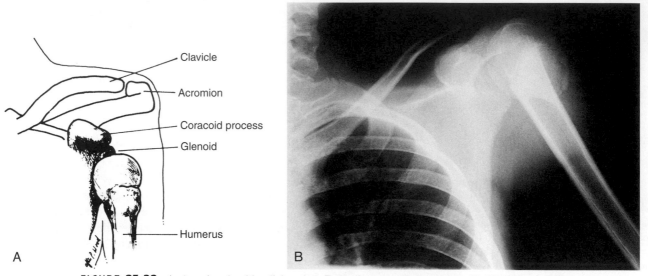

FIGURE **25-32.** **A,** Anterior shoulder dislocation. **B,** Radiograph. (**B** from Marx JA, Hockberger RS, Walls RM: *Rosen's emergency medicine: concepts and clinical practice,* ed 6, St. Louis, 2006, Mosby.)

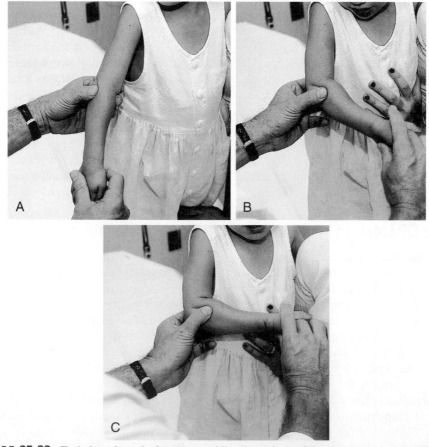

FIGURE **25-33.** Technique for reducing nursemaid's elbow. **A,** Applying pressure to the radial head. **B,** Supinating the forearm. **C,** Flexing elbow, in one continuous motion. (From Marx JA, Hockberger RS, Walls RM: *Rosen's emergency medicine: concepts and clinical practice,* ed 6, St. Louis, 2006, Mosby.)

Wrist Dislocation

Dislocation of the wrist (Figure 25-34) is seen most frequently in athletes but does occur in all age-groups from a fall on an outstretched hand. The patient complains of severe pain in the wrist with swelling, deformity, and point tenderness. The wrist is placed in a splint in the position of comfort, then a cold pack is applied. Radiographic studies are obtained, the joint is relocated, and a cast is applied. Complications include neurovascular compromise, especially median nerve damage.

Hand or Finger Dislocation

Hand or finger dislocations (Figure 25-35) are usually seen in athletes secondary to a fall on an outstretched hand or finger and may also result from direct trauma to the tip of the finger. The patient presents with pain in the area of the injury, inability to move the joint, deformity, and swelling. The patient is sent for radiographs of both the anterior and lateral view of the dislocated finger. After reviewing the films and making certain that a fracture is not present, the patient is given a digital block and reduction is done by emergency care providers. A postreduction film is obtained to confirm successful reduction. The injured area is splinted to immobilize the joint.

Hip Dislocation

Hip dislocations occur in all age-groups, usually when the leg is extended before an impact. The injury is common with head-on, frontal impact MVCs when the leg is extended with the foot on the brake pedal just before impact or when the knee jams into the dashboard. Injury also occurs with falls and crush injuries. Hip dislocations can also result from a failed or displaced implant in patients who have previously undergone surgical interventions for joint replacement or hip fracture (Figure 25-36). Dislocation may be anterior or posterior. The patient complains of pain in the hip and knee and arrives with the hip flexed, adducted, and internally rotated (posterior dislocation) or flexed, abducted, and externally rotated (anterior dislocation). The joint feels locked, and the patient cannot move the leg.

The extremity is splinted in the presenting position or position of greatest comfort. Other injuries are assessed. Necrosis of the femoral head may occur if the joint is not relocated within 4 to 6 hours. After the hip joint is relocated, the patient begins a period of bed rest with traction. Children may be placed in a spica cast. Complications from this type of injury are femoral artery and nerve damage.

Knee Dislocation

Knee dislocations are common in all age-groups and are usually caused by major trauma. The patient complains of severe pain in the knee, inability to move the leg, swelling,

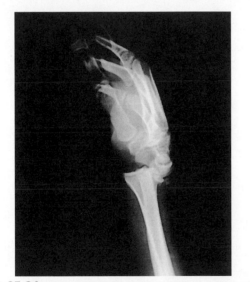

FIGURE **25-34.** Wrist dislocation. (From Ballinger PW: *Merrill's atlas of radiographic positions and radiologic procedures,* ed 8, St. Louis, 1995, Mosby.)

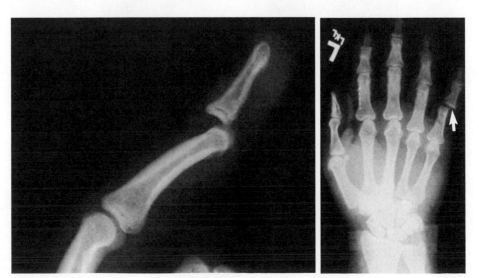

FIGURE **25-35.** Finger dislocation.

and deformity (Figure 25-37). Immediate therapeutic intervention includes splinting the limb in position of comfort or presenting position. A fractured tibia is frequently associated with a knee dislocation. Almost all people with dislocation of the knee joint have associated damage to the joint capsule.

After reduction the patient is admitted to the hospital for bed rest with the knee elevated and intermittent cold packs for 24 to 48 hours. A cast is usually applied after this time. Knee dislocations are associated with a high incidence of injury to the popliteal artery; vascular integrity needs to be evaluated. Other complications include peroneal and tibial nerve damage.

Patellar Dislocation

Dislocation of the patella occurs in all age-groups, usually during athletic events secondary to direct trauma to the lateral aspect of the knee or rapid rotation on a planted foot. Patients usually have severe pain, keep the affected knee in a flexed position, and are unable to use the knee (Figure 25-38). Significant tenderness and swelling in the patellar area is evident. The patella can usually be observed or palpated outside of its normal position. The leg is splinted in the presenting position and a cold pack applied. After

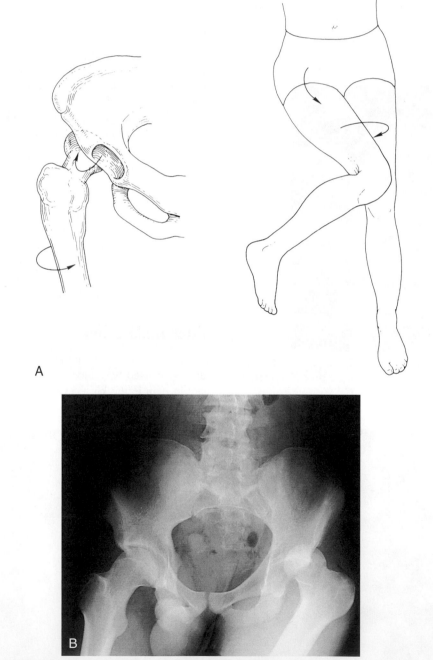

A

B

FIGURE **25-36.** **A,** Hip dislocation. **B,** Radiograph: dislocation of the femoral prosthesis in a patient with a total hip arthroplasty. (From Marx JA, Hockberger RS, Walls RM: *Rosen's emergency medicine: concepts and clinical practice,* ed 6, St. Louis, 2006, Mosby.)

radiographs, if spontaneous reduction does not occur with extension of the leg, the patella is reduced. After relocation, the knee is placed in a compression bandage and knee immobilizer or cylinder cast.

Ankle Dislocation

Ankle dislocation is usually the result of athletic injury and is commonly associated with a fracture. Dislocation results from lateral stress motion when normal range of motion for the ankle is exceeded (Figure 25-39). Patients complain of severe pain in the ankle, inability to move the joint, swelling, and deformity. The ankle and foot are splinted in a position of comfort, and an ice pack is applied. The ankle may be relocated by a closed or open method, depending on the degree of injury and associated fractures. Primary complication of this injury is neurovascular compromise, including the tibial artery.

Foot Dislocation

Dislocations of the foot can occur in all age-groups but are rare. Injury is often the result of an automobile or motorcycle collision in which a combination of forces occurs simultaneously. Foot dislocation is almost always associated with an open wound. The patient complains of severe pain in the foot with point tenderness and inability to use the foot. Significant swelling and deformity are evident. If present, an open wound is covered with a sterile dressing before a soft splint is applied. After the foot is relocated, a cast is applied. The patient is instructed to elevate the limb and apply cold packs for 24 hours. No weight bearing is permitted.

Toe (Metatarsophalangeal) Dislocation

Dislocations of the metatarsophalangeal joints (toes) are rare; when they do occur, they are often associated with open fractures. Toe dislocations should be reduced immediately because delay can result in swelling, making closed reduction more difficult to perform. The patient complains of pain and

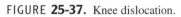

FIGURE **25-37.** Knee dislocation.

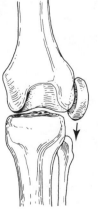

FIGURE **25-38.** Patella dislocation.

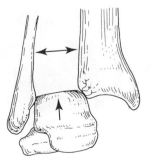

FIGURE **25-39.** Ankle dislocation.

point tenderness in the joint area with significant swelling and noticeable deformity. The area should be covered with a bulky dressing to prevent further damage. After radiographs have been obtained, the dislocation is reduced and then the foot and toes are immobilized.

REDUCTION ISSUES

The goal for reduction of fractures and dislocations is to restore anatomic alignment, allow bone healing, and preserve function. Fractures that do not require anatomic alignment for healing include an impacted fracture of the humeral neck, fractured clavicle (particularly in children), and pediatric nonangulated femur. Conversely, reduction is particularly important for intraarticular fractures, especially for weight-bearing bones.

Reduction methods are described as closed or open (surgical). Closed reduction uses traction-countertraction, angulation, and rotation (i.e., the reverse force of what caused the injury). A finger trap and weights may be used for forearm reduction (Figure 25-40). Manipulation may require local anesthesia, IV sedation, pain medications, or general anesthesia. Reduction should be accomplished as soon as possible after stabilization of other injuries because swelling can impede successful reduction. Postreduction radiographs are done after casting to verify acceptable bone alignment.

Open reduction is used for open fractures; multiple injuries; major fractures; and fractures involving intraarticular joints, epiphysis, or femoral neck. Surgical reduction is also used for soft-tissue entrapment; major nerve, arterial, or ligament injuries; pathologic fractures; unsatisfactory or failed closed reduction; or delayed union. Open reduction employs internal fixation or external fixation devices.

TRACTION

Skin or skeletal traction may be initiated in the ED. A traction splint (e.g., Hare or Sager) can be used until more definitive stabilization is available. Buck's traction uses a wrapped dressing or boot to provide temporary immobilization before surgery for a hip or femur fracture and to reduce muscle spasm. Traction is set up on a hospital bed that is brought to the ED. This eliminates painful and possibly injurious removal of traction with transfer of the patient from the ED stretcher.

Steinman Pin

Skeletal traction may be applied in the ED with a Steinman pin (Figure 25-41). This provides temporary reduction of long-bone fractures until open reduction and internal fixation can be done. The pin is a round stainless steel rod drilled perpendicularly into the distal femur or proximal tibia for connection to a stirrup with traction (15 to 40 pounds). After pin placement, sterile dressings are placed around insertion sites. Osteomyelitis is a potential complication of pin insertion.

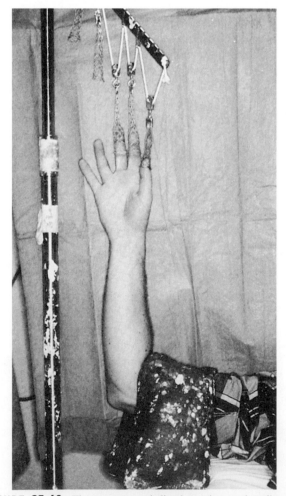

FIGURE 25-40. Finger traps and distal traction at the elbow to distract and reduce fracture dislocations. (From Rosen P, Barkin RM, Rockberger RS at al: *Emergency medicine: concepts and clinical practice,* ed 4, St. Louis, 1998, Mosby.)

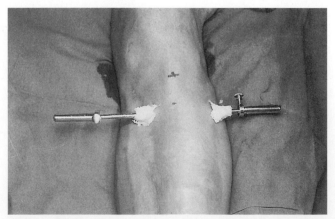

FIGURE 25-41. The pin is passed through the tibia to project equally medially and laterally. Points are protected with covers. (From Mills K, Morton R, Page G: *Color atlas and text of emergencies,* ed 2, London, 1995, Times Mirror International.)

Casts

In the ED the decision to immobilize an injury with a cast versus a splint or fiberglass mold is based on the actual amount of edema and potential swelling that is likely to occur. The goal is to prevent neurovascular compromise (and compartment syndrome) from a restrictive immobilization device. A brief overview of casting and care of casts is presented here. An orthopedic or medical-surgical text should be consulted for complete description of techniques and types of casts/molds.

Before a cast is applied, any particulate matter is removed and the skin completely dried. Any skin abnormalities are documented. Casting equipment includes plaster or fiberglass, stockinette and padding, a bucket of cool-to-warm water, gloves, and a gauze or elastic bandage if a splint is applied.

After the cast is applied, the patient should remain immobile with the limb placed on a plastic-coated pillow for at least 20 minutes to avoid pressure and indentations to allow the cast to set. A plaster cast generally requires 24 hours or more to dry thoroughly; a fiberglass cast dries in about an hour. Box 25-1 lists aftercare instructions for a patient with a cast.

Complications associated with casting include compartment syndrome, pressure sores, and infection. Symptoms of compartment syndrome include severe pain disproportionate to the injury with accompanying neurovascular compromise. An elevated temperature accompanied by a foul odor from the cast suggests infection from a possible pressure sore. Interventions include immediate cast removal. Cast removal or a bivalve procedure is accomplished with an electric cast saw. The saw blade cuts by vibrating rapidly back and forth. The patient should be reassured that the blade does not cut the skin, but heat, vibration, or pressure may be felt. Burns secondary to the blade are rare. After the cast is cut, a cast spreader is used to widen the split and allow removal. Padding beneath the cast should be cut with bandage scissors.

Box 25-1   AFTERCARE INSTRUCTIONS FOR PATIENTS WITH CASTS

Keep cast dry and elevated above heart 24 hours after injury.
Apply cold packs or sealed ice bags over injured area for 30 minutes every 2 to 3 hours for 1 to 2 days.
See your doctor immediately with a change in temperature of fingers or toes (digits are very cold or very hot), a change in color of fingers or toes (they are blue), or loss of feeling in fingers or toes.
Wiggle fingers or toes at least once each hour.
See a physician immediately if a foreign object is dropped into the cast.
Do not put anything inside your cast.
If swelling returns or a foul odor is present, see your physician.
Make an appointment to see a private physician or orthopedic physician for follow-up care.

ASSISTED AMBULATION: CRUTCHES, CANE, AND WALKER

When a patient is fitted for crutches, a cane, or a walker, measurement is ideally taken with the patient wearing shoes that will be worn for ambulating. The shoes should be sturdy, fit well, have low heels, and fasten with a tie, buckle, or Velcro.

Axillary Crutches

Axillary crutches should fit so that each arm piece is 2 inches or two to three finger widths below the axilla with no weight placed on the axilla. Tips of the crutches should be placed 6 inches to the side (or with enough room for the patient's hips to swing through) and 6 inches to the front. Taller individuals require a broader base, so crutches may be placed up to 12 inches to the side for these patients. Each hand piece should be fitted so that the elbow is flexed 30 degrees. For most people, this can be accomplished by having the patient place the crutch in the correct position and extend the arm along the crutch—the hand piece should hit at the level of the wrist.

Cane

A cane should be fitted so that when it is held next to the heel, the elbow is at a 30-degree angle of flexion. A cane should be used for minimal support during ambulation and

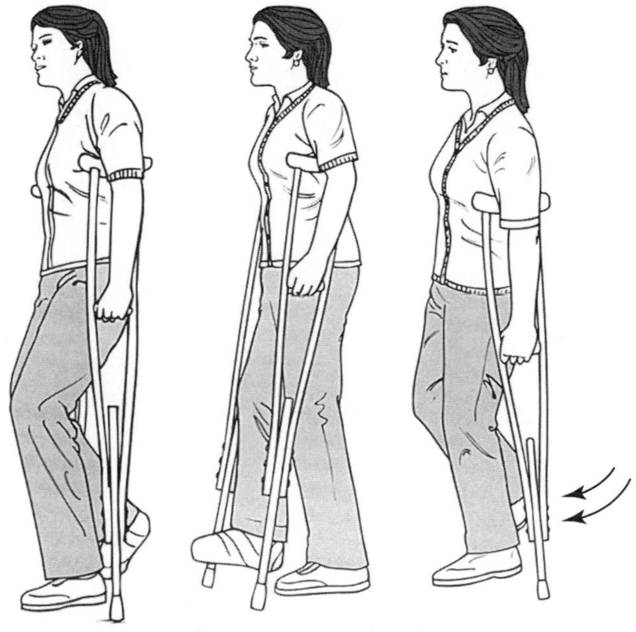

FIGURE **25-42.** Three-point gait. **A,** Standing with crutches, all weight is on the good leg. **B,** Move crutches and injured leg forward simultaneously. **C,** Bearing weight on the palms of the hands, step forward onto the good leg. (From Proehl JA, Jones LM: *Mosby's emergency department teaching guides,* St. Louis, 1997, Mosby.)

to assist with balance and stability. A cane should be used on the side opposite the injury.

Walker

A walker may be chosen for patients who are unsteady on crutches and those who can bear full weight on at least one leg. A walker is measured to fit with the arms bent at 30 degrees. Patients having difficulty ambulating with assist devices may require physical therapy for training, using a

wheelchair temporarily until able to ambulate safely. A walker is not ideal for use on stairs.

Gait Training

A three-point gait is used when minimal or no weight bearing is desired, making this gait ideal for ED patients. Figure 25-42 shows this gait. Figures 25-43 and 25-44 illustrate movement on stairs and changing from a sitting to standing position using crutches.

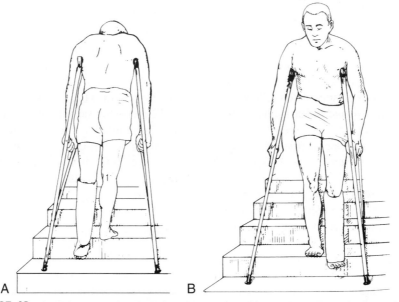

FIGURE **25-43.** **A,** Going up stairs. **B,** Going down stairs with crutches. (From Barber J, Stokes L, Billings D: *Adult and child care,* ed 2, St. Louis, 1977, Mosby.)

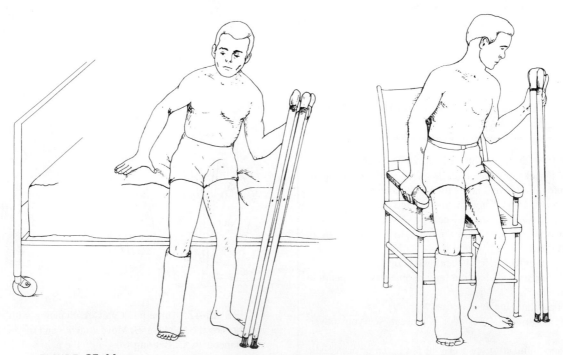

FIGURE **25-44.** Transferring from sitting to standing with crutches. (From Barber J, Stokes L, Billings D: *Adult and child care,* ed 2, St. Louis, 1977, Mosby.)

SUMMARY

Advances in surgical and orthopedic treatments have improved outcome for patients with soft-tissue injuries and fractures. However, the best outcomes occur if injury never happens. Trauma prevention through education and legislation should be the primary goal of overall trauma management.

The main objective for nursing care of the patient with an orthopedic or soft-tissue injury is to preserve or restore normal neurovascular status and motor function. Attention to these injuries is a secondary priority to ABCs. The emergency nurse must assess and intervene as soon as possible and monitor for developing complications to prevent further harm to the extremity.

REFERENCES

1. American College of Surgeons: Committee on Trauma: Shock. In *Advanced trauma life support for doctors: instructor course manual*, ed 7, Chicago, 2004, The College.
2. Black JM, Hawks-Hokanson J: *Medical-surgical nursing*, ed 7, St. Louis, 2005, Saunders.
3. Crowther CL: *Primary orthopedic care*, ed 2, St. Louis, 2004, Mosby.
4. Frank ED, Long BW, Smith BJ: *Merrill's atlas of radiographic positioning and procedures*, ed 11, St. Louis, 2007, Mosby.
5. Griffin Yurko L: *Essentials of musculoskeletal care*, ed 3, Rosemont, Ill, 2005, American Academy of Orthopaedic Surgeons.
6. Hoyt SK, Selfridge-Thomas J: *Emergency nursing core curriculum*, ed 6, St. Louis, 2007, Saunders.
7. Maher AB, Salmond SW, Pellino T: *Orthopaedic nursing*, ed 3, Philadelphia, 2002, WB Saunders.
8. Marx JA, Hockberger RS, Walls RM: *Rosen's emergency medicine: concepts and clinical practice*, ed 6, St. Louis, 2006, Mosby.
9. Moore EE, Feliciano DV, Mattox KL: *Trauma*, ed 5, New York, 2004, McGraw-Hill.
10. Moore W, Smith T: Salter-Harris fractures, 2006, *eMedicine*. Retrieved October 25, 2006, from http://www.emedicine.com/radio/topic613.htm.
11. Roberts JR, Hedges JR: *Clinical procedures in emergency medicine*, ed 4, Philadelphia, 2004, Saunders.
12. Schnell ZB, Leeuwen AVM, Kranpitz TR: *Davis's comprehensive handbook of laboratory and diagnostic tests with nursing implications*, Philadelphia, 2003, FA Davis.
13. Simon RR, Sherman SC: Koeningsknecht: *Emergency Orthopedics*, ed 5, New York, 2007, McGraw-Hill.
14. Thomas-Ojanen D, Bernardo LM, Herman B: *Core curriculum for pediatric emergency nursing*, Sudbury Mass, 2003, Jones & Bartlett.
15. Tintinalli JE, Kelen GD, Stapczynski JS: *Emergency medicine: a comprehensive study guide*, ed 6, New York, 2004, McGraw-Hill.

CHAPTER 26

Burns

Cheryl Wraa

Burn trauma continues to be an immense challenge to caregivers in the emergency department (ED), playing a critical role in the care of the burn patient. Every year in the United States an estimated 500,000 patients are treated in the ED for burn injury. Of these, approximately 4000 die with the majority of deaths, approximately 3500, due to residential fires. The majority of deaths, approximately 75%, occur at the scene or during initial transport. Admissions to the hospital due to burn injury number approximately 40,000 annually in the United States with more then 60% being admitted to hospitals with specialized burn centers. Decreases of burn incidence and hospitalization are attributed to fire and burn prevention education, regulation of consumer products, and implementation of occupational safety standards. The recent decline in mortality is attributed to early excision and closure of the burn wound. Other factors contributing to the decline are management of burn patients in specialty burn units, improved resuscitation, control of infection, and support of the hypermetabolic response. A significant portion of morbidity and mortality associated with burn injuries is due to associated injuries. Pulmonary pathology from inhalation injury is the major cause of burn trauma death, with the majority of deaths at the extremes of age. Burn injury and deaths associated with fires are the third leading cause of accidental death in children between the ages of 1 and 14 years.[2-5,7,14,16]

More than 90% of all burns are considered preventable. Education, particularly in the school-age population, combined with legislative efforts is helping decrease the number of burn injuries. The American Burn Association has developed effective public education programs. Legislation has been enacted that requires smoke alarms and sprinkler systems in public buildings, hotels, apartments, and new homes. For the caregiver an accurate classification of injury, timely intervention, and rapid transport to an appropriate burn facility significantly reduces burn injury mortality and morbidity.[5]

ETIOLOGY

Not all burns are caused by fire. Tissue damage may be secondary to chemicals, hot liquids, tar, electricity, lightning, or frostbite. The location and duration of exposure to the source affects outcome, regardless of the specific source of burn injury. Specific mechanisms of burn injury are described in the following sections.

Thermal Burns

Thermal injuries represent the majority of all burns. They may result from flame, flash, steam, or scalding liquid. Figure 26-1 presents example of one cause of burn injury.

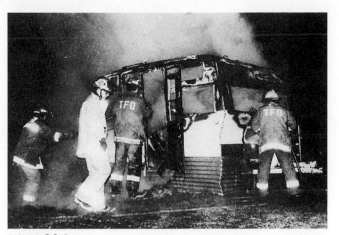

FIGURE **26-1.** Burn injuries occur as a result of exposure to flame and smoke. (Courtesy Tacoma Fire Department, Tacoma, Wash.)

Scald Burns

Scalds from hot liquids are the most common cause of all burns. Exposure to water at 140° F (60° C) for 3 seconds can cause a deep partial-thickness or full-thickness burn. If water is 156° F (69° C), the same type of burn occurs in only 1 second. As a comparison, fresh brewed coffee is about 180° F (82° C). Tap water scalds occur within seconds and often happen during routine activities, involve large body surface area (BSA) burns, and are the most common source of scald-related deaths.[14] Soups and sauces, which are a thicker consistency, remain in contact longer with the skin and cause deeper burns. Other liquids that cause scalds are cooking oil and grease. When used for cooking, oil and grease may reach 400° F (204° C). Immersion burns are usually deep and severe because of prolonged contact with a scalding liquid.

Specific groups of patients at risk for scald burns include those with preinjury comorbidities such as neurologic impairment, diabetes, and the extremes of ages. Adults older than 60 years disproportionately suffer burns from hot liquids.[1] The fact that older patients are at high risk for burn injury and experience worse prognoses than younger patients is well documented. This has been attributed to their compromised physical health status with chronic, debilitating conditions that increase the risk, exacerbate the extent of the injury, and impair recovery.[14]

Flame Burns

Burns from flames are the next most common cause of burns. Fortunately, the number of house fires has decreased with increased use of smoke detectors. Most flame burns are caused by careless smoking, motor vehicle crashes, and clothing ignited from stoves or space heaters. Flame burns that occur outdoors are usually secondary to misuse of cooking stoves fueled by white gasoline, lanterns in tents, smoking in a sleeping bag, and gasoline or kerosene used in a charcoal fire.[4]

Flash Burns

Explosions of natural gas, propane, gasoline, or other flammable liquids cause flash burns—the third most common type of thermal burn. The explosion causes intense heat for a very brief time. Flash burns are usually partial thickness, although depth is dependent on the amount and kind of fuel that explodes. Flash burns can be large and are often associated with significant thermal damage to the upper airway.[4]

Contact Burns

Contact with a hot object such as metal, plastic, glass, or hot coals results in contact burns. The burns are usually not extensive but tend to be deep. People involved in industrial accidents often have contact burns associated with crush injuries from machine presses or hot, heavy objects. An increased incidence of contact burns has been seen in toddlers secondary to the increased use of wood-burning stoves. The most common injury is to the palm when a child falls against the stove with hands outstretched.[4]

Electrical Burns

As electricity passes through the body and meets resistance from body tissues, it is converted to heat in direct proportion to amperage and the body's electrical resistance. It initially passes through the skin, causing an external burn at the entry and exit sites, with extensive damage internally between these sites. Nerves, blood vessels, and muscle are less resistant and more easily damaged than bone or fat. The heart, lungs, and brain can sustain immediate damage. The nervous system is particularly sensitive to electrical burns. Damage to the brain, spinal cord, and myelin-producing cells causes devastating transverse myelitis. Autonomic dysfunction can cause pupils to appear fixed and dilated, but this finding should not cause resuscitation efforts to stop. The smaller the body part through which the electricity passes, the more intense the heat and the less it is dissipated. Consequently, extensive damage can occur in the fingers, hands, forearms, toes, feet, and lower legs. If the path is near or through the heart, damage to the heart's electrical conduction system can cause spontaneous ventricular fibrillation or other dysrhythmias. Papillary muscle damage may lead to sudden valvular incompetence and cardiac failure. Alternating current is more likely to induce ventricular fibrillation than direct current.

Most lightning injuries do not traverse the body but flow around it, creating a shock wave capable of causing fractures and dislocations. Close to two thirds of patients sustain a ruptured eardrum. About 70% of patients who survive a lightning strike complain of paresthesia or paralysis. Fortunately, both conditions are usually temporary.[2,4,16]

Chemical Burns

Chemicals cause a denaturing of protein within the tissues or a desiccation of cells. Chemical concentration and duration of exposure determine extent of the burn. Alkali products usually cause more tissue damage than acids. A wet chemical should be removed as soon as possible by flushing with copious amounts of water. Dry substances should be brushed off the skin before the area is flushed. Care must be taken not to expose the caregiver to the chemical during this procedure. All fluids used to decontaminate the patient should be contained; the fluid should not be allowed to drain into the general drainage system. Chemical burns can be deceiving as to depth; appearances can be similar in surface discoloration until tissue begins to slough days later. Consequently, all chemical burns should be considered deep partial thickness or full thickness until proven otherwise. After chemical removal, wounds are managed in the same manner as thermal burns.[3,4]

Frostbite

Frostbite is actual freezing of tissue from exposure to freezing or below-freezing temperatures. In a cold environment the body attempts to maintain heat by vasoconstriction of peripheral blood vessels to reduce heat exchange. The longer the period of exposure, the more peripheral blood flow is reduced. When extremities are left unprotected, intracellular and extracellular fluids can freeze, forming crystals that damage local tissues. Blood clots may form and impair circulation to the area.

Signs, symptoms, and classification of frostbite are the same as thermal burns. The affected extremity should be rapidly rewarmed using warm water. Use of excessive heat such as steam is dangerous and can cause unnecessary damage. Dress the rewarmed extremity and immobilize it with a padded splint. As with flame burns, frostbite can be very painful, so pain management is needed.[3,4] For a more extensive review of frostbite, see Chapter 40.

Cold immersion of the foot or hand is a nonfreezing injury that occurs from chronic exposure to wet conditions at temperatures just above freezing. The extremity may appear black, but deep tissue destruction may not be present. Initially there is an alternating arterial vasospasm and vasodilation with the tissue first cold and numb, progressing to hyperemia in 24 to 48 hours. As the injury progresses to hyperemia, the patient experiences intense burning sensation and dysesthesia. Tissue damage occurs with resultant edema, blistering, redness, ecchymosis, and ulcerations. Attention to hygiene will prevent local infection, cellulitis, or gangrene.[3]

Patients who have exposure to chronic repetitive damp cold may develop chilblain, or pernio. This is a dermatologic condition that usually occurs on the face, dorsum of the hands and feet, or any area chronically exposed to a cold environment. Signs and symptoms include pruritic, reddened skin lesions that with continued exposure, ulcerate or develop hemorrhagic lesions that progress to scarring, fibrosis, or atrophy with itching, tenderness, and pain. Symptoms are controlled by protection from further exposure, and the use of antiadrenergics or calcium channel blockers.[3]

BURN ASSESSMENT

Burn depth and extent are assessed to determine the severity of burn injury. In many cases final determination is not made for several days.

Depth of Burn

Burns are described as partial thickness or full thickness. Identification of the depth of injury may be difficult initially because depth may actually increase over time as edema forms and circulation to the area of injury is compromised. This process usually peaks at 48 hours; therefore a more accurate determination of depth can be made between 48 and 72 hours. Depth determination is not a priority during initial resuscitation.

Extent of Burn

Extent of injury for thermal and chemical injuries is assessed by using formulas such as the rule of nines (Figure 26-2), Berkow formula, or Lund and Browder table (Figures 26-3 and 26-4). The caregiver should remember that the rule of nines must be modified for children. As noted in Figure 26-2, *B,* the head and neck of an infant represent 18% of BSA, whereas legs represent 14% for each lower extremity. To correct for age 1% is subtracted from the head for each year of age through 10 years, and 0.5% is added to each lower extremity. To estimate scatter burns, the size of the patient's palm (including fingers) is used to represent 1% of total BSA (TBSA). The palm is visualized over the burned areas. To obtain a more accurate estimate of the extent of burns, both burned and unburned areas are calculated. The two estimates should then be compared. If the total is more or less than 100%, the areas should be reestimated. Assessing extent of injury in electrical burns is more difficult because surface damage is minimal when compared with underlying damage. When discussing an electrical injury, describing the injury anatomically is more important than calculating percentage of BSA burned.

Severity of Burn

The severity of burn injury is based on assessment of extent and depth of injury, patient age, presence of concomitant injuries, smoke inhalation, and preexisting diseases. The American Burn Association's guidelines for classification of severity of burn injuries are listed in Table 26-1.

Care of patients with burns of different severity is determined by availability of specialized care facilities. Initial stabilization of the burn patient should be available in any community hospital with 24-hour emergency capabilities. Patients with minor burns may be treated as outpatients or admitted to the community hospital. Patients with moderate burns may be treated in a community hospital with appropriate staff and facilities to deliver burn care or transferred to a specialized burn care facility. Patients with major burns

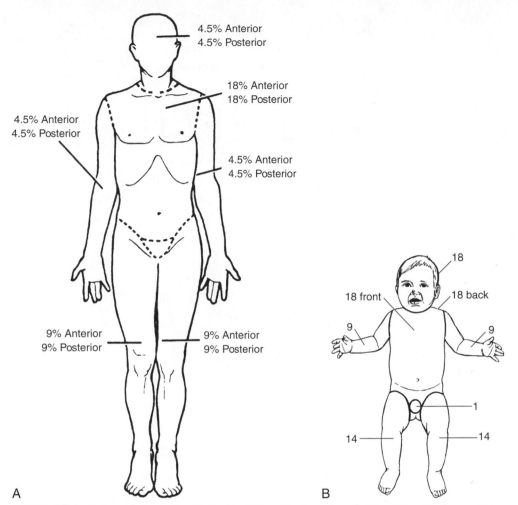

4.5% Anterior
4.5% Posterior

18% Anterior
18% Posterior

4.5% Anterior
4.5% Posterior

4.5% Anterior
4.5% Posterior

9% Anterior
9% Posterior

9% Anterior
9% Posterior

18

18 front   18 back

9   9

1

14   14

A   B

FIGURE **26-2.** Rule of nines. **A,** Adult. **B,** Child. (**A** from Ignatavicius DD, Workman LM: *Medical-surgical nursing: critical thinking for collaborative care,* ed 5, Philadelphia, 2006, WB Saunders. **B** from Sole ML, Klein DG, Moseley MJ: *Introduction to critical care nursing,* ed 4, Philadelphia, 2005, WB Saunders.)

require care in a specialized burn care facility. Transfer agreements with special-care units should be developed in advance to facilitate timely and uneventful transfer. [11] Box 26-1 summarizes criteria for transfer to a burn center. Any patient with concomitant trauma that poses increased risk for morbidity or mortality should be treated in a trauma center until he or she is stable and then transferred to a burn center as appropriate.

PATHOPHYSIOLOGY

Burn injury occurs when skin is exposed to more energy than it can absorb. The cause of the burn may vary, but local and systemic responses are generally similar. To understand the pathophysiology of burns, one must first understand the functions of the skin, which consists of two layers: the epidermis and the dermis. The epidermis, the outer layer of the basement layer of cells, consists of cells that migrate upward to become surface keratin. The dermis, or inner layer, consists of collagen and elastic fibers and contains hair follicles, sweat and sebaceous glands, nerve endings, and blood vessels. The skin is the largest organ of the body and acts as an infection barrier, vapor barrier, and a heat regulator.[4,5]

Three zones of tissue damage occur at the burn site. First is the central zone of coagulation, an area of irreversible damage. Concentrically surrounding this area is the zone of stasis, where capillary and small vessel stasis occurs. The ultimate fate of the burn wound depends on resolution or progression of the zone of stasis. Edema formation and prolonged compromise of blood flow to this area cause a deeper, more extensive wound; therefore depth and severity of burn wounds may not be known for 2 or more days after the initial injury. The third zone of damage is the zone of hyperemia, an area of superficial damage that heals quickly on its own.[5]

The body responds to the burn injury with varying degrees of tissue damage, cellular impairment, and fluid shifts. A brief decrease in blood flow to the affected area is followed by a marked increase in arteriolar vasodilation. Damaged tissues release mediators that initiate an inflammatory response. Histamine, serotonin, prostaglandin derivatives, and the complement cascade are all activated. Release of proinflammatory mediators combined with vasodilation causes

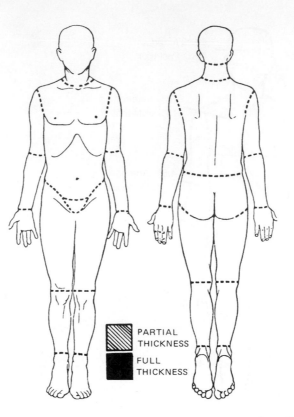

Percent Surface Area Burned

AREA	1 YEAR	1-4 YEARS	5-9 YEARS	10-14 YEARS	Y 15 YEARS	ADULT	2°	3°
Head	19	17	13	11	9	7		
Neck	2	2	2	2	2	2		
Ant. Trunk	13	13	13	13	13	13		
Post Trunk	13	13	13	13	13	13		
R. Buttock	2½	2½	2½	2½	2½	2½		
L. Buttock	2½	2½	2½	2½	2½	2½		
Genitalia	1	1	1	1	1	1		
R. U. Arm	4	4	4	4	4	4		
L. U. Arm	4	4	4	4	4	4		
R. L. Arm	3	3	3	3	3	3		
L. L. Arm	3	3	3	3	3	3		
R. Hand	2½	2½	2½	2½	2½	2½		
L. Hand	2½	2½	2½	2½	2½	2½		
R. Thigh	5½	6½	8	8½	9	9½		
L. Thigh	5½	6½	8	8½	9	9½		
R. Leg	5	5	5½	6	6½	7		
L. Leg	5	5	5½	6	6½	7		
R. Foot	3½	3½	3½	3½	3½	3½		
L. Foot	3½	3½	3½	3½	3½	3½		
TOTAL								

FIGURE **26-3.** Lund and Browder formula. (From Cornwell P, Gregory C: Management of clients with burn injury. In Black J, Hawks J, editors: *Medical-surgical nursing,* ed 7, St. Louis, 2005, Elsevier.)

increased capillary permeability, leading to intravascular fluid loss and wound edema. For burn injuries less than 20% TBSA, these actions are usually limited to the burn site with 90% of the edema present by 4 hours. The edema tends to reside within the dermis, and resorption is complete by 4 days. As the affected TBSA goes beyond 20%, local response becomes systemic. With large burns the overwhelming inflammation, coagulation, and fibrinolysis can continue and constantly be reactivated. The cytokine activity creates a state of exaggerated or reactivated inflammation that includes organ involvement such as acute respiratory distress syndrome (ARDS), systemic inflammatory response syndrome (SIRS), and multiple organ dysfunction syndrome (MODS). Large burns cause a hypermetabolic state that has multiple harmful physiologic derangements associated with it. Derangements noted are muscle catabolism, hepatic dysfunction, and immunosuppression. Treatments such as tight glycemic control and beta blockade may be used to attenuate the hypermetabolic state.[15] Basal metabolic rate increases from insensible fluid loss, which, along with fluid

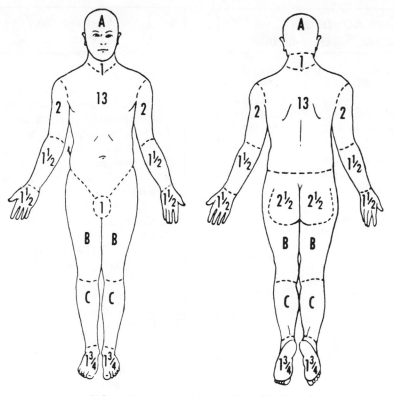

Relative Percentage of Areas Affected by Growth

	Age in Years					
	0	1	5	10	15	Adult
A—½ of head	9½	8½	6½	5½	4½	3½
B—½ of one thigh	2¾	3¼	4	4¼	4½	4¾
C—½ of one leg	2½	2½	2¾	3	3¼	3½

FIGURE **26-4.** Lund and Browder formula. (From Artz CP, Moncrief JA: *The treatment of burns,* ed 2, Philadelphia, 1979, WB Saunders.)

shift, produces hypovolemia. Hypoproteinemia resulting from increased capillary permeability aggravates edema in nonburned tissue. Capillary permeability increases for 2 to 3 weeks with the most significant changes occurring in the first 24 to 36 hours.[5,8,10,16]

Initially blood viscosity increases when hematocrit rises secondary to vascular fluid shifts into the interstitium. Because of a marked increase in peripheral vascular resistance, decreased intravascular fluid volume, and increased blood viscosity, cardiac output falls. Capillary leakage and depressed cardiac output can depress central nervous system function, causing restlessness, followed by lethargy, and finally coma. Decreased cardiac output, decreased blood volume, and intense sympathetic response cause a decreased perfusion to the skin, viscera, and kidneys. Levels of thromboxane A2, a potent vasoconstrictor, are significantly increased in burned patients and contribute to mesenteric vasoconstriction and decreased splanchnic blood flow. Decreased flow can convert a zone of stasis to a zone of coagulation, which increases depth of the burn. Decreased circulating plasma with increased hematocrit can cause hemoglobinuria, which can lead to renal failure. Immediate hemolysis of red cells

occurs, with the life span of remaining red cells reduced by approximately 30% of normal. Platelet count and platelet survival time initially drop drastically then continue to decrease for 5 days after injury. This period is followed by a rebound increase in platelets over the next 2 to 3 weeks.[5,8,16]

Cardiovascular changes begin immediately after a burn; their extent varies with burn size and presence of additional injuries. Patients with an uncomplicated burn less than 15% TBSA can usually be treated with oral fluid resuscitation. Burn patients who surpass 20% TBSA have massive shifts of fluid and electrolytes from intravascular to extravascular spaces. This shift begins to resolve in 18 to 36 hours; however, normal extracellular volume is not completely restored until 7 to 10 days after the burn injury. If intravascular volume is not replenished, hypovolemic shock occurs. If untreated, the patient can die of cardiovascular collapse. Inadequate treatment may lead to renal failure from acute tubular necrosis.

The vasoconstriction of the mesentery mentioned above predisposes the patient to gastric distension, aspiration, and ulceration (Curling's ulcer). A patient with a burn greater than 20% TBSA should have a gastric tube placed to decompress

Table 26-1. AMERICAN BURN ASSOCIATION'S CLASSIFICATION OF SEVERITY OF INJURY

Classification	Characteristics	Treatment Facility
Minor	SPT DPT, <15% TBSA adult <40 years of age DPT, <10% TBSA adult >40 years of age <10% TBSA burn in children <10 years of age *With* <2% TBSA full-thickness burn and no cosmetic or functional risk to the face, eyes, ears, hands, feet, or perineum	Outpatient or inpatient (for 24 hr)
Moderate	DPT, 15% to 25% TBSA adult <40 years of age DPT, 10% to 20% TBSA adult >40 years of age 10% to 20% TBSA burn in children <10 years of age *With* <10% TBSA full-thickness burn without cosmetic or functional risk to the face, eyes, ears, hands, feet, or perineum	Community hospital
Major	DPT, 25% TBSA adult <40 years of age DPT, 20% TBSA adult >40 years of age 20% TBSA burn in children <10 years of age Burns of face, eyes, ears, hands, feet, and perineum Burns with concomitant inhalation injury or major trauma All major electrical injuries	Burn center

Data from Cornwell P, Gregory C: Management of clients with burn injury. In Black J, Hawks J, editors: *Medical-surgical nursing*, ed 7, St. Louis, 2005, Elsevier.
DPT, Deep partial thickness; *SPT,* shallow partial thickness; *TBSA,* total body surface area.

Box 26-1 CRITERIA FOR TRANSFER TO A BURN CENTER

1. Partial-thickness and full-thickness burns greater than 10% total body surface area (TBSA) in patients less than 10 years or over 50 years of age.
2. Partial-thickness and full-thickness burns greater than 20% TBSA in other age groups
3. Burns that involve the face, eyes, ears, hands, feet, genitalia, perineum, or major joints.
4. Full-thickness burns greater than 5% TBSA in any age-group.
5. Electrical burns, including lightning injury.
6. Significant chemical burns.
7. Inhalation injury.
8. Burn injury in patients with preexisting medical disorders that could complicate management, prolong recovery, or affect mortality.
9. Any patient with a burn injury that has concomitant trauma poses an increased risk of morbidity or mortality, and may be treated initially in a trauma center until stable before being transferred to a burn center.
10. Children with burn injuries in hospitals without qualified personnel or equipment for the care of children.
11. Burn injury in patients who will require special social, emotional, or long-term rehabilitative intervention, including cases involving suspected child abuse and neglect.

Data from American College of Surgeons: *Advanced trauma life support student manual,* Chicago, 2008, The College.

the stomach and avoid aspiration. Admission orders will include medication to reduce gastric secretion and early enteral feedings (within 24 hours of injury) to meet basic energy needs.[15]

The hypermetabolic response after burn trauma far exceeds the response seen in other forms of trauma. The patient's metabolic rate can increase as much as two to three times the normal rate. Release of catabolic hormones, including catecholamines, cortisol, and glucagon, initiates a persistent hypermetabolic response. This response causes accelerated breakdown of skeletal muscle, decreased protein synthesis, increased peripheral lipolysis, and increased utilization of glucose, which rapidly depletes glycogen stores. It manifests clinically as severe muscle wasting, decreased muscle strength, and increased liver fat with hepatomegaly and functional impairment. The hypermetabolic response is commensurate with the size of the burn. The adverse effects of the response are managed through nutritional and pharmacologic intervention to improve net nitrogen balance, preserve lean body mass, decrease cardiac work, and decrease hepatic fatty infiltration.[16]

Burn injuries can affect every organ system in the body, causing cerebral perfusion abnormalities, impaired coronary blood supply, renal insufficiency, and acid-base imbalance.[4] Realization of these broad effects can enhance management of the burn patient.

Pulmonary Response to Smoke Inhalation

Inhalation injury or smoke inhalation is a syndrome comprising three distinct problems: carbon monoxide intoxication, upper airway obstruction, and chemical injury to the lower airways and lung parenchyma. The majority of deaths from fires are due to smoke inhalation rather than the burn injury or its sequelae. A burn injury with associated inhalation injury increases the mortality rate. Pulmonary complications associated with inhalation injury directly contribute to death in up to 77% of patients with combined cutaneous and inhalation injury.[12]

Carbon monoxide intoxication is the most common killer of victims of fire. Of the patients admitted to burn centers, approximately 10% to 20% have inhalation injuries. This incidence increases with the size of the burn.[14] Most people who die in a fire have been overcome by carbon monoxide before they sustain a burn injury. In the body, carbon monoxide has a 240-times greater affinity for hemoglobin than oxygen, which causes inadequate oxygen delivery to the tissues. Carbon monoxide combines with myoglobin in muscle cells, causing muscle weakness. Tissue hypoxia and the resultant confusion and muscle weakness may be the major reasons for most fire fatalities. Carbon monoxide poisoning is characterized by pink to cherry-red skin, tachypnea, tachycardia, headache, dizziness, and nausea. An arterial blood gas sample is drawn to measure the carboxyhemoglobin level. Levels below 15% are rarely associated with symptoms of carbon monoxide poisoning and can be normal for a heavy smoker. Levels of 15% to 40% are associated with varying disturbances such as headache and confusion. Levels greater than 40% are associated with coma. Reliance on pulse oximetry or an oxygen saturation of arterial blood (SaO_2) that is calculated from the partial pressure of oxygen (PO_2) rather than measured on a CO oximeter may result in failure to diagnose carbon monoxide poisoning. Most pulse oximeters cannot reliably differentiate between oxygenated hemoglobin and hemoglobin with carbon monoxide and will give a false high measurement. All patients with suspected carbon monoxide poisoning should be placed on 100% oxygen.[3,5,12]

Cyanide poisoning may also occur during a fire and can rapidly result in death. Hydrogen cyanide is highly toxic and can be formed in high-temperature combustion from materials such as polyurethane, acrylonitrile, wool, cotton, and nylon. Cyanide binds to a variety of iron-containing enzymes, one of which plays a critical role in electron transport during oxidative phosphorylation. Even minute amounts of bound cyanide can inhibit aerobic metabolism and rapidly result in death.

The patient with cyanide poisoning will rapidly develop coma, apnea, cardiac dysfunction, and severe lactic acidosis. Diagnosis can be difficult when combined with carbon monoxide poisoning, and the patient can have sublethal levels of carbon monoxide and cyanide and still die due to the combination. The two are synergistic because carbon monoxide primarily affects oxygen delivery and cyanide affects oxygen utilization.

Thermal injury to the upper airway is usually associated with facial burns. Upper airway obstruction is the result of intrinsic or extrinsic edema that may lead to airway occlusion at or above the vocal cords Edema progresses rapidly, totally occluding the airway in minutes to hours (Figure 26-5). This injury is primarily a thermal injury, resulting in tissue damage in the posterior pharynx. Figure 26-6, *B,* shows radiographic evidence of epiglottitis secondary to thermal/chemical injury. Upper airway edema will usually manifest within 24 hours of the injury. Management for airway edema is early intubation or tracheostomy if intubation is not possible. If the patient exhibits dyspnea, stridor, or cyanosis, suspect impending airway obstruction and be prepared to assist with intubation that may be difficult.

Actual thermal injury below the vocal cords is rare because the posterior pharynx is such an efficient heat exchange system. True thermal injury below the vocal cords is usually the result of superheated steam in which water vapor carries heat into the lungs. Injuries that occur in an oxygen-enriched atmosphere or one in which the person was inhaling explosive gases (e.g., during inhalation anesthesia) also cause true thermal injury below the vocal cords. True thermal injury to the lungs is almost always fatal.

Chemical injury to the lower airway is a common problem with inhalation of smoke. Many lower-molecular-weight constituents of smoke are toxic to the mucosa and alveoli because of their pH or the ability to form free radicals. Chemical injury, from acids and aldehydes in the smoke, may damage the lung parenchyma. These chemicals, attached to carbon particles in the smoke, are heavier than air, so they are readily inhaled and find their way down the bronchi into alveoli. This chemical injury causes hemorrhagic tracheobronchitis, increased edema formation, decreased surfactant levels, and decreased pulmonary macrophage function. Although the compounds produce acute neutrophilic airway inflammation, the symptoms, cough, bronchorrhea, dyspnea, and wheezing, may not appear for 12 to 26 hours. Many centers perform early bronchoscopy to determine if there is injury to the lower airways. The bronchoscopy will reveal erythema, edema, carbonaceous debris, and ulceration of the airways. This condition may lead to rapid development of ARDS over 24 to 48 hours. Severe inhalation injury may increase the patient's fluid needs in the first 24 hours by as much as 50% of calculated values.[12,13]

PATIENT MANAGEMENT

The burn patient may have other injuries in addition to the burn; therefore the patient should be initially evaluated using the ABCDE survey for trauma.[3] The cervical spine is protected while assessing for an adequate airway. Assessment of specific burn injuries should be done after the primary assessment is completed. A history is obtained as time and patient condition permit. How did the injury occur? What caused the injury—flame, scald, etc? Was smoke involved? Did injury occur in a confined space? What was the patient doing before the injury? Did the patient have a stroke or myocardial infarction before the injury? Does the patient have any medical problems or allergies? General assessment and interventions for the burn patient are described in this section.

Airway

A primary trauma survey should be performed with appropriate management. Look for evidence of respiratory distress and smoke inhalation injury. A high index of suspicion

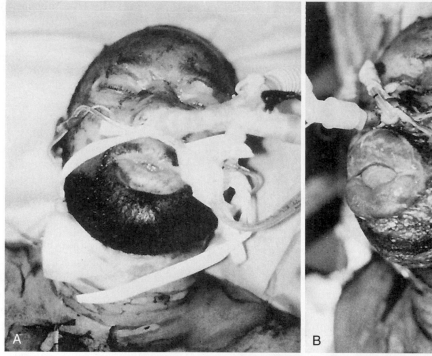
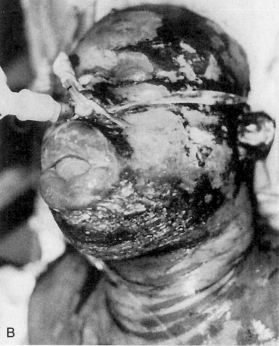
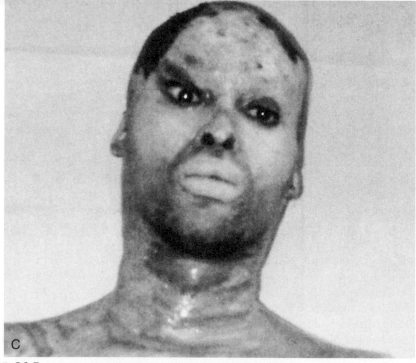

FIGURE **26-5.** Facial edema. **A,** Four to 5 hours after burn. **B,** Thirty hours after burn, showing distortion of facial features and necessity of intubation before the full extent of burn edema development. **C,** Facial contour 3 months after burn. (Courtesy Anne E. Missavage, MD, UC Davis Regional Burn Center, Sacramento, Calif.)

for smoke inhalation is essential for these patients. Burns that occur in small spaces are often associated with smoke inhalation. Administration of high-flow oxygen should be started in an attempt to reverse tissue hypoxia resulting from a low fraction of inspired oxygen (FiO_2) at the fire and to begin displacing carbon monoxide and cyanide from their protein-binding sites. If the patient has a history of chronic obstructive pulmonary disease and is a suspected carbon dioxide retainer, immediate intubation is recommended to prevent progressive carbon dioxide retention.

The half-life of carboxyhemoglobin on room air is approximately 240 minutes. When the patient is placed on 100% FiO_2, the half-life is reduced to approximately 75 to 80 minutes. Hyperbaric oxygen at 2.0 atm decreases the

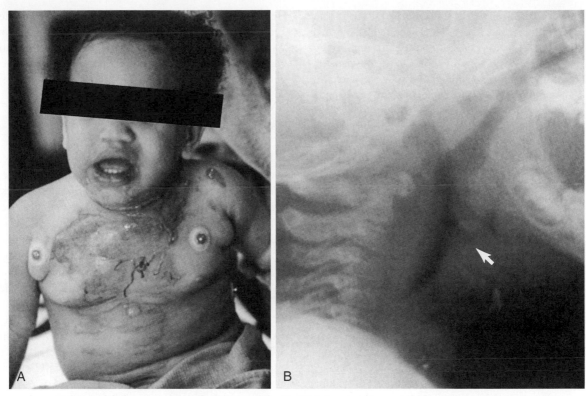

FIGURE **26-6.** **A,** Photograph of 22-month-old child showing burn primarily to the anterior chest wall. **B,** Lateral airway radiograph of the same child demonstrating effects of thermal or chemical epiglottitis. (From Barkin RM: *Pediatric emergency medicine: concepts and clinical practice,* ed 2, St. Louis, 1997, Mosby.)

half-life of carboxyhemoglobin to approximately 20 minutes and appears to hasten the resolution of symptoms. The use of hyperbaric oxygen in the treatment of carbon monoxide poisoning is controversial. Centers that advocate hyperbaric oxygen use it for patients with a carboxyhemoglobin level greater than 40%, loss of consciousness, or in pregnant women with a carboxyhemoglobin level greater than 20% or evidence of fetal distress.

Hyperbaric chambers are limited in availability and most are small and hold only the patient. Larger multiplace chambers allow an attendant to dive with the patient, but even then, complex medical interventions are difficult to perform in this setting. Therefore an unstable patient who may require intensive therapy should not be placed in a chamber. A complication of hyperbaric therapy is barotrauma to the ear due to the inability of the patient to equalize the pressure within the ear as the atmospheric pressure increases. Myringotomy with tube placement has been used as a preventative measure because the pressure difference that leads to barotrauma cannot occur with a hole in the tympanic membrane.[12,14]

If the patient has suspected cyanide poisoning, antidotal treatment includes induction of methemoglobinemia, use of sulfur donors, and binding of cyanide. Outside the United States the combination of sodium thiosulfate and hydroxocobalamin has been successful in the treatment of severe poisoning. In the United States the Taylor cyanide antidote package is used and includes amyl nitrate and sodium nitrite

to induce methemoglobinemia and sodium thiosulfate to act as a sulfur donor. The kit will treat two adult patients. If the patient also has carbon monoxide poisoning, the treatment with amyl nitrite or sodium nitrite is contraindicated until normal carbon monoxide levels can be confirmed. Pending test results for carboxyhemoglobin, sodium thiosulfate may be given intravenously.[6]

The oropharynx and vocal cords should be inspected for redness, blisters, and carbonaceous particles. The patient is observed for increasing restlessness, dyspnea, difficulty swallowing, increasing hoarseness, and rapid, shallow respirations. The patient may have increasing difficulty managing secretions with a significant risk for impending airway obstruction. Early intubation is recommended before complete obstruction occurs. Tracheostomies should be avoided initially because edema of the neck makes this procedure difficult.

Breathing

Circumferential full-thickness burns of the chest can impair breathing by limiting chest wall excursion and preventing adequate gas exchange. The chest should be visually inspected for tight, leathery eschar that circles the chest. Evidence of breathing compromise includes inadequate chest expansion, restlessness, confusion, decreased oxygenation, decreased tidal volume, and rapid, shallow respirations.

Escharotomy is indicated for circumferential burns that compromise breathing. Surgical incisions are made in burned tissue on the chest to release eschar and expose underlying subcutaneous tissue. Improvement in chest wall expansion should occur immediately after incisions are made. General anesthesia is not required because the incisions are made in a full-thickness burn. Intravenous (IV) narcotic analgesia is usually adequate to relieve any pain associated with escharotomy.

The patient with a burn injury is also at risk for carbon monoxide poisoning. Altered breathing patterns such as decreased respirations or apnea may be evident, as may the characteristic cherry-red skin, or the skin can appear slightly cyanotic. Confusion, irritability, or coma may be present. Carboxyhemoglobin level and chest radiograph are obtained to assess for carbon monoxide poisoning and the presence of pulmonary damage or associated injuries. High-flow oxygen with a nonrebreather mask or bag-mask device is administered as appropriate. If the patient does not respond after 1 to 1½ hours of regular oxygen therapy, hyperbaric oxygen therapy may be used.

ARDS occurs in patients with carbon monoxide poisoning but is usually not a problem until approximately 18 hours after injury. Clinical findings associated with ARDS include decreased oxygenation, increased secretions, rapid respirations, confusion, and increasing patchy infiltrates on the radiograph. Treatment includes intubation and ventilation with positive end-expiratory pressure (PEEP). Bronchodilators may be indicated; however, corticosteroids are not. Giving corticosteroids to patients with burns and smoke inhalation can increase morbidity and mortality. Refer to Chapter 30 for additional information on ARDS.

The burn patient should be assessed for other injuries that can affect breathing, such as pneumothorax, hemothorax, tension pneumothorax, and flail chest. These problems can occur with a burn injury from a motor vehicle crash or explosion. Additional injuries may be present when a patient has jumped to escape the fire. Preexisting health problems that may affect respiratory functions (e.g., chronic obstructive pulmonary disease, asthma) should be noted.

Circulation

The patient with a burn injury is at significant risk for hypovolemia from actual fluid loss and fluid movement from increased capillary permeability and vasodilation. Assess the patient for increased respirations, increased pulse, decreased blood pressure, decreased urine output, diminished capillary refill, restlessness, confusion, nausea, and vomiting. Additional indications of volume compromise include central venous pressure less than 3 cm H_2O, hematocrit greater than 50 mg/dL, presence of an ileus, and urine output less than 0.5 mL/kg/hr.

One or two large-bore IV catheters should be started. A single IV catheter is adequate for a burn less than 40% TBSA. Two peripheral access sites are established if the burn is greater than 40% TBSA or the patient will be transferred. Leg veins are avoided because of increased risk for thrombophlebitis. The IV catheter can be inserted into burned tissue if no other access is available, but this should be considered a last resort. Fluid volume requirements are calculated using an accepted formula such as the Parkland or Baxter formula (Table 26-2). These formulas are guidelines for fluid replacement type and volume and should be adjusted to the patient's response to the fluid. Ideally, fluid resuscitation is adequate if pulse and blood pressure are within normal limits for age and urine output is 0.5 mL/kg/hr for adults and 1 to 1.5 mL/kg/hr for infants.

Table 26-2. FLUID REPLACEMENT FORMULAS

Formula	Electrolyte Solution	Colloid	Water	Rate	Example: 70 kg/45% TBSA (per 24 hr)
Evans	1 mL/kg/% TBSA of NS	1 mL/kg/%	2000 mL	½ in first 8 hr; ½ in next 16 hr	3150 mL NS 3150 mL colloid 2000 mL water 8300 mL total
Brooke	1.5 mL/kg/% TBSA of LR	0.5 mL/kg/%	2000 mL	½ in first 8 hr; ½ in next 16 hr	4725 mL LR 1575 mL colloid 2000 mL water 8300 mL total
Modified Brooke	2-3 mL/kg/% TBSA of LR	None	None	½ in first 8 hr; ½ in next 16 hr	6300-9450 mL LR
Parkland (Baxter)	4 mL/kg/% TBSA of LR	None	None	½ in first 8 hr; ½ in next 16 hr	12,600 mL LR
Hypertonic formula (Warden)	4 mL/kg/% TBSA of LR plus 50 mEq $NaHCO_3$ (180 mEq of Na) per liter for first 8 hr	None	None	Switch to LR when pH normalizes or at 8 hr Adjust rate based on urine output	Unknown

Modified from Greenhalgh D: Burn resuscitation, *J Burn Care Res* 28:4, 2007.
LR, Lactated Ringer's solution; *NS*, normal saline; *TBSA*, total body surface area.

No formula exists for calculating fluid resuscitation in electrical injuries. An infusion of lactated Ringer's solution is administered at 1 to 2 L/hr in the average adult until he or she shows signs of adequate resuscitation. Urine output should be maintained at two to three times the normal volume to facilitate excretion of myoglobin. After urine output is established, an osmotic diuretic such as mannitol may be given to increase urine flow and aid in excretion of myoglobin. Significant acidosis can occur, so repeated administration of sodium bicarbonate may be required to prevent dysrhythmias. Once fluid therapy corrects acidosis, repeated administration may not be necessary.

Disability and Exposure

If not yet done, all clothing and jewelry should be removed and a head-to-toe assessment done to check for any concomitant trauma and to estimate burn depth and size. Refer to the earlier section on burn assessment for estimate of burn depth and size. Because the burn patient has lost ability to control body temperature, it is important to increase the temperature in the room and to monitor the patient. Body temperature below 35° C should be avoided.

Diagnostic Procedures

Diagnostic procedures that may assist during the resuscitation of the burn patient are the following:
Laboratory
 1. Complete blood count with differential
 2. Serum electrolytes
 3. Carboxyhemoglobin
 4. Type and crossmatch/screen blood
 5. Urinalysis, pregnancy test in females of childbearing age
 6. Arterial blood gas
Radiography
 1. Chest
 2. Other x-ray examinations as indicated for associated trauma
Other special studies as indicated for associated trauma
 1. Focused assessment sonography for trauma (FAST)
 2. Computed tomography (CT) scan as indicated by assessment findings
 3. Possible peritoneal lavage
 4. 12-lead electrocardiogram (ECG) if electrical or lightning injury

Protection Against Infection

The patient with a burn injury has lost the greatest protection against invasion by various pathogens and must be protected with scrupulous aseptic technique. Gloves, masks, caps, and gowns must be worn. Sterile technique is necessary for all procedures. Wounds are kept covered with clean sheets while other care is provided. If the patient is transferred, sterile sheets are used to cover the patient. If treatment is followed by discharge, the nurse should debride the burn, apply a topical antibiotic, and cover the wound with a fluffy dressing. Systemic antibiotics are rarely indicated even in severe burns until infection is confirmed by culture. Exceptions to this guideline may include young children, older adult patients, diabetic patients, or those with immune system compromise.

For minor or moderate burns, tetanus immunization is given if the patient has not been immunized within the past 10 years. In major burns or grossly contaminated burns, tetanus immunization is given if previous immunization has occurred within 5 years. If the patient has never been immunized or no clear history of immunization exists, tetanus hyperimmune globulin (HyperTET) and tetanus immunization is given.

Pain Management

Burn wounds are exquisitely painful and deserve special consideration. The pain of primary tissue damage and nerve damage may be worsened by primary and secondary hyperalgesia. Intravenous opioid administration should be the prime treatment for burn pain. During initial resuscitation, analgesics or anesthetics should be titrated to effect.[9] After 24 hours, decreased plasma protein levels increase bioavailability of free drugs, especially those that are protein bound. Giving pain medication as needed may increase the patient's awareness of pain and other symptoms. Administering opioids on a schedule, based on drug half-life or by continuous infusion, can facilitate the patient's ability to cope with the pain. The opioid of choice has been IV morphine at 25 to 50 mcg/kg/hr, titrating to avoid respiratory depression. Fentanyl may also be used for some patients. For the burn victim, pain can be made worse by fear of pain or disfigurement, anxiety related to loss of control, and distress over losing family members or material possessions at the time of injury. Anxiety decreases pain tolerance. Reducing anxiety minimizes interplay between acute pain and sympathetic arousal. For the burn patient, anxiolytics may help decrease anxiety and improve pain tolerance. They are especially helpful during painful procedures. The most commonly used anxiolytics are benzodiazepine drugs. Diazepam has a long half-life and high lipid solubility. After repeated use in the burn patient, prolonged mental impairment may occur when the drug is stopped. Therefore short-term administration of lorazepam and midazolam are preferred.

Patients with burn-induced or traumatic nerve injury may develop neuropathic pain. Pain is usually described as tingling, burning, shooting, or numbing. When a postburn patient comes to the ED with this type of pain, it is because the pain did not respond to opiate analgesics. Drugs that decrease neuronal excitability by mechanisms other than opiate receptors are useful for this type of pain. Tricyclic antidepressants in low doses are often successful in relieving neuropathic pain. Sodium channel–blocking drugs such as IV lidocaine, carbamazepine, phenytoin, and mexiletine have also produced successful analgesia.[16]

Wound Care

Wound care should be delayed until the patient's condition is stabilized; however, initial management must include removal of jewelry and constrictive clothing. Wounds must be kept covered with clean sheets until more definitive care can be provided. All patients with full-thickness burns are assessed for circulatory problems. Capillary refill and the presence of paresthesia are evaluated with distal pulses checked by Doppler ultrasonography. Because burn tissue does not

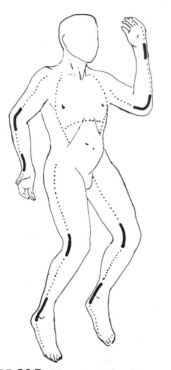

FIGURE **26-7.** Placement of escharotomies.

stretch, swelling beneath burned tissue compromises circulation because of lack of elasticity. If the patient has signs of compromise, escharotomy is indicated. Figure 26-7 illustrates placement of these surgical incisions. Significant bleeding that occurs with escharotomy can be controlled with an electrocautery unit or small hemostats (Figure 26-8). After the procedure is completed, a topical antibacterial agent is applied to the open wound, a light pressure dressing is applied, and the extremity is slightly elevated.

Thermal burns may be secondary to flame, flash, scalds, or hot objects. Figure 26-9 shows an example of a thermal burn. Thermal burns are cleaned with mild soap and water. The use of skin disinfectant, such as povidone-iodine (Betadine), has been shown to inhibit the healing process and is discouraged. Ruptured blisters should be removed, but intact blisters may be left alone and should never be aspirated with a needle because this increases the chance of infection. The wound is covered immediately with a topical antibacterial agent such as silver sulfadiazine (Silvadene) or bacitracin. Burns of the face should be left open and covered by a topical antibiotic ointment such as bacitracin, which is reapplied every 6 hours after gently washing the skin.

Chemical burns should be immediately irrigated with tap water or normal saline for at least 5 to 10 minutes to remove the chemical. Clothing and jewelry are removed, and unburned areas adjacent to the burned areas are rinsed. These areas can be injured but may not hurt, blister, or turn red immediately. If the chemical is dry, it can be brushed from the patient before irrigating. After the wound is thoroughly irrigated, it is treated like a thermal burn. Chemical burns of the eye are an ophthalmologic emergency. The eye must be irrigated thoroughly with copious amounts of water or saline. (Refer to Chapter 45 for additional discussion of chemical eye injuries.)

Electrical injuries are different from thermal and chemical burns. These wounds may have little superficial tissue

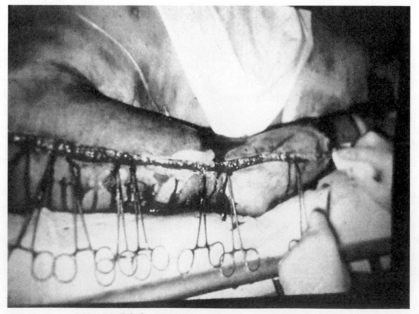

FIGURE **26-8.** Control of bleeding from escharotomy.

loss; however, massive muscle injury may be present beneath normal-looking skin or minor to severe exit wounds (Figures 26-10 and 26-11). Wounds should be cleaned gently with a 0.25% povidone-iodine solution using sterile water or 0.9% sodium chloride; they rarely need immediate debridement. Topical agents such as mafenide acetate (Sulfamylon) solution that deeply penetrate tissue are used to cover the wound. Light dressings may be applied to cover these often grotesque wounds; however, dressings must not interfere with assessment for circulatory compromise and

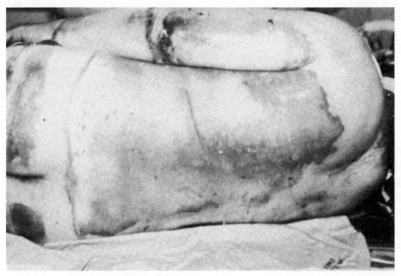

FIGURE **26-9.** Flame burns to back.

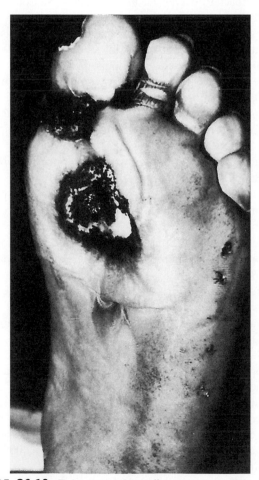

FIGURE **26-10.** Exit wound from direct current. (From Air & Transport Nurses Association: *Air & surface patient transport: principles and practice,* ed 4, St. Louis, 2019, Mosby.)

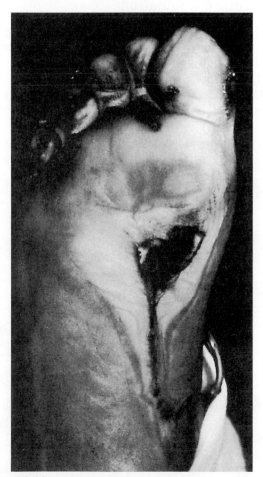

FIGURE **26-11.** Exit wound from alternating current. (From Air & Transport Nurses Association: *Air & surface patient transport: principles and practice,* ed 4, St. Louis, 2019, Mosby.)

possible compartment syndrome. High-voltage injuries are associated with severe muscle contractions, so radiographs of the cervical spine may be indicated.

Electrical injuries of the extremities cause significant damage that leads to tissue swelling. Consequently, these patients are at risk for compartment syndrome. Symptoms associated with this condition include pain, pallor, paresthesia, pulselessness, paralysis, and pressure in the affected area. Fasciotomies are used to relieve compartment syndrome.

Tar or asphalt burns may be deep or superficial depending on the temperature of the tar, which may range from 150° F to more than 600° F, as well as the length of time the skin was in contact with it. Figure 26-12 shows a tar burn before tar removal. Immediate treatment of a tar burn is to cool the tar, but do not try to peel it off the patient's skin. Using mineral oil, petroleum jelly, or a solvent such as Medi-Sol loosens the tar. In areas where the burn is not circumferential, oil or ointment is applied and the burn is covered with a light dressing. Dressings are removed in 4 to 12 hours, oil or ointment reapplied, and a new dressing applied. For areas with circumferential tar, oil or ointment can be applied with light dressings and changed every 20 to 30 minutes until tar is removed. After the tar is removed, the burn is treated as a thermal injury.

Temperature Regulation

The patient with a burn injury has lost a major control mechanism for temperature regulation. This heat loss is worsened by administration of room temperature IV fluids, irrigation of burned tissue, and environmental coolness often encountered in the ED. The patient's temperature should be documented as soon as possible after arrival in the ED and rechecked within 1 hour. Keeping the patient covered, using warmed IV fluids, and increasing room temperature minimizes heat loss.

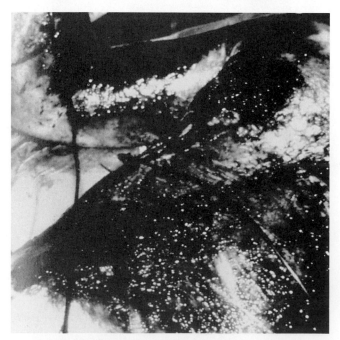

FIGURE 26-12. Tar burns of chest before removal of tar.

SUMMARY

Burn injury can be devastating to the patient and family; for the caregiver, it can also be visually disturbing. Regardless of how severe the burn may be, a primary survey should be performed for potentially life-threatening injuries. Resuscitation of the burn patient includes evaluation of the burn, replacement of fluid losses, wound care, protection against contamination, maintenance of body temperature, and pain control. A multidisciplinary approach to burn care can reduce mortality and morbidity. Appropriate application of burn center transfer criteria ensures the best outcome for the patient with a major burn injury.

REFERENCES

1. Alden N, Bessey P, Rabbitts A et al: Tap water scalds among seniors and the elderly: socio-economics and implications for prevention, *Burns* 33(5):666, 2007.
2. American Burn Association: *Fact sheet.* Retrieved August 20, 2007, from http://www.ameriburn.org/resources_factsheet.php.
3. American College of Surgeons: *Advanced trauma life support student manual,* Chicago, 2008, The College.
4. Auerbach P: *Wilderness medicine,* ed 4, St. Louis, 2001, Mosby.
5. Cornwell P, Gregory C: Management of clients with burn injury. In Black J, Hawks J, editors: *Medical-surgical nursing,* ed 7, St. Louis, 2005, Elsevier.
6. Desai S, Su M: *Cyanide intoxication.* Retrieved August 20, 2007, from http://www.uptodate.com.
7. Fagenholz P, Sheridan R, Harris N et al: National study of emergency department visits for burn injuries, 1993 to 2004, *J Burn Care Res* 28:1, 2007.
8. Greenhalgh D: Burn resuscitation, *J Burn Care Res* 28:4, 2007.
9. Hackenschmidt A: Burn trauma priorities for a patient with 80% total body surface area burns, *J Emerg Nurs* 33:4, 2007.
10. Hershberger R, Hunt J, Arnoldo B et al: Abdominal compartment syndrome in the severely burned patient, *J Burn Care Res* 28:1, 2007.
11. Mandal A: Quality and cost-effectiveness: effects in burn care, *Burns* 33(4):414, 2007.
12. Mandel J, Hales C: *Smoke inhalation.* Retrieved August 20, 2007, from http://www.uptodate.com.
13. Marek K, Piotr W, Stanislaw S et al: Fibreoptic bronchoscopy in routine clinical practice in confirming the diagnosis and treatment of inhalation burns, *Burns* 33(5):554, 2007.
14. Palmieri T: Inhalation injury: research progress and needs, *J Burn Care Res* 28:4, 2007.
15. Rice P: *Emergency care of moderate and severe thermal burns in adults.* Retrieved December 14, 2007, from http://www.uptodate.com.
16. Sona C: Burns. In Urdan L, Stacy K, Lough M, editors: *Thelan's critical care nursing,* ed 5, St. Louis, 2006, Mosby.

CHAPTER 27

Maxillofacial Trauma

Chris M. Gisness

Maxillofacial trauma involving injury of the facial bones, neurovascular structures, skin, subcutaneous tissue, muscles, and glands is a common injury in patients treated in the emergency department (ED). Facial trauma is a complicating factor in the management of patients with multisystem injuries.

Motor vehicle crashes (MVCs) are the most common cause of facial injury in the United States; however, facial trauma from assaults and personal altercations is increasing. Domestic violence and child abuse are among the increasing number of personal assaults. Handguns also cause facial injury. With bullet trajectory above the mandible, intracranial injury should also be considered. Facial injury from falls is common among older adults and children. In children, skull and facial bone flexibility absorb energy associated with deceleration injuries such as MVCs and falls. Lack of and incorrect use of seat belts and helmets can also cause injury to the maxillofacial area.

When a patient presents with facial trauma, a thorough assessment of the eyes is a priority after life-threatening injuries have been addressed. Globe disruption and blindness can occur with facial trauma that involves the eyes. Damage to the optic nerve or retina may also occur.

The use of air bags and seat belt restraints in vehicles can save lives but not without some risk. Facial injuries involving abrasions and chemical burns to the eyes have occurred with the deployment of air bags. Pediatric occupants are at significant risk for life-threatening injuries when seated in the front seat if an air bag deploys.[2,7] Infants weighing less than 40 pounds should be placed in the rear seat, with those less than 20 pounds or 1 year of age placed in a rear-facing car seat. Children should also be placed in the rear seat with a size- and weight-appropriate car seat or booster seat.[3]

Assessment and treatment of facial injuries—regardless of severity—does not take priority over recognition and treatment of life-threatening injuries. Rapid, thorough assessment using a systematic approach with emphasis on airway, breathing, circulation (ABCs), and cervical spine stabilization is essential.

ANATOMY AND PHYSIOLOGY

Principal facial bones include the frontal, nasal, maxilla, zygoma, and mandible. The frontal bone articulates with the frontal process of the maxilla and nasal bone and laterally with the zygoma. The orbital complex is composed of the frontal bone superiorly, zygoma laterally, maxilla inferiorly, and processes of the maxilla and frontal bone medially. Paired nasal bones form the bridge of the nose and articulate with the frontal bone above and maxilla below. The nasal cavity is divided by the nasal septum; the lateral wall has ridges, or conchae, that affect phonation.

The midface, or maxilla, forms the upper jaw, anterior hard palate, part of the lateral wall of the nasal cavity, and part of the orbital floor. Below the orbit, the maxilla is perforated by the infraorbital foramen to allow passage of the infraorbital nerve and artery. Projecting downward, the alveolar process joins the opposite side to form the alveolar arch, which houses the upper teeth. Sinus cavities in the midface decrease weight and act as resonating chambers.

The zygoma forms the cheek and the lateral wall and floor of the orbital cavity. Articulations with the maxilla, frontal bone, and zygomatic process of the temporal bone form the zygomatic arch.

The mandible is a horizontal horseshoe body with two rami, anterior coronoid processes, and posterior condyloid processes.[11] The mandibular notch lies medial to the zygomatic arch and separates the two processes. The mandible articulates with the temporal bone to form the temporomandibular joint (TMJ), whereas the upper body of the mandible, called the alveolar part, contains the lower teeth.

The facial nerve (cranial nerve VII) provides sensory and motor innervation to the side of the face. It originates in the brainstem, then divides into five branches to innervate the scalp, forehead, eyelids, facial muscles for expression, cheeks, and jaw. Specific functions for each branch are listed in Table 27-1. Other cranial nerves that may be affected by facial trauma are the oculomotor, trochlear, and trigeminal. Function and testing for each are described in Table 27-2.

The parotid gland is located adjacent to the anterior ear and drains into the oral cavity through the parotid duct. These structures are located adjacent to branches of the facial nerve on top of the masseter muscle.[1] Lacerations near this area

can be quite concerning if they breach the parotid duct near the facial nerve; they must be evaluated for injuries to the parotid duct and facial nerve.

PATIENT ASSESSMENT

Once the primary and secondary assessment has been completed, the patient is now ready for a more focused assessment. An organized approach to patient assessment is essential for identification and stabilization of facial injuries. Regardless of injury or mechanism of injury, the first priority is a clear, secure airway. Damaged facial structures can cause airway obstruction. If the mandible is displaced, the tongue loses anatomic support and may occlude the airway. Foreign objects (e.g., dentures or avulsed teeth) can obstruct the airway, whereas fractures of the nasoorbital complex may compromise the airway secondary to hemorrhage. Gunshot wounds to the face cause significant swelling and hematoma formation, which can obstruct the airway. When airway compromise is recognized, the chin lift–head tilt method should be used unless cervical spine injury is suspected, in which case the jaw-thrust maneuver is indicated. Altered mental status from alcohol, drugs, or head injury can diminish the patient's gag reflex and leave the airway unprotected. Frequent reassessment of the neurologic status is necessary. Suctioning of the oropharynx or nasopharynx is required when bleeding or excessive secretions are present. A tonsil-tip suction catheter can be provided for an alert patient to self-suction. If cervical spine injury is not a consideration or the cervical spine has been cleared, allow the patient to sit upright or elevate the head of the bed to promote drainage.

Excessive bleeding and swelling of the mouth and facial structures, coupled with inability to clear the airway, requires aggressive airway control. Supplemental oxygen and assisted ventilations can be accomplished with a bag-mask device; however, swelling and facial fractures can make use of a bag-mask device difficult with some patients. An oropharyngeal airway can be used in an unconscious patient with obstruction from the tongue. A nasopharyngeal airway

Table 27-1. F ACIAL N ERVE B RANCH F UNCTIONS

Branch	Function
Buccal	Wrinkle nose
Cervical	Wrinkle skin of neck
Mandibular	Purse and depress lips
Temporal	Raise eyebrows, wrinkle forehead
Zygomatic	Close eyelids

Table 27-2. C RANIAL N ERVES I NVOLVED IN F ACIAL T RAUMA

Nerve	Name	Function	Description	Assessment
III	Oculomotor	Motor	Eyeball movement; supplies five of seven ocular muscles	Pupil response; ocular movement to four quadrants
IV	Trochlear	Motor	Eyeball movement (superior oblique)	Same as above
V	Trigeminal	Motor and sensory	Facial sensation; jaw movement	Assessing pain, touch, hot and cold sensations, bite, opening mouth against resistance
VII	Facial	Motor and sensory	Facial expression; taste from anterior two thirds of tongue	Zygomatic branch: have patient close eyes tightly; temporal branch: have patient elevate brows, wrinkle forehead; buccal branch: have patient elevate upper lip, wrinkle nose, whistle

can be used in the conscious patient with no nasal or midface fractures. Noisy breathing suggests an obstructed airway.

Orotracheal intubation is preferred in patients with facial injuries; blind nasotracheal intubation should be avoided in facial fractures. Cribriform plate fractures increase the risk for cerebral penetration by an endotracheal tube. Rapid-sequence induction facilitates intubation and has the added benefit of protecting the patient from increases in intracranial pressure.[4] If rapid-sequence induction is used, equipment to perform a surgical airway opening must be available should cricothyrotomy or tracheostomy be needed. Pulse oximetry is an essential adjunct for monitoring the airway patency and breathing. Cervical spine injury should be considered in all facial trauma patients with plain radiographs or computed tomography (CT) scan used to rule out injury.

After a patent airway is established, the next priority is hemorrhage control. Adult patients with facial injury can develop shock because of profuse bleeding because the face is highly vascularized. Facial bleeding can be controlled with direct pressure and pressure dressings. Bleeding vessels on the face should be carefully assessed before ligation to prevent accidental clamping of facial nerve branches. A large cotton-tip swab can be used to apply direct pressure to bleeding vessels; ice packs and direct nasal pressure usually stop bleeding from the nose. A nasal tampon may be inserted to control anterior bleeding; a nasal catheter can be used to control posterior bleeding. Severe facial trauma, such as Le Fort II or III fractures, requires manual reduction of the face to control bleeding. With closed fractures, bleeding from lacerated arteries and veins into sinus cavities can cause significant posterior pharyngeal bleeding; ligation of arteries and veins or embolization is necessary to control blood loss.

Once the primary assessment has been completed and life-threatening conditions addressed, a more focused assessment of the face should be completed. Palpate facial structures before edema and hematomas obscure bony landmarks. Use both hands simultaneously to palpate for step-off irregularities and crepitus of the supraorbital ridges and zygoma. Inspect the face by looking down on the face from the eyebrows to compare height of the malar eminences, then look up from below the chin. Gently palpate nasal bones and look intranasally for septal hematoma. Palpate laterally for depressions in the zygomatic arch, and visualize the mouth for gross dental malocclusion. Ask the patient if the teeth close and fit together properly, and then check the patient's ability to completely open the jaw. Upper and lower jaws should be carefully palpated intraorally (wearing gloves). Check midface stability by attempting to move the upper teeth and hard palate.

Evaluate the facial nerve and its branches. Loss of sensation over the lower lip may indicate injury to the inferior alveolar nerve and possible mandibular fracture. Numbness over the upper lip occurs with fracture in the maxilla and injury to the infraorbital nerve. Assessment of the eye should be done early, before increasing lid edema makes it more difficult. Visual acuity is determined with use of the Snellen chart, hand-held card, or standard chart. If the patient is unable to count fingers, check for light perception and document findings before other testing is done.[9,12] Assess eyes for loss of vision, visual acuity, pupillary reactivity, symmetry, and extraocular movements. Ensure that pupils are on the same facial plane and observe closely for enophthalmos and proptosis. A teardrop-shaped pupil suggests a ruptured globe. Hyphema and subconjunctival hemorrhage often indicate a serious eye injury. In some patients with periorbital injuries, widening of the distance between the medial canthus (called telecanthus) may indicate serious orbital injury. Raccoon eyes (i.e., periorbital ecchymosis) suggests anterior basilar skull fracture, Le Fort fracture, or nasoethmoid injury, whereas nasal or ear drainage positive for cerebrospinal fluid (CSF) occurs with cribriform plate fracture or basilar skull fracture. Appearance of a bull's eye or halo when bloody drainage from the nose or ear is placed on white paper indicates the presence of CSF. Clear fluid positive for glucose or clear fluid that does not crust also indicates CSF. A ruptured tympanic membrane or laceration of the external ear canal can occur with mandibular fractures. Deep lacerations of the cheek should be carefully evaluated for injury to the parotid gland, parotid (Stenson's) duct, and branches of the facial nerve. Diagnostic evaluation for maxillofacial injury includes radiographs, CT, and magnetic resonance imaging.

SPECIFIC MAXILLOFACIAL INJURIES
Soft Tissue Trauma

For soft-tissue injuries to the face, the goal is to retain function and have good cosmesis. It is important that repair of facial wounds occur is a timely manner. Because of the highly vascular nature of the face, the length of time for wound closure can be extended to 20 hours from the time of injury, although it is preferable to delay no longer than 8 to 12 hours. In a healthy patient the face is considered to be at low risk for infection. Deeper lacerations and lacerations associated with fractures can be conservatively debrided, irrigated, and closed before reduction. With tissue that is considered viable, excessive debridement should be avoided. Repair of facial lacerations in uncooperative patients is extremely difficult and may injure other important structures. Delaying repair until the patient is more cooperative usually results in better outcome. Figure 27-1 shows contusions, abrasions, and lacerations of the face.

Lacerations caused by animal or human bites are highly contaminated because of the bacteria and debris found in the mouth. All bites should be meticulously cleaned with soap and water and irrigated with warmed saline (preferred) because the warm temperature is more appealing to the patient. Detergent, hydrogen peroxide, and concentrated povidone-iodine solutions should be avoided because they are considered toxic to the tissues.[8] There are many factors to consider when deciding whether to close a facial laceration caused by a bite. Human and animal bite wounds on the face can be disfiguring, so suturing is more commonly done; however, cat bites, which are most often puncture wounds, are left open. Extensive or gaping wounds on the face present cosmetic problems, so consultation with a plastic surgeon is recommended. Most experts recommend closing the wound after meticulous irrigation and debridement. Both human and animal bites should be inspected for tooth fragments. Extensive animal bites, usually caused by large dogs, frequently require surgical exploration and repair. A helpful mnemonic for dealing with animal bites is RATS (rabies, antibiotics, tetanus, and soap). All patients should be covered for tetanus and rabies prophylaxis as indicated. Patients with animal and human bites should receive prophylactic antibiotics that cover streptococcus, staphylococcus, *Eikenella corrodens*, and *Pasteurella multocida*.[8]

Road rash or friction injuries present a unique problem because of potential tattooing or epidermal staining. Debridement should be done as soon as possible to avoid accidental, but permanent, tattooing from grease and asphalt. After the area has been injected with local anesthetic, skin should be vigorously scrubbed with mild soap. Gunpowder can cause permanent discoloration of skin with subsequent cosmetic disfigurement; therefore black powder fragments embedded in facial skin should be removed by using a local anesthetic and scrubbing with a hard brush or hard-bristle toothbrush in the first hour whenever possible. Gunpowder penetrating the skin is very hot and continues to burn epithelial and collagen layers. The longer it is allowed to remain,

the greater the risk for permanent discoloration.[8,13] When glass fragments are visible, tape applied to the face may help remove the glass.

Lacerations of eyebrows and eyelids should be repaired before swelling occurs so borders can be matched. Eyebrows should never be shaved because landmarks are eliminated and the brow is unlikely to grow back. When suturing the brow, hairs are aligned so they slant in a downward and outward direction.

Vermillion borders or margins are important anatomic landmarks in repair of lip lacerations. Borders must be perfectly aligned to prevent development of step-off deformity of the lip. Figure 27-2 illustrates closure of this type of laceration. Tissue loss from the lip requires reconstruction by a plastic surgeon.

Intraoral injuries should be carefully inspected for debris, crushed tissue, and tooth fragments. Injuries should be meticulously cleaned and irrigated. Gaping intraoral lacerations tend to bleed and become infected, so they should be closed. Antibiotics are usually prescribed. Encourage the patient to use a mild antiseptic mouthwash to swish and spit several times a day.

When the tongue is lacerated, inspect the mouth carefully for other lacerations from teeth. Gaping or bleeding lacerations are sutured, and antibiotic therapy is indicated. Children are prone to hard and soft palate lacerations, usually from falling with a sharp object in the mouth.

Ear injuries are categorized into three groups: hematomas, lacerations, and avulsions. Hematomas must be properly drained and dressed to prevent a scar deformity that resembles a cauliflower (Figure 27-3). Follow-up with plastic surgery is necessary because hematomas tend to recur. Lacerations may involve skin or skin and cartilage. Wounds to the ear require minimal debridement and are usually closed in two layers; however, avulsion injuries of the ear require skin preservation; otherwise grafts from other body sites are required. Anesthetics containing epinephrine should not be used on

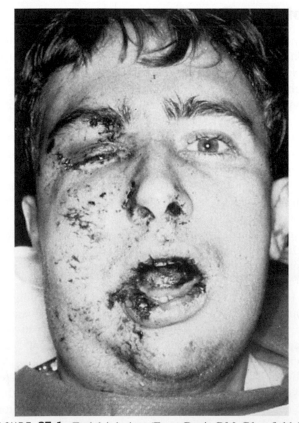

FIGURE **27-1.** Facial injuries. (From Danis DM, Blansfield JS, Gervasini AA: *Manual of clinical trauma care: the first hour*, ed 4, St. Louis, 2007, Mosby.)

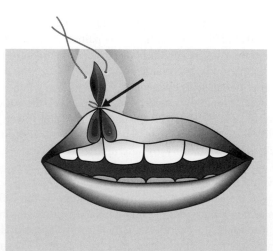

FIGURE **27-2.** Lip laceration through the vermillion border. Closure requires proper alignment with first suture placed at the vermillion-cutaneous border.

the ear because of the deleterious effects of vasoconstriction. Antibiotics are prescribed to prevent cartilage infection. Cartilage necrosis can occur if bandages are left unpadded or unchecked for long periods.

Deep cheek lacerations can damage the parotid gland, parotid duct, and branches of the facial nerve, a motor nerve that governs muscles of facial expression. Injury to the temporal branch causes forehead asymmetry because the patient cannot wrinkle the forehead on the affected side. With injury to the temporal or zygomatic branch, the patient is unable to fully close the eyelids on the affected side. Buccal branch injury keeps the patient from pursing the lips to whistle, and injury to the mandibular branch causes inability to lower or depress the lower lip. At rest, elevation of the lower lip occurs on the affected side. Injury to the facial nerve can be easily missed if the patient is unconscious or has numerous facial dressings. Facial paralysis after blunt facial trauma has a good prognosis for complete recovery if minimal soft-tissue damage occurs. Lacerations of the parotid duct or the parotid gland are an infrequent occurrence. Duct cannulization is used to determine patency when injury is suspected.

Nasal Fractures

Nasal fractures are the most common facial fracture because the nose offers the least resistance. The mechanism of injury is usually blunt trauma. Overlooked nasal injury can lead to permanent deformity and airway obstruction. Clinical findings include swelling, deformity, bleeding, and crepitus. In children the nose is more elastic and resistant to fractures; however, dislocations are common. Nasal fractures can usually be diagnosed by physical examination. If radiographs are needed, the lateral view is usually the best. Unrecognized or untreated nasal fractures can lead to abnormal nasal bone growth that affects nasal contour.

Nasal bones are lined with mucoperiosteum. A nasal fracture with an overlying laceration is considered an open fracture. Fractures caused by a frontal blow can damage

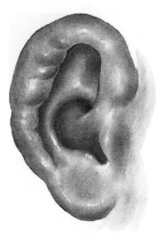

FIGURE 27-3. Cauliflower ear. (From Sheehy SB, Jimmerson CL: *Manual of clinical trauma care*, ed 4, St. Louis, 2007, Mosby.)

the ethmoid and frontal sinuses, lacrimal duct, and orbital margins. If the cribriform plate is affected and the dura torn, CSF leak or rhinorrhea occurs. Careful examination of each naris can identify septal hematomas, lacerations, and ability of the patient to breathe through his or her nose.[11,12] A septal hematoma appears as a bulging tense bluish mass that feels doughy when palpated. Septal hematomas should be emergently drained to prevent airway obstruction and necrosis of septal cartilage. The patient should be placed on an antistaphylococcal antibiotic. An untreated septal hematoma causes a permanent nasal deformity called saddle deformity.[10]

Initial interventions focus on controlling bleeding with direct pressure. Bleeding may be intranasal and in the pharynx. Ice compresses applied to the bridge of the nose aid hemostasis and help relieve pain. Anterior or posterior nasal packing may be required to control bleeding. Splinting maintains position, ensures alignment, and prevents further edema and injury. In some cases the physician may not set the fracture until the swelling subsides. When the fracture involves the nasal mucosa of the lacrimal system, blowing the nose causes intracranial air or subcutaneous emphysema that can cause localized infection or meningitis.

Nasoorbital-Ethmoidal Fracture

Nasoorbital-ethmoidal (NOE) fracture occurs with a direct blow to the face that results in fractures of the medial orbital wall, nose, and ethmoid sinus. Most bones in this area are thin, fragile, and have low tolerance to impact. Injury to this area can result in direct ocular injury. Fractures can extend through the cribriform plate and result in CSF leak (rhinorrhea) from the nose. This fracture is usually the result of high-impact MVCs. The presenting symptoms include pain and visual abnormalities.[6] Clinical presentation shows massive periorbital and upper facial edema with ecchymosis, epistaxis, traumatic telecanthus, foreshortening of the nose with telescoping and associated intracranial injuries. Diagnostic findings on CT scan may include disruption of interorbital space and comminution of nasal pyramid; frontal, zygomatic, orbital, and maxillary fractures are a common concomitant finding. Complications of NOE fracture are residual upper midface deformity ("dish face"); telecanthus; and frontal sinus–nasolacrimal system pathology with mucocele, mucopyocele and dacryocystitis.

Maxillary Fractures

Maxillary, or midface, fractures are caused by significant force and are usually a combination of fractures involving several facial structures. Maxillary fractures are classified as Le Fort I, II, and III (i.e., lower third, middle third, and orbital complex). Plain radiographs of the face with emphasis on Waters' view have been used in the past, but CT is used for definitive diagnosis and identification of the fractures. Maxillary fractures are rarely seen in children because of the flexible and pliable nature of their maxillofacial structures.

Patients with maxillary fractures complain of severe facial pain, anesthesia or paresthesia of the upper lip, and some visual disturbances. Clinically the patient has severe facial swelling, ecchymosis, periorbital or orbital swelling, subconjunctival hemorrhage, elongation of the face, facial asymmetry, epistaxis, and malocclusion and may occasionally exhibit complete airway obstruction.[9] CSF may leak from the nose (rhinorrhea).

Le Fort I, or lower third fracture (Figure 27-4, *A*), is a horizontal fracture in which the body of the maxilla is separated from the base of the skull above the palate but below the zygomatic process attachment. Separation may be unilateral or bilateral. There is a free-floating segment of the upper teeth and lower maxilla; however, the fracture may not be displaced. The hard palate and upper teeth are mobile when moved by grasping the alveolar process and anterior teeth. The presenting symptoms are pain in the upper jaw and numbness in the upper teeth. Clinical presentation includes midface edema and ecchymosis, epistaxis, malocclusion, and mobility of maxillary dentition. Diagnosis is best determined

Lateral view

Frontal view

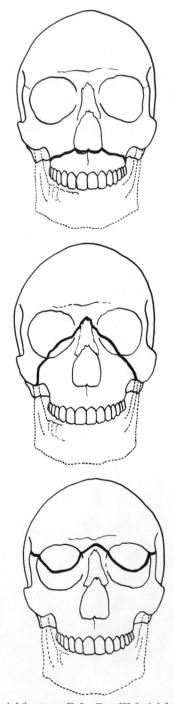

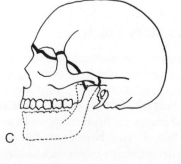

FIGURE **27-4.** **A,** Le Fort I facial fracture. **B,** Le Fort II facial fracture. **C,** Le Fort III facial fracture.

by CT scan, but a Waters' and Panorex radiographic view may still be used. Findings demonstrate opaque maxillary sinus, displacement of fragments of alveolus if comminuted, and fracture through maxillary sinus and pterygoid plates. Complications of Le Fort I fractures include loss of teeth, infection, and malocclusion.

Le Fort II, or middle third fracture (Figure 27-4, *B*), involves the pyramidal area, including the central maxilla, nasal area, and ethmoid bones. This portion of the face is a tripod shape with the apex at the nose. Grasping the front teeth and palate causes movement of the nose and upper lip, with no movement of the orbital complex. Significant force is required to fracture this area, and the patient should be carefully evaluated for other injuries. The presenting symptoms are pain in the midface, numbness in the upper lip and lower lid, malocclusion, mobility of midface, nasal flattening, anesthesia, and the infraorbital nerve territory. The nose, mouth, and eyes are usually edematous with subconjunctival hemorrhage and epistaxis frequently noted. The presence of rhinorrhea suggests an open skull fracture. CT scan remains the diagnostic gold standard, although the Waters' radiographic view is still used. CT scan findings consistent with a midface fracture include opaque maxillary sinuses and separation through frontal process, lacrimal bones, floor of orbits, zygomaticomaxillary suture line, lateral wall of maxillary sinus, and pterygoid plates. Complications of Le Fort II fractures include nonunion, malunion, lacrimal system obstruction, infraorbital nerve anesthesia, diplopia, and malocclusion.

Le Fort III, or orbital complex fracture (Figure 27-4, *C*), causes total cranial facial separation. The nose and dental arch move without frontal bone involvement. Massive edema, ecchymosis, epistaxis, and malocclusion are present with a spoonlike appearance of the face noted in side profile. Early ocular examination is necessary to prevent unrecognized ocular injuries secondary to extensive swelling. Fractures of the cribriform plate and bleeding from the middle meningeal artery threaten airway patency; cervical spine fracture-dislocation may also occur.[6]

Presenting symptoms are facial pain and difficulty breathing. Clinical signs are "donkey-face" deformity and rhinorrhea. CT scan findings demonstrate separation of the mid third of the face at zygomaticotemporal and nasofrontal sutures, and across orbital floors; and opaque maxillary sinuses. Complications of Le Fort III fractures include nonunion, malunion, malocclusion, lengthening of midface, and lacrimal system obstruction.[10]

Management of maxillary fractures includes aggressive airway control. Endotracheal intubation may be difficult because of edema and loss of normal anatomic contour. Nursing care should include anticipating potential cricothyroidotomy or tracheotomy. Excessive secretions and bleeding require frequent suctioning; therefore allow the patient to use a tonsil-tip suction when appropriate.[9] Position the patient upright and leaning forward (once the cervical spine is cleared) to promote drainage and decrease swelling. Apply ice compresses for pain relief and to decrease swelling, and administer prophylactic antibiotics and tetanus immunization as appropriate.

Zygoma Fractures

Fractures of the zygoma usually occur in two patterns: zygomatic arch fracture and tripod fracture. Fracture of the orbital floor may also be present with zygomatic fractures. Injury is usually caused by blunt trauma to the front and side of the face. With a tripod fracture the zygoma fractures in three places: zygomatic arch, posterior half of the infraorbital rim, and frontozygomatic suture. A step deformity is palpated at the infraorbital rim and frontozygomatic suture area with flattening or asymmetry of the cheek, periorbital edema, circumorbital or subconjunctival ecchymosis, and pain exacerbated by jaw motion. A zygoma fracture that occurs at the arch presents with pain in the lateral cheek and inability to close the jaw. There is swelling and crepitus over the arch and obvious asymmetry. Complications that may occur with a zygomatic arch fracture are contour irregularities of the arch area and flattening of the arch. A fracture that occurs at the body of the zygoma or a tripod fracture presents with pain, trismus, diplopia, numbness of the upper lip, lower lid, and bilateral nasal area. Clinical signs include swelling, ecchymosis of malar and periorbital areas, palpable infraorbital rim step-off, entrapment of extraocular muscles with disconjugate gaze, scleral ecchymosis, and displacement of the lateral canthal ligament. Entrapment of the inferior rectus muscle causes double vision and asymmetry of ocular levels and anesthesia of the upper lip, cheek, teeth, and gums. Interventions focus on pain control and decreasing swelling. Complications include residual malar deformity, enophthalmos, diplopia, infraorbital nerve anesthesia, and chronic maxillary sinusitis.

A CT scan is the preferred diagnostic test, but a Waters' or submentovertex radiograph is acceptable. Diagnostic findings may show clouding, air/fluid level in the maxillary sinus, and separation of the zygomaticomaxillary, zygomaticofrontal, and zygomaticotemporal suture lines.[10] Plain radiographs with a "jughandle" view demonstrate zygomatic arch fracture, whereas CT scans are often needed to demonstrate extent of a tripod fracture.

Orbital Blowout Fractures

Zygoma fractures and orbital blowout fractures can occur independently but are often found in combination. Orbital blowout fracture occurs when blunt trauma to the globe causes abrupt rise in orbital pressure. The orbital floor is the weakest part of the bony orbit, so increased pressure causes orbital contents to prolapse into the maxillary sinus (Figure 27-5).[4] Inferior rectus muscle, inferior oblique muscle, infraorbital nerve, orbital fat, and connective tissue become entrapped in the orbital floor, so extraocular movements should be carefully evaluated. The globe may also become entrapped. This fracture frequently results from sports, such as a baseball thrown at the eye, and altercations such as fist fights. Golf balls can extend past the protective orbital rim and rupture the globe. If the globe is perforated, manipulating the eyes or nose blowing can lead to intraorbital air.

Presenting symptoms include binocular diplopia, orbital pain, periorbital edema and ecchymosis, enophthalmos, extraocular muscle entrapment, dysconjugate gaze, hyphema, subluxation of lens, retinal detachment, and rupture of the globe.

Subcutaneous orbital emphysema suggests fracture in the sinus arch. Nose blowing, coughing, sneezing, vomiting, and straining can force air from sinuses through the fracture into the orbital space. Proptosis, or bulging of the eye, and limitation of extraocular motion suggest orbital involvement (Figure 27-6). Double vision, pupil asymmetry,

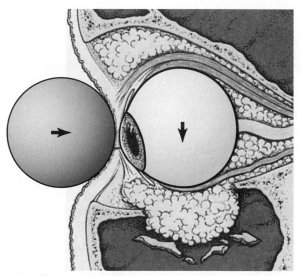

FIGURE 27-5. Mechanism of a blowout fracture caused by the impact of a ball. The periorbital fat is forced through the floor of the orbit. (From Ragge N: *Immediate eye care,* London, 1990, Wolfe Medical Publications.)

enophthalmos (sunken appearance), anesthesia of the cheek and upper lip, and ptosis (drooping of the lid) are clinical manifestations of blowout fracture. Extreme swelling may occur after a blowout fracture has occurred, making it difficult to obtain a good eye examination, so it is important to remember to assess the eye early, before more swelling develops. Globe injuries may occur concurrently with blowout fractures. Ruptures usually occur at the weakest area of the globe or opposite the side of impact.[4] If a ruptured globe is suspected, an eye shield or plastic cup should be used over the eye to prevent further injury. A ruptured globe is an ophthalmologic emergency. Emergent ophthalmologic consultation is indicated. Complications of an orbital floor fracture are enophthalmos, diplopia, recurrent orbital cellulitis with implant (alloplastic), and extrusion.

Plain radiographs with Waters' view can help distinguish these injuries, but CT scan is able to define the fracture site and determine the size of the defect. Findings reveal air/fluid levels in the maxillary sinus, herniated adnexa, and/or orbital floor fragments in the maxillary sinus.

Surgical intervention is usually postponed until swelling diminishes, usually several days. Ice compresses and elevating the head of the bed decrease swelling and relieve pain. Broad-spectrum antibiotics and nasal decongestants are used. The patient should be reminded to avoid straining and nose blowing.[5]

Mandibular Fractures

Mandibular fractures are the second most common facial fracture. Blunt force, such as a severe blow to the face during contact sports, altercations, and MVCs, is the usual mechanism of injury. Mandibular fractures can be a significant life-threatening injury if loss of bony support displaces the tongue posteriorly and obstructs the airway. Malocclusion is a cardinal indication of mandibular fracture (Figure 27-7).

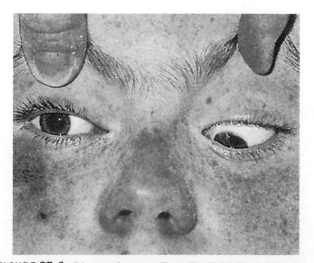

FIGURE 27-6. Blowout fracture. (From Zitelli BJ, Davis HW: *Atlas of pediatric physical diagnosis,* ed 5, St. Louis, 2007, Mosby.)

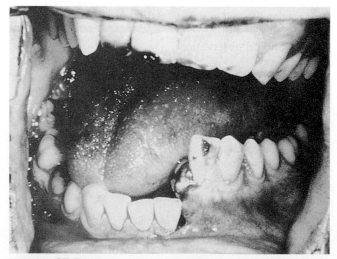

FIGURE 27-7. Malocclusion caused by fracture. (From Danis DM, Blansfield JS, Gervasini AA: *Manual of clinical trauma care: the first hour,* ed 4, St. Louis, 2007, Mosby; courtesy Dr. Daniel Cheney.)

Signs and symptoms vary with fracture site; however, point tenderness and crepitus may be palpated and step-off deformity found. Trismus and decreased range of motion are usually noted. The face may be asymmetric with swelling and ecchymosis. Paresthesia in the lower lip and chin imply injury to the inferior alveolar nerve. The oral cavity should be assessed for broken or loose teeth, lacerations, or ecchymosis. Sublingual hematoma can compromise the airway. Inspect ears for tears in the external canal and tympanic membrane.

Mandibular fractures are classified according to the region of the jaw injured. The most common sites for fracture are the angle of the mandible, condyle, and molar and mental regions, with the symphysis the least common injury site. Reciprocal fractures can occur on the side opposite the point of impact. Specific symptoms related to a condyle fracture are pain at the fracture site with referred pain to the ear. Other symptoms might include crepitus, excessive salivation, swelling of the condylar region, deviation of the jaw toward the fracture, cross-bite, or open bite deformity. Plain radiographs with anteroposterior and oblique views, Waters' view, or Panorex show a nondisplaced or displaced (anteriorly and medially) condyle fracture. Complications include ankylosis of the TMJ and or chronic TMJ disorders.

For a fracture at the angle of the mandible, there is pain at the fracture site and inability to close the mouth. Assessment findings may include swelling at the angle of the jaw, ecchymosis, crepitus, and malocclusion. Mandibular radiographic series or Panorex reveal a nondisplaced (favorable) fracture or a posterior fragment displaced upward and medially (nonfavorable) fracture. Complications of fractures of the angle of the mandible include nonunion, malunion, and osteomyelitis.

The clinical presentation for a fracture of the body of the mandible includes pain at the fracture site and limitation of jaw movement with edema, ecchymosis, crepitus, and malocclusion. A mandibular radiographic series or Panorex might reveal a nondisplaced (favorable) fracture or a posterior fragment displaced upward and medially, anterior fragments rotated lingually (nonfavorable) fracture. Complications of this type of fracture include osteomyelitis and infection of the tooth in the fracture line.

Lastly, a fracture of the symphysis of the mandible might produce symptoms of pain, malocclusion, and soft-tissue wounds of the lower lip or tongue. A mandibular series or submentovertex view would find a nondisplaced or lingual rotation, or anterior fragments, and may be associated with angle or condyle fractures. Complications of this type of fracture include residual malocclusion, loss of chin projection, asymmetry, and osteomyelitis.

Treatment consists of surgical intervention with open reduction and internal fixation or wiring the jaw, depending on the location of the fracture. Nursing care in the ED includes allowing the patient to sit upright as soon as the cervical spine is cleared and applying ice compresses to the face to minimize swelling and relieve pain. Oral saline rinses for the mouth may also be used. Intravenous antibiotics are indicated for open fractures, and repair of lacerations should occur as soon as possible.

SUMMARY

Maxillofacial injuries are a common occurrence in the ED. Special attention should be given to stabilizing the cervical spine, maintaining a patent airway, and controlling hemorrhage. The goal of treatment is life, function, and aesthetics.

REFERENCES

1. Agur A, Lee M: *Grant's atlas of anatomy*, ed 10, Philadelphia, 1999, Lippincott Williams & Wilkins.
2. Costello B, Papadopoulas H, Ruiz R: Pediatric craniomaxillofacial trauma, *Clin Pediatr Emerg Med* 6(1):32, 2005.
3. Emergency Nurses Association: *Emergency nurses pediatric core course manual*, ed 6, Des Plaines, III 2007, The Association.
4. Emergency Nurses Association: *Trauma nurses core course manual*, ed 6, Des Plaines, Ill, 2007, The Association.
5. Eurele B, Kelly B: Maxillofacial injuries: clinical characteristic and initial management, *Trauma Rep* 6(3):1, 2005.
6. Eurele B, Kelly B: Maxillofacial injuries: imaging, management and disposition, *Trauma Rep* 6(4):1, 2005.
7. Kim G, Wong M: Ocular trauma: an evidence based approach to evaluate and manage in the ED, *Pediatr Emerg Med Pract* 3(11):1-15, 2006.
8. McManas JG, Wedmore I, Shwartz RB, editors: Emergency department wound management, *Emerg Med Clin North Am* 25(1):xvii, 2007.
9. Newberry L, Criddle L, editors: *Sheehy's manual of emergency care*, St. Louis, 2005, Mosby.
10. Rogers L, editor: *Radiology of skeletal trauma*, ed 3, Philadelphia, 2002, Churchill Livingstone.
11. Snell R, Smith M: *Clinical anatomy for emergency medicine*, St. Louis, 1993, Mosby.
12. Tintinalli JF, Kelen GD, Stapczynski JS, editors: *Emergency medicine*, ed 6, New York, 2004, McGraw-Hill.
13. Trott AT: *Wounds and lacerations*, ed 3, Philadelphia, 2005, Mosby.

CHAPTER 28

Pediatric Trauma

Autumne Bailey Mayfield and Kate Copeland

Despite scientific advances in injury prevention and treatment, traumatic injury continues to be the leading cause of death in children older than 1 year of age. Each year approximately 20,000 children and teenagers die as a result of injury. For every child who dies from an injury, 40 others are hospitalized and 1120 are treated in emergency departments (EDs). An estimated 50,000 children acquire permanent disabilities each year, most of which are the result of closed head injury. Pediatric trauma continues to be one of the major threats to the health and well-being of children.[1]

Several factors influence childhood injuries, including age, sex, behavior, and the surrounding environment. Of these, age and sex are the most important factors affecting the patterns of injury. Male children younger than 18 years have higher injury and mortality rates, most likely due in part to their more aggressive behavior and exposure to contact sports. In the infant and toddler age-group, falls are a common cause of severe injury. The most common scene of pediatric injuries is the home environment, where approximately 35% of significant injuries occur.[1]

The frequency of childhood injuries compels the emergency nurse to participate in primary, secondary, and tertiary prevention of pediatric injuries. This chapter highlights anatomic and physiologic differences in pediatric patients, describes patient assessment, reviews essential interventions, discusses treatment of selected traumatic injuries, and identifies specific injury prevention strategies.

EPIDEMIOLOGY

Blunt force trauma is the most common mechanism of pediatric morbidity and mortality, including motor vehicle crashes (MVCs), all-terrain and off-road vehicles, falls, pedestrian incidents, and bicycle crashes.[1] MVCs are the leading cause of death from blunt force trauma,[18] with most fatalities resulting from head injuries.[16] In 2005, MVCs killed 1946 child occupants under 14 years of age, with an average of 640 children injured every day.[35] Penetrating trauma accounts for 10% to 20% of all pediatric trauma admissions. Gunshot wounds are responsible for most penetrating injuries and carry a significantly higher mortality compared with blunt mechanism injury.[1] A rising incidence of pediatric penetrating trauma has occurred because of the proliferation of handguns and increased violence.[1] Access to firearms in the home increases the risk for unintentional firearm-related death and injury among children. Unintentional shootings cause more than 20% of all firearm-related deaths among children ages 14 and under. These two mechanisms of injury, blunt and penetrating, are interrelated in that blunt mechanical force can result in penetrating injury, such as that caused by fender edges, door handles, or shrapnel.[1]

For children between the ages of 4 and 14, unintentional injury-related deaths occur most often when riding in a car. Children are most often injured, suffer more severe injuries, or die in MVCs when they are not properly restrained. Within this age-group, children 4 to 8 years of age are especially at risk for injury because of the improper use of safety belts in motor vehicles. Safety seats are the most effective protection against fatal injury to child motor vehicle passengers. Rear-facing infant safety seats reduce the risk for death in an MVC by 71%, forward-facing seats for toddlers reduce risk for death by 54%, and safety belts reduce risk for death by 45%.[36] However, parents must know how to correctly install and use child safety seats to achieve the most protection for their children. The American Academy of Pediatrics is a valuable resource for car safety seats for families.[8] As many as 85% of child safety seats are found to be improperly installed. Infants should be placed in rear-facing seats until they are at least 1 year of age and weigh at least 9 kg (20 pounds) because they have large heads, proportionally, and weak neck muscles, which place them at risk for cervical distraction and dislocation during frontal crashes.[39] Children do not fit in adult shoulder and lap belts (without a booster seat) until they are 58 inches tall and weigh 36 kg (80 pounds). However, children between the ages of 4 and 8 years who have outgrown their child safety seat often are placed too soon in adult lap and shoulder belts without a booster seat. It is estimated that only 5% of children in this age-group are properly restrained with booster seats in motor vehicles. Children restrained with a lap belt and shoulder harness are susceptible to certain injuries. Young children have a shorter sitting height than adults and a higher center of gravity above the lap belt. A greater proportion of body mass is located above the safety belt, which may cause more forward motion and increase the risk for head and neck injury. Children can jackknife over restraints, causing an airway or hanging injury. Similarly, a child can "submarine" under the restraint system, leading to neck and airway injuries. The lap belt itself can also cause injuries. During sudden deceleration, children are thrown forward with their full body weight going into the lap belt. Resulting injuries include lumbar spine fractures, small bowel injuries, and abdominal bruising.

Sitting in the rear seat of a car offers significant protection during an MVC. Restraint use enhances this effect[4]; therefore parents must be encouraged to restrain children with proper child safety devices in the vehicle's rear seat for optimal protection in the event of an MVC.

Other high-risk motor vehicle situations are trunk entrapment and leaving children unattended in cars. Unintentional trunk entrapment leads to death in 35% to 40% of cases. When left unattended, children may be able to start the vehicle or put the vehicle in neutral. In addition, they can suffer from hypothermia and hyperthermia dependent on environmental temperature.

In 2005, a total of 414, or 21%, of the fatalities among children age 14 and younger occurred in crashes involving alcohol. Over half were passengers in vehicles with drivers who had blood alcohol levels of 0.01 g/dL or higher. An additional 48 children under the age of 14 were killed by drinking drivers when they were pedestrians or on bicycles.[35]

Annually approximately 1000 16-year-old drivers are involved in fatal crashes, and traffic injury is the leading cause of death of adolescents. Graduated driver-license programs, which place restrictions on new drivers, have reduced the incidence of fatal crashes by 11%. The more comprehensive programs have the greatest effect on decreasing fatalities and injuries among this age-group.[14]

Children and adolescents sustain injuries as passengers or operators of all-terrain vehicles, two-wheeled off-road vehicles, and go-carts/buggies. These children had a mean age of 12.7 years, and 77% were male. Most injuries occur from disruptions in the driving surface, such as bumps, holes, and uneven terrain.[10] Young children riding as passengers can be crushed by the adult driver on impact with a stationary or moving object. Older children who are not the appropriate size or weight to operate such vehicles can flip vehicles onto themselves and sustain serious multisystem injuries.

Falls are the most common mechanism of injury in children and the leading cause of nonfatal injuries in children below the age of 14.[1] Many serious falls among children occur on playgrounds and during sports and recreational activities. Falls in the youngest children happen more often in the home environment, on stairs, furniture, and out of windows, from varying heights.[21] They also fall while running, playing, and participating in sports. Injuries sustained from falls vary from mild to severe single-system or multisystem trauma.

Injuries associated with shopping carts occur especially among children younger than 5 years. Injuries to children occur via several mechanisms, including falling from carts, carts tipping over, becoming entrapped in a cart, and being run over by a cart.[33] Head injuries account for approximately two thirds of all injuries associated with falls from shopping carts.[32]

Pedestrian injuries are a common cause of morbidity and mortality in the pediatric population. As pedestrians, children are struck by moving vehicles while playing, walking, running, crossing the street, or entering or exiting a school bus. Rates of childhood pedestrian injuries have been reported as 2.5 times higher on one-way streets compared to two-way streets.[37] Most injuries occur in the afternoon and early evening hours on urban streets. Lower socioeconomic status and urban domicile have also been implicated in pedestrian incidents, with a rate three times higher for children from poorer neighborhoods compared with those from wealthier neighborhoods.[37]

Young children struck by motor vehicles in driveways are at risk for severe injury and death. During 2001-2003, an estimated 7475 children between the ages of 1 and 14 years were treated for nonfatal motor vehicle back-over injuries.[21] Approximately 100 children suffer fatal injuries per year in driveways or parking lots, often when relatives or family friends back over them.[31] Children younger than 5 years of age struck in their driveway had a higher Injury Severity Score (ISS), were more likely to sustain a closed-head injury, and were more likely to die compared with children older than 5 years of age struck in their driveway.[27]

Bicycle crashes are a common mechanism of fatal and nonfatal injuries. Approximately 373,000 children are treated in hospital EDs for bicycle-related injuries each year in the United States. More than 40% of all bicycle-related deaths are due to head injuries with the largest percentage among children under the age of 14. Other injuries associated with bicycle crashes are long bone fractures and abdominal, thoracic, and facial injuries. Wearing a bicycle helmet can reduce the likelihood of head injury by 85% and brain injury by 88%. Universal use of bicycle helmets by children ages 4 to 15 would prevent between 135 and 155 deaths, between 39,000 and 45,000 head injuries, and between 18,000 and 55,000 scalp and facial injuries annually. Helmet use significantly reduces morbidity and mortality associated with bicycle-related head injuries. Primary and secondary prevention are equally important in the use of helmets among children. Children who present following a minor injury provide an opportunity for educating the child and family on the importance of proper helmet use.[18]

Children can sustain injuries from skateboards and scooters. Children have a high center of gravity, which limits their ability to break a fall. The American Academy of Pediatrics recommends that children under the age of 10 years should not use skateboards without close supervision by an adult or responsible adolescent. Children younger than 5 years should not use skateboards.[34] These children do not have a well-developed neuromuscular system, do not have good judgment, and cannot protect themselves from injury. Skateboards should not be ridden in traffic. Proper protective wear, including helmets, elbow pads, and knee pads, should be worn. Skateboard-related injuries account for an estimated 50,000 ED visits and 1500 hospitalizations each year. Nonpowered scooter–related injuries accounted for an estimated 9400 ED visits; 90% of these were for children under the age of 15 years.[34] Proper protective gear for scooter safety includes a helmet, knee pads, and elbow pads; wrist guards are not recommended because they make it difficult to grip the handle and steer the scooter. Children less than 8 years of age should not use scooters without close adult supervision. Children should not ride scooters in streets, in traffic, or at night.[34]

Drowning and near-drowning injuries resulted in 1178 deaths for all ages in 2002.[21] In 2003 approximately 4200 children ages 14 and under were treated in EDs for accidental drowning incidents. Bathtub drowning is most common in children younger than 1 year of age. In the preschool-age child, drowning occurs most commonly in residential swimming pools. Young adults typically drown in ponds, lakes, rivers, and oceans. Alcohol use has been involved with 25% to 50% of adolescent drownings associated with water recreation.[23] Children should never be unsupervised when in or around water.

ANATOMY AND PHYSIOLOGY

Children differ from adults developmentally, anatomically, and physiologically. Recognizing differences and implementing appropriate interventions to support these differences can result in increased survivability of the pediatric trauma patient.

Respiratory System

Crucial anatomic and physiologic differences exist between the adult and pediatric airway. The child's oropharynx is relatively small; therefore the airway is easily obstructed by the large tongue. The U-shaped epiglottis protrudes into the pharynx, with the tonsils and adenoids often enlarged. Vocal cords are short and concave, with the larynx relatively cephalad and easily collapsible if the neck is hyperflexed or extended. In a child younger than 10 years of age, the narrowest portion of the airway is the cricoid cartilage.[28] Lower airways are smaller and supporting cartilage less developed in infants and small children, so airways are easily obstructed by mucus and edema.[28]

Ribs are pliable and do not provide adequate protection and support for the lungs; therefore blunt trauma to the chest causes pulmonary contusions rather than rib fractures. If rib fractures are present, a high index of suspicion for severe internal trauma should be raised. The mediastinum is more mobile, causing greater susceptibility to great-vessel damage. Retractions are more likely when the child is in respiratory distress. These can be suprasternal, supraclavicular, infraclavicular, intercostal, or substernal. Breathing is primarily diaphragmatic or abdominal in children younger than 7 or 8 years of age. Crying children are more prone to swallowing air, which causes gastric distension and hampers respiratory excursion. A thin chest wall transmits breath sounds easily from one location or side of the thorax to another, which can make an accurate respiratory assessment difficult; it is challenging to detect the presence of a pneumothorax by auscultation alone in younger children. Respiratory rates are higher in children because of higher metabolic rates. Oxygen consumption in infants is 6 to 8 mL/kg/min compared with 3 to 4 mL/kg/min in adults; therefore hypoxemia can occur rapidly.[28]

Cardiovascular System

The child's estimated blood volume is 80 mL/kg. Although this absolute blood volume is small, it is larger than an adult's on a milliliter per kilogram basis. Seemingly small amounts of blood loss can impair perfusion and decrease circulating blood volume. Because of their large cardiac reserve and catecholamine response, children can maintain a high to normal blood pressure even with significant blood loss. Hypotension is not observed until the child has lost 20% to 25% of circulating blood volume.[28] Hypotension is a late sign of hypovolemia in children and signals imminent cardiac arrest. The best assessment of perfusion is skin parameters (color, temperature, moisture) and capillary refill—normal is 2 seconds or less on all four extremities and checked at frequent intervals. Other assessment factors include the presence of bradycardia or tachycardia with decreased urinary output.

Children have a higher metabolic rate and oxygen requirement that requires a higher cardiac output per kilogram.[28]

Tachycardia is the initial response to decreased oxygenation. When tachycardia fails to increase oxygen delivery, tissue hypoxia and hypercapnia occur, followed by bradycardia.[28] Bradycardia is a late sign of cardiac decompensation.

Children can present with a variety of congenital heart defects (e.g., tetralogy of Fallot, large ventricular septal defect) that may impair circulatory status. If a child has had a shunting surgical procedure to redirect blood flow, blood pressure readings are unattainable in the arm from which the subclavian artery was used because that arm is perfused by collateral circulation. Children may also have functional or nonfunctional heart murmurs. Children with congenital heart defects may also experience heart failure and dysrhythmias.

Neurologic System

An infant's head is larger in proportion to the rest of the body than an adult's. The skull is more malleable, providing less protection to the brain. The posterior fontanel closes at age 4 months; the anterior fontanel is normally closed by age 18 months. Although open fontanels allow for release of increased intracranial pressure (ICP), they may allow direct injury to the brain or cause extensive bleeding. Infants bleed significantly from a scalp laceration because of the large surface area and increased vascularity. Finally, a young child has a higher center of gravity, which, together with the larger head, makes the child prone to head injuries.

Children's cerebral tissues are thin, soft, and flexible compared with those of adults. Sulci are still deepening during childhood, and myelinization is still occurring. These differences make brain tissues more easily damaged, especially from shearing injuries. Several features make the cervical spine vulnerable to injury in children younger than 9 years of age[12]:

- The head is disproportionately large, making the child vulnerable to flexion-extension injury.
- The neck muscles are underdeveloped.
- The vertebral bodies are wedge shaped.
- The articulating facets are angled horizontally, resulting in subluxation from minimal force.
- The end plates are cartilaginous.
- The interspinous ligaments are elastic and lax, leading to increased spinal mobility.

Gastrointestinal and Genitourinary Systems

Young children have protuberant abdomens as a result of underdeveloped abdominal musculature.[29] Because solid abdominal organs are relatively larger in children compared with adults, there is an increased risk for direct organ injury following blunt and penetrating kinetic forces.[29] A pliable rib cage does not afford adequate protection to abdominal organs and can predispose children to further internal injuries. The large size of the organs in a relatively small space predisposes children to have multiple organ injury with trauma. Though partially protected by the flexible rib cage, the liver is still vulnerable to injury because of its large size and fragility.

The transverse diameter of the abdomen is small, and lower abdominal organs are not well protected by the pelvis.[25] Renal injuries occur because the relatively large kidneys are not protected by the small amount of perinephric fat, weak abdominal muscles, and elastic rib cage. The kidneys also retain fetal lobulations, which may predispose these organs to separation and fracture.[29] Congenital abnormalities such as hydronephrosis, horseshoe kidneys, and ectopic kidneys make the child more susceptible to renal trauma. Many congenital anomalies are not diagnosed until abdominal trauma has occurred. Greater elasticity makes ureteral tearing rare. Ureteral injuries are suspected with penetrating trauma to the abdomen or flank area. The bladder is an abdominal organ and not well protected. In girls the bladder neck is also less protected. Tissues of a prepubescent girl are more rigid because of a lack of estrogen; they do not become more pliable until adolescence, when estrogen is released.

Musculoskeletal System

The periosteum in a growing child is stronger, thicker, and more osteogenic compared with the periosteum in an adult, which results in decreased fracture displacement and fewer open fractures.[21] Consequently, four unique bone fracture patterns are found in children: plastic deformity (the bone is deformed but not broken); torus (buckle) fracture (compression forces applied at the metaphysis and diaphysis cause bone to buckle rather than break because of its porous nature); greenstick fracture (an incomplete fracture in which the compressed side's cortex and periosteum are intact); and physis fractures (injury to the growth plate, which can lead to angulation deformities if not diagnosed and treated properly).[21] Bone osteogenicity allows rapid callus formation, permitting bones to heal quickly. Even though bone is strong, fractures occur more frequently than muscle sprains or ligament tears because these structures are stronger than the bones themselves.

Another unique feature of the pediatric musculoskeletal system is the presence of a physis or growth plate. This area of bone, which is responsible for longitudinal bone growth, is found between the epiphysis and metaphysis. The physis is cartilaginous and does not ossify until puberty; therefore treatment to attain proper anatomic alignment is critical to optimize bone growth and reduce the risk for deformity.[21]

Integumentary System

Children have a larger ratio of body surface area to weight, which makes them prone to convective and conductive heat loss. Having less subcutaneous fat for insulation can increase heat loss through radiation, convection, conduction, and evaporation. Infants younger than 6 months of age do not have the fine-motor coordination to shiver and are unable to keep themselves warm. Nonshivering thermogenesis does occur in infants, in which brown fat is broken down slowly to produce warmth. Shivering is a high-energy-consuming, nonproductive muscular activity initiated for thermogenesis.[7]

Shivering may not be possible in injured children receiving sedation or neuromuscular blocking agents.[7]

PATIENT ASSESSMENT

Each ED should be equipped with personnel and supplies necessary to treat an injured child effectively and efficiently. Equipment should be readily available and prepared before patient arrival.

Initial assessment and stabilization of the pediatric trauma patient requires knowledge of developmental and physiologic differences among infants, children, and adolescents. Injured children are frightened—strange, painful things are happening. The patient may feel he or she is being punished for a real or imagined wrongdoing. Talking with the child in language he or she understands is essential for relieving anxiety and developing trust.

Initial assessment consists of a primary and secondary assessment. During primary assessment, airway with cervical spine protection, breathing, circulation, and disability (neurologic status) are assessed. Life-threatening injuries are identified and treated. Table 28-1 describes the primary survey in the preferred order. During secondary assessment, all other body systems are assessed and other injuries are treated. Table 28-2 details the secondary survey. Throughout the initial assessment and stabilization, airway, breathing, and circulation are continually reassessed.

Initial Stabilization

Airway/Cervical Spine

The tongue is the most common cause of airway obstruction in the child. Opening the airway with the jaw-thrust technique to prevent hyperextension of the cervical spine is the initial step in relieving airway obstruction. Suction the oropharynx with a tonsil suction device if vomitus, blood, or loose teeth are present.

Place an oropharyngeal airway to help maintain airway patency in the child with altered level of consciousness who does not have an intact gag reflex. Oropharyngeal airways are measured from the corner of the mouth to the tragus of the ear. An oropharyngeal airway that is too small or too large will obstruct the airway, so correct size is critical. Use a tongue depressor to insert the airway directly. Do not rotate 90 degrees as in the adult patient because a child's oropharyngeal tissues can be damaged and the tongue inadvertently pushed posteriorly, causing obstruction. A nasopharyngeal airway may be used for airway patency if there is no evidence of head and midface trauma. This airway is measured from the nares to the tragus of the ear.

In a child who requires continuous airway maintenance, endotracheal intubation using rapid-sequence induction (RSI) is necessary. RSI is "a technique in which a potent sedative or induction agent is administered virtually simultaneously with a paralyzing dose of a neuromuscular blocking agent to facilitate rapid tracheal intubation."[9] This procedure must be undertaken by a health care professional skilled in pediatric intubation. The orotracheal route is preferred because the nasotracheal route can be difficult or contraindicated in severe facial trauma or basilar skull fracture.

Before the intubation attempt, cardiac and pulse oximetry monitoring devices are placed on the child. Sedating medications followed by paralyzing agents are administered while the child's lungs are ventilated with 100% oxygen. After the trachea is intubated, observe for rise and fall of the chest, auscultate breath sounds bilaterally in the midaxillary line, then over the epigastrium; listen high in the axilla because breath sounds are easily transmittable across the thin chest wall. Right mainstem bronchus intubations are a common complication with pediatric intubation; therefore bilateral chest

Table 28-1.	PRIMARY SURVEY OF THE PEDIATRIC TRAUMA PATIENT
Component	**Actions**
Airway	Assess for patency; look for loose teeth, vomitus, or other obstruction; note position of head.
	Suspect cervical spine injury with multiple trauma; maintain neutral alignment during assessment; evaluate effectiveness of cervical collar, cervical immobilization device, or other equipment used to immobilize the spine.
	Open cervical collar to evaluate neck for jugular vein distension and tracheal deviation.
Breathing	Auscultate breath sounds in the axillae for presence and equality.
	Assess chest for contusions, penetrating wounds, abrasions, or paradoxical movement.
Circulation	Assess apical pulse for rate, rhythm, and quality; compare apical and peripheral pulses for quality and equality.
	Evaluate capillary refill; normal is 2 seconds or less.
	Check skin color and temperature.
Disability	Assess level of consciousness; check for orientation to person, place, and time in the older child.
	In a younger child, assess alertness, ability to interact with environment, and ability to follow commands. Is the child easily consoled and interested in the environment? Does the child recognize a familiar object and respond when you speak to him or her?
	Check pupils for size, shape, reactivity, and equality.
	Remove clothing to allow visual inspection of entire body.
Expose	Note open wounds or uncontrolled bleeding.

wall movement should be observed during ventilation with a bag-mask device. Movement is best assessed by standing at the foot of the bed and watching the chest rise and fall during ventilation. Correct endotracheal tube placement is determined through auscultation of equal, bilateral breath sounds in all fields; observation of condensation in the endotracheal tube; and assessment of end-tidal carbon dioxide measurements with pediatric-specific equipment, while evaluating the child's response. Final confirmation is made by chest radiograph. The tube must be secured with commercially available holders, tape, or ties and the measurement of the tube at the lip line documented. The tube should not press on the corner of the mouth (nares with nasotracheal intubation) because of the potential for tissue breakdown. Frequent suctioning may be necessary if aspiration is suspected or injury to the airway or lung tissue has occurred.

Children are diaphragmatic breathers, so compression on the diaphragm impedes lung expansion. A gastric tube is inserted to relieve gastric distension. The preferred method is to insert the tube orally. The tube should not be inserted nasally if the child has obvious facial trauma or signs of a basilar skull fracture. After the tube is inserted, it is taped to the child's face and connected to low intermittent suction.

Cricothyrotomy and tracheostomy are reserved for severe cases of airway instability from facial, head, and neck trauma. Fortunately, these procedures are rarely required in children.

Strategies to protect the cervical spine in the multiply injured child include application of a rigid cervical collar and cervical immobilization devices. Care must be taken to prevent cervical spine flexion from the cervical collar or backboard (Figure 28-1). Movement can worsen spinal cord injury (SCI) and compromise the airway. Spinal protection is maintained until radiographic and clinical evidence demonstrate that SCI is not present.

Use of an appropriately sized cervical collar is essential to prevent SCI and airway compromise. A collar that is too large pushes the jaw backward, causes airway obstruction,

Table 28-2. SECONDARY SURVEY OF THE PEDIATRIC TRAUMA PATIENT	
Component	**Actions**
Head, eye, ear, nose	Assess scalp for lacerations or open wounds; palpate for step-off defects, depressions, hematomas, and pain.
	Reassess pupils for size, reactivity, equality, and extraocular movements; ask the child if he or she can see.
	Assess nose and ears for rhinorrhea or otorrhea.
	Observe for raccoon eyes (bruising around the eyes) or Battle's sign (bruising over the mastoid process).
	Palpate forehead, orbits, maxilla, and mandible for crepitus, deformities, step-off defect, pain, and stability; evaluate malocclusion by asking child to open and close mouth; note open wounds.
	Inspect for loose, broken, or chipped teeth as well as oral lacerations.
	Check orthodontic appliances for stability.
	Evaluate facial symmetry by asking child to smile, grimace, and open and close mouth.
	Do not remove impaled objects or foreign objects.
Neck	Open cervical collar, and reassess anterior neck for jugular vein distension and tracheal deviation; note bruising, edema, open wounds, pain, and crepitus.
	Check for hoarseness or changes in voice by asking child to speak.
Chest	Obtain respiratory rate; reassess breath sounds in anterior lobes for equality.
	Palpate chest wall and sternum for pain, tenderness, and crepitus.
	Observe inspiration and expiration for symmetry or paradoxical movement; note use of accessory muscles.
	Reassess apical heart rate for rate, rhythm, and clarity.
Abdomen/pelvis/genitourinary	Observe abdomen for bruising and distension; auscultate bowel sounds briefly in all four quadrants; palpate abdomen gently for tenderness; assess pelvis for tenderness and stability.
	Palpate bladder for distension and tenderness; check urinary meatus for signs of injury or bleeding; note priapism and genital trauma such as lacerations or foreign body.
	Have rectal sphincter tone assessed, usually by physician.
Musculoskeletal	Assess extremities for deformities, swelling, lacerations, or other injuries.
	Palpate distal pulses for equality, rate, and rhythm; compare to central pulses.
	Ask child to wiggle toes and fingers; evaluate strength through hand grips and foot flexion/extension.
Back	Logroll as a unit to inspect back; maintain spinal alignment during examination; observe for bruising and open wounds; palpate each vertebral body for tenderness, pain, deformity, and stability; assess flank area for bruising and tenderness.

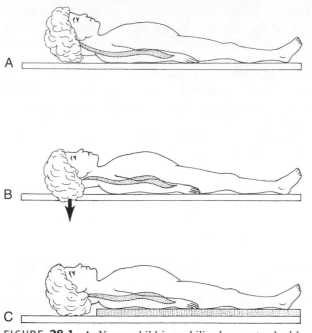

FIGURE **28-1. A,** Young child immobilized on a standard backboard; note how the large head forces the neck into flexion. Backboards can be modified by an occiput cutout (**B**) or a double mattress pad (**C**) to raise the chest. (From Roberts JR, Hedges JR: *Clinical procedures in emergency medicine,* ed 4, Philadelphia, 2004, WB Saunders.)

and allows the child to move the head from side to side, which prevents cervical spine control. A collar that is too small does not provide appropriate alignment and may cause airway compromise from constriction. A cervical collar fits properly if the chin rests securely in the chin holder, the collar is beneath the ears, and the upper part of the sternum is not covered.

Infants and young children may arrive in the ED secured in their car safety seat. Children can initially remain in their car seats if there are no signs of distress and the car seat is intact.[11] Cervical protection with a collar, if possible, and towel rolls should be completed.[20] Although no evidence-based guidelines indicate that car seat immobilization is effective, it may be an option for emergency medical services personnel to transport stable, injured children.[11]

Cervical spine radiographs from C1 through T1 are obtained in the anterior-posterior and lateral views to evaluate for vertebral fractures. The radiograph is assessed for vertebral symmetry, alignment, and spacing. Spinal protection can be discontinued if there is no radiographic evidence of cervical spine injury and the child has normal neurologic findings.

Breathing

Supplemental oxygen is administered to any child with multiple trauma. First, auscultate breath sounds at the mid-axillary line. The child breathing spontaneously with effective air exchange can receive humidified oxygen via nasal cannula, partial nonrebreather face mask, or nonrebreather face mask.

Flow rate for a nasal cannula should be no more than 6 L/min of oxygen; higher flow rates will irritate the nasopharynx. A nasal cannula is used in children with minimal oxygen requirements. With infants and young children, it is important to secure the cannula in the nares and then initiate oxygen flow. (Remember that oxygen flow may frighten the child.) The final oxygen delivery to the patient is usually 30% to 40% through a nasal cannula.[24] A partial rebreathing mask set at a flow rate of 10 to 12 L/min delivers an inspired oxygen concentration of 50% to 60%. Blow-by oxygen can be used for children who do not tolerate the cannula or mask.

Nonrebreather oxygen masks are used for a child with greater oxygen requirements; flow rate is set at 10 to 12 L/min. A properly fitting face mask fits snugly on the face, covering nose and mouth without covering eyes or cheeks. In the child who is not breathing spontaneously or effectively, ventilations are assisted with a bag-mask device set at 15 L/min, which allows oxygen delivery up to 90%.[24] A bag-mask device needs to be self-inflating, in case there is no oxygen source available. Bag-mask devices are equipped with pop-off valves to avoid delivery of high pressures while bagging the patient.[24] When ventilations are assisted with a bag-mask device, the bag is squeezed until enough air volume is delivered to allow easy rise and fall of the chest. Care must be taken not to ventilate with extreme force because pneumothorax can occur.

A pulse oximeter sensor is applied to the child's finger, earlobe, or toe to determine oxygen saturation. Pulse oximetry readings should be 95% or more (at sea level).

Circulation

To assess adequacy of circulation, palpate central versus peripheral pulses for quality, and assess capillary refill and skin temperature. Continuous cardiopulmonary and blood pressure monitoring devices are connected to the child immediately in a trauma situation. Vital signs should be measured every 5 minutes until the child's condition stabilizes. Blood pressure readings should be evaluated against other vital signs. A properly fitting blood pressure cuff fits two thirds of the upper arm. A cuff that is too small gives false-high readings, whereas a cuff that is too large gives false-low readings.

It is important to apply direct pressure to open, bleeding wounds. Tourniquets are not recommended because direct tissue damage may occur.

Two large-bore intravenous (IV) catheters are inserted, preferably in the antecubital fossae, for venous access and fluid replacement. Catheter size is determined by the size of the child's veins. If peripheral venous access is not readily available, the intraosseous route should be used.[28] Central venous access through the jugular, subclavian, or femoral vein may be obtained by an experienced practitioner. It is important to obtain blood for laboratory analysis and initiate crystalloid fluid replacement. Central venous pressure monitoring or arterial pressure monitoring is reserved for severely injured children and should be performed only under controlled circumstances by experienced providers.

Hypovolemic shock is suspected in the child with tachypnea, tachycardia, decreased level of consciousness, decreased urinary output, and prolonged capillary refill. Isotonic crystalloid fluid bolus of 20 mL/kg normal saline or lactated Ringer's solution should be administered rapidly, with effectiveness determined by reassessment. Stopcocks connected to IV tubing allow easy administration of fluid boluses. If there is no improvement, a second bolus can be administered followed by a third bolus. Warmed O-negative blood may be given at 10 mL/kg if there is no improvement after two to three fluid boluses.[28] Excessive fluid administration in the child with a head injury may increase ICP; therefore strict intake and output of trauma patients should be documented.

Routine blood tests include complete blood count (CBC) and differential, electrolytes, blood urea nitrogen, creatinine, glucose, venous blood gas, type and screen, prothrombin time, partial thromboplastin times, and less frequently toxicology screening. If abdominal trauma is suspected, amylase, lipase, and liver enzymes may be obtained. In suspected cardiac or muscle damage, creatine phosphokinase levels are also obtained. Urine may be sent for complete urinalysis and toxicology testing. Pregnancy testing should be considered in the postmenarcheal female.

Pneumatic antishock garments are not routinely used in pediatric trauma but can be used as a splint for pelvic fractures or femur fractures when other forms of splinting are not available.

An indwelling urinary catheter is placed if there is no sign of genitourinary trauma (i.e., no blood at the meatus). A urimeter on the urine collection bag allows monitoring of hourly urinary output. Decreased output can indicate hypovolemic shock. Hematuria suggests genitourinary trauma; however, the first urine specimen may test negative for blood because of urine in the bladder before injury. Therefore a subsequent urine specimen may be necessary. Normal urinary output for infants and children should be 2 mL/kg/hr; for older children and adolescents, 1 mL/kg/hr is optimal.[28]

Children may arrive in the ED following a traumatic arrest. Children with traumatic injuries who are found to be asystolic or hypotensive by prehospital personnel have a poor prognosis. If the patient survives to hospital discharge, there are almost always neurologic side effects.[3]

Disability

Serial neurologic assessments are necessary to identify changes in mental status. Changes in level of consciousness can indicate hypovolemia or increased ICP. Early signs of increased ICP are vomiting and irritability. In infants, a bulging fontanel is a late sign of increasing ICP. Another important assessment finding during disability is the pupil examination. Check pupils for symmetry, size, reactivity, and shape.

In older children the first sign of increased ICP is disorientation to time, place, and familiar people, then to self. This description is not applicable to the younger child, who has no concept of time or place. The Glasgow Coma Scale

(GCS) can be slightly modified for children (Table 28-3). Children as young as 3 months old should recognize their parents/caregivers; toddlers should know the names of their pets and may also recognize popular cartoon or television characters or favorite toys.

In a child with severe head trauma, ventilation with 100% oxygen is initiated. Mannitol may be administered at 0.5 to 1 g/kg to decrease cerebral swelling; controlled hyperventilation may be employed to maintain arterial carbon dioxide pressure ($PaCO_2$) between 30 and 35 mm Hg if herniation is impending.[15]

Exposure/Environmental Control

The child's temperature is recorded initially and monitored throughout initial stabilization to detect and treat hypothermia. Common temperature measurement routes are tympanic, temporal artery, oral, rectal, and bladder. Factors to consider when selecting a route for temperature measurement in pediatric trauma patients include safety, accuracy, and compliance.

Numerous factors during the child's initial ED care increase the risk for hypothermia, including transfusion of large amounts of unwarmed IV fluids or blood products[26]; clothing removal during assessment and treatment; large, open wounds; neurologic or multisystem injuries; administration of paralytic or sedative agents; and treatment in cold trauma rooms and diagnostic suites. Therefore measures to prevent heat loss and promote thermoregulation should be initiated. Passive warming measures include increasing ambient temperature by using overhead lights and applying warm blankets. Active warming measures include administering warmed IV fluids and blood products. In a study of eight injured children randomized to receive either warmed IV fluids or a convective warming blanket, there was no statistically significant difference in temperatures for either group on ED discharge—all patients maintained body temperature in the normothermic range.[5] No evidence-based practice is defined for nursing interventions to prevent heat loss in injured children during initial ED treatment. Further, measures effective in adults cannot be extrapolated for application in injured children.[6]

Full Set of Vital Signs

Vital signs (temperature, heart rate, respiratory rate, blood pressure) are measured on ED arrival and throughout initial ED treatment. Vital signs should be measured continuously and recorded every 5 minutes in unstable patients and every 15 minutes in stable patients. Documenting patient care on a trauma flow sheet allows visual inspection of trends in patient vital signs and permits rapid interventions as needed. Weight should be determined through actual measurement or by estimation with a length-based resuscitation tape (Figure 28-2).

Family Presence

The presence of a supportive parent does wonders for a frightened child. Allow parents to see the child as soon as possible after stabilization is complete. Explain to the parents beforehand what they will see and why because this allows

Table 28-3.   PEDIATRIC MODIFICATION OF GLASGOW COMA SCALE

GCS Score		Pediatric Modification
EYE OPENING		
≥1 year	**0-1 year**	
4 Spontaneously	4 Spontaneously	
3 To verbal command	3 To shout	
2 To pain	2 To pain	
1 No response	1 No response	
BEST MOTOR RESPONSE		
≥1 year	**0-1 year**	
6 Obeys		
5 Localizes pain	5 Localizes pain	
4 Flexion—withdrawal	4 Flexion—withdrawal	
3 Flexion—abnormal (decorticate rigidity	3 Flexion—abnormal (decorticate rigidity	
2 Extension (decerebrate rigidity)	2 Extension (decerebrate rigidity)	
1 No response	1 No response	
BEST VERBAL RESPONSE		
0-2 years	**2-5 years**	**>5 years**
5 Cries appropriately, smiles, coos	5 Appropriate words and phrases	5 Oriented and converses
4 Cries	4 Inappropriate words	4 Disoriented and converses
3 Inappropriate crying/screaming	3 Cries/screams	3 Inappropriate words
2 Grunts	2 Grunts	2 Incomprehensible sounds
1 No response	1 No response	1 No response

From Barkin RM, Rosen P: *Emergency pediatrics: a guide to ambulatory care,* ed 6, St. Louis, 2003, Mosby.
*Score is the sum of the individual scores from eye opening, best verbal response, and best motor response, using age-specific criteria. GCS score of 13-15 indicates mild head injury. GCS score of 9-12 indicates moderate head injury, and GCS score of ≤8 indicates severe head injury.

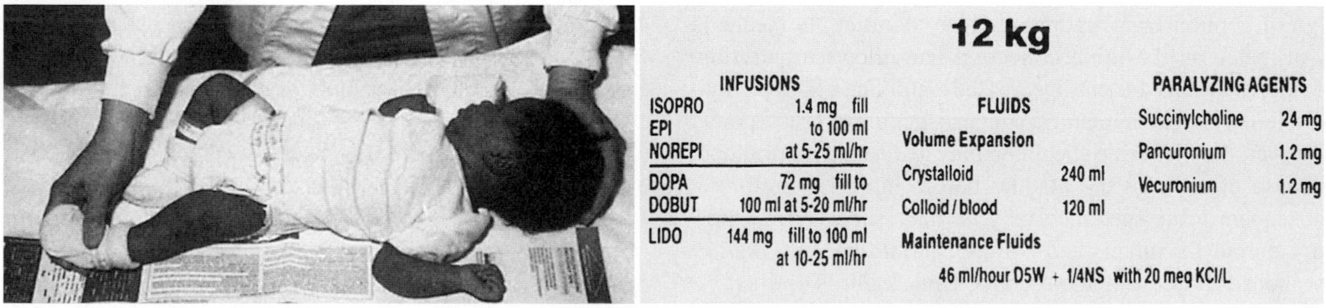

12 kg

INFUSIONS		FLUIDS		PARALYZING AGENTS	
ISOPRO	1.4 mg fill			Succinylcholine	24 mg
EPI	to 100 ml	Volume Expansion		Pancuronium	1.2 mg
NOREPI	at 5-25 ml/hr			Vecuronium	1.2 mg
DOPA	72 mg fill to	Crystalloid	240 ml		
DOBUT	100 ml at 5-20 ml/hr	Colloid / blood	120 ml		
LIDO	144 mg fill to 100 ml	Maintenance Fluids			
	at 10-25 ml/hr	46 ml/hour D5W + 1/4NS with 20 meq KCl/L			

FIGURE **28-2.** The Broselow tape can be used as a rapid method for generating drug and fluid doses, as well as endotracheal tube and suction catheter sizes. The tape uses the principle that length correlates with body surface area and weight. The patient is measured with the tape in the supine position, and the line on which the foot of the patient reaches contains the precalculated drug doses and equipment sizes appropriate for the patient. (From Barkin R et al: *Pediatric emergency nursing,* ed 2, St. Louis, 1997, Mosby.)

them to look at the child and not become overwhelmed with the medical equipment involved in the care of their child. Parents may believe they need permission to touch or talk to their child, so encourage them to do so.

Controversy exists as to whether parents should be present during resuscitation. If parents are present, a designated support person must stay with them and explain what is happening to their child. The Emergency Nurses Association advocates parental presence during resuscitation. Such presence may be beneficial to the child and the family members. A designated emergency nurse or social worker can stay with the family and explain treatment that is taking place.

While parents are waiting to see their child, a social worker, emergency nurse, or designated patient advocate should keep them apprised of the situation and serve as a support person. If the decision is made to transfer the child to another facility, parents should see their child before departure. If the child dies before parents arrive at the accepting institution, they may feel guilty because they were not able to see the child or agreed to have their child transferred elsewhere. When the child leaves, say "Mommy will see you later" rather than "goodbye" because "goodbye" implies that they may never see each other again. Most flight programs have policies in place for transport of a family member with a patient. Many factors influence the decision to have a parent or other family member accompany a child in a helicopter, so the decision to do so ultimately rests with the pilot and flight crew and should be respected.[13]

Give Comfort Measures

The injured child has a number of fears—mutilation, losing control, getting in trouble with his or her parents for engaging in a forbidden activity, death, disfigurement, and pain. It is the responsibility of the emergency nurse to help the child cope effectively with these fears during trauma resuscitation. Children who are hearing impaired or require a translator should have an interpreter other than a family member present during the examination.

Assign one nurse as the child's support person. While the child remains in cervical protection, the nurse should stand at the child's side and down from his or her face, about chest level, so the child is able to see the person. Standing directly over the child's face is frightening, especially when different faces keep appearing and reappearing. Hold the child's hand or stroke his or her hair to provide tactile comfort. Talk softly and slowly, using words he or she can understand (e.g., "The doctor is going to listen to your heartbeat," "You will feel a pinch in your right arm. You can scream, but you must keep your right arm still."). Avoid words such as "take" or "cut out" because they imply mutilation. Use words such as "make it better." If the child requires general anesthesia, avoid telling the child he or she will "be put to sleep." If the child had a pet that was "put to sleep," this statement may create death fears. Instead, tell the child he or she will get "special medicine to help you take a short nap." The child understands "nap" is a short time. Tell the child what will happen before it happens. Children do not like surprises any more than adults do. Prepare them by using feeling terms, that is, "This will feel cold; this will feel heavy; this will smell sweet." If a procedure will hurt, tell the child. Lying will only cause him or her to mistrust you. A child life specialist is a professional trained to work with children in medical settings. They serve as a resource to help patients and families adjust and understand the hospital and medical situation.

Children cope in a variety of ways. Because young children are mobile, crying and kicking are ways for them to cope. Being restrained removes one of their coping mechanisms, which can increase their fear. School-age children and adolescents cope by seeking information; they may ask the same questions over and over again. Be patient. Scolding or threatening the child is fruitless and will only increase fear and resistance.

Severe injuries should be shielded from the child's visual field. Refrain from discussing the magnitude of an injury in the child's presence. It is not known if unconscious children remember discussions in their presence, so it is best to avoid talking about other family members or the child's condition in his or her presence. Talk to the child who is comatose or unresponsive just as if he or she were awake.

Pain management is of utmost importance when treating the injured child; however, it may be neglected. Recent requirements from The Joint Commission require that all patients receive pain assessment and appropriate pain-relief measures. The awake child may be able to use a pain scale to rate the pain. Various pain scales are available to measure pain in preverbal and verbal children. The appropriate pain scale should be used according to the age and development of the child. The most common pain scales are FACES, FLACC (face, legs, activity, cry, and consolability), and the number scale for older children. Analgesics may be administered after all injuries are identified and the child is determined to be physiologically and neurologically intact. Pharmacologic management of pain includes narcotic and nonnarcotic analgesics. Nonpharmacologic management of pain includes comfort measures such as distraction techniques, progressive relaxation, positive self-talk, and deep-breathing exercises. Allowing an infant to suck a pacifier promotes comfort, whereas allowing a toddler to hold a transitional object such as a blanket or toy promotes security. Reevaluation is necessary after any pain relief measures are initiated.

Head-to-Toe-Assessment

The secondary survey is outlined in Table 28-2. Each body area is inspected and palpated to identify signs of injury; auscultation is performed while assessing the chest and abdomen. In addition, frequent monitoring of the neurovascular status of an injured extremity is necessary to identify impairment of circulation or possible compartment syndrome. An injured extremity can be splinted for protection and comfort until definitive care is provided. After the extremity is splinted or casted, frequent reevaluation is necessary because edema may develop and impede circulation.

Inspect the Posterior Surface

The child is logrolled as a unit to inspect the posterior surface for contusions, abrasions, open wounds, and impaled objects; the spine and flank are palpated for tenderness and pain. The child is logrolled back into the supine position with spinal protection resumed or removed at that time.

History

History allows the trauma team to prepare for the patient and anticipate interventions that may be required. However, this information is not always available because the injury may not have been witnessed. The awake, nonverbal child cannot relate circumstances surrounding the injury. Such situations require special attention, because child neglect or abuse may be involved (see Chapter 48). In all injuries it is important to ascertain if loss of consciousness occurred.

The AMPLE mnemonic (Box 28-1) is helpful for organizing and obtaining an adequate patient history. This information may be obtained from the parent, family member, or an awake, older child or adolescent. In addition to this information, it is important to determine the need for vision or hearing aids, such as eyeglasses, contact lenses, or hearing aids. These may or may not be with the child on arrival.

Additional Interventions

Additional interventions undertaken during emergency management of the injured child include radiologic testing, medication administration, management of pain, and provision of emotional support.

RADIOLOGIC TESTING. Along with cervical spine radiographs, other radiographic testing may be undertaken relative to suspected injuries. A head computed tomography (CT) scan is indicated for a child with suspected brain injury, an abdominal CT scan may be indicated in a child with abdominal trauma, whereas chest, spine, and pelvis films may be indicated for the child with multiple injuries. Specific radiographs with views of injured extremities before definitive treatment is administered may also be performed. Radiographs may be obtained in the trauma room, or the child may be transported to the radiology department. A nurse should remain with the child to explain procedures and monitor the child's condition.

A CT scan of the abdomen and pelvis is performed as indicated and serves as the "gold standard" imaging technique to verify presence or absence of free fluid in the abdomen. The focused assessment sonography for trauma (FAST) examination currently cannot replace CT scanning in the pediatric patient.[21] Although detection of free fluid in the abdomen may be possible using sonography, additional research is needed to validate usefulness of this diagnostic tool in the initial care of children with abdominal injuries.

A CT scan is indicated in children with head, chest, spinal, or abdominal trauma. Mechanism of injury should also be used in determining the need for radiologic testing. In the absence of identifying injuries, type of injury should factor into the need for further studies. Again, a nurse must accompany the child for continuous monitoring. Appropriate equipment should be readily available in case there is a change in the child's status. Sedation may be required for stable children undergoing a CT scan of the head after head injury. Sedation practices vary widely among health care providers. Emergency nurses should follow hospital policies for sedation for all trauma patients undergoing diagnostic procedures.

MEDICATIONS. Antibiotics may be administered to the child with large, open contaminated wounds; open fractures; or arterial injury. Determine the child's immunization status to ensure appropriate tetanus prophylaxis. Children bitten by domestic or wild animals may require rabies prophylaxis, in which case local health department guidelines should be followed.

LABORATORY TESTING. Baseline tests are a routine component of the trauma evaluation. A type and screen, CBC, serum chemistries, and urinalysis are typically obtained, and liver function tests and pancreatic enzymes may be included for abdominal organ injuries.

SPECIFIC CONDITIONS
Traumatic Brain Injuries

Traumatic brain injury (TBI) is the leading cause of trauma-related death in children. The central nervous system is the most commonly injured isolated system and is the principal determinant of outcome. Head injuries, either alone or in association with multiple system injuries, are the most severe and cause the most deaths.[18] TBI often results from blunt trauma from MVCs, bicycle crashes, falls, and maltreatment. Children are susceptible to brain injury because of their larger head-to-body ratio, thin cranial bones, and less-myelinated brain. These factors leave the brain relatively unprotected and vulnerable to injury.[15] The thinner cranium allows injury forces to be transmitted directly to the brain itself.[15] Unmyelinated brain tissue in infants and young children appears to be more susceptible to shearing forces when compared with older children and adults.[15] Furthermore, cranial sutures remain open in early infancy, with the anterior fontanel open until 18 months. These features increase the child's susceptibility to head injury but also serve as an outlet for swollen cerebral tissues, allowing greater tolerance for increases in ICP.

When determining the severity of brain trauma, the GCS score is used to differentiate between mild, moderate, and severe injuries. A GCS score of 13 to 15 indicates mild head injury, GCS score of 9 to 12 indicates moderate head injury, and GCS score of less than 8 indicates severe head injury.[1] Mild to moderate head injuries are more common than severe head injuries.[15] Brain injuries are divided into primary and secondary injuries. Primary injury results from mechanical damage from traumatic forces applied to the brain where the brain contacts the interior skull or foreign bodies that cause direct brain injury.[15] Diffuse axonal injury, skull fractures, contusions, and hemorrhage can result. Secondary injury occurs from the resultant changes in the brain caused by the initial injury; for example, cerebral edema, hypoxia, ICP, and decreased cerebral blood flow.[15]

Mild to Moderate Traumatic Brain Injury

Mild to moderate TBI may cause persistent vomiting, post-traumatic seizure, and loss of consciousness. Persistent vomiting (over a few hours) warrants further observation and evaluation with possible hospital admission.[38] Children who experience posttraumatic seizures require a CT scan and hospital admission, especially children older than 5 years of age when seizures occur late after the injury, reoccur, persist, or if other symptoms suggest severe injury.[38] Loss of consciousness immediately after injury may not be known because no witnesses may have been present. The child may arrive in the ED awake and alert or unconscious. In either situation, further assessment and evaluation are warranted.

Children with mild to moderate TBI must receive serial neurologic evaluations to determine if ICP is increasing. Serial evaluations include measurement of level of consciousness, pupillary response, motor and sensory response, and vital signs. Making a game of assessment may elicit cooperation from the young, awake, and frightened child. Having the awake child touch the nose and move the heels down the shins tests cerebellar function, whereas having the child squeeze the nurse's fingers and "push on the gas pedal" tests motor strength. The awake infant and toddler should be able to focus on and reach for a toy or object. This child should recognize the parent and be easily consoled. Any changes in the child's level of consciousness should be reported immediately to avoid subsequent deterioration and possible brainstem herniation from increased ICP. The child should be evaluated for clinical signs of TBI, including hemotympanum, cerebrospinal fluid (CSF) otorrhea, CSF rhinorrhea, orbital bruising (raccoon eyes), or mastoid bruising (Battle's sign), that may indicate a basilar skull fracture.[38] Other clinical findings that may be evident are altered level of consciousness, altered pupillary responses, speech deficits, and sensory motor deficits.

A CT scan without contrast may be obtained if intracranial pathology is suspected. Skull radiographs may be obtained to detect location and extent of skull fractures in infants and young children. Toxicology screening is considered in children with altered level of consciousness. In general, children with mild to moderate TBI are admitted to the hospital for observation if they have any neurologic deficits, seizures, vomiting, severe headache, fever, prolonged loss of consciousness, skull fracture, altered level of consciousness, or suspected child maltreatment.[15]

Children with mild TBI may be discharged home if parents or guardians understand the required home care. Parents should be instructed to return to the ED if the child has persistent vomiting, changes in vision, unequal pupil size, persistent headache or drowsiness, changes in level of consciousness, unequal strength or gait, or seizures. Be sure parents understand the child may sleep and that sleeping is not an indication of a problem. They should be instructed to observe for nose or ear drainage on the pillow and to return to the ED if this is observed. Acetaminophen may be administered for headache.

Infants with skull fractures may be admitted for 24-hour observation. Among 101 infants hospitalized with an isolated skull fracture, the median length of hospital stay was 1 day, with 88% (89) staying less than 24 hours.[16] Among this series of infants, neurologic symptoms and signs of head injury, such as loss of consciousness, vomiting, lethargy, irritability, focal neurologic abnormalities, and seizures, were not sensitive predictors of isolated skull fractures. However, physical examination revealed that the majority of these infants had local signs of injury at the fracture site location.[16] Infants with isolated skull fractures may not require hospitalization if they can be cared for by reliable parents, child maltreatment is not suspected, and neurologic symptoms are not present.[16]

Skull fractures that occur in one of the suture lines should create a high index of suspicion for epidural hematomas. A complication of these fractures is growth of the fracture. This expansion of the fracture is usually observed in infants and children younger than 3 years of age and is thought to result from cerebral tissue or arachnoid membrane herniation through a dural laceration[15] causing a pulsatile mass. Surgery may be indicated for these situations; therefore infants and young children with this type of fracture must receive follow-up treatment. Infants can sustain significant blood loss from scalp lacerations, so they require close observation for development of hypovolemic shock.

Severe Traumatic Brain Injury

Severe TBI is characterized by decreased level of consciousness, posturing, combative behavior, and abnormal neurologic findings. This catastrophic injury can be caused by severe shaking, falls, or MVCs.

In severe TBI the airway is secured using RSI and followed by controlled ventilation. A quick neurologic assessment should be completed before administering sedative and paralytic agents. Because carbon dioxide is a potent cerebral vasodilator, $PaCO_2$ should be maintained between 35 and 40 mm Hg to allow adequate cerebral blood flow.[15] Arterial oxygen saturation should be maintained at greater than 90% with mean arterial pressure slightly higher than age-appropriate norms. Current treatment of elevated ICP includes CSF drainage, sedation, neuromuscular blockade, mannitol, and hypertonic saline. The only recommended role for hyperventilation is in the setting of acute herniation, to briefly assist while definitive measures are being pursued.[34]

Laboratory analyses, including type and crossmatch, toxicologic testing, and clotting times (prothrombin time and partial thromboplastin time) should be performed in the event surgery is required. A CT scan without contrast is performed emergently as soon as the patient is stabilized to determine location and extent of the injury. Operative management may be indicated, followed by admission to an intensive care unit for ongoing nursing and medical care.

Generally children have better outcomes than adults after TBI, although the reasons are not clear. Neurologic deficits are the most common complications of TBI and are relative to the area of brain injury. For example, frontal brain injury results in cognitive deficits. Children may require rehabilitation for speech, motor, and cognitive improvements.

Maxillofacial Injuries

The incidence of maxillofacial injuries in children older than 5 years and younger than 16 years is estimated at 1% to 14% and 0.87% to 1% for children younger than 5 years of age.[17] MVCs account for the largest proportion of maxillofacial injuries.[17] The most frequently fractured facial area is the mandible, followed by the midface and upper face.[29]

One concern in the young pediatric population is damage to growing facial structures, such as incomplete calcification of bone or developing dentition, as well as injury to cartilaginous and soft tissue. Facial injuries are diagnosed by clinical assessment and confirmed by diagnostic tests such as CT scan. Plain or panoramic radiographs are not effective in detecting facial injuries[17] because of the aforementioned composition of facial structures.

Dental injuries are the most common orofacial injuries sustained during sports activities.[30] More than 5 million teeth are avulsed annually.[30] Avulsed primary teeth should not be replaced, but avulsed adult (permanent) teeth should be reimplanted within 2 hours (preferably 30 minutes).[17] The avulsed tooth should be handled by the crown and placed in milk, saline, or tooth preservative solution. Tissues attached to the teeth are left in place and not scrubbed away.[30] Consultation with a maxillofacial surgeon should be considered for children with severe facial injuries. It is important to pay close attention to potential airway compromise in patients with facial injuries.

Spinal Cord Injuries

SCIs are relatively uncommon in the pediatric population. When these injuries do occur, rapid acceleration-deceleration forces and hyperflexion-hyperextension forces are suspected. Children younger than 9 years of age are susceptible to cervical spine injuries because of their larger head size, weaker neck muscles and ligaments, and horizontal facets.[12] Laxity of the pediatric spine contributes to SCI without radiographic abnormality (SCIWORA). This phenomenon occurs because of inherent elasticity of the pediatric spine, shaping of vertebral bodies, and level of flexion in the cervical spine.[22] Hyperflexion or hyperextension of the spinal cord can lead to injury or transection. The spinal cord then returns to normal length and the vertebrae to normal alignment. The child may exhibit signs of SCI, such as numbness, tingling, or weakness; however, subsequent radiographs show no evidence of bony abnormality. Although SCIWORA is most often diagnosed at the cervical level, thoracic SCIWORA is also possible. The most common mechanism of injury for SCI in children is MVCs. The second most common cause in children less than 8 years of age is falls, whereas older children are more likely to sustain SCI from sports-related injuries.[22]

Signs and symptoms of SCI are the same in children as in adults. Numbness, tingling, weakness, and spasticity or flaccidity may be observed. The child may complain of pain in the back or neck with tenderness on palpation. Priapism suggests neurogenic shock. The awake child with an SCI may feel helpless and afraid, so continuous reassurance is essential. If the caregiver is present, the child's anxiety can be decreased by allowing the caregiver to stay close to the patient.

Spinal injuries should always be suspected in children with multiple injuries. Spinal protection is maintained until it is clinically determined that SCI is not present. Endotracheal intubation and mechanical ventilation are indicated in children with high cervical SCIs. Children with lower cervical injuries require close observation for changes in their respiratory status. IV fluids should be administered at one half to two thirds of maintenance requirements. The use of high-dose steroids continues to be a controversial treatment in SCI.[40] There is limited research in children younger than 13 years of age; however, they may benefit from this protocol.[40] If used, steroids are administered within 8 hours of injury: methylprednisolone 30 mg/kg IV is administered over 15 minutes followed by normal saline over the next 45 minutes; a continuous infusion of 5.4 mg/kg/hr is then run for 23 hours if the injury occurred within 8 hours. Lateral, anterior-posterior, and open mouth (odontoid) radiographic views of the cervical spine are obtained. Anterior-posterior views of the thoracic or lumbar spine are obtained as needed. Serial neurologic assessments are performed to identify changes in neurologic function such as level of sensation and movement resulting from increasing cord swelling.

Unconscious children with suspected SCI should remain in spinal protection until they are awake and able to complete a neurologic examination. Advanced diagnostic tests, such as magnetic resonance imaging and somatosensory evoked potentials, may be indicated to determine the presence or extent of SCI. Operative management may be needed for children with unstable vertebral fractures or dislocations.

Complications or sequelae of SCI range from mild neurologic deficits to complete hemiplegia, paraplegia, or quadriplegia. Autonomic areflexia, bowel and bladder incontinence, and ventilator dependence occur relative to the level of the cord lesion. Rehabilitation assists the child to maximize his or her potential for recovery.

Thoracic Injuries

Most thoracic injuries are caused by blunt trauma. With infants and young children these injuries are usually caused by falls, whereas older children sustain these injuries as pedestrians or passengers in motor vehicles. Penetrating chest trauma is seen in adolescents as a result of violence—intentional or self-inflicted. Common thoracic injuries in the pediatric population are pulmonary contusion, cardiac contusion, and pneumothorax.

Children are susceptible to transmission of blunt forces to underlying thoracic structures (heart, lungs, great vessels) because soft cartilage and developing bones make the thorax pliable.[19] Rib fractures should raise a high index of suspicion for severe blunt forces. Similarly, when flail segments are present, severe parenchymal pulmonary injury should be suspected.[19] The mediastinum is easily displaced by air or fluid. As the mediastinum shifts, venous return, cardiac output, and lung volume are severely compromised.[19]

Rib Fractures

Rib fractures are associated with chest pain, tenderness on palpation, and respiratory distress.[19] Flail segments lead to paradoxical chest wall movement during respiration. Changes in pulse oximetry and respiratory rate and effort may occur. Children should receive supplemental oxygen as needed and analgesics for pain relief. A chest radiograph is obtained to determine location and extent of fractures. Evaluate carefully for spleen or liver injury with lower rib fractures.

Pneumothorax and Hemothorax

Pneumothorax may be open, closed, or tension. Clinical signs and symptoms vary with severity of injury but can include respiratory distress, air hunger, decreased or absent breath sounds on the affected side, and anxiety. In a tension pneumothorax, the above symptoms are combined with hypotension and tracheal deviation (a late sign) away from the affected side; jugular vein distension may be observed, although this sign is difficult to detect in young children with short necks. Hemothorax from severe blunt or penetrating chest trauma is characterized by hypovolemic shock, decreased or absent breath sounds on the affected side, and respiratory distress.

Pneumothoraces are treated relative to severity. Chest radiographs confirm the presence of air in the pleural space but should not delay treatment in a symptomatic child. Children in no acute distress with a small pneumothorax receive supplemental oxygen and are observed for worsening symptoms. Large pneumothoraces/hemothoraces require chest tube placement, usually inserted at the fourth intercostal space midaxillary line, attached to water seal drainage and suction. In tension pneumothoraces, needle decompression is the immediate treatment: a large IV catheter is inserted into the second intercostal space, midclavicular line and left in place until a chest tube has been inserted. Needle decompression precedes chest radiograph because this situation is an immediate threat to life. After needle decompression, chest tubes are inserted and a chest radiograph is obtained. Similarly, in hemothoraces chest radiographs may be delayed until chest tubes are inserted. Autotransfusion should be considered for these patients when there are no contraindications; for example, enteric contamination or wound greater than 6 hours old. Surgical intervention is indicated with ongoing blood loss into the chest drainage system greater than 100 mL/hr or immediate blood loss greater than 20% of the child's estimated circulating blood volume.[19] Local anesthetic, and preferably sedatives, should be administered before insertion of chest tubes.

Pulmonary Contusion

Pulmonary contusions should be suspected in children with respiratory distress after blunt chest trauma without abnormal radiographic findings. Pulmonary contusion is usually not diagnosed until after hospital admission. Signs and symptoms include increasing respiratory distress, hemoptysis, and decreased pulmonary function. Chest radiographs show changes from the initial film. Management of these patients in the ED begins with supplemental oxygen. Endotracheal intubation and subsequent ventilation with positive end-expiratory pressure is usually reserved for severe injuries. Fluids may be limited if the child is not hypovolemic.

Tracheobronchial Injury

Tracheobronchial rupture, although rare, can occur with blunt or penetrating forces to the neck and chest. The child may have respiratory distress, subcutaneous emphysema, and cyanosis. Severe tracheobronchial rupture causes massive subcutaneous emphysema, persistent air leak, mediastinal air, tension pneumothorax, and failure of the lung to expand after chest tube insertion. Airway management with endotracheal intubation or tracheostomy is imperative. Chest tubes may also be required. Ongoing reassessment is essential in this fragile situation.[7]

Diaphragmatic Injury

Diaphragmatic rupture can occur after blunt trauma. In this case, diminished breath sounds are auscultated (usually on the left side), bowel sounds are heard within the chest cavity, or a scaphoid abdomen (Gibson's sign) is present.[29] Diaphragmatic rupture requires early identification, operative management, and repair—mortality increases with delayed identification and treatment.

Cardiac Injury

In general, cardiac injuries are suspected in children with chest bruising, upper body cyanosis, unexplained hypotension, and dysrhythmias. Injuries include cardiac tamponade, blunt cardiac injury (formerly termed cardiac contusion), and great vessel injuries. Management of cardiac injuries includes initial and ongoing evaluations of electrocardiograms, cardiac enzymes, and echocardiographic studies.

Abdominal Injuries

Blunt force is the most common cause of abdominal trauma in children, with subsequent hemorrhaging a common cause of traumatic death. Because of the child's smaller abdomen, injuries can occur to multiple organs. The spleen followed by the liver are the most commonly injured abdominal organs in blunt trauma,[21] whereas the stomach and intestines are the most commonly injured abdominal organs in penetrating trauma.[29] Trauma can result from pedestrian MVCs, falls or forces applied to the abdomen, bicycles, and child maltreatment. Penetrating abdominal trauma usually results from acts of violence. The lap belt complex—small bowel contusion/laceration, lumbar flexion-distraction injury (Chance fracture), and cutaneous bruising—may occur in restrained passengers in an MVC.

The alert child who sustains abdominal trauma may complain of tenderness with palpation. Deep palpation should be avoided to prevent guarding.[25] For young infants and toddlers, placing a warm hand on the abdomen for a few seconds before palpation may avoid startling or frightening the patient.[25] Abdominal distension, abrasions, or contusions may be noted. Hypovolemic shock suggests internal hemorrhaging. CT can identify injury to solid abdominal organs.

Children with blunt abdominal trauma are treated according to their hemodynamic stability. A gastric tube (nasogastric tubes should be avoided in the child with TBI) is inserted to decompress the stomach and avoid aspiration. Serial CBCs are obtained to monitor for ongoing blood loss. A CT scan with contrast is used to determine extent of the injuries in the hemodynamically stable child. This is preferred over diagnostic peritoneal lavage because of accuracy in detecting specific abdominal organ involvement and retroperitoneal injury. Many injuries are treated conservatively with serial reevaluation; however, surgical intervention is indicated for persistent hemorrhaging or peritonitis. The hemodynamically unstable child who does not respond to fluid and blood boluses must be prepared for immediate surgery.

Splenic injury is suspected in children with tenderness in the left upper quadrant. Pain in the left shoulder may be elicited with abdominal palpation (Kehr's sign). Splenic injury is suspected in children with altered level of consciousness, altered vital signs, low blood count, left lower rib fractures, abdominal pain, or grunting.[37] Children with splenic injuries who are hemodynamically stable are admitted to the hospital and managed with bed rest and serial reevaluation. Hemodynamically unstable patients (those who are hypotensive even with fluid and blood administration) require operative management.

Liver injuries are suspected in children who sustain any blunt force trauma to the abdomen. Right upper quadrant pain, tenderness, or diffuse pain are symptoms of liver injury.[29] Levels of serum aspartate aminotransferase (AST, formerly called SGOT) and serum alanine aminotransferase (ALT, formerly called SGPT) are obtained and evaluated, with a threshold of 200 units/L for each test indicative of hepatic injury.[25] Large liver lacerations cause significant blood loss and require immediate surgical repair, whereas smaller lacerations without signs of hypovolemia can be managed conservatively.

Pancreatic injuries cause abdominal pain that radiates to the back and persistent epigastric tenderness or vomiting; however, these injuries may not be noted until several days after injury.[25] Serum amylase and lipase levels are obtained, and the patient is hospitalized for further evaluation.

Intestinal injury is suspected in MVC passengers with abdominal bruising from the seat belt, bicycle riders who strike the handlebars, and those sustaining penetrating trauma.[29] Pain can be the only symptom, but free air may be noted on radiographs in some patients. These patients require a CT scan, hospitalization, and observation for possible intestinal perforation and subsequent surgical repair.[29] Intestinal perforation should be suspected in children with lap belt injuries. Symptoms include fever, increasing pain, hypotension, and peritoneal signs.[29]

All children who sustain high-velocity abdominal trauma (e.g., gunshot wounds) should undergo surgical exploration.[29] Children sustaining low-velocity injuries (e.g., stab wound to the anterior torso) and who are hemodynamically stable are hospitalized and observed.

Genitourinary Injuries

Genitourinary injuries result from pedestrian or passenger MVCs, sledding, sports activities, falls, and altercations. Bladder and urethral injuries result mostly from blunt trauma and are often associated with pelvic fractures. Blunt and penetrating injuries to the kidneys and ureters also occur. Renal injuries may be minor or so severe that surgical intervention is necessary.

Renal Injury

Renal injury should be considered in children who sustain fractures to the lower ribs or the transverse process of the vertebrae. In such cases, there may be direct flank trauma or rapid deceleration forces that crush the kidney against the rib cage or vertebral column.[29] Symptoms of renal trauma include abdominal, back, or flank tenderness. The awake, stable child may be able to provide a urine specimen by voiding spontaneously, or an indwelling bladder catheter can be inserted to measure urine output and obtain urine specimens for testing. A catheter should not be passed in suspected urethral trauma. Physical signs include localized abrasions or lacerations and hematuria. Hematuria is an important indicator of both severe and nonsevere renal injury, with the degree of hematuria correlating to a higher risk for renal injury.[29] Hematuria may also occur without substantial renal injury resulting from capillary disruption after blunt force trauma.[29] In the presence of gross hematuria, CT scan of the abdomen is indicated because there is an association between gross hematuria and severe intraabdominal injury.[29] Bedside urine screening may be performed to identify blood in the urine. Urinalysis testing with a threshold of more than 50 red blood cells (RBCs) per high-power field (hpf) indicates the need for further genitourinary tract evaluation; a threshold of more than 10 RBCs/hpf is used in children with high-risk injuries such as pelvic or proximal lower extremity fractures.[25]

A CT scan with contrast dye is usually obtained. Treatment is specialized relative to the type of injury and may range from observation and bed rest to surgical exploration for patients with pedicle injuries or renal pelvis rupture.[29]

Ureteral Injury

Ureteral injuries are rare, so recognition may be delayed unless the possibility for this injury is entertained. Hematuria or urinary leak may present as a flank mass; iliac pain may be present. Symptoms may not be noted until 7 to 10 days after the initial injury. Urine may appear at entrance or exit wounds or on a surgical dressing. If no wound is present, signs of retroperitoneal abscess such as chills, fever, lower abdominal pain, palpable mass, pyuria, and frequency may occur. Surgical repair is indicated for ureteral injuries, with a ureteral stent required in some patients.

Bladder Injury

Symptoms of bladder injuries vary with sustained injury. Suprapubic tenderness, urgency to void, inability to void, hematuria, and palpable abdominal mass may be observed with a ruptured bladder. Children with an extraperitoneal rupture may be able to pass small amounts of sanguineous urine but with significant discomfort. If severe hemorrhaging is present, signs of shock are observed. Most bladder contusions are minor and managed conservatively with observation and reevaluation. Large extraperitoneal injuries and intraperitoneal bladder ruptures with pelvic fractures necessitate surgical intervention for most patients.[29]

Urethral Injury

Urethral injury should be suspected in patients with vaginal bleeding; penile, scrotal, perineal, and prostate trauma; or the inability to advance an indwelling bladder catheter.[29] No attempt should be made to insert a urinary bladder catheter when there is blood at the meatus because the child may have a partial urethral tear. Inserting a catheter may convert a partial tear to a complete tear. Urethrography is indicated with cystography and CT cystography/CT scan of the abdomen and pelvis may be performed for some patients.[29] Partial urethral tears are managed conservatively with a suprapubic catheter or indwelling urethral catheter inserted under fluoroscopy. Complete urethral tears require surgical repair.

Genital Injuries

Injuries to female genitalia can result from falls, straddle type of injuries (e.g., falls on monkey bars, picket fences, or diving boards), and sexual abuse or assault. Testicular trauma can also result from straddle type of injuries. The most common cause of penile injuries is direct forces such as zipper injuries and trauma from toilet seats. Infants can sustain a tourniquet injury from threads, bands, rings, or human hair lodged in the coronal groove, which forms a constricting ring and lacerates the penile shaft. Sexual abuse must be considered in any child with genital trauma, particularly when injuries are inconsistent with the history. In children with suspected sexual abuse or assault, proper evidence collection is critical (see Chapter 48).

Musculoskeletal Injuries

Musculoskeletal injuries are common occurrences in the pediatric population. Long-bone fractures occur from falls, sports activities, and motor vehicle and pedestrian crashes.

Strong ligaments account for the prevalence of fractures rather than ligamentous injury.

The most unique feature of the child's musculoskeletal system is the epiphyseal growth plate (physis) located at the articulating ends of bones between the epiphysis and metaphysis. The epiphyseal growth plate is responsible for longitudinal bone growth; therefore injury can cause growth disturbance or arrest. In general, growth is completed in boys by age 16 years and in girls by 14 years of age. If a patient has a long-bone fracture, it is important to assess radiographs of the closest physis for concurrent injury.[20] Growth plate fractures are categorized with the Salter-Harris classification (Table 28-4).

Signs of musculoskeletal trauma include point tenderness, soft-tissue swelling, discoloration, limitations in range of motion, loss of function, altered sensory perception, and changes in pulses, temperature, or capillary refill distal to the injury.[2] An obvious deformity may be noted, or an actual open fracture may be observed. The child may complain of pain and splint the injured extremity by holding the broken arm with the other hand, for example.

Musculoskeletal trauma is rarely life threatening, so the child's airway, breathing, circulation, and neurologic status are usually intact. The injured extremity is elevated, and ice is applied. A splint or sling and swath can be applied, provided neurovascular status is assessed before and after splint application. A sterile dressing is applied to any open fracture. Prophylactic antibiotics are given for open fractures, and tetanus prophylaxis is administered as needed. Analgesia is required during splinting and during any reduction measures.

Radiographs of the anteroposterior and lateral views of the injured extremity should be obtained, including the joints above and below the injury.[2] Comparative views of the injured and uninjured extremities may be obtained. Child maltreatment should be investigated in nonambulatory children with spiral fractures in the lower extremities or upper

Table 28-4.	SALTER-HARRIS CLASSIFICATION, FRACTURE DESCRIPTIONS, AND OUTCOME	
Type	Description of Fractures	Treatment and Outcome
Type I	Horizontal separation of epiphysis and metaphysis; point tenderness; radiographs may be normal; mild soft-tissue swelling produced by shearing forces	No disturbance in growth if properly diagnosed; favorable prognosis; treated with closed reduction and casting
Type II	Separation of epiphysis and metaphysis with some avulsion of the metaphysis produced by shearing forces	No disturbance in growth if properly diagnosed; favorable prognosis; treated with closed reduction and casting
Type III	Produced by intraarticular shearing forces; intraarticular fracture; fracture extends through epiphyseal plate into the metaphysis	Angular deformities may occur; requires good reduction; variable-poor prognosis
Type IV	Fracture starts at the articular surface and extends through the epiphysis, epiphyseal plate, and metaphysis; intraarticular fracture produced by shearing forces	Open reduction and external fixation is needed; variable-poor prognosis; angular deformity may result
Type V	Epiphyseal plate is crushed without fracture or displacement; radiographic diagnosis virtually impossible; produced by crushing force	Poor prognosis, even when correctly identified and treated

From Bernardo LM, Trunzo R: Pediatric trauma. In Kitt S, Selfridge-Thomas J, Proehl J et al, editors: *Emergency nursing: a physiologic and clinical perspective,* ed 2, Philadelphia, 1995, WB Saunders.

arms, toddlers with femur fractures, young children with multiple fractures, fractures with different stages of healing, or in circumstances in which the injury does not match the history.

Most children require a simple cast when the fracture is nondisplaced. Casting may be performed in the ED or deferred until swelling has subsided; the injury may be stabilized in a splint or fiberglass mold. Parents or guardians are given discharge instructions to observe for swelling of the toes or fingers, odor from the cast/splint/mold, and changes in skin color and temperature. Parents should contact the ED with any of these complaints or if the child complains of sharp pain or numbness.

Displaced fractures require manipulation to realign the fractured bone(s). In such situations the ED physician or orthopedic surgeon may attempt closed reduction in the ED. Procedural sedation is administered using analgesics and sedatives such as midazolam, fentanyl, or ketamine. The nurse must carefully monitor the child throughout the procedure for adverse effects of the sedation. After the fracture is reduced, sedatives are stopped, the cast/splint/mold is applied, and postreduction radiographs are obtained. If reduction is not successful, the child may require open reduction and internal fixation in the operating room.

Treatment for femoral fractures varies with age. Infants are placed in spica casts, often in the ED. Reamed- and nonreamed-intramedullary rodding used in older children allows early mobilization. Tibial skeletal traction, external fixation, and plating techniques are also used depending on the type of fracture and the child's age. Children with pelvic fractures require admission to the hospital and subsequent bed rest. Unstable pelvic fractures may require application of an external fixation device.

SUMMARY

Pediatric trauma patients provide a unique challenge for the emergency nurse. The ability to identify potentially life-threatening conditions is essential. Emergency nurses are in a unique position to offer anticipatory guidance to families concerning primary injury prevention. Becoming actively involved in trauma prevention and safety education is another opportunity for emergency nurses to promote safety through education, engineering, and enforcement strategies. Educating parents and children during ED visits using posters, pamphlets, one-on-one discussions, and videos provides families with opportunities for discussion with nurses and with each other regarding their safety practices. Volunteer to speak with students and parent-teacher groups about safety on such topics as wearing bicycle helmets, firearm safety, or wearing safety belts. Engineering efforts include becoming a car seat safety inspector with the National Safe Kids Campaign to check proper installation and security of car safety seats. Write to manufacturers to express concerns about product safety. Report unsafe products or patients injured by products to the Consumer Product Safety Commission. Enforcement includes promoting safety laws in one's community. Become politically aware, and support legislators who favor legislation aimed at reducing injuries (e.g., mandatory bicycle, motorcycle, and skateboard helmet use). Educate legislators and government officials about unsafe road conditions, traffic problems, and other community hazards that cause injuries in children.

Emergency nurses can become involved in organizations such as the National Safe Kids Campaign and the Emergency Nurses Association's Injury Prevention Institute. Emergency nurses can minimize the effects of pediatric trauma by providing quality patient care to injured children and their families. Participating in injury prevention activities helps reduce the incidence of pediatric trauma and enhances the professional image of nursing.

REFERENCES

1. Alterman DM: Consideration in pediatric traumas, 2006, *eMedicine.* Retrieved August 26, 2007, from http://www.emedicine.com/med/topic3223.htm.
2. Bachman D, Santora S: Orthopedic trauma. In Fleisher G, Ludwig S, editors: *Textbook of pediatric emergency medicine*, ed 4, Philadelphia, 2000, Lippincott Williams & Wilkins.
3. Bennett M, Kissoon N: Is cardiopulmonary resuscitation warranted in children who suffer cardiac arrest post trauma? *Pediatr Emerg Care* 23:4, 2007.
4. Berg M, Cook L, Corneli H et al: Effect of seating position and restraint use on injuries to children in motor vehicle crashes, *Pediatrics* 105:831, 2000.
5. Bernardo L, Gardner M, Lucke J et al: The effects of core and peripheral warming methods on temperature and physiologic variables in injured children, *Pediatr Emerg Care* 12(2):138, 2001.
6. Bernardo L, Henker R, O'Connor J: Treatment of trauma-associated hypothermia in children: evidence-based practice, *Am J Crit Care* 9:227, 2000.
7. Bingol-Kologlu M, Fedakar M, Yagmurlu A et al: Tracheobronchial rupture due to blunt chest trauma: report of a case, *Surg Today* 36:9, 2006.
8. *Car safety seats: a guide for families 2008.* Retrieved May 20, 2008, from http://www.aap.org/FAMILY/carseatguide.htm.
9. Clinical Policies Committee: Rapid-sequence intubation, *Ann Emerg Med* 29:573, 1997.
10. Committee on Injury and Poison Prevention: All-terrain vehicle injury prevention: two-, three-, and four-wheeled unlicensed motor vehicles, *Pediatrics* 105:1352, 2000.
11. Dietrich A, Shaner S, Campbell J: *Pediatric basic trauma life support,* Oakbrook Terrace, Ill, 2002, Basic Trauma Life Support International.
12. Eleraky M, Theodore N, Adams M et al: Pediatric cervical spine injuries: report of 102 cases and review of the literature, *J Neurosurg Spine* 92:12, 2000.
13. Fultz J: Tips for helping the families of patients transported by helicopter, *J Emerg Nurs* 25:132, 1999.

14. *Graduated driver licensing reduces fatal crashes by 11 percent,* July 3, 2006, Public Health News Center. Retrieved August 26, 2007, from http://www.jhsph.edu/publichealthnews/press_releases/2006/baker_gdl.html.

15. Greenes D, Madsen J: Neurotrauma. In Fleisher G, Ludwig S, editors: *Textbook of pediatric emergency medicine,* ed 4, Philadelphia, 2000, Lippincott Williams & Wilkins.

16. Greenes D, Schutzman S: Infants with isolated skull fracture: what are their clinical characteristics, and do they require hospitalization? *Ann Emerg Med* 30:253, 1997.

17. Haug R, Foss J: Maxillofacial injuries in the pediatric patient, *Oral Surg Oral Med Oral Pathol Oral Radiol Endodontics* 90:126, 2000.

18. Hsu A, Slonim A: Preventing pediatric trauma: the role of the critical care professional, *Crit Connections,* p 10, February 2006. Retrieved August 30, 2007, from http://www.sccm.org.

19. Kadish H: Thoracic trauma. In Fleisher G, Ludwig S, editors: *Textbook of pediatric emergency medicine,* ed 4, Philadelphia, 2000, Lippincott Williams & Wilkins.

20. Kay R, Skaggs D: Pediatric polytrauma management, *J Pediatr Orthop* 26:2, 2006.

21. Kliegman Robert M, Jenson H et al: *Nelson textbook of pediatrics,* ed 18, Philadelphia, 2007, WB Saunders.

22. Koestner A, Hoak S: Spinal cord injury without radiographic abnormality (SCIWORA) in children, *J Trauma Nurs* 8:4, 2001.

23. Liller KD: Unintentional injuries in children, *APHA 2006,* 2006. Retrieved September 2, 2007, from http://www.medscape.com/viewarticle/553273?rss.

24. Ludwig S: Resuscitation—pediatric basic and advanced life support. In Fleisher G, Ludwig S, editors: *Textbook of pediatric emergency medicine,* ed 4, Philadelphia, 2000, Lippincott Williams & Wilkins.

25. Meyer M, Burd R: The top 10 things to evaluate in children with suspected blunt abdominal injuries, *J Trauma Nurs* 7:98, 2000.

26. Moulton S: Early management of the child with multiple injuries, *Clin Orthop Relat Res* 376:6, 2000.

27. Partrick D, Bensard D, Moore E et al: Driveway crush injuries in young children: a highly lethal, devastating, and potentially preventable event, *J Pediatr Surg* 33:1712, 1998.

28. Ralston M, Hazinski M, Zaritsky A, et al: *Pediatric advanced life support provider manual,* Dallas, 2006, American Heart Association.

29. Rothrock S, Green S, Morgan R: Abdominal trauma in infants and children: prompt identification and early management of serious and life-threatening injuries. I. Injury patterns and initial assessment, *Pediatr Emerg Care* 16:106, 2000.

30. Rudy C: Dental trauma, *School Nurse News* 18:33, 2001.

31. Schneider G: Safety advocates decry back-over deaths: solutions sought for blind spots, *Washington Post,* April 28, 2005. Retrieved September 2, 2007, from http://www.highbeam.com/doc/1P2-30576.html.

32. *Shopping cart injury,* 1999, Firehouse.com Safe Kids. Retrieved September 2, 2007, from http://www.firehouse.com/safekids/factsheets/cart_inj.html.

33. Shopping cart related injuries to children, *Pediatrics* 118(2):825, 2006. Retrieved September 2, 2007, from http://www.pediatrics.org/cgi/doi/10.1542/peds.2006-1215.

34. Skateboard and scooter injuries, *Pediatrics* 109(3):542, 2002. Retrieved September 2, 2007, from http://aappolicy.aappublications.org/cgi/content/full/pediatric:109/3/542.

35. *Traffic safety facts 2005* data. Retrieved August 26, 2007, from http://www.nhtsa.gov.

36. U.S. Department of Transportation, National Highway Traffic Safety Administration: *Child restraint systems safety plan (draft),* Washington, DC, 2000, U.S. Department of Transportation.

37. Wazana A, Rynard V, Raina P: Are child pedestrians at increased risk of injury on one-way compared to two-way streets?, *Can J Public Health* 91:201, 2000.

38. Wiley P: Paediatric head injuries: a literature review, *Aust Emerg Nurs J* 1:20, 1997.

39. Winston F, Durbin D: Buckle up! Is not enough: enhancing protection of the restrained child, *JAMA* 281:2070, 1999.

40. Woodward G: Neck trauma. In Fleisher G, Ludwig S, editors: *Textbook of pediatric emergency medicine,* ed 4, Philadelphia, 2000, Lippincott Williams & Wilkins.

CHAPTER 29

Obstetric Trauma

Terri McGowan Repasky

The actual incidence of obstetric trauma is unknown, but it has been estimated that injuries occur in 6% to 7% of all pregnancies.[5] Trauma is the leading cause of maternal death from nonobstetric causes for women during their childbearing years. Most obstetric trauma involves minor injury, although significant trauma-related injuries can occur. Nursing priorities for the pregnant and nonpregnant trauma patient are the same, but interventions are intended to benefit two patients, the mother and the fetus.

Like their nonpregnant counterparts, pregnant patients sustain blunt, penetrating, burn, and submersion injuries. Blunt trauma is the most common, often due to motor vehicle crashes (MVCs), falls, and assaults.[5] Trauma secondary to battering is more common in pregnant patients. During the first 4 months of pregnancy 154 per 1000 women are assaulted by their partners. During the fifth through ninth month 170 per 1000 are assaulted.[4] Overexertion may also lead to injuries during pregnancy.[6]

Most maternal deaths from trauma are secondary to head injury or hemorrhagic shock. Pelvic fracture is the most common maternal injury that results in fetal death. Abruptio placentae and premature delivery are the most common trauma-related causes of fetal demise.

Primary and secondary assessment and initial nursing priorities for the pregnant trauma patient are essentially the same as for a nonpregnant patient. However, anatomic and physiologic differences related to the gravid state must be considered during all stages of the trauma nursing process.

ANATOMY AND PHYSIOLOGY

Normal respiratory and circulatory changes during pregnancy can mask the typical signs and symptoms that emergency nurses rely on to guide care of their trauma patient. Optimal outcome for mother and fetus is based on sound knowledge of maternal anatomy and physiology and implications for interventions.

Uterine

Uterine size and blood flow are a concern in the gravid trauma patient. The uterus enlarges from a 7-cm and 70-g structure to a 36-cm and 1100-g walled organ (similar in size and weight to a bowling ball). As the uterus grows, its wall becomes thinner. Through the first 12 weeks of pregnancy the uterus remains a small, self-contained intrapelvic organ protected from abdominal injury by the bony pelvis. After 12 weeks the uterus becomes an intraabdominal organ as it enlarges and ascends, encroaching on the peritoneal cavity and confining the intestines to the upper abdomen. Figure 29-1 shows uterine size for various gestational periods. During the second trimester the uterus is susceptible to abdominal injury, although the fetus remains small and relatively

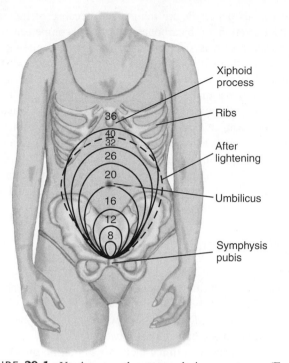

FIGURE **29-1.** Uterine growth patterns during pregnancy. (From Murray SS, McKinney ES: *Foundations of maternal-newborn nursing*, ed 4, Philadelphia, 2006, WB Saunders.)

cushioned by large amounts of amniotic fluid. By the third trimester the uterus is large and thin walled. During the last 2 to 8 weeks' gestation, the fetus descends and the fetal head engages in the pelvis. The fetus occupies most of the intra-uterine and abdominal space when the head becomes fixed in the pelvis. Maternal pelvic fractures during this trimester may be associated with fetal skull fractures and intracranial hemorrhage, as well as significant maternal blood loss.

Uterine blood flow increases from a baseline of 60 mL/min to 600 mL/min during the third trimester. Uterine blood flow has no autoregulation and depends solely on maternal perfusion pressure. Uterine veins may dilate up to 60 times their prepregnant state; uterine injury may be a major source of blood loss. In response to trauma, maternal catecholamines are released by the sympathetic nervous system and cause uteroplacental constriction, which shunts blood to the mother and away from the fetus and leads to fetal distress. By the third trimester, vessels of the uterus and placenta have reached maximum vasodilatation and cannot increase blood flow in response to decreased perfusion.

Cardiovascular

Anatomically, the heart is elevated and rotated forward by the ascending diaphragm and pushed up by the enlarging uterus. This cardiac displacement causes a 15-degree left axis deviation that is considered a normal change of pregnancy. An electrocardiogram may also show a flattened or inverted T wave in lead III and Q waves in III and aVF. Ectopic beats are also common during pregnancy.

Cardiovascular physiology is profoundly altered during pregnancy. Maternal blood volume increases by the tenth week of gestation and increases 40% to 50% by the twenty-eighth week, remaining at that level until delivery. Uterine blood flow increases to 600 mL/min by the end of pregnancy. Increased blood flow and volume increase maternal cardiac output by 1 to 1.5 L/min. After approximately 20 weeks' gestation, cardiac output can decrease with compression of the vena cava and aorta by the fetus when the mother is in a supine position. This event is called inferior vena cava syndrome or supine hypotensive syndrome. Because the uterus at 20 weeks has grown and risen to the level of the inferior vena cava, compression of the vena cava by the uterus may decrease cardiac output by 28% and systolic blood pressure by 30 mm Hg. Sequestering blood in the venous system may decrease perfusion to the uterus; when maternal systolic blood pressure is below 80 mm Hg, the uterus and fetus will not be perfused. Displacing the gravid uterus to the side by placing the pregnant patient in a lateral decubitus position or manual displacement reverses aortocaval compression. When spinal injury is suspected, maintain spinal protection and tilt the patient 15 degrees laterally or manually displace the uterus.

Resting heart rate increases until the second trimester and remains 10 to 20 beats/min above baseline for the duration of the pregnancy. Systolic and diastolic blood pressures decrease in the first trimester, reach their lowest levels in the second trimester, then rise toward prepregnancy levels during the final 2 months of gestation. A decrease of 15 mm Hg for systolic and diastolic pressure is normal in the second trimester.

Hemodynamic measurements may be misleading. Signs of shock such as tachycardia and hypotension may be normal physiologic changes of pregnancy. Conversely, "normal" findings may mask an underlying shock state. Hypervolemia of pregnancy enables a woman to tolerate acute blood loss of 10% to 15% or gradual loss of 30% (1500 mL) without a change in vital signs.[5]

Catecholamine release, caused by maternal hypovolemia, leads to vasoconstriction of peripheral and uterine vascular beds and shunting of blood to vital maternal organs. A 15% to 30% reduction of uterine blood flow can occur without obvious change in maternal blood pressure. Uterine hypoperfusion and fetal hypoxia can occur before evidence of maternal shock. Signs of fetal distress include fetal bradycardia, fetal tachycardia, and decreased or increased fetal movement.

Gravid women in shock may not have the cool, clammy skin typical of shock because of maternal vasodilatation during the first and second trimester. Vasoconstriction in response to stress occurs predominantly in the third trimester.

Adequate and appropriate fluid replacement is necessary to restore maternal and uteroplacental perfusion. Isotonic crystalloid solutions (e.g., normal saline or lactated Ringer's) are acceptable for initial resuscitation. Blood transfusions should be given with Rh-compatible blood. In cases of impending shock, only O-negative or type-specific blood is acceptable. Vasopressors are not indicated for initial management of hypovolemic shock but may be used in management of cardiogenic shock secondary to cardiac contusion or distributive shock resulting from spinal cord injury.

Hematologic

Cautious interpretation of laboratory values is required. Dilutional anemia in pregnancy is caused by the disproportionate increase of plasma volume relative to erythrocyte volume. Dilutional states can decrease the hematocrit level to 31% to 34% and reduce hemoglobin to 11.0 g/dL. These changes are referred to clinically as "physiologic anemia of pregnancy."[2]

Platelet levels may be normal or slightly decreased. Physiologic leukocytosis occurs during the second and third trimesters. An increase in white blood cells of 15,000/mm[3] may occur by term and rise even higher during stress or labor. Sedimentation rate also increases during pregnancy. These increased levels may mask or falsely indicate an infectious process.

Fibrinogen levels start to rise in the third month and double by term. An increase in clotting factors VII, VIII, IX, X, and XII produces hypercoagulability and increased thromboembolic risk. Deep vein thrombosis and pulmonary embolism are a significant risk, especially when the gravid woman is inactive. The pregnant woman who sustains trauma is at a high risk for disseminated intravascular coagulopathy if abruptio placentae or amniotic fluid embolism occur.

Pulmonary

Significant anatomic and physiologic alterations occur in the pulmonary system during pregnancy. Capillary engorgement of the mucosal lining of the respiratory tract predisposes gravid women to nosebleeds and airway obstruction. Gentle suction and intubation may be necessary to control epistaxis and prevent airway compromise. Complications of pregnancy such as pregnancy-induced hypertension (PIH) and gestational diabetes exacerbate normal airway engorgement, making intubation more difficult. Often a smaller-than-expected endotracheal tube is required.

The diaphragm elevates as the uterus enlarges, up to 4 cm with associated flaring of the ribs. During the third trimester, chest tubes, when needed, should be inserted in the third or fourth intercostal space to avoid diaphragm injury.

Diaphragmatic elevation reduces pulmonary functional reserve capacity by 20% at the end of pregnancy. Reduction is associated with increased maternal oxygen consumption and diminished oxygen reserve. Maternal tidal volume and minute ventilations decrease to 40% by late pregnancy. Respiratory rates will increase. Arterial oxygen pressure (PaO_2) levels increase to 101 to 104 mm Hg. Arterial carbon dioxide pressure ($PaCO_2$) levels decrease to approximately 30 mm Hg by the end of the second trimester and remain at this level until delivery.[5]

The maternal respiratory center is especially sensitive to minute changes in $PaCO_2$ levels. Although normal arterial and venous pH levels are maintained because of increased renal excretion of bicarbonate, partially compensated respiratory alkalosis occurs during pregnancy, making the pregnant patient less able to cope with respiratory distress and acidosis associated with trauma. A diminished maternal oxygen reserve makes the gravid uterus vulnerable to hypoxia. Because maternal hypoxia affects fetal oxygenation, fetal compromise may occur with minimal maternal distress. Fetal heart rate changes are frequently the first indicator of maternal hypoxia. Maternal trauma may require blood gas analysis to determine hypoxia and acidosis. Supplemental oxygen at 100% FIO_2 is essential until maternal and fetal hypoxia are ruled out or resolved.

Gastrointestinal

Various anatomic and physiologic gastrointestinal (GI) changes occur during pregnancy. The small bowel is pushed up into the upper abdomen by the uterus, and the large bowel moves posteriorly. Diminished bowel sounds may be a normal finding in pregnancy or indicate intraperitoneal injury. Stretching of the abdominal wall due to uterine growth can impair maternal sensitivity to peritoneal irritation, so muscle guarding, rigidity, or rebound tenderness may be dulled or absent.

Increased progesterone and estrogen affect the GI tract, reducing motility and tone and relaxing the gastric sphincter. Gastric emptying is delayed, and gastroesophageal reflux occurs frequently. The lower esophageal sphincter is displaced into the thorax. Risk for aspiration is increased. As with all trauma patients, the pregnant patient is always considered to have a full stomach. A gastric tube should be considered early in the resuscitation to minimize risk for aspiration; nasal insertion of gastric tubes should be performed cautiously (to minimize the risk for epistaxis) using a smaller-size tube.

Genitourinary

Maternal susceptibility to traumatic bladder injury increases as the bladder moves from a pelvic organ to an intraabdominal position by 12 weeks' gestation. Urinary frequency increases in the third trimester because of bladder compression by the uterus. Dilation of the ureters, renal calyces, and pelvis from compression by the ovarian plexus can result in urinary stasis. Glomerular filtration rate increases, causing a decrease in blood urea nitrogen and creatinine.

Musculoskeletal

The pelvis becomes more flexible during pregnancy in preparation for fetal delivery. Hormonal changes loosen ligaments of the symphysis pubis and sacroiliac joints. By 7 months' gestation, there is considerable widening of the pelvis. An unsteady gait, usually caused by the widening pelvis and heavy abdomen, predisposes the gravid female to falls.

Neurologic

Changes in the central nervous system (CNS) related to pregnancy are abnormal findings. PIH (formerly referred to as preeclampsia) may occur after 20 to 24 weeks' gestation and is characterized by hypertension, proteinuria, and edema. CNS irritability can lead to seizures (eclampsia). Hypoxia from seizure activity places the mother and fetus at risk. Altered mentation, seizures, and hypertension may also indicate head injury; therefore meticulous neurologic assessment of the pregnant trauma patient is essential.

Endocrine

The pituitary gland doubles in size and weight by term, requiring a greater blood supply. Hypoperfusion causes ischemia and can lead to pituitary necrosis. Hemorrhage within the gland can occur with reperfusion. Sheehan's syndrome, which is necrosis of the anterior pituitary gland, produces long-term complications related to decreased hormone levels.[5] Aggressive and rapid treatment of shock is required to prevent these serious complications.

PATIENT ASSESSMENT

The anatomic and physiologic changes of normal pregnancy can obscure the mother's response to trauma. Maternal compensatory mechanisms preserve vital maternal functions at the expense of the fetus. Fetal survival depends on adequate gas exchange and uterine perfusion. Rapid and efficient assessment and appropriate intervention for specific abnormalities provides for an optimal maternal-fetal outcome.

The primary survey focuses on airway, breathing, and circulation. Repositioning the airway by chin-lift or jaw-thrust maneuvers may be enough to establish patency and should not interfere with cervical spine protection. Airway adjuncts should be used as needed to prevent secondary injury from hypoxia; nasal airways should be used with caution because the mother may be predisposed to nasopharyngeal bleeding that can lead to further airway obstruction.

Cervical spine protection is maintained until the neck is cleared. If injury is suspected, spinal protection should be maintained with a rigid cervical collar; the patient should be logrolled off the backboard as soon as possible and pillows or foam wedges used to tilt the patient 15 degrees laterally to deflect the uterus from the vena cava.

All trauma patients need supplemental oxygen. Injury can exacerbate existing pulmonary alterations related to pregnancy, such as decreased pulmonary reserve and increased maternal oxygen consumption, compromising the mother and fetus. Oxygen is critical for fetal survival because of fetal inability to tolerate hypoxia.

Assessment and intervention for external and internal hemorrhage is necessary to ensure maternal-fetal survival. Apply direct pressure to sites of uncontrolled external bleeding. The mother can lose 1500 mL of blood before signs of shock are evident. Retroperitoneal and uteroplacental injury can be sources of occult blood loss. Venous access with two large-bore catheters and aggressive fluid volume replacement optimize maternal blood volume and oxygen-carrying capacity. Initiate blood replacement with Rh-compatible blood if crystalloids do not stabilize circulatory status. Aortocaval compression can occur by 20 weeks' gestation; therefore displacing the uterus can increase cardiac output by 20%. Insertion of an arterial line or central venous line provides accurate monitoring of circulation and response to treatment and may be used in some centers.

Primary assessment includes a brief neurologic assessment. If neurologic deficits are found, both PIH and trauma should be considered as potential causes.

Secondary assessment involves identification of other injuries. Thorough history includes standard trauma history and obstetric history—last menstrual period (LMP), expected date of delivery, parity, problems and complications of current or past pregnancies, presence of uterine contractions, and current fetal activity. Focused obstetric assessment in the secondary survey includes evaluation of the abdomen, uterus, and fetus.

Abdomen

The abdomen may be difficult to assess because of blunted signs of intraperitoneal irritation. Severe occult intraabdominal hemorrhage may occur without signs of impending shock. Liver and splenic injuries are common in MVCs and may be a source intraperitoneal hemorrhage.

Inspect the abdomen for signs of injury, including ecchymosis, abrasions, and contusions. Note the shape and contour of the abdomen. Irregularity or deformity may indicate uterine rupture. Inspect for fetal movement. Palpate for masses, abdominal tenderness, contractions, and fetal movement. Remember abdominal rigidity, guarding, and rebound tenderness may be blunted by the stretched abdominal wall.

Ultrasonography (US) is beneficial in determining intraabdominal injury and fetal status; some centers use focused assessment sonography for trauma (FAST) examinations routinely in the initial assessment of each trauma patient. Abdominal computed tomography (CT) is used to determine abdominal injuries in the stable trauma patient. Diagnostic peritoneal lavage (DPL) has been safely and accurately used to detect intraperitoneal hemorrhage in obstetric trauma.

Fetus and Uterus

Assessment of the fetus and uterus should occur early in the secondary survey. Signs of abdominal pain, uterine tenderness, or contractions may indicate uteroplacental injury and maternal-fetal compromise.

Determining gestational age is critical because this guides fetal assessment and intervention. The best indicator of gestational age is LMP. If the woman is unsure or unresponsive, she is assumed pregnant until a negative human chorionic gonadotropin (hCG) is documented. Normal gestation is 40 weeks, with the uterus usually palpable by 12 to 14 weeks' gestation. The fundus generally reaches the umbilicus by 20 weeks' gestation. Fundal height just below the xiphoid indicates a term fetus. Fetal gestational age is frequently estimated by US. If emergency US is not available, an estimate of gestational age of a single fetus can be accomplished by measuring fundal height. A measurement midline from the symphysis pubis to the top of the uterus correlates gestational age with the height of the fundus in centimeters. A fundal height of 25 cm corresponds to gestational age of 25 weeks. Fetal viability is generally considered 24 to 25 weeks' gestation, although fetal survival has occurred earlier with advanced neonatal resuscitation and treatment in a neonatal intensive care unit. Serial fundal measurements are beneficial; increased fundal height may indicate occult intrauterine bleeding or uterine injury.

The fetus should be assessed as soon as possible, but this assessment should not interfere with maternal resuscitation and stabilization. Evaluation of fetal well-being begins with a baseline fetal heart rate (FHR) or evaluation of fetal heart tones (FHTs). Fetal heart tones are audible with Doppler testing by 10 to 12 weeks' gestation. Normal FHR ranges from 100 to 160 beats/min at term and post term (gestational age 37 weeks or more) and 120 to 160 beats/min in a preterm fetus (less than 37 weeks).[8] FHR will initially increase in response to hypoxia or hypotension; however, severe hypoxia is associated with fetal bradycardia (less than 100 to 120 beats/min) Fetal bradycardia indicates serious fetal stress and decompensation. Another indicator of fetal well-being is fetal movement and activity. Maternal report of approximately 10 "kicks" in 2 hours may be considered a sign of fetal well-being.[8]

The gravid trauma patient may require continuous fetal monitoring or cardiotocography based on gestational age of the fetus. Cardiotocography consists of continuous electronic monitoring of FHR, patterns, and uterine contractions. When possible, early continuous monitoring should be initiated for patients greater than 20 weeks' gestation. Fetal tachycardia (rate greater than 160 beats/min), bradycardia (rate less than 100 to 120 beats/min), decreased variability in fetal heart rate, and/or fetal heart rate decelerations associated with contractions are indicators of fetal distress. Significant FHR patterns such as late deceleration are ominous signs of fetal distress. Monitoring FHR and contractions should be continued for 4 to 6 hours in the absence of uterine tenderness, vaginal bleeding, fetal distress, or serious maternal injury or complications.[1] If FHR abnormalities or maternal complications are detected, monitoring should continue for at least 24 hours or until fetal well-being is established. Fetal monitoring should be performed and interpreted by a clinician skilled in use of the equipment, interpretation of the data, and requisite interventions; ideally a nurse from the labor and delivery unit should perform this monitoring. Box 29-1 summarizes signs of fetal distress.

Assessment includes inspection of the perineum for blood or amniotic fluid. Presence of amniotic fluid indicates a leaking or ruptured amniotic membrane and places the fetus at risk for infection and early delivery. Microscopic examination of vaginal fluid can determine presence of amniotic fluid. Fluid

---

Box 29-1	SIGNS OF FETAL DISTRESS

- Fetal heart rates consistently below 100 beats/min in known term or postterm fetus (37 weeks or greater gestational age)[8]
- Fetal heart rates consistently below 120 beats/min in a preterm fetus (gestational age less than 37 weeks)
- Fetal heart rates consistently above 160 beats/min
- No fetal movement reported by mother or per nursing examination (approximately 10 "kicks" in 2 hours may be considered a sign of fetal well-being)
- Bloody or meconium-stained amniotic fluid

---

is placed on a slide and allowed to air dry; if the specimen contains amniotic fluid, a fern pattern appears on the slide. Some centers use point-of-care tests that use vaginal swabs and color cards to detect amniotic fluid. In the absence of blood or urine, nitrazine paper can be used to differentiate amniotic fluid from vaginal fluid. Fluid should be obtained as close to the cervical os as possible to avoid a false-positive test. Normal vaginal fluid has a pH of 4.5 to 5.5. Amniotic fluid has a pH of 7.0 to 7.5, which turns nitrazine paper blue. If blood is detected, the source of bleeding must be determined.

A general pelvic examination identifies crowning, fetal presentation, blood, and fluids. The necessity for speculum examination is determined by the trauma physician and may be deferred to the attending obstetrician. Direct visualization allows assessment of cervical dilation, locates the source of blood or fluids, and identifies uterine or fetal injury. Bimanual examination is avoided unless delivery is imminent or genital tract injury is present. Urinary catheter placement is indicated to empty the bladder and to assist in monitoring fluid resuscitation. Return of blood or hematuria suggests genitourinary (GU) injury.

Diagnostics

Ultrasonography

US, and in some centers FAST, is used to identify acute problems with the pregnant trauma patient. US can determine fetal cardiac activity, body movement, placental location, estimated gestational age, and volume of amniotic fluid. Fetal death may also be diagnosed by US. Maternal intraabdominal and intrapericardial fluid can be detected during a FAST examination.

Laboratory

Laboratory studies include standard trauma profiles; however, results should be interpreted cautiously because of hematologic changes with pregnancy. Standard laboratory studies include complete blood count, serum electrolytes, amylase, coagulation profile, arterial blood gas, type and screen or type and crossmatch, toxicology screen, and urinalysis. Hospital policy and the attending physician determine the need for hepatitis B and human immunodeficiency virus screening. hCG levels should be obtained for all women of childbearing age if LMP is unknown or greater than 4½ weeks before admission. Special attention to antibody screening is needed for Rh immune status because maternal Rh sensitization can occur when an Rh-negative mother carries an Rh-positive fetus. Administration of Rho (D) immune globulin (Rho-GAM or Rhophylac) can prevent maternal sensitization. A Kleihauer-Betke (KB) test is used to identify the mixing of fetal blood in maternal circulation and should be performed on all patients over 12 weeks' gestation.[1] A positive KB test is useful in predicting the risk for preterm labor after maternal trauma.[7] This test is particularly important when the mother is determined to be Rh negative. KB test results can be used to determine the dose of Rh immune globulin administered to inhibit formation of maternal antibodies against an Rh-negative fetus. Some hemoglobinopathies such as sickle cell can result in a positive KB test; the presence of a positive KB test alone does not necessarily indicate pathologic trauma and should not be used to diagnose placental abruption.[3]

Radiographic Evaluation

Radiodiagnostic procedures necessary for trauma evaluation should not be omitted in the presence of a gravid uterus. Studies should be performed with a vigilant attempt to minimize fetal irradiation. Need for radiographic studies is determined by clinical examination and physician suspicion of injury.

Every effort should be made to minimize fetal risk. An expert radiology technician can avoid duplicate films, shield the uterus whenever possible, and perform only essential radiodiagnostics. Consulting with an obstetrician or geneticist may be beneficial when fetal radiation exposure is a concern and if there is time. Though magnetic resonance imaging (MRI) scans are generally more detailed and involve no ionizing radiation, MRI is less commonly employed in the emergent setting.

Diagnostic Peritoneal Lavage

Although DPL can effectively assess abdominal injury for hemoperitoneum and is considered safe and accurate for the gravid trauma patient, it is rarely used since the development of FAST. DPL does not assess retroperitoneal or intrauterine injury, and CT assessment is used more often. If CT is not available, DPL may be indicated in a symptomatic patient after blunt or multiple traumatic injury. Before the procedure an indwelling urinary catheter should be inserted to decompress the bladder and decrease the risk for perforation. Decompression of the stomach with an orogastric or nasogastric tube decreases the risk for perforation and aspiration. Further diagnostics are required to locate the source and extent of injury. Immediate, delayed, or deferred laparotomy is determined by maternal and fetal condition.

INJURIES

Blunt Trauma

Blunt abdominal trauma can cause minor or severe life-threatening injuries to mother and fetus. The most common causes of abdominal trauma are MVCs, falls, and assaults,[2] with falls the most common cause of minor maternal injury. Hormonal changes soften joints and relax pelvic ligaments, which decreases stability in balance and gait. These changes in combination with a protruding abdomen and easy fatigue increase the mother's susceptibility to falls. Many falls occur during the third trimester and are the second most common cause of maternal injury.[2]

Injury to the abdomen can result from direct force during an MVC as the abdomen impacts the dashboard or steering wheel or from a direct blow to the mother during an assault. Abdominal injury can also be secondary to organ displacement and hemorrhage from a coup-contrecoup event. Injury to the uterus can cause severe complications for the fetus, including premature labor, abruptio placentae, uterine rupture, fetal head injury, and fetal-maternal hemorrhage. Treatment varies depending on injuries sustained and status of the mother and fetus.

Seat Belts

MVCs are one of the most common causes of maternal injury or mortality. Ejection from the vehicle with resulting head trauma accounts for most deaths. Fetal death rates are also high when the mother is ejected. Combined lap and shoulder restraints (i.e., three-point restraints) reduce maternal ejection and risk for fetal injury. Lap belts without shoulder harnesses also decrease ejection from the vehicle; however the lap restraint alone can cause intraabdominal injuries. Elevation of the small bowel during pregnancy exposes the protuberant uterus and increases the risk for uterine or fetal injury from the lap belt. The two-point shoulder harness without lap restraint does not prevent ejection. Proper use of three-point restraints is advocated to reduce maternal mortality and fetal risk. The lap belt should be worn snugly across the pelvis below the abdomen and uterus; the shoulder harness should be worn in the normal position across the chest and between the breasts.

Premature Uterine Contractions

A frequently occurring complication of obstetric trauma is uterine contractions. Damage to myometrial (muscular layer of the uterus) and decidual (epithelial lining of the uterus) cells releases prostaglandins, which stimulate the uterus. The extent of uterine damage, release of prostaglandins, and fetal age determine labor progression. Uterine contractions greater than six to eight per hour may indicate preterm labor. Usually contractions are self-limiting and tocolysis is not indicated. Tocolysis, pharmacologic suppression of contractions, may be effective in halting preterm labor of the injured but hemodynamically stable gravida. Pharmacology is determined by physician discretion.

Adequate fluid volume replacement and positioning the mother in the lateral tilt position can minimize uterine irritability. Cardiotocographic monitoring should be initiated early to assess uterine activity and fetal response.

Abruptio Placentae

Abruptio placentae is premature separation of the normally implanted placenta from the uterine wall. Major abruptions may cause fetal anoxia, exsanguination, or premature delivery and are the most common cause of fetal death with a surviving mother.[5] As illustrated in Figure 29-2, the abruption may be partial, marginal, or complete. Hemorrhage may be concealed. Blood trapped behind the separating placenta is old blood and appears dark when expelled. Fresh bleeding is usually bright red, whereas a port-wine color is seen when blood is mixed with amniotic fluid. In addition to blunt trauma, predisposing factors for abruptio placentae are related to PIH, glomerulonephritis, diabetes, increased maternal age, cigarette smoking, alcohol consumption, or possible dietary deficiencies.

Abdominal trauma is a direct force that can trigger abruptio placentae. Energy from a blunt force is dissipated to the elastic uterus, causing the placenta, which is relatively inelastic, to shear away from the uterine lining. Risk for abruptio placentae is usually immediately after injury. Bleeding

can be severe enough to cause immediate maternal circulatory shock. Lack of oxygenation from impaired maternal-fetal gas exchange can lead to infant mortality resulting from hypoxia or intracranial hemorrhage.

Classic signs of abruption include vaginal bleeding, uterine tenderness, abdominal pain, back pain, and uterine hyperactivity with poor relaxation between contractions. Presentation may be vague or severe. Other indications of abruption include preterm labor, maternal shock, increasing fundal height, and fetal distress. Vaginal bleeding may be absent with concealed retroplacental bleeding. Fetal distress may be the first indication of uteroplacental injury and potential abruption. Rapid deterioration can occur in both mother and fetus, so intensive monitoring is indicated. Two large-bore intravenous catheters should be started with isotonic crystalloid solution. A complete blood count and type and crossmatch should be immediately sent to the laboratory. Fetal monitoring is essential. A small abruption may be compatible with fetal survival; however, a viable fetus in distress requires immediate surgical delivery.

Uterine Rupture

Rupture of the uterus is an uncommon catastrophic injury resulting from blunt abdominal trauma. Previous cesarean section is a predisposing factor because rupture can occur at the healed incision site. Rupture of the posterior aspect of the uterus usually occurs in an unscarred uterus and is likely to involve bladder injury; urine may contain blood or meconium. Increased maternal blood volume and perfusion increases the risk for maternal hypovolemic shock with uterine rupture. The patient may initially have acute pain followed by no pain. The uterus will be tender, and fetal limbs may be palpated outside the uterine borders with uterine rupture. Uterine contour may be abnormal and fundal height difficult to assess. There may be vaginal bleeding. Fetal distress may be evident. Early detection and repair of minor lacerations may prevent maternal hemorrhage and fetal compromise,[2] but rarely can the uterus be repaired; hysterectomy is indicated for almost all patients with uterine rupture. Fetal mortality is almost 100%.

Direct Fetal Injury

Blunt trauma infrequently results in direct fetal injury, with fetal skull fractures and intracranial hemorrhage the most common injuries noted. Injuries usually occur in association with maternal pelvic fractures. Later in pregnancy, when the head is engaged in the pelvis, the fetal skull can become trapped and injured by the fractured pelvis. Compression of the fetal skull may occur between the maternal spine and restraining lap belt or a striking object. Other fetal fractures from direct injury may include clavicle and long-bone injury.

Penetrating Injury

Increasing size and position make the gravid uterus susceptible to penetrating trauma. Fetal injury after penetrating trauma to the mother is a frequent occurrence with a high

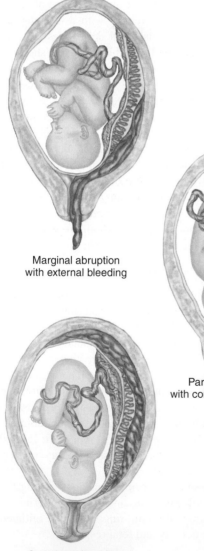
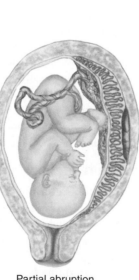

Marginal abruption
with external bleeding

Partial abruption
with concealed bleeding

Complete abruption
with concealed bleeding

FIGURE 29-2. Types of abruptio placentae. (From Murray SS, McKinney ES: *Foundations of maternal-newborn nursing,* ed 4, Philadelphia, 2006, WB Saunders.)

rate of fetal mortality. Gunshot wounds to the abdomen are more common than stab wounds. Degree of injury depends on type, caliber, and range of the weapon. Upper abdominal wounds involve bowel perforation or retroperitoneal injuries to the mother caused by compartmentalization by the gravid uterus. Lower abdominal entry wounds cause direct injury to the fetus. Indirect injury to the fetus may be caused by trauma to the umbilical cord, placenta, or membrane. All abdominal gunshot wounds require exploratory laparotomy.

Stab wounds have a better prognosis for the mother and fetus. Visceral organs can slide away from the penetrating object, so fewer organs are injured. Surgical exploration is usually required in cases of upper abdominal trauma from a bullet or stab wound. Conservative management of lower abdominal injuries is indicated if the patient is stable or there is no evidence of GI or GU trauma. Diagnostic options include local exploration of wounds and CT, US, or DPL of the abdomen. Emergency exploratory laparotomy is indicated for the pregnant patient with penetrating trauma and unstable vital signs or fetal distress. The decision to deliver the fetus depends on (1) gestational age, (2) evidence of penetration of the amniotic sac, (3) evidence of fetal death or distress, and (4) maternal injuries requiring abdominal exploration. Otherwise, vaginal delivery can be anticipated as the fetus continues to grow and mature.

Burns

Most burn injuries in pregnant women occur in the home, with extremities, face, and neck burned most often. Fortunately, the majority of burn injuries are minor. Pregnancy does not appear to affect maternal outcome; however, fetal outcome is affected by maternal condition. Total body surface area (BSA) involved and severity of burn affect maternal outcome, premature delivery, and fetal death. Fetal mortality is close to 90% when maternal burns are greater than 50% BSA but drops to approximately 20% if maternal burns are less than 50% BSA. Fetal mortality results from hypoxia, hyponatremia, sepsis, and prematurity. Spontaneous abortion usually occurs within the first week after a severe burn event. Occasionally delivery of a healthy term infant is possible.

One potential complication associated with burn injury and smoke exposure is carbon monoxide (CO) poisoning. Fetal hemoglobin has a higher affinity for CO than maternal hemoglobin; when measuring maternal carboxyhemoglobin it must be kept in mind that the fetus's level will be higher. Hyperbaric oxygen therapy should be considered if elevated carboxyhemoglobin levels are detected in the gravid patient.

Immediate care of the burned pregnant woman is the same as that of the nonpregnant patient. Severe burns require treatment at a burn center. Aggressive and appropriate fluid resuscitation, electrolyte therapy, supplemental oxygen, ventilation, and prevention of infection are critical. Sterile, dry dressings should be applied. Avoid wet or cool dressings. Antibiotics should be used if necessary; however, silver sulfadiazine cream should be avoided because it can displace

bound bilirubin in fetal plasma, resulting in an increase in circulating fetal bilirubin. Elevated fetal bilirubin can cross the fetal blood-brain barrier and interfere with neuronal development, leading to fetal kernicterus or brain damage.[5]

Electrical Injury

Few cases of electrical injury during pregnancy are reported; however, fetal mortality has been associated with even minor electrical shock. Most electrical incidents occur at home. Alternating current found in the home usually follows a hand-to-foot route. Consequently, the fetus lies in the direct path of the current. Fetal injury can result from cardiac conduction changes or uteroplacental lesions. If the fetus survives, oligohydramnios or growth retardation can develop. Pregnant women should report all incidents of electrical shock to the obstetrician. Baseline fetal monitoring and close, frequent follow-ups are necessary to evaluate fetal well-being.

SPECIAL CONSIDERATIONS
Maternal Cardiac Arrest

Objectives for cardiopulmonary resuscitation (CPR) during pregnancy are to sustain circulation and perfusion for both patients—the mother and fetus. Basic and advanced life support should be initiated early and performed with only slight variations. The maternal heart is located more cephalad and laterally rotated; therefore compressions are performed slightly higher on the sternum. Prompt, gentle intubation may reduce risk for nasoesophageal or oroesophageal bleeding and aspiration. In the presence of maternal hypoxia and acidemia, vasoconstriction occurs in the uteroplacental vascular bed. Monitoring blood gas levels and serum pH levels is vital to determining maternal acidosis and response to treatment. Renal excretion of sodium bicarbonate increases during pregnancy; therefore bicarbonate administration is determined by blood gas results. Aggressive ventilation with supplemental oxygen and fluid loading with isotonic crystalloids and possibly blood products are necessary for resuscitation. Vasopressors should be used with caution because of uteroplacental vasoconstriction and deleterious effects on the fetus. There are no contraindications to external defibrillation during pregnancy; however, if an internal fetal monitor has been inserted, it should be removed before use of electrical intervention.

From about 20 weeks until delivery, supine hypotension can occur from compression of the inferior vena cava, abdominal aorta, and pelvic veins by the gravid uterus. Cardiac output and venous return may be significantly reduced. Displacing the uterus laterally during chest compressions minimizes this effect and increases cardiac output; it may be all that is needed to restore maternal pulses. At gestation greater than 24 weeks, fetal viability and survival must be considered. Perimortem cesarean section (PMCS) promotes survival of the mother and fetus; however, there are few documented cases of maternal recovery with return to the preresuscitation state after cesarean delivery. After the need for perimortem cesarean section is determined, the procedure must be performed quickly, with a neonatal resuscitation team immediately available.

Perimortem Cesarean Section

The injured mother may require emergency delivery of a potentially viable fetus. Indications for cesarean delivery include fetal distress, placental abruption, uterine rupture, unstable pelvic or lumbosacral fracture during labor, or impending maternal death.

A PMCS is delivery of the neonate before maternal death. Fetal survival depends on the interval between maternal arrest and fetal delivery, gestational age, fetal condition, and cause of maternal arrest. Gestational age is best determined by LMP; however, measurement of fundal height can be used to estimate fetal age. A fundal height above the umbilicus suggests a viable fetus.

The interval between maternal arrest and fetal delivery is the most important factor predictive of fetal survival. Most infants that survive are delivered within 5 minutes of maternal arrest.[6] As the interval increases, neonatal survival decreases. PMCS should be initiated while maternal CPR is performed to ensure uteroplacental perfusion. The "4-minute rule" (that is, PMCS should be initiated within 4 minutes after maternal cardiac arrest and the infant delivered by the fifth minute) promotes best maternal and fetal outcome. Maternal recovery may occur after cesarean section secondary to release of aortocaval compression, increased cardiac output, and increased tissue perfusion. Two resuscitation teams should be in attendance, one for the mother and one for the infant.

Evidence of FHTs and viability are often considered as primary indications for PMCS; however, PMCS is sometimes completed in an attempt to resuscitate the mother even if the fetus is not viable. PMCS is recommended if maternal death is imminent, regardless of presence or absence of FHTs. After the uterus is emptied, there can be a 25% to 56% increase in maternal circulating blood volume. Releasing the weight of the gravid uterus off the maternal vena cava may restore maternal vital signs.

Neonatal Resuscitation

Emergency delivery of a neonate is performed because of maternal or fetal stress or both. Compromised fetal condition secondary to maternal arrest or other stressors may necessitate aggressive resuscitation. A neonatal team skilled in assessment and treatment of the newborn should be prepared with equipment necessary to resuscitate the fetus. Assessment and resuscitation should be performed simultaneously in a stepwise fashion. Drying, warming, positioning, suctioning, and providing tactile stimulation are the first interventions, required of all neonates. The apneic neonate will require positive-pressure ventilation with a bag-mask device. Oxygen is needed by a compromised neonate if central cyanosis is present. Chest compressions should be initiated when heart rate is absent or the neonate has a heart rate less than 60 beats/min after 30 seconds of adequate assisted ventilation. Intubation may be performed at various steps in the resuscitation effort; medication administration is the final phase of neonatal resuscitation, rarely needed by most newborns. Figure 29-3 summarizes neonatal resuscitation. Apgar scoring, an objective method of quantifying the newborn's condition based on the newborn's color, heart rate, reflex irritability, muscle tone, and respirations, is calculated at 1 minute after delivery and repeated at 5 minutes. Resuscitation should not be delayed awaiting the 1-minute Apgar score.

Patient Transport

Prehospital care and transport of the pregnant woman are influenced by several factors. As with any trauma patient, the initial focus is on spinal integrity, basic life support assessment, and emergency interventions. Supplemental oxygen benefits the mother and fetus because the pregnant woman is at higher risk for respiratory compromise than a nonpregnant woman and the fetus cannot tolerate hypoxia. Supplemental oxygen is required throughout transport until respiratory and circulatory status is thoroughly evaluated. Intravenous access is needed for fluid replacement to treat maternal hypovolemia and ensure uterine perfusion. To avoid serious maternal-fetal complications, appropriate maternal positioning during transport is vital. The lateral decubitus position is advocated to avoid aortocaval compression in gestation greater than 20 weeks. If spinal protection is needed, a cervical collar and backboard with a lateral tilt of 15 degrees should maintain spinal protection and minimize compression of the great vessels.

SUMMARY

Obstetric trauma, although rare, can be a catastrophic event. Two patients, the mother and the fetus, must be considered during assessment and treatment of the obstetric patient. Clinical management requires a team approach. The emergency physician, emergency nurse, trauma surgeon, obstetrician, perinatologist, labor and delivery nurse, and neonatal nurse may be key members of the trauma team during resuscitation of an obstetric trauma patient.

Optimal fetal outcomes are dependent on maternal survival. Aggressive resuscitation and stabilization of the mother promotes the best maternal and fetal outcomes. Concern for both maternal and fetal condition produces elevated stress levels in the patient and family. Keeping the family informed and providing emotional support for the patient and family is essential during trauma intervention.

Prevention efforts can decrease the incidence and severity of obstetric trauma. Public and private education about proper use of seat belts, accidental poisoning, and avoidance of overexertion during pregnancy can reduce maternal and fetal injury. Violence, especially intimate partner violence, should be assessed in the emergency department. Appropriate intervention may prevent a repeat attack and avoid

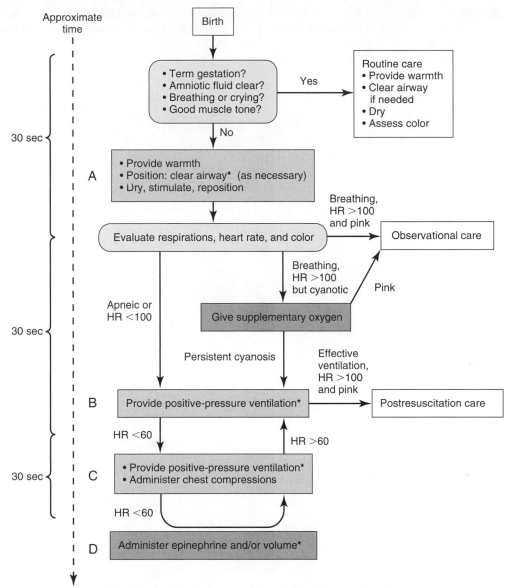

FIGURE **29-3.** Neonatal resuscitation flow diagram. (From 2005 American Heart Association guidelines for cardiopulmonary resuscitation and emergency cardiovascular care. XIII. Neonatal resuscitation guidelines, *Circulation* 112:IV188, 2005.)

maternal injury. Education and discharge teaching that fetal condition basically depends on maternal condition may help the mother choose actions that promote fetal well-being.

REFERENCES

1. Barraco R, Chiu W, Clancy T et al: *Practice management guidelines for the diagnosis and management of injury in the pregnant patient: the EAST management guidelines work group,* 2005, Eastern Association for the Surgery of Trauma (EAST). Retrieved July 13, 2007, from http://www.east.org.

2. Emergency Nurses Association: Special populations: pregnant, pediatric, and older adult trauma patients, In: *Trauma nursing core course provider manual,* ed 6, Park Ridge, Ill, 2007, The Association.

3. Dhanraj D, Lambers D: The incidences of positive Kleihauer-Betke test in low-risk pregnancies and maternal trauma patients, *Am J Obstet Gynecol* 190(5):1461, 2004.

4. *Domestic violence fact sheet.* Retrieved July 13, 2007, from http://www.athealth.com/consumer/disorders/DomViolFacts.html.

5. Knudson M, Paquin M, Rozycki GS: Reproductive system trauma. In Mattox KL, Feleciano DV, Moore EE, editors: *Trauma,* ed 5, New York, 2001, McGraw-Hill.

6. Kuo C, Jamieson D, McPheeters M et al: Injury hospitalizations of pregnant women in the United States, 2002, *Am J Obstet Gynecol* 196(2):161. el, 2007.

7. Muench MV, Baschat AA, Reddy UM et al: Kleihauer-Betke testing is important in all cases of maternal trauma, *J Trauma* 57(5):1094, 2004.

8. Murray M: *Antepartal and intrapartal fetal monitoring*, New York, 2007, Springer.

9. Sperry J, Casey B, McIntire D et al: Long term fetal outcomes in pregnant trauma patients, *Am J Surg* 192(6):715, 2006.

UNIT V

Medical and Surgical Emergencies

CHAPTER 30

Respiratory Emergencies

Paula Works and Sharon A. Graunke

Patients present to the emergency department (ED) with a variety of respiratory complaints. Their symptoms will range from mild to life threatening. It is crucial to recognize early warning signs of respiratory compromise and to intervene before further respiratory deterioration occurs.

This chapter will discuss the basic anatomy and physiology of the respiratory system, as well as frequent respiratory emergencies that occur in the adult population, including asthma, bronchitis, emphysema, pulmonary edema, pulmonary embolus, near-drowning, and spontaneous pneumothorax. Epiglottitis, bronchiolitis, and other respiratory emergencies seen more frequently in the pediatric population will be addressed in Chapter 47.

ANATOMY AND PHYSIOLOGY

The respiratory system can be divided into two parts: the upper airway and the lower airway. The upper airway includes the nasopharynx, oropharynx, and laryngopharynx. The structures within the upper airway are supported by cartilaginous rings to prevent collapse during respiration. Cartilaginous rings are replaced with smooth muscle fibers in the lower airways for stability and support. Connecting the upper and lower airways is the larynx, which acts as a gate to prevent aspiration. The lower airway comprises the larynx, trachea, bronchi, bronchioles, and alveoli. The functional unit of the pulmonary system is the alveolus, which interacts with adjacent capillaries to ensure oxygen transport from alveolus into blood.

Within the pleural cavity there is a negative intrathoracic pressure, which causes a vacuum effect, pulling air into the lungs during inspiration. During expiration, this negative pressure decreases and the air is passively expelled. During inspiration, air is filtered, warmed, and humidified as it travels through the upper and lower airways. Cilia, hairlike structures within the passageways, help to move air toward the alveoli. Cilia also help to move mucus and debris out of the pulmonary system, keeping the lower airways from being contaminated. The sterility of the lower airway is achieved with the help of mucus-secreting goblet cells. Mucus traps debris and keeps the airway moist. Gas exchange occurs in the alveoli and pulmonary capillaries. Oxygen and carbon dioxide are exchanged at this cellular level.

Cellular oxygenation is dependent upon several factors: (1) an adequate supply of oxygen carried to the cell, (2) the affinity of hemoglobin for oxygen, and (3) the ease with which hemoglobin releases oxygen to cells. The affinity of hemoglobin for oxygen is described by the oxygen-hemoglobin dissociation curve. If the curve shifts to the left, hemoglobin picks up oxygen more easily in the lungs but does not easily release oxygen to tissues. When the curve shifts to the right, oxygen uptake by hemoglobin is less rapid, but oxygen delivery to cells is easier. Oxygen dissociation is affected by temperature, acid-base balance, and carbon dioxide pressure (PCO_2) levels.

Normal gas exchange depends on adequate ventilation and perfusion. Respiration is divided into pulmonary ventilation, diffusion of oxygen and carbon dioxide across the alveolar capillary membrane, transport of oxygen and carbon dioxide to and from the cells, and regulation of ventilation. Ventilation refers to the mechanical flow of air into and out of the lungs. Respiration is the actual exchange of oxygen and carbon dioxide at the cellular level. Diffusion is a process in which particles in a fluid move from an area of higher concentration to an area of lower concentration, resulting in an even distribution of particles in the fluid. Perfusion relates to the transport of blood to the tissues. Ventilation/perfusion (V/Q) mismatch occurs when either ventilation or perfusion is inadequate. When there is an extreme imbalance, inadequately oxygenated blood is shunted into the arterial system.

PATIENT ASSESSMENT

When assessing a patient with a respiratory emergency, begin with airway patency. The patient must have a patent airway before proceeding. Once patency has been established, assess the patient's work of breathing, looking for nasal flaring, retractions, accessory muscle use, tracheal tugging, or dyspnea. Be alert to other signs of distress, including abnormal color such as pallor or cyanosis, grunting, difficulty speaking in complete sentences, tripod positioning, or decreased mental status. Changes in the patient's mental status can be an early warning sign of deterioration. Once airway, breathing, and circulation have been assessed, then perform a quick head-to-toe assessment. Listen for adventitious breath sounds, and obtain a full set of vital signs. While performing the assessment, observe the patient's appearance. Physical characteristics such as a barrel chest and club fingers are often associated with chronic obstructive pulmonary disease (COPD). Although these findings can be normal in some patients, they can also indicate cardiovascular abnormalities, valvular heart disease, or congenital defects.

The patient history should include when the symptoms began, what occurred just before the event, history of similar episodes, past medical history, any treatments that have been used before arrival, smoking history, orthopnea, and nocturnal dyspnea. Not every patient will be able to provide a history because of his or her degree of breathing difficulty. Observe for silent clues such as use of accessory muscles or leaning over a bedside table. While obtaining the history, inquire about occupational hazards the patient may have been exposed to such as asbestos, beryllium dust, bird droppings, coal dust, iron oxide, or silica dust. These agents are associated with the following lung diseases, respectively, asbestosis, berylliosis, bird handler's lung, black lung, siderosis, and silicosis.

If the patient smokes, determine how much the patient smokes and how long he or she has been smoking. Smoking decreases lung compliance because it damages the elastin and collagen fibers. Patients who smoke usually have a decreased sense of taste and smell along with increased secretions and cough. Cigarette smoke negatively affects the functions within the pulmonary system that are used to keep it clear. Smoking increases the likelihood of cancer, chronic bronchitis, emphysema, and the incidence of infection.

Patients who present with respiratory emergencies should be placed on a bedside monitor for continuous monitoring of oxygen saturation, cardiac rhythm, and vital signs. The patient's oxygen saturation will often be decreased in respiratory emergencies. Always treat the patient—do not rely simply on a number on the bedside monitor. Many factors (e.g., artificial fingernails, nail polish, and cold extremities) can skew the numbers displayed on the bedside monitor. If the patient is having difficulty breathing, administer oxygen using the device (e.g., nasal canula, nonrebreather, bag-mask device) that is most appropriate for the situation. Chest radiograph, complete blood count (CBC), and arterial blood gas (ABG) levels should be obtained.

SPECIFIC PULMONARY EMERGENCIES

Acute Bronchitis

Acute bronchitis is an inflammatory process that is usually caused by a virus. Some of the common offenders include influenza virus A or B, parainfluenza virus, respiratory syncytial virus, rhinovirus, Coxsackie virus, and adenovirus.[1] Acute bronchitis is more common during cold and flu season and does not have age boundaries. Secondary infections are possible from organisms such as *Mycoplasma pneumoniae*, *Haemophilus influenzae*, pneumococci, and streptococci. The highest incidence of acute bronchitis occurs in smokers, older adults, young children, and during the winter months. Patients complain of sore throat, stuffy nose, and cough. Initially the cough will be dry and nonproductive and may worsen at night. Aggravating factors include exposure to cold, talking, deep breathing, and laughing. After a few days the patient's cough usually becomes productive. Other symptoms can include low-grade fever, chest discomfort, and fatigue.

Diagnosis is based on the clinical presentation. Chest radiograph is needed to distinguish between acute bronchitis and pneumonia. Treatment of acute bronchitis includes increasing fluid intake, avoiding smoke or other irritants, cough preparations, and using a vaporizer to add moisture to the air. Antibiotics are not helpful except for secondary infections.

Pneumonia

Pneumonia is an inflammatory reaction usually caused by an acute bacterial, viral, or fungal infection. It may be preceded by an upper respiratory tract infection, ear infection, or eye infection. Pneumonia occurs primarily in young children, debilitated individuals, and those with an underlying chronic disease. It is the leading cause of death among older adults[4] and is the sixth leading cause of death in the United States.[1]

There are certain conditions that may lead to recurrent cases of pneumonia, including underlying cardiac or pulmonary disorder, compromised immune function, cystic fibrosis, esophageal abnormalities, bronchial obstruction, and bronchiectasis.[1] Patients who are immobile or bedridden and patients with rib fractures are at an increased risk. Other risk factors for pneumonia include smoking, steroids, immunosuppressive therapy, diabetes mellitus, and exposure to extreme changes in environmental temperature.

Patients present with complaints of fever, malaise, cough, hemoptysis, dyspnea, and pleuritic chest symptoms. On physical examination the patient will have crackles that do not clear with coughing, as well as consolidation. Older adult patients may not exhibit the classic symptoms of pneumonia. Instead, these patients may have a sudden mental status change.[1] Some patients with pneumonia experience abdominal distension, vomiting, and headache.

Treatment for patients with pneumonia includes humidified oxygen, antibiotics, and monitoring of fluid and electrolyte balance. Diagnostic assessment includes sputum culture and Gram stain, chest radiograph, and CBC. Pulse oximetry is obtained initially and monitored over time to determine changes in the patient's oxygenation. ABG values may be obtained as a baseline. Teaching should include the importance of pneumonia vaccinations to reduce the likelihood of future occurrences, as well as flu shots. Smoking cessation information should also be provided.

Hospital Core Measures for patients with community-acquired pneumonia (CAP) have been created by The Joint Commission as a means to improve patient outcome.[10] Each year, close to 3 million cases of CAP lead to physician visits, hospitalizations, and death.[10] *Streptococcus pneumoniae* is one of the leading infectious causes of illness and death for young children, those with chronic conditions, and older adults. Patients who present to the ED with symptoms suggestive of pneumonia need to have an oxygen assessment either via pulse oximetry or ABG measurement. Most often pulse oximetry is used because it is less invasive and more cost-effective. During triage the patient's pneumococcal vaccination and smoking history should be determined. Smoking cessation information should be provided to all patients with a smoking history. Blood cultures should be performed on all patients admitted with CAP before the first antibiotic dose, although this is still controversial. Antibiotic administration should not be delayed for blood cultures. Through the implementation of these core measures it has been found that those patients with CAP who receive antibiotics within 4 hours of arrival to the hospital have improved hospital course and 30-day mortality.[10]

Asthma

Asthma is an obstructive disease of the lungs characterized by airway inflammation and hyperreactivity. Symptoms can range from mild to severe. Asthma can be controlled, not cured, and has an unpredictable course with increasing prevalence and hospitalizations. The majority of asthmatic patients are children with males being affected more than females. Thirty percent of those diagnosed with asthma

during childhood will have it as adults. There is positive family history in more than one third of asthmatic patients.[3]

Airway inflammation and hyperresponsiveness occur in response to certain triggers (Box 30-1). Immunologic triggers cause a humoral immune response with complex multicellular activation, including mast cells, eosinophils, and immunoglobulin E (IgE) antibodies (Figure 30-1). Inflammatory mediators cause smooth muscle contraction, vasodilation, mucosal edema, increased mucus secretion, and macrophage eosinophil infiltration. Acetylcholine directly increases airway resistance and bronchial secretions. This cholinergic response further stimulates histamine and inflammatory mediator release, with the exception of IgE.

Nonimmunologic triggers stimulate the autonomic nervous system and cause mast cell and inflammatory mediator response. The pathway of emotional triggers is through the parasympathetic nervous system and stimulation of the hypothalamus. Aspirin sensitivity exacerbates asthma through reaction to prostaglandin synthesis. Exercise-induced asthma occurs after 10 to 20 minutes of vigorous exercise because of airway cooling secondary to decreased warming, reduced

BOX 30-1   TRIGGERS OF ACUTE ASTHMA ATTACKS

Allergen inhalation
  Animal dander
  House dust mite
  Pollens
  Molds
Air pollutants
  Exhaust fumes
  Perfumes
  Oxidants
  Sulfur dioxides
  Cigarette smoke
  Aerosol sprays
Viral upper respiratory infection
Sinusitis
Exercise and cold, dry air
Stress
Drugs
  Aspirin
  Nonsteroidal antiinflammatory drugs
  β-Adrenergic blockers
Occupational exposure
  Metal salts
  Wood and vegetable dusts
  Industrial chemicals and plastics
  Pharmaceutical agents
Food additives
  Sulfites (bisulfites and metabisulfites)
  Beer, wine, dried fruit, shrimp, processed potatoes
  Monosodium glutamate
  Tartrazine
Hormonesmenses
Gastroesophageal reflux
Emotional stress

From Lewis SM, Heitkemper MM, Dirksen SR: *Medical-surgical nursing: assessment and management of clinical problems,* ed 7, St. Louis, 2007, Mosby.

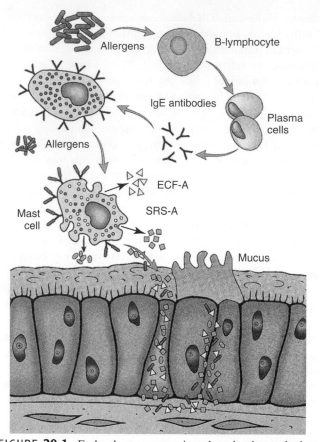

FIGURE 30-1. Early-phase response in asthma is triggered when an allergen or irritant cross-links immunoglobulin E receptors on mast cells, which are then activated to release histamine and other inflammatory mediators. *ECF-A,* Eosinophil chemotactic factor of anaphylaxis; *IgE,* immunoglobulin E; *SRS-A,* slow-reacting substance of anaphylaxis. (From Lewis SL, Heitkemper MM, Dirksen SR et al: *Medical-surgical nursing: assessment and management of clinical problems,* ed 7, St. Louis, 2007, Mosby.)

humidification, and increased respiratory rates. Exercise may be the only trigger for some patients and is usually limited to the early phase. Gastroesophageal (GE) reflux, a common condition associated with asthma, involves esophageal spasm with reflux of gastric acid causing spasm of nearby bronchial and esophageal structures.

Immunologic and nonimmunologic triggers cause increased mucus production, airway hyperresponsiveness, airway narrowing, and chronic inflammatory airway changes. These triggers can cause either an early or late response in asthmatic patients. Early-phase reactions involve rapid bronchospasms, whereas late-phase reactions involve inflammatory epithelial lesions, increased mucosal edema, and increased secretions. Complex interactions among lung cells cause a chronic inflammatory process that irritates airways. An acute exacerbation involves airway obstruction caused by spasms, inflammation, and mucus plugging.

There are no definitive tests to diagnose asthma. The diagnosis should be based on careful history, examination, and laboratory studies. The history should include symptoms, patterns, usual triggers, family history, and allergies the

patient may have. Physical examination may reveal upper airway rhinitis, sinusitis, or nasal polyps, as well as wheezes and prolonged expiratory phase. Laboratory studies should include CBC with differential, nasal smears, and sputum specimen. The CBC may have elevated eosinophils. There may be increased hilar or basilar infiltrates or areas of atelectasis secondary to mucus plugging and alveolar collapse on chest radiographs. To aid in the diagnosis of asthma, patients over the age of 5 years should have spirometry, which evaluates the air capacity of the lungs using a spirometer and measures the volume of air inhaled and exhaled. Spirometry can demonstrate obstruction and assess reversibility of airway narrowing. Peak expiratory flow rate (PEFR) is the greatest flow velocity produced during forced expiration after fully expanding lungs during inspiration. It is measured using a peak flowmeter. PEFR is used to monitor response to therapy in acute episodes but is not designed as a diagnostic tool.[8] PEFR measurement is effort dependent, so the results need to be duplicated.

The 2007 National Asthma Education and Prevention Program (NAEPP) *Expert Panel Report 3: Guidelines for the Diagnosis and Management of Asthma* expanded the 2002 guidelines and recommended some updates based on new evidence. There are new focus areas for monitoring asthma control and looking at impairment (i.e., the frequency and intensity of symptoms) and risk (i.e., the likelihood of exacerbations, progressive decline in lung function, or risk for adverse effects from the medication). There is a modification to the stepwise approach to long-term asthma management focusing on different age-groups. There is a new emphasis on patient education and control of environmental factors or comorbid conditions that affect asthma. There are also modifications to treatment strategies for managing asthma exacerbations, which include the following: simplifying the classification of severity of exacerbations; encouraging the development of prehospital protocols to allow administration of albuterol, oxygen, and with medical oversight, anticholinergics and oral systemic corticosteroids; adding levalbuterol; adding magnesium sulfate or heliox for severe exacerbations unresponsive to initial treatment; emphasizing oral corticosteroids; emphasizing that anticholinergics are used in emergency care, not hospital care; and considering initiation of inhaled corticosteroids at discharge.[7]

Inhaled allergens are common triggers, particularly for patients less than 30 years of age. For patients who have persistent asthma, skin testing to assess sensitivity to indoor allergens is recommended.[7] Although patients may have positive skin reactions to food allergens, these usually do not lead to acute exacerbations. In addition to inhaled allergens, other triggers such as occupational exposures, viral illnesses, and GE reflux can stimulate an asthma attack. Gastroesophageal reflux disease (GERD) is associated with nocturnal exacerbations that do not respond well to inhaled nebulizers. When GERD is suspected, a thorough gastrointestinal workup is indicated.

Occupational asthma initially presents with rhinitis or eye irritation along with evening or nocturnal cough. With prolonged exposure the patient will note increased symptoms, such as coughing, wheezing, and dyspnea. These symptoms will diminish with time away from exposure to irritants. Smokers have a higher incidence of occupational asthma because of increased airway irritation.

Clinical manifestations of asthma include cough, wheezing, prolonged expiratory time, and reduced peak expiratory flow. Patients may also experience increased work of breathing and accessory muscle use. When a patient presents to the ED with decreased air movement, low oxygen saturation, altered level of consciousness, and increased work of breathing, immediate interventions are required. These patients require high-flow oxygen and continuous pulse oximetry, along with nebulizer therapy, in an effort to provide some relief of symptoms. Close observation is required because their symptoms can lead to respiratory failure if rapid interventions are not provided. Severity can be assessed by determining type and frequency of home medications required to control symptoms, prior intubation, recent hospitalizations, spirometric indexes of air flow obstruction, nocturnal symptoms, and number of prior ED visits. ABG values initially indicate reduced arterial oxygen pressure (PaO_2) and arterial carbon dioxide pressure ($PaCO_2$) from hyperventilation. $PaCO_2$ eventually rises, which creates further V/Q mismatching.

Management goals are to maintain near-normal pulmonary function and exercise levels, prevent chronic symptoms and acute exacerbations, and avoid adverse effects of medications. Therapy includes objective measurement of lung function, environmental control, avoidance of triggers, select drugs, and comprehensive patient education.

PEFR provides objective data for management, documents personal best and daily variations, detects impending exacerbation, guides medicine therapy, and helps identify triggers. To correctly obtain peak expiratory flow measurements the patient should stand, if able, take a deep breath, and forcefully blow out all inspired air. The highest of three readings is recorded. A diary of peak expiratory flow measurements, along with documentation of viral infections, weather, medicine changes, environments, and other possible triggers aids in management of asthma.

Avoidance and environmental control of allergens such as dust mite antigens, animal dander, pollens, and molds can greatly reduce symptoms. Encasing pillows and mattresses in dust mite–proof covers, washing bedding every week in water temperatures greater than 130° F, and carpet removal or antimite treatment aid in the reduction of dust mites. Keep pets outside the house to decrease dander allergens, outdoor pollens, and mold. Asthma patients should remain inside with air conditioning during early morning and midday hours to further reduce exposure.

Drugs for asthma reduce bronchial spasms, airway inflammation, mucosal edema, and airway hyperreactivity. These medications can be given orally, intravenously, subcutaneously, or inhaled. There are several forms of inhaled therapy, such as nebulizers and inhalers (Table 30-1). Advantages of inhaled therapy include smaller drug amounts, rapid onset of action, direct delivery to respiratory system, fewer side effects, and painless, convenient administration.

Asthma exacerbation can be defined as an episode of progressively worsening shortness of breath, cough, wheezing, and chest tightness. The most severe exacerbations require admission to the intensive care unit for optimal monitoring and treatment. Special attention should be given to infants and those who are at increased risk for death associated with asthma.[7] Patients with a history of recent (within the last year) intubation or admission to the intensive care unit, two or more admissions to the hospital because of asthma exacerbation, three or more visits to the ED, or those who have been to the ED within the last month for asthma exacerbation are at an increased risk for death.[7] Patients who use more than two canisters of short-acting β_2-agonists (SABAs) per month are also at increased risk.[10] Other risk factors include low socioeconomic status, illicit drug use, major psychosocial problems, cardiovascular disease, chronic lung disease in addition to asthma, and chronic psychiatric disease.[7]

In the ED, patients with moderate to severe exacerbations will present with a variety of symptoms. The best way to determine the extent of the exacerbation is based upon objective measures such as lung function.[7] Objective measurements are a more reliable indicator of the severity than the symptoms alone.[7] Treatment options in the ED are aimed at relieving hypoxemia and airflow obstruction and decreasing airway inflammation. Some of these treatments include oxygen therapy, SABAs, and the addition of inhaled ipratropium bromide and systemic corticosteroids.[7] In addition, treatment options should look at adjunct therapy such as intravenous magnesium sulfate or heliox in those patients with severe exacerbation who are not responding to other treatment options[7] (Figure 30-2). Successfully relieving the exacerbation is the goal in the ED, but good follow-up care needs to be provided in an effort to prevent a relapse of the exacerbation. Patients should be instructed to have follow-up asthma care within 1 to 4 weeks along with specific instructions about any medications that are prescribed while in the ED.[7] Teaching should be done with regard to increasing medication or seeking medical care if the patient's symptoms become worse. Current guidelines also encourage that inhaler technique be reviewed and initiating inhaled corticosteroids should also be considered.

Chronic Obstructive Pulmonary Disease

COPD is a progressive and irreversible syndrome characterized by diminished inspiratory and expiratory capacity of the lungs. COPDs include emphysema and chronic bronchitis.[4] Almost every case of COPD is associated with a history of smoking, both active and passive. Cessation of smoking may prevent the development of COPD. There are four stages of COPD. Stage I is mild COPD. With this the patient may not even realize he or she has abnormal lung functioning. Stage II is considered moderate COPD. At this point the patient may seek treatment because of chronic respiratory symptoms and exertional dyspnea. With stage III the patient will have

Table 30-1.	Common Pulmonary Drugs		
Medication	**Actions**	**Strength/Dosage (Adults)**	**Side Effects/ Comments/Precautions**
BRONCHODILATORS	Stimulate β-receptors for bronchodilation		
Epinephrine (Adrenalin, Primatene Mist)	As above	IM or subcutaneous: 0.2-1 mg (0.2-1 mL) of 1:1,000 solution; may repeat every 20 min (maximum three doses) IV: 0.1-0.25 mg (1-2.5 mL) of 1:10,000 solution slowly Inhaler: 1-2 deep inhalations using a hand-bulb nebulizer q 3 hr as needed	Tremors, palpitations, increased blood pressure, headache, nervousness, dizziness, nausea
Racemic epinephrine	As above	2.25% solution Inhaled: 0.25-0.75 mL with 2-3 mL normal saline	Has half the cardiac effects of epinephrine
Terbutaline (Brethaire, Brethine)	As above	Subcutaneous: 0.25 mg; may repeat in 15-30 min; maximum 0.5 mg in 4 hr Oral: 2.5-5 mg 3 times a day; maximum 15 mg daily	
Long-Acting β₂-Agonists (LABAs)	Inhaled bronchodilators with a duration of at least 12 hr		
Salmeterol xinafoate (Serevent Diskus)	As above Can be used to prevent exercise-induced bronchospasm	50 mcg/blister; 1 puff q 12 hr or 30 min before exercise To prevent exercise-induced bronchospasm, give 30 min before exercise Do not use more than every 12 hr	Shaking, headache, nervousness, cough, runny or stuffed nose, dry mouth, sore throat, fast or pounding heartbeat Not for use during acute episodes
Formoterol (Foradil Aerolizer, Perforomist)	As above Can be used to prevent exercise-induced bronchospasm	12-mcg capsule for inhalation; one capsule q 12 hr via Aerolizer inhaler To prevent exercise-induced bronchospasm, give 30 min before exercise Do not use more than every 12 hr	Nervousness, headache, dry mouth, nausea, sore throat, difficulty falling or staying asleep, hoarseness, difficulty swallowing
Short-Acting β₂-Agonists (SABAs)	Inhaled bronchodilators that relax smooth muscles		Treatment of choice for relief of acute symptoms Can cause paradoxical bronchospasm
Albuterol (Proventil, Ventolin, Salbutamol)	As above	Nebulizer: 2.5 mg 3 times a day or 4 times a day Inhaler: 90-100 mcg per inhalation; 2 inhalations every 4-6 hr for acute episodes Tablets: 2-4 mg oral 3 times a day or 4 times a day	Uncontrollable shaking, nervousness, headache, nausea, vomiting, cough, throat irritation, fast or pounding heartbeat, chest pain
Levalbuterol (Xopenex, Xopenex HFA)	As above	Nebulizer: 0.63 mg-1.25 mg 3 times a day Inhaler: 2 inhalations (90 mcg) q 4-6 hr	Headache, dizziness, nervousness, shaking, heartburn, cough, vomiting, diarrhea, fever, chest pain, fast or pounding heartbeat

Table 30-1. Common Pulmonary Drugs—cont'd

Medication	Actions	Strength/Dosage (Adults)	Side Effects/ Comments/Precautions
Pirbuterol (Maxair Autoinhaler)	As above	Inhaler: 0.2 mg/metered dose; 1 or 2 inhalations every 4-6 hr; do not exceed 12 inhalations per day	Tremor, nervousness, dizziness, weakness, headache, nausea, diarrhea, cough, dry mouth, rapid or irregular heartbeat
Methylxanthines	Smooth muscle dilation, CNS stimulation, cerebral vasoconstriction, vasodilation of periphery and cardiac vessels, cardiac stimulation, diuresis		
Theophylline (100% theophylline) (Theolair, Theo-Dur, Elixophyllin, Slo-bid)	As above	Dosages vary based on whether patient is currently on a theophylline drug. Each 0.5 mg/kg of IV or oral theophylline will increase drug level by 1 mcg/mL	Nausea, abdominal pain, diarrhea, headache, restlessness, insomnia
Aminophylline (79% theophylline)	As above	Dosages vary based on whether patient is currently on aminophylline	Nausea, abdominal pain, diarrhea, headache, restlessness, insomnia
ANTICHOLINERGICS	Antimuscarinic action: block acetylcholine by occupying receptor sites and block PSNS bronchoconstriction effects, inhibit mast cell release (decreased mucus and chemotaxis), block cough receptors		
Atropine	As above	Nebulizer: 1-2.5 mg with normal saline; 3 or 4 times a day	Rarely used
Ipratropium (Atrovent, Atrovent HFA)	As above	17-18 mcg/metered dose; 2 inhalations 4 times a day; do not exceed 12 inhalations per day	Dizziness, nausea, heartburn, constipation, dry mouth, difficulty or pain with urinating, urinary frequency
CORTICOSTEROIDS	Decrease inflammation of inflamed epithelial cells in asthma		
Inhaled			Considered the most effective medications for long-term control of asthma
Dexamethasone (Decadron)	As above	Oral: 0.75-9 mg daily; IV/IM: 0.5-9 mg daily	Infection of the mouth, cough, hoarseness, headache
Beclomethasone (Beclovent, Vanceril)	As above	Inhaled: 40-80 mcg twice a day when used alone or 40-160 mcg twice a day when used with inhaled corticosteroids	Infection of the mouth, cough, hoarseness, headache
Flunisolide (AeroBid)	As above	Inhaler (CFC): 2 inhalations (total of 500 mcg) twice a day; maximum 8 inhalations per day. Inhaler (HFA): 2 inhalations (total of 160 mcg); maximum 320 mcg twice daily	Infection of the mouth, cough, hoarseness, headache

(Continued)

Table 30-1.	COMMON PULMONARY DRUGS—CONT'D		
Medication	**Actions**	**Strength/Dosage (Adults)**	**Side Effects/ Comments/Precautions**
Fluticasone propionate (Flovent Diskus, Flovent HFA)	As above	Flovent Diskus inhaled: 500-1000 mcg twice a day Flovent HFA inhaled: 88-440 mcg twice a day	Infection of the mouth, cough, hoarseness, headache
Triamcinolone (Azmacort)	As above	75 mcg/spray Inhaler: 2 inhalations 3 or 4 times a day; maximum 16 inhalations per day	Infection of the mouth, cough, hoarseness, headache
Oral			
PrednisolonePrednisolone sodium phosphate (Orapred, Pediapred, Prelone)		Prednisolone oral: 2.5-15 mg 2-4 Prednisolone sodium phosphate oral: 4-60 mg daily	Euphoria, insomnia, seizures, heart failure, arrhythmias, peptic ulcers, pancreatitis, menstrual irregularities, growth suppression in children, adrenal insufficiency, hyperglycemia, hypokalemia, hirsutism
Prednisone (Winpred, Liquid Pred)		Oral: 5-60 mg daily	Euphoria, insomnia, seizures, heart failure, arrhythmias, peptic ulcers, pancreatitis, menstrual irregularities, growth suppression in children, adrenal insufficiency, hyperglycemia, hypokalemia, hirsutism
ANTIASTHMATICS	Inhibit mast cell degranulation— block release of chemical mediators of inflammation		
Cromolyn sodium (Intal)	As above	Inhaler: 3-4 times per day; may take within 1 hr before activities to prevent exercise-induced asthma	Sore throat, bad taste in mouth, abdominal pain, cough, itchy or burning nasal passages, sneezing, headache May take up to 4 weeks to work
LEUKOTRIENE MODIFIERS	Interfere with the pathway of leukotrienes (inflammatory mediators of bronchoconstriction and airway inflammation)		
Montelukast (Singulair)	As above	Oral: 10 mg once daily in the evening	Headache, dizziness, heartburn, abdominal pain, fatigue
Zafirlukast (Accolate)	As above	Oral: 20 mg twice a day taken 1 hr before or 2 hr after meals	Headache, nausea, loss of appetite, excessive fatigue, itching, yellowing of sclera, rash
Zileuton (Zyflo CR)	As above	Oral: 1200 mg (2 tabs) twice a day	Headache, nausea, heartburn, vomiting, constipation, nervousness, insomnia
IMMUNOMODULATORS	Prevent binding of IgE to the high-affinity receptors on basophils and mast cells		Be prepared and equipped to identify and treat anaphylaxis should it occur

Table 30-1.	COMMON PULMONARY DRUGS—CONT'D		
Medication	Actions	Strength/Dosage (Adults)	Side Effects/Comments/Precautions
Omalizumab (anti-IgE) (Xolair)	Monoclonal antibody	Subcutaneous: 150-375 mg every 2-4 weeks	Pain, redness, swelling, etc. at the injection site; joint pain; fatigue; ear pain Divide doses larger than 150 mg into more than one injection site
HELIOX	Heliox is less dense than air, allowing molecules to diffuse faster than through an oxygen-nitrogen mixture; air flow is less turbulent and work of breathing decreases	Can be given by high-flow nasal cannula, hood, or face mask	Mixture of helium and oxygen There are no contraindications to the administration of heliox
MAGNESIUM SULFATE	Inhibits smooth muscle contraction; decreases histamine release; inhibits acetylcholine release	Varies by practitioner	IV magnesium sulfate seems to be effective for patients with severe asthma—no benefit has been found for those with mild or moderate asthma

Data from Doyle RM, editor: *Nursing 2008 drug handbook*, ed 28, Philadelphia, 2008, Wolters Kluwer/Lippincott Williams & Wilkins; and MedlinePlus: *Drugs and supplements.* Retrieved January 2008 from http://www.nlm.nih.gov/medlineplus/druginfo/medmaster.
CFC, Chlorofluorocarbon; *CNS,* central nervous system; *HFA,* hydrofluoroalkane (an environmentally friendly propellant); *IM,* intramuscular; *IV,* intravenous; *PSNS,* parasympathetic nervous system.

increased shortness of breath and reduced exercise capacity, and the quality of life may be affected because of repeated exacerbations. Stage IV is very severe COPD. There are serious airway limitations at this point. The quality of life is greatly affected, and exacerbations of COPD may be life threatening.

When patients present to the ED, it is important to differentiate between other possible causes of respiratory difficulty. Differential diagnoses for COPD include asthma, congestive heart failure, bronchiectasis, tuberculosis, obliterative bronchiolitis, or diffuse panbronchiolitis. Patients with an acute exacerbation of COPD will complain of worsening dyspnea, an increase in sputum production, and an increase in sputum purulence. Typically patients with COPD will have a barrel chest, chronic cough, distant breath sounds, and tachypnea. During times of acute exacerbation these patients may also have an upper respiratory infection, fever, wheezing, tachycardia, and tachypnea.[3]

On physical examination, rhonchi and/or wheezes may be noted. If the patient has an acute infection, crackles may be present. Note the patient's respiratory pattern and work of breathing. Signs of distress include pursed lips, nostril flaring, and use of accessory muscles. The patient may want to lean or sit forward to help his or her work of breathing.

Sometimes these patients will be referred to as "blue bloaters" or "pink puffers." With the "blue bloater," chronic bronchitis is the more dominant disease process. These patients appear edematous and cyanotic. They have increased mucus production and inflammation from bronchitis and panlobular emphysema. Decrease in ventilation and increase in cardiac output cause a V/Q mismatch, which leads to polycythemia

and hypoxemia. "Pink puffers" are markedly dyspneic and have a pink skin color. Alveolar cell destruction decreases oxygen exchange; however, the body compensates with hyperventilation and decreased cardiac output. "Pink puffers" have highly oxygenated blood with decreased cardiac output.

COPD patients are taught how to manage their disease at home. These patients must avoid irritants and practice good bronchial hygiene, which includes adequate hydration, humidification, and postural drainage. These patients routinely use bronchodilators, expectorants, and mucolytics to control their symptoms.[7] Anticholinergic bronchodilators may have better results than intermittent nebulizer treatments for these patients. Corticosteroids are used sparingly, although infections should be treated aggressively. Viral and bacterial infections play a major role in exacerbations of COPD and contribute to disability. Patients should receive influenza and pneumococcal vaccines. Changes in cough and sputum production and characteristics require prompt antibiotic therapy. Proper education, patient compliance, adequate nutrition, and exercise are important parts of therapy.

In advanced disease, chronic respiratory failure with severe hypoxemia and hypercapnia are present; serum carbon dioxide levels no longer provide the drive for respiration. Hypoxia, or low serum oxygen, becomes the drive for respiration. Chronic oxygen delivery is necessary if PaO_2 falls below 55 mm Hg. Management in the ED includes oxygen therapy, nebulized medications, bronchodilators, and steroids. Low-flow oxygen may be administered with nasal cannula or Venturi mask. High-flow oxygen should not be withheld when the patient is in respiratory failure.

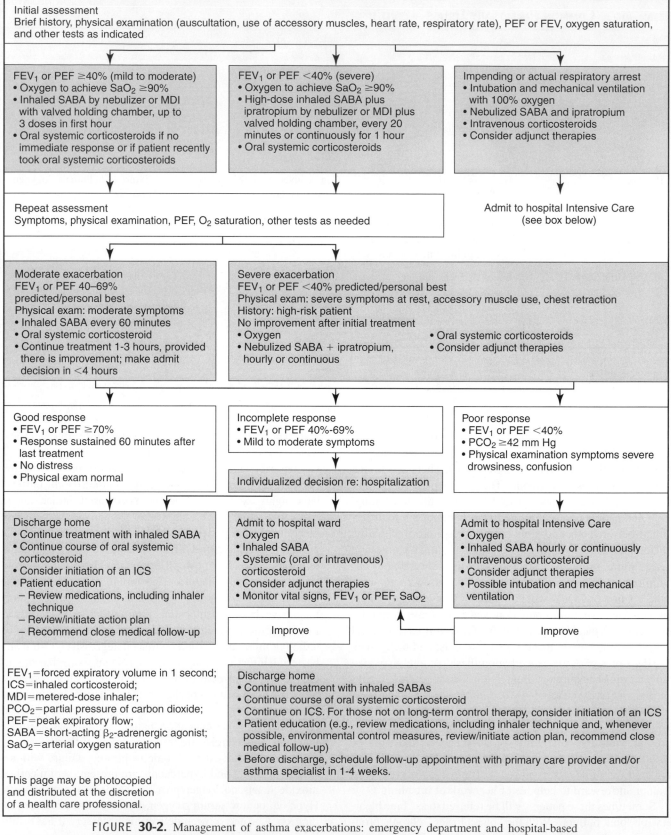

FIGURE **30-2.** Management of asthma exacerbations: emergency department and hospital-based care. (From Cydulka RK: Managing acute exacerbations and influencing future outcomes in the emergency department: update on the 2007 National Asthma Education and Prevention Program guidelines, *ACEP News,* p 1, 2007.)

Emphysema

Emphysema is the permanent abnormal enlargement of the respiratory tract distal to the terminal bronchioles and associated destructive changes of the alveolar wall.[1] The pathologic changes leading to alveolar destruction are associated with the release of proteolytic enzymes from inflammatory cells.[1] Alveolar damage results from inflammation of the parenchyma and the inactivation of α_1-antitrypsin. α_1-Antitrypsin protects the lung parenchyma. With the loss of alveolar walls, there is also a marked reduction in the pulmonary capillary bed, which is essential for exchange of oxygen and carbon dioxide between the alveolar air and capillary blood. The loss of elastic tissue within the lung leads to diminished smaller bronchioles. Increased pressure around the outside of the airway lumen leads to increased airway resistance and decreased airflow.

Within a person's lungs there are 25,000 acini, airways that are distal to the terminal bronchiole, and 3 million alveoli. There are three categories of emphysema, which are dependent on the area of lung tissue involved, including centrilobular, panlobular, and bullous. Centrilobular emphysema involves the upper lung fields and occurs in the center of lobules, corresponding to the enlargement of the respiratory bronchioles. It is associated with chronic bronchitis. Centrilobular emphysema rarely occurs in nonsmokers. Panlobular emphysema is less common, associated more with familial α_1-antiprotease deficiency.[1] Panlobular emphysema occurs primarily in lower and anterior fields and is not directly associated with cigarette smoking. Entire acini and many bullae (airspaces less than 1 mm in diameter in distended state) are involved. Bullous emphysema is characterized by isolated emphysemic changes within the bullae without generalized emphysema.

There is a direct correlation between smoking, chronic bronchitis, and emphysema, but it should be noted that not all smokers develop emphysema. Genetic or familial trait may predispose patients to this disease process. A small minority of patients have a genetic deficiency of serum α_1-antiprotease or α_1-antitrypsin, which inhibits protease that digests proteins such as elastin and collagen fibers of the lung. Protease is found in macrophages and polymorphonuclear leukocytes during inflammatory processes. The inhibitors are inactivated by irritants such as smoke and pollutants.

The end result is destruction of elastic properties of the lung and loss of natural recoil and support. During expiration, increased intrathoracic pressure causes collapse with premature closure of airways, whereas decreased support of the lung causes large residual volumes and decreased flow rates. Inspiratory rates are normal unless there is airway obstruction from chronic bronchitis, air trapping, and overdistended airspaces. Eventually the area for gas exchange at the alveolar capillary membrane decreases because of destruction of the alveolar wall causing V/Q mismatch with patchy emphysemic changes, increased physiologic dead space, and abnormal ABG values.

Patients may exhibit signs of chronic bronchitis in the beginning of the disease process. There will be exertional dyspnea that slowly progresses to dyspnea at rest. Primary emphysema presents with dyspnea. There is no associated cough or sputum production. The severity of dyspnea does not correlate with severity of destructive changes within the lung. Increasing dyspnea indicates increasing airway obstruction. As the disease progresses, there may be structural changes that become evident such as an increased anteroposterior diameter of the chest, dorsal kyphosis, elevated ribs, flare at the costal margin, and widening of the costal angle. Upon auscultation, diminished breath sounds and expiratory wheezes will be noted, as well as hyperresonance. Radiography will reveal hyperinflation of the lungs. Other evidence of emphysema includes decreased vascular markings, hyperlucency, and deeper space between the sternum and heart. Pulmonary function tests reveal hyperinflation, increased residual volume, reduced vital capacity, and increased total lung capacity with decreased expiratory flow rates.[1] Emphysema may be differentiated from asthma or bronchitis because of the reduction in diffusion capacity. ABG values may be normal in mild cases of emphysema with the exception of decreased PaO_2. As the disease progresses, $PaCO_2$ becomes elevated.

Treatment regimens for patients with emphysema include the use of bronchodilators. Inhaled sympathomimetics and ipratropium bromide are the treatment of choice. Patients need to practice good bronchial hygiene to mobilize secretions. All patients should be encouraged to stop smoking. Smoking cessation programs should be offered to patients at each visit. In addition, with each visit question the patient about smoking habits and evaluate his or her readiness to stop. Patients should be encouraged to participate in graded aerobic exercise. Abdominal diaphragmatic breathing exercises with pursed-lip breathing will improve muscle conditioning for breathing and promote exhalation of more air from the lungs. All patients with emphysema should avoid pollution and irritants—especially cigarette smoke. As the disease progresses, the patient may need home oxygen therapy during exercise, only at nighttime, or for continuous use. During times of exacerbation the patient should be managed in the ED with continuous pulse oximetry, oxygen therapy, bronchodilators, and steroids. Any patient with decreased oxygen saturation should receive a high triage priority and have treatment initiated immediately.

Chronic Bronchitis

Chronic bronchitis is a COPD of the larger airways. It is most often associated with cigarette smoking but has been associated with other environmental pollutants.[2] Inflammation of the bronchial mucous membranes causes increased mucus production and is a direct result of various irritants such as cigarette smoke, fumes, and dust. This increased mucus production leads to swelling and enlargement of the submucosal glands and may result in obstruction of the airways.

Chronic bronchitis is diagnosed when the patient has a productive cough lasting at least 3 consecutive months annually for at least 2 years.[3] This disease is most often diagnosed in patients from 40 to 55 years of age.[4] Patients with chronic bronchitis will often have a hacking cough, rhonchi that clear with coughing, barrel chest, and prolonged expiration. As the disease progresses, patients will exhibit wheezing and dyspnea at rest. Patients generally will not seek treatment until they have difficulty breathing or notice increased sputum production, which can vary in color.

When assessing patients with chronic bronchitis, elicit a history from them regarding how they function at home, issues with fatigue, sleep patterns, and sleep positions. Patients may sleep in an upright position for comfort. On examination, patients may be using accessory muscles and appear cyanotic.[9] These patients are often referred to as "blue bloaters." As the disease progresses, patients will retain carbon dioxide. If their $PaCO_2$ levels are too high, patients may be confused and complain of a headache and light sensitivity. Patients with chronic bronchitis may have peripheral edema and jugular vein distention. Adventitious lung sounds such as scattered crackles and wheezing will be present, as well as a prolonged expiration. In the late stages, chest radiography will reveal hyperinflation of the lungs.

Interventions include low-flow oxygen therapy, bronchodilators, and possibly steroids. If patients are on home oxygen therapy, remind them of the dangers of smoking near oxygen. Antibiotics may be given if there is an infection present. It is important to discuss smoking cessation with these patients.

Pulmonary Embolus

A pulmonary embolus (PE) is an undissolved piece of material that occludes a vessel and obstructs the circulation distally. Approximately 10% of patients with a fatal PE die within 1 hour after symptoms begin. About 650,000 patients will be diagnosed with PE annually. PE is commonly underdiagnosed.

Generally the presenting symptoms will depend on the size of the blockage. They can be nonspecific and lead the emergency nurse to think of other causes. The most common symptom is dyspnea. Patients may also exhibit tachycardia, tachypnea, signs of restlessness, apprehension, and anxiety. Patients may complain of sudden shortness of breath and severe chest pain. The pain may worsen with inspiration. On examination the patient may be diaphoretic and have crackles on auscultation. The patient may also complain of cough, hemoptysis, fever, or syncope. Petechiae may be seen on the patient's chest wall; this is most likely associated with fat emboli (commonly associated with long-bone fractures). If the embolism occludes a large vessel, symptoms may be more severe and include hypotension and signs of right ventricular failure. The diagnosis of PE can be quite challenging because the clinical presentation is often nonspecific.

Approximately 90% of pulmonary thromboemboli originate in the deep veins of the legs. The most common risk factors for a venous thromboembolus include immobility, trauma, surgery, long-bone fractures, pregnancy, cancer,

heart failure, and estrogen use. It is also seen with obesity, decreased peripheral circulation, congestive heart failure, and thrombophlebitis. Sometimes congestive heart failure or myocardial infarction can lead to pulmonary emboli.

Stasis of blood, damage to epithelium of the vessel wall, and alterations in coagulation, known as Virchow's triad, can lead to formation of venous thrombi. An embolus becomes dislodged and travels through the venous system and through the right side of the heart, finally lodging in a pulmonary vessel, obstructing blood flow, and decreasing perfusion to a portion of the lungs. If the embolism lodges in a large pulmonary vessel, pulmonary vascular resistance increases and cardiac output is decreased. The embolism causes the body to respond by releasing serotonin, histamine, prostaglandins, and catecholamines, which trigger bronchospasms and vasoconstriction. The production of surfactant ceases, and alveoli collapse.

There are no simple diagnostic tests for a PE. To determine if there is a V/Q mismatch, a V/Q scan or spiral (also called helical) computed tomography (CT) scan will be performed. A diagnosis of PE is confirmed if there is adequate ventilation with impaired blood flow to the pulmonary vasculature on the V/Q scan or if there is a filling defect in the pulmonary arterial tree on the spiral CT scan. Additional tests include ABG measurement, 12-lead electrocardiogram (ECG), chest radiograph, and cardiac enzymes. Laboratory studies are completed to rule out other possible causes. The chest radiograph may be normal. The 12-lead ECG will have nonspecific T wave and ST segment changes along with T-wave inversion. Additional ECG changes include new-onset right bundle branch block and right axis deviation with peaked P waves in limb leads and depressed T waves in right precordial leads (V_1 to V_3). The ABG values will have decreased PaO_2 and $PaCO_2$. The only conclusive test for PE is pulmonary arteriography. This invasive procedure is usually reserved for last. Duplex ultrasonography of both lower extremities should be completed.

Patients who present to the ED with these clinical symptoms should have continuous cardiac monitoring and supplemental oxygen therapy. Analgesics may be given for patient comfort. Intravenous fluids and vasopressors should be used to maintain pressure. Once a diagnosis is made, intravenous anticoagulants are initiated to prevent further clot formation. Weight-based heparin protocols or home therapy with low-molecular-weight heparin are the preferred anticoagulant options for these patients. If there are no contraindications, fibrinolytic therapy (urokinase or tissue plasminogen activator) should be started immediately in the unstable patient and should be considered in the ED for any patient with a diagnosed pulmonary embolus. Surgical intervention may be necessary and may include an embolectomy or placement of an inferior vena caval umbrella filter.

Pulmonary Edema

Pulmonary edema is not a primary disease process, but rather the result of an acute event. Pulmonary edema is a life-threatening complication that is manifested by severe dyspnea, diaphoresis, hypertension, tachycardia, anxiety, and tachypnea. Many times the patient will have pink, frothy sputum production.

There are two types of pulmonary edema: cardiogenic and noncardiogenic. Cardiogenic pulmonary edema occurs when there is inadequate left ventricular pumping, which leads to increased fluid pressure. Increased left ventricular pressure inhibits left atrial emptying, blood backs up into alveolar-capillary membranes, and pulmonary capillary filtration increases. Fluid from the pulmonary circulation floods the alveolar-capillary membrane and fills alveolar spaces that normally contain air. The end result is increased fluid in the lungs. Potential causes of cardiogenic pulmonary edema include acute coronary syndromes and heart failure.

Noncardiogenic pulmonary edema is the result of primary damage to the alveolar-capillary membrane. Loss of integrity increases membrane permeability, which causes fluid and protein accumulation in interstitial spaces that eventually flood the alveoli, causing significant fluid accumulation in the lungs. Acute respiratory distress syndrome (ARDS) is a cause of noncardiogenic pulmonary edema that results from acute lung injury. Damage to the alveolar epithelium and pulmonary vasculature leads to edema from an increased capillary permeability.[5] The patient with ARDS will have decreased lung compliance, refractory hypoxemia, severe acute respiratory distress, and pulmonary parenchymal consolidations. There are three stages of ARDS.[3] Stage I occurs immediately after the initial injury. During this time there will be pulmonary capillary congestion, endothelial cell swelling, and extensive microatelectasis.[3] During stage II, days 1 to 5 following initial injury, airspace ossification begins and progresses to a uniform appearance on chest radiograph. Stage III is characterized by hyperplasia of type II alveolar cells and collagen deposition. The overall mortality rate associated with ARDS is approximately 50%.[5] There are a multitude of conditions such as trauma, sepsis, and fluid overload that predispose patients to ARDS.

Excessive extracellular fluid volume can result in pulmonary edema as increased pressure at the arterial capillary membranes pushes fluid into surrounding tissues. Fluid shifts across the alveolar-capillary membrane into the alveoli, resulting in pulmonary edema. Fluid overload inhibits left ventricular pumping, and excess fluid backs up into the left atrium with the same effect as cardiogenic pulmonary edema. Excessive fluid volume may be caused by increased sodium intake such as with packaged foods, abuse of tap water enemas, or overload of intravenous fluids high in sodium. Renal disorders and cirrhosis can also cause fluid overload.

Patients with pulmonary edema exhibit cardiovascular and respiratory symptoms. Cardiovascular symptoms result from generalized fluid overload. Poor left ventricular function is generally followed by poor right ventricular function, leading to heart failure with engorged neck veins, sacral edema when the patient is sitting with legs not in a dependent position, lower extremity pitting edema, weight gain, rapid and bounding pulse, and S_3 and S_4 heart sounds. If the condition is left untreated, the pulse will become weak and thready. The skin is cool, pale, and moist and may appear cyanotic or mottled in some patients. Blood pressure initially increases in an attempt to pump the excess fluid but decreases as the condition worsens.

Respiratory symptoms occur because increased alveolar fluid impairs oxygen exchange across the alveolar-capillary membrane. The patient develops dyspnea, and respiratory rate increases in an effort to increase oxygenation. Increased respiratory rate decreases PCO_2, causing respiratory alkalosis. As the condition worsens, metabolic acidosis occurs in an effort to rid the body of metabolic waste products. Respiratory effort becomes labored as the patient tires from the effort of breathing. Fluid in the lungs causes crackles and productive cough with frothy, white sputum. Sputum can have a pink tinge in fulminate pulmonary edema. Cyanosis may be present, and oxygen saturation decreases as hypoxia increases. Bronchospasms may develop, causing wheezing, crackles, and rhonchi. Chest radiographs usually show bilateral interstitial and alveolar infiltrates. The left ventricular wall is usually enlarged, which gives the heart a water-bottle shape.

Treatment focuses on improving oxygenation through administration of high-flow oxygen, improving cardiac function, and decreasing cardiac workload. Bronchodilators may be given via aerosol inhalation treatments to decrease bronchospasms. Positive end-expiratory pressure is indicated when hypoxia continues despite aggressive oxygen therapy. Most patients with hypoxemia refractory to maximum ventilation have a poor prognosis because of secondary multiple-system organ failure.

Heart rate increases in an attempt to manage excess fluid; however, this leads to decreased filling time and decreased contractility. Digoxin is given via intravenous push to increase contractility and decrease heart rate. Dobutamine is given intravenously to increase contractility and reduce peripheral vascular resistance. Dopamine is indicated for hemodynamically significant hypotension, whereas nitroprusside is used to decrease afterload by vasodilation. Cardiac workload is also decreased through diuretic therapy (e.g., furosemide, bumetanide) and positioning the patient in high-Fowler's position with legs dependent. Dependent-leg position results in venous distension in lower extremities or pooling of blood, which decreases circulatory volume. Intravenous morphine causes vasodilation, which increases venous pooling and decreases preload. Preload is the result of blood volume in the left ventricle. In pulmonary edema, treatment is given to decrease volume so backflow into the atria is decreased and to increase strength of contraction by preventing overstretch of muscle fibers (Starling's law). Nitroglycerin may be administered to increase venous distension and venous pooling, which decreases blood return to the heart. Other interventions include using a urinary catheter to monitor urine output and the effects of diuretics.

Lung Transplants

Lung transplants are given to people as a last resort treatment for irreversible lung failure. Lung failure occurs when the lungs are no longer able to exchange oxygen and carbon dioxide. Lung transplant patients now have longer survival rates and are more likely to seek emergency care. The most common complications include pleural space complications, pulmonary parenchymal complications, opportunistic infections, and immunosuppression-induced complications. Early postoperative complications of the pleural space include pneumothorax or hemothorax. Other complications include chylothorax and empyema. At any time the patient may present with an episode of acute rejection or a pulmonary embolism. Opportunistic infections can be caused by bacterial, viral, mycotic, or parasitic organisms, and antibiotics should be started as soon as possible in the ED. Other complications may be related to the patient's chronic medication regimen. Transplant patients presenting to the ED have an increased risk for infection because of their immunocompromised state and should be placed in protective precautions (positive-pressure-flow environment is essential) while in the ED.

Spontaneous Pneumothorax

Spontaneous pneumothorax may occur with or without an underlying pulmonary condition. Primary spontaneous pneumothorax occurs in individuals who do not have known pulmonary disease, whereas a secondary spontaneous pneumothorax occurs in those with a history of pulmonary conditions, such as COPD or pulmonary fibrosis. Generally, primary spontaneous pneumothorax occurs in males 20 to 40 years of age who are tall and thin. Older males will more likely experience a secondary spontaneous pneumothorax. Smokers have an increased risk for developing a spontaneous pneumothorax. With spontaneous pneumothorax the cause is usually rupture of an apical, subpleural emphysematous bleb. Iatrogenic pneumothorax can result from invasive procedures, such as insertion of a subclavian catheter or transthoracic needle aspiration, or from trauma secondary to mechanical ventilation and cardiopulmonary resuscitation.

Patients with a pneumothorax experience dyspnea and chest pain on the affected side. The larger the pneumothorax, the more acute the symptoms will be. With a larger pneumothorax there may be subcutaneous emphysema noted, as well as cyanosis, hypotension, and severe dyspnea. Monitor the patient's oxygen saturation closely. Interventions are based upon the clinical presentation and the degree of collapse. Asymptomatic patients with less than 15% pneumothorax may be observed on an inpatient or outpatient basis. Other treatment options include needle aspiration and tube thoracostomy. These patients are more likely to return to the ED for the same complaint.

Inhalation Injury

There are three factors to be considered when evaluating a patient who has suffered an inhalation injury: exposure to asphyxiants (or asphyxiation), thermal or heat injury, and smoke poisoning (or pulmonary irritation). Exposure to asphyxiants is the most frequent cause of early mortality. Carbon monoxide (CO) is the most frequent asphyxiant from a fire.

Carbon Monoxide Poisoning

Hemoglobin has a greater affinity for CO than for oxygen, resulting in oxygen being displaced from the hemoglobin. This displacement leads to hypoxia within the tissues. Carboxyhemoglobin (COHb) levels greater than 10% indicate CO exposure. Smokers or individuals exposed to automobile exhaust can have baseline COHb levels of 10% to 15%. Fetal hemoglobin binds even more quickly with CO, so a fetus is at greater risk for injury from CO poisoning. As the COHb levels increase, symptoms worsen. Patients whose COHb levels are 5% to 10% may complain of a mild headache or vertigo. COHb levels of 10% to 20% cause headache, nausea, vomiting, loss of coordination, and dyspnea, and the patient may appear flushed. At 20% to 30% patients will be confused and lethargic; they may also complain of visual disturbances. Cardiac complications include ST depression due to profound myocardial hypoxia. With COHb levels of 40% to 60% the patient may be comatose, have seizures, or ectopy may be noted on the cardiac monitor. COHb levels above 60% are incompatible with life. Pulse oximetry readings may be deceiving because the oximeter cannot distinguish between oxygenated hemoglobin and carboxyhemoglobin. Hyperbaric oxygen therapy may need to be considered for patients with COHb levels above 25% to 30%.

An additional consideration with CO poisoning is the potential for exposure to other asphyxiants. For example, cyanide can be produced with combustion of wool, silk, paper products, rubber, plastics, and polyurethane; the risk for exposure to these increases when in a confined space. Cyanide impedes cellular metabolism, causing anaerobic metabolism resulting in lactic acidosis and decreased oxygen consumption. Clinical presentation of cyanide poisoning may include multiple symptoms because cyanide inhalation affects the respiratory, cardiovascular, and central nervous systems. Treatment in the ED will include administration of a cyanide antidote containing amyl nitrate, sodium nitrate, and thiosulfate or use of the newer Cyanokit.

Thermal or Heat Injury

Unless the cause of heat injury is from steam, explosive or volatile gases, or hot liquid aspiration, it is rare to have heat injury below the oropharyngeal airway. The respiratory tract's ability to efficiently exchange heat, combined with closure of the glottis, protects lower airways from extreme heat. Extreme heat on the upper airway initially causes erythema, edema, and blisters of the mucosa. These patients should be closely monitored for the first 24 to 48 hours after injury because the airway can become obstructed from increasing mucosal edema.

Smoke Poisoning

Inhalation of toxic gases, such as hydrogen chloride, phosgene, ammonia, and sulfur dioxide define smoke poisoning. These toxins damage pulmonary endothelial cells and destroy epithelial cilia, leading to mucosal edema. Surfactant production decreases, followed by atelectasis. Pulmonary edema can develop within 24 to 48 hours of the initial injury. Interventions for these patients include humidified oxygen, vigorous pulmonary toilet, and bronchodilators. Intubation and mechanical ventilation may be necessary to maintain airway patency should severe pulmonary edema occur.

When assessing patients with a potential inhalation injury it is crucial to obtain a detailed history. Determine if the patient was in an enclosed space, how long the patient was exposed to toxic gases, and what was the general environment where the incident occurred. Mortality increases with age and physical and cognitive disabilities, so it is crucial to obtain a detailed medical history. Initial interventions include protecting and maintaining a patent airway while supporting the patient's hemodynamic status. Patients with carbonaceous sputum, singed facial or nasal hair, or burns of the neck or face should be carefully evaluated for inhalation injury. Hoarseness, wheezing, dyspnea, and restlessness may also be present. These patients may require early intubation to maintain the airway before excessive edema occurs. Patients with smoke poisoning should be placed on 100% oxygen. COHb half-life is 320 minutes on room air. This time can be cut to 75 to 80 minutes with administration of 100% oxygen and approximately 20 minutes in a hyperbaric chamber.

Foreign Body Aspiration

Foreign body aspiration can have a variety of presentations. It most often occurs in children and older adults. With children, coins are the most frequent culprit. Foreign body aspiration in the upper airway will present with obvious clinical symptoms and may be immediately life threatening. When a foreign body is aspirated into the lower airways, the presentation can vary. Commonly there will be a new onset of sudden coughing, gagging, and choking. Unless the airway is completely obstructed, the patient may become asymptomatic for a period of time.

The treatment depends on the severity of the case. If there is foreign body occlusion of the upper airway, follow basic life support (BLS) measures in an attempt to clear the airway. If BLS measures fail to clear the airway, then direct visualization with a laryngoscope should be performed. If all attempts fail to clear the airway, then needle or surgical cricothyroidotomy should be performed.[6] Chest and/or neck radiography may reveal the foreign body. The foreign body will have to be removed via direct visualization. Lower airway obstruction usually requires bronchoscopy to relieve the airway obstruction.

Submersion Injury

Each year approximately 8000 deaths due to drowning occur, making submersion-related injuries the fifth leading cause of accidental death in the United States.[8] Submersion deaths are more common in children under the age of 4 years and in young adult males. Risk factors can include lack of supervision, poor swimming skills, poor judgment, and alcohol or substance abuse.

The cause of death in all drowning victims, whether freshwater or saltwater, is profound hypoxia. Aspiration of water floods the alveoli, causing a loss of surfactant, which leads to impaired gas exchange. Contaminants such as chlorine, algae, sand, and mud worsen the pulmonary injury. The most significant physiologic effect of drowning is hypoxemia from laryngospasms. In some individuals, asphyxiation results in relaxation of the airways, allowing water to enter the lungs. This is referred to as wet drowning. In approximately 10% to 20% of patients, aspiration of water does not occur because the airway does not relax until cardiac arrest and cessation of respiratory attempts. This is referred to as a dry drowning.

Clinically patients may present with respiratory distress, bronchospasm, loss of consciousness, pulmonary edema, hypothermia, poor perfusion, hypotension, dysrhythmias, metabolic acidosis, electrolyte abnormalities, and associated injuries such as spinal cord damage. Spinal cord injuries are more common in adolescents and young adults injured when diving or falling headfirst into water. The outcome of submersion injuries is determined by age, length of submersion, type of liquid medium, fluid temperature, and associated injuries. Submersion injury in cold, icy waters is associated with better neurologic recovery. In young children, cold water submersion creates a response known as the mammalian diving reflex. Bradycardia, apnea, and vasoconstriction occur during cold water submersion, causing shunting of blood and oxygen to the coronary and cerebral vasculature. With submersion injuries the earlier the victim regains consciousness, the greater the likelihood of return to prior level of function. Most patients who are alert and conscious on arrival survive without neurologic deficits.[8]

Care for the patient with a submersion injury includes maintaining a patent airway and stabilizing the cervical spine. Assess the patient's ventilatory status. Administer supplemental oxygen to maintain adequate oxygen saturation levels. If oxygen saturation cannot be maintained with supplemental oxygen, then proceed with intubation and mechanical ventilation. If the patient is hypothermic, rewarm him or her slowly. Begin fluid resuscitation with an isotonic crystalloid solution if needed. Obtain laboratory studies (CBC, electrolytes, and ABG) and chest radiograph. Other nursing interventions include placement of a gastric tube to decompress the stomach and minimize risk for aspiration and a urinary catheter to monitor output and volume status. Early recognition of associated injuries is important. Additional treatments such as diuretic therapy, intracranial pressure monitoring, and neuromuscular blocking agents may be indicated for some patients. Prophylactic antibiotics and steroids are not recommended.[8]

SUMMARY

Respiratory emergencies can result in rapid clinical deterioration. Accurate assessment skills and knowledge of signs and symptoms associated with respiratory compromise are both vital in the role of the ED nurse. Without rapid intervention, respiratory compromise can lead to respiratory failure and death.

REFERENCES

1. Bongaard F, Sue D: *Current critical care diagnosis and treatment*, ed 2, New York, 2002, McGraw-Hill.
2. Buttaro T, Trybulski J, Bailey P et al: *Primary care: a collaborative practice*, ed 2, St. Louis, 2003, Mosby.
3. Copstead L, Banasik J: *Pathophysiology*, ed 3, St. Louis, 2005, Saunders.
4. Dains J, Baumann L, Scheibel P: *Advanced health assessment and clinical diagnosis in primary care*, ed 2, St. Louis, 2003, Mosby.
5. Global Initiative for COPD: *Pocket guide to COPD diagnosis, management, and prevention: a guide for healthcare professionals*, 2006. Retrieved September 4, 2007, from http://www.goldcopd.org.
6. Holleran R: *Air and surface patient transport principles and practice*, St. Louis, 2003, Mosby.
7. National Heart Lung and Blood Institute: *NHLBI guidelines for the diagnosis and treatment of asthma*. Retrieved October 16, 2007, from http://www.nhlbi.nih.gov.
8. Shepherd S, Martin J: *Submersion injury, near drowning*. Retrieved August 30, 2007, from http://www.emedicine.com/emerg/topic744.htm.
9. Sommers M, Johnson S: *Diseases and disorders: a nursing therapeutics manual*, ed 2, Philadelphia, 2002, FA Davis.
10. The Joint Commission: *A comprehensive review of development for core measures*. Retrieved October 24, 2007, from http://www.jointcommission.org.

CHAPTER 31

Cardiovascular Emergencies

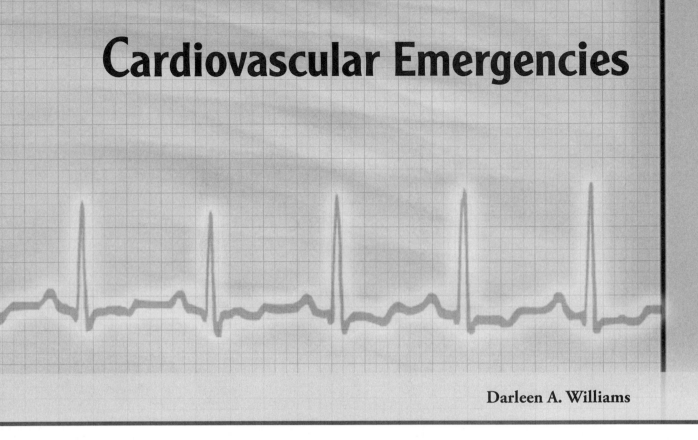

Darleen A. Williams

The American Heart Association (AHA) estimates that in 2004 there were 15,800,000 Americans age 20 and older with some form of coronary heart disease (CHD).[3] Fifty percent of men and 64% of women who die suddenly of CHD do so without having had or recognizing any early warning signs. Using 2004 data, the AHA calculates that "every 26 seconds an American will suffer a coronary event and every minute someone will die from one." Approximately 83% of those who die of CHD are age 65 or older; however, this is not a disease exclusive to our senior citizens. Data have shown that sudden cardiac death accounts for 19% of sudden deaths in children ages 1 to 13 and 30% between 14 and 21 years of age.[3] For many years organizations such as the AHA and the American Red Cross have worked to educate the public to become more aware of the warning signs and risk factors related to heart disease and heart attacks. The generally accepted risk factors that contribute to the development of CHD include elevated blood cholesterol levels; untreated hypertension; tobacco use; diabetes; obesity; lack of regular physical activity; poor dietary intake, including low intake of daily fruits and vegetables; and overindulgence in alcohol. In addition to the great loss of life, it is estimated by the AHA that the 2007 direct and indirect financial cost to American society was $151.6 billion.

Evidence has shown that prevention is the key to reducing complications associated with heart disease. In CHD, time really is muscle. The earlier that interventions begin, the greater the opportunity for the patient to experience a positive outcome and return to a productive life. Regulatory agencies and third-party payers are focused on ensuring that appropriate timely care is delivered. Clinical practice guidelines have been the end result of studies such as the Thrombolysis in Myocardial Infarction (TIMI-IIB), Efficacy and Safety of Subcutaneous Enoxaparin in Non–Q-Wave Coronary Events (ESSENCE), and Platelet Receptor Inhibition in Ischemic Syndrome Management in Patients Limited by Unstable Signs and Symptoms (PRISM-PLUS).[4]

Core measures have been identified by the Centers for Medicare and Medicaid Services (CMS) to ensure that patients with acute coronary syndrome (ACS) receive appropriate evidence-based standards of care.[21] Health care facilities must meet the standards associated with the core measures or face serious sanctions and loss of financial reimbursement. Although evidence-based practice is the gold standard for care, challenges continue to arise and facilities struggle to change their policies, procedures, and practices to meet the increasing complex requirements. Data associated with core measure compliance are available for review on public access Web sites.

It is important to remember that patients affected by cardiovascular diseases do not always have obvious signs and symptoms before presenting or even during their evaluation in the emergency department (ED). Understanding basic anatomy and physiology along with disease development and its impact is imperative for those providing emergency care.

The focus of this chapter is on cardiovascular emergencies secondary to disease processes and their progression. Cardiovascular emergencies related to trauma are discussed in Chapter 23, whereas pediatric-specific cardiovascular emergencies will be covered in Chapter 47.

ANATOMY AND PHYSIOLOGY

The heart is a muscular four-chambered organ with valves that separate each chamber. The primary function of these valves is to prevent backflow of blood (Figure 31-1). Despite being a two-pump system, the heart works in synchrony. Deoxygenated blood from the venous system enters the right atrium through the inferior and superior vena cavae. Blood is then pumped from the right ventricle into the pulmonary vasculature, where it becomes oxygenated in the lungs. After the exchange of carbon dioxide and oxygen occurs, the oxygenated blood moves to the left atrium via the pulmonary veins. The left ventricle then pumps this blood, via the arterial system, to the body. Figure 31-2 illustrates blood flow through the heart. The left ventricle is stronger than the right and has the ability to pump 4 to 8 L of blood per minute. Oxygenation of the heart muscle is provided by blood from the right and left coronary arteries. The coronary arteries lie on the surface of the heart and are filled during ventricular diastole.[17]

The heart is divided into three distinctive layers: epicardium, myocardium, and endocardium. The epicardium, also known as the visceral pericardium, serves as the outer layer of the heart and is where the coronary arteries lie. Next is the myocardium, the thick and muscular portion of the heart. It is composed of concentric muscular fiber rings. It is the contraction of these concentric rings that facilitates blood flow into and out of the ventricles. Finally, the endocardial layer is the innermost portion of both the atria and ventricles and is made of smooth tissue. This endocardial layer also functions as the surface for the heart valves. The entire heart is surrounded by a fibrous sac called the pericardium. This sac holds the heart in place and has fluid inside to lubricate the heart and prevent friction from occurring during contractions.

One of the most unique characteristics of cardiac tissue is its automaticity, the ability to initiate electrical activity. Figure 31-3 shows the heart's electrical conduction system. The sinoatrial (SA) node has the highest rate of automaticity, spontaneously depolarizing between 60 and 100 times per minute. The impulses generated by the SA node are carried to the atrioventricular (AV) node by intraatrial tracts (i.e., Bachmann's Bundle, Wenckebach's, and Thorel's tracts). Electrical stimulation of heart muscle begins in the atria and causes the mechanical event of atrial contraction. At the AV node there is a slight delay in the impulse transmission, which allows for atrial contraction to be completed before ventricular stimulation begins. From the AV node the electrical impulse is carried to the ventricles by the bundle of His, which includes the right and left bundle branches. The bundles terminate at the Purkinje fibers, where the impulses are delivered to the ventricular muscle, resulting in ventricular contraction.

The mechanical events of the cardiac cycle are called diastole and systole. Approximately 60% of the cardiac cycle is diastole, the time when the ventricles are filling. During diastole the aortic and pulmonic valves close while the mitral and tricuspid valves open. Electrically this corresponds

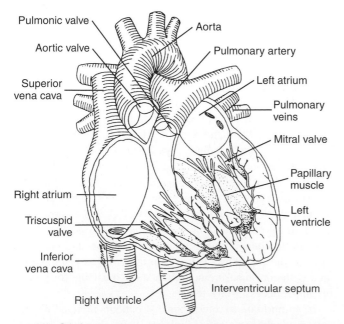

FIGURE 31-1. Anatomy of the heart. (From Lounsberry P, Frye SJ: *Cardiac rhythm disorders: a nursing process approach*, ed 2, St. Louis, 1992, Mosby.)

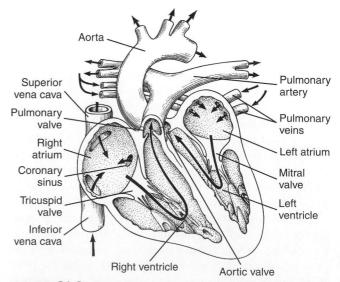

FIGURE 31-2. Circulation of blood through the heart. Arrows indicate direction of flow. (From Atkinson LJ, Fortunato NM: *Berry and Kohn's operating room technique*, ed 8, St. Louis, 1996, Mosby.)

to electrical stimulation and mechanical contraction of the atria. As the atria contract, the pressure in the atria becomes greater than in the ventricles, causing the AV valves to open and allowing blood to flow from an area of greater pressure to an area of lower pressure (Figure 31-4). The systolic phase of the cardiac cycle corresponds with ventricular contraction and opening of pulmonic and aortic valves. During contraction, AV valves close and chordae tendineae contract to prevent any regurgitation of blood. Figure 31-5 depicts the relationship between electrical and mechanical components of the cardiac cycle.

The pressures within the cardiovascular system are affected by both preload and afterload and greatly affect cardiac output. Preload refers to the volume of blood entering the right side of the heart. Afterload refers to pressure in the arterial system that the heart must overcome to pump out its ventricular blood volume.

Cardiac activity is regulated by branches of the autonomic nervous system, and the specific effects of each branch are described in Table 31-1. Receptors in the heart and great vessels respond to signals from the sympathetic nervous system (Table 31-2). Their stimulation affects heart rate, contractility, automaticity, conduction, and vascular smooth muscle. These receptors help prepare the body for the fight-or-flight response to either perceived threats or actual physiologic changes, including blood volume loss.

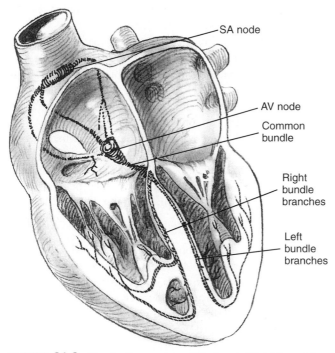

FIGURE **31-3.** Conduction system of the heart. *AV,* Atrioventricular; *SA,* sinoatrial. (From Davis JH, Drucker WR et al: *Clinical surgery,* vol 1, St. Louis, 1987, Mosby.)

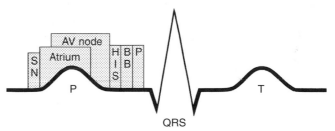

FIGURE **31-5.** Schematic drawing of cardiac activation related to the surface electrocardiogram (ECG). The timing of activation of the components of the conduction system is superimposed on the surface ECG. *AV,* Atrioventricular; *BB,* bundle branches; *HIS,* common bundle of His; *P,* Purkinje network; *SN,* sinus node. (From Lounsberry P, Frye SJ: *Cardiac rhythm disorders; a nursing process approach,* ed 2, St. Louis, 1992, Mosby.)

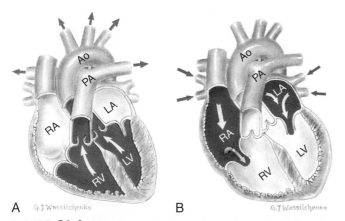

FIGURE **31-4.** Blood flow during (**A**) systole and (**B**) diastole. *Ao,* Aorta; *LA,* left atrium; *LV,* left ventricle; *PA,* pulmonary artery; *RA,* right atrium; *RV,* right ventricle. (From Canobbio MM: *Mosby's clinical nursing series, cardiovascular disorders,* vol 1, St. Louis, 1990, Mosby.)

Table 31-1.	**PARASYMPATHETIC AND SYMPATHETIC STIMULATION OF THE HEART**	
Nerve Activation	**Cardiac Effect**	**Clinical Manifestations**
Parasympathetic	Slows SA node discharge	Symptomatic bradycardia
	Slows AV node conduction and increases refractoriness	Transient heart block
Sympathetic	Heart rate increases	Tachycardia
	Enhances AV node function	Hypertension
	Shortens His-Purkinje and ventricular muscle refractoriness	Increased cardiac output
	Increased ventricular contraction	
	Increased peripheral vascular resistance	

AV, Atrioventricular; *SA,* sinoatrial.

Table 31-2.	SYMPATHETIC NERVOUS SYSTEM RECEPTORS	
Sympathetic Receptor	**Location**	**Clinical Response**
α	Vascular smooth muscle	Vasoconstriction
β₁	Myocardium	Increased heart rate, contraction, automaticity, and conduction
β₂	Peripheral vasculature and lungs	Vasodilation of peripheral vasculature and bronchodilation
Dopaminergic	Renal, mesenteric, cerebral, and coronary arteries	Vasodilation

SPECIFIC CARDIOVASCULAR EMERGENCIES

The following specific emergencies will be discussed: cardiac arrest, ACS, dysrhythmias, heart failure (HF), pericarditis, aortic aneurysm, and hypertensive crisis.

Cardiac Arrest

Sudden cardiac arrest is defined as death from a sudden loss of heart function.[23] More than 700,000 American adults die annually from cardiovascular disease; of these, approximately 850 die every day from sudden cardiac arrest.[2] A common cause of sudden cardiac arrest in adults is ventricular tachycardia (VT) that, if left untreated, deteriorates into ventricular fibrillation (VF). These lethal dysrhythmias are usually the end result of an evolving myocardial infarction; however, these dysrhythmias and resulting cardiac arrest may also be associated with aneurysm rupture, cardiomyopathies, rheumatic heart disease, mitral valve prolapse, and cardiac surgery. Sudden cardiac arrest can also be associated with many other conditions or events. Table 31-3 reviews some of the other potential causes of cardiopulmonary arrest, their causes, signs, symptoms, and therapeutic interventions. In addition, the health care team should gather information related to the events of the arrest. Determining the cause of the cardiac arrest event may assist the health care team in preventing a reoccurrence.

In a cardiac arrest situation immediate interventions begin with initiation of basic life support. Effective cardiopulmonary resuscitation is essential for a positive outcome to occur. Advanced life support measures should not be initiated until the basics have been addressed. The steps involved in both basic and advanced life support evolve based on ongoing research; therefore all health care providers must stay abreast of the changes in order to provide patients with the best evidence-based care possible.

Basic life support begins with the primary survey and appropriate interventions. Initial measures begin with establishing an airway (remember to use techniques that also stabilize the cervical spine if mechanisms suggest a potential injury). Airway management and oxygenation are discussed in greater detail in Chapter 30. Once the airway has been established, evaluate the patient's breathing status and provide artificial ventilations as indicated. While providing ventilations, it is important for the rescuer to ensure that the rate and volume are sufficient to oxygenate the patient. Once breathing has been ensured, chest compressions should be started, if appropriate. When performed properly, chest compressions provide and perhaps even restore cardiac circulation. Properly performed chest compressions produce approximately 30% of normal cardiac output, which is enough blood flow through the heart and brain to sustain tissue viability for a short time. Cerebral blood flow must be at least 50% of normal volume to maintain consciousness.[1] Chest compressions are best accomplished with the pulseless patient supine on a firm surface. This positioning allows for even compression of the chest cavity. Compressions should be smooth, even, and strong enough to generate a central pulse—either carotid or femoral. Defibrillation is the last step in the initial resuscitation effort. Evidence has clearly shown the need for early defibrillation in an effort to restore a viable heart rhythm. The use of electricity in resuscitation, both defibrillation and synchronous cardioversion, will be discussed in more detail later in this chapter.

Mechanical cardiopulmonary resuscitation devices have been available for years. There are many versions available; some devices simply provide chest compressions, whereas others are capable of providing both chest compressions and synchronous ventilations for the patient. There are devices available that will record the resuscitation activities, including the patient's rhythm, compressions being performed, and any attempts at defibrillation or cardioversion provided. Advantages of using such a device are that it can assist in providing consistent chest compressions and reduce or prevent rescuer fatigue during long resuscitation events or extended transport times for rural emergency medical services units. In addition, in the absence of multiple staff to participate in the resuscitation, using a chest compression device may allow the rescuer to begin providing advanced life support measures while the basics are being done using the mechanical device. Use of these devices should be restricted to adult patients, and they should be used by specially trained and experienced personnel only. Some current animal studies have shown promise in improving the hemodynamic status of the cardiac arrest victim when a mechanical compression device was used.[17]

Indications for an open thoracotomy and cardiac massage in the ED are limited to patients who are in full cardiopulmonary arrest secondary to penetrating chest trauma. Generally, patients who have sustained blunt trauma have very poor outcomes following resuscitative efforts that include an open thoracotomy. Open thoracotomy and cardiac massage are rarely performed and should be attempted only

Table 31-3. DIFFERENTIAL DIAGNOSIS OF CARDIOPULMONARY ARREST*

Causes	Specific Cause	Signs and Symptoms	Therapeutic Intervention	Notes
Metabolic	Hypoglycemia	Loss of consciousness, Physical signs of insulin or oral hypoglycemic agent usage; tachydysrhythmias; seizures; aspiration	Dextrose, 50% IVP or if unable to obtain an IV give glucagon IM	Consider hypoglycemia a strong possibility in patients who have a history of diabetes
	Hyperkalemia	ECG: Prolonged QT interval; peaked T waves; loss of P waves; wide QRS complexes	IV calcium chloride or calcium gluconate, sodium bicarbonate, insulin, and glucose	Often seen in hemodialysis and renal failure patients; also seen in patients taking potassium-sparing diuretics and patients with rhabdomyolysis
Drug-induced	Tricyclic antidepressants, amitriptyline (Elavil), amitriptyline and perphenazine (Etrafon, Triavil), imipramine (Tofranil), doxepin (Sinequan), protriptyline (Vivactil)	Tachydysrhythmias Prolonged QT/ torsade de pointes	Sodium bicarbonate IV	Causes direct cardiac toxicity; often delayed toxicity in adults
	Opiates	Bradydysrhythmias; heart blocks	Naloxone (Narcan) IV	Street drugs may be mixed with multiple substances
	β-Blockers	Cardiac: Heart blocks; bradydysrhythmias; PVCs	Atropine	PVCs may be caused by slow rate
		Respiratory: Bronchospasm	Aminophylline	
Pulmonary (any disease causing severe hypoxia)	Asthma	Severe bronchospasm causing hypoxia and respiratory acidosis ECG: Tachydysrhythmias (especially ventricular fibrillation)	Endotracheal intubation and ventilatory support	Abuse of sympathomimetic inhalants
	Pulmonary embolus	Pleuritic chest pain; shortness of breath in high-risk patients (postoperative, those taking birth control pills); syncope (recent study shows 60% have syncope as part of initial complaint); tachydysrhythmias	Good ventilatory support; consider fibrinolytic agents	Pathophysiology; acute hypoxia and cor pulmonale leading to tachydysrhythmias
	Tension pneumothorax	Distended neck veins; tracheal deviation; asymmetric chest expansion ECG: Often PEA	Needle thoracostomy; chest tube	Often seen in patients with blunt chest trauma; often occurs during CPR because of chest compressions (especially in patients with COPD)

(Continued)

Table 31-3.	DIFFERENTIAL DIAGNOSIS OF CARDIOPULMONARY ARREST*—CONT'D			
Causes	**Specific Cause**	**Signs and Symptoms**	**Therapeutic Intervention**	**Notes**
Neurogenic	Increased intracranial pressure from any cause (e.g., subarachnoid hemorrhage, subdural hematoma)	Central neurogenic breathing; dilated pupil(s); abnormal posturing (decerebrate/decorticate) ECG: Wide range of dysrhythmias, especially heart blocks	Central neurogenic hyperventilation (causes respiratory alkalosis, which results in cerebral vasoconstriction); steroids; diuretic agents; surgery	Damage to brainstem and autonomic centers
Hypovolemic	Anything that causes volume loss such as gastrointestinal bleeding, severe trauma with organ damage, ruptured ectopic pregnancy, dissecting or leaking aneurysm	Tachycardia; decreasing blood pressure; skin cool, clammy, pale; obvious signs of external blood loss	IV fluids; shock; position; surgery	A major cause of cardiopulmonary arrest that may be unrecognized
Other cardiac causes	Pericardial tamponade	Distended neck veins; decreasing blood pressure; distant heart sounds; widening pulse pressure ECG: PEA; bradydysrhythmias	IV fluids: Atropine; isoproterenol; pericardiocentesis; thoracotomy	Look for this especially in patients with blunt chest trauma or prolonged CPR

COPD, Chronic obstructive pulmonary disease; *CPR*, cardiopulmonary resuscitation; *ECG*, electrocardiogram; *IM*, intramuscular; *IV*, intravenous; *IVP*, intravenous push; *PEA*, pulseless electrical activity; *PVC*, premature ventricular contraction.

*There are many causes of cardiopulmonary arrest other than primary cardiac abnormalities, and it is for this reason that the health care provider must be very familiar with these potential causes and their associated signs and symptoms. Timely accurate identification of the cause of the patient's problem via the use of diagnostic testing in conjunction with assessment findings will determine the definitive therapeutic interventions needed. This table lists some of these nonprimary cardiac abnormalities that may result in cardiopulmonary arrest. Also listed in the table are therapeutic interventions for each condition that in addition to basic and advanced cardiac life support measures may be necessary with these patients. SPECIAL NOTE: Accurate, rapid assessment and interventions are the patient's best chance for having a good outcome.

when the facility has the appropriate resources available to manage the patient if a pulse returns after open thoracotomy is performed.

Family Presence During Resuscitation

Allowing a family member to be present during resuscitation is not only a common occurrence, it is supported by many organizations, including the Emergency Nurses Association and the American Association of Critical Care Nurses. Providing the option for family presence during resuscitation is discussed in detail in Chapter 13.

Therapeutic Electrical Interventions

The use of electricity in the treatment of patients with heart disease is a common therapeutic intervention. Whether it is pacing, defibrillation, or cardioversion, electricity is frequently the lifesaving intervention for this patient population. The goal is to restore normal electrical conduction within the heart, which in turn should initiate contractions and restore essential cardiac output. Patients who are in cardiopulmonary arrest require a prompt and accurate assessment to determine their current cardiac rhythm followed by implementation of the appropriate evidence-based algorithm and emergency care. Health care providers should be aware

of basic defibrillator safety concepts to avoid injury to both the patient and staff. Some noteworthy safety points to be aware of before any therapeutic electrical intervention use include the following:

- Remove all medication patches; if left on they can cause arcing during shock delivery and burn the patient.
- When paddles are used with conductive gel, ensure that just enough gel is placed on each paddle to lightly cover its surface. Excess conductive medium can run across the patient's chest and potentially cause arcing during shock delivery, resulting in burns to both the patient and the rescuer.
- Maintain firm contact between paddles and the chest wall to deliver the desired energy and prevent arcing.
- Do not place patches/paddles directly over implanted devices.
- When hands-free adhesive pads/patches are being used, carefully inspect wires regularly for any fraying or cracking.

Always loudly announce "I'm clear, everybody clear" before delivering each shock, and physically look to ensure that everyone is clear of the patient.

DEFIBRILLATION. Defibrillation has been defined as "the arrest of fibrillation of the cardiac muscle (atrial or ventricular) with restoration of the normal rhythm if successful."[1] For practical purposes defibrillation is a definitive way in which the rescuer uses electricity in an attempt to convert a patient's lethal rhythm into a viable one. Although exact statistics are not available, the AHA estimates that with early defibrillation (within 5 to 7 minutes) only 30% to 45% of cardiac arrest patients will survive the event, but without it 95% will die before reaching the hospital.[2]

In addition to being able to recognize dysrhythmias, the emergency nurse must be knowledgeable of current evidence-based interventions for each abnormal rhythm. The first step is to be familiar with the equipment used at your facility. Is the defibrillator monophasic or biphasic? Does it function as hands-off only or paddles only? Can it pace, defibrillate, and synchronize cardiovert, or is it only an automated external defibrillator (AED)? Before using the defibrillator it is important to be sure that the machine either is plugged in or has a fully charged battery. This maintenance procedure should be performed daily to ensure that the defibrillator will be fully functional in the event of an emergency.

Previously the standard monophasic defibrillators allowed electrical current to flow in only one direction. With the advancement of technology, biphasic defibrillators have evolved, which allow the energy to flow in both directions. With biphasic energy delivery the amount of energy required to convert a lethal rhythm is significantly reduced. When deciding on the energy needed for defibrillation or synchronized cardioversion, confirm if the defibrillator is monophasic or biphasic and be aware of the manufacturer's recommendations for energy delivery.

After confirming that the patient's rhythm requires defibrillation, place the adhesive electrode pads (if the hands-off device is being used) on the patient's bare chest. One pad goes to the upper chest just right of the sternum and the other at the apex of the heart on the patient's left lateral chest, under the left breast. If paddles are used, they are held firmly in the same locations after being covered with conduction gel or placed on commercially prepared defibrillator pads (Figure 31-6).

Anterior/posterior placement may also be used with the hands-free method and is indicated when repeated or long-term placement may be necessary. If the patient has any implanted devices, pad/paddle placement may need to be slightly altered. Do not place the pad/paddle directly over the implanted device, and external devices should be at least 1 inch away. To deliver the defibrillation the machine must be turned on and the desired mode selected. It is important to be sure that the "defib" mode is engaged. Next the energy level must be selected/programmed in and the machine charged. When fully charged the machine will sound an alert. It is at this time that the rescuer will loudly announce that a shock is going to be delivered, "I'm clear, everybody clear," and physically look to verify that all personnel are free from contact with the patient. To deliver the energy via the pads, press and hold the appropriate button on the device until the shock is delivered; with the paddles, press the discharge buttons on the paddle handles simultaneously. In the defibrillation mode the shock will be delivered immediately;

Defibrillator electrode placement

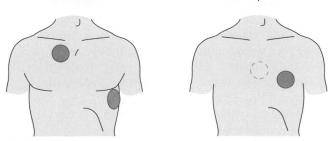

FIGURE **31-6.** Standard and anterior-posterior electrode placement for defibrillation. (From Rosen R, Barkin R: *Emergency medicine: concepts and clinical practice,* ed 4, St. Louis, 1998, Mosby.)

rescuers should resume chest compressions immediately after the shock is delivered.

Another electrical delivery device available is the AED. There are many versions of this self-contained defibrillator available, and it is an integral part of the public access defibrillation program. Some health care facilities have chosen to place these lifesaving devices throughout their buildings and on low-acuity units where need is infrequent and staff are not trained in advanced resuscitation skills. The vast majority of AEDs use biphasic technology; some are fully automated with no oscilloscope, whereas others are semiautomated and require the user to have rhythm-recognition skills. Both types of AED use only "hands-free" defibrillation. Once properly placed on the patient, the device will analyze the rhythm and decide if a shock is needed. The fully automated AED will deliver the shock automatically, whereas the semiautomated AED requires the rescuer to follow the audible instructions step-by-step to deliver the shock. Introduction and training for AEDs are done in basic life support classes. In an effort to assist people with remembering the steps, the PAAS mnemonic was developed: power, attach, analyze, shock. As with all electrical devices, use the safety concepts discussed earlier.

Successful defibrillation depends on multiple factors. The reason the patient arrested is important. Determining the cause will be instrumental in correcting the issue and preventing reoccurrence. Using the AHA advanced cardiac life support (ACLS) guidelines, health care providers should consider reasons for the initial arrest (Table 31-4) and perhaps identify the reason for an unsuccessful defibrillation.

CARDIOVERSION. Synchronized cardioversion is used when either the patient has become hemodynamically unstable or pharmacologic interventions have been unsuccessful in managing sustained ventricular tachycardia, supraventricular tachycardia, atrial fibrillation, or atrial flutter. In synchronized cardioversion, energy is timed with the QRS complex and avoids shock delivery during the relative refractory period, which could produce ventricular fibrillation. Synchronized cardioversion decreases potential energy delivery during the vulnerable period of repolarization, that is, the T wave of the electrocardiogram (ECG) (Figure 31-7).

The procedure for cardioversion is the same as for defibrillation with three important distinctions: (1) the machine must be set on synchronous mode; (2) sedation should be given for the conscious patient if time allows; and (3) when the delivery button is pushed, there will be a slight delay in firing because the machine is sensing the R wave in order to deliver the energy at the precise moment. Anxiolytics such as diazepam (Valium) or midazolam (Versed) should be administered intravenously (IV) in small, incremental doses before energy delivery. The procedure should be explained to the patient and informed consent obtained whenever possible.

As has been previously discussed, it is important to determine the cause of the patient's current condition. Potential treatable causes of cardiac arrest are found in Table 31-4. When possible a baseline 12-lead ECG should be obtained before and after the attempted cardioversion. Immediately after the procedure the patient's cardiac rhythm, vital signs, and level of consciousness should be assessed and closely monitored until the patient is hemodynamically stable and returns to an acceptable rhythm. Complications of cardioversion include asystole, junctional rhythms, premature ventricular contractions (PVCs), ventricular tachycardia, ventricular fibrillation, embolization, and return to the original dysrhythmia.

Another method to convert a patient's rhythm is through manual stimulation of the vagus nerve using a Valsalva maneuver such as causing the patient to gag or vomit. Stimulation of the vagus nerve will slow the heart rate and may terminate the dysrhythmia. In the past, ocular pressure and application of ice water to the patient's face have been used; however, these methods are no longer recommended.

The physician may try carotid sinus massage to convert the rhythm. This is accomplished by placing pressure on the carotid bodies, which stimulates the baroreceptors and therefore the parasympathetic branch of the autonomic nervous system. This stimulation decreases blood pressure and heart rate. Only one side should be done at a time. Before attempting this procedure the physician should auscultate the carotid arteries for bruits. Bruits are produced by turbulent flow through the carotid arteries and are suggestive of atherosclerotic plaque in the artery. If any of this plaque were dislodged during the procedure, the patient would be at risk for a stroke. If a bruit is heard, carotid massage is contraindicated. If no bruits are heard and the procedure will be attempted, the patient should be supine on supplemental oxygen and have at least one patent IV access. Before, during, and after the attempt the patient should be closely monitored. In more than 75% of the population, preferential massage of the right carotid body affects the SA node, whereas left carotid body massage affects the AV node. Even when the SA node is completely shut down, the AV node can provide pacemaker activity. If the left side is massaged first, complete block of the AV node could occur and lead to a slow ventricular rate. Pressure must be applied gently to the carotid artery just below the mandible and in small, circular motions, rotating the fingers backward and medially. Carotid massage should not exceed 5 to 10 seconds and should be discontinued sooner if the rhythm changes. Even when properly performed, carotid massage may cause asystole for 15 to 30 seconds, followed by a few idioventricular complexes before a new pacemaker site becomes active. Emergency resuscitation equipment and medications should be readily available whenever carotid massage is performed. If carotid massage is successful, continue to monitor the patient for several hours. Complications of carotid massage include further dysrhythmias (e.g., ventricular tachycardia, ventricular fibrillation, asystole), stroke, cerebral anoxia, and seizures.[1]

PACEMAKERS. A pacemaker is an electrical device that may restore an adequate heart rate and cardiac output. It can be used either via the transvenous or transcutaneous routes. A transcutaneous pacemaker (TCP) is a temporary intervention for patients experiencing symptomatic, unstable bradycardia, and second- or third-degree heart blocks because it is easily applied and managed until the patient can receive definitive treatment. The TCP can be applied by

Table 31-4.	POTENTIAL CAUSES TO CONSIDER FOR CARDIAC ARREST	
H's	**T's**
Hypovolemia (bleeding or dehydration)	Thrombosis (coronary or pulmonary)
Hypoxia	Tension pneumothorax
Hypokalemia/ hyperkalemia	Tamponade (cardiac)
Hypothermia	Tablets (overdose or ingestion)
Hydrogen ion (acidosis)	Toxins
Hypoglycemia	Trauma

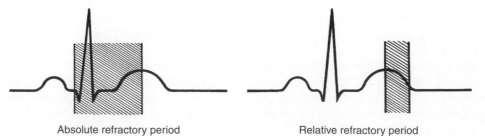

Absolute refractory period   Relative refractory period

FIGURE 31-7. Absolute and relative refractory periods on the electrocardiogram.

following these steps: (1) place the pacing electrodes on the patient's bare chest as recommended by the manufacturer; (2) turn the pacemaker on, and set the demand rate as ordered by the physician (usually between 60 and 70 beats/min); and (3) turn up the milliamperes (mA) current slowly, increasing the dose until capture occurs with pacer spikes noted on the patient's monitored rhythm. Keep the pacer's mA at the lowest level possible that still maintains electrical capture (pacer spikes) and mechanical capture (patient's pulse) and at a rate that keeps the patient clinically stable. Continuous pacing can be uncomfortable; therefore analgesia or anxiolytics should be considered.

Patients with complete heart block may be unable to electrically or mechanically respond to the pacemaker stimulus. Successful pacing depends on the condition of the myocardium. Mechanical capture is evaluated by the presence of a pulse consistent with paced beats. Both types of capture (electrical and mechanical) must be present for pacing to be considered effective. Two major reasons for lack of capture are acidosis and hypoxemia. Evaluate the patient's oxygen saturation and acid-base levels to determine if further airway or ventilatory interventions are needed. If there is a lack of pacer spikes, begin by checking the TCP electrodes followed by inspecting all the wires and connections. If necessary replace electrodes to ensure contact between external pacing electrodes and skin surface is adequate. Skin should be clean and dry before electrode application. Tincture of benzoin may be used to improve adherence to the skin if the patient has been diaphoretic.

IMPLANTABLE CARDIOVERTER-DEFIBRILLATOR. The implantable cardioverter-defibrillator (ICD) is a small generator that is used in patients at risk for life-threatening dysrhythmias—especially ventricular dysrhythmias. The ICD device is surgically placed under the skin in the chest wall just below the clavicle or in the abdominal cavity. This minigenerator monitors the patient's rhythm, providing pacing, cardioversion, or defibrillation based on the patient's needs, device capability, and programming.

When a patient with an ICD requires external defibrillation because the implanted device has malfunctioned or failed, it is important to know how to perform this intervention in a safe and effective manner. Defibrillator paddles or hands-free adhesive patches must not be placed directly over the ICD device. If standard paddle/patch placement and defibrillation attempts are unsuccessful, the resuscitation team should try the anterior-posterior placement for defibrillation. Health care professionals who have direct physical contact with the patient may experience a slight harmless tingling sensation when the ICD device fires. If the ICD fires inappropriately, the device can be deactivated by placing a magnet over the ICD generator.[1]

Resuscitation Interventions

FLUID RESUSCITATION. The use of IV fluids during resuscitation must be determined on an individual patient basis. Some patients may need crystalloid fluid boluses secondary to volume loss, whereas others may be in a fluid overload state and need to have intake strictly limited. In addition to the patient's current status, it is important to gather as much of the health history as possible because this information will influence the amount, rate, and type of IV fluids administered. After every intervention it is necessary to reassess and evaluate the patient's response. Because of adverse effects on cerebral tissue, dextrose-containing solutions are not recommended during resuscitation; instead the fluids of choice are normal saline or lactated Ringer's solution.

PHARMACOLOGIC THERAPY. Emergency drug therapy depends on the patient's cardiac rhythm, 12-lead ECG, and hemodynamic status. Table 31-5 provides an overview of commonly used emergency medications. The first-line drug in management of cardiac arrest, specifically asystole, pulseless electrical activity (PEA), VF, and pulseless VT is either epinephrine or vasopressin.[1] It is important to remember that the management of VF and pulseless VT requires immediate defibrillation followed by chest compressions before the administration of medications.

Patients with ventricular dysrhythmias associated with cardiopulmonary arrest may benefit from amiodarone (Cordarone) administration. Other antidysrhythmic agents considered for management of patients with VF or pulseless VT include lidocaine (Xylocaine), magnesium, and procainamide (Pronestyl). After the ventricular dysrhythmia is controlled, an infusion of the converting agent is necessary to maintain therapeutic drug levels. Antidysrhythmics should not be given to patients with third-degree AV block, with an escape rhythm, or with bradycardia and PVCs. Ectopic beats may contribute to the patient's cardiac output; therefore lidocaine could effectively reduce output and cause further decompensation or asystole.

Bradycardic dysrhythmias are initially managed with atropine, which blocks stimulation of the vagus nerve. Atropine may also be used for asystole and PEA. Atropine may not be effective for high-degree AV block dysrhythmias. Isoproterenol (Isuprel) is a β-adrenergic agonist and may be used to increase cardiac output in bradydysrhythmias. Routine use of isoproterenol is not recommended because of effects on ventricular irritability; however, it is considered a first-line drug for the heart transplant patient with symptomatic bradycardia. Atropine is not used for heart transplant patients because the vagus nerve is not reattached during the transplant. Bradycardic rhythms that affect hemodynamic stability may ultimately require cardiac pacing.

Supraventricular rhythms impair effective cardiac output by decreasing cardiac filling time and may decrease the patient's hemodynamic stability. Adenosine (Adenocard) is used to treat reentry dysrhythmias. It is an extremely fast-acting drug with a half-life of less than 10 seconds. For this reason it must be given rapidly and in a proximal vein, then followed with a 20-mL saline bolus. Side effects include flushing, dyspnea, hypotension, chest pain, transient bradycardia, transient asystole, and ventricular ectopy. These side effects will usually terminate spontaneously without further medical or nursing interventions. Other pharmacologic agents such as ibutilide, β-adrenergic blocking drugs

Table 31-5. DRUGS COMMONLY USED IN CARDIOPULMONARY RESUSCITATION

Drug	Category	Actions	Indications	Dose	Comments
Adenosine (Adenocard)	Unclassified antidysrhythmic	Slows conduction through the AV node; also can interrupt the reentry pathways through the AV node to decrease the heart rate	PSVT	**PSVT:** 6 mg IV/IO rapid push over 1-3 seconds; may give an additional 12 mg IV/IO rapid push if first dose is not effective; may repeat a second 12 mg IV/IO rapid push after 1-2 min. It is helpful to administer 20 mL of normal saline by rapid bolus after giving adenosine to clear the IV tubing	May cause brief heart block or transient asystole; may cause other dysrhythmias (e.g., PVC, PAC, sinus bradycardia, sinus tachycardia) during time of conversion from PSVT. These symptoms are usually brief because of the short half-life of the drug (i.e., <10 seconds). Contraindications include second- or third-degree AV block or sick sinus syndrome
Amiodarone (Cordarone)	Combined β-adrenergic blocker and calcium channel blocker	Prolongs myocardial cell action potential duration and refractory period; decreases AV conduction and sinus node function	Recurring ventricular fibrillation and unstable ventricular tachycardia	**Cardiac arrest:** 300 mg IV/IO push diluted in 20-30 mL of D_5W. If no response in 3-5 min may be followed by 150 mg IV/IO push. **Nonarrest:** Initial infusion: 150 mg over 10 min; can repeat every 10-15 min as needed. Early maintenance: 1 mg/min for 6 hours. Late maintenance: 0.5 mg/min. Do not exceed 2.2 g in 24 hours, including initial dose	May cause hypotension, nausea, bradycardia
Atropine sulfate	Parasympatholytic; anticholinergic	Increases the rate of SA node firing; increases conduction through AV node; decreases vagal tone	Hemodynamically significant bradycardia; asystole; high-degree AV blocks	**Bradycardia:** 0.5-1 mg IV every 3-5 min max dose 0.04 mg/kg. **Asystole/PEA:** 1 mg IV/IO push repeat every 3-5 min up to a total of 3 mg. **ACS:** 0.06-1 mg IV repeated every 5 min to max 0.04 mg/kg. **Endotracheal:** 2-3 mg diluted in 10 mL water or NS	In symptomatic patients do not delay pacing to administer medication. May cause paradoxic slowing of heart rate when given slowly or in doses of less than 0.5 mg

Table 31-5.	DRUGS COMMONLY USED IN CARDIOPULMONARY RESUSCITATION—CONT'D				
Drug	**Category**	**Actions**	**Indications**	**Dose**	**Comments**
Epinephrine (Adrenalin)	Sympathomimetic	Both α- and β-adrenergic effects; increases mean arterial pressure; decreases fibrillatory threshold; stimulates heart in asystole and idioventricular rhythms	Allergic reaction; cardiac arrest; bronchoconstriction or bronchospasm	**Cardiac arrest:** 1 mg IV/IO push; or endotracheally at 2-2.5 mg, repeat either dose every 5 min when needed and follow with 20 mL NS flush	Available as 1:10,000 solution (1 mg in 10 mL) May cause tachycardia, palpitations, PVCs, angina
Isoproterenol (Isuprel)	Sympathomimetic	Nonspecific β-adrenergic stimulation	Hemodynamically significant bradycardia refractory to atropine Refractory torsades de pointes Temporary treatment of bradycardia in heart transplant patients	**Bradycardia:** 1 mg in 250 mL D$_5$W (4 mcg/mL); 2-10 mcg/min IV titrate to achieve desired heart rate	Causes an increased workload on the heart; use with extreme caution: exacerbates ischemia and extends infarct
Lidocaine (Xylocaine)	Category IB antidysrhythmic	Decreases automaticity; suppresses ventricular ectopy; depresses conduction through reentry pathways; elevates VF threshold	PVCs, VT, VF, preintubation for patients with suspected increased intracranial pressure or laryngospasm	**Pulseless VF and VT:** 1-1.5 mg/kg IV/IO push; may repeat in 3-5 min; do not exceed 3 mg/kg; endotracheal 2-4 mg/kg **PVCs and VT:** 0.5-0.75 mg/kg IV push up to 1-1.5 mg/kg every 5-10 min; maximum total not to exceed 3 mg/kg **IV infusion:** 1 g in 250 mL D$_5$W (4 mg/mL) at 2-4 mg/min (30-60 μgtt/min) **RSI preintubation:** 1.5-2 mg/kg IV over 30-60 seconds, wait 90 seconds then intubate	May cause central nervous system depression, drowsiness, dizziness, confusion, and anxiety Contraindications include bradycardia and related PVCs, idioventricular rhythm; if given too rapidly, may cause seizures
Procainamide (Pronestyl)	Category IA antidysrhythmic	Suppresses PVCs; suppresses reentry dysrhythmias; may elevate VF threshold; negative chronotrope and dromotrope; mild negative inotrope; potent peripheral vasodilator	PVCs and VT refractory to lidocaine; hemodynamically significant SVT	**IV push:** 100 mg slow IV push 20 mg/min; may repeat every 5 min; dose not to exceed 17 mg/kg **IV infusion:** 1 g in 250 mL D$_5$W (4 mg/mL) at 1-4 mg/min (15-60 μgtt/min)	May cause hypotension, bradycardia Contraindications: Third-degree AV block, digoxin toxicity

(Continued)

Table 31-5. DRUGS COMMONLY USED IN CARDIOPULMONARY RESUSCITATION—CONT'D

Drug	Category	Actions	Indications	Dose	Comments
Sodium bicarbonate	Alkalotic agent	Buffers or neutralizes metabolic acidosis	Suspected acidosis in cases of cardiac arrest	1 mEq/kg IV push; repeat 0.5 mEq/kg every 10 to 15 min when required	May inactivate catecholamines when given together in the same IV line; when possible use arterial blood gas levels to guide administration
Vasopressin			An alternative to epinephrine	40 units IV/IO push May be given via endotracheal tube but no evidence-based dose recommended at this time	.
Verapamil (Calan, Isoptin)	Category IV anti-dysrhythmic	Blocks entry of Ca^{2+} into cells; negative dromotrope and depresses atrial automaticity; negative chronotrope; negative inotrope; vasodilator	SVT	2.5-5 mg IV over 2 min Over 3 min in older adults; Second dose 5-10 mg if needed Maximum dose 20 mg	May cause hypotension

AV, Atrioventricular; *D₅W,* 5% dextrose in water; *gtt,* drops, *IO;* intraosseous; *IV,* intravenous; *NS,* normal saline; *PAC,* premature atrial contraction; *PSVT,* paroxysmal supraventricular tachycardia; *PVC,* premature ventricular contraction; *RSI,* rapid sequence intubation; *SA,* sinoatrial; *SVT,* supraventricular tachycardia; *VF,* ventricular fibrillation; *VT,* ventricular tachycardia.

(e.g., metoprolol [Lopressor]), and calcium channel blocking agents (e.g., verapamil [Calan] and diltiazem [Cardizem]) can be used for controlling ventricular response rate in patients with supraventricular tachycardias (e.g., atrial fibrillation, atrial flutter, supraventricular tachycardia, atrial tachycardia). Monitor for bradycardia and hypotension when administering these medications.

Other miscellaneous drugs that may be used during cardiac arrest include sodium bicarbonate, calcium, and magnesium sulfate. Sodium bicarbonate is reserved for specific clinical situations including hyperkalemia, preexisting bicarbonate-responsive acidosis, and tricyclic antidepressant overdose. Magnesium is considered useful in the treatment of torsades de pointes, suspected hypomagnesaemia, and refractory ventricular fibrillation. Calcium, an ion essential for myocardial contractions and impulse formation, is recommended for hyperkalemia, hypocalcemia, and calcium channel blocker toxicity.

During cardiopulmonary arrest, hemodynamic status is unstable and requires intervention to stabilize not only the patient's cardiac rhythm but also the cardiovascular system. Table 31-6 reviews vasoactive drugs more commonly used during cardiopulmonary emergencies.[1,9,22] Refer to Table 31-7 for an overview of cardiovascular drugs that can be given via the endotracheal tube or intraosseous route when IV access cannot be established.[1,9,22]

Post–Cardiac Arrest Therapeutic Hypothermia

Recent evidence has demonstrated that the postarrest patient may benefit from controlled hypothermia. The AHA has endorsed the use of therapeutic hypothermia in the comatose post–cardiac arrest patient for 12 to 24 hours after resuscitation. This support is based on research results that have demonstrated improved neurologic status in survivors in whom cooling has been used. If it is used, the postarrest patient's body temperature should be closely monitored and maintained between 90° and 95° F (32° and 35° C). Many facilities have protocols and order sets for this procedure. Regardless of the cooling method employed, great care should be taken to prevent unintentional overcooling.[1]

Acute Coronary Syndrome

Acute coronary syndrome is a general term used to describe a group of coronary artery diseases and their clinical symptoms. These include unstable angina; ST elevation myocardial infarction (STEMI), also called a Q-wave myocardial infarction; and non-STEMI, also referred to as the non–Q-wave myocardial infarction. Initial presenting symptoms are very similar and require prompt, thorough assessments and diagnostic testing to determine the most appropriate treatment. It is estimated that in 2008 about 770,000 Americans had

Text continued on page 427.

Table 31-6. COMMONLY USED PARENTERAL VASOACTIVE DRUGS FOR CARDIOVASCULAR EMERGENCIES

Drug	Category	Actions	Indications	Dose	Comments
Esmolol (Brevibloc)	β-Adrenergic blocker Class II antiarrhythmic	Depresses AV conduction and myocardial automaticity, especially in the SA node; prolongs the refractory period	SVT (e.g., PAT, atrial fibrillation/flutter, sinus tachycardia)	**IV push:** Initial loading dose of 500 mcg/kg given over 1 min, followed by 50 mcg/kg over 4 min. May repeat initial loading dose followed by the 4 min infusion increased at increments of 50 mcg/kg/min. Do not give over 200 mcg/kg/min. **IV infusion:** Follow loading dose with an infusion of 100 mcg/kg/min	May cause significant bradycardia, hypotension, bronchospasm, heart failure. Contraindications: Heart block, CHF, severe asthma. Has an immediate onset of action. Duration of action approximately 30 min after end of infusion
Calcium chloride	Electrolyte replacement	Improves vascular tone and myocardial contractility	Rapid electrolyte replacement. In seriously hypotensive patients who respond poorly to fluid/vasopressors when hypocalcemia suspected	**IV push:** For Ca^{2+} replacement: 500 mg to 1 g (i.e., 7 to 14 mEq). For hyperkalemic ECG changes: 100 mg to 1 g. For hypocalcemic tetany: 300 mg to 1.2 g. For hypotension associated with Ca^{2+} channel blockers: 500 mg to 2 g. Administer slowly at a rate not to exceed 0.7 to 1.4 mEq/min. **IV infusion:** Administer diluted solution over 30-60 min (i.e., dilute calcium chloride in 50-100 mL D_5W, LR, or 0.9% NS)	May cause hypotension, bradycardia, dysrhythmias. Contraindications: Hypercalcemia, ventricular fibrillation
Diazoxide (Hyperstat)	Antihypertensive vasodilator	Direct relaxation of arteriolar smooth muscle. Inhibits release of pancreatic insulin	Significant hypertension	**IV push:** 1-3 mg/kg (e.g., approx. 50-150 mg). May repeat every 5-15 min as needed. Maintenance dose: 50-150 mg every 4-24 hours	Inject drug rapidly because slow administration reduces hypotensive effects. Onset of action <1 min, with peak in 2-5 min. May cause hypotension, CHF, dysrhythmias, myocardial and cerebral ischemia, and hyperglycemia

(Continued)

Table 31-6. COMMONLY USED PARENTERAL VASOACTIVE DRUGS FOR CARDIOVASCULAR EMERGENCIES—CONT'D

Drug	Category	Actions	Indications	Dose	Comments
Diltiazem HCL (Cardizem)	Calcium channel blocker	SA node automaticity decreased; AV conduction prolonged; increased refractoriness of AV node; and vasodilation including coronary arteries	SVT (e.g., atrial fibrillation/flutter, PSVT)	**IV push:** 0.25 mg/kg to be administered over 2 min. May give additional dose in 15 min of 0.35 mg/kg if initial dose inadequate to control HR. **IV infusion:** 5-15 mg/hr	May cause hypotension, bradycardia, AV heart block. Has an immediate onset when given IV, with peak effect in 15 min. Contraindications: Heart block, accessory conduction pathways or preexcitation syndromes
Dobutamine HCL (Dobutrex)	Sympathomimetic, β_1-adrenergic receptor agonist	Positive inotropic effects (e.g., increases force of myocardial contraction); increases heart rate at higher doses	To optimize cardiac output; may be used as concurrent therapy with afterload-reducing agents to also increase cardiac output	**IV infusion:** Initially 2.5 mcg/kg/min; continue titration to maintain effective cardiac output. Maintenance dose usually 2.5-10 mcg/kg/min. Maximum dose: 5-20 mcg/kg/min	May cause tachycardia, dysrhythmias (e.g., ventricular). Consider dose reduction of dobutamine if heart rate 10% above baseline
Dopamine HCL (Intropin, Dopastat)	Sympathomimetic, β_1- and α-adrenergic agent; also a dopaminergic stimulator	At low doses: Vasodilates mesenteric and cerebral blood flow. At intermediate doses: Increased myocardial contractility and peripheral vasodilation. At high doses: Increased peripheral/renal vascular resistance and increased myocardial contractility	At low doses: To increase urinary output. At intermediate doses: To increase cardiac output. At high doses: To increase BP in nonhypovolemic shock	**IV infusion:** *Low dose:* 0.5-2 mcg/kg/min. *Intermediate dose:* 2-10 mcg/kg/min. *High dose:* >10 mcg/kg/min. Maximum dose: 5-20 mcg/kg/min	May cause dysrhythmias. Extravasation of the drug may cause tissue sloughing and necrosis
Enalapril and enalaprilat (Vasotec)	ACE inhibitor	Reduces vascular tone	Significant hypertension. Adjunct to digitalis and diuretics for acute CHF	**IV push:** Initial dose 0.625 mg IVP; may repeat in 1 hour. Maintenance dose: 1.25 mg every 6 hours IVP	May cause hypotension, pulmonary edema
Ibutilide (Corvert)	Class III antiarrhythmic	Slows conduction; delays repolarization by activation of slow, inward current (mostly sodium) resulting in prolongation of atrial and ventricular action potentials	Recent onset atrial fibrillation or atrial flutter	**IV:** ≥60 kg: 1 mg administered over 10 min, may repeat dose in 10 min if not effective in converting rhythm. <60 kg: 0.01 mg/kg over 10 min, may repeat dose in 10 min if needed	May have proarrhythmic effects—monitor closely for torsades de pointes or polymorphic ventricular tachycardia; especially within 4-6 hours after administration

Labetalol (Normodyne, Trandate)	Selective α-adrenergic blocker and non-selective β-adrenergic blocker	Blocks sympathetic stimulation, thereby causing vasodilation	Hypertension	**IV push:** 20 mg (0.25 mg/kg) IV to be administered over 2 min Additional doses of 40-80 mg of the drug can be given at 10-min intervals up to maximum dose of 300 mg total	May cause hypotension, bradycardia, heart block, bronchospasm
Magnesium sulfate	Electrolyte replacement	Adequate Mg^{2+} is needed for normal cardiac automaticity, excitability, conduction, and contractility	Supraventricular and ventricular dysrhythmias	**IV push:** 1-3 g of magnesium sulfate (concentration of magnesium should *not* exceed 200 mg/mL; also Mg^{2+} should not be administered faster than 150 mg/min) **IV infusion:** Follow initial IV dose with 1-2 g of Mg^{2+} per hour	Rapid injection may cause hypotension, heart block, cardiac/respiratory arrest Onset of action is immediate when given IV Observe for hyper-magnesemia: Flushing, hypotension, bradycardia, confusion, weakness, depressed deep tendon reflexes, respiratory depression
Metoprolol tartrate (Lopressor)	β-Adrenergic blocker	Selectively blocks β_1-adrenergic receptors, which slows sinus heart rate, decreases cardiac output, decreases BP	Hypertension; AMI in hemodynamically stable patient	**IV push:** 5 mg IVP for hypertension **Treatment for AMI:** 3 IV injections of 5 mg; give 50 mg metoprolol "orally" every 6 hours after last dose IV metoprolol	May cause bradycardia, hypotension, bronchospasm
Nicardipine (Cardene)	Calcium channel blocker	Significantly decreases peripheral vascular resistance	Hypertensive emergency	**IV infusion:** 5 mg/hr to be titrated to desired effect—up to 15 mg/hr	May cause tachycardia, angina, hypotension
Nitroglycerin (Tridil)	Vasodilator	Relaxation of vascular smooth muscle, promoting venous and coronary artery vasodilation; reduces venous return	Angina, hypertension	**IV infusion:** Initiate infusion at 5-10 mcg/min Increase infusion by 5-10 mcg/min every 5-10 min Maximum dose: 200 mcg/min	May cause hypotension, headache, dizziness Nitroglycerin is absorbed by many soft plastics; therefore dilute the concentrate in a glass bottle and consider using non-absorbing, non–polyvinyl chloride tubing, or flush tubing with 20-25 mL before starting infusion

(Continued)

Table 31-6. COMMONLY USED PARENTERAL VASOACTIVE DRUGS FOR CARDIOVASCULAR EMERGENCIES—CONT'D

Drug	Category	Actions	Indications	Dose	Comments
Nitroprusside, sodium (Nipride)	Vasodilator	Relaxes vascular smooth muscle—lowering both arterial and venous BP	Significant hypertension	**IV infusion:** Initiate infusion at 0.3-0.5 mcg/kg/min Increase infusion by 1-2 mcg/kg/min to attain desired hemodynamic effects Maximum infusion rate: 10 mcg/kg/min	May cause hypotension, angina, increased ICP, seizures The IV solution needs to be protected from the light by using a light-resistant covering (e.g., aluminum foil, opaque plastic) Onset of action immediate, with peak action of 1-2 min
Norepinephrine bitartrate (Levophed)	Vasopressor	Peripheral venous/arterial vasoconstriction; cardiac stimulation	Short-term use for hypotension or shock	**IV infusion:** Initiate infusion at 2 mcg/min and titrate to desired BP Usual range: 2-12 mcg/min	May cause ventricular tachycardia/ fibrillation (i.e., secondary to increased myocardial oxygen consumption) Extravasation of the drug may cause tissue sloughing and necrosis
Phenylephrine (Neo-Synephrine)	Vasopressor	Potent postsynaptic α-adrenergic agonist	Short-term use for hypotension/ shock	**IV push:** 0.1-0.5 mg to be given over 1 min **IV infusion:** Dilute to yield solution of 0.1 mg/mL and titrate gtt every 10-15 min to achieve and to maintain BP >90 mm Hg	May cause hypertension, dysrhythmias, reflex bradycardia, cerebral hemorrhage Extravasation of the drug may cause tissue sloughing and necrosis
Propranolol HCL (Inderal)	Nonselective β-adrenergic blocker and class II antidysrhythmic	Blocks sympathetic stimulation of β₁-adrenergic receptors	Control of hypertension and suppression of rapid-rate cardiac dysrhythmias	**IV push:** 0.5 to 3 mg Give slowly 1 mg/min; may repeat dose after 2 min	May cause bronchospasm, hypotension, heart block, angina
Vasopressin (Pitressin)	Vasopressor	Directly stimulates contraction of smooth muscles; causes vasoconstriction with reduced blood flow to coronary, peripheral, cerebral, and pulmonary vessels	Short-term use for hypotension or shock Alternative to epinephrine in cardiac arrest resulting from VF or pulseless VT in patients without CV disease	**IV infusion:** Dilute with 5% dextrose in water or 0.9% NaCl to a concentration of 0.1 to 1.0 units/mL titrate gtt every 10-15 min to achieve and to maintain BP >90 mm Hg **Cardiac arrest:** 40 units IV push	May cause hypertension, dysrhythmias Contraindicated in preexisting CV disease; IV dose same as IO and ET dose

ACE, Angiotensin-converting enzyme; *AMI,* acute myocardial infarction; *BP,* blood pressure; *CHF,* congestive heart failure; *CV,* cardiovascular; *ECG,* electrocardiogram; *ET,* endotracheal; *HCL,* hydrochloride; *ICP,* intracranial pressure; *IVP,* intravenous push; *LR,* lactated Ringer's; *PAT,* paroxysmal atrial tachycardia; see Table 31-5 for other definitions.

Table 31-7. **ALTERNATE ROUTES FOR DRUG ADMINISTRATION IN CARDIOVASCULAR EMERGENCIES**

Route	Nursing Management
ENDOTRACHEAL (ET)	
When IV access not available, can administer selected emergency drugs: Epinephrine Atropine Lidocaine Naloxone	Dilute drug in sterile saline or sterile water (i.e., 10 mL for adults and 1 to 2 mL for children) Administer medications as far down ET tube as possible; consider inserting intracatheter in ET tube and advancing to give medication
Consider dose 2.0 to 2.5 times recommended IV dose (for above medications) Vasopressin (ET dose same as IV dose)	Administer drug quickly down ET tube, follow with three to four rapid insufflations of bag-mask device to aerosolize medication in tracheobronchial tree
INTRAOSSEOUS (IO)	
May be used in patients of any age IO needle usually placed in proximal tibia or distal femur Can be placed in any portion of the tibia excluding the epiphyseal plates (e.g., distal tibia, midanterior distal one third of the femur, iliac crest, humerus); the sternum can be used as a site in patients age 3 years or older Use for medications, fluids, and blood and blood products	Use sterile technique to insert an IO needle; alternative methods include using 16- or 18-gauge rigid spinal or bone marrow needle Be sure to follow manufacturer's guidelines when using devices to insert IO (e.g., EZ-IO) Confirm placement by aspiration of bone marrow, and freely flowing fluid without evidence of infiltration Secure firmly with sterile dressing and tape to prevent dislodgement Monitor for extravasation of IV fluids at, below, or distal to the site; confirm patency before giving any fluids or medications. Flush with dilute saline to maintain patency Dilute hypertonic-alkaline solutions before administration

IV, Intravenous.

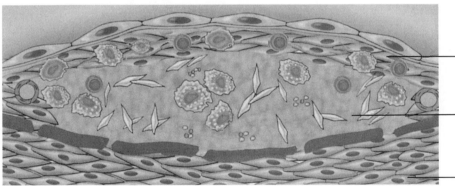

FIGURE 31-8. Major components of well-developed atheromatous plaque. (From Kumar V, Abbas AK, Fausto N: Robbins and Cotran: *pathologic basis of disease,* ed 7, Philadelphia, 2005, WB Saunders.)

a primary myocardial infarction and another 430,000 had a recurrent myocardial infarction.[20] A significant number of patients die within the first 2 hours after onset of a myocardial infarction. Mortality from the infarction can be reduced significantly if the patient receives prompt and definitive care in the early phases of the infarction. ACS evolves from inflammation, rupture, or erosion of atheromatous plaque within the coronary arteries. The resulting platelet activation changes the membranes, allowing aggregation of the platelets, resulting in interruption of coronary blood flow.

Pathogenesis of atherosclerosis includes accumulation of lipids on the intimal lining of the arteries, calcification and sclerosis of the medial layer of arteries, and thickening of the walls of the arteries (Figure 31-8). Generally atherosclerosis affects the aorta and the coronary, cerebral, femoral, and other large or middle-size arteries. Risk factors for atherosclerosis include smoking, hyperlipidemia, hypertension, diabetes mellitus, stress, lack of exercise, aging, diet high in fat and cholesterol, gender, and family history. Multiple existing risk factors increase the individual's chance of developing ACS.[20,24]

Overview of Acute Coronary Syndrome

As discussed above, the major cause of acute myocardial infarction (AMI) is thrombosis formation in a narrowed coronary artery from a ruptured or fissured atherosclerotic plaque and platelet activation. Subsequent vessel occlusion and thrombosis cause myocardial hypoxia and necrosis. Myocardial hypoxia may also be caused by coronary artery spasm or a dissecting aortic aneurysm. Complete necrosis occurs in 4 to 6 hours. The area surrounding the zone of necrosis is ischemic. Damage to the myocardium predisposes the patient to pump failure and various dysrhythmias secondary to conduction defects and irritability of myocardial tissue. Location and size of the infarct depend on which coronary artery is affected and where the occlusion occurs (Table 31-8). AMI often results from blockage of the left anterior descending coronary artery, which causes involvement of the anterior wall of the myocardium.[6,24]

Non-STEMI is usually related to intermittent occlusive thrombosis causing distal myocyte necrosis of the region supplied by the related coronary artery. As the clot enlarges around the thrombus, it may embolize and eventually occlude the coronary microvasculature, resulting in small elevations of cardiac enzymes. The underlying pathologic change for

unstable angina is partial occlusion by a thrombus of atherosclerotic plaque. Patients with either non-STEMI or unstable angina are at high risk for progression to transmural myocardial infarction.[12,24]

When the coronary artery(s) becomes narrowed or occluded, the myocardium becomes hypoxic, often resulting in classic retrosternal chest discomfort or angina pectoris. Pain is frequently described as crushing, burning, sharp, or heavy. It is important to remember that not all patients will present with classic signs and symptoms. Some have vague complaints that by themselves would not be readily associated with cardiac disease; therefore it is imperative to perform a rapid assessment and health history. This information will be invaluable in performing risk stratification and appropriately treating the patient in a timely manner. The pain can last several minutes to several weeks and may vary in location. Local hypoxia, lactate buildup, and sensory response of the hypoxic myocardium contribute to the amount of pain experienced. The pain may localize in the substernal area or

Table 31-8. CORONARY ARTERIES IN MYOCARDIAL INFARCTION

Right Coronary Artery	Left Coronary Artery

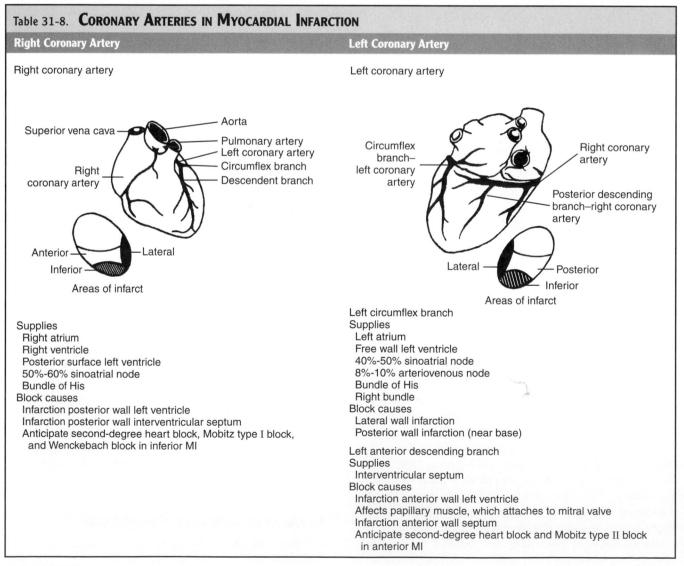

Right coronary artery

Supplies
 Right atrium
 Right ventricle
 Posterior surface left ventricle
 50%-60% sinoatrial node
 Bundle of His
Block causes
 Infarction posterior wall left ventricle
 Infarction posterior wall interventricular septum
 Anticipate second-degree heart block, Mobitz type I block,
  and Wenckebach block in inferior MI

Left coronary artery

Left circumflex branch
Supplies
 Left atrium
 Free wall left ventricle
 40%-50% sinoatrial node
 8%-10% arteriovenous node
 Bundle of His
 Right bundle
Block causes
 Lateral wall infarction
 Posterior wall infarction (near base)

Left anterior descending branch
Supplies
 Interventricular septum
Block causes
 Infarction anterior wall left ventricle
 Affects papillary muscle, which attaches to mitral valve
 Infarction anterior wall septum
 Anticipate second-degree heart block and Mobitz type II block
  in anterior MI

MI, Myocardial infarction.

radiate to the jaw and down the left arm. Associated symptoms include nausea, vomiting, diaphoresis, and hiccups if the phrenic nerve is stimulated.

With AMI the patient's blood pressure may decrease because of poor pump action that decreases cardiac output. Sodium and water retention may also occur as a result of decreased cardiac output and increased venous pressures. When AMI occurs, ventricular failure can occur. Severe ventricular failure causes stroke volume to decrease and ventricular diastolic pressure to increase, whereas the sympathetic response

decreases blood flow to the periphery. Decreased blood flow to the kidneys slows glomerular filtration rate (GFR). Decreased GFR stimulates renal cells to produce renin, causing angiotensin levels to rise and aldosterone to be secreted. Increased aldosterone and decreased GFR cause sodium and water retention and formation of interstitial edema.[19]

Patient Assessment for Acute Coronary Syndrome

Immediate assessment of patients experiencing symptoms of ACS is crucial due to the increased incidence of ventricular fibrillation during the first hour after onset of symptoms. It is not uncommon for patients to delay seeking treatment secondary to denial that what they are experiencing is serious. Most patients are resting or engaged in only moderate activity when their symptoms begin. Chest pain indicative of AMI is usually severe, lasts longer than 30 minutes, and is not relieved with rest or vasodilators such as nitroglycerin. Ironically, up to 20% of patients with AMI do not experience chest pain. Patients with diabetes mellitus are more prone to neuropathy and may not experience any pain. Among patients older than 85 years, the classic symptom of AMI is shortness of breath. Heart transplant patients also do not experience chest pain because pain receptors are denervated during their transplant procedure.

Doing risk stratification after obtaining a brief but accurate history of the patient's chest pain is crucial; the PQRST mnemonic is an organized and systematic way to get all the necessary information (Table 31-9). In addition, patients suspected of having angina should have a differential diagnosis made between angina pectoris and AMI.[20,24] There are two types of angina: stable and unstable (Table 31-10). Stable angina, known as typical angina, occurs as a predictable occurrence during or after exercise or straining activities. There are two categories of unstable angina: typical unstable angina and Prinzmetal's angina. Attacks of typical unstable angina, also called preinfarction angina, are usually prolonged, occur more frequently, and worsen with each episode. Typical unstable angina is associated with higher incidence of left main and proximal left anterior descending coronary arterial disease. Half the patients with typical unstable angina have total or near-total occlusion (70% to 100% stenosis)

Table 31-9. PQRST MNEMONIC FOR CHEST PAIN ASSESSMENT

Factor	Description Questions
P Provokes, palliates, precipitating factors	What provoked the pain? What makes the pain better? What makes the pain worse? Have you had this type of pain before? What were you doing when the pain occurred?
Q Quality	What does the pain feel like? Is it burning? Crushing? Tearing? Sharp?
R Region, radiation	Show me where the pain is. How large an area is involved? Does the pain radiate? If so, where?
S Severity, associated symptoms	How severe is the pain? If you were to rate the pain on a scale from 0 to 10 with 10 being the most severe pain you can imagine, how would you rate your pain? What else did you feel besides the pain?
T Time, temporal relations	When did the pain start? How long did it last? Does it come and go? Were you awakened by the pain? Is the pain always present?

Table 31-10. DIFFERENTIAL DIAGNOSIS OF ANGINA

Characteristic	Stable Angina	Unstable (Preinfarction) Angina
Location of pain	Substernal; may radiate to jaws, neck, and down arms and back	Substernal; may radiate to jaws, neck, and down arms and back
Duration of pain	1-5 min	5 min; occurring more frequently
Characteristic of pain	Aching, squeezing, choking, heavy burning	Same as stable angina but more intense
Other symptoms	Usually none	Diaphoresis; weakness
Pain worsened by	Exercise; activity; eating; cold weather; reclining	Exercise; activity; eating; cold weather; reclining
Pain relieved by	Rest; nitroglycerin; isosorbide	Nitroglycerin; isosorbide may give only partial relief
ECG findings	Transient ST-segment depression; disappears with pain relief	ST-segment depression; often T-wave inversion; ECG may be normal

ECG, Electrocardiogram.

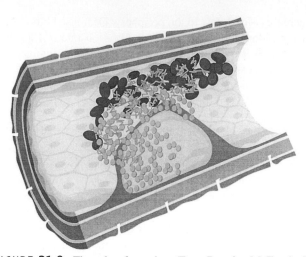

FIGURE **31-9.** Thrombus formation. (From Roetting M, Tanabe P: Emergency management of acute coronary-syndromes, *J Emerg Nurs* 26(suppl 6):S1, 2000.)

of a coronary artery (Figure 31-9). Prinzmetal's angina, or variant angina, occurs when the patient is at rest and usually at the same time each day.

In addition to assessing the patient's pain, determine if there are any associated symptoms such as diaphoresis, nausea, vomiting, indigestion, dyspnea, palpitations, or dizziness. Obtaining pertinent medical history and an accurate list of all medications (prescription, nonprescription, and herbal preparations) is very important. Knowing all the medications the patient may be taking can provide valuable information when considering other possible causes for the chest pain (differential diagnosis). For example, drugs such as H_2 blockers, antacids, sucralfate (Carafate), and nonsteroidal antiinflammatory medications can assist in differentiating cardiac pain from gastrointestinal problems such as hiatal hernia, gastric or peptic ulcers, pancreatitis, esophageal spasms, Mallory-Weiss syndrome, Boerhaave's syndrome, and/or musculoskeletal discomfort secondary to trauma, degenerative disk disease, xiphoidalgia, costochondritis, Mondor's disease, and postherpetic syndrome. Table 31-11 lists common etiologic factors that may be associated with chest pain.

Assessment findings associated with AMI are usually consistent with a patient who is acutely ill. Because of the hemodynamic effects of AMI, the patient may have a variable heart rate and multiple dysrhythmias. These patients may be hypertensive secondary to low cardiac output and sympathetic stimulation or as a result of pump failure. The first heart sound may be decreased because of decreased myocardial contractility, whereas the second heart sound may be increased because of increased pulmonary artery pressure. An S_3 sound (gallop) may be present as the result of ventricular dilation and increased ventricular fluid pressure. The presence of a new systolic murmur indicates ischemic mitral regurgitation or a ventricular septal defect.

A transient pericardial friction rub may occur secondary to the inflammatory response of an evolving necrosis. There may also be an alternating pulse rate caused by left-sided HF. Jugular vein distention can also develop as pressures increase from congestion, causing backflow of blood into jugular veins. This can be seen when the patient is sitting at a 45-degree angle. These patients may also have an elevated temperature caused by inflammation and necrosis of the myocardial tissue.

The patient is often diaphoretic and anxious. Diaphoresis is related to the autonomic nervous system response, whereas anxiety may be due to pain, fever, or fear; it is not uncommon for patients to have an intense sense of doom or dread. Cyanosis may be present and is caused by decreased oxyhemoglobin concentration and reduced blood supply to the peripheral vascular system.

ELECTROCARDIOGRAM. Changes in the ECG provide information regarding the location of coronary artery occlusion, myocardial ischemia, and the presence of tissue necrosis. Lead placement of the ECG determines which area of the heart the ECG signal is representing (Figures 31-10 and 31-11). Changes in the ECG occur when alterations in electrical current flow are seen secondary to myocardial injury or ischemia (Figure 31-12). When current flows toward a lead, an upward ECG deflection occurs; when the current flows away from a lead, a downward deflection occurs. If the current flows perpendicular to a lead, a biphasic ECG deflection occurs.[18] Figures 31-13 through 31-16 illustrate ECG changes with myocardial infarction. Serial ECGs are an important tool used in conjunction with patient assessment, history, and other diagnostic measures to confirm the diagnosis of AMI. A single ECG cannot be used exclusively. ECG findings are sensitive only 50% of the time, and ECG changes can occur with other conditions. Patients with stable angina can have ST-segment depression, whereas ST-segment elevation can occur with unstable angina and Prinzmetal's angina. Pericarditis may cause ST-segment elevation in many leads, hemorrhagic stroke is associated with T-wave inversion, and ventricular aneurysms may be associated with ST elevation.[11,16,18]

Elevation of the segment between the end of the S wave and the beginning of the T wave (ST segment) is indicative of myocardial injury and occurs minutes after occlusion of a coronary artery. A probable new transmural AMI has occurred if there is 1 mm or greater elevation of the ST segment in at least two leads or if there are abnormal Q waves noted in two or more leads. The ST segment can remain elevated for 24 hours after the event. Pathologic Q waves, measuring more than 0.04 second in width and at least 25% or more of overall QRS height, occur within 24 hours and indicate irreversible myocardial cell death. T-wave inversion occurs 6 to 24 hours after an ischemic event and can persist for months to years. Hypoxia should also be considered when T-wave inversion is present. ST-segment depression 1 mm or greater may also be associated with an AMI. Reciprocal changes (ST-segment depression and peaked T wave) may be seen in ECG leads that view regions opposite the damaged area. Hyperkalemia should be eliminated as a cause of tall, peaked T waves (Box 31-1).

Table 31-11. ETIOLOGIC FACTORS TO BE CONSIDERED IN THE DIFFERENTIAL DIAGNOSIS OF CHEST PAIN

Etiologic Factors	P Precipitating/Palliating	Q Quality	R Radiating/Region	S Severity/Symptoms	T Time/Temporal
Ischemic/Anginal	Precipitating factors: Effort-related activity, large meals, emotional stress Palliation: Ceases with activity abatement, relief with nitroglycerin, relief with rest	Tightness, burning, deep, constrictive	Retrosternal, area affected the size of the palm of the hand Pain may radiate to left shoulder, left hand (e.g., especially the fourth and fifth fingers), epigastrium, trachea, larynx Never involves region above the level of the eye	Associated symptoms: Profuse diaphoresis, weakness, shortness of breath, nausea, vomiting	Gradual onset of pain builds up to maximum pain intensity; usually anginal pain lasts 1-5 min
Myocardial infarction	Precipitating factors: Effort-related activity, large meals, emotional stress	Severe chest pain	Chest pain; may have radiation of pain to back, jaw, or left arm	Associated symptoms: Palpitations, dyspnea, diaphoresis, nausea, vomiting, dizziness, weakness, sense of impending doom	Usually pain has lasted 30 min or more
Pericarditis	Precipitating factors: May occur after AMI, may also be related to viral, collagen, or vascular disorders	Chest pain may be dull to severe and crushing type of pain	Anterior chest pain with radiation to the neck, arms, or shoulders; pain may be intensified by deep inspiration	Associated symptoms: Fever (i.e., 101°-102° F or 38.3°-38.9° C); pericardial friction rub; ECG: ST-segment elevation in all leads except V_1 and aV_R	May be hours to days
Dissecting aortic aneurysm	Sudden onset	Severe, ripping, tearing type pain	Anterior and posterior chest Often radiates from anterior chest to intrascapular region or to abdomen Pain may move with progression of aortic dissection	Associated symptoms: Dyspnea, tachypnea, CHF (i.e., secondary to aortic regurgitation caused by dissection); also CVA, syncope, paraplegia, and pulse loss associated with dissecting aneurysm	Sudden onset
Esophageal disorders (esophageal reflux, esophageal spasm)	Precipitating factors: Often triggered by exercise, or by food (large meal, spicy foods, acidic foods, cold foods) or ethanol intake	Burning or pressurelike pain May be severe	May radiate to neck, ear, jaw or lower abdomen	Associated symptoms: Dysphagia, aspiration	Minutes to days
Cocaine induced	Precipitating factors: Cocaine use Palliation: Relieved with nitroglycerin	Sharp, heaviness, pressure of the chest Severe type of pain	Substernal location, with radiation to both arms	Associated symptoms: Tachycardia, palpitations, diaphoresis, nausea, dizziness, syncope, dyspnea	Occurs 1-6 hours after cocaine use
Postoperative coronary artery bypass graft (CABG) due to harvest of internal mammary artery (IMA)	Precipitating factors: Use of IMA for graft of CABG patient	Mild to severe chest pain, burning, prickling, and dull type of sensations	Anterior chest, may radiate over entire chest wall and particularly over the site of the graft, may radiate to neck or axilla	Associated symptoms: Numbness, tenderness on palpation of the sternum, hyperesthesia along the incision line, delayed healing of the sternum	Persistent type of pain Shooting type of pain may last for several seconds and occur several times per day

(Continued)

Table 31-11. **ETIOLOGIC FACTORS TO BE CONSIDERED IN THE DIFFERENTIAL DIAGNOSIS OF CHEST PAIN—CONT'D**

Etiologic Factors	P Precipitating/Palliating	Q Quality	R Radiating/Region	S Severity/Symptoms	T Time/Temporal
Mitral valve prolapse	Palliation: Relief in recumbent position, no relief with nitroglycerin	Dull and aching, although may also be sharp	Nonretrosternal chest pain	Associated symptoms: Systolic murmur, unexplained dyspnea, weakness, midsystolic (apical) click	Onset may be sudden or recurrent May last for a few seconds or be persistent for days
5-Fluorouracil (5-FU) therapy	Precipitating factors: Following infusion of 5-FU Palliation: relief with nitroglycerin	Mild to severe pain	Central chest pain; radiates to left shoulder and left arm	Associated symptoms: Nausea, vomiting, tachycardia, hypertension	Occurs several hours after IV bolus or infusion of 5-FU No chest pain between treatment
Spontaneous pneumothorax	COPD, chronic asthma	Sharp or stabbing; described as moderate to severe	Usually pain of entire lung region (hemithorax), may radiate to back and neck	Associated symptoms: Decreased or absent breath sounds; pneumothorax per chest radiograph	Continuous pain until treated
Tachydysrhythmias	Precipitating factors: anxiety, digitalis toxicity, exercise, organic heart disease Palliation: terminated by antiarrhythmics, direct current shock, vagal maneuvers	Sharp, stabbing type of chest pain May have palpitations, "skipped beats"	Precordial chest pain	Associated symptoms: Weakness, fatigue, lethargy, palpitations, dizziness, vertigo	Paroxysmal in onset Lasts briefly to hours
Anxiety disorders	May have history of depression or anxiety	Pain may be vague, diffuse; may be further described as disabling	Anterior chest and abdomen	Associated symptoms: Dyspnea, fatigue, anorexia	Variable; often continuous for hours to days
Monosodium glutamate	Occurs with food ingestion high in monosodium glutamate	Burning type of chest pain	Retrosternal chest pain	Associated symptoms: Facial pain, nausea, vomiting	Occurs shortly after meals or up to several hours after meal
Musculoskeletal	Precipitating factors: pain with inspiration or with musculoskeletal movement	Generalized aching, stiffness with point tenderness, swelling	Tenderness of the anterior chest wall	Persistent chest pain without relief with rest	Duration of pain is longer than pain generally associated with angina

AMI, Acute myocardial infarction; *CHF*, congestive heart failure; *COPD*, chronic obstructive pulmonary disease; *CVA*, cerebrovascular accident; *ECG*, electrocardiogram.

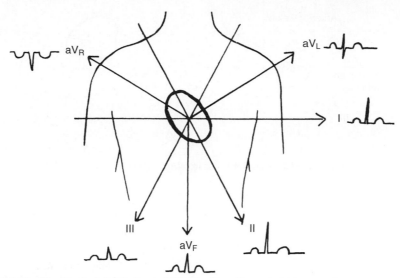

FIGURE **31-10.** Six limb leads (leads I, II, III, aV$_R$, aV$_L$, and aV$_F$) normally appear as shown.

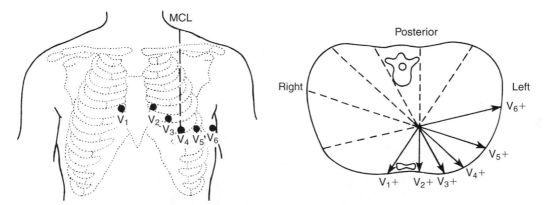

FIGURE **31-11.** Precordial or chest (V$_1$ through V$_6$) leads. *MCL,* modified chest lead

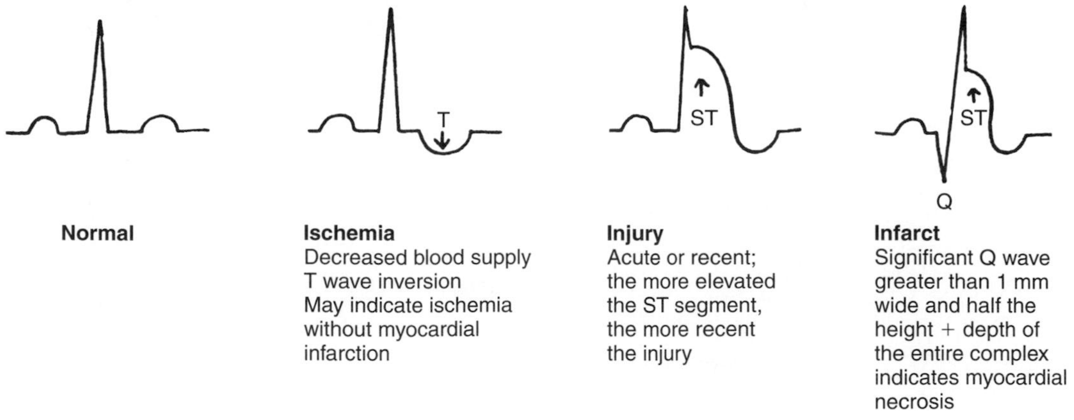

Normal

Ischemia
Decreased blood supply
T wave inversion
May indicate ischemia
without myocardial
infarction

Injury
Acute or recent;
the more elevated
the ST segment,
the more recent
the injury

Infarct
Significant Q wave
greater than 1 mm
wide and half the
height + depth of
the entire complex
indicates myocardial
necrosis

FIGURE **31-12.** Electrocardiogram changes.

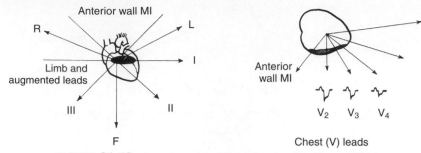

FIGURE **31-13.** Anterior myocardial infarction (V₂, V₃, and V₄).

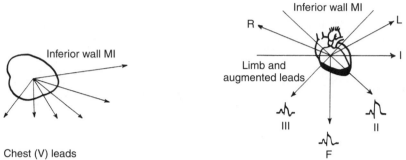

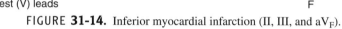

FIGURE **31-14.** Inferior myocardial infarction (II, III, and aV$_F$).

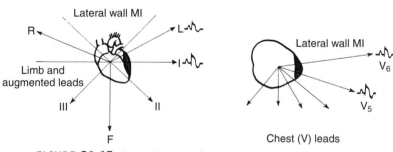

FIGURE **31-15.** Lateral myocardial infarction (I, aV$_1$, V$_5$, and V$_6$).

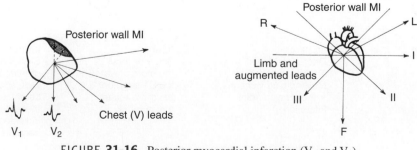

FIGURE **31-16.** Posterior myocardial infarction (V$_1$ and V$_2$).

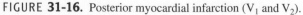

AMI, Acute myocardial infarction; *ECG,* electrocardiogram.

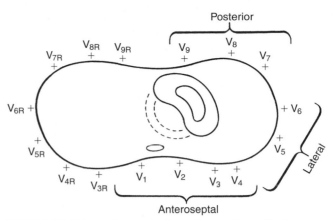

FIGURE **31-17.** Right ventricular and posterior wall electrocardiogram lead placement. (Modified from Hearns PA: Differentiating ischemia, injury, infarction: expanding the 12-lead electrocardiogram, *Dimens Crit Care Nurs* 13:176, 1994.)

Presence of a Q wave has been associated with transmural AMI; however, studies now demonstrate that both Q-wave (STEMI) and non–Q-wave (non-STEMI) infarcts can be transmural or subendocardial. In general, Q-wave infarctions are associated with a larger region of myocardial necrosis, higher enzyme levels, fresh coronary thrombosis, frequent vomiting, congestive HF, conduction defects, dysrhythmias, and less collateral circulation. When ST-segment depression occurs in the inferior (II, III, aV_F), lateral (I, aV_L, V_5, V_6), or anterior (V_1 through V_6) leads and cardiac enzymes are elevated, diagnosis of non-STEMI is supported. ST elevation is most frequently associated with Q-wave infarctions and almost 50% of non-STEMIs.[11,12,16,18]

All patients with suspected inferior or lateral AMI should be evaluated for right ventricular infarction. Right ventricular infarct is present in up to 40% of patients with inferior myocardial infarctions resulting from occlusion of the right coronary artery. Changes noted on the ECG may include isolated ST-segment elevation in V_1 or ST elevation in V_1 through V_4. A more reliable method of determining right ventricular infarct is the use of right ventricular leads (V_{3R} through V_{6R}). Figure 31-17 and Box 31-2 illustrate right ventricular lead placement. Use of lead V_{4R} has a high degree of sensitivity for right coronary artery occlusion.[8]

ECG changes in a posterior infarct (ST depression in V_1 to V_4) represent reciprocal changes of the anterior wall, the portion of the heart opposite the posterior portion. Other changes include R waves longer than 0.04 second in V_1 and V_2 and R wave to S wave ratio larger in V_1 and V_2.[8] Further evaluation may include posterior ECG leads (V_7 to V_9) (Box 31-2).

Continuous ECG monitoring in one or more leads is essential for the AMI patient. Dual-lead or continuous ST-segment monitoring is available to detect changes in the ECG and identify dysrhythmias. The best leads to use for diagnosing wide-complex QRS rhythms are MCL_1 and MCL_6 (Figure 31-18). This combination of a limb lead and precordial lead is valuable both in detecting ST-segment changes associated with further blockage of coronary arteries and for dysrhythmia detection. If bedside monitoring permits, the combination of leads V_1, I, and aV_F allows quick evaluation

of ECG axis. Figure 31-19 provides an overview of axis based on leads I and aV_F. Evaluation of axis during wide-complex QRS rhythms or dysrhythmias assists in differentiating supraventricular from ventricular dysrhythmias. In one study, three lead combinations were 100% sensitive for ischemic changes in the major coronary vessels.[4] Leads III, V_3, and V_5 reflect left anterior descending artery.[1] Leads II, III, and aV_F reflect the right coronary artery. Leads V_1 to V_6 reflect the left anterior descending artery. Leads V_5 and V_6 reflect the left anterior descending or the left circumflex artery. Leads I and aV_L reflect the left circumflex artery and the left anterior descending artery. Multilead ECG monitoring and continuous ST-segment monitoring have become more common, and it is essential that the emergency nurse be able to accurately interpret these readings.[14]

CARDIAC BIOMARKERS. In addition to ECG monitoring, cardiac biomarkers are measured as part of the diagnostic workup for ACS. Myoglobin is a nonspecific protein associated with muscle oxygen transport. Myoglobin levels elevate about 1 hour sooner than creatine kinase (CK) after myocardial injury and peak in 2 to 4 hours. Myoglobin is found in the striated muscle of the heart and in skeletal muscle; thus elevations can be associated not only with AMI

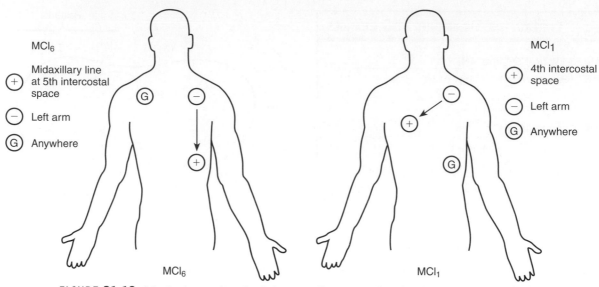

FIGURE **31-18.** Monitoring on three-lead electrocardiogram monitor. Leads MCI$_6$ and MCI$_1$ are the best leads for monitoring dysrhythmias.

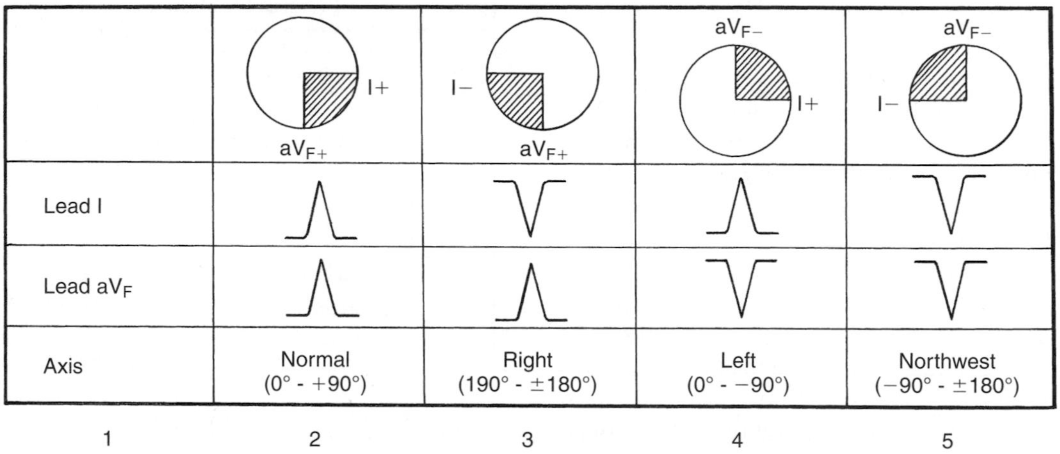

			aV$_{F-}$	aV$_{F-}$
	I+ aV$_{F+}$	I− aV$_{F+}$	I+	I−
Lead I	ʌ	v	ʌ	v
Lead aV$_F$	ʌ	ʌ	v	v
Axis	Normal (0° - +90°)	Right (190° - ±180°)	Left (0° - −90°)	Northwest (−90° - ±180°)
	1	2	3	4	5

FIGURE **31-19.** Determination of QRS axis. *(1)* Note predominant QRS polarity in leads I and aV$_F$. *(2)* If QRS during tachycardia is primarily positive in I and aV$_F$, axis falls within normal quadrant from 0 degrees to 90 degrees. *(3)* If complex is primarily negative in I and positive in aV$_F$, right axis deviation is present. *(4)* If complex is predominantly positive in I and negative in aV$_F$, left axis deviation is present. *(5)* If QRS is primarily negative in both I and aV$_F$, markedly abnormal "northwest" axis is present that is diagnostic of ventricular tachycardia. (Modified from Drew BJ: Bedside electrocardiographic monitoring, *Heart Lung* 20:610, 1991.)

but also with conditions such as neuromuscular disorders, strenuous exercise, and renal failure.

Cardiac-specific troponin is also a protein found in the myofibrils of muscle. There are two subforms of cardiac-specific troponin: troponin I and troponin T. Both are very specific for the cardiac muscle because of their role in myocardial muscle contractions. Troponin T is detectable 3 to 12 hours after an AMI, peaks at 12 to 48 hours, and returns to baseline in 10 to 14 days. Troponin I can be measured as early as 3 to 12 hours as well, peaking at 10 to 24 hours after AMI and returning to baseline in 3 to 7 days.

Additional cardiac biomarkers released from necrotic myocardium include CK and CK-MB. These once were the "gold standard" for a definitive diagnosis of AMI; however, CK-MB can take 4 to 12 hours to elevate. Therefore biomarkers that elevate earlier, such as myoglobin and troponin, result in a more timely diagnosis. Table 31-12 describes markers released with myocardial tissue necrosis.

Further evaluation of the patient with ACS includes a chest radiograph to rule out other causes of chest pain such as pneumonia, pneumothorax, trauma, and malignancy. A chest radiograph is also valuable in determining the presence of cardiomegaly and pulmonary congestion. In some situations an echocardiogram may be used to evaluate myocardial wall motion, valve abnormalities, and septal wall defect. Although not diagnostic of AMI, an echocardiogram is

Table 31-12.	CARDIAC BIOMARKERS FOR ACUTE MYOCARDIAL INFARCTION		
Cardiac Biomarker	Initial Elevation After Acute Myocardial Infarction	Mean Peak Time	Time to Return to Baseline
Myoglobin	1-4 hours	6-7 hours	18-24 hours
Troponin I (cardiac specific)	3-12 hours	10-24 hours	3-7 days
Troponin T (cardiac specific)	3-12 hours	12-48 hours	10-14 days
Creatine kinase-MB (CK-MB)	4-12 hours	10-24 hours	48-72 hours

useful in determining the extent of damage to the myocardium. Extensive myocardial damage puts the patient at risk for complications such as HF and cardiogenic shock. Research is being conducted to determine the role of coronary computed tomography angiography (CCTA) in evaluating patients with symptoms of ACS. The goal of this diagnostic procedure is to rule out acute coronary artery atherosclerosis in patients who have normal ECGs and negative biomarkers.

Patient Management

The approach to the patient suspected of having an AMI should be one of professional efficiency. Obtaining the patient's history while simultaneously assessing the patient's current status and beginning basic interventions and diagnostic procedures is imperative if definitive care is to be initiated in a timely manner; remember, time is muscle. One easy way to remember some of the basic medications used in AMI patients is to use the mnemonic MONA: morphine, oxygen, nitroglycerin, and aspirin.[1,4,20]

All patients suspected of having an AMI should be placed on oxygen to maintain saturations greater than 95%. If oxygenation cannot be maintained or the patient is acidotic, intubation and mechanical ventilation are indicated.

After oxygen therapy is initiated, establish IV access for potential medications and fluid therapy. Insert at least two large-caliber (18-gauge) IV catheters, and infuse normal saline as needed. Ongoing assessments include frequent blood pressure measurements, continuous ECG, and pulse oximetry monitoring. In addition, assessment and reassessments of pain, its intensity, location, and radiation are important components of the patient's care. After every intervention it is important to assess the patient's response to determine if the desired outcome has been achieved.

After the initial evaluation, aspirin should be given orally (to be chewed) unless contraindicated (e.g., allergy, active gastrointestinal bleeding). If the patient is unable to tolerate oral aspirin, one rectal suppository (300 mg) may be administered. The recommended oral dose of aspirin ranges from 160 to 325 mg of non–enteric-coated tablets. If the patient is "allergic" to aspirin, other oral antiplatelet agents such as ticlopidine (Ticlid) or clopidogrel (Plavix) can be considered.[1,4] Further treatment options for anticoagulation to be considered are IV administration of standard heparin or low-molecular-weight heparin such as enoxaparin (Lovenox).

Nitroglycerin is the initial drug of choice for treatment of chest pain related to angina pectoris and AMI. Nitroglycerin can be administered sublingually in 0.3- or 0.4-mg tablets or in a metered-dose spray.[1] One tablet or spray is administered every 5 minutes, up to three doses. Nitroglycerin dilates coronary arteries, reduces afterload by dilating peripheral venous circulation, and reduces preload by decreasing venous return to the heart. Nitroglycerin is not usually given unless systolic blood pressure (SBP) is at least 100 mm Hg because of potential decreased blood pressure that can occur. If sublingual nitroglycerin is not effective, IV nitroglycerin (e.g., Tridil) can be used. Initiate nitroglycerin infusion at 10 to 20 mcg/min, and titrate in increments of 5 to 10 mcg/min up to a total of 50 to 180 mcg/min.[1]

If nitroglycerin fails to relieve chest pain, the next drug of choice is morphine sulfate. This narcotic analgesic relieves both chest pain and anxiety, thereby decreasing myocardial oxygen consumption.[1,22] If SBP is greater than 100 mm Hg, administer morphine 2 to 4 mg IV every 5 to 10 minutes until pain is relieved. Monitor respiratory status and hemodynamic response carefully after each morphine administration.

PERCUTANEOUS CORONARY INTERVENTION. Percutaneous coronary intervention (PCI) is a general term used to describe a host of invasive procedures performed in the cardiac catheterization laboratory to reestablish blood flow in the occluded coronary artery or arteries in the patient experiencing an AMI. Evidence has demonstrated that the use of PCI has improved outcomes for patients over the previous standard of fibrinolytic therapy.[1,4] Current standard time from arrival in the ED to intervention is 90 minutes for patients with diagnosed STEMI.

The emergency nurse should be knowledgeable about the PCI procedure and the placement of stents. Patients may return to the ED after stent placement with symptoms of ACS from stent occlusion if they do not comply with the pharmacologic regimen to maintain stent patency. Most patients will receive an IV glycoprotein IIb/IIIa inhibitor (Integrilin, ReoPro, Angiomax) before the procedure and for 24 hours after the procedure. This therapy will be followed by a course of oral antiplatelet agents (Ticlid, Plavix).

FIBRINOLYTIC THERAPY. The frequency of fibrinolytic therapy for the patient with AMI is decreasing because evidence is now supporting improved patient outcomes with the use of early PCI. The goal of fibrinolytic therapy is to lyse coronary thrombi, restore blood flow to a hypoperfused myocardium, and abort or prevent complete evolution of the infarction process. Treatment with fibrinolytics is recommended to be initiated within 12 hours of onset of symptoms.

Fibrinolytic therapy targets elements of the clotting process to cause fibrinolysis, the process of clot degradation. Lysis of the clot begins with activation of plasminogen, which converts to plasmin. Plasmin degrades or breaks down fibrin in the clot, circulating fibrinogen, factor V, and factor VIII. Fibrinolytic agents are an exogenous source of plasminogen. Refer to Table 31-13 for a comparison of fibrinolytic agents.[1,22]

Fibrinolytic agents greatly increase the risk for bleeding complications; therefore it is crucial that a thorough assessment and accurate health history be obtained before administration. Absolute contraindications for fibrinolytic therapy include any history of previous cerebrovascular accident or intracerebral hemorrhage within the last year. Complications that may occur in the patient receiving fibrinolytic therapy include reperfusion dysrhythmias, bleeding from puncture sites, reocclusion/reinfarction, and hemorrhagic stroke.

During and after infusion it is important to monitor the patient closely for hypotension, decreased hemoglobin and hematocrit, and tachycardia. Another significant complication that may occur is an allergic reaction, particularly with use of streptokinase or anistreplase. Monitor for respiratory distress, rash, or urticaria. Minimize tissue trauma by keeping the patient on bed rest, limiting arterial and venous punctures, and limiting use of noninvasive blood pressure cuffs. Reperfusion cannot be absolutely determined without benefit of cardiac angiography; however, markers of reperfusion that can be assessed by the emergency nurse include resolution of chest pain, normalizing of ST changes, and occurrence of reperfusion dysrhythmias such as accelerated idioventricular rhythms.

Patients less than 75 years old can be considered for rescue PCI or emergency coronary bypass surgery if they have not improved after the administration of fibrinolytic therapy.

ADDITIONAL PHARMACOLOGIC THERAPY. A heparin infusion is recommended in conjunction with fibrinolytic therapy to prevent formation of a new clot and reocclusion of the coronary vessel. The recommended dose is 60 units/kg as a bolus at the same time as initiating fibrinolytic therapy. A maintenance infusion of 12 units/kg/hr is titrated to maintain the patient's partial thromboplastin time (PTT) at 1.5 to 2 times the control levels. Heparin is also recommended for patients who receive nonselective fibrinolytic agents (e.g., anistreplase); however, before initiation of antithrombotic therapy, heparin should be withheld for 6 hours and appropriate diagnostic studies performed such as an International Normalized Ratio (INR) or activated PTT.

Heparin is also indicated for use in patients with non–ST-elevation ACS. Options for heparin include IV heparin, subcutaneous unfractionated heparin (7500 units twice daily), or low-molecular-weight heparin (e.g., enoxaparin [Lovenox], dalteparin [Fragmin]) at 1 mg/kg twice daily.[1,4]

Nitroglycerin IV infusions are recommended for the first 24 to 48 hours after an ACS, especially an acute anterior myocardial infarction. Nitroglycerin dilates coronary arteries, increases collateral blood flow, reduces myocardial oxygen demand, and decreases preload and afterload.

Angiotensin-converting enzyme (ACE) inhibitor agents for patients with AMI (e.g., enalapril, captopril, lisinopril) should be started within 24 hours of AMI. Use of ACE inhibitors has been associated with reduced mortality. Known contraindications to ACE inhibitor therapy include allergies, history of renal failure, or bilateral renal artery stenosis.[9,22]

β-Blockers are recommended within 24 hours of an AMI because they help decrease mortality and morbidity by decreasing myocardial oxygen demands and reducing the possibility of ventricular fibrillation. Use of β-blockers is contraindicated in patients who are bradycardic or hypotensive with a SBP less than 100 mm/Hg. In addition, patients with chronic obstructive pulmonary disease and those who have symptoms of heart blocks or HF should not be given

Table 31-13. **COMPARISON OF FIBRINOLYTIC AGENTS**			
Agent	**Action**	**Dose**	**Comments**
Alteplase (Activase, Activase rt-PA)	Proteolytic enzyme; direct activator of plasminogen; high degree of clot specificity	**IV:** 15 mg IV bolus over 1-2 min; then 50 mg over 30 min, then 35 mg over 60 min	Half-life in plasma is 5-7 min; may cause sudden hypotension; inline IV filters can remove as much as 47% of the drug
Reteplase (Retavase)	Activates the conversion of plasminogen to plasmin; high degree of clot specificity	**IV:** 10 units over 2 min; then repeat 10 units in 30 min after initiation of first bolus	Give normal saline fluid before and after administration of reteplase (Retavase) Reconstitute just before administration and use within 4 hours after reconstituting
TNK-tissue plasminogen activator (TNKase)	Activates clot-bound plasminogen to plasmin	**IV:** 30-50 mg bolus over 5 sec Dosing based on patient weight: <60 kg = 30 mg TNK ≥60 to <70 kg = 35 mg TNK ≥70 to <80 kg = 40 mg TNK ≥80 to <90 kg = 45 mg TNK ≥90 mg = 50 mg TNK	More fibrin specificity and less incidence of bleeding than rt-PA

IV, Intravenous.

β-blockers. Once it is decided to administer β-blockers, the emergency nurse must monitor the patient closely for side effects, including hypotension, bradycardia, and heart blocks.

Glycoprotein IIb/IIIa inhibitors are another potential option to manage non–ST-elevation ACS. Platelet adhesion, activation, and aggregation play major roles in development of thrombus, which can potentiate evolution of this ACS into an AMI. Glycoprotein IIb/IIIa inhibitors antagonize or inhibit the receptor sites, which inhibits platelet aggregation. It has been demonstrated that these medications reduce the risk for development of thrombus independent of aspirin and heparin therapies. Refer to Table 31-14 for an overview of these agents.[1,4,9,22]

Dysrhythmias

Blood flow deprivation to the myocardium as a result of CHD can affect the heart's electrical conduction system, causing various dysrhythmias. Table 31-15 summarizes dysrhythmias and categories of antidysrhythmics according to modified Vaughan-Williams classification schema. By understanding drug classifications, the emergency nurse can anticipate expected action of the drug and nursing implications for drug administration and patient assessment.[9,22]

Bradycardia

Bradycardia is defined as a heart rate less than 60 beats/min and frequently occurs in AMI patients, particularly those with inferior wall infarctions. Bradycardic dysrhythmias include AV blocks. Four different types of blocks occur, depending on the area and degree of damage to the conduction system. These AV blocks are referred to as first-degree, second-degree Mobitz I (Wenckebach), second-degree Mobitz II, and third-degree or complete heart block. Blocks in conduction may be caused by myocardial infarction, infection, degenerative changes in the conduction system, rheumatic heart disease, or medications such as β-blockers, calcium channel blockers, and cardiac glycosides. Management of symptomatic bradycardias and heart blocks includes drugs such as atropine and epinephrine. An external pacemaker or transvenous pacemaker may also be used. Second-degree Mobitz I heart block is associated with a conduction defect through the AV node and is usually benign and transient. This rhythm is commonly associated with inferior infarctions because the right coronary artery supplies this area of the heart and AV node. Second-degree Mobitz II AV block occurs when conduction through the bundle branches is impaired, usually secondary to blockage of the left coronary artery, which supplies the anterior wall and bundle branches.[17] This form of second-degree block is more likely than the other form to progress to third-degree block.

Long QT Syndrome

Long QT syndrome is a disorder affecting the mechanisms of ion channels within the heart causing slowed ventricular repolarization (Figure 31-20). With the alteration of ion movement, polymorphic ventricular tachycardia, also known as torsades de pointes, can occur. This disorder can develop after using any medications that prolong the QT interval, such as particular diuretics, antibiotics, antihistamines, antifungals, antidepressants, heart, cholesterol-lowering, or diabetic medications. This syndrome can also be a congenital abnormality of the heart's electrical conduction system and is now found in at least nine genes. Treatment for long QT syndrome depends on the severity of the patient's symptoms. It can be as simple as lifestyle modifications and medications such as β-blockers to implanted devices such as ICDs and pacemakers. The main goals are to prevent any severe symptoms or sudden death.

Other Dysrhythmias

Other dysrhythmias that commonly occur are supraventricular tachycardias, which may be indicative of myocardial ischemia or anterior wall infarct. Often associated with chest pain, tachycardias are dangerous because they increase myocardial oxygen consumption and may extend an infarct. Treatment depends on clinical findings from initial and frequently repeated assessments. For hemodynamically unstable patients, therapy may include pharmacologic agents such as adenosine, verapamil, and procainamide. Vagal maneuvers or synchronized cardioversion may also be used. Evaluation of dysrhythmias requires a systematic approach (Box 31-3).

Heart Failure

According to the AHA, in 2004 there were more than 1 million acute HF patients hospitalized.[15] HF occurs when the myocardium (one or both ventricles) fails to function adequately as a pump. This inadequacy can also be classified as systolic (impaired pumping) or diastolic (impaired filling

Table 31-14.	OVERVIEW OF GLYCOPROTEIN IIB/IIIA INHIBITORS	
Glycoprotein IIb/IIIa Inhibitor	**Dosage**	**Potential Side Effects**
Abciximab (ReoPro)	0.25 mg/kg over 10-60 min 0.125 mg/kg/min for 12 hours	Potential for increased bleeding, hypotension, bradycardia, nausea and vomiting, diarrhea
Eptifibatide (Integrilin)	180 mcg/kg over 1 to 2 min 2 mcg/kg/min for up to 72 hours	Potential for increased bleeding, hypotension
Tirofiban HCL (Aggrastat)	0.4 mcg/kg/min for 30 min 0.1 mcg/kg/min for 12-24 hours	Potential for increased bleeding, nausea, bradycardia

Table 31-15. ANTIDYSRHYTHMIC PHARMACOLOGIC AGENTS AS CLASSIFIED BY MODIFIED VAUGHAN–WILLIAMS CLASSIFICATION SCHEMA

Class	Pharmacologic Action	Electrophysiologic Effects	Indications	Drug Examples	Comments
I	Sodium channel blockade (stabilizes cell membrane)	Decreases conduction velocity; prolongs PR and QRS intervals	Ventricular dysrhythmias	Moricizine (Ethmozine)	Risk for proarrhythmia potential
IA		Blocks and delays repolarization, thereby lengthening the action potential duration and the effective refractory period	Atrial and ventricular dysrhythmias	Quinidine sulfate (Quinidex) Procainamide HCL (Pronestyl) Disopyramide (Norpace)	Observe for heart block, hypotension, prolonged PR/QRS/QT intervals
IB		Shortens the action of potential duration	Ventricular dysrhythmias	Lidocaine HCL (Xylocaine) Tocainide HCL (Tonocard) Mexiletine HCL (Mexitil)	Potential toxicity: Dizziness, vertigo, confusion, seizures
IC		Slows conduction of electrical impulses in atria, AV node, and ventricular/His–Purkinje fibers	Ventricular dysrhythmias	Flecainide acetate (Tambocor) Propafenone (Rythmol)	Risk for proarrhythmia potential
II	β-Adrenergic blockade	Inhibition of the sympathetic stimulation—reduces heart rate and decreases myocardial irritability and shortens action potential	Supraventricular and ventricular dysrhythmias	Propranolol HCL (Inderal) Esmolol HCL (Brevibloc) Acebutolol (Sectral)	Observe for hypotension, bradycardia, heart block
III	Potassium channel blockade	Delayed repolarization and prolongation of the action potential, thus decreasing myocardial irritability	Ventricular tachycardia and ventricular fibrillation	Amiodarone HCL (Cordarone) Dofetilide (Tikosyn) Ibutilide fumarate (Corvert)	Observe for exacerbation of dysrhythmias, hypotension Pulmonary fibrosis may occur with amiodarone use
IV	Calcium channel blockade	Slows conduction of electrical impulses and decreases rate of impulse initiation	SVT and atrial dysrhythmias	Verapamil (Calan) Diltiazem (Cardizem) Nifedipine (Procardia)	Observe for hypotension, bradycardia, heart block
Unclassified	Potassium channel opener	Slows conduction through AV node and increases refractory period in AV node	SVT	Adenosine (Adenocard)	Has very rapid effect, short half-life

AV, Atrioventricular; *HCL,* hydrochloride; *SVT,* supraventricular tachycardia.

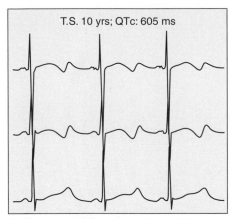

T.S. 10 yrs; QTc: 605 ms

FIGURE **31-20.** Long QT syndrome. (From Libby P, Bonow RO, Mann DL, Zipes, DP: *Braunwald's heart disease : a textbook of cardiovascular medicine, ed. 8,* Philadelphia, 2008, Saunders.)

Box 31-3	SYSTEMATIC EVALUATION OF CARDIAC RHYTHMS

RATE

Bradycardia: Under 60 beats/min
Normal rate: 60 to 100 beats/min
Tachycardia: Over 100 beats/min

RHYTHM

Is the rhythm regular or irregular?

P WAVES

Are P waves present? Does one P wave appear before each QRS? Is P wave deflection normal?

QRS COMPLEX

Normal is 0.06 to 0.12 second. Are the QRS complexes normal shape and configuration?

P/QRS RELATIONSHIP

Does QRS complex follow every P wave?

PR INTERVAL

Normal is 0.12 to 0.2 second. Is the interval prolonged? Shortened?

of the ventricles), resulting in venous congestion, decreased stroke volume, decreased cardiac output, and increased peripheral systemic pressure. Onset may be gradual or sudden. The primary precipitating event for HF is some type of myocardial damage that activates many compensatory mechanisms which, over time, are exhausted and result in the occurrence of symptoms. HF can be seen alone or in conjunction with pulmonary edema. HF is a symptom of underlying damage from ACS or a problem such as hypertension, fluid overload, valvular heart disease, dysrhythmias, cardiomyopathy, hyperthyroidism, fever, and adult respiratory distress syndrome.[17] HF may also occur with oxygen toxicity syndrome, pneumothorax, and drugs such as methotrexate (Rheumatrex), busulfan (Mylaran), and nitrofurantoin (Furadantin).

Symptoms of HF are characterized by severe dyspnea, orthopnea, fatigue, weakness, abdominal discomfort (secondary to ascites or hepatic engorgement), dependent edema, distended neck veins, bilateral rales, and a third heart sound (gallop). Assessment and reassessments of the patient should be organized and systematic, beginning with airway, breathing, and circulation (ABCs), to ensure that the patient has a patent airway, that breathing is effective, and that circulation is adequate. This patient's vital signs must be watched closely and the ECG rhythm monitored for potential dysrhythmias. Monitoring oxygen saturation, auscultating lung and heart sounds, and observing for distended neck veins and peripheral edema are also important components of nursing care for this patient.

Interventions include diagnostic tests such as a serum B-type natriuretic peptide (BNP). This is a cardiac hormone secreted in response to ventricular wall stretch. Measurement of BNP assists the health care team in determining the severity of the patient's HF and treating causes as they are identified. It is important that interventions and diagnostics be simultaneously coordinated. Initial interventions include having the patient in a high-Fowler's position, applying oxygen, and administering medications as appropriate (e.g., ACE inhibitors to decrease systemic vascular resistance, dobutamine [Dobutrex]) to increase cardiac output. Left ventricular assistive devices may also be used in these patients as a temporary measure. Lastly, it is very important to maintain IV access with strict control of infused fluids and accurate documentation of intake and output.

Pericarditis

Pericarditis is inflammation of the pericardial sac and can be caused by AMI, trauma, infection, or neoplasms. Among younger patients, causes of pericarditis include infectious processes such as Coxsackie virus, streptococci, staphylococci, tuberculosis, and *Haemophilus influenzae.* An early pericardial friction rub may be auscultated with pericarditis in conjunction with AMI. Friction rub occurs when the inflamed area over a transmural infarction causes the pericardial surface to lose its lubricating fluid. Pericarditis is most evident 2 to 3 days after an AMI.

Patients with pericarditis experience fever, chills, dyspnea, and severe chest pain that increases during inspiration and increased activity. Tachycardia or other dysrhythmias may also be present. Pericardial friction rub increases in intensity when the patient leans forward. The patient may complain of general malaise, and ST-segment elevation 1 to 3 mm will be seen in all ECG leads except aV_R and V_1. Therapeutic interventions include oxygen via nasal cannula, sedation, analgesia, and bed rest. Antiinflammatory agents and steroids may also be indicated.[5,17]

Aortic Aneurysm

An aneurysm is a dilated area of the artery (at least 1.5 times its normal size) caused by weakness of the arterial wall. Aneurysms can occur anywhere along the aorta and are generally caused by atherosclerosis and related factors such as infection, smoking, hypertension, trauma, hyperlipidemia, diabetes, syphilis, and heredity. Abdominal aortic aneurysms occur four times more often than thoracic aneurysms and are seen more often in men than women. Aneurysms account for more than 15,000 deaths each year.[9]

The atherosclerotic process contributes to weakening and eventual destruction of the medial wall of the artery. Over time the hemodynamic forces of blood flow cause thickening of the wall and replacement of muscle fibers with fibrous tissue and calcium deposits. The aneurysm enlarges over time, and the wall tension of the aneurysm increases. Dilation of the aneurysm allows development of a thrombus, which may be dislodged and cause thromboembolism distally in the patient's circulation, for example, in the lower extremities.[7,10,25]

Three types of aneurysms are fusiform, saccular, and dissecting. Fusiform aneurysms are characterized by a segment of artery dilated around the entire circumference of the artery, whereas a saccular aneurysm dilates only a portion of the artery. A dissecting aneurysm actually results in a tear of the artery's intimal layer, which allows blood to flow between the intimal and medial layers (Figure 31-21). Dissecting aneurysms are further classified by the extent of the tear and location. Type 1 dissection occurs in the ascending aorta and extends beyond the aortic arch. Type 2 dissection occurs only in the ascending aorta, and a type 3 dissection begins distal to the left subclavian artery.[9]

As the aorta dissects, major vessels (e.g., myocardial, cerebral, mesenteric, and renal) that branch off the aorta may be occluded. Rupture of the dissection can cause pericardial tamponade or hemorrhage into the thoracic cavity, resulting in exsanguination, shock, and imminent death.

Patient Assessment

Signs and symptoms depend on the location and size of the aneurysm; it is very uncommon for patients to have early symptoms, and some may be totally asymptomatic until a rupture occurs. An abdominal aortic aneurysm may be discovered during the physical examination when a pulsating mass is felt while palpating the abdomen; this may be difficult to feel in the obese patient. Patients who present to the ED with a leaking or rupturing abdominal aortic aneurysm may have a classic presentation characterized by extreme back pain accompanied by abdominal pain and tenderness with palpation. Back pain may radiate to the legs, groin, or lower back secondary to stretching of the anterior spinal ligament. Patients with a dissecting thoracic aneurysm may complain of excruciating, "ripping," substernal chest pain with radiation to the back, dyspnea, and stridor or cough secondary to pressure on the trachea. Rupture of the aneurysm compromises hemodynamic stability and blood flow distal to the aneurysm. Regardless of aneurysm location, patients may have severe apprehension, tachycardia, unilateral absence of major pulses, bilateral blood pressure differences, hypertension, hemiplegia, or paraplegia. Accurate initial and reassessments of vital signs, including comparing

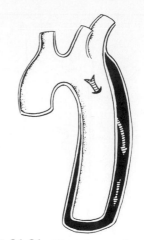

FIGURE **31-21.** Dissecting aortic aneurysm.

blood pressures and pulses bilaterally, can give the health care provider valuable information regarding the aneurysm status.

Diagnostic tests can include a portable chest radiograph, magnetic resonance imaging, computed tomography scan with contrast of the suspected area (chest or abdomen), sonogram, transesophageal echocardiogram, and angiogram.

Patient Management

All patients should be placed in a high-Fowler's position (if hemodynamically stable), given high-flow oxygen, and have two large-caliber IV catheters initiated. The main goals in treating these patients are control of pain, anxiety, and blood pressure. Close monitoring of blood pressure is critical; if hypertension is present, drugs such as nitroprusside sodium (Nipride) can be used to maintain blood pressure at the desired level. Dissecting aneurysms are often managed with a β-blocker such as esmolol (Brevibloc) to control heart rate and blood pressure as low as possible (systolic 90 to 120 mm Hg). If the patient has signs of hypovolemic shock, interventions then focus on maintaining ABCs, fluid resuscitation, and preparing for emergency surgery.

Hypertensive Crisis

Blood pressure ranges are now evidence based and have the following categories and ranges[6]:
- Prehypertension: systolic pressure of 120 to 139 mm Hg and/or diastolic pressure of 80 to 89 mm Hg
- Stage I hypertension: systolic pressure of 140 to 159 mm Hg and/or a diastolic pressure of 90 to 99 mm Hg
- Stage II hypertension: systolic pressure greater than 160 mm Hg and/or diastolic pressure greater than 100 mm Hg

When blood pressure becomes abruptly elevated to extreme levels, the patient has a life-threatening situation. An estimated 50 million people in the United States have hypertension.[13]

Hypertensive crisis is categorized by the degree of acute-target end-organ damage and the rapidity with which the blood pressure must be lowered. Hypertensive crisis has been further categorized into hypertensive emergencies and hypertensive urgencies. Hypertensive emergencies are those clinical situations in which excessively high blood pressure must be lowered quickly, within 1 to 2 hours, to prevent new or worsening organ damage. Hypertensive urgencies may develop over days to weeks and generally demonstrate an elevated diastolic blood pressure (DBP) without signs of end-organ damage; treatment should occur within 24 to 48 hours after identification.

Regardless of the underlying mechanism of hypertension, elevated blood pressure increases systemic or peripheral vascular resistance and cardiac output. These increases perpetuate the cycle by stimulating release of catecholamines, which increases a sympathetic activity and activates the renin-angiotensin system. The net result is continued increases in blood pressure. Hypertensive crisis usually occurs in patients with a history of hypertension. Other conditions that may cause or precipitate hypertensive crisis include renal parenchymal disease (e.g., acute glomerulonephritis, vasculitis), endocrine problems (e.g., pheochromocytoma, Cushing's syndrome), use of sympathomimetic drugs (cocaine, amphetamines, phencyclidine, lysergic acid diethylamide, diet pills), and food-drug interactions (e.g., monoamine oxidase inhibitors and tyramine interaction).[8]

Patient Assessment

Patients with hypertensive crisis usually have an SBP greater than 240 mm Hg or a DBP greater than 140 mm Hg. Primary symptoms are consistent with new or evolving end-organ damage. Increase in systemic peripheral vascular resistance and sympathetic stimulation imposed by the significant hypertension causes an increase in myocardial workload and myocardial oxygen consumption. Cardiovascular manifestations include congestive heart failure, chest pain, angina, and AMI. Neurologic changes include headache, nausea, vomiting, dizziness, visual disturbances (e.g., blurred vision, temporary visual loss, decreased visual acuity, photophobia), altered mental states (e.g., agitation, confusion, lethargy, coma), and seizures.[1] Other neurologic symptoms include focal cranial nerve palsy, sensory deficits, motor deficits, aphasia, and hemiparesis. Funduscopic evaluation may reveal papilledema from effects of hypertension on the retina.

Patient Management

In addition to closely monitoring for any ECG changes and dysrhythmias, frequent and accurate vital sign measurements must be performed. IV access should be established, and if possible an arterial line should be initiated for the most accurate blood pressure readings. If insertion of an arterial line is not possible, a noninvasive blood pressure device can also be used for continuous blood pressure monitoring. Caution must be taken to ensure that the right cuff size is used and applied correctly for these readings to be accurate. The goal of management is to lower DBP to parameters appropriate for the patient. Previously it was believed that the goal for DBP was 100 to 110 mm Hg. However, more recent data suggest that the SBP should be lowered to about 160 mm Hg because lower pressures may compromise cerebral blood flow. IV pharmacologic agents such as nitroprusside sodium (Nipride), nitroglycerin (Tridil), clevidipine (Cleviprex), fenoldopam mesylate (Corlopam), enalapril and enalaprilat (Vasotec), labetalol hydrochloride (Normodyne), nicardipine hydrochloride (Cardene), and esmolol hydrochloride (Brevibloc) are used because they can be titrated for safe, effective reduction of SBP. Assess the patient's response to these agents (i.e., presenting symptoms improved or new symptoms not present).

SUMMARY

Cardiac disease is a major health threat to American society. Emergency nurses are challenged to stay current not only with research and the evidence-based practice changes it brings, but also with the rapid advancements in technology that affect the diagnostic and interventional tools available to care for this patient population.

REFERENCES

1. American Heart Association: *Advanced cardiac life support provider manual*, Dallas, 2006, The Association.
2. American Heart Association: *American Heart Association scientific position: sudden cardiac death*, 2007. Retrieved March 8, 2008, from http://www.american-heart.org/print_presenter.jhtml?identifier=4741.
3. American Heart Association: *Heart disease and stroke statistics—2007 update*, Dallas, 2007, The Association.
4. Antman EM, Hand M, Armstrong PW et al: 2007 Focused update of the ACC/AHA 2004 guidelines for the management of patients with ST-elevation myocardial infarction: a report of the American College of Cardiology/American Heart Association Task Force on Practice Guidelines, *Circulation* 117:296, 2008.
5. Carter T, Riegel B: Care of patients with pericardial disease. In Moser D, Riegel B, editors: *Cardiac nursing: a companion to Braunwald's heart disease*, St. Louis, 2008, Elsevier.
6. Chobanian AV, Bakris GL, Black HR et al: Seventh report of the Joint National Committee on Prevention, Detection, Evaluation, and Treatment of High Blood Pressure, *Hypertension* 42:1206, 2003.
7. Christman SK: Care of the patient with peripheral vascular disease. In Moser D, Riegel B, editors: *Cardiac nursing: a companion to Braunwald's heart disease*, St. Louis, 2008, Elsevier.
8. Drew BJ: ST Segment monitoring. In Moser D, Riegel B, editors: *Cardiac nursing: a companion to Braunwald's heart disease*, St. Louis, 2008, Elsevier.
9. Fahey VA: *Vascular nursing*, ed 4, Philadelphia, 2004, WB Saunders.
10. Fleming C, Whitlock EP, Beil TL et al: Screening for abdominal aortic aneurysm: a best-evidence systematic review for the US Preventive Health Services Task Force, *Ann Intern Med* 142:203, 2005.

11. Futterman LG: Electrocardiography: abnormal electrocardiogram. In Moser D, Riegel B, editors: *Cardiac nursing: a companion to Braunwald's heart disease*, St. Louis, 2008, Elsevier.

12. Gibler WB, Cannon CP, Blomkains AL et al: Practical implementation of the guidelines for unstable angina/non–ST-segment elevation myocardial infarction in the emergency department: a scientific statement from the American Heart Association, *Circulation* 111:2699, 2005.

13. Hajjar I, Kotchen TA: Trends in prevalence, awareness, treatment and control of hypertension in the United States, 1988-2000, *JAMA* 290:199, 2003.

14. Howard PK: Emergency department care of the cardiac patient. In Moser D, Riegel B, editors: *Cardiac nursing: a companion to Braunwald's heart disease*, St. Louis, 2008, Elsevier.

15. Hunt SA, Abraham WT, Chin MH et al: ACC/AHA 2005 guideline update for the diagnosis and management of chronic heart failure in the adult—summary article: a report of the American College of Cardiology/American Heart Association Task Force on Practice Guidelines (Writing Committee to Update the 2001 Guidelines for the Evaluation and Management of Heart Failure), *Circulation* 112:1825, 2005.

16. Leonard A: Care of patients with stroke. In Moser D, Riegel B, editors: *Cardiac nursing: a companion to Braunwald's heart disease*, St. Louis, 2008, Elsevier.

17. McCance KL, Huether SE: *Pathophysiology: the biologic basis for disease in adults and children*, ed 5, St. Louis, 2006, Mosby.

18. Pelter MM: Electrocardiography: normal electrocardiogram. In Moser D, Riegel B, editors: *Cardiac nursing: a companion to Braunwald's heart disease*, St. Louis, 2008, Elsevier.

19. Piano MR: Pathophysiology of heart failure. In Moser D, Riegel B, editors: *Cardiac nursing: a companion to Braunwald's heart disease*, St. Louis, 2008, Elsevier.

20. Rosamond W, Flegal W, Furie K et al: Heart disease and stroke statistics—2008 update: a report from the American Heart Association Statistics Committee and Stroke Statistics Subcommittee, *Circulation* 117:e25, 2008.

21. Ross M, Lesikar S, Peacock F et al: Chest pain center accreditation is associated with better performance of Center for Medicare and Medicaid Services core measures for acute myocardial infarction, *Acad Emerg Med* 14(5 suppl 1):s55, 2007.

22. Spratto GR, Woods AL: *PDR nurse's drug handbook*, Clifton Park, NY, 2008, Delmar Learning.

23. Springhouse: *Nursing 2008 drug handbook*, Philadelphia, 2008, Lippincott Williams & Wilkins.

24. Thygesen K, Alpert JS, White HD et al: Universal definition of myocardial infarction, *Circulation* 116:2634, 2007.

25. US Preventive Health Services Task Force: Screening for abdominal aortic aneurysm: recommendation statement, *Ann Intern Med* 142:198, 2005.

CHAPTER 32

Shock Emergencies

Reneé Semonin Holleran

Shock is a clinical manifestation of inadequate tissue perfusion. It is a life-threatening, generalized maldistribution of blood flow that results in failure of the delivery and utilization of oxygen. There are multiple causes of shock; however, the pathophysiology of shock is generally the same. It is important to remember that vital sign changes do not define shock. Evidence of inadequate tissue perfusion based on physical examination and suspicion based on history are the best methods of identifying shock.[1,12]

The shock state is also associated with systemic inflammatory response syndrome (SIRS). The causes of shock, such as an infection or volume loss, serve as a primary insult, or the body's response to hemorrhage or infection as a secondary response, that triggers SIRS. Inflammatory markers can be detected in the blood of all patients in shock. However, biomarker levels and the significance of these levels vary depending on the cause of the shock state.[1]

This chapter will discuss the pathophysiology of shock, the categories of shock, shock management in the emergency department (ED), and the effects of shock on selected patient populations.

PATHOPHYSIOLOGY

Shock results from inadequate tissue perfusion that leads to failure of the delivery and/or use of oxygen, causing tissue dysoxia.[1] In the presence of hypoxia and inadequate tissue perfusion, cells do not receive oxygen and nutrients (especially glucose), nor are they able to remove waste products. Cellular damage and eventual death ensues when cellular oxygen demands exceed the tissue's oxygen supply.

Normal cell metabolism requires an aerobic environment to break down glucose and oxidize substrates. Enzyme-mediated chemical reactions transfer energy from this process into adenosine triphosphate (ATP). Oxidative energy synthesis of ATP is necessary for cell survival and is a fundamental characteristic of life. This process is also referred to as cellular respiration.

Cellular respiration occurs within organelles known as mitochondria, which are located in the cell's cytoplasm. Mitochondria are the site of ATP synthesis and energy production. Lysosomes in the cytoplasm store hydrolytic or digestive enzymes that mediate chemical reactions within the cell.

The production of cellular energy and synthesis of ATP is dependent on a continuous oxygen supply. Availability of oxygen is influenced by blood flow, oxygen saturation, and cardiac output. Oxygen consumption (VO_2) is the amount of oxygen removed by the tissues for metabolism. Oxygen debt refers to the difference between cellular demand for oxygen and cellular consumption of available oxygen. A continuous oxygen debt related to tissue hypoxia creates an anaerobic environment that adversely affects cellular metabolism. Oxygen delivery (DO_2) depends on the oxygen content of arterial blood and the cardiac output.

Anaerobic metabolism leads to the accumulation of lactate, hydrogen ions, and inorganic phosphates within the cell. ATP production is diminished, and protein production is compromised, which results in damage to the mitochondria of the cell. Damage to the mitochondria triggers problems with electron transport and the activation of apoptosis (programmed cellular destruction). Intracellular enzymes that are activated by these changes release enzymes that further deplete ATP stores (cellular energy) and damage cellular membranes, including noninjured cells.

A shift of sodium into the cell to increase cellular fluid causes the displacement of potassium outside of the cell. When cells swell from the absorption of interstitial fluid, this swelling narrows the capillary lumens and further decreases the supply of oxygen and nutrients to the cells. Changes in potassium interfere with nervous, cardiovascular, and muscular cell function. Eventually, energy-dependent potassium channels fail, causing arterioles to dilate and lead finally to uncompensated shock.

The cause of shock serves as a trigger to initiate a systemic inflammatory response. Whether it is direct tissue damage, for example, a brain contusion or liver laceration, or an infection from burn wounds, the body initiates an immune response that releases proinflammatory cytokines and phospholipids. This sets off a cascade of changes that assist in protecting the body. Proinflammatory cytokines activate cells that function within the immune system. This results in a hyperinflammatory response (i.e., SIRS). One function of the immune system is to stop the programmed cell death (apoptosis) that occurs with SIRS. If the cause of shock is not recognized and managed early, SIRS will continue and result in the production of arachidonic acids, prostaglandins, thromboxanes, and other metabolites that will continue the inflammatory response.[10]

In an effort to maintain homeostasis, antiinflammatory mediators are produced. Unfortunately, these mediators are responsible for immunosuppression that leaves the patient at risk for further infection and/or septic complications. The body's ability to successfully balance proinflammatory and antiinflammatory responses so that it can heal or fight off an infection depends on early and appropriate interventions to manage and treat the cause of the shock state.

The activation of cytokines, arachidonic acid metabolites, and other toxins instigates the plasmatic cascade system, which plays a role in endothelial and parenchymal cell death and in coagulation. This can result in an inability to heal, as well as development of disseminated intravascular coagulation (DIC),[10] and becomes a vicious cycle that must be stopped as early as possible.

Glucose metabolism is also impaired. The stress of the shock state triggers gluconeogenesis to provide fuel for system functioning and healing. In addition, the liver and kidneys produce more glucose in response to the secretion of epinephrine, norepinephrine, glucagon, and cortisol as part of the body's stress response. Even though the body produces more glucose as a response to stress, insulin resistance occurs because of increased production of serum cytokines.[20]

Increased production of glucose and insulin resistance actually impair cellular growth and metabolism. This has lead to the development of protocols to use insulin therapy in the care of patients in shock, particularly sepsis.[19,20]

Figure 32-1 provides a summary of impaired cellular metabolism that occurs as a result of inadequate tissue perfusion and impaired oxygen and glucose use.

Stages of Shock

Regardless of the cause of the shock state, the body mobilizes a series of responses to compensate. Compensatory responses are stimulated by decreasing tissue perfusion. Ideally the outcome of these compensatory mechanisms is restoration of cardiac output and tissue perfusion. To accomplish this, blood is shunted from the kidneys, gastrointestinal tract, liver, and skin to vital organs (the heart, lungs, and brain). Key compensatory responses include the baroreceptors, sympathetic nervous system, fluid shifts, and endocrine system. Without these compensatory mechanisms, shock progresses and ultimately death occurs. Table 32-1 summarizes the progression of the shock state.

Compensatory Mechanisms

When the patient "goes into shock," there are multiple compensatory mechanisms that are triggered within the body in an attempt to compensate and maintain a state of homeostasis. The following is a discussion of these.

Baroreceptors

Baroreceptors are a collection of specialized neural tissues located in the aortic arch and bifurcation of the common carotid arteries. Baroreceptor reflexes respond to small changes in vascular tone or pressure. Inhibition of baroreceptors by the vasomotor center of the brain in response to decreasing cardiac output results in sympathetic stimulation followed by peripheral vasoconstriction in an effort to increase circulating volume and maintain blood pressure. Similarly, the resulting decrease in vagal tone decreases coronary resistance in an attempt to improve myocardial oxygen supply.[12]

Sympathetic Nervous System

Stimulation of the sympathetic nervous system by decreases in circulating volume and cardiac output results in release of epinephrine, norepinephrine, and other catecholamines that stimulate α- and β-receptors. Stimulation of α-receptors is followed by arteriolar and venous vasoconstriction, which shunts blood to organs. Other effects include stimulation of the adrenal glands, which ultimately leads to fluid retention by the kidneys. The chronotropic effect is tachycardia. β-Receptor stimulation has a positive inotropic effect, increasing myocardial contractility and improving coronary artery blood flow. The α- and β-adrenergic effects augment venous return, increasing ventricular filling or preload, heart rate, and myocardial contractility, which facilitates ventricular emptying and improves cardiac output and blood pressure.[6]

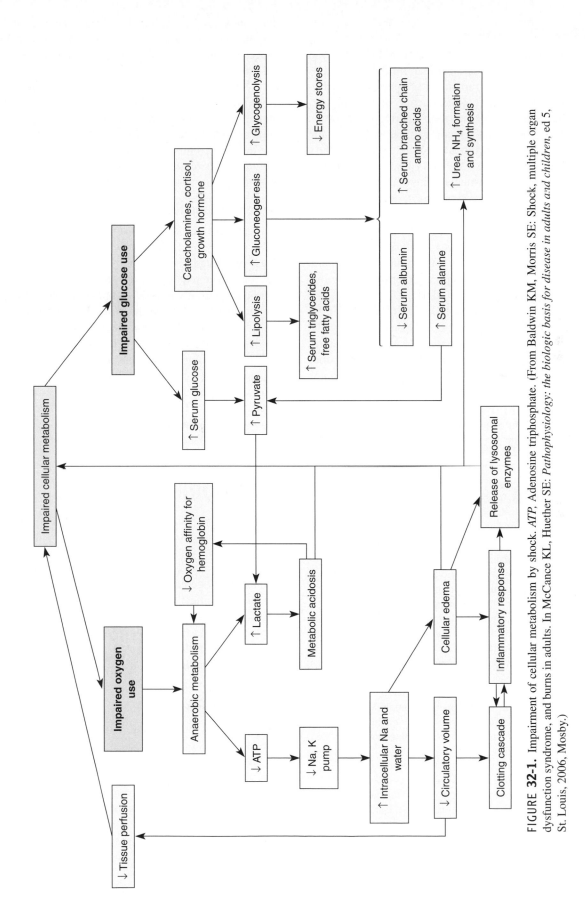

FIGURE 32-1. Impairment of cellular metabolism by shock. *ATP,* Adenosine triphosphate. (From Baldwin KM, Morris SE: Shock, multiple organ dysfunction syndrome, and burns in adults. In McCance KL, Huether SE: *Pathophysiology: the biologic basis for disease in adults and children,* ed 5, St. Louis, 2006, Mosby.)

Shift of Interstitial Fluid

Normal distribution of body fluid is 75% intracellular and 25% extracellular. Of the extracellular fluid, one third is located intravascularly; the remainder is interstitial. Hydrostatic pressure and plasma colloid oncotic pressure (COP) are forces that maintain normal fluid distribution between the intravascular and interstitial compartments. Hydrostatic pressure pushes fluid from the arterial end of the capillary bed into the interstitial space. COP pulls fluid into the venous capillary bed because of plasma proteins such as albumin.

Endocrine Response

The endocrine system response to decreased circulating volume or decreased cardiac output is a result of the interaction of the adrenal glands, the kidneys, the pituitary gland, and the lungs. Components are the renin-angiotensin-aldosterone system and antidiuretic hormone (ADH).

RENIN-ANGIOTENSIN-ALDOSTERONE SYSTEM. Renal hypoperfusion and mediation of β-receptors by the sympathetic nervous system secondary to shock causes release of renin. Renin activates conversion of angiotensinogen to angiotensin I, which is then converted by the lungs into angiotensin II and causes release of aldosterone and produces vasoconstriction. Aldosterone promotes sodium reabsorption within the renal tubule. Water follows reabsorption of sodium, so the net effect is water movement from the interstitial space into the intravascular space. Ideally, circulating volume and cardiac output increase. There is a corresponding decrease in urinary output as a result of this response.

ANTIDIURETIC HORMONE. ADH is released by the posterior pituitary gland in response to increased plasma osmolarity, altered circulating volume, and in response to angiotensin. ADH causes sodium and water reabsorption from the distal renal tubules in an attempt to increase circulating volume and cardiac output. Urine output decreases, and urine specific gravity increases as a result of this process.

Adrenal Gland Response

The adrenal glands are stimulated by the sympathetic nervous system when a patient is in shock. This causes the release of epinephrine and norepinephrine as part of the stress response. The release of these catecholamines causes tachycardia and initially improves cardiac output to focus on end-organ perfusion. Both epinephrine and norepinephrine cause peripheral vasoconstriction to increase peripheral vascular resistance and increase blood return to the heart.

The triggering of the stress response stimulates the hypothalamus to secrete corticotropin-releasing hormone, which stimulates the pituitary to release adrenocorticotropic hormone (ACTH). This causes the release of cortisol (another stress-response hormone) from the adrenal glands. Cortisol will elevate blood glucose and renal retention of water and sodium.[6]

CATEGORIES OF SHOCK

Shock has been categorized or classified in a number of ways. The one most commonly used is based on the cause of shock, for example, hemorrhagic because of blood loss. Shock may also be described by type, including hypovolemic, cardiogenic, distributive, and obstructive. Finally, another classification looks at alterations in circulating volume, alterations in the capability of the heart to move the circulating volume, and alterations in peripheral vascular resistance. The following is a description of the categories of shock based on the cause.

Hypovolemic Shock

Hypovolemic shock results from loss or redistribution of blood, plasma, or other body fluids, which ultimately leads to overall reduction in intravascular volume. Hypovolemic shock is primarily an alteration in circulating volume. Hemorrhagic shock is a form of hypovolemic shock. Hypovolemic shock is the type of shock seen most frequently by the emergency nurse. It is a direct result of reduction in intravascular volume. Decreased circulating volume can be caused by loss or redistribution of whole blood, plasma, or other body fluids. Loss of volume in the intravascular space causes a reduction in preload. Preload describes the force that stretches the cardiac ventricles to an initial length. The resting force on the heart is determined by the pressure in

Table 32-1. STAGES OF SHOCK	
Stage	**Pathophysiology**
Compensated (nonprogressive) stage	Various receptors sense the drop in systemic pressure and initiate a cascade of physiologic changes. Homeostatic compensatory mechanisms, mediated by the sympathetic nervous system, increase end organ perfusion. Aerobic metabolism changes to anaerobic metabolism and lactic acid is produced.
Uncompensated (progressive) stage	Compensatory mechanisms begin to fail. Mechanisms initially helpful, now cause more injury. Cellular derangement occurs which causes organ death. Severe lactic acidosis and inflammatory/immune system activation contribute to this.
Irreversible (refractory) stage	In refractory shock, no treatment can reverse the shock process. The cause of the shock is indistinguishable. The clinical progression of the shock state is unique to the patient and is influenced by factors such as the cause of the shock, the age of the patient, severity and duration of the hypoperfused state, and presence of preexisting diseases.

Modified from Holleran RS: Shock emergencies. In Hoyt KS, Selfridge TJ, editors: *Emergency nursing core curriculum*, ed 6, St. Louis, 2007, Mosby.

ventricles at the end of diastole. When blood or volume is lost, there is inadequate fluid returning to the heart and that has an impact on preload. Redistribution, or third-space sequestration, occurs when fluid shifts from the intravascular compartment to the interstitial space. This can occur with changes in capillary permeability or capillary fluid pressures, as in burn injuries or sepsis, and can also have an impact on preload. Actual volume loss is associated with traumatic injury, posterior nasal bleeds, intraabdominal hemorrhage, significant vaginal bleeding, gastrointestinal bleeding, or excessive vomiting and diarrhea. Table 32-2 illustrates the physiologic response to hemorrhage based on a 70-kg male.

Cardiogenic Shock

Cardiogenic shock occurs when the heart fails as a pump, causing a significant reduction in ventricular effectiveness. Cardiac output decreases and tissue perfusion diminishes, while left ventricular end-diastolic pressure increases. Injury to the myocardium impairs contractility, which decreases ventricular emptying. Cardiogenic shock continues to carry a high mortality rate; most patients die within 24 hours; others may live only a few days. Cardiogenic shock is caused by myocardial infarction with damage to greater than 40% of the left ventricle, severe myocardial contusion, valvular heart disease, cardiomyopathies, ruptured papillary muscle, ruptured ventricular septum, and dysrhythmias such as third-degree heart block. Myocardial damage may occur as the result of a single infarction or subsequent to multiple events.

When pump failure occurs, the myocardium cannot forcibly eject blood. Stroke volume decreases because of decreased contractility, which decreases cardiac output and blood pressure. Subsequent alterations in tissue perfusion precipitate myocardial ischemia and extend the region of injury, further compromising cardiac contractility. Myocardial contractility is also affected by hypoxemia, metabolic acidosis, ventricular diastolic volume, and sympathetic nervous system stimulation. Poor myocardial contractility causes inadequate emptying of the left ventricle.

Incomplete emptying of the left ventricle during diastole elevates pressures in the left ventricle, left atrium, and pulmonary vessels. There is a corresponding increase in pulmonary pressures as pulmonary capillaries leak fluid into the alveolar spaces, causing pulmonary edema. Elevated pulmonary pressures increase right ventricular and atrial pressures, which contribute to right-sided heart failure.

Increased myocardial performance as a compensatory response to shock translates to increased myocardial oxygen demand and increased myocardial ischemia, which further compromises cardiac output and eventually progresses to cardiovascular collapse.

Neurogenic Shock

Neurogenic shock is most often associated with acute spinal cord disruption from trauma or spinal anesthesia. Other causes of neurogenic shock are brain injury, hypoxia, depressant drug actions, and hypoglycemia associated with insulin shock. In neurogenic shock, outflow from the vasomotor center in the medulla is inhibited or depressed, causing loss of sympathetic vasomotor regulation. Uncontested parasympathetic responses cause vasodilatation and loss of sympathetic tone. Inhibition of sympathetic innervation impedes release of norepinephrine and interferes with the body's ability to vasoconstrict. Consequently, venous return and cardiac output decrease.

Septic Shock

Septic shock is defined as the presence of sepsis with refractory hypotension.[14] Septic shock is caused by an infectious agent or infection-induced mediators. The body responds through both hyperinflammatory and antiinflammatory means. Endotoxins released by the invading organisms prompt release of hydrolytic enzymes from weakened cell lysosomes, which causes cellular destruction of bacteria and normal cells. When the body is unable to control the proinflammatory mediators, it produces a systemic inflammatory response. As a result, there is widespread cellular dysfunction that brings about acute respiratory distress syndrome (ARDS), DIC, multiple organ dysfunction syndrome (MODS), and eventually death. The mortality rate from septic shock is 50% and increases when patients have comorbid problems such as immunosuppression, diabetes, or cardiovascular disease.

Table 32-2. PHYSIOLOGIC RESPONSES TO HEMORRHAGE (BASED ON 70-KG MALE)

Class % Blood Loss	Pulse	Blood Pressure	Pulse Pressure	Level of Consciousness	Respiratory Rate	Urinary Output
Class One (I) Up to 15% (up to 750 ml)	<100	Normal	Normal or increased	Slightly anxious	14-20	>30 ml/hr
Class Two (II) 15%-30% (750-1500 ml)	>100	Normal	Decreased	Mildly anxious	20-30	20-30 ml/hr
Class Three (III) 30%-40% (1500-2000 ml)	>120	Decreased	Decreased	Anxious, confused	30-40	5-15 ml/hr
Class Four (IV) >40% (>2000 ml)	>140	Decreased	Decreased	Anxious, confused	30-40	5-15 ml/hr

From Emergency Nurses Association: *Trauma nursing core course (TNCC)*, ed 6, Des Plaines, Ill, 2007, The Association.

Anaphylactic Shock

Anaphylaxis is an acute immune and inflammatory response to an allergen. An allergen is an antigen to which someone has become sensitized, for example, insect venom, pollens, shellfish, and antibiotics. Anaphylactic shock is a profound hypersensitivity reaction with a systemic antigen-antibody response. Antibodies are formed on initial exposure to a foreign protein. Current research suggests that the pathophysiology of anaphylactic shock results from a profound reduction in venous tone and extravasation of fluid, which causes reduced venous return and depressed myocardial function.[3] Clinical manifestations are usually acute and sudden and include hypotension, altered mental status, and in some cases cardiac arrest. The release of histamine causes peripheral skin flushing, hypotension, and tachycardia. The initial clinical manifestations of anaphylactic shock may include anxiety, shortness of breath, nausea, vomiting and diarrhea, hives, urticaria, and sensations of burning and itching of the skin.[12]

Obstructive Shock

Obstructive shock occurs from mechanical obstruction or compression of the great veins, pulmonary arteries, aorta, or the myocardium itself, which prevents adequate circulating volume. Inadequate cardiac output and tissue hypoperfusion occur when the obstruction prevents adequate emptying of the myocardium during systole or filling during diastole. Pulmonary embolus prevents right ventricular emptying when a large portion of the pulmonary artery lumen is obstructed. Incomplete right ventricular emptying causes decreased cardiac output, right ventricular failure, and increased right atrial pressure. Air embolus obstructs flow from the right atrium to the pulmonary outflow tract, preventing emptying of the right ventricle during systole. Pericardial tamponade compresses the heart and prevents filling of the atria and ventricles, leading to a reduction in stroke volume.

CLINICAL MANIFESTATIONS OF SHOCK

Although shock occurs at the cellular level, manifestations of the shock state are evident at the systemic level. A thorough physical examination is needed to identify clinical findings such as hypotension, tachycardia, altered mental status, delayed capillary refill, decreased urinary output, and pale, cool skin and extremities, which have been found to be some of the most reliable physical signs of shock.[1] The following is a discussion of some of the other clinical findings of shock.

Respiratory

During shock, respiratory effectiveness is affected by hypoxia. Evaluation of respiratory rate, rhythm, and work of breathing should be performed. Tachypnea is a common finding and occurs in an effort to decrease carbon dioxide and compensate for cellular acidosis. Adequate oxygenation may be indicated by pulse oximetry, but in reality, inadequate circulating volume perpetuates cellular hypoxia and anaerobic cellular metabolism. Therefore gradual increases in depth and rate of respiration may be early signs of impending shock. Breath sounds may also be absent, unequal, or diminished. Wheezes, crackles, or coarse breath sounds indicating pulmonary congestion occur with cardiogenic shock.

Circulatory

Cardiac output is determined by preload, afterload, contractility, and heart rate. Preload is the volume in the right and left ventricles at the end of diastole. It is affected by circulating volume, right arterial pressure, and intrathoracic pressure. Preload affects myocardial stretch and the force of myocardial contractility. Afterload is the arterial pressure or resistance the ventricles must overcome with each contraction, that is, the amount of pressure necessary for the left ventricle to contract. Afterload is affected by aortic pressure, pulmonary arterial pressure, and systemic vascular resistance. An increase in afterload decreases stroke volume and subsequently decreases cardiac output. Contractility refers to the heart's contractile force.

The pulse rate increases when the sympathetic nervous system responds to decreased cardiac output in shock. A corresponding decrease in stroke volume results in weak, thready pulses. It is important to remember that in young children the only way they can increase their cardiac output is to increase their pulse rate. This also leads to increased oxygen consumption by the heart. If allowed to continue, this compensatory mechanism will eventually fail. Bradycardia is an ominous sign of impending arrest in the child.

The older adult patient may have limited ability because of preexisting cardiac disease or failure to maintain an increased heart rate. Medications such as β-blockers will impede the heart's ability to increase its rate.

Evaluate and compare peripheral pulses to central pulses for presence, rate, equality, and quality.

A drop in systolic blood pressure occurs from decreased cardiac output or decreased venous return. In early shock the diastolic blood pressure rises because of sympathetic effect on peripheral vascular resistance, which causes vasoconstriction. Consequently, pulse pressure narrows in the presence of decreased systolic blood pressure. As shock progresses, sympathetic activity becomes less effective and diastolic blood pressure begins to fall.

A reduction in arterial distension caused by decreased cardiac output and a proportionate decrease in stroke volume causes flattened jugular veins when the patient is supine. However, the patient in obstructive shock or cardiogenic shock can have neck veins that appear full as a result of right-sided ventricular failure or increased pulmonary pressures. Flat neck veins are an indication of decreased systemic volume.

Auscultate heart sounds to evaluate rate, quality, and the presence of abnormal sounds such as S_3 or S_4 and to identify irregularities such as murmurs, friction rubs, or a gallop. Distant heart tones may indicate cardiac tamponade, a cause of obstructive shock. Cardiac dysrhythmias develop frequently as a result of injury to the myocardium or metabolic acidosis. Stimulation of the sympathetic nervous system causes tachycardia. Progression of shock and depletion of epinephrine stores lead to bradycardia, heart blocks, and ventricular dysrhythmias, including ventricular fibrillation.

Level of consciousness is a sensitive assessment of shock and its progression. Decreased cerebral perfusion and hypoxia are initially manifested by restlessness, anxiety, or confusion. Continued progression of shock with significant cerebral hypoperfusion and hypoxia leads to an obtunded, unresponsive patient.

Other Organ Systems

When tissue perfusion decreases, the body considers only three organs essential: the brain, heart, and lungs. All others (the kidneys, intestines, and skin) are nonessential for self-preservation. Blood is shunted away from these nonessential organs in an attempt to maintain cardiac output and cerebral perfusion. Sympathetic nervous system activity and peripheral vasoconstriction shunt blood from the skin, causing cool skin, pallor, cyanosis, and diaphoresis. Children develop mottled extremities. Capillary refill is greater than 2 seconds. Skin perfusion and capillary refill may be altered by hypothermia or preexisting peripheral vascular disease. Delayed capillary refill should be considered in light of other assessment findings for determining shock or impending shock.

Normal urinary output is 0.5 to 1 mL/kg/hr. In shock, urinary output falls secondary to renal hypoperfusion and release of ADH. Urine specific gravity increases with reabsorption of water in the renal distal tubules. Reduction in hourly urine output with a rise in specific gravity may signify shock. Blood urea nitrogen (BUN) and creatinine levels increase as renal perfusion decreases.

Vasoconstriction leads to hypoperfusion of the gastrointestinal tract. Clinical manifestations include hypoactive or absent bowel sounds, leakage of pancreatic enzymes with an elevated serum amylase level, and inability of the liver to metabolize substrates such as lactic acid. In addition, peristalsis ceases and increases the risk for a paralytic ileus or necrosis of the gastrointestinal tract. Concurrently, there is hypoperfusion of the liver and alteration of hepatic function that result in decreased conversion of lactate to bicarbonate and mobilization of glycogen stores, resulting in increased blood glucose levels. These effects worsen the metabolic acidosis found in the patient in shock.

MANAGEMENT OF THE PATIENT IN SHOCK
Patient Assessment

The assessment of a patient who is in shock is composed of clinical, historical, and laboratory findings. The emergency nurse must maintain a high index of suspicion that a patient may be at risk for developing shock based on a significant history or if the patient is exhibiting one or more of the following clinical findings: hypotension, tachycardia, altered mental status, delayed capillary refill, decreased urinary output, and pale cool skin and extremities.

History

History related to the patient's illness or injury needs to be rapidly collected. The emergency nurse should consider factors that would place the patient at risk for shock, including mechanisms that may cause injuries to organs such as the liver, spleen, or long bones that can cause blood loss; recent exposure to an infectious agent; or presence of an invasive device such as a urinary catheter, peripherally inserted central catheter, or feeding tube. Any patient who is human immunodeficiency virus (HIV)-positive, has had an organ transplant, or is receiving chemotherapy is at risk for sepsis and septic shock. A history of diabetes, cardiovascular disease, or hematologic disorder are a few of the medical conditions that can place a patient at greater risk for complications from inadequate tissue perfusion.

Medications such as corticosteroids, antibiotics, and immunosuppressants may produce additional risk factors for shock complications. Anticoagulants such as warfarin sodium may cause excessive blood loss, even from minor injuries, and lead to hemorrhagic shock.

Normal physiologic differences or changes associated with the very young and the very old may interfere with the body's ability to cope with some of the causes of shock such as volume loss.

Finally, recent surgery or immobility can be risk factors for obstructive shock from a pulmonary embolus.

The more information that can be gathered from the patient, family, or significant others, the more likely the cause of shock can be identified and appropriate treatment begun in the ED.

Box 32-1 contains a summary of some of the pertinent pieces of history related to shock.

Resuscitation

The resuscitation of any patient begins with the primary assessment and implementation of the critical and correct interventions. Early recognition of the cause of the shock and goal-directed therapies are critical for a positive patient outcome. Adequate oxygenation and circulatory support to correct hypoxia and inadequate tissue perfusion are essential. An effective airway should be obtained or maintained along with support of effective ventilation. Supplemental oxygen should be applied to the patient, generally a nonrebreather mask at a high flow rate. Endotracheal intubation and mechanical ventilation may be needed to maintain adequate ventilation.

Resuscitation End Points

Over the past two decades, shock resuscitation has been extensively evaluated. Using evidence-based methods, resuscitation end points have been identified to manage patients with specific shock syndromes, including hemorrhagic and septic shock.[18] The objectives for the use of resuscitation endpoints are the following:

- Identification of the severity of the physiologic derangement of the shock state
- The ability to predict the risk for developing MODS or death
- To determine end points that would predict whether the patient may or may not survive without multiple organ dysfunction
- To improve patient survival by using the appropriate resuscitation end points

Suggested resuscitation end points have included oxygen delivery measured by the monitoring of mixed venous oxygen saturation (SVO_2), hemodynamic profiles measured by central venous pressure (CVP) and pulmonary capillary wedge pressure, and acid-base status measured by monitoring base deficits and lactate levels.

Management of Circulation and Perfusion

Management of circulation is directed toward identification of fluid or blood loss in hypovolemic/hemorrhagic shock. Active bleeding must be controlled through direct pressure, embolization, or operative management. The emergency care team must recognize what capabilities are available for patient management and appropriately transfer a patient if resources are not offered at the current care facility. Peripheral veins should be cannulated with the largest-caliber intravenous catheter possible. Central venous access may be necessary, but careful consideration must be given to the risk for infection. Intraosseous access may be necessary for a patient with profound shock and can provide a method of fluid and drug administration until adequate resuscitation has occurred to obtain other venous access.

There is limited evidence that guides fluid resuscitation.[1] Aggressive fluid resuscitation should be avoided in a patient with penetrating trauma until the bleeding can be surgically controlled. Evidence-based guidelines recommend that target blood pressures during shock resuscitation should be maintained in the following way[18]:

- For uncontrolled hemorrhage due to trauma: mean arterial pressure (MAP) of 40 mm Hg until bleeding is controlled
- For traumatic brain injury without systemic hemorrhage: MAP of 90 mm Hg
- For all other shock states: MAP greater than 65 mm Hg

CIRCULATION AND PERFUSION IN HEMORRHAGIC SHOCK. Controversy continues about resuscitation of the patient in hemorrhagic shock.[2,6] The major themes are related to fluid type, amount, the use of blood, and the role of permissive hypotension. As previously discussed, research continues to demonstrate that during active hemorrhage, the blood pressure should be managed based on the patient's response, not on a specific number. Aggressive fluid resuscitation has been associated with dislodgement of blood clots, dilation of the venous system, dilution of clotting factors, exacerbation of coagulopathies, and hypothermia.[2,6]

Administration of blood and blood products (including massive transfusion) have also come under question. Massive blood product use has been associated with coagulopathies, the development of ARDS, multiple organ failure, and death. In addition, blood supplies in most parts of the world (including the United States) are limited and expensive. Triggers for blood transfusions for hemorrhagic shock need to be in place in all institutions that use blood as part of the resuscitation of hemorrhagic shock.[13] Future control of hemorrhage may include the administration of recombinant factor VIIa, hemoglobin-based oxygen carriers, and blood substitutes.[1]

CIRCULATION AND PERFUSION IN CARDIOGENIC SHOCK. Options to enhance cardiac output and myocardial contractility include administration of sympathomimetic agents; however, these should be used only after hypovolemia has been corrected and preload optimized. Some of the agents include dopamine, dobutamine, norepinephrine, epinephrine, and phenylephrine. Mechanical support may need to be initiated to provide support for a failing heart. Devices that may be used include intraaortic balloon pumps, right ventricular assist devices, and left ventricular assist devices.

CIRCULATION AND PERFUSION IN NEUROGENIC SHOCK. Spinal cord injuries may be managed initially by fluid resuscitation. If there is no response and other sources of hypotension have been ruled out, vasopressors may be used to maintain an adequate MAP.

CIRCULATION AND PERFUSION IN SEPTIC SHOCK. The management of sepsis and septic shock has received a great deal of attention over the past 10 years.[14] The ED plays a key role in the initiation of goal-directed therapy for the management of severe sepsis and septic shock. Research has demonstrated better outcomes when there is a seamless and organized continuum of care from the ED to the critical care unit.[15] Hypotension should be managed through crystalloid or colloid-equivalent at a rate of 20 mL/kg. If the patient's hypotension does not respond to fluid resuscitation, vasopressors should be initiated to maintain an MAP greater than 65 mm Hg.

CIRCULATION AND PERFUSION IN ANAPHY-LACTIC SHOCK. Profound hypotension and cardiovascular collapse can be sudden and rapid in the patient with anaphylaxis. This requires aggressive fluid resuscitation to restore volume to the heart. It is important to remember a quick and simple intervention that can be performed is laying the patient flat and raising the legs. Epinephrine is administered to increase cardiac output through its direct β-effect on the heart. When the patient is in profound shock, only the intravenous infusion of epinephrine is found to be effective.[3]

CIRCULATION AND PERFUSION IN OBSTRUC-TIVE SHOCK. In order to restore circulation and adequate perfusion in obstructive shock, the source of the obstruction must be identified and proper critical interventions performed. For example, for a tension pneumothorax, an emergent needle thoracentesis should be performed, followed by insertion of a chest tube.

ACID-BASE BALANCE

Inadequate tissue perfusion and hypoxia lead to acidosis. The body will attempt to compensate for this acidosis in multiple ways. The lungs and the kidneys play a key role in acid-base balance for the patient who is in shock. The major body buffer systems are found in the interstitial fluids, the blood, intracellular fluid, urine, and bone.

In early shock, respiratory alkalosis occurs because of tachypnea, the body's attempt to increase oxygen levels and decrease carbon dioxide levels in the body's tissues. Increased carbon dioxide and hydrogen ions in tissues stimulate respiratory centers in the brain and increase the rate and depth of the patient's respirations. Anaerobic metabolism increases serum lactic acid, which culminates in metabolic acidosis. Base deficit is also a sensitive indicator of shock. Both of these values can be easily measured. It is important to remember that lactate levels and base deficit can also be influenced by other factors such as liver and renal diseases. It has been found that a persistently high base deficit and low pH may be an early indicator of complications. Metabolic acidosis is corrected by providing adequate oxygenation and perfusion through ventilation, fluids, and medications. The cause of the shock state needs to be quickly identified and appropriate management initiated to correct the origin of the anaerobic process. If the pH is less than 7.1, administration of sodium bicarbonate may be needed to correct the pH. However, sodium bicarbonate should not be administered before adequate ventilation and fluids have been established.

HEMODYNAMIC MONITORING

Hemodynamic monitoring is available in many EDs. These monitoring avenues can play a role in caring for the patient in shock; however, it is important to correlate these modalities with patient assessment and weigh the risk for additional complications such as infection before using invasive monitoring devices. In 2006 an international consensus conference published evidence-based guidelines for hemodynamic monitoring in shock.[1] The group recommended the following for hemodynamic monitoring of goal-directed therapy in the management of the patient in shock:

- Frequent measurement of blood pressure and physical examination of signs of hypoperfusion, including mental status, urinary output, and skin color and temperature, should be used to monitor the patient in shock.
- Invasive blood pressure monitoring should be used only in refractory shock states.
- Routine use of pulmonary artery catheters is not recommended for patients in shock.

Pulse Oximetry

Pulse oximetry is a noninvasive method of determining hypoxia through measurement of arterial hemoglobin saturation. Light is transmitted through tissue to a light detector attached to the patient's fingertip, toes, or ear. Variability of transmission is determined by pulsated arterial flow. The light absorption abilities of oxyhemoglobin and deoxyhemoglobin are calculated by the monitor to determine the percentage of arterial saturation. Changes in peripheral circulation, use of vasoactive medications, and hypothermia will affect the usefulness of pulse oximetry monitoring for the patient in shock.

Central Venous Pressure

CVP is used to indirectly measure circulating volume, cardiac pump effectiveness, and vascular tone through measurement of pressures on the right side of the myocardium. Normal CVP measurements range from 4 to 10 cm H_2O pressure. CVP measurements lower than 4 cm H_2O indicate decreased circulating volume. A measurement greater than 10 cm H_2O signifies excessive pressures on the right side of the myocardium—often the result of pulmonary edema, fluid overload, or obstruction such as pericardial tamponade or tension pneumothorax. CVP monitoring has been found to be a useful tool to measure the effectiveness of early goal-directed therapies in shock management.[1]

Arterial Lines

Arterial pressure may be measured directly using an invasive, arterial line or indirectly using noninvasive blood pressure monitoring. Normal MAP is between 70 and 90 mm Hg. A mean arterial pressure less than 70 mm Hg indicates inadequate circulating volume with inadequate perfusion of the brain, kidneys, and coronary arteries. This may result from hypovolemia, pump failure, obstruction, or loss of systemic vascular resistance. Arterial lines can be useful for continuous monitoring of blood pressure when vasoactive drugs are being used. They also decrease the number of punctures required for the measurement of laboratory values, which is particularly important for a patient with coagulopathies.

SVO$_2$ Monitoring

The measurement of SVO$_2$ may be used as an indirect method of measuring tissue oxygenation.[4] SVO$_2$ monitoring is used to monitor the imbalance between oxygen delivery and oxygen consumption that is seen in the global hypoxia that occurs with inadequate tissue perfusion. When there is an imbalance between oxygen delivery and oxygen consumption, compensatory mechanisms are initiated. Increased cardiac output and increased oxygen extraction are triggered to increase the amount of oxygen delivery to hypoxic tissues. When the body's oxygen demand exceeds the body's ability to supply oxygen, an imbalance in SVO$_2$ is seen. If the body cannot meet these demands, anaerobic metabolism, lactic acidosis, and global hypoxia develop.[7] SVO$_2$ can be monitored by using a fiberoptic, pulmonary artery catheter. The normal range of the venous oxygenation measured from the pulmonary artery catheter is 60% to 80%. The SVO$_2$ reflects tissue use of oxygen, tissue perfusion, and cardiac output.

A fiberoptic catheter may be placed into the superior vena cava so that vena cava oxygen saturation (SVcO$_2$) can be monitored. This reflects the oxygen saturation of the blood returning from the upper body—particularly the brain. There is a limited correlation between the SVO$_2$ and SVcO$_2$; however, they have been shown to trend when the patient is in shock. SVcO$_2$ monitoring is easier to use in the ED when a pulmonary artery catheter may not be available. An SVcO$_2$ of 70% is used to guide therapy in such critical illnesses as sepsis and septic shock. The advantage of SVcO$_2$ monitoring during and after shock resuscitation is that the measurement of vital signs may indicate that the resuscitation has been successful, but the patient still suffers tissue hypoxia.[4] There are specific protocols that have been developed for goal-directed management of hypoxia that can be guided by the use of SVcO$_2$ in the ED.[7,16]

Currently, Edwards LifeSciences manufactures the Pre-Sep Central Venous Oximetry Catheter, which has multiple functions including continuous venous oxygen saturation monitoring, pressure monitoring, for high flow rates for rapid fluid administration and administration of blood products or other therapeutic medications.[5]

SVcO$_2$ and SVO$_2$ monitoring can be used to monitor goal-directed therapy for sepsis and septic shock, as well as monitoring the resuscitation of patients after hemorrhagic shock, especially when it is related to trauma.[7]

LABORATORY AND DIAGNOSTIC TESTING FOR SHOCK EMERGENCIES

Diagnostic and laboratory testing is directed at finding the cause of shock. A complete blood count; type and screen or crossmatch; serum chemistry values, including glucose, blood urea nitrogen, and creatinine; liver function tests; and a coagulation profile are some of the routine tests that may be obtained for all shock emergencies. If the source of the shock is cardiac injury, a cardiac profile should be evaluated. Serum lactate levels, arterial blood gas values, and base deficit levels can provide a "measurement" of the oxygen debt in hypoperfused patients.

Based on the patient's history, specific radiographic studies may be ordered. All patients should have a chest radiograph. If the patient has suffered a traumatic injury, radiographs of affected areas where blood loss may occur, such as the pelvis or long bones, should be obtained. The focused assessment sonography for trauma (FAST) can assist in identifying abdominal bleeding. A computed tomography or magnetic resonance imaging scan may also aid in identifying areas of blood loss or possible sources of infection causing septic shock.

Other diagnostic procedures may include 12- to 18-lead electrocardiogram, diagnostic peritoneal lavage, bronchoscopy, paracentesis, and gastroscopy or endoscopy.[9]

EMERGENCY NURSING MANAGEMENT OF THE PATIENT WITH A SHOCK EMERGENCY

The emergency nursing care for any patient with a shock emergency begins with a history and physical examination. Any potential source for shock needs to be quickly identified from the patient's history and chief complaint. The general appearance of the patient is evaluated, including the patient's level of consciousness and behaviors. Anxiety and confusion are signs of inadequate tissue perfusion and hypoxia.

High-flow oxygen should be administered. Intubation may be required to assist with oxygenation.

Color and temperature of the patient's skin needs to be assessed. Pink, pale, mottled, warm, cool, or moist are descriptors for skin perfusion. Purpuric lesions and petechiae may be hidden under clothing or mistaken for bruising.

A primary assessment should be performed and critical interventions initiated. Any signs of obvious bleeding must be controlled.[9] The appropriate use of a tourniquet is once again recommended for selected serious bleeding. Several steps can be taken to avoid injury from a tourniquet. These include the following[11,16]:

- Placing the tourniquet as distally as possible, but at least 5 cm proximal to the wound
- Avoiding application over a joint
- Applying the tourniquet directly to the exposed skin because this can prevent unnecessary movement or slipping
- Releasing the tourniquet as soon as it is medically safe. Generally, if the tourniquet is in place less than 2 hours, there should be little damage
- Never applying a tourniquet directly over a foreign object

Obtaining a blood pressure can be difficult because of vasoconstriction and low cardiac output. An ultrasonic stethoscope should be used to obtain a pressure. Central and peripheral pulses should be palpated. Capillary refill has been found to be of value in the pediatric patient to assess perfusion. However, the influence of temperature should be considered. Breath sounds, heart tones, and bowel sounds should be auscultated.

Intravenous fluids need to be administered until adequate perfusion is attained. Blood and blood products may be required for hemorrhage. O-negative packed red blood cells may be used before a patient is typed and screened. If large amounts of blood and blood products are needed for resuscitation, massive transfusion protocols should be instituted to ensure that the patient receives the appropriate blood products to prevent the additional stress of hypothermia and coagulopathy. O-positive packed red blood cells are sometimes used for male patients when O-negative is limited. If blood needs to be administered to a premenopausal female whose blood type is unknown, $Rh_O(D)$ immune globulin should be considered in the future.[6]

Pharmacologic management of shock may include medications that are used to maintain peripheral perfusion. These include dopamine, epinephrine, and norepinephrine bitartrate. These medications require close monitoring for effect and possibility of inadvertent injury if they infiltrate into tissues. Most are administered through central lines, which require meticulous care to prevent infection.

Even for the hypotensive patient, providing comfort and pain management should not be ignored. Patients may be anxious and fearful and may also require sedation. Allowing the family to be present with the patient may also provide comfort for both the patient and family.

COMPLICATIONS ASSOCIATED WITH SHOCK

Unfortunately, there are multiple complications that can occur with shock states. The most deadly is MODS, which ranges from multiple organ impairment to failure and death.[8] The sequential organ failure assessment score (SOFA) was developed to describe the degree of organ failure and how it progresses. Included in the assessment are respirations, coagulation (platelets), liver function (bilirubin), cardiovascular (inotrope use), central nervous system, and renal function (creatinine).

The definition of DIC, developed by the Scientific Subcommittee on DIC of the International Society of Thrombosis and Hematostasis, states that "DIC is an acquired syndrome characterized by intravascular activation of coagulation with loss of localization arising from different causes. It can originate from and cause damage to the microvasculature, which if sufficiently severe, can produce organ dysfunction."[17] DIC is widespread microvascular coagulation followed by depletion of clotting factors. Microthrombi form and are distributed to the microvasculature of various organs, producing infarction, tissue ischemia, and hemorrhagic necrosis when secondary fibrinolysis fails to lyse the fibrin quickly. Secondary fibrinolysis reduces clotting factors and impairs the release of fibrin degradation products

that act as anticoagulants. These processes contribute to serious bleeding tendencies. The DIC syndrome may occur after massive transfusion with blood products or in association with acute lung injury. Other factors that place the patient at risk for the development of DIC include polytrauma, neurotrauma, and fat emboli. Severe toxic or immunologic reactions to snake bites may also initiate DIC. The primary intervention for DIC is early identification and interventions to correct or manage the primary cause. For the patient with a shock emergency, that would include detection of the source of bleeding or infection. Continuous bleeding from intravenous sites or wounds serves as an important signal of DIC. Patients should be observed for obvious or occult bleeding, hematuria, petechiae, and ecchymosis.

SPECIAL POPULATIONS

It is important for the emergency nurse to recognize that pediatric, older adult, and pregnant patients respond differently to volume depletion and other causes of shock. These varied responses are due to normal growth and physiologic differences found in these patients. Table 32-3 highlights some of these differences. Emergent conditions in these populations are covered in greater detail in other chapters of this text.

Table 32-3.	SHOCK IN THE PEDIATRIC, OLDER ADULT, OR PREGNANT PATIENT
Patient	**Description**
Pediatric	Increases cardiac output by increasing heart rate; fixed stroke volume; sustains arterial pressure despite significant volume loss; loses 25% of circulating volume before signs of shock occur; hypotension and lethargy are ominous signs: early clinical manifestations are tachycardia, tachypnea, pallor, cool mottled skin, and delayed capillary refill; volume replaced with 20 mL/kg bolus of crystalloid
Older adult	Shock progression often rapid; normal physiologic changes of aging reduce compensatory mechanisms; predisposed to hypothermia; preexisting disease states contribute comorbidities
Pregnant	Hypervolemia of pregnancy means patient can remain normotensive with up to a 1500-mL blood loss; compression of inferior vena cava by gravid uterus reduces circulating volume by 30%; place patient on left side, manually displace uterus to the left, or elevate right hip with towel; risk for aspiration resulting from decreased gastric motility and decreased gastric emptying; treat suspected hypovolemia to prevent placental vasoconstriction associated with catecholamine release; potential for fetal distress exists despite maternal stability

SUMMARY

Shock is a progressive, pervasive process caused by inadequate tissue perfusion and oxygenation. Regardless of cause, the cellular effects of shock are the same. Nursing assessment, early recognition, and appropriate management are essential to prevent or reverse the shock process and ensure a positive patient outcome.

REFERENCES

1. Antonelli M, Levy M, Andrews PJ et al: Hemodynamic monitoring in shock and implications for management, *Intensive Care Med* 33:575, 2007.
2. Berry R: Management of shock in trauma, *Anesth Intensive Care Med* 6(9):308, 2005.
3. Brown SG: The pathophysiology of shock in anaphylaxis, *Immunol Allergy Clin North Am* 27:165, 2007.
4. Dickens JJ: Central venous oxygenation saturation monitoring: a role for critical care? *Curr Anesth Crit Care* 15:378, 2004.
5. Edwards LifeSciences: *Sepsis: find it fast, manage it early*, Edwards PreSep central venous oximetry catheter. Retrieved October 24, 2007, from http://www.edwards.com.
6. Emergency Nurses Association: *Trauma nursing core course (TNCC)*, ed 6, Des Plaines, Ill, 2007, The Association.
7. Goodrich C: Continuous central venous oximetry monitoring, *Crit Care Nurs Clin North Am* 18:203, 2006.
8. Gupta S, Jonas M: Sepsis, septic shock and multiple organ failure, *Anesth Intensive Care Med* 7(5):143, 2006.
9. Holleran RS: Shock emergencies. In Hoyt KS, Selfridge TJ, editors: *Emergency nursing core curriculum*, ed 6, St. Louis, 2007, Mosby.
10. Keel M, Trentz O: Pathophysiology of polytrauma, *Injury* 36:691, 2005.
11. Langley D, Criddle L: The tourniquet debate, *J Emerg Nurs* 32(4):354, 2006.
12. McCance KL, Huether S, editors: *Pathophysiology: the biologic basis for disease in adults and children*, ed 5, St. Louis, 2006, Mosby.
13. Mitra B, Mori A, Camerin P et al: Massive blood transfusion and trauma resuscitation, *Injury* 38:1023, 2007.
14. Nguyen HB, Rivers EP, Abrahamian FM et al: Severe sepsis and septic shock: review of the literature and emergency department management guidelines, *Ann Emerg Med* 48(1):28, 2006.
15. Rivers E: Early goal directed therapy in severe sepsis and septic shock, *Chest* 129(2):217, 2006.
16. Schreiber MA, Tieu B: Homeostasis in Operation Iraqi Freedom III, *Surgery* S61, 2007.
17. Taylor F, Toh CH, Hoots WK: *Towards a definition, clinical laboratory criteria, and a scoring system for disseminated intravascular coagulation*, posted at the ISTH website. Retrieved October 26, 2007, from http://www.med.unc.edu/isth/welcome.
18. Tisherman S, Barie P, Bokhari F et al: *Clinical practice guideline: endpoints of resuscitation*, National Clearinghouse, 2007, http://www.guideline.gov. Retrieved August 10, 2008.
19. Van den Berghe G: Insulin therapy for the critically ill patient, *Clin Cornerstone* 5(2):56, 2003.
20. Zauner A, Nimmerrichter P, Anderwald C et al: Severity of insulin resistance in critically ill medical patients, *Metabolism* 56:1, 2007.

CHAPTER 33

Neurologic Emergencies

Amy Brown and Diana King

The emergency nurse encounters a variety of neurologic emergencies related to illness or injury, including stroke, head trauma, spinal cord trauma, headache, and meningitis. Regardless of cause, a neurologic emergency is one that causes severe temporary or permanent disability or is an immediate threat to the patient's life. This chapter focuses on assessment and treatment of neurologic conditions caused by disease or pathologic abnormality. Patient assessment, anatomy, and physiology are also reviewed. Neurologic emergencies secondary to injury (i.e., head trauma and spinal cord trauma) are covered in Chapters 21 and 22, respectively.

ANATOMY AND PHYSIOLOGY

The nervous system coordinates, interprets, and controls interactions between the individual and the surrounding environment. The central nervous system (CNS) and the peripheral nervous system regulate most body systems.

Central Nervous System

The CNS consists of the brain and spinal cord. Functional units of the CNS are neurons, cells that relay signals between the body and the brain. More than 100 billion neurons relay signals that control the body's various systems.[2] Signal relay between neurons is controlled by neurotransmitters located at the synapse, or junction, between two neurons. Examples of neurotransmitters include acetylcholine, dopamine, norepinephrine, epinephrine, histamine, insulin, glucagon, serotonin, and angiotensin II. Signal movement along the neuron itself is an electrical phenomenon enhanced by the presence of myelin.

Brain

The adult brain weighs approximately 3 pounds, or 2% of total body weight. Brain tissue is the most energy-consuming tissue in the body, receiving approximately 20% of the cardiac output and using approximately 20% of the body's oxygen supply. Structurally the brain consists of external gray matter and internal white matter. The brain has three distinct parts: cerebrum, brainstem, and cerebellum. The cerebrum, divided into two hemispheres, represents almost 90% of the brain's weight. Bands of connective tissue, called the corpus callosum, relay information between the two hemispheres. Each hemisphere consists of lobes named for the adjacent portion of the skull (i.e., frontal, temporal, parietal, and occipital). The brainstem, consisting of the midbrain, pons, and medulla, is continuous with the spinal cord and serves as an important relay and reflex center for the CNS. Nuclei for the cranial nerves are found in the brainstem. The brainstem also controls respiration, the cardiovascular system, gastrointestinal functions, equilibrium, and eye movement.[2] The cerebellum controls activities below the level of consciousness (e.g., posture, equilibrium). Within the brain, there is a series of interconnected cavities called ventricles. Most cerebrospinal fluid (CSF) is produced within the ventricles by the choroid plexus and the ependymal cells.

In addition to the cranium, three layers of connective tissue, called meninges, surround and protect the brain. The dura matter, the outermost layer, is a double-layered fibrous membrane that lines the skull. One layer of the dura forms a tent over the brain and separates the cerebrum from the cerebellum. (This is the basis for the term supratentorial.) Below the thin middle subarachnoid mater is the subarachnoid space, which contains sinuses that collect venous blood from the brain and return blood to the internal jugular veins. CSF also flows in the subarachnoid space. The pia mater, the innermost layer, covers the brain and spinal cord and extends below the conus medullaris of the spinal cord to form the filum terminale.

Cranial Nerves

Twelve pairs of cranial nerves arise directly from the brainstem. Each nerve is identified with a Roman numeral and name. Cranial nerves may be sensory, motor, or both. Cranial nerve functions are not consciously controlled; therefore assessment of cranial nerves provides an accurate picture of brainstem activity and neurologic function. Table 33-1 lists cranial nerves and their functions.

Cerebral Blood Flow

Two pairs of arteries connect to form the circle of Willis, the brain's major blood supply. The terminal branches of each internal carotid artery branch into the posterior communicating artery and the middle and anterior cerebral arteries. This is commonly called the anterior circulation. The internal carotid arteries supply most of the cerebral hemispheres, basal ganglia, and the upper two thirds of the diencephalon (a division of the cerebrum). Two vertebral arteries unite to form a single basilar artery, which then divides into two posterior cerebral arteries. This artery complex supplies the cerebellum, brainstem, spinal cord, the occipital lobes, portions of the temporal lobes, and the posterior diencephalon. The anterior circulation supplies 80% of the blood to the brain, and the posterior circulation carries 20%. Figure 33-1 illustrates arterial blood supply to the brain. Venous blood drains from the brain through sinuses in the dura mater into the internal jugular veins.

The brain occupies 80% of the cranium. Vascular volume and CSF account for the remaining 20%. Cranial rigidity limits the brain's ability to tolerate volume expansion. If one component increases, the other components must decrease to prevent pressure on the brain. Cerebral blood flow is altered by changes in cerebral perfusion pressure (CPP). CPP is the difference between mean arterial pressure (MAP) and intracranial pressure (ICP) (MAP – ICP = CPP). The normal CPP is 60 mm Hg. Normal ICP is 10 to 15 mm Hg and is measured with invasive monitoring. Responses in fluid alterations can result in CSF reabsorption, shunting to the spinal subarachnoid space, or a decrease in cerebral blood volume into the sinus cavity. The

Table 33-1.	CRANIAL NERVES AND THEIR FUNCTIONS	
Number	Name	Function
I	Olfactory	Smell
II	Optic	Vision
III	Oculomotor	Elevate upper lid, pupillary constriction, most extraocular movements
IV	Trochlear	Downward, inward movement of the eye
V	Trigeminal	Chewing, clenching the jaw, lateral jaw movement, corneal reflexes, face sensation
VI	Abducens	Lateral eye deviation
VII	Facial	Facial motor, taste, lacrimation, and salivation
VIII	Acoustic	Equilibrium, hearing
IX	Glossopharyngeal	Swallowing, gag reflex, taste on posterior tongue
X	Vagus	Swallowing, gag reflex, abdominal viscera, phonation
XI	Spinal accessory	Head and shoulder movement
XII	Hypoglossal	Tongue movement

body's compensatory mechanisms allow for minimal changes in cranial volumes with minimal increases in ICP.[1]

Cerebrospinal Fluid

CSF is produced in the ventricles by the choroid plexus at a rate of 7 to 10 mL/hr. CSF protects the brain and spinal cord by forming a shock-absorbing cushion, providing nutrition via glucose transport, and removing metabolic waste products. CSF also compensates for changes in pressure and volume within the cranium. Table 33-2 summarizes normal CSF characteristics.

Spinal Cord

The spinal cord lies in the spinal canal of the vertebral bodies and is covered by meningeal layers. The adult spinal cord is approximately 16 to 18 inches long and extends from the brainstem to the intervertebral disk between L-1 and L-2. Sensory and motor neurons in the spinal cord conduct impulses to and from the brain. Unlike the brain, the spinal cord has white matter on the exterior and gray matter on the interior. Reflex arcs into the spinal cord operate without voluntary or conscious control. Table 33-3 lists these reflexes.

Peripheral Nervous System

The peripheral nervous system consists of 31 spinal nerves and the autonomic nervous system. Spinal nerves innervate skeletal muscle and a segment of skin called a dermatome. In

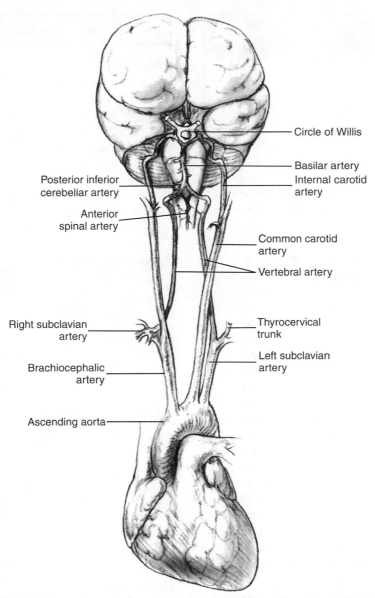

FIGURE **33-1.** Origin and course of arterial supply to the brain. (From Davis JH, Drucker WR, Foster RS et al: *Clinical surgery,* vol 1, St. Louis, 1987, Mosby.)

certain areas spinal nerves form a network called a plexus; for example, the brachial plexus innervates the upper extremity.

Autonomic Nervous System

The autonomic nervous system controls the body's visceral functions. There is no sensory component; functions are entirely motor. The cerebral cortex, hypothalamus, and the brainstem regulate activity. Two major divisions, the sympathetic and parasympathetic nervous systems, respond to stressors such as fear or blood loss to provide extra energy or conserve existing energy stores. The sympathetic nervous system provides the body energy, creating the fight-or-flight response. Receptors are scattered throughout the body, including the skin. Parasympathetic nervous system receptors distributed primarily in the head, chest, abdomen, and pelvis conserve the body's energy.

Table 33-2.	NORMAL CEREBROSPINAL FLUID
Quality	**Value/Description**
Appearance	Clear, colorless, odorless
Cell count	WBC count 5/mm³
	RBC count 0/mm³
Pressure	80-180 mm H$_2$O
Glucose	60-80 mg/100 mL (two-thirds serum glucose value)
Protein	15-45 mg/100 mL (lumbar)
pH	7.35-7.40
Sodium	140-142 mEq/L
Chloride	120-130 mEq/L
Volume	125-150 mL

WBC, White blood cell; *RBC,* red blood cell.

Table 33-3. SPINAL REFLEXES	
Reflex	**Segmental Level**
Biceps	C5-6
Brachioradialis	C5-6
Triceps	C7-8
Knee	L2-4
Ankle	S1-2
Superficial abdominal	T8-10
Superficial abdominal	T10-12
Cremasteric	L1-2
Plantar	L4-5, S1-2

Box 33-1. GLASGOW COMA SCALE	
EYE OPENING	
Spontaneous	4
To verbal command	3
To pain	2
No response	1
BEST MOTOR RESPONSE	
Obeys commands	6
Localizes pain	5
Withdraws from pain	4
Abnormal flexion	3
Abnormal extension	2
No response	1
BEST VERBAL RESPONSE	
Oriented	5
Confused	4
Inappropriate words	3
Incomprehensible sounds	2
No response	1
TOTAL	3-15

PATIENT ASSESSMENT

The most reliable indicator of neurologic function is the patient's level of consciousness (LOC). LOC must be reassessed and compared with the baseline to monitor the patient's neurologic status. Question the patient's family and significant other about changes in behavior, mood, or physical ability. Evaluate for signs of increasing ICP such as headache, nausea, vomiting, or altered LOC. Assess cranial nerve function and pupil size, equality, reactivity, and accommodation. The pupil dilates when increased ICP causes pressure on cranial nerve III; however, this is a late indicator of increasing ICP. Serial assessment is essential to identifying subtle changes that may indicate impending herniation. A universal tool such as the Glasgow Coma Scale is recommended (Box 33-1). Evaluating motor strength requires comparison of the patient's dominant hand with the evaluator's dominant hand. Sensory evaluation should include differentiation of dull and sharp objects. Assessment should also include identification of existing deficits such as muscle weakness, pupil abnormality, and gait disturbances.

Stabilization of the patient with a neurologic emergency begins with the airway, breathing, and circulation (ABCs). Specific interventions depend on patient complaint and acuity. The patient with a severe migraine headache has different priorities than does a comatose patient. A patient with severe migraine requires pain management; the comatose patient needs support of the ABCs, management of increased ICP, and monitoring for impending herniation. Herniation occurs when increased ICP forces the brain downward through the foramen magnum. Compression of the brainstem impairs respiratory and cardiovascular function, ultimately causing death. Figure 33-2 illustrates this process. Controlling increased ICP includes use of medications such as osmotic diuretics, sedatives, and analgesics. Elevating the patient's head facilitates venous drainage and decreases ICP; however, cervical spine injury must be ruled out before elevation. Decreasing stimulation such as noise and certain procedures such as suctioning can also affect ICP.

SPECIFIC NEUROLOGIC EMERGENCIES

Specific neurologic emergencies represent a threat to the patient's life, integrity of specific functions such as vision, or quality of the patient's life. Specific emergencies include headache, seizures, stroke, meningitis, Guillain-Barré syndrome, and myasthenia gravis. A brief review from the emergency nurse's perspective is presented.

Headache

Headache is one of the most common complaints seen in the emergency department (ED), with only 1% to 2% not related to trauma.[6] It is important for the emergency nurse to remember that headache is a symptom of an underlying disorder rather than a diagnosis. The headache may be minor or represent a life-threatening situation such as subarachnoid hemorrhage; therefore careful assessment is essential.

Key points to identify during the patient assessment are time of onset, duration, intensity, and location of the headache. A brief history should include any injury, vision changes, seizure activity, recent infection, and/or diagnosis of hypertension. "The worst headache ever" should be viewed as a red flag for further evaluation.

Headaches may be caused by an extracranial or intracranial condition. Extracranial causes include acidosis, dehydration, hypoglycemia, uremia, and hepatic disorders. Ophthalmic causes of headache include glaucoma, refractory errors, inflammation, or allergic reactions (see Chapter 45). Poisoning and toxicologic emergencies can also cause headache (see Chapters 42 and 52). Other extracranial causes include

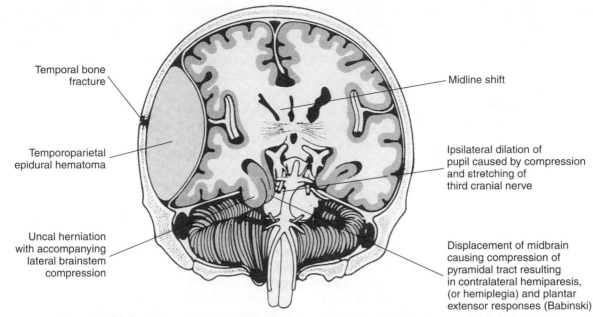

Temporal bone fracture

Temporoparietal epidural hematoma

Uncal herniation with accompanying lateral brainstem compression

Midline shift

Ipsilateral dilation of pupil caused by compression and stretching of third cranial nerve

Displacement of midbrain causing compression of pyramidal tract resulting in contralateral hemiparesis, (or hemiplegia) and plantar extensor responses (Babinski)

FIGURE **33-2.** Cross-section showing herniation of lower portion of temporal lobe (uncus) through tentorium caused by temporoparietal epidural hematoma. Herniation may occur also in the cerebellum. Note mass effect and midline shift. (From Meeker MH, Rothrock JC: *Alexander's care of the patient in surgery,* ed 10, St. Louis, 1995, Mosby.)

ear infection, upper respiratory infection, sinus congestion, facial trauma, temporomandibular joint syndrome, toothache, anemia, polycythemia, electrolyte imbalance, and systemic infection. Women have reported headaches associated with the start of menses or during the premenstrual period. Identification and treatment of extracranial causes should relieve the headache.

Specific headaches related to intracranial conditions include migraine headache, tension headache, and temporal arteritis. Traumatic headaches may occur as an emergency or nonemergency. Nonemergency conditions include postconcussion or contusion headaches. Emergent conditions that cause severe headache include intracranial injury (see Chapter 21).

Migraine Headache

Twenty-three million Americans suffer migraine headaches.[7] Diagnosis of migraine headache is based on the patient's history and presenting symptoms. Headache is rarely the only symptom. Before the diagnosis is made, other causes should be ruled out. Migraine symptoms include nausea, vomiting, and visual disturbances. Approximately 12% of the U.S. population has migraine headaches, and almost 70% of those with migraines have a positive family history.[7]

Migraine headaches are classified as vascular or nonvascular. Muscular contraction or tension headache is an example of a nonvascular migraine headache. Skeletal muscle contraction in the head or neck produces steady, pulsatile pain and limited motion of the head, neck, and jaw. Pressure over contracted muscles worsens the pain. Pain also worsens with vasoconstrictive drugs such as ergotamines. Treatment includes mild analgesia with identification and treatment of the underlying cause.

Vascular headaches occur suddenly and are described as intense, sharp, and piercing or pounding and throbbing. Vascular migraine headaches have three distinct phases. During the prodromal phase the patient may experience an aura. Fifteen percent of migraine patients experience an aura.[7] Author Lewis Carroll saw the distorted figures in *Alice in Wonderland* as part of a migraine attack. Most auras are visual; however, any sign or symptom of brain dysfunction can be a feature of an aura. During the second phase, inflammation and cerebral vasodilation cause the characteristic headache—unilateral with throbbing, which may progress to bilateral and dull. Nausea and vomiting are also common during this phase. The third phase, or recovery phase, is characterized by extreme temporal and cranial tenderness. Migraines can be caused by changes in sleep patterns, physical exertion, sudden changes in barometric pressure, increased stress, dieting, heat, lights, cyclic estrogen levels, and certain foods, such as alcohol, caffeine, monosodium glutamate, ripened cheeses, and coffee.

Pharmacologic therapy used during a migraine attack includes analgesics, antiinflammatory agents, β-adrenergic blockers, serotonin antagonists, vasoconstrictors, and antidepressants. Diuretics, antihistamines, anticonvulsants, and short courses of steroids may also be used. Female patients with migraines should avoid oral contraceptives. Other interventions include biofeedback, relaxation training, assertiveness training, family counseling, dietary counseling, allergy testing, and education.

Temporal Arteritis

Temporal arteritis is inflammation of branches of the carotid artery that usually occurs in patients older than 50 years of age. Women are affected four times more often than men. Headache is the most frequent and severe symptom of temporal arteritis. Pain is severe and stabbing in one or both temporal regions, with decreased visual acuity. The patient may have difficulty sleeping and opening or closing the mouth because of pain. Weight loss, night sweats, aching joints, fever, and red nodules over the temporal region also occur. Untreated, this condition can result in blindness. Definitive diagnosis is biopsy of the temporal artery. ED management includes steroids and pain management with antiinflammatory drugs or stronger agents as necessary.[7]

Seizures

Approximately 2.3 million Americans are diagnosed with a seizure disorder yearly.[7] Seizure is a symptom of an underlying problem rather than an independent diagnosis. Defined as an abnormal neuronal function due to excessive or oversynchronized neuronal discharges within the brain, seizures are classified as partial, generalized, or unclassified. Unclassified seizures are seizures that do not fall into other categories. The manifestations of a seizure reflect the area of the brain in which neurons are discharging. Seizures are often described by phases such as preictal, prodromal, aura, postictal, tonic, clonic, and atonic.

Seizure management is dependent on the type and duration of seizure activity. Most seizures are self-limiting and do not require immediate intervention. Initial treatment focuses on maintaining airway patency and prevention of injury during the seizure. Oxygen therapy should be initiated and intravenous access obtained. Glucose level should be checked immediately because hypoglycemia can cause seizures. Additional treatment depends on the type of seizure and the underlying cause.

Partial Seizures

Partial or focal seizures involve one of the hemispheres of the brain. Partial seizures are limited to one specific body part and may be further classified as simple or complex. The patient's mental status is not affected in a simple partial seizure, whereas in a complex partial seizure there is a loss of consciousness. A partial seizure may consist of focal motor activity, somatic sensory symptoms, or disturbances in the patient's vision, hearing, smell, or taste. Focal motor activity can occur in a specific area or begin in one area and progress to surrounding areas in an organized manner (jacksonian seizure). Somatic sensory symptoms include tingling or numbness.

Temporal lobe seizures are often preceded by an aura, such as foul smell, metallic or bitter taste, buzzing, ringing, or hissing sounds, or vague visceral feelings in the chest and abdomen. Feelings of familiarity in an unfamiliar setting (déjà vu) or unfamiliarity in a familiar setting (jamais vu) have been reported. The most characteristic symptom of temporal lobe seizure is semipurposeful patterns of movement (automatism) such as lip smacking, chewing, patting hands, or facial grimacing.

Partial seizures can occur with secondary generalized seizures. Seizure activity originates locally and progresses until the entire body is involved. There is an associated loss of consciousness. Partial seizures are often seen in adults and generally are less responsive to medical treatment.

Generalized Seizures

There are two major types of generalized seizures—absence (petit mal) and tonic-clonic (grand mal) seizures. Generalized seizures may involve both hemispheres of the brain. Generalized seizures involve loss of consciousness and may be accompanied by bilateral tonic-clonic movements.

Absence seizures usually occur in children 4 to 12 years of age and tend to run in families. Episodes are characterized by abrupt cessation of activity with momentary loss of consciousness, duration less than 15 seconds, and may be accompanied by automatism. The patient returns to baseline immediately after the seizure.

Tonic-clonic seizures begin with sudden loss of consciousness followed by major tonic contractions of large muscle groups. Arms and legs extend stiffly as the person falls to the ground. A shrill cry may precede the event. During the tonic phase the person is apneic, pupils are dilated and unresponsive, and bowel and bladder incontinence occur. The individual may also bite his or her tongue. During the clonic phase strenuous, rhythmic muscle contractions occur. Hyperventilation, profuse sweating, tachycardia, and excessive salivation with frothing are usually present. A postictal phase follows as muscles relax. Deep breathing and a depressed level of consciousness are present. The person awakens confused with complaints of headache, muscle aching, and fatigue. There is generalized amnesia concerning the event, and the person may sleep for hours afterward.

Status Epilepticus

Seizures occurring in greater intensity, number, or length than the patient's usual seizures are considered acute and life threatening. Status epilepticus is a series of consecutive seizures without the person's regaining consciousness in between or a single seizure that does not respond to conventional therapy or lasting more that 30 minutes. Some of the known causes of status epilepticus are sudden withdrawal from antiepileptic drugs, head trauma, and acute alcohol withdrawal. Uncontrolled seizure activity increases the patient's temperature, blood pressure, and pulse; interferes with cerebral blood flow; and increases the risk for hypoxic brain damage. Control of seizure activity is critical.

Therapeutic interventions begin with the ABCs. Endotracheal intubation is used to maintain the airway and oxygenate the patient. The patient should be protected from injury with seizure precautions. Naloxone, dextrose 50%, and thiamine may be given. Sedation medications (e.g., midazolam [Versed] and lorazepam [Ativan]) are used initially to stop the seizure. However, patients should be monitored frequently because of side effects of respiratory depression and hypotension. Anticonvulsant medications (e.g., phenobarbital, fosphenytoin and phenytoin) are then given until seizure activity is controlled. Possible side effects of these medications are cardiac arrhythmias and hypotention.[6] If these medications fail, general anesthesia is considered. Drug therapy is the major component of long-term management. Medications must be adjusted to achieve therapeutic blood levels without causing side effects. Medications need to be taken at the same time each day to achieve therapeutic blood levels and prevent the recurrence of seizures. The treatment goal with generalized seizures or status epilepticus is to control seizures with the fewest side effects.

Stroke

Each year in the United States almost 700,000 people suffer from a stroke.[5] Stroke is a sudden loss of neurologic function resulting from an acute disruption of blood flow to the brain.[7] This leads to cellular ischemia and ultimately, cerebral infarction. Strokes may be ischemic or hemorrhagic with ischemic strokes counting for 88% of all strokes.[7] Ischemic strokes are caused by occlusion of cerebral vessels by a thrombus or embolus. A decrease in blood flow by approximately 25% causes a decrease in the amount of oxygen and glucose available to the cerebral cells, resulting in cellular ischemia.[7] The most common location for occlusion is the bifurcation of the common carotid artery into the internal and external carotid arteries. Hemorrhagic strokes occurs when an intracranial blood vessel ruptures, leaking blood into the brain tissue, ventricles, or subarachnoid space. Modifiable factors that increase the patient's risk for stroke are hypertension, diabetes mellitus, obesity, substance abuse, atherosclerosis, cardiac valve disease, and smoking. Nonmodifiable factors include age, gender, race/ethnicity, and family history of cerebrovascular or cardiovascular disease.[5]

Approximately half of all strokes are caused by cerebral thrombosis. Thrombotic strokes occur because atherosclerotic plaque accumulates within the vessel, leading to decreased blood flow through the vessel. Carotid stenosis is a major cause of thrombotic stroke. Symptoms occur slowly as cerebral blood flow gradually decreases. Neurologic deficits depend on the area of the brain affected. Embolic strokes occur when a free-floating substance travels to the brain and occludes a vessel. Substances tend to fragment as they float, so multiple areas of the brain may be affected, causing multifocal neurologic deficits. Free-floating substances include blood clots, tumor particles, fat, air, or vegetation from a diseased heart valve. Patients with atrial fibrillation are at risk for embolic stroke because of clot formation on the mitral valve.

Cerebral infarction, or stroke, may occur anywhere in the brain. Symptoms and lethality are determined by location and size of the infarction. Surrounding the area of infarction is an area of ischemia called the penumbra.[6] Recognition and treatment of stroke focus on preservation and reperfusion of this ischemic area to prevent further cellular destruction. Rapid reperfusion is a crucial factor in reducing cellular infarction. Common clinical manifestations of an acute stroke include unilateral paralysis or weakness; difficulty with speech, gait, or coordination; and headache. Other symptoms may include facial droop, altered vision, sensory impairment, or thought-process problems.

Strokes are classified according to duration of symptoms. Transient ischemic attack (TIA) is a temporary disturbance of blood flow that results in no permanent neurologic damage. About 15% of strokes occur within 90 days of a TIA.[5] Reversible ischemic stroke causes minimal neurologic damage. Both TIAs and reversible ischemic strokes are considered warning signs of an impending stroke and may possibly result from cerebral vasospasms. A stroke in evolution has progressive neurologic deterioration with residual deficits. A completed stroke will have permanent and unchanging neurologic deficits. Table 33-4 summarizes stroke classifications.

Treatment of stroke patients begins with the assessment of airway patency. Breathing rate and rhythm is controlled within the brainstem and can be affected by brain swelling. It is critical that oxygen-saturated blood be provided to the affected area early during a stroke. Supplemental oxygen is beneficial for patients without overt hypoxia, but with suboptimal oxygen saturation. The unconscious patient or one who is unable to manage oral secretions is also at risk for respiratory compromise. Endotracheal intubation may be required to ensure a patent airway. If the patient is hypertensive (greater than 220 mm Hg systolic or 120 mm Hg diastolic), antihypertensive agents such as nitroprusside (Nipride) should be used. Rising blood pressure can increase perfusion to the brain for a short time; it may also lead to edema and increased ICP. However, precipitous reduction of blood pressure is not recommended. Sudden rapid decrease in blood pressure can impair cerebral perfusion and reduce perfusion to the penumbra, thereby converting an area of ischemia to an area of infarction.[7] An approach of "permissive hypertension," based on the need to maintain perfusion to brain cells, may be followed dependent on the patient's symptoms.[6] CPP should be maintained at a level above 50 mm Hg to obtain adequate blood flow to brain tissue. The exception is in patients who receive recombinant tissue plasminogen activator (r-tPA). Blood pressure will need

Table 33-4.	STROKE CLASSIFICATION
Type	**Description**
Transient ischemic attack (TIA)	Temporary disturbance of blood supply causes transient neurologic deficit; symptoms present less than 24 hours; no permanent neurologic deficit
Reversible ischemic stroke	Neurologic deficits last a few days or weeks; minimal permanent neurologic deficits
Stroke in evolution	Progressive neurologic deterioration occurs; residual neurologic deficit present
Completed stroke	Patient appears stable with neurologic deficit permanent and unchanging

to be lowered to prevent complications from the medication during reperfusion. Lower blood pressure is also the goal in patients with hemorrhagic stroke, because higher pressures lead to more bleeding and cellular irritation. A general neurologic examination, including a Glasgow Coma Scale, must be performed to establish a patient baseline.

Identification of stroke type is critical to successful treatment. Several prehospital scores (the Cincinnati Prehospital Stroke Scale and the Los Angeles Stroke Screen) have been successfully used to identify possible stroke patients before they arrive in the ED. The National Institutes of Health Stroke Scale (NIHSS) is a quantitative measure of stroke-related neurologic deficits.[5] NIHSS has been commonly used to detect patient outcomes. The NIHSS (Box 33-2) provides a standardized baseline and consistent set of parameters that can be repeated throughout the hospital stay. Initiating this screen in the ED allows for a more accurate assessment of the stroke patient. A true baseline can be established and used for patient evaluation and to improve continuity of care.

Patients exhibiting signs of an acute stroke need emergent evaluation because the treatment window for cerebral viability is narrow. Prehospital recognition of a suspected acute stroke is crucial and can greatly decrease the door-to-computed-tomography (CT) time. CT scans must be done quickly to determine if the stroke is hemorrhagic or ischemic. A normal CT scan allows patients who have neurologic deficits consistent with acute stroke to receive fibrinolytic therapy. Currently the only fibrinolytic agent that is Food and Drug Administration (FDA) approved for use in ischemic stroke is alteplase, recombinant tissue plasminogen activator (r-tPA). An abnormal CT scan, particularly a hemorrhagic stoke, is a contraindication for fibrinolytic therapy. There is a very narrow window of opportunity for use of r-tPA therapy. Box 33-3 highlights fibrinolytic administration.[3] The agent is given intravenously in most centers across the nation but is also given intraarterially in a small number of centers. There is some controversy as to the effectiveness of r-tPA therapy—reversal of symptoms may simply be due

---

Box 33-2   NATIONAL INSTITUTES OF HEALTH STROKE SCALE

1a. Level of Consciousness
0 = alert
1 = not alert
2 = not alert (requires repeated stimulation)
3 = reflex motor/autonomic/unresponsive

1b. LOC Questions
Answers must be correct
0 = 2 correctly
1 = 1 correctly
2 = neither correctly

2. Best Gaze
Only horizontal eye movements will be tested
0 = normal
1 = partial gaze palsy
2 = forced deviation

3. Visual
Visual fields are tested by confrontation
0 = no visual loss
1 = partial hemianopia
2 = complete hemianopia
3 = bilateral hemianopia

4. Facial Palsy
0 = normal
1= minor paralysis
2 = partial paralysis
3 = complete paralysis

5. Motor Arm
Drift is scored if the arm falls before 10 seconds
0 = no drift
1 = drift
2 = some effort against gravity
3 = no effort against gravity
4 = no movement

6. Motor Leg
Drift is scored if the leg falls before 10 seconds
0 = no drift
1 = drift
2 = some effort against gravity
3 = no effort against gravity
4 = no movement

7. Limb Ataxia
Tests are done on both sides upper and lower extremities
0 = absent
1 = present in one limb
2 = present in two limbs

8. Sensory
Tests done to as many body areas as needed for accuracy
0 = normal
1 = mild to moderate sensory loss
2 = severe to total sensory loss

9. Best Language
Describe scenario in picture, name items shown, and read
sentences
0 = no aphasia
1 = mild to moderate aphasia
2 = severe aphasia
3 = mute, global aphasia

10. Dysarthria
Read or repeat words from the list
0 = normal
1 = mild to moderate dysarthria
2 = severe dysarthria
3 = intubated

11. Extinction and Inattention
0 = no abnormality
1 = visual/tactile/auditory/spatial/personal

Modified from *NIH Stroke Scale*, http://www.Ninds.nih.gov/disorders/stroke/strokescales.htm.
NIH, National Institutes of Health.

to resolution of a TIA. Hemorrhagic stroke usually requires surgical intervention to control hemorrhage and manage increased ICP.

A hemorrhagic stroke or aneurysm is a weak spot, usually at the junction of two arteries. Once the aneurysm ruptures, blood is forced into the subarachnoid space and then spreads to the basal cistern, following the flow of CSF. After the diagnosis of subarachnoid hemorrhage is made, a cerebral angiogram can confirm the location, size, and shape of the aneurysm. Early (within the first 48 hours) securing of the aneurysm is recommended.[1] The best treatment for the aneurysm depends upon patient condition, anatomy, and the location and history of the aneurysm. The goal of treatment is to minimize the risk for neurologic deficits related to aneurysm rupture. Currently two procedures are used to treat aneurysms. Clipping of the aneurysm has been the standard treatment for the last 60 years.[1] This involves placing a clip around the "neck" of the aneurysm, where it bulges off from the artery, which steers blood flow away from the weakened walls of the aneurysm so that it will not break open. This requires general anesthesia and a craniotomy. In 1995 the FDA approved the use of the Guglielmi Detachable Coil for endovascular therapy for aneurysms of nonsurgical candidates.[1] This procedure involves coiling a thin strand of wire inside the aneurysm. Blood clots in and around the coil instead of pushing on the weak walls of the aneurysm. This procedure is performed within the vascular system and does not require general anesthesia or a craniotomy. A catheter is manipulated through the blood vessels from the groin to the head. Management of the aneurysm patient regardless of clipping or coiling focuses on neurologic assessment and blood pressure management.

A number of neuroprotective agents have been approved for use in cases of ischemic stroke. These agents preserve cerebral function by increasing perfusion of the penumbra.[5] Mechanism of action varies with type of agent. Some agents remove oxygen free radicals, whereas others increase movement of calcium across the cell membrane. Agents are usually time limited and must be given within 6 to 12 hours of symptom onset. As more research occurs in this area, additional agents with a longer window of opportunity for administration are anticipated. The mechanical embolus removal device is a new retrieval mechanism used to remove clots related to cerebral ischemia.[5]

In 2003 The Joint Commission developed standardized performance measures for stroke.[5] Hospitals designated as primary stroke centers must launch disease-specific care certification programs for stroke patients based on recommendations. Initial implementation of 4 of the 10 identified measures must occur to be verified as a primary stroke center. These include r-tPA use, patients discharged with antithrombotics, deep vein thrombosis prophylaxis, and anticoagulation therapy for patients diagnosed with atrial fibrillation.

Meningitis

Meningitis is inflammation of the meningeal layers surrounding the brain and spinal cord; it is a neurologic emergency and an infectious disease emergency. Infection may be viral, bacterial, or fungal. Viral meningitis is usually less acute, with gradual onset of symptoms. Bacterial meningitis has acute onset of symptoms and is fatal in 50% of patients. Common bacterial agents include *Streptococcus pneumoniae*, *Neisseria meningitides*, *Haemophilus influenzae*, group B streptococci, and *Listeria monocytogenes*. Fungal meningitis usually occurs in immune-compromised individuals; agents include *Aspergillus* and *Candida* organisms. Noninfectious causes of meningitis include drugs, toxic exposure, and neoplasms.

Symptoms of meningitis are fever, headache, photophobia, nuchal rigidity, lethargy, seizures, vomiting, and chills. The classic triad of fever, stiff neck, and altered LOC is noted in approximately two thirds of adult patients but rarely in infants.[7] The clinical presentation in patients with acquired immunodeficiency syndrome (AIDS) is not as dramatic. The patient may have isolated fevers and a chronic headache.[7] The patient may arrive at the ED with mild headache and severe confusion or comatose with shock. Patients with meningococcemia can have purpura, petechiae, splinter hemorrhages, and pustular lesions. The clinical progression is characterized by rapid deterioration in the patient with meningococcal meningitis.

Diagnosis is confirmed with lumbar puncture (LP) and CSF cultures. Analysis of CSF includes white blood cell count, glucose, protein, and leukocyte differential. Results vary with the cause of the meningitis. Latex agglutination may also be ordered. This test is useful for patients on previous antibiotic therapy but is not effective in ruling out bacterial infection.[7] If a brain abscess is suspected, LP is contraindicated because of the potential for herniation. A CT scan may be obtained before the LP. Treatment includes support of the patient's ABCs, immediate administration of appropriate antibiotics, antipyretics, and anticonvulsants as indicated. Serial neurologic assessment is critical to identify changes in level of consciousness. The patient with bacterial

Box 33-3	FIBRINOLYTIC THERAPY FOR ISCHEMIC STROKE
MEDICATION	**ADMINISTRATION**
Alteplase	**IV Administration**
Total dose 0.9 mg/kg IV	Must be started within 3 hours
Maximum IV dose is 90 mg	of symptom onset
Bolus is 10% of the total dose—	**Intraarterial Administration**
given IV over 1 minute	May be given up to 6 hours
Remainder of the total dose is	after symptom onset
given IV over 60 minutes	Given by the radiologist
	Requires cannulization of the
	femoral or brachial artery

Data from Hazinski MF, Cummins RO, Field JM: *Handbook of emergency cardiovascular care for health care providers*, Dallas, 2000, American Heart Association.
IV, Intravenous.

meningitis should be isolated. Prophylactic antibiotics are given for intimate contact or documented exposure such as needle stick. The vaccine Menomune is available for meningococcal meningitis.

Guillain-Barré Syndrome

Guillain-Barré syndrome is an acute, idiopathic paralytic disease caused by decreased myelin at the nerve roots and in peripheral nerves. Individuals in their 20s and 30s are affected most often. Symptoms usually follow an acute febrile episode—usually respiratory or gastrointestinal.[5] Signs and symptoms include tingling sensation in the extremities lasting for hours to weeks, severely decreased deep tendon reflexes, and a symmetric paralysis that begins in the lower extremities and ascends. This classic pattern is seen in 90% to 95% of patients diagnosed with Guillain-Barré syndrome.[7] Paralysis eventually affects the diaphragm and intercostal muscles, causing respiratory paralysis and death if not treated. Emergency management focuses on support of the ABCs. Endotracheal intubation and ventilator support are often required. Use of succinylcholine is contraindicated because of the potential for lethal hyperkalemia. Therapy is initially plasmapheresis, with immunoglobulin considered as a secondary therapy. Provide general supportive care until the disease has run its course. Patients who survive this disease usually require a long program of rehabilitation.

Myasthenia Gravis

Myasthenia gravis (MG), a chronic autoimmune disease caused by a defect in neuromuscular transmission, occurs more frequently in women. The disease can occur at any age but is predominant in adults age 20 to 30 years (an estimated 5 to 10 cases per 100,000 population).[4] Ocular dysfunction is the most common initial symptom, seen in 70% of the cases.[7] Ocular symptoms include ptosis, diplopia with sustained directional gaze, and difficulty keeping the eye closed. It is important to note that MG never affects the pupil. An MG crisis has a sudden onset, causing respiratory paralysis and arrest. Patients experience increasing fatigue; delayed muscle strength recovery; weak eye, facial, and jaw muscles; weak pharyngeal muscles; diplopia; dysphagia; and inability to swallow. Therapeutic intervention is support of ABCs, with possible endotracheal intubation and ventilator management. Pharmacologic therapy is pyridostigmine bromide (Mestinon), barbiturates,

opiates, quinidine, quinine, corticotropin, corticosteroids, aminoglycosides, antibiotics, and muscle relaxants. Differentiation of "myasthenic crisis" from "cholinergic crisis" may be accomplished with administration of edrophonium (Tensilon), an anticholinesterase inhibitor. If the patient's condition worsens after edrophonium, cholinergic crisis should be suspected.[7]

SUMMARY

Neurologic emergencies represent a significant challenge for the emergency nurse. Life-threatening neurologic emergencies require rapid, organized assessment with simultaneous intervention. Patients with neurologic problems that are not life threatening may fear loss of function or cognitive ability, or pain. Patients require supportive, therapeutic care to minimize discomfort and facilitate recovery.

Management of neurologic emergencies is undergoing rapid change. Old treatments such as hyperventilation to decrease ICP are being questioned. Research in management of stroke and preservation of cerebral function in other neurologic problems—for example, head injury—is rapidly changing. Changes represent an opportunity for improved patient outcomes with decreased mortality and morbidity. Diligence by the emergency nurse is essential to maintaining a current knowledge base in the face of this rapidly changing information.

REFERENCES

1. Fulgham JR, Kallmes DF, Manno EM et al: Subarachnoid hemorrhage: neurointensive care and aneurysm repair, *Mayo Clin Proc* 80(4):550, 2005.
2. Guyton AC, Hall JE: *Textbook of medical physiology*, ed 10, Philadelphia, 2000, WB Saunders.
3. Hazinski MF, Cummins RO, Field JM: *2000 Handbook of emergency cardiovascular care for health care providers*, Dallas, 2000, American Heart Association.
4. Ignatavicius DD, Workman ML: *Medical-surgical nursing: critical thinking for collaborative care*, St Louis, 2006, WB Saunders.
5. Lopez A, Emirose O, Yamamoto L: Challenges in seizure management, *Top Emerg Med* 26(3):212, 2004.
6. Rosen P, Barkin R: *Emergency medicine: concepts and clinical practice*, ed 4, St. Louis, 1998, Mosby.
7. Tintinalli JE, Ruiz E, Krome RL: *Emergency medicine: a comprehensive study guide*, ed 4, New York, 1996, McGraw-Hill.

CHAPTER 34

Gastrointestinal Emergencies

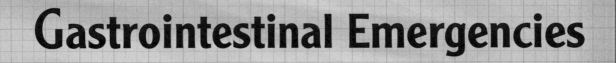

Amy Herrington

Gastrointestinal (GI) emergencies vary from minor problems to more serious, potentially life-threatening problems. Complaints of a GI nature are a common reason for visits to the emergency department (ED). Clinical indications of a problem in the GI system include heartburn, nausea, vomiting, constipation, diarrhea, bloating, chest pain, abdominal pain, and blood in stool or vomitus. This chapter focuses on those conditions seen most often in the ED. A brief review of anatomy and physiology is followed by discussion of specific GI conditions (e.g., gastroenteritis, GI bleeding, bowel obstruction, diverticulitis, gastroesophageal reflux disease [GERD], appendicitis, cholecystitis, and pancreatitis). Trauma of the GI system is discussed in Chapter 24.

ANATOMY AND PHYSIOLOGY

Normal GI function requires ingestion of nutrients and fluids and is followed by elimination of waste products formed from metabolic actions. Major organs and structures of the GI system are the esophagus, stomach, intestines, liver, pancreas, gallbladder, and peritoneum.

Esophagus

The major function of the esophagus is movement of food. The esophagus, a straight, collapsible tube approximately 25 cm long and up to 3 cm in diameter, extends from the pharynx to the stomach. Distinct esophageal layers are the mucous membrane, submucosa, and muscular layer. Secretions from mucous glands spread throughout the submucosa keep the inner lining moist and lubricated. Striated muscle in the upper esophagus is gradually replaced by smooth muscle in the lower esophagus and GI tract. The upper esophageal sphincter is at the proximal end of the esophagus, and the lower esophageal sphincter (LES) (also called the cardiac sphincter) is at the distal junction of the esophagus and stomach. The LES prevents regurgitation from the stomach into the esophagus.

Stomach

The stomach is a J-shaped organ located below the diaphragm between the esophagus and small intestine. Stomach functions include food storage and combining food with gastric juices. Limited absorption occurs in the stomach before the movement of food into the small intestine. Recognized regions of the stomach are the pylorus, fundus, body, and antrum. The pyloric sphincter controls food movement from stomach to duodenum. Distinct layers of the stomach wall are outer serosa, muscular layer, submucosa, and mucosa. The mucosal layer contains multiple wrinkles called rugae that straighten as the stomach fills to accommodate more volume. Completely relaxed, the stomach holds up to 1.5 L.[8] Gastric juices containing pepsin, hydrochloric acid, mucus, and intrinsic factor are secreted by glands in the submucosa. These agents begin food breakdown. Acids in the stomach maintain the pH of gastric juices at 1.0.

Intestines

The small intestine is a tubular organ extending from the pyloric sphincter to the proximal large intestine. Secretions from the pancreas and liver complete the digestion of nutrients in chyme—the semiliquid mixture of food and gastric secretions. The small intestine absorbs nutrients and other products of digestion and transports residue to the large intestine. Segments of the small intestine are the duodenum, jejunum, and ileum. The duodenum attaches to the stomach at the pyloric sphincter in the retroperitoneal space and represents the only fixed portion of the small intestine. The duodenum is approximately 25 cm long and 5 cm in diameter. The jejunum and ileum are mobile and lie free in the peritoneal cavity.

Segments of the large intestine are the cecum, colon, rectum, and anal canal. The large intestine is approximately 1.5 m long, beginning in the lower right side of the abdomen where the ileum joins the cecum. The colon is divided into ascending colon, transverse colon, descending colon, and sigmoid colon. Primary functions of the large intestine are absorption of water and electrolytes, formation of feces, and storage of feces.

Liver

The liver, located in the right upper quadrant of the abdomen, is divided into right and left lobes. Functional units of the liver called lobules contain sinusoids and Kupffer cells. Each lobule is supplied by a hepatic artery, sublobular vein, bile duct, and lymph channel. The liver is extremely vascular; approximately 1450 mL of blood flow through the liver each minute. Sinusoids in lobules act as a reservoir for overflow of blood and fluids from the right ventricle. A thick capsule of connective tissue known as Glisson's capsule covers the liver. The liver is involved in hundreds of metabolic functions, including metabolism of nutrients, gluconeogenesis, and drug metabolism. Production of bile is a major function of the liver; 600 to 1200 mL of bile are secreted each day. Bile is essential for digestion and absorption of fats and fat-soluble vitamins and excretion of bilirubin and excess cholesterol. Bilirubin is an end product of hemoglobin destruction.

Pancreas

The pancreas is a lobulated organ behind the stomach that contains endocrine and exocrine cells. The organ is divided into the head, body, and a thin, narrow tail. Cells in the islets of Langerhans secrete insulin and regulate glucose levels. Exocrine cells called pancreatic acini secrete pancreatic juices for digestion of fats, carbohydrates, proteins, and nucleic acids. Pancreatic enzymes (i.e., lipase and amylase) enter the intestines through the pancreatic duct at the same juncture as the bile duct from the liver and gallbladder. Pancreatic and bile ducts join at a short dilated tube called the ampulla of Vater. A band of smooth muscles called the sphincter of Oddi surrounds this area and controls exit of pancreatic juices and bile.

Gallbladder

The gallbladder is a pear-shaped sac located in a depression on the inferior surface of the liver. The organ's main functions are the collection, concentration, and storage of bile. Maximum volume is 30 to 60 mL; however, input from the liver can reach 450 mL over 12 hours. Concentration of bile in the gallbladder can be 5 to 20 times that of bile in the liver.[5] Bile is 80% water, 10% bile acids, 4% to 5% phospholipid, and 1% cholesterol.[8]

Peritoneum

The peritoneum is a serous membrane covering the liver, spleen, stomach, and intestines that acts as a semipermeable membrane, contains pain receptors, and provides proliferative cellular protection. Technically, all abdominal organs are behind the peritoneum and therefore are retroperitoneal; however, the liver, spleen, stomach, and intestines are suspended into the peritoneum and considered intraperitoneal organs. Omenta are folds of peritoneum that surround the stomach and adjacent organs. The greater omentum drapes the transverse colon and loops of small intestine. It is extremely mobile and spreads easily into areas of injury to seal off potential sources of infection. The lesser omentum covers parts of the stomach and proximal intestines but is not as movable as the greater omentum.

The peritoneum is permeable to fluid, electrolytes, urea, and toxins. Somatic afferent nerves sensitize the peritoneum to all types of stimuli. In acute abdominal conditions the peritoneum can localize an irritable focus by producing sharp pain and tenderness, voluntary or involuntary abdominal muscle rigidity, and rebound tenderness.

PATIENT ASSESSMENT

Assessment of a patient with a GI emergency should initially focus on airway, breathing, and circulation (ABCs) with the primary survey completed before the focused assessment. Determination of chief complaint, social and medical history, reason for seeking treatment, and treatment before arrival follows the initial assessment. Information may be obtained from the patient, family members, significant other, friends, emergency medical services personnel, or previous medical records. Historical assessment should include questions related to gynecologic and genitourinary (GU) symptoms because many gynecologic or GU conditions cause abdominal pain, nausea, and vomiting. Information related to food intake and alcohol consumption should be obtained during assessment of patient history.

Evaluate the patient for abnormal skin color, abdominal wall abnormalities, pain, and alterations in bowel patterns. Abdominal pain is a common chief complaint in the ED that may be caused by an acute event or related to a chronic process. Abdominal pain may be visceral, somatic, or referred.

Visceral pain is caused by stretching of hollow viscus and is described as cramping or a sensation of gas. Pain intensifies, then decreases, and is usually centered at the umbilicus or below the midline. Diffuse pain makes localization of pain difficult. Diaphoresis, nausea, vomiting, hypotension, tachycardia, and abdominal wall spasms may be present. Conditions associated with visceral pain are appendicitis, acute pancreatitis, cholecystitis, and intestinal obstruction.

Somatic pain is produced by bacterial or chemical irritation of nerve fibers. Pain is sharp and usually localized to one area. A patient may be found lying with legs flexed and knees pulled to the chest to prevent stimulation of the peritoneum and subsequent increase in pain. Associated findings include involuntary guarding and rebound tenderness.

Referred pain occurs at a distance from the original source of the pain and is thought to be caused by development of nerve tracts during fetal growth and development. Biliary pain can be referred to the subscapular area, whereas a peptic ulcer and pancreatic disease can cause back pain.

Individual and cultural variations in expressions of pain must be considered when assessing abdominal pain. Each person reacts differently—older adult patients may not exhibit the same level of pain as younger patients; men may hide pain because expression of pain is not considered masculine in many cultures. Conversely, dramatic expression of pain may be expected in some cultures. Emergency nurses must remember that pain is a symptom—not a diagnosis. Interventions should focus on identification and treatment of the source of pain.

A systematic approach is recommended for assessment of abdominal pain. The PQRST mnemonic can be used to obtain appropriate historical information and identification of essential characteristics of pain. *Provocation*—Is there an action or movement that increases or changes the pain? *Quality* or character of pain—Is the pain sharp, dull, intermittent? *Radiation* or referral of pain—Does the pain stay in the right lower quadrant or move to the left lower quadrant as well? Using an age-appropriate pain scale such as a numeric rating of 0 (no pain) to 10 (worst pain ever) can identify the intensity or *Severity* of the pain. Question the patient regarding how long the pain has lasted to determine the *Time* of pain onset. It is important to consider the anatomy of the patient and to correlate the location of pain with the organ or system located in that region. For example, right lower quadrant pain in a female is often associated with ovarian or appendix conditions. The next step would be evaluating the descriptive information using the mnemonic discussed earlier. Final diagnosis would occur following serial examinations and diagnostics to evaluate or rule out each organ of potential disease or injury.

Another common finding with most GI emergencies is nausea and vomiting. Specific treatment varies with the underlying cause and physician preference. Abdominal assessment uses a sequence of inspection, auscultation, percussion, and palpation. Patient position should be noted because patients assume positions of comfort. Observe facial expression for signs of discomfort. Note skin color, temperature, and moisture. Inspect the abdominal wall for pulsations, movement, masses, symmetry, or surgical scars.

Auscultate bowel sounds in all four quadrants, determining frequency, quality, and pitch. Normal bowel sounds are irregular, high-pitched gurgling sounds occurring 5 to 35 times per minute. Decreased or absent bowel sounds suggest peritonitis or paralytic ileus, whereas hyperactive bowel sounds associated with nausea, vomiting, and diarrhea suggest gastroenteritis. Frequent, high-pitched bowel sounds may occur with bowel obstruction. Vascular sounds such as venous hums or bruits are abnormal findings. Auscultation should always be done before palpation because palpation may create false bowel sounds. The presence of hypoactive or hyperactive bowel sounds can be found in patients without abdominal pathologic processes. Thus bowel sounds must be evaluated in association with other abdominal findings such as guarding and tenderness with palpation. Factors such as stress and last food intake can affect bowel sounds.

Percussion is performed in all four quadrants. Dull sounds occur over solid organs or tumors, whereas tympanic sounds occur over air masses. Dull sounds may also be heard over a distended bladder or an area of bowel distended with stool. Tympany is the predominant sound heard when percussing the abdomen.

Palpation is the last step in abdominal assessment. Begin palpation away from painful sites, noting areas of tenderness, guarding, or rigidity. Assess for abnormal masses and rebound tenderness.

Concurrent findings such as fever and chills are usually found with bacterial infection, appendicitis, or cholecystitis. Other signs associated with pain are nausea, vomiting, and anorexia. Intractable vomiting or feces in emesis suggest bowel obstruction. Blood in emesis occurs with gastritis or upper GI bleeding. Assess bowel patterns for abnormalities such as diarrhea or constipation, noting stool color and consistency. Diarrhea can occur with gastroenteritis; black, tarry stools suggest upper GI bleeding; and clay-colored stools are found with biliary tract obstruction. Fatty, foul-smelling, frothy stools occur with pancreatitis.

SPECIFIC GASTROINTESTINAL EMERGENCIES

Infection, structural abnormalities, or pathologic processes may cause GI emergencies. Heredity and lifestyle also play a role. For example, excessive alcohol consumption can lead to GI bleeding, cirrhosis, or esophageal varices. Regardless of cause, nontraumatic GI emergencies are a common occurrence in any ED—ranging from minor inconvenience to life-threatening problems.

Gastrointestinal Bleeding

Bleeding can originate anywhere in the GI tract and can occur at any age. Bleeding is functionally categorized by location—upper or lower GI bleeding. Upper GI bleeding is more common in males, whereas lower GI bleeding is seen more often in females. Symptoms associated with bleeding in the GI tract include bright-red blood and/or black, "coffee grounds" material in vomitus, as well as bright-red blood from the rectum and/or black, tarry stools. Bleeding stops spontaneously in the majority of hospitalized patients.

Upper Gastrointestinal Bleeding

Upper GI bleeding refers to blood loss between the upper esophagus and duodenum at the ligament of Treitz. Bleeding is categorized as variceal or nonvariceal.[10] The risk for death is greater with variceal bleeding because of the occurrence of massive hemorrhage in these patients. Gastroesophageal varices are enlarged, venous channels that are dilated by portal hypertension. The common causes of portal hypertension in the United States are alcoholic liver disease and chronic active hepatitis.[8] As portal hypertension increases, varices continue to enlarge and eventually rupture, causing hemorrhage. Systemic manifestations of cirrhosis vary depending on the stage of the disease. Early symptoms include generalized weakness and fatigue; intermittent low-grade fevers; ankle edema; right upper quadrant abdominal pain; and various (GI) symptoms, including anorexia, nausea and vomiting, dyspepsia, and changes in bowel pattern. As the disease progresses, jaundice, mental status changes, muscle wasting, weight loss, ascites, epistaxis, spontaneous bruising, and hypotension may occur.[6] It is during this later stage that GI bleeding becomes prevalent. Bleeding from varices requires immediate intervention and close observation following initial control of bleeding. The risk for rebleeding is high until the varices are obliterated.

Nonvariceal bleeding occurs because of the disruption of esophageal or gastroduodenal mucosa with ulceration or erosion into an underlying vein or artery. Ulcerations or erosions occur when hyperacidity, pepsin, or aspirin inhibit mucosal prostaglandins and overwhelm protective factors of the esophagus (i.e., esophageal motility, salivary secretions, and the LES) and gastric mucosa (i.e., mucus, rapid epithelial renewal, and tissue mediators). Peptic ulcer disease, an infectious process caused by *Helicobacter pylori*, renders the underlying mucosa more vulnerable to gastric acid damage by disrupting the mucosal layer and initiating an inflammatory response that perpetuates tissue damage. Peptic ulcer disease may account for more than 50% of upper GI bleeding cases.[2] Other causes of upper GI bleeding include drug-induced erosions and severe or prolonged retching and vomiting such as with bulimia. Mallory-Weiss syndrome occurs from longitudinal tears or lacerations in the distal esophagus and proximal stomach.[18] The lacerations

may result in bleeding from submucosal arteries. This syndrome is usually associated with severe retching. Mallory-Weiss syndrome has also been reported in patients with a history of straining with stools, coughing, lifting, and grandmal seizures. Patients with a hiatal hernia are at greater risk for Mallory-Weiss syndrome.

Clinical signs and symptoms of GI bleeding are variable. Hematemesis, the vomiting of blood or coffee grounds–like material, confirms upper GI bleeding. Abdominal pain, nausea, vomiting, hematemesis, or melena (black, tarry stools) can be present. Other presenting symptoms may include pallor, dizziness, weakness, and lethargy. Signs of hypovolemia such as tachycardia, orthostatic hypotension, and syncope may also occur. Mental confusion, jaundice, or ascites are often observed in patients associated with variceal bleeding.

Management begins with maintenance of the ABCs. Administer high-flow oxygen via nonrebreather mask for patients with hemodynamic compromise or indicators of hypovolemic shock. Fluid replacement begins with normal saline or lactated Ringer's solution followed by blood (packed red blood cells [PRBCs] or whole blood) replacement if the patient's condition does not improve. Using a cardiac monitor and continuous pulse oximetry is recommended for patients with significant blood loss or bright-red bleeding. Older adult patients can experience myocardial infarction secondary to ischemia caused by hypovolemia. Monitor vital signs and level of consciousness for signs of hemodynamic compromise. A nasogastric tube is inserted for gastric lavage with saline solution to remove blood clots. Lavage also serves to clear the GI tract, which facilitates endoscopy. A urinary catheter is inserted to monitor output and fluid status.

Determine if the patient has a history of nonsteroidal antiinflammatory drug or aspirin use, and alcohol or liver disease. Baseline laboratory studies include complete blood count (CBC), type and crossmatch, electrolytes, blood urea nitrogen (BUN), creatinine, and serum glucose. Normal creatinine level with increased BUN suggests bleeding with breakdown of blood in the gut or dehydration. Liver function and coagulation studies are also recommended to rule out coagulopathies or liver disease. An upright chest radiograph can provide valuable information if perforation is suspected; however, this is not feasible if significant hemodynamic compromise is present. An electrocardiogram should be obtained to assess for dysrhythmias or cardiac ischemic changes related to blood loss.

A variety of endoscopic methods are available to control upper GI bleeding. Endoscopic injection of sclerosing agents or cautery/thermal techniques have been used to control bleeding from peptic ulcer disease. Endoscopic band ligation and sclerotherapy are frequently used to control variceal bleeding.[9] Treatment modalities include medications and surgical interventions. Medical therapy for nonvariceal bleeding includes intravenous (IV) infusion of proton pump inhibitors such as pantoprazole. Gastroesophageal variceal bleeding is treated with IV vasopressin (20 units in 200 mL saline at 0.25 to 0.5 units/min) or octreotide.[7] A Sengstaken-Blakemore, Minnesota, or Linton balloon tube can be used to tamponade bleeding. Surgical intervention may be necessary in cases when the bleeding cannot be controlled via other methods. Complications related to upper GI bleeding include aspiration, pneumonia, respiratory failure, and hypovolemic shock.

Lower Gastrointestinal Bleeding

Lower GI bleeding is bleeding that occurs below the ligament of Treitz. Common causes are hemorrhoids, diverticulum, angiodysplasia, colonic polyps, colon cancer, or colitis.[17] The cardinal sign of lower GI bleeding is hematochezia, the passage of bright-red blood, maroon colored blood, or blood clots per rectum. Diverticulum and angiodysplasia are common causes of lower GI bleeding in older adults, whereas hemorrhoids, anal fissures, and inflammatory bowel disease occur most often in younger patients. A diverticulum is a pouch or saclike protrusion of the colonic wall (Figure 34-1). Diverticulitis represents inflammation and possible perforation of a diverticulum. Diverticular bleeding can be severe and life threatening because diverticula often form at the site of arterial vascular penetration. Hemorrhoids are dilated submucosal veins in the anus located above (internal) or below (external) the dentate line. Figure 34-2 depicts internal and external hemorrhoidal veins, where hemorrhoids often erupt. Serious lower GI bleeding from hemorrhoids is uncommon. The risk for bleeding is increased in patients with a coagulopathy. Internal hemorrhoids are rarely associated with pain, whereas external hemorrhoids can cause significant discomfort. Angiodysplasia refers to dilated tortuous submucosal vessels. Lower GI bleeding from angiodysplasia is from a venous source and most often originates from the cecum or ascending colon.

Colitis refers to mucosal inflammation and can have an infectious or inflammatory cause. Inflammatory bowel disease includes both Crohn's disease and ulcerative colitis. Hematochezia is a more common initial finding in patients with ulcerative colitis. However, it is not necessary to differentiate between the two in the ED because the treatment is similar for both conditions.[17] Colon cancer is a relatively less common but serious cause of lower GI bleeding. The bleeding tends to be less severe but can occur multiple times.

Many patients with lower GI bleeding experience acute bleeds that are self-limiting and do not cause significant changes in hemodynamic status. Most patients with mild lower GI bleeding who are hemodynamically stable may be evaluated on an outpatient basis. Patients with severe symptomatic lower GI bleeding require hospital admission for resuscitation, diagnosis, and treatment. Colonoscopy should be performed to determine the source of bleeding after the patient is stabilized.

Blood originating from the left colon is typically bright red in color. Anemia may be present in patients with low-grade bleeding over a period of time. Crampy abdominal pain may be present. Painless bleeding also occurs. Tachycardia, pallor, diaphoresis, and other indicators of hypovolemic shock indicate significant bleeding. Orthostatic changes in pulse or blood pressure occur in many patients.

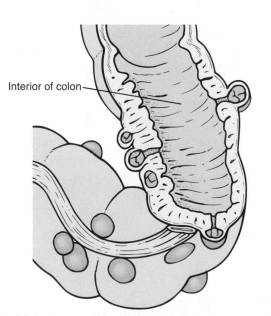

FIGURE 34-1. Diverticula are outpouchings of the colon. When they become inflamed, the condition is diverticulitis. The inflammatory process can spread to the surrounding area in the intestine. (From Lewis SM, Heitkemper MM, Dirksen SR: *Medical-surgical nursing: assessment and management of clinical problems,* ed 7, St. Louis, 2007, Mosby.)

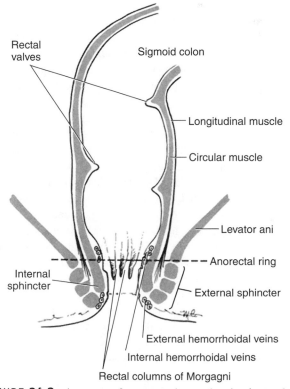

FIGURE 34-2. Anatomy of rectum and anus showing internal and external hemorrhoidal veins. (From Price SA, Wilson LM: *Pathophysiology: clinical concepts of disease processes,* ed 6, St. Louis, 2003, Mosby.)

Baseline laboratory studies include CBC, platelet count, and coagulation studies. The first priority is management of the ABCs followed by IV fluid resuscitation with normal saline or lactated Ringer's solution via large-bore catheter. Administration of PRBCs may be necessary in cases of significant blood loss. Treatment to correct coagulopathies or thrombocytopenia should be initiated. The ideal hematocrit depends on the patient's age, past medical history, and the presence of significant medical problems. For example, a young adult may tolerate a hematocrit of 25. However, the same hematocrit could be detrimental in an older adult patient with coronary artery disease.[16] Determining the source of bleeding is a priority. Colonoscopy, radionuclide imaging, or mesenteric angiography may be performed. Colonoscopy is the initial examination of choice in the majority of cases. Endoscopic therapy and interventions can be used to treat diverticula, angiodysplasia, and hemorrhoids. Surgical intervention may be required in some patients with exsanguinating lower GI bleeding. Barium studies have no role in the evaluation of lower GI bleeding.[4]

Gastroesophageal Reflux Disease

GERD applies to patients with symptoms or mucosal damage produced by the abnormal reflux of gastric contents into the esophagus. The typical symptoms are heartburn, chest pain, regurgitation, and dysphagia.[5] Some patients report the sensation of a lump in the throat that is not relieved with swallowing or coughing. Nausea may also be present. Bronchospasm, chronic cough, and laryngitis have also been associated with GERD. Conditions associated with GERD are decreased LES pressure, decreased esophageal motility, and increased gastric emptying time. Many foods such as fatty foods, chocolate, tea, coffee, alcohol, and foods/drinks containing caffeine can exacerbate symptoms. Some medications can also worsen or lead to GERD, and these include calcium channel blockers, theophylline, nitrates, and valium. The emergency nurse needs to be vigilant when reviewing home medication lists and past medical history. Look for medications or conditions that could lead to delay in gastric emptying and predispose the patient to GERD. Examples include pregnancy or the use of hormones, diabetes mellitus, scleroderma, diabetic gastroparesis, use of anticholinergics, and gastric outlet obstruction. It is of interest that acid secretion does not increase in patients with GERD. Complications associated with GERD include esophagitis and peptic stricture.

GERD-related chest pain may mimic cardiac-related chest pain and is typically described as squeezing or burning. Chest pain may be the only reported symptom. The pain may radiate to the neck, jaw, or abdomen. Similarities to the clinical presentation of ischemic heart disease require thoughtful consideration. The emergency nurse should pay close attention to patient history and to the patient for changes in condition. Other symptoms associated with GERD are nocturnal choking, sleep apnea, recurrent pneumonia, recurrent ear, nose, and throat infections, loss of dental enamel, and chronic halitosis.

Management of GERD begins with elimination of other conditions that are more lethal (e.g., ischemic heart disease and esophageal perforation). Studies such as electrocardiogram, chest radiograph, and CBC are primarily used to rule out other conditions. Additional imaging studies include endoscopy. Specific treatment in the ED includes symptomatic relief through use of antacids, H_2-blockers, and proton pump inhibitors.[11] Antacids are given with viscous lidocaine to increase effectiveness. Table 34-1 highlights specific medications and their expected outcomes.

Appendicitis

The appendix is a hollow organ. Obstruction of the appendiceal lumen appears to be the most common mechanism for the development of appendicitis. Once obstructed, the lumen becomes distended. Obstruction and distension decrease blood flow, resulting in ischemia and bacterial invasion. Untreated, inflammation progresses so that the appendix becomes nonviable and gangrenous, eventually rupturing into the peritoneal space. The incidence of appendicitis is higher in males than in females. It is also higher in the 10- to 19-year-old age-group. The diagnosis of appendicitis is challenging in young children and older adults. Approximately 6% to 8% of the population will develop appendicitis during their lifetime.

Patients may have abdominal pain or abdominal cramping, nausea, vomiting, tachycardia, malaise, and anorexia.

Table 34-1. DRUG THERAPY FOR GERD	
Mechanism of Action	**Examples**
INCREASE LOWER ESOPHAGEAL SPHINCTER PRESSURE	
Cholinergic	Bethanechol (Urecholine)
Dopamine antagonist	Metoclopramide (Reglan)
Serotonin antagonist	Cisapride (Propulsid)
ACID NEUTRALIZING	
Antacids	Gelusil, Maalox, Mylanta
ANTISECRETORY	
Histamine H_2-receptor antagonists	Ranitidine (Zantac)
	Cimetidine (Tagamet)
	Famotidine (Pepcid)
	Nizatidine (Axid)
Proton pump inhibitors	Omeprazole (Prilosec)
	Lansoprazole (Prevacid)
	Pantoprazole (Protonix, Pantoloc)
	Rabeprazole (Aciphex)
CYTOPROTECTIVE	
Alginic acid–antacid	Gaviscon
Antacids	Gelusil, Maalox, Mylanta
Acid-protective	Sucralfate (Carafate)

From Lewis SM, Heitkemper MM, Dirksen SR: *Medical-surgical nursing: assessment and management of clinical problems*, ed 7, St. Louis, 2007, Mosby.
GERD, Gastroesophageal reflux disease.

Chills and fever also occur. Abdominal pain may be initially diffuse and periumbilical in location; later the pain may become intense and localized to the lower right quadrant. Classic pain associated with appendicitis is located just inside the right iliac crest at McBurney's point. Older adult patients are often afebrile and do not exhibit this classic pain. Pressure on the lower left abdomen intensifies pain in the right lower quadrant (Rovsing's sign). Pain may not always occur in this classic location because of normal variations in the location of the appendix (Figure 34-3). The position of comfort for most patients is supine with hips and knees flexed.

If the appendix ruptures, peritoneal signs increase and involuntary guarding develops. Increased fever and rebound tenderness occur when the appendix abscesses or ruptures. Diagnosis is made by assessment of clinical signs and symptoms in concert with physical examination. Diagnostic data include elevation of white blood cell (WBC) count greater than 10,000 cells/mm^3 with increased neutrophils, specifically bands. Although leukocytosis is common, 30% of patients may have a normal WBC. Ultrasonography may occasionally demonstrate an enlarged appendix or collection of periappendiceal fluid. Computed tomography (CT) scan is considered a more accurate diagnostic imaging test in the diagnosis of acute appendicitis. A CT scan of the abdomen or "appendiceal CT scan" with rectal contrast may be obtained.[19] Urinalysis should be performed to rule out GU problems.

Definitive therapy for appendicitis is surgical intervention with the laparoscopic approach as the preferred method. Obtain IV access, administer a prophylactic broad-spectrum antibiotic, and instruct the patient not to eat or drink. Complications such as perforation, peritonitis, and abscess formation can occur when treatment is delayed.

Cholecystitis

Acute cholecystitis involves inflammation of the gallbladder and is usually associated with gallstone disease. However, approximately 10% of patients who present with acute cholecystitis will not have gallstones (acalculous cholecystitis).[1] Acalculous cholecystitis is more common in critically ill patients and is associated with a high morbidity and mortality.

Secondary infection and distension can occur if the cystic duct becomes obstructed. The most common organisms associated with the secondary infection include *Escherichia coli*, enterococcus, and *Klebsiella*. Complications of acute cholecystitis include gangrene.[12] Perforation, though rare, may occur if gangrene develops. Cholecystitis can occur in both males and females. Obese, fair-skinned women of increasing age and parity may be at greater risk.

Symptoms include sudden onset abdominal pain—usually after ingestion of fried or fatty foods. Pain is usually located in the epigastrium and/or right upper quadrant and may be referred to the right shoulder or supraclavicular area. Patients often describe the pain as steady and severe. Marked

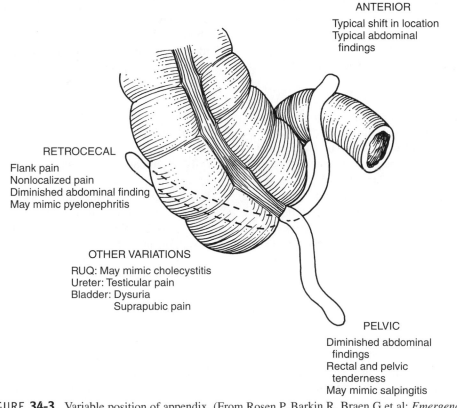

ANTERIOR
Typical shift in location
Typical abdominal
   findings

RETROCECAL
Flank pain
Nonlocalized pain
Diminished abdominal finding
May mimic pyelonephritis

OTHER VARIATIONS
RUQ: May mimic cholecystitis
Ureter: Testicular pain
Bladder: Dysuria
       Suprapubic pain

PELVIC
Diminished abdominal
   findings
Rectal and pelvic
   tenderness
May mimic salpingitis

FIGURE **34-3.** Variable position of appendix. (From Rosen P, Barkin R, Braen G et al: *Emergency medicine,* vol 2, ed 3, St. Louis, 1992, Mosby.)

tenderness, inspiratory limitation on deep palpation under the right subcostal margin (Murphy's sign), and local and rebound tenderness may also be present. Low-grade fever (100.4° F [38° C]), tachycardia, nausea, vomiting, and flatulence are common findings. If the common bile duct is obstructed, the patient may appear slightly jaundiced. Clinical signs associated with obstructed bile flow include but are not limited to dark amber urine that foams when shaken, clay-colored stools, pruritus, and bleeding tendencies.

Diagnostic tests include urinalysis, CBC, serum electrolytes, BUN, creatinine, serum glucose, and serum bilirubin levels. A WBC with differential often reflects leukocytosis with an increased number of band forms. The serum bilirubin level may be elevated. An elevated amylase level suggests pancreatitis rather than cholecystitis. Ultrasonography is extremely useful in the emergency setting for detection of a thickened gallbladder wall, gallstones, and pericholecystic fluid, but it may not detect smaller gallstones or sludge. A CT scan may reveal gallbladder wall edema and is useful when perforation is suspected or other diagnoses are considered. Patients with acute cholecystitis frequently require hospitalization. In these cases a hepatobiliary iminodiacetic acid (HIDA) scan, also called cholescintigraphy, may be performed if the ultrasound scan is negative.

Treatment of cholecystitis includes administration of IV crystalloid solution and medications for nausea and vomiting. Opioids or ketorolac may be ordered for pain control.[20] A nasogastric tube may be necessary for patients with persistent vomiting. Monitor vital signs and intake and output. Broad-spectrum antibiotics are indicated for potential microbial infection. Definitive treatment for cholecystitis is surgery with traditional laparotomy or laparoscopic cholecystectomy.

Acute Pancreatitis

Acute pancreatitis is defined as an acute inflammatory process of the pancreas. The exact mechanism is not clear. Theories include bile or duodenal reflux, bacterial infection, pancreatic enzyme activation with autolysis, and ductal hypertension. Seventy to eighty percent of pancreatitis cases are due to gallstone disease or alcoholism.[4] Gallstone disease can result in ductal hypertension and pancreatic enzyme activation. Alcohol abuse causes toxic metabolites that injure the pancreas, leading to inflammation. Other causes include malignant strictures obstructing the pancreatic duct, chronic hypercalcemia, abdominal trauma, infections (e.g., mumps, cytomegalovirus infection), drugs such as antimetabolites, or toxins (e.g., organophosphate insecticides, scorpion venom). Regardless of mechanism, pancreatitis is characterized by the release of activated digestive enzymes into the pancreas and surrounding tissues. This leads to tissue damage in the pancreas, surrounding fat, and adjacent structures that results in a chemical type of burn and fluid loss, also known as third-space fluid loss. In response to the inflammation, inflammatory mediators are released into the circulation. This can also lead to systemic inflammatory response syndrome (SIRS). Complications of pancreatitis can include necrosis to segments of the pancreas, abscess formation, pseudocyst, and pulmonary capillary leak syndrome, resulting in respiratory distress syndrome.

A clinical hallmark found in 95% of patients with pancreatitis is abdominal pain, originating in the epigastric region and radiating to the back. Abdominal tenderness, rebound, and guarding are common. Nausea, vomiting, and abdominal distention may be present. Patients may have a low-grade fever. Tachycardia and hypotension may be present due to the third-space fluid loss. Tachypnea is often the result of muscle splinting secondary to pain. Decreased gastric motility causes hypoactive or absent bowel sounds.

Certain laboratory values aid in the diagnosis of acute pancreatitis. Serum amylase and lipase values should be obtained in patients who are suspected of having pancreatitis. Additional serum assessments include blood glucose and triglycerides. Elevated serum amylase and lipase levels are frequently seen in pancreatitis. Amylase levels three times greater than the upper normal limit are highly suggestive of pancreatitis.[3] The amylase level may be normal in some patients with acute alcoholic pancreatitis. The lipase level is considered useful because it will stay elevated for several days after the onset of symptoms. The amylase level will lower at a faster rate compared with lipase. Leukocytosis, decreased hematocrit, hyperglycemia, and hypocalcemia may also be present. In some cases, the hematocrit may be high due to hemoconcentration from substantial third-space fluid loss.

Radiographic studies are useful in diagnosing acute pancreatitis. A chest radiograph may reveal pleural effusions or pulmonary infiltrates, and an ileus may be detected on abdominal radiographs. Abdominal ultrasonography can identify gallstones as an underlying cause. Abdominal CT scan may also contribute to the diagnosis of acute pancreatitis by identification of pancreatic edema or fluid around the pancreas.

Management includes maintaining strict NPO (nothing by mouth) status. Obtain IV access for fluid and electrolyte replacement with normal saline. Fluid resuscitation is a priority in patients with indicators of hypovolemia. Antiemetics are administered for nausea, vomiting, and to minimize further fluid loss. Pain control with IV analgesics, usually narcotic, is a high priority for the patient with pancreatitis (Table 34-2). Nasogastric suction helps alleviate nausea, vomiting, and abdominal distension. Ongoing monitoring of respiratory, cardiovascular, and renal functions is recommended. Antibiotic administration is generally limited to patients with some necrosis of the pancreas because they are at greater risk for infection.[3]

Diverticulitis

Diverticula are small pouches that develop in the large intestines secondary to aging (see Figure 34-1). This condition, called diverticulosis, occurs in about half of all Americans age 60 to 80 years and is found in almost all Americans

Table 34-2. DRUGS USED IN TREATMENT OF ACUTE PANCREATITIS	
Drug	**Expected Outcomes**
Meperidine (Demerol)	Relief of pain
Nitroglycerin or papaverine	Relaxation of smooth muscles and relief of pain
Antispasmodics (e.g., dicyclomine [Bentyl], propantheline bromide [Pro-Banthine])	Decrease in vagal stimulation, motility, and pancreatic outflow (inhibition of volume and concentration of bicarbonate and enzymatic secretion); contraindicated in paralytic ileus
Carbonic anhydrase inhibitor (acetazolamide [Diamox])	Reduction in volume and bicarbonate concentration of pancreatic secretion
Antacids	Neutralization of gastric secretions; decrease in hydrochloric acid stimulation of secretin, which stimulates production and secretion of pancreatic secretions
Histamine H_2-receptor antagonists (cimetidine [Tagamet], ranitidine [Zantac])	Decreases hydrochloric acid by inhibiting histamine (hydrochloric acid stimulates pancreatic activity)
Calcium gluconate	Treatment of hypocalcemia and to prevent or treat tetany
Corticosteroids	Use only for seriously ill patients with hypotension or shock. NOTE: Corticosteroids can be used to treat autoimmune pancreatitis. Additionally, corticosteroids have been noted to be a class of drugs that may cause acute pancreatitis.
Glucagon	Reduction in pancreatic inflammation and decrease in serum amylase, suppression of pancreatic secretions
Somatostatin	Inhibition of pancreatic secretions

Modified from Lewis SM, Heitkemper MM, Dirksen SR: *Medical-surgical nursing: assessment and management of clinical problems,* ed 7, St. Louis, 2007, Mosby.

older than age 80 years. Weakened areas that predispose the colon to herniation of inferior tissue layers in combination with a low-fiber diet lead to this primarily painless disorder. Less than 10% of patients with diverticulosis experience pain. However, pain is the most-reported complaint when diverticula become inflamed and diverticulitis develops. Inflammation develops when fecal material is trapped in the pouches, causing trauma to the intestinal lining, which ultimately leads to inflammation. Persistent pain associated with diverticulitis is localized in the left lower quadrant. Fever, chills, nausea, and vomiting are seen when infection is present. Other symptoms include cramping and constipation. Complications of diverticulitis include intestinal obstruction, hemorrhage, perforation, abscess, stricture, and fistula.[16]

Diagnostic evaluation includes CBC and urinalysis. Results of the CBC show a left shift resulting from infection. The presence of WBCs and red blood cells (RBCs) in urine is also a common finding. Supine and upright abdominal radiographs are obtained to rule out perforation or obstruction. Abdominal CT is the preferred diagnostic modality because it is more effective in identification of processes outside the colon's lumen (i.e., diverticulitis). Barium enema, endoscopy, and ultrasonography may also be used.

Treatment of patients with diverticulitis includes rehydration with a saline solution, resting the bowel by making the patient NPO, and inserting a gastric tube if persistent vomiting is present. Anticholinergics are used to reduce colonic spasms, with opiates reserved for more aggressive pain management. Oral or parenteral antibiotics may be given depending on clinical presentation. Emergent surgery is required when there is evidence of peritonitis.

Bowel Obstruction

Bowel obstruction occurs in either sex, at any age, and from a variety of causes. The most common cause is adhesions from previous abdominal surgery, followed by incarcerated inguinal hernia. Postoperative adhesions account for approximately three fourths of small bowel obstructions.[13] Other causes include foreign bodies, volvulus, intussusception, strictures, tumors, congenital adhesive bands, and fecal impaction.

Bowel obstructions are classified as mechanical or nonmechanical. Mechanical obstruction results from a disorder outside the intestines or blockage inside the lumen of the intestines. Intussusception, telescoping of the bowel within itself by peristalsis, is an example of a mechanical obstruction. The peak age for intussusception to occur is 5 to 9 months of age.[13] Nonmechanical obstruction results when muscle activity of the intestine decreases and movement of contents slows (e.g., paralytic ileus) (Figure 34-4).

When obstruction occurs, bowel contents accumulate above the obstruction. This leads to rapid accumulation of anaerobic and aerobic bacteria, which causes an increase in methane and hydrogen production. The more proximal the obstruction is, the quicker the onset of discomfort. Peristalsis increases, which leads to the increased release of secretions. These events worsen distension, cause bowel edema, and increase capillary permeability. Plasma leaks into the peritoneal cavity while fluid is trapped in the intestinal lumen, causing a decrease in the absorption of fluid and electrolytes.

Obstruction can be partial or complete. Strangulation with ischemia and necrosis almost always occurs in the setting of complete obstruction of the small intestines. Necrosis and perforation lead to peritonitis and sepsis.

Clinical signs vary with the location of the obstruction. Symptoms include colicky, crampy, intermittent, and wavelike abdominal pain. At times pain may be severe. Abdominal distension may also be present. Patients may have diffuse abdominal tenderness, rigidity, and constipation. Hyperactive

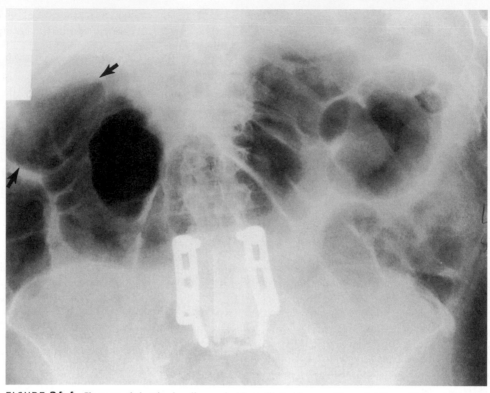

FIGURE 34-4. Ileus on abdominal radiograph. Note dilated loops of bowel. (From Dettenmeier PA: *Radiographic assessment for nurses,* St. Louis, 1995, Mosby.)

bowel sounds or absent bowel sounds may be noted. The patient may also be febrile, tachycardic, and hypotensive with nausea and vomiting. Emesis usually has an odor of feces from proliferation of bacteria. Patients may pass some stool and flatus because the colon requires 12 to 24 hours to empty after the onset of a bowel obstruction.

Laboratory studies include CBC, BUN, serum glucose, electrolytes, serum creatinine, and arterial blood gas measurements. Leukocytosis with a left shift indicates strangulation and necrosis. The BUN may be elevated secondary to dehydration from vomiting and decreased oral intake. Metabolic acidosis can result if the bowel becomes ischemic. Metabolic alkalosis can occur in patients who have frequent emesis.[12] Upright abdominal radiographs may reveal dilated, fluid-filled loops of bowel with visible air-fluid levels. A CT scan may also be useful in determining the level and cause of obstruction. Management includes IV access for fluid and electrolyte replacement using crystalloid solution to maintain hemodynamic values and renal perfusion. Intake, output, and patient response to therapy should be monitored to prevent fluid overload. Frequently assess the abdomen for distension, tenderness, and guarding to identify changes. A nasogastric tube is inserted to decompress the stomach and reduce vomiting. Evaluate pain for worsening of the condition. Prophylactic administration of antibiotics is recommended. Surgical intervention may be required for some patients. Adults with intussusception and strangulated bowel will frequently have a laparotomy after fluid resuscitation and hemodynamic stability has been achieved. Life-threatening

complications of bowel obstruction include peritonitis, bowel strangulation or perforation, renal insufficiency, aspiration, hypovolemia, intestinal ischemia or infarction, and death. Untreated obstruction that progresses to shock has a high mortality rate.[14]

Gastroenteritis

Acute gastroenteritis is one of the most common illnesses in children and adults. Gastroenteritis is an inflammation of the stomach and intestinal lining caused by viral, protozoal, bacterial, or parasitic agents. Viruses account for the majority of cases. Bacterial infection also accounts for acute diarrheal disease. Gastroenteritis may be caused by an imbalance of normal flora *(E. coli)* resulting from the ingestion of contaminated food. Patients have nausea, vomiting, diarrhea, and abdominal cramps. Hyperactive bowel sounds, fever, and headaches are also present. Anal excoriation occurs with frequent episodes of diarrhea.

Laboratory data include CBC, electrolytes, stool for ova and parasites, and stool culture. Obtain IV access for replacement of fluid and electrolytes. Administer antiemetics as ordered. Antibiotics are determined by patient history and presenting symptoms. Successful treatment is based on identifying the causative agent and resting the intestinal tract. Oral hydration with clear liquids is possible in most patients. Suggested fluids include cola, ginger ale, apple juice, tea, broth, and electrolyte replacement drinks such as Gatorade. Fluid replacement in children is critical to prevent dehydration. The BRAT diet (bananas, rice, applesauce, and toast) can be started as soon as diarrhea subsides. Feeding should begin as soon as possible in children and adults.

SUMMARY

GI emergencies can be minor or life threatening. Most GI emergencies present with similar clinical manifestations. Triage history and physical assessment play an important role in management of these patients. Reassessment of signs and symptoms such as quality and intensity of pain, vital signs, intake and output, and/or level of consciousness should lead to rapid intervention by emergency nurses providing care for patients with GI emergencies. The ability to differentiate GI emergency conditions that require immediate attention is a requisite skill for the emergency nurse.

REFERENCES

1. Barie PS, Fischer E: Acute acalculous cholecystitis, *J Am Coll Surg* 180:232, 1995.
2. Boonpongmanee S, Fleischer DE, Pezullo JC et al: The frequency of peptic ulcer as a cause of upper GI bleeding is exaggerated, *Gastrointest Endosc* 59:788, 2004.
3. Daragonov P, Forsmark CE: Diseases of the pancreas, *ACP Medicine*, 2007. Retrieved October 12, 2007, from http://www.acpmedicine.com/acpmedicine/institutional/tableOfContent.action#.
4. Davila RE, Rajan E, Adler DG et al: ASGE guideline: the role of endoscopy in the patient with lower GI bleeding, *Gastrointest Endosc* 62:656, 2005.
5. Devault KR, Castell DO: Updated guidelines for the diagnosis and treatment of gastroesophageal reflux disease,, *Am J Gastroenterol* 100:190, 2005.
6. Fenimore GS, Manno MS: Control cirrhosis complications, *Nurs Crit Care* 3:44, 2008.
7. Gotzsche PC: Somatostatin or octreotide for acute bleeding esophageal varices, *Cochrane Database Syst Rev* 2000. Retrieved October 12, 2007, from http://www.eboncall.org/CATs/2192.html.
8. Guyton AC, Hall GE: *Textbook of medical physiology*, Philadelphia, 2006, Elsevier.
9. Jutabha R, Jensen DM, Martin P et al: Randomized study comparing banding and propranolol to prevent initial variceal hemorrhage in cirrhotics with high risk esophageal varices, *Gastroenterology* 128:870, 2005.
10. Matsui S, Kamisake T, Kudo M et al: Endoscopic band ligation for control of nonvariceal upper GI bleeding, *Gastrointest Endosc* 55:214, 2002.
11. Numan ME, Lau J, deWitt NJ et al: Short term treatment with proton-pump inhibitors as a test for gastroesophageal reflux disease, *Ann Intern Med* 140:518, 2004.
12. Papi C, Catarci M, D'Ambrosio L: Timing of cholecystectomy for acute calculus cholecystitis: a meta-analysis, *Am J Gastroenterol* 99:147, 2004.
13. Quickel R, Hodin RA: Clinical manifestations and diagnosis of small bowel obstruction, *UpToDate*, 2007. Retrieved October 12, 2007, from http://www.uptodate.com/online/content/topic.do?topicKey=gi_dis/22094&selectedTitle=1~150&source=search_result.
14. Quickel R, Hodin RA: Treatment of small bowel obstructions, *UpToDate*, 2007. Retrieved October 12, 2007, from http://www.uptodate.com/online/content/topic.do?topicKey=gi_dis/23412.
15. Rafferty J, Shellito P, Hyman NH et al: Practice parameters for sigmoid diverticulitis, *Dis Colon Rectum* 49:939, 2006.
16. Saab S, Jutabha R: Approach to the adult patient with lower gastrointestinal bleeding, *UpToDate*, 2007. Retrieved October 12, 2007, from http://www.uptodate.com/online/content/topic.do?topicKey=gi_dis/14838&selectedTitle=1~150&source=search_result.
17. Saab S, Jutabha R: Etiology of lower GI bleeding in adults, *UpToDate*, 2007. Retrieved October 12, 2007, from http://www.uptodate.com/online/content/topic.do?topicKey=gi_dis/14450&selectedTitle=1~79&source=search_result.
18. Shok P: Fatal hemorrhage from a Mallory-Weiss tear, *Endoscopy* 35:345, 2003.
19. Teresawa T, Blackmore CC et al: Systematic review: computed tomography and ultrasonography to detect acute appendicitis in adults and adolescents, *Ann Intern Med* 141:537, 2004.
20. Zakko SF, Afdhal NH: Treatment of acute cholecystitis, *UpToDate*, 2007. Retrieved October 12, 2007, from http://www.uptodate.com/online/content/topic.do?topicKey=biliaryt/8379&selectedTitle=1~98&source=search_result.

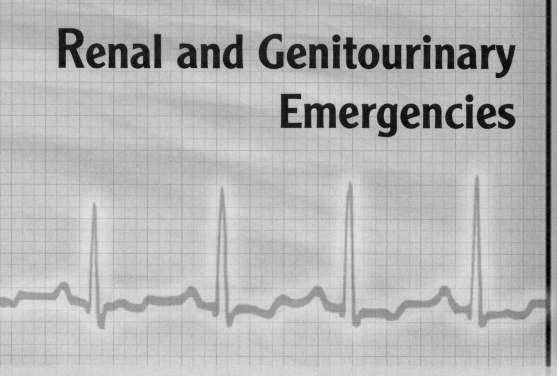

CHAPTER 35

Renal and Genitourinary Emergencies

Cynthia S. Baxter

Genitourinary (GU) problems are a common complaint in the emergency department (ED). According to the National Institutes of Health (NIH), urinary tract infections (UTIs) are the second most common infection in the body and affect women more often than men. Up to one in five females will have at least one UTI in their lifetime; many will experience multiple UTIs.[5] Kidney stones are one of the most common disorders of the urinary tract. In 2000, kidney stones resulted in 2.7 million visits to health care providers and more than 600,000 visits to EDs.[10] Approximately 18.9 million new cases of sexually transmitted infections (STIs) occured in the United States in 2000. According to an incidence and prevalence study, 48% were among persons age 15 to 24 years, and three STIs (human papilloma virus, trichomoniasis, and *Chlamydia*) accounted for 88% of all new cases among this age-group.[12] Incidence of end-stage renal disease (ESRD) is rising in all industrialized nations, although the cause of this increase is not clear. ESRD affects African Americans three times more often than whites and is most prevalent in those with diabetes or hypertension, occurring six times more often in those with hypertension. In people 65 years of age or older, incidence of renal failure increases sixfold; however, 66% of all diabetes-induced renal failure occurs before age 64. Males account for 65% of the ESRD population.[7] Acute tubular necrosis, the most common type of acute renal failure

(ARF), accounts for 5% of all hospital admissions. Patients with compromised renal function often arrive at the ED with life-threatening fluid and electrolyte imbalances.

ANATOMY AND PHYSIOLOGY

The GU tract consists of the kidneys, ureters, urinary bladder, urethra, and external genitalia. Urine is produced by the kidneys as a way to regulate fluid volume and electrolyte balance. Ureters transport urine to the bladder for temporary storage. The urine is drained from the bladder to the outside by the urethra. External structures of the male GU system have reproductive functions.

The kidneys are located on the posterior abdominal wall behind the peritoneum on either side of the vertebral column inside the rib cage. The medial aspect of each kidney contains the hilum, where the renal artery and nerve enter and the renal vein and ureter exit. Blood flow to the kidney is supplied by the renal artery, which branches off the abdominal aorta and enters the kidney through the renal sinus. Blood leaves the kidney through the renal vein, which empties into the abdominal inferior vena cava.

The nephron, the functional unit of the kidney, is composed of the renal corpuscle, proximal convoluted tubule, Henle's loop, distal convoluted tubule, and collecting ducts. Each kidney contains an estimated 1 million nephrons that are individually capable of producing urine. These nephrons cannot be reproduced once destroyed. The renal corpuscle contains the glomerulus, a web of tightly convoluted capillaries, and Bowman's capsule, which surrounds and supports these structures. Blood flows through the afferent arteriole into the glomerulus and out the efferent arteriole. Renal blood flow accounts for 21% of cardiac output, or 1200 mL/min. Without adequate renal blood flow the kidneys are unable to function adequately. Specialized cells called juxtaglomerular cells are located at the entrance to the glomerulus of the afferent arteriole in 15% of nephrons. These specialized cells sense changes in pressure and sodium concentration and play a role in the renin-angiotensin-aldosterone (RAA) system.

Filtration of plasma in the renal corpuscle is the first step in urine production and helps the kidneys rid the body of wastes and retain water and essential solutes. Pressure generated as blood courses through the tight web of capillaries in the glomerulus, along with oncotic pressure within the blood, is greater than pressure created by Bowman's capsule, so plasma or filtrate and small solutes cross the semipermeable epithelial capillary lining. Injury to the glomerulus, such as ischemia or inflammation, increases permeability of the capillary membrane and allows larger molecules (red blood cells [RBCs], epithelial casts, protein, or white blood cells [WBCs]) to cross. Decreased oncotic pressure, often the result of decreased serum albumin levels, or decreased pressure within the glomerulus produced by systemic hypotension decreases glomerular filtration rate (GFR) and eventually urine output. GFR in the average adult is 125 mL/min or 180 L/day.

Tubules, Henle's loop, and collecting ducts excrete waste products (e.g., urea, nitrogen, creatinine, drug metabolites), reabsorb water and solutes (potassium, sodium, chloride, hydrogen, glucose, and amino acids) from filtrate, and secrete excess solutes the body does not need into filtrate. Osmosis, diffusion, and active transport occur between the nephron and surrounding capillaries. Hormonal control regulates reabsorption and secretion in the nephron.

The RAA system and antidiuretic hormone (ADH) are feedback-loop systems within the body that maintain homeostasis. Serum osmolarity increases and causes stimulation of the hypothalamus, which releases ADH. Nephron permeability increases, so additional water is absorbed, serum osmolarity returns to normal, and ADH release stops. Pressure changes in the glomerulus are overcome by vasodilation and constriction of the afferent arteriole by a process called autoregulation. This autoregulation keeps pressure in the glomerulus within a wide range of systolic blood pressures. When range is exceeded, autoregulation fails and epithelial damage occurs with eventual scarring and sclerosis followed by decreased permeability, GFR, and urine output. Inadequate nephron perfusion stimulates the juxtaglomerular apparatus to secrete renin that converts angiotensinogen to angiotensin I, which stimulates aldosterone release from the adrenal cortex and reabsorption of sodium and water by the nephron. Conversion of angiotensin I to angiotensin II by an enzyme in the lung causes peripheral vasoconstriction. Perfusion increases to the nephron, and the cycle is altered.

Without a functioning kidney and adequate urine production, homeostasis is severely impaired. Fluid and electrolyte imbalance, accumulation of urea and creatinine, decreased excretion of drug metabolites, and inadequate reabsorption of amino acids and glucose occur. The kidneys help convert vitamin D into its active form to ensure calcium absorption from intestines and secrete erythropoietin for stimulation of RBC production in bone marrow. Consequently, altered renal function decreases bone mineralization and oxygen-carrying capacity of the blood.

The renal pelvis narrows to enter the ureter, where urine is moved to the bladder by peristaltic contractions. The muscular bladder stores urine until release to the urethra by the micturition reflex.

External genitalia are also part of the GU system. Female genitalia consist of the vestibule, the space into which the urethra and vagina open, and surrounding labia minora and majora. Anatomic position and the short length of the female urethra are responsible for the high frequency of UTIs in females.

Male external genitalia include penis, scrotum, and scrotal contents. Scrotal contents include the testes, tubules that carry developing sperm cells and secrete testosterone, and the epididymis, which lies along the posterior testes and is the final maturation area for sperm. The prostate is glandular muscle tissue that surrounds the urethra at the base of the bladder. Enlargement of the prostate can cause outlet obstruction and urinary retention. The penis consists of three columns of erectile tissue that become engorged with blood, producing erection. Two columns of corpora cavernosa form the dorsum and sides of the penis and the corpus spongiosum forms the base and glans. Clinical manifestations of GU disease frequently involve external genitalia.

PATIENT ASSESSMENT

Assessment of the GU system should determine history of hypertension, diabetes, previous infections, prostatitis, urethritis, bladder or urethral damage during childbirth, history of renal calculi, and recurrent UTIs. A detailed drug list, including prescription, over-the-counter (OTC), herbal preparations, and illicit drugs should be obtained. Identification of any history of exposure to occupational chemicals or toxins may identify contact with substances that could cause nephrotoxicity. Sexual history should include discussion of risk factors that can cause GU symptoms (e.g., use of contraceptive jellies or creams, multiple partners, abnormal penile or vaginal discharges, unsafe sexual practices, history of STIs). GU complaints often arise from changes in urinary patterns; for example, frequency, dysuria, urgency, dribbling, or incontinence.

Urinary disorders can be identified by the patient's own subjective interpretation (e.g., changes in output, voiding pattern, location of pain). Obtaining a urine sample for analysis can validate the nurse's suspicions. Gross visual examination for color, clarity, and amount should be done before urine is sent to the laboratory. Palpation and percussion of the kidneys may reveal costal vertebral tenderness, structural asymmetry, or the presence of masses.

Female patients, particularly those of reproductive age, warrant additional assessment for a broad spectrum of complaints. One should always consider the possibility of an unknown pregnancy and take a careful menstrual history, including use of contraceptives. If the patient is pregnant, fetal heart tones are assessed for presence, location, and rate. When a woman has a specific genital concern, a vaginal examination is indicated. Any discharge or bleeding should be noted and described by character and amount.

Males should be assessed for problems specific to their GU anatomy, including presence of a slow stream, inability to void, penile discharge, or warts.

Hematuria, the presence of blood in the urine, may be the primary complaint or may accompany other symptoms. A detailed medication and diet history may uncover other causes for discoloration of urine—foods such as beets, rhubarb, and blackberries and medications such as phenytoin are common nonhematuric causes of red or dark urine. Hematuria can be confirmed by urinalysis (UA); however, microscopic hematuria on a single test is common. Early-stream hematuria suggests bleeding from the urethra, hematuria throughout the stream indicates upper GU tract bleeding, and bleeding at the end suggests bladder neck or urethral bleeding. Complete urinalysis and urine cytologic study may indicate the need for further diagnostic testing for urologic cancer, renal disease, infection, or renal calculi as the source of hematuria.

Pain should be assessed using the PQRST mnemonic—provocation, quality, region or radiation, severity, and time. The most severe pain associated with the GU system is renal colic caused by calculi. Increased pressure and dilation of the kidney and urinary collecting system cause sudden, unbearable pain. The patient usually presents with restlessness and pallor and complains of flank pain that often radiates to the abdomen and groin. If the stone lodges in the bladder, urinary frequency and urgency develop. Pain can cause tachypnea and tachycardia with elevated blood pressure. Oliguria, defined as urine output less than 400 mL in 24 hours, or anuria, less than 75 mL in 24 hours, may be the presenting symptom. The cause is usually obstruction; however, blood chemistry values should be evaluated for azotemia, which indicates renal failure from prolonged obstruction leading to hydronephrosis or other causes. If the patient has a urinary catheter in place, patency should be assessed. A physical examination can identify urinary retention by palpating the bladder as a firm mass above the symphysis pubis, with an urge to void on palpation; bladder scanning using ultrasonography may also be used to detect bladder distention. History should be obtained to identify drugs that contribute to retention, including OTC nasal decongestants containing anticholinergic ingredients. A neurologic examination should be performed to rule out spinal cord injury or disease that can interfere with the micturition reflex. The prostate is

examined for enlargement as the cause of obstruction. After the patient has attempted to void, a urethral catheter may be inserted for residual volume. Bedside bladder ultrasonography may avoid the need for catheterization and allow assessment of prevoid and postvoid volume. If the catheter cannot be inserted without resistance, a suprapubic bladder tap or assistance from a urologist may be necessary. With a residual volume greater than 500 mL, the catheter may be left in place to allow the bladder to regain muscle tone. If residual volume is minimal, further diagnostic evaluation is aimed at identifying the cause.

SPECIFIC CONDITIONS
Acute Renal Failure

Until recently, a systemic definition of ARF was lacking. In 2004 the Acute Dialysis Quality Initiative (ADQI) group published the RIFLE criteria for classification of ARF (Table 35-1). Because baseline values may not be available, the Crockcroft-Gault equation is used most often in the ED: GFR mL/min equals (140 − age in yrs)(weight in kg)(0.85 if female) divided by (72 × serum creatinine mol/L). Azotemia, or uremia, refers to accumulation of nitrogen waste products in the blood. Acute azotemia generally refers to the patient with ARF, which usually develops over a period of days; however, chronic renal failure (CRF) patients can experience acute episodes because of noncompliance or other medical conditions.

ARF has prerenal, intrarenal, or postrenal causes. Prerenal causes include syndromes that decrease blood flow to the kidney and therefore alter its ability to function. Those include hypovolemia, decreased cardiac output, decreased peripheral vascular resistance or obstruction of the renal vascular system. Intrarenal causes are those that cause

Table 35-1.	**RIFLE CRITERIA FOR ACUTE RENAL FAILURE CLASSIFICATION**
Risk (R)	Increase serum creatinine level × 1.5 or decrease in GFR by 25%, or UO <0.5 mL/kg/hr for 6 hours
Injury (I)	Increase serum creatinine level × 2 or decrease in GFR by 50%, or UO <0.5 mL/kg/hr for 12 hours
Failure (F)	Increase serum creatinine level × 3 or decrease in GFR by 75%, or serum creatinine level ≥4 mg/dL; UO <0.3 mL/kg/hr for 24 hours, or anuria for 12 hours
Loss (L)	Persistent ARF, complete loss of kidney function >4 weeks
End-stage kidney disease (E)	Loss of kidney function >3 months

ARF, Acute renal failure; *GFR,* glomerular filtration rate; *UO,* urine output.
Modified from Kellum JA, Ronco C, Mehta, R, Bellomo, R: Consensus development in acute renal failure: The Acute Dialysis Initiative, *Curr Opin Crit Care* 11:530, 2005.

damage to the kidney tubules (acute tubular necrosis) and include nephrotoxic agents (aminoglycosides, nonsteroidal antiinflammatory agents, contrast dye, crush injury, and rhabdomyolysis) or diseases that damage the vascular or interstitial tissue (hypertension, diabetes, lupus, and infectious processes). Postrenal causes are those diseases resulting in obstruction of the urinary tract such as calculi, prostatic hypertrophy, tumors, strictures, or neurologic causes affecting emptying of the urinary system. ARF is largely preventable.

Symptoms of ARF include short-term weight gain or loss, nausea and vomiting, hematemesis, melena, dysrhythmias, dyspnea, stupor, or coma. Compromise of airway, breathing, circulation, and neurologic function requires intervention. Fever may be associated with infectious or inflammatory events. Fever reduction measures should be instituted to prevent continued rise of nitrogenous waste products by catabolic effect of fever.

Hyperkalemia, hyponatremia, hypocalcemia, hyperphosphatemia, and volume overload are the most common fluid and electrolyte imbalances resulting from loss of the kidney's ability to excrete potassium and phosphorus, conserve sodium, and eliminate excess volume. Calcium is inversely related to phosphorus. In renal failure, calcium levels decrease because of the rise in phosphorus and the inability of the kidney to convert vitamin D to its active form, which facilitates calcium absorption from the gut. The electrocardiogram (ECG) may reveal tall peaked T waves, widened QRS, and prolonged PR interval secondary to hyperkalemia. Administration of intravenous (IV) calcium may be needed to antagonize the membrane and improve cardiac conductivity until removal of excess potassium by emergency dialysis can be initiated. IV calcium works within minutes, but duration is short, as evidenced by return of ECG changes. Administration of IV sodium bicarbonate ($NaHCO_3$), glucose, and insulin redistributes extracellular potassium into the intracellular fluid, works within 15 to 30 minutes, and lasts approximately 4 hours. Potassium can also be removed by cation exchange resin (e.g., sodium polystyrene sulfonate [Kayexalate]), but onset of action is 60 minutes when given rectally and 120 minutes after oral administration. Nebulized albuterol may also be administered to manage hyperkalemia.

Urine output may be increased or decreased. If ARF is nonoliguric, large volumes of fluid can be lost, so the patient may be dehydrated and hypotensive. Volume replacement with normal saline or volume expanders is guided by monitoring jugular vein distention, lung auscultation, and vital signs or by invasive lines such as central venous pressure and pulmonary artery catheters to monitor fluid status, avoiding further ischemic injury to renal tissue. If ARF presents with oliguria, the patient may be volume overloaded and hypertensive, so minimal fluid is given until the volume can be removed by diuretics or through hemodialysis. Metabolic acidosis occurs because renal tubules can no longer regulate concentration of hydrogen ions. IV $NaHCO_3$ may be used unless contraindicated by volume status.

Indications for emergency dialysis include stupor or coma (caused by rising nitrogen waste products in the blood and metabolic changes), volume overload and pulmonary edema, dangerous hyperkalemia, and acidosis. Emergency hemodialysis requires vascular access (usually a temporary femoral or subclavian dual-lumen catheter or internal shunt) and an artificial kidney (dialyzer) to act as a semipermeable membrane. The dialysate must be low in ions that the body needs to excrete and high in those to be reabsorbed. Hemodynamically unstable patients may require continuous renal replacement therapy, also called continuous extracorporeal renal therapy.

After initial stabilization, history and diagnostic testing focus on identifying the cause of ARF. Tests include serial blood chemistry values, UA with sodium and potassium concentrations, chest radiograph, renal ultrasonography and Doppler studies, or computed tomography (CT) scan. Imaging procedures are usually done without contrast media because of toxic effects of the media on renal tubules. When contrast is needed, acetylcysteine (Mucomyst) may be administered before and after the contrast study in patients with altered renal function to minimize toxic renal effects.

Dialysis Access Complications

Chronic renal failure requiring dialysis is known as end-stage renal disease. Renal replacement therapy may be provided by peritoneal dialysis or hemodialysis. Peritoneal dialysis involves instilling 1 to 2 L of dialysate fluid containing varying amounts of glucose, magnesium, calcium, chloride, and lactate into the abdomen. The peritoneal membrane acts as a semipermeable pathway for exchange of solutes and water between the vascular peritoneal space and dialysate by osmosis and diffusion. Access to the peritoneal cavity is achieved through a plastic catheter held in place by a Dacron cuff. Peritonitis and exit site infections may bring the patient to the ED with complaints of abdominal pain, nausea and vomiting, fever, and cloudy dialysate fluid. Antibiotics may be given IV and added to dialysate. If this is unsuccessful, the catheter should be removed and hemodialysis initiated until peritonitis clears. Unless scarring impairs permeability of the peritoneal membrane, the catheter can be surgically replaced and peritoneal dialysis reinitiated. Care in the ED may include obtaining a sample of peritoneal fluid after installation of dialysate. During access of the peritoneal catheter, careful adherence to aseptic technique, limiting and masking persons present in the room, and use of sterile gloves to prevent contamination during access of the peritoneal catheter are extremely important to prevent infection and resultant peritonitis.

Clotted vascular access frequently brings patients with CRF to the ED. Arteriovenous fistulas are surgical connections of a native artery and vein in an extremity or insertion of Gore-Tex graft material to form the connection (Figure 35-1). Available sites suitable for vascular access become exhausted, so permanent subclavian dual-lumen catheters are placed for hemodialysis. Clotted vascular access should be emergently declotted with use of locally instilled or infused fibrinolytics or surgery. Grafts, fistulas, and insertion

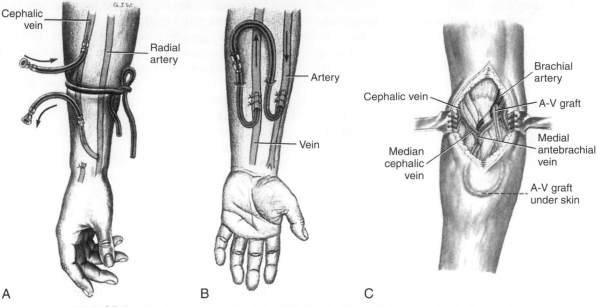

FIGURE 35-1. Circulatory access for hemodialysis. **A,** External (temporary) arteriovenous cannula (shunt). **B,** Internal (permanent) arteriovenous fistula. **C,** Internal (permanent) arteriovenous (A-V) graft. (From Thompson JM, McFarland GK, Hirsch JE et al: *Mosby's clinical nursing,* ed 5, St. Louis, 2002, Mosby.)

sites also become infected and may progress to septicemia. Local symptoms include redness, drainage, or edema. Blood cultures and a complete blood count (CBC) should be obtained to rule out systemic infection. Access removal may be necessary, so temporary subclavian or femoral access (replaced every 2 or 3 days) can be used until blood is free of infection. Some type of anticoagulant will reside in the lumens of a dual-lumen dialysis catheter to prevent clotting. When accessing the catheter, failure to withdraw this anticoagulant could cause serious bleeding complications due to alteration of coagulation status.

Rhabdomyolysis

Skeletal muscle destruction with subsequent release of myoglobin into the circulatory system causes rhabdomyolysis, which can lead to ARF from hypovolemia and tubular necrosis. There are many different causes, including crush injuries, drug or toxin ingestion (including the statin drug class for hypercholesterolemia), infection, burns, or metabolic disturbances. Crush injuries may be caused by entrapment, such as prolonged compression of the abdomen or a limb after a motor vehicle crash. Fluid shifts from the intravascular space into the interstitial space in the area of injury or systemically and can cause the patient to become profoundly hypovolemic, leading to decreased blood flow to the kidneys and resultant decrease in function. Electrolyte imbalances are also associated with the fluid shift. Hyperkalemia is predominant, but hypocalcemia and hyperuricemia are also present. There is an increase in serum creatine kinase (CK), blood urea nitrogen (BUN), creatinine, phosphate (PO_4), uric acid, aspartate aminotransferase (AST), and alanine aminotransferase (ALT). Urine will have a reddish brown color as a result of myoglobinuria (brown urine and clear serum). Proteinuria and hematuria are noted on urinalysis; however, few or no RBCs are seen during microscopic examination.

Presenting signs and symptoms include complaints of muscle aches or acute muscle pain. General malaise, fever, and muscle tenderness may occur. Other symptoms will be present based on the cause of rhabdomyolysis.

Treatment of rhabdomyolysis consists of volume replacement, monitoring, and maintenance of electrolyte balance. Increasing the urine output helps flush myoglobin through the kidneys. Correcting volume depletion and use of an osmotic diuretic such as mannitol will increase the urine output and help flush myoglobin through the kidneys. Treatment also includes preventing myoglobin precipitation in the urine; therefore sodium bicarbonate is added to IV fluids to raise the pH of the urine and help increase excretion of myoglobin. If the patient progresses to ARF, hemodialysis may be considered.

Urinary Tract Infections

Most UTIs result from contamination with *Escherichia coli* and are more common in women.[5] Any abnormality in the urinary tract that obstructs flow of urine, such as urinary calculi, enlarged prostrate gland, or congenital abnormalities in children, also increases the risk for infection. *Chlamydia trachomatis* or *Neisseria gonorrhoeae* should be considered with infections limited to the urethra and reproductive system with pyuria that has a negative culture on standard media. Common symptoms of UTI include signs of bladder irritability such as frequency, dysuria, and urgency, as well as microscopic hematuria, suprapubic discomfort, and cloudy urine. With renal involvement (pyelonephritis), dull flank pain and costovertebral angle tenderness may also be present along with pyuria, gross hematuria, malodorous urine, chills and fever, leukocytosis, nausea, and vomiting. UTIs in children are not common but should be considered with irritability, decrease in appetite, and fever. Diagnosis is made by history, presenting signs, UA, urine culture and sensitivity (C&S), and CBC with differential. A kidneys-ureters-bladder (KUB) radiograph or ultrasound evaluation may show a hazy outline of the kidney secondary to edema. BUN, creatinine, and electrolyte values are obtained to rule out alteration in renal function. Persistent microscopic or gross hematuria, symptoms of obstruction, or persistent positive cultures or symptoms require workup with renal ultrasonography, cystogram, or intravenous pyelogram (IVP). Table 35-2 compares common GU infections that are seen in the ED.

Interstitial Cystitis

The signs and symptoms of interstitial cystitis vary from person to person and may vary over time but include a persistent urgent need to void; minimal urine volumes with urination; suprapubic, perineal, or pelvic pain; and pain during intercourse. Women are affected more than men or children, and they may have other chronic pain syndrome diagnoses such as irritable bowel syndrome or fibromyalgia.[2,8] Interstitial cystitis is difficult to diagnose because other disorders, including UTIs, kidney stones, cancer, and STIs, are usually excluded before a diagnosis is made. Diagnosis occurs most often in women in their 30s or 40s. Tests for UTIs will be negative, and cystoscopy may be required, as well as a potassium sensitivity test, before diagnosis is made. Although the cause is unknown, it is thought that there may be a defect in the epithelial lining of the bladder that allows leakage and irritation of toxic substances into the bladder. Current treatment revolves around combinations of antiinflammatory agents and antidepressants to relax the bladder and ease pain; starting the patient on pentosan polysulfate sodium (Elmiron), a mild anticoagulant whose action is unknown but may restore bladder lining; nerve stimulation; bladder distention techniques; instillation of medications into the bladder; and dietary changes. Treatment in the ED focuses on acute pain management and appropriate specialty referral.

Urinary Calculi

A primary risk factor for calculi is hypercalciuria; however, there is also an association with UTI, gout, excessive ingestion of certain foods, family history, dehydration, pregnancy, immobility, and warmer climates, which tend to produce more concentrated urine. Seventy-five percent of stones are composed of calcium combined with oxalate or phosphate; the remaining 25% are composed of struvite (associated with infection) or uric acid (associated with gout) and rarely cystine.[10] Calculi are asymptomatic until movement causes intermittent painful backache with radiation to the lower abdomen or groin, urge to void, dysuria, renal colic, and hematuria. Bacteremia and proteinuria may also be present. Diagnostic studies include CBC, BUN, creatinine, electrolytes, uric acid, UA with C&S, and helical CT scans. Helical CT has a 94% to 100% positive predictive value for urinary calculi and is currently the gold standard testing for diagnosis.[3] KUB, IVP, and ultrasound can also be used. Figure 35-2 shows staghorn calculus on a KUB radiograph. Ninety percent of stones exit spontaneously; however, if unpassed, they may be removed by extracorporeal shock wave lithotripsy, percutaneous nephrolithotomy, or uteroscopy.

Nursing interventions include intake and output measurement, straining all urine, sending solid material for laboratory analysis, and increased fluids. Pain assessment and management are critical in these patients because of the severity of their pain. Narcotics such as morphine and hydromorphone hydrochloride (Dilaudid) may be used alone; however, combination with nonnarcotics such as ketorolac (Toradol) increases the effectiveness for most patients. Complications include ischemia at obstructive site, altered elimination, and UTI. Criteria for admission include need for frequent pain medicine, large-diameter stones, solitary kidney, ileus, bladder stones, and infection. If the patient is discharged, information should be provided about returning to the ED in case of increasing pain, vomiting, or fever and chills. Dietary restrictions should also be included for foods and drinks that contain high levels of calcium oxalate such as beets, chocolate, coffee, cola, nuts, rhubarb, spinach, strawberries, tea, and wheat bran. Patients should be encouraged to drink large amounts of liquid, especially water, in order to facilitate passage of the remaining stones.

Testicular Torsion

Testicular torsion, the sudden twisting of the spermatic cord (usually internally), causes vascular compromise of the testes within 4 to 6 hours and can lead to infarction with resultant atrophy and loss of spermiogenesis. Time for testis salvage decreases with number of turns: about 6 hours with one turn, 2 hours with three turns.[4] Most cases occur in adolescent males; 50% occur during sleep and are associated with a congenital abnormality of the tunica vaginalis, the canal from which the testes descend; and they can be associated with trauma or sudden rapid movement. Clinical manifestations include upwardly retracted testes with redness and edema at the site of the torsion, abdominal pain, and nausea and vomiting. Figure 35-3 compares normal testicular structures with testicular torsion. Manual detorsion under local anesthesia or surgery must be performed emergently to promote salvage of the involved testes. Prehn's sign may be helpful in differentiating testicular torsion from epididymitis. To assess for Prehn's sign, the scrotum is gently elevated to the level of the symphysis. In testicular torsion, pain increases; however, in epididymitis, a decrease in pain is noted. Prehn's sign is not always reliable, and definitive diagnosis is made with color Doppler ultrasonography showing decrease or

Table 35-2. COMMON GENITOURINARY INFECTIONS

Type	Description	Additional Signs and Symptoms	Interventions	Complications and Comments
Pyelonephritis	Involves renal parenchyma and pelvis Usually unilateral Kidneys enlarged by edema More prevalent in women and persons with diabetes Most commonly caused by ascending *Escherichia coli* infection from lower GU tract, to a lesser extent group D streptococci		Antibiotics specific to C&S Antipyretics and antiemetics Adequate hydration Monitor intake and output Treat fever Bed rest	Complications uncommon but may include septicemia, abscess Follow-up urine C&S to ensure effective antibiotic therapy Recurrence may require continuous antibiotic prophylactic suppression Risk factors for acute pyelonephritis in healthy women age 18-49 years: • Sexual intercourse 3 or more times per week in previous 30 days • Recent UTI • Diabetes • Recent incontinence • New sexual partner in previous year • Recent spermicide use • Maternal family history of UTI
Urethritis	More common in women; *E. coli* most common organism, to a lesser extent group D streptococci Associated behavioral factors include sexual intercourse, diaphragm and/or spermicide use, not voiding within 10-15 minutes after intercourse		Short-term antibiotics May need continuous antibiotic, prophylactic suppression, or postcoital antibiotic	Associated behaviors: • UTIs • Direction of wiping after defecation • Tampon use • Bubble bath • Douche • Tight clothing • Carbonated beverages, coffee, alcohol • Resisting urge to void • Decreasing PO fluids • Synthetic underwear
Epididymitis	Retrograde passage of infected urine from the prostatic urethra to the epididymis via ejaculatory ducts and vas deferens Obstruction of prostate or urethra Congenital abnormalities causing obstruction may result in sterile epididymitis Usually *Neisseria gonorrhoeae* or *Chlamydia trachomatis* in sexually active heterosexual men <35 years of age, Enterobacteriaceae in those >35 years of age (older men with voiding dysfunction) Usually preceded by STI or urethritis in young men Reflux induced by Valsalva or strenuous exertion with full bladder	Gradual onset of scrotal pain and swelling Dysuria, frequency, urgency Fever, chills in 25% acute epididymitis May have urethral discharge preceding Scrotum red, swollen, and warm Bilateral in only 5%-10% of cases Prehn's sign: decrease in pain with elevation of scrotum	Antibiotics and antiinflammatory agents Posttreatment culture Bed rest Scrotal support Avoid heavy lifting and straining	Teach safe sex and condom use, complete antibiotic regimen 3%-11% of patients on amiodarone will have epididymitis limited to the head of the epididymis

Table 35-2.	COMMON GENITOURINARY INFECTIONS—CONT'D			
Type	Description	Additional Signs and Symptoms	Interventions	Complications and Comments
Prostatitis	Usually gram-negative enteric bacteria—*E. coli* (most common), *Klebsiella, Enterobacter, Serratia, Proteus, Pseudomonas, Enterococcus* Occasionally other bacteria— *Staphylococcus aureus, Streptococcus faecalis, Bacteroides* species *Chlamydia* and *Ureaplasma* are bacteria but may be considered "nonbacterial" causes because of lack of growth on standard bacterial cultures Radiation (e.g., therapy for malignant pelvic disease) Expressed prostate secretions have more WBCs than urine (prostate massage contraindicated)	May have bladder outlet obstruction and retention Constant or intermittent: low back pain; perineal, suprapubic, or rectal pain; ejaculatory pain Tender, boggy, hot prostate on manual examination	Antibiotics, urine C&S and expressed prostate fluid C&S	Associated with other UTIs Most cured with antibiotic therapy, only 20% have recurrence or chronic prostatitis

Data from National Institutes of Health: *Kidney stones in adults,* updated December 2004. Retrieved August 26, 2007, from http://kidney.niddk.nih.gov/kudiseases/pubs/stone-sadult/index.htm; and Dynamed: *Nephrolithiasis,* updated July 1, 2007. Retrieved August 26, 2007, http://dynamed101.ebscohost.com/Detail.aspx?style=1&docid=/dynamed/627411efceefa03b852562d3007fc1f6.

C&S, Culture and sensitivity; *GU,* genitourinary; *PO,* oral; *STI,* sexually transmitted infection; *UTIs,* urinary tract infections; *WBCs,* white blood cells.

absence of vascular flow. Management of the patient in the ED includes pain management, facilitation of diagnostic and surgical interventions, education about the plan of care, and reassurance.

Epididymitis

Epididymitis results from inflammation of the epididymis predominately secondary to an STI. It is most common in sexually active males younger than 35 years. The causative organism is most often *C. trachomatis* or *N. gonorrhae*.[6] Extreme physical strain or exertion can also cause epididymitis. Signs and symptoms of epididymitis include severe scrotal pain, which can radiate into the abdomen, tenderness along the spermatic cord, edema, fever, pyuria, and possibly, urethral discharge. A positive Prehn's sign may also be observed. On laboratory assessment of the CBC, an elevated WBC count will be present, and UA will reveal bacteria.

Treatment of epididymitis includes administration of antibiotics, antipyretics, and analgesics. Bed rest is indicated for approximately 3 to 4 days. A scrotal support should be worn to assist in pain relief. Sexual activity and physical strain should be avoided.

Priapism

Priapism is a persistent, painful erection not associated with sexual desire. Engorgement is limited to the two corpora cavernosa; the corpus spongiosum and glans are not involved.

Obstruction of venous drainage causes buildup of viscous deoxygenated blood, interstitial edema, and eventual fibrosis. Pain severity increases with duration. With urinary obstruction and bladder distention, pain can last as long as 24 hours. Causes include sickle cell crisis, spinal cord injury, cerebrovascular accident, multiple sclerosis, psychotropic or erectile dysfunction medications, or prolonged sexual activity.

Local anesthesia through a dorsal nerve block using 1% lidocaine without epinephrine may be helpful. Pharmacologic management of priapism may include parenteral vasodilators such as terbutaline or papaverine.[9] Acute detumescence is accomplished surgically with a large-bore needle after a regional nerve block by removing aspirate and injecting an adrenergic agent such as 5% phenylephrine. Surgical stenting may be necessary by tissue removal to relieve obstruction or by anastomosis of veins between glans and cavernosa. CBC with increased reticulocyte count may identify sickling cells as the underlying cause, so supplemental oxygen along with transfusion may be effective. Fifty percent of cases require a urinary catheter for bladder obstruction and distention. Development of fibrosis and scarring in cavernous spaces related to the duration of priapism and decompression can cause impotence.

Sexually Transmitted Infections

STIs spread through intimate sexual contact can present with a variety of symptoms. History should include location, color, smell, character, and quantity of discharge. Pruritus

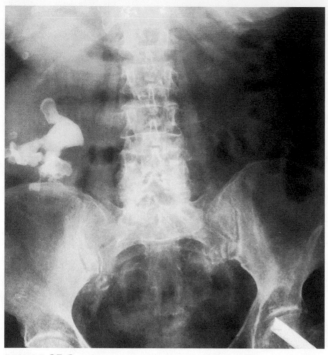

FIGURE 35-2. Radiograph of a staghorn calculus. (Courtesy Harborview Medical Center, University of Washington, Seattle.)

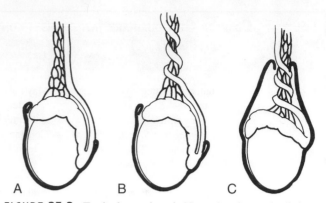

FIGURE 35-3. Testicular torsion. **A,** Normal tunica vaginalis insertion. **B,** Extravaginal torsion. **C,** Intravaginal torsion with abnormally high vaginal insertion. (From Price SA, Wilson LM: *Pathophysiology: clinical concepts of disease processes,* ed 6, St. Louis, 2003, Mosby.)

and burning at the urethra, vagina, perineum, or pharynx can be mild to severe, and with associated lesions. Sexual activity, medical history, and date of the last menstrual period should be obtained. A pelvic examination may be performed with warm water employed as the only lubricant. A rectal examination and sigmoidoscopy may also be indicated. Diagnostic studies include C&S of lesions or drainage, serum Venereal Disease Research Laboratory (VDRL) test, wet mount (saline and KOH), UA with C&S, and cytology smear. Along with antibiotics, discharge teaching should include abstinence until treatment is completed and lesions are healed, need for partner treatment, use of condoms (avoid "natural" or "lambskin" because they are not effective protection against STIs)[1], 7- to 10-day follow-up, and consideration of human immunodeficiency virus testing. Complications of untreated STIs include endocarditis, arthralgias, meningitis, salpingitis, chronic pelvic inflammatory disease, severe proctitis, and sterility. Table 35-3 compares common STIs, excluding acquired immunodeficiency syndrome.

PREVENTION

Disturbances involving the GU system range from life and tissue threats to communicable infections. One common denominator many of these emergencies share is that they are preventable. Safe-sex practices decrease the incidence of STIs; dietary modifications may reduce the number of recurrent urinary calculi and UTIs; and changes in hygienic practices may also be helpful. Individuals who control their diabetes, hypertension, and heart failure reduce their risk for developing ESRD. ED nurses play a pivotal role in initiating strategies that protect patients from ARF: maintaining adequate intravascular volume, supporting/normalizing blood pressure, and minimizing exposure to nephrotoxic agents. Evidence exists that the prophylactic use of acetylcysteine (Mucomyst) before radiocontrast-media procedures decreases the incidence of ARF as does infusion of sodium bicarbonate.[11]

SUMMARY

GU emergencies require evaluation of renal function to rule out renal involvement. The GU system functions to maintain homeostasis, so disruption of renal function interrupts almost all organ systems. Emerging strains of resistant bacteria are challenging health care professions in treatment and prevention. Public education regarding safe sexual practice should be included in all discharge teaching for STIs. The emergency nurse has many opportunities to play an important role in the detection and prevention of GU diseases.

Table 35-3. COMMON SEXUALLY TRANSMITTED INFECTIONS

Diseases	Epidemiology	Clinical Presentation	Diagnosis	Treatment
DISEASES CHARACTERIZED BY GENITAL ULCERS OR LESIONS				
Chancroid	Caused by *Haemophilus ducreyi* 3-14 days' incubation 10% coinfected with *Treponema pallidum* (syphilis) or HSV	Acute painful ulcers that are nonindurated with nonspecific edges Inguinal tender lymphadenopathy Dysuria	Culture of lesion (<80% sensitivity) Absence of *T. pallidum* and HSV in exudate culture	Azithromycin 1 g PO for one dose **OR** Ceftriaxone 250 mg IM for one dose **OR** Ciprofloxacin 500 mg PO 2 times a day for 3 days **OR** Erythromycin base 500 mg PO 3 times a day for 7 days
Herpes simplex	Most common cause of nongonococcal proctitis in sexually active homosexual men Incubation 1-12 days for first episode Recurrence in 60% of cases, usually less severe HSV1 can occur genitally but HSV2 is more common; both can occur orally	Pain, itching, dysuria, vaginal or urethral purulent discharge Classic small painful vesicles on erythematous base that may ulcer Crusting of vesicles indicates healing Lymph enlargement occurs with primary infection 33% develop meningitis	Virologic or serologic culture of lesions or spinal fluid if neurologic involvement suspected	*First clinical episode* Acyclovir 400 mg PO 3 times a day or 200 mg 5 times a day for 7-10 days **OR** Famciclovir 250 mg PO 3 times a day for 7-10 days **OR** Valacyclovir 1 g PO 2 times a day for 7-10 days *Suppressive therapy (>6 recurrences per year)* Acyclovir 400 mg PO 2 times a day **OR** Famciclovir 250 mg PO 2 times a day **OR** Valacyclovir PO 500 mg to 1 g once a day *Episodic therapy for recurrence* Acyclovir PO 400 mg 3 times a day or 800 mg 2 times a day to 3 times a day for 5 days **OR** Famciclovir PO 125 mg 2 times a day for 5 days or 1 g 2 times a day for 1 day
Syphilis	Spirochete infection with *T. pallidum* Transmitted via sexual contact with moist skin lesions 3-6 weeks' incubation for the primary stage (chancre) 6-8 weeks later secondary stage with disseminated bacteremia Tertiary stage (if untreated) with endocarditis and granuloma formation	Papule that progresses to indurated ulcer that is painless and associated with lymphadenopathy	VDRL serology Lesion culture Some availability of urine or vaginal/penile swab quick tests	*Adult regimen* Benzathine PCN G 2.4 million units IM in a single dose Latent phase: 2.4 million units IM once weekly × 3 weeks (7.2 million units total) *Pediatric regimen* Benzathine PCN G 50,000 units/kg IM (maximum 2.4 million units) Latent phase: 50,000 units/kg once weekly × 3 weeks (maximum 2.4 million units per dose) NOTE: CDC recommends desensitizing to PCN or doxycycline 100 mg PO 2 times a day or tetracycline 500 mg PO 4 times a day for 28 days

(Continued)

Table 35-3.   COMMON SEXUALLY TRANSMITTED INFECTIONS—CONT'D

Diseases	Epidemiology	Clinical Presentation	Diagnosis	Treatment
Human papilloma virus (HPV) infection and genital warts	More than 100 types of HPV exist, more than 30 can infect the genital area Infection is common and generally self-limiting Types 6 and 11 are associated with genital warts Types 16, 18, 31, 33, and 35 are associated with cervical neoplasia	No discharge Pink-gray soft lesions, singular or grouped Lesions are tall and may bleed	Diagnosis of genital warts is made by visual inspection, confirmed by biopsy (uncommon) Management of neoplasia is per histopathologic findings in follow-up	*External wart treatment* Patient applied treatment: Podofilox 0.5% solution 2 times a day × 3 days (may repeat after a 4-day no-therapy cycle) **OR** Imiquimod 5% cream once daily at bedtime 3 times a week for 16 weeks (removed with soap and water after 6-10 hours) Provider administered treatment: Podophyllum resin 10%-25% in tincture of benzoin, repeatedly weekly as needed **OR** Trichloroacetic or bichloroacetic acid (TCA/BCA) in 10%-90% solution, repeatedly weekly as needed **OR** Surgical removal, intralesional interferon or laser removal NOTE: Internal warts, provider administered: Cryotherapy, TCA or BCA, podophyllin, or surgical removal

DISEASES CHARACTERIZED BY URETHRITIS, CERVICITIS, OR VAGINAL DISCHARGE

Diseases	Epidemiology	Clinical Presentation	Diagnosis	Treatment
Gonorrhea	Gram-negative diplococcus bacteria *Neisseria gonorrhoeae* Asymptomatic carriage in pharynx, urethra, rectum, and cervix common 3- to 5-day incubation Up to 50% of patients may be coinfected with *Chlamydia*	Urethritis in men with dysuria and mucoid drainage Endocervicitis usual form of infection in women with dysuria, frequency, abnormal discharge Anorectal infection from pruritus to proctitis Pharyngitis may occur Yellow mucopurulent drainage May be asymptomatic	Culture swab transported directly to laboratory (will plate on modified Thayer-Martin agar, which suppresses growth of other gram-negative bacteria to allow for identification of *N. gonorrhoeae*) Strains resistant to quinolones increasing in incidence Some availability of urine or vaginal/penile swab quick tests	Ceftriaxone drug of choice 125 mg IM in a single dose **OR** Cefixime 400 mg PO single dose **OR** Ciprofloxacin 500 mg PO in single dose **OR** Ofloxacin 400 mg PO in single dose **OR** Levofloxacin 250 mg PO in single dose **PLUS** Treatment for chlamydia if not ruled out
Chlamydia	Intracellular parasitic infection with *Chlamydia trachomatis* 5-10+ days' incubation period Up to 50% of patients may be coinfected with gonorrhea	Pelvic inflammatory disease in women Epididymitis in men Urethritis with mucopurulent drainage May be asymptomatic	Swab of discharge by various laboratory methods Some availability of urine or vaginal/penile swab quick tests	*Recommended regimen:* Azithromycin 1 g PO × one dose **OR** Doxycycline 100 mg 2 times a day for 7 days *Alternative regimen:* Erythromycin base 500 mg PO 4 times a day for 7 days **OR** Erythromycin ethylsuccinate 800 mg PO 4 times a day for 7 days **OR** Ofloxacin 300 mg PO 2 times a day for 7 days **OR** Levofloxacin 500 mg PO once daily for 7 days

Table 35-3. COMMON SEXUALLY TRANSMITTED INFECTIONS—CONT'D				
Diseases	**Epidemiology**	**Clinical Presentation**	**Diagnosis**	**Treatment**
Trichomoniasis vaginalis	Caused by protozoan *T. vaginalis* Incubation period of 1 week	Copious, thin, frothy, yellow, greenish, gray, foul-smelling discharge Severe pruritus Edema and redness of vagina Worse following menstrual bleeding	Culture and sensitivity Wet prep slide	Metronidazole 2 g PO in a single dose **OR** Tinidazole 2 g PO in a single dose **OR** Alternative treatment: Metronidazole 250 mg PO 3 times a day or 375 mg 2 times a day for 7 days
Bacterial vaginosis	Caused by *Gardnerella vaginalis* or *Mycoplasma hominis* Incubation period 5-10 days Most common cause of vaginal discharge or malodor Associated with multiple sex partners or douching, unclear if bacterial vaginosis results from sexually transmitted pathogen	Fishy odor Thin, white discharge in lesser amounts than with *T. vaginalis* Mild itching	Culture and sensitivity Fishy odor with 10% KOH (whiff test)	Metronidazole 500 mg PO 2 times a day for 7 days **OR** Metronidazole gel 0.75% intravaginally once daily for 5 days **OR** Clindamycin cream 2% intravaginally at bedtime for 7 days

Data from Centers for Disease Control and Prevention: Sexually transmitted diseases treatment guidelines, 2006, *MMWR Morb Mortal Wkly Rep* 55(RR-11), 2006, http://www.cdc.gov/std/treatment/2006/rr5511.pdf.

CDC, Centers for Disease Control and Prevention; *HSV*, herpes simplex virus; *IM*, intramuscularly; *PCN*, penicillin; *PO*, orally; *VDRL*, Venereal Disease Research Laboratory.

REFERENCES

1. Centers for Disease Control and Prevention: Sexually transmitted diseases treatment guidelines, *MMWR Morb Mortal Wkly Rep* 55(RR-11), 2006, http://www.cdc.gov/std/treatment/2006/rr5511.pdf

2. Dynamed: *Interstitial cystitis*, updated July 5, 2007. Retrieved August 26, 2007, from http://dynamed101.ebscohost.com/Detail.aspx?id=116429.

3. Dynamed: *Nephrolithiasis*, updated July 1, 2007. Retrieved August 26, 2007, from http://dynamed101.ebscohost.com/Detail.aspx?style=1&docid=/dynamed/627411efceefa03b852562d3007fc1f6.

4. Dynamed: *Testicular torsion*, updated June 25, 2007. Retrieved August 26, 2007, from http://dynamed101.ebscohost.com/Detail.aspx?id=114645.

5. Dynamed: *Urinary tract infection (UTI) in adults*, updated August 21, 2007. Retrieved August 26, 2007, from http://dynamed101.ebscohost.com/Detail.aspx?id=116894.

6. Konety B, Franks M: *Epididymitis*, February 2, 2006. Retrieved August 26, 2007, from http://www.emedicine.com/Med/topic704.htm.

7. Krause R: *Renal failure, chronic and dialysis complications*, June 14, 2006. Retrieved August 26, 2007, from http://www.emedicine.com/emerg/topic501.htm.

8. Mayo Clinic: *Interstitial cystitis*, updated January 2007. Retrieved August 26, 2007, from http://www.mayoclinic.com/health/interstitial-cystitis/DS00497.

9. McCollough M, Ghazala S: Renal and genitourinary tract disorders, In Marx JA, Hockberger RS, Walls RM, editors: *Rosen's emergency medicine: concepts and clinical practice*, ed 5, St. Louis, 2002, Mosby.

10. National Institutes of Health: *Kidney stones in adults*, updated December 2004. Retrieved August 26, 2007, from http://kidney.niddk.nih.gov/kudiseases/pubs/stonesadults/index.htm.

11. Needham E: Management of acute renal failure, *Am Fam Physician* 72(9):1739, 2005.

12. Weinstock H, Berman S, Cates W Jr: Sexually transmitted disease among American youth: incidence and prevalence estimates, 2000. *Persp Sex Reprod Health* 36(1):6-10, 2004.

CHAPTER 36

Fluids and Electrolytes

Betty Kuiper

W ater is the most abundant fluid medium in the body, composing 60% of total body weight for the average adult, 80% in a full-term infant, and as little as 45% to 55% in an older adult.[6] In a healthy physiologic state this fluid medium has a constant balance of electrolytes controlled by a unique system of checks and balances. Effects of fluid and electrolyte disturbances are often a primary or secondary reason for many emergency department (ED) visits. Fluid and electrolyte abnormalities may be caused by gastrointestinal (GI), urologic, cardiac, respiratory, and endocrine diseases and many forms of traumatic injury.

This chapter describes the interrelationship of water, water metabolism, and electrolyte composition. Fluid and electrolyte control mechanisms, signs and symptoms, etiology, and treatment of specific fluid and electrolyte abnormalities are discussed.

PATHOPHYSIOLOGY

Water and electrolytes are interdependent. The pathophysiology of one affects the function and value of the other. Normal fluid and electrolyte levels are the result of structural, physiologic, and environmental factors.

Water

Water has many important metabolic functions, including transport of nutrients and other essential substances, removal of metabolic waste products, normal cellular metabolism, and maintenance of normal body temperature. Age, weight, body fat, gender, and environmental factors such as ambient temperature determine individual fluid requirements. Fat is virtually water free; therefore increases in body fat are associated with decreases in the percentage of body water. The average adult ingests 1500 to 2000 mL of water per day.[2] In addition, the body produces 250 mL of water per day as a result of oxidation of food.[3]

The most common areas of the body for fluid excretion are the bowels, skin, lungs, and kidneys. The kidneys are the primary regulators of fluid and electrolyte balance.[6] Approximately 180 L of plasma are filtered daily by the kidneys of a healthy adult.[6] From this volume, approximately 1500 mL of urine is excreted daily.[6]

Total body water (TBW) is distributed between extracellular and intracellular compartments. Extracellular fluid (ECF) constitutes one third of TBW, or approximately 15 L in the average (70-kg) adult male.[6] Plasma, interstitial fluid, cerebrospinal fluid, intraocular fluid, fluids of the GI tract, and fluids of potential spaces (i.e., pleural space, peritoneal space) are examples of ECF.[6] Intracellular fluid (ICF) accounts for two thirds of TBW and represents the sum of fluid content for all the cells in the body, approximately 27 L in the average (70-kg) adult male.[6]

Two regulatory mechanisms influential in maintaining normal water volume and tonicity or osmotic pressure are thirst and renal function. Thirst is the primary regulator for intake of water. It is triggered by receptors in the anterolateral hypothalamus that respond to increased plasma osmolality (as little as 2%) or decreased body fluid volume.[1] Thirst ensures adequate replacement of fluid losses and is stimulated by ECF hypertonicity and decreased ICF volume.[4] Similarly, thirst is depressed by ECF hypotonicity and increased ICF volume. Because the thirst mechanism is triggered by increased osmolality, thirst is not effective in hypotonic or hyponatremic dehydration, in which water and sodium losses are equal. Hypothalamic dysfunction also decreases the capacity for thirst.[1] Other factors that adversely affect the thirst mechanism include brain injury and psychosocial factors such as depression, confusion, and fear of incontinence.

Renal regulation of water balance is twofold, affecting both tonicity and body water. When glomerular filtrate is hypertonic, osmoreceptors in the hypothalamus are stimulated, and antidiuretic hormone (ADH) is released by the pituitary gland. ADH makes renal collecting tubules more permeable to water, so water is reabsorbed into the body, diluting blood and concentrating urine. If plasma or glomerular filtrate is hypotonic, ADH secretion is inhibited and collecting tubules reabsorb less water. Blood becomes concentrated and the urine is diluted as more water exits the kidneys.

The kidneys, through the renin-angiotensin-aldosterone system, regulate the volume of body water. When ECF volume, specifically blood volume, is low, receptors in the kidneys secrete an enzyme called renin. Renin stimulates angiotensinogen (a normal plasma protein) to release angiotensin I, which is then converted to angiotensin II by another enzyme, primarily in the lungs. Angiotensin II stimulates the adrenal cortex to secrete aldosterone, which increases sodium reabsorption from glomerular filtrate in exchange for potassium and hydrogen ions. This exchange increases plasma tonicity, which leads to ADH secretion, water retention, and increased volume. With excessive ECF volume (blood volume), aldosterone secretion is depressed, so tubular reabsorption of sodium and water decreases.

Electrolytes

An electrolyte is a substance capable of carrying an electrical charge. An electrolyte with a positive charge is called a cation, whereas an electrolyte with a negative charge is an anion.[5] Electrolytes are found in varying concentrations in ECF and ICF (Figure 36-1).

For the purposes of this chapter, serum electrolyte measurements are equivalent to extracellular electrolyte values

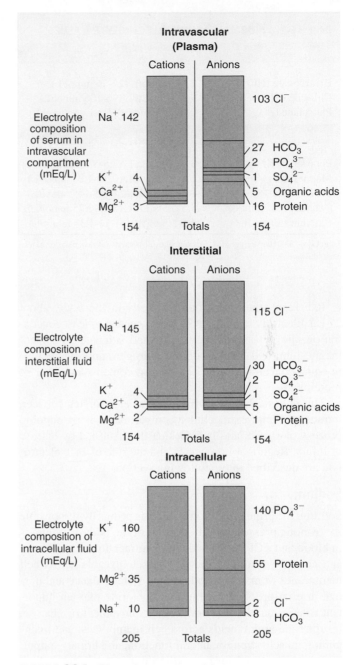

FIGURE 36-1. Electrolyte content of fluid compartments. (From Lewis SL, Heitkemper MM, Dirksen SR et al: *Medical-surgical nursing: assessment and management of clinical problems*, ed 7, St. Louis, 2007, Mosby.)

(Table 36-1). Direct measurement of intracellular electrolyte concentrations in the clinical setting is not yet feasible, so ICF electrolyte concentrations must be inferred from serum electrolyte values.

All fluids outside the cells are collectively referred to as the ECF. Electrolytes in the ECF, from greatest to least concentration, are sodium, chloride, potassium, bicarbonate, and hydrogen. ECF also contains oxygen, carbon dioxide, proteins, and a few miscellaneous anions.

Table 36-1. NORMAL SERUM ELECTROLYTE VALUES	
Anions	**Normal Value**
Bicarbonate (HCO_3^-)	22-26 mEq/L (22-26 mmol/L)
Chloride (Cl^-)	96-106 mEq/L (96-106 mmol/L)
Phosphate (PO_4^{3-})	2.8-4.5 mg/dL (0.90-1.45 mmol/L)
Cations	**Normal Value**
Potassium (K^+)	3.5-5.0 mEq/L (3.5-5.0 mmol/L)
Magnesium (Mg^+)	1.5-2.5 mEq/L (0.75-1.25 mmol/L)
Sodium (Na^+)	135-145 mEq/L (135-145 mmol/L)
Calcium (Ca^+) (total)	4.5-5.5 mEq/L (2.25-2.75 mmol/L)
Calcium (ionized)	4.5-5.5 mg/dL (1.13-1.38 mmol/L)

From Lewis SM, Heitkemper MM, Dirksen SR et al: *Medical-surgical nursing: assessment and management of clinical problems,* ed 7, St. Louis, 2007, Mosby.

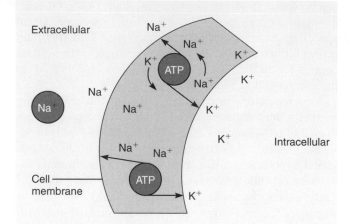

FIGURE **36-2.** Sodium-potassium pump. As sodium diffuses into the cell and potassium out of the cell, an active transport system supplied with energy delivers sodium back to the extracellular compartment and potassium to the intracellular compartment. *ATP,* Adenosine triphosphate. (From Lewis SL, Heitkemper MM, Dirksen SR et al: *Medical-surgical nursing: assessment and management of clinical problems,* ed 7, St. Louis, 2007, Mosby.)

ICF represents fluid found in cells in the body, about 27 L.[2] Electrolytes in the ICF, from greatest to least concentration, are potassium, phosphate, and sulphate combined; magnesium; and lastly sodium, hydrogen, and bicarbonate in equal concentrations. The ICF also contains a number of proteins.

The delicate balance of water and electrolytes between intracellular and extracellular compartments is an ongoing process of checks and balances easily disturbed by disease or injury. Regulatory processes and the role of each electrolyte are described in the following sections.

Sodium

Sodium, the principal cation in ECF, is primarily responsible for osmotic pressure.[6] Forty percent of the body's sodium is in blood and ECF; the remainder is intracellular and in bone and connective tissue. Sodium is exchangeable across cell membranes to maintain sodium and water balance and normal arterial pressure. Sodium and chloride play an important role in maintaining body water; movement of glucose, insulin, and amino acids across cell membranes; and maintaining muscle strength, neural function, and urinary output. Sodium is essential for the sodium-potassium pump, which moves sodium and potassium across the cell membrane during repolarization (Figure 36-2). As sodium diffuses into the cell and potassium out of the cell, an active transport system supplied with energy delivers sodium back to the extracellular compartment and potassium to the intracellular compartment.[8]

Sodium levels are maintained through the renin-angiotensin-aldosterone system, sympathetic nervous system, and a less well-defined system mediated by atrial natriuretic factor.[6] Decreased fluid volume decreases blood flow and arterial pressure, which stimulate baroreceptors in the kidneys (Figure 36-3). Baroreceptors stimulate the sympathetic nervous system, which leads to vasoconstriction of renal arterioles, decreased glomerular filtration rate, and retention of sodium and water. The opposite sequence of events occurs when fluid intake (or blood volume) rises above normal.

Atrial natriuretic hormone (ANH), released from the atria in response to increased arterial pressure, produces natriuresis (excretion of abnormal amounts of sodium in the urine), diuresis, vasodilation, and antagonistic effects on ADH release, renin, and aldosterone.[5] The resulting increase in sodium excretion eliminates excess volume.

Chloride

Chloride, the principal anion of blood and ECF, is secreted in various body fluids along with other electrolytes. Sodium and chloride are excreted in sweat, bile, pancreatic fluids, and intestinal fluids. Gastric juice contains chloride and hydrogen. As with sodium, chloride plays a cooperative role in maintaining acid-base balance and takes part in the exchange of oxygen and carbon dioxide in red blood cells.[3] Serum chloride levels are passively regulated by serum sodium levels. When serum sodium increases, serum chloride also increases. However, chloride levels are inversely related to bicarbonate levels because chloride is sacrificed in the kidneys to produce more bicarbonate.

Potassium

Potassium is the most abundant cation in the body, with 98% in the ICF and 2% in the ECF.[3] Potassium is primarily responsible for cell membrane potential and is the counterpart to sodium in the sodium-potassium pump. Potassium governs cell osmolality and volume and is secreted in sweat, gastric juice, pancreatic juice, bile, and fluids of the small intestine.

Potassium level is primarily controlled through secretion of potassium by the distal and collecting tubules in the kidney. Potassium secretion increases in response to increased ECF potassium concentration, aldosterone levels, and distal tubular flow. A rise in ECF potassium stimulates the sodium-potassium pump located in the renal tubules. This

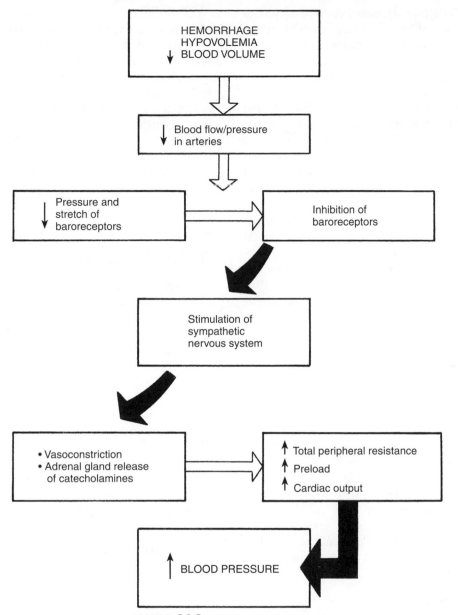

FIGURE **36-3.** Baroreceptor response.

pump maintains a low intracellular sodium concentration through exchange of potassium across the cell membrane. Increased extracellular potassium also triggers aldosterone secretion by the adrenal cortex. Aldosterone increases the rate at which tubular cells secrete potassium and the permeability of the renal tubular lumen for potassium. This is a negative feedback system regulated by the serum potassium level. Finally, increased distal tubular flow causes rapid secretion of potassium into the urine.

Alkalosis temporarily decreases serum potassium by driving potassium into the cells in exchange for hydrogen ions.[3] Conversely, acute acidosis is the major factor that decreases potassium secretion and increases serum potassium. Acute acidosis increases hydrogen ion concentration in the ECF, causing potassium to move out of the cell in exchange for excess hydrogen ions.[3]

Calcium

Approximately 99% of the body's calcium is found in bone, with 1% in ICF and 0.1% in ECF.[3] Bone acts as a large reservoir for calcium when ECF calcium levels fall. Calcium is transported in the blood in two forms. Half is bound to plasma proteins, usually albumin, and a small amount of nonionized calcium forms complexes with anions such as phosphate, citrate, and sulfate. The rest exists as an ionized form that is free and metabolically active. Most ionized calcium is found in the ECF. Because of the large amount of calcium bound to plasma proteins, assessment of total serum calcium without simultaneous measurement of serum proteins has limited value in determining hypocalcemia or hypercalcemia.

Calcium has many important functions—smooth and skeletal muscle contraction, bone and brain metabolism, blood clotting, and as a primary ingredient in lung surfactant.[5] Calcium is essential for membrane polarization and depolarization, action potential generation, neurotransmission, and muscle contraction. Calcium channels in myocardial cells allow transmembrane calcium transport.

The most important regulatory factors for calcium homeostasis are parathyroid hormone (PTH), calcitonin, and vitamin D.[5] When ECF calcium falls below normal levels, parathyroid glands release PTH, which acts directly on bones to stimulate the release of large amounts of calcium into ECF. When calcium ion concentration is elevated, PTH secretion decreases, causing excess calcium to deposit in the bones.

Bones rely on proper intake and absorption of calcium to maintain calcium stores. Calcium absorption in the GI tract and kidneys is regulated by PTH levels. In hypocalcemic states PTH activates vitamin D_3, the form of vitamin D necessary to increase intestinal calcium reabsorption. PTH also directly stimulates the kidneys to increase renal tubular calcium reabsorption, which prevents loss of calcium in the urine.

Another factor that influences calcium reabsorption is plasma concentration of phosphate. Serum calcium levels are inversely related to serum phosphate levels. Increases in plasma phosphate may indirectly stimulate PTH, which increases calcium reabsorption by renal tubules and reduces calcium loss in the urine.[3]

In response to elevated calcium levels, the thyroid gland secretes a hormone called calcitonin. The effect of calcitonin on plasma calcium levels is directly opposite that of PTH. Calcitonin decreases plasma calcium levels by increasing calcium deposits in bone and decreasing formation of new osteoclasts, the cells responsible for breakdown and removal of bone.[3] Calcitonin also has minor effects on calcium absorption in the renal tubules and GI tract.

Phosphate and Phosphorus

Phosphorus, the major anion in the ICF, is essential for metabolism of carbohydrates, lipids, and proteins. Phosphate also plays a role in hormonal activities and acid-base balance and has a close relationship to calcium in maintaining homeostasis. Clinical studies have shown that changing the phosphate level in ECF far below or far above normal levels does not cause immediate effects on the body. However, even minute increases or decreases in calcium ions in ECF cause significant physiologic effects.

Renal tubules maintain a normal phosphate level by an "overflow" mechanism. When the phosphate level in the glomerular filtrate falls below the normal level, essentially all filtered phosphate is reabsorbed. When extra phosphate is present in the glomerular filtrate, excess phosphate is excreted in the urine.

PTH also plays a significant role in phosphate regulation. When PTH is present, bones dump phosphate salts and calcium into the ECF. PTH then stimulates the kidneys to dump more phosphate into the urine.

Magnesium

Magnesium is the second most important intracellular cation.[3] More than half the body's magnesium is stored in bones, with the rest in cells, particularly muscle. Only a small fraction of the body's magnesium is found in the ECF. Magnesium is involved in numerous biochemical processes in the body, so normal concentrations must be carefully maintained. Although the exact mechanism is unclear, magnesium excretion is probably regulated by altering renal tubular reabsorption. With excess magnesium, renal tubules allow excretion of extra magnesium in the urine. In magnesium depletion, renal excretion dramatically decreases.

FLUID AND ELECTROLYTE ABNORMALITIES

Imbalances in fluid and electrolytes may be due to physiologic abnormalities, injury, or stress. Fluid and electrolyte levels are closely related. For example, sodium losses are almost always associated with water losses, just as sodium retention is associated with water excess.

Fluid and electrolyte therapy has three objectives—maintain daily requirements, restore previous losses or excesses, and prevent further losses or excesses. Oral electrolyte replacement is preferred. However, most patients who present to the ED with vomiting, diarrhea, and other fluid losses can no longer treat losses orally. Treatment of electrolyte abnormalities focuses on slowly restoring previous balance and carefully correcting the underlying cause. Electrolyte levels, hydration, and cardiovascular, renal, and neurologic function should be carefully monitored.

Water Abnormalities

Water abnormalities may be due to underlying disease, iatrogenic causes, environmental factors, or psychologic abnormalities. ECF imbalances may be caused by an extracellular volume deficit, which includes an increase in insensible water loss or perspiration (high fever, heatstroke), diabetes insipidus, osmotic diuresis, hemorrhage, GI losses (vomiting, gastric suction, diarrhea, fistula drainage), overuse of diuretics, inadequate fluid intake, and third-space fluid shifts (burns and intestinal obstruction).[8] An extracellular volume excess may be caused by an extreme intake of isotonic or hypotonic intravenous (IV) fluids, heart failure, renal failure, primary polydipsia, syndrome of inappropriate antidiuretic hormone (SIADH), Cushing's syndrome, and the long-term use of corticosteroids.[8] Determining the cause should occur concurrently with fluid replacement.

Water Depletion

Water depletion may be due to reduced water consumption, diarrhea, vomiting, excessive sweating, excessive respiration, renal disease, ADH deficiency (i.e., diabetes insipidus), excessive diuretic use, and diabetic ketoacidosis (DKA). Water deficiency is almost always associated with loss of sodium. True water deficiency without concurrent sodium loss is rarely seen in the ED.

Signs and symptoms of water deficiency include thirst, loss of eyeball and skin turgor, dry mucous membranes, flushed skin, decreased urinary output, increased urine specific gravity, increased temperature, tachycardia, delirium, and coma. Most patients with water deficiency are also deficient in sodium and other electrolytes, so oral or parenteral fluid replacement must be determined on an individual basis. Frequently selected fluids to replenish water and sodium loss include normal saline (0.9%) and hypotonic half-normal saline (0.45%). Serial electrolyte and plasma osmolarity levels are required to determine appropriate fluid replacement.

Water Excess

Water excess is characterized by weight gain, muscle twitching and cramps, pulmonary and peripheral edema, hyperventilation, confusion, hallucination, coma, and convulsions. Water excess may be due to increased water ingestion, excessive IV therapy, renal disease, excess ADH, and inadequate water transport to the kidney (e.g., shock, congestive heart failure).[10]

The goal of treatment for fluid volume excess is removal of fluid without producing abnormal changes in the electrolyte composition.[8] The primary cause of water excess must be identified and treated. Diuretics and fluid restriction are the primary forms of treatment.[8] Other treatments that may be used by the clinician include restriction of sodium intake, abdominal paracentesis for ascites, and thoracentesis for a pleural effusion.

Electrolyte Abnormalities

Electrolyte abnormalities may be caused by an underlying disease or may be the result of starvation, therapeutic drugs, drug overdose, or other iatrogenic causes. Electrolyte abnormalities are almost always associated with some degree of neuromuscular dysfunction (e.g., weakness, paralysis, cramps, restless legs, tetany, areflexia, hyperreflexia, and myotonia).[8] Cardiac abnormalities are another common occurrence with many electrolyte abnormalities. Ventricular dysrhythmias may be seen with hypokalemia and hypercalcemia, and cardiac arrest may be seen with hyperkalemia; torsades de pointes has been seen with hypocalcemia. Dysrhythmias associated with hypomagnesemia include ventricular ectopy, torsades de pointes, and atrial fibrillation. Hypermagnesemia may cause atrioventricular block.

Anion Gap

The balance between positive and negative electrolytes is measured by calculating the anion gap: $Na^+ - (Cl^- - HCO_3^-)$. Some formulas may include potassium with the sodium. This measurement is particularly useful in determining whether metabolic acidosis is due to acid excess or bicarbonate loss. The reference range for the anion gap is 10 to 14 mmol/L.[6] Abnormalities in the anion gap may be due to a change in

unmeasured anions or cations or an error in measurement of sodium, chloride, or bicarbonate.

Causes of high-anion-gap metabolic acidosis are lactic acidosis, ketoacidosis (diabetic, alcoholic, starvation), toxins (ethylene glycol, methanol, salicylates), and renal failure (acute and chronic).[7] A normal anion gap is seen in diarrhea, lower GI fistulas, renal tubular acidosis, ureterosigmoidostomy, early renal insufficiency, and metabolic acidosis caused by diuretics.[6] Albumin administration causes a falsely elevated anion gap.[7] A decreased anion gap may be due to error in electrolyte measurement.

Sodium Abnormalities

Sodium and chloride travel together across most membranes, so sodium abnormalities are usually associated with chloride abnormalities. For the purpose of this discussion, abnormalities are described separately.

HYPONATREMIA. Hyponatremia is probably the most common electrolyte imbalance seen in the clinical arena. Hyponatremia is characterized by vague signs and symptoms, so diagnosis can rarely be made from clinical evaluation. Clinical manifestations are due to decreased osmolarity and cerebral edema and include anorexia, nausea, weakness, confusion, agitation, and disorientation. When serum sodium levels fall below 110 mEq/L, seizures, coma, or death can occur.

Mild hyponatremia does not require treatment. If the primary cause of hyponatremia is fluid imbalance, normal saline is the treatment of choice. In severe symptomatic hyponatremia, hypertonic (3%) saline solution may be cautiously administered with an infusion pump.[2] The patient should be carefully monitored for fluid overload secondary to sodium replacement. Furosemide may be administered concurrently to reduce the likelihood of fluid overload. Any potassium deficits that occur as a result of treatment should be corrected.

HYPERNATREMIA. Hypernatremia is a significant risk for infants, older adults, and the debilitated because of their inability to independently replace fluid losses. Clinical signs and symptoms are similar to those seen with hyponatremia but are secondary to hyperosmolarity and cellular dehydration. The patient will be thirsty and appear dehydrated. Early symptoms include anorexia, nausea, and vomiting. As serum sodium levels rise above 160 mEq/L, neurologic symptoms such as agitation, irritability, lethargy, coma, muscle twitching, and hyperreflexia may occur. Intracranial hemorrhages can result from shrunken brain tissue or engorged vasculature.

Treatment of sodium excess focuses on restoring normal fluid volume and osmolarity. Fluid replacement is the first step when hypovolemia is the cause of sodium excess. If oral fluids cannot be ingested, IV solutions of 5% dextrose in water or hypotonic saline may be given initially.[8] Serum sodium levels must be reduced gradually to prevent too rapid a shift of water back into the cells.[8] Rapid overcorrection of hypernatremia can result in cerebral edema and seizures.

Chloride Abnormalities

Chloride abnormalities rarely occur independently but usually occur in conjunction with sodium or potassium abnormalities.

HYPOCHLOREMIA. Hypochloremia occurs in conjunction with hyponatremia and may also be seen with hyperkalemia caused by excretion of potassium chloride. Symptoms of chloride deficiency are basically the same as hyponatremia with the additional problems of profound muscle weakness, twitching, tetany, slow shallow respirations, and respiratory arrest. Treatment includes chloride and sodium replacement with careful monitoring of serum levels to determine effectiveness.

HYPERCHLOREMIA. Hyperchloremia produces all the signs and symptoms seen with hypernatremia but also causes deep, labored breathing. Causes of hyperchloremia are the same factors that cause hypernatremia, with two exceptions: ammonium chloride ingestion and salicylate intoxication cause hyperchloremia but do not affect serum sodium. Treatment of hyperchloremia is essentially the same as for hypernatremia.

Potassium Abnormalities

Potassium is subject to multiple influences within the body. Alkalosis, aldosterone, insulin, and β_2-agonists drive potassium into the cell, whereas acidosis and hyperosmolarity cause potassium to leave the cell.[6] Potassium abnormalities are almost always associated with electrocardiogram (ECG) changes, which may or may not correlate with severity.

HYPOKALEMIA. Hypokalemia is characterized by muscle weakness, cramps, paralysis, hyporeflexia, paralytic ileus, paresthesia, latent tetany, cardiac dysrhythmias, hyposthenuria (inability to form urine with a high specific gravity), and a serum potassium level of less than 3.5 mEq/L [mmol/L].[6] Muscle weakness is usually more pronounced in the lower extremities and proximal muscle groups. Respiratory muscle weakness may lead to respiratory failure and arrest. Rhabdomyolysis may also occur.[10] ECG changes such as flattened or inverted T waves and U waves do not correlate well with clinical severity. The ECG may demonstrate ST-segment depression, presence of U wave, and bradycardia. Ventricular ectopy is the most common dysrhythmia. Hypokalemia is the result of decreased potassium intake or shifts of potassium from the ECF to the cells. Vomiting, diarrhea, intestinal obstruction, fistulas, GI suctioning, renal insufficiency and renal losses such as the use of diuretics, hyperaldosteronism, and magnesium depletion are associated with hypokalemia. Nephritis, dialysis, DKA, diuretics, Cushing's syndrome, and steroid therapy are also associated with hypokalemia.

Treatment is recommended when potassium level is lower than 3.5 mEq/L. Potassium supplements added to IV solutions should never exceed 60 mEq/L.[8] The preferred level is 40 mEq/L.[8] Administer potassium through a large-bore peripheral site or through a central line at a rate not to exceed 10 to 20 mEq/hr to prevent hyperkalemia and cardiac arrest.[8] An infusion pump is always recommended. Cardiac monitoring and serial evaluation of potassium levels are recommended to prevent inadvertent hyperkalemia secondary to potassium replacement. In less acute situations, oral potassium may be used or potassium may be added to enteral feedings. Serum magnesium levels should be checked because both electrolytes can be depleted with persistent hypokalemia.

HYPERKALEMIA. Hyperkalemia is characterized by prominent cardiac changes and neuromuscular effects such as paresthesia and muscle weakness leading to flaccid paralysis, and a serum potassium level greater than 5.0 mEq/L [mmol/L]. Various ECG changes correlate well with severity in hyperkalemia. Elevated T waves occur when serum potassium reaches 5.0 to 6.6 mEq/L, whereas prolonged PR interval and widened QRS complexes are evident when the level reaches 6.5 to 8.0 mEq/L.[10] Dysrhythmias include sinus bradycardia, sinus arrest, first-degree heart block, nodal rhythm, idioventricular rhythm, and ventricular fibrillation. Asystole may also occur. Hyperkalemia may be due to increased oral or IV intake, acute renal disease, potassium-sparing diuretics, potassium-containing salt substitute, crush injuries, tumor lysis syndrome, renal disease, angiotensin-converting enzyme (ACE) inhibitors, adrenal insufficiency, acidosis, anoxia, and hyponatremia.[10]

IV calcium chloride or calcium gluconate is the most rapid method for neutralizing neuromuscular effects of hyperkalemia. Serum potassium is rapidly reduced by administration of glucose, insulin, and sodium bicarbonate, which drives potassium into the cell in exchange for sodium. However, this intervention provides only temporary reduction in serum potassium. Urinary potassium excretion is promoted with loop or osmotic diuretics. If these efforts fail, renal dialysis may be needed for significant hyperkalemia. Ion exchange resins such as sodium polystyrene sulfonate (Kayexalate, oral or rectal) may be used in nonemergency situations. Continuous cardiac monitoring and serial potassium levels are essential for the patient with hyperkalemia.

Calcium Abnormalities

Calcium abnormalities may be due to diet, medications, injury, or disease. Bones provide a large reservoir of calcium; however, adequate dietary intake is necessary to maintain stores. Calcium abnormalities are often associated with phosphorus and magnesium abnormalities.

HYPOCALCEMIA. Hypocalcemia makes the nervous system more excitable, which can lead to cardiac dysrhythmias, constipation, and lack of appetite. In skeletal muscle, excitability can lead to tetanic muscle contractions. Seizures are occasionally seen as a result of increased excitability of brain tissue. Clinical signs include a positive Trousseau's sign (carpal spasms induced by inflating a blood pressure cuff on the upper arm) and a positive Chvostek's sign (abnormal facial spasms elicited by light taps on the facial nerve).

Other manifestations include muscle twitching and cramping; facial grimacing; numbness and tingling of fingers, toes, nose, lips, and earlobes; hyperactive deep tendon reflexes; and abdominal pain. The ECG may show a prolonged QT interval, and the patient may appear anxious, irritable, and even psychotic. More severe symptoms include laryngospasms, bronchospasms, seizures, and cardiac failure.

Calcium abnormalities occur with hypoparathyroidism, hypovitaminosis D, malabsorption syndrome, malnutrition, chronic nephrotic syndrome, chronic nephritis, Cushing's syndrome, and metastatic carcinoma of the bone. Overdose of calcium channel blockers can also cause hypocalcemia. Multiple blood transfusions, usually more than 10 units, are associated with hypocalcemia because citrate in banked blood binds with calcium, making it inactive.

Before treatment for hypocalcemia is started, hypomagnesemia should be excluded because patients with low serum magnesium levels respond poorly to calcium replacement. Hypocalcemia is easily managed with IV calcium. For adults, one to two ampules of 10% calcium gluconate (each containing 93 mg of elemental calcium) mixed in 5% dextrose in water (D_5W) is administered over 10 to 20 minutes.[9] In severe deficits a continuous infusion may be necessary after the initial bolus. Calcium levels, cardiac rhythm, and blood pressure should be carefully monitored during calcium administration.

HYPERCALCEMIA. Hypercalcemia is characterized by vague symptoms such as headache, irritability, fatigue, malaise, difficulty concentrating, anorexia, nausea, vomiting, and constipation. Neurologic effects are often the primary symptoms. Patients may be lethargic, confused, and have a depressed level of consciousness. Deep tendon reflexes may be depressed, the QT interval may be shortened, and the patient may have polyuria, polydipsia, or an ileus. Chronic hypercalcemia is associated with renal lithiasis, peptic ulcer, and pancreatitis.

Although rarely seen in the ED, serum calcium levels that exceed 13.5 mg/dL require immediate attention.[6] Correction of hypercalcemia includes treating the underlying cause and increasing renal excretion of calcium with IV hydration and loop or osmotic diuretics. Other therapeutic options depend on the specific clinical situation and include glucocorticoid administration to decrease intestinal calcium absorption and increase urinary calcium excretion. Administration of calcitonin or phosphate inhibits bone reabsorption.

Phosphate Abnormalities

Phosphate abnormalities are associated with a reciprocal calcium abnormality. Phosphate elevations occur with calcium losses, whereas phosphate depletion occurs with calcium excess. The patient with a phosphate abnormality should be carefully monitored for the effects of calcium abnormality.

HYPOPHOSPHATEMIA. Hypophosphatemia has a variable clinical presentation ranging from no symptoms to anorexia, muscle weakness, rhabdomyolysis, respiratory failure, hemolysis, and altered mental status. Causes include hyperparathyroidism, vitamin D deficiency, intestinal malabsorption, and renal tubular acidosis.

Management of a mild phosphorus deficiency may involve oral supplements and ingestion of foods high in phosphorus.[8] Severe hypophosphatemia can be serious and may require IV administration of sodium phosphate or potassium phosphate.[8] Frequent monitoring of serum phosphate levels is necessary to guide the therapy.[8] Sudden symptomatic hypocalcemia, secondary to increased calcium phosphorus binding, is a potential complication of IV phosphorus administration.[8]

HYPERPHOSPHATEMIA. Hyperphosphatemia is associated with a reciprocal fall in serum calcium and the resultant clinical effects of hypocalcemia. Hyperphosphatemia is also associated with and can even produce acute renal failure. The most serious effect of excess phosphate relates to precipitation of calcium phosphate crystals in soft tissues such as the cornea, lung, kidney, and blood vessels. Causes include hypoparathyroidism, chronic renal disease, Addison's disease, leukemia, sarcoidosis, osteolytic metastatic bone tumor, and milk-alkali syndrome.

Treatment includes limiting phosphate intake, using oral phosphate-binding agents such as aluminum hydroxide, and increasing excretion. IV hydration with saline is followed by diuretics to enhance excretion.

Magnesium Abnormalities

Magnesium abnormalities are frequently associated with other electrolyte abnormalities. Clinically, hypomagnesemia and hypermagnesemia have the same effect on release of PTH and calcitonin as hypocalcemia and hypercalcemia. Calcium and magnesium excretion are interdependent. A sudden calcium load causes excretion of both calcium and magnesium.

HYPOMAGNESEMIA. Hypomagnesemia may result from malabsorption syndrome, ulcerative colitis, ileal bypass, cirrhosis, alcoholism, chronic renal disease, DKA, diuretic therapy, and malnutrition. Symptoms include nausea, vomiting, sedation, increased deep tendon reflexes, and muscle weakness.[6] With significant hypomagnesemia, hypotension, bradycardia, coma, respiratory paralysis, and cardiac arrest may occur.[5] Severe hypomagnesemia can also exist in the absence of clinical symptoms. When symptoms do occur, they are usually confined to the neuromuscular and cardiovascular systems. Generalized weakness, muscle fasciculations, and positive Trousseau's and Chvostek's signs may be seen. Dysrhythmias such as torsades de pointes, ventricular tachycardia, and ventricular fibrillation have been associated with hypomagnesemia.

Treatment depends on severity of symptoms. Mild magnesium deficiencies can be treated with oral supplements and increased dietary intake of foods high in magnesium.[8] If the condition is severe, IV or intramuscular magnesium sulfate should be administered.[8] Vital signs, deep tendon reflexes, fluid intake, urinary output, and magnesium levels should be carefully monitored, because too-rapid administration of magnesium can lead to cardiac or respiratory arrest.

HYPERMAGNESEMIA. Hypermagnesemia may result from reduced excretion secondary to advanced renal failure, adrenocortical insufficiency, overdose of therapeutic magnesium, or routine doses of magnesium in the patient with renal compromise. Treatment of hypermagnesemia also depends on severity of symptoms. Calcium chloride, 100 to 200 mg, is given every 3 to 5 minutes until symptoms are reversed and is then followed by a continuous infusion.[9] Saline diuresis and furosemide may also be used. In severe cases hemodialysis may be required. Serial magnesium levels, vital signs, and deep tendon reflexes should be closely monitored.

SUMMARY

Whether caring for a trauma patient, chronically ill geriatric patient, or previously healthy person with acute simple gastroenteritis, the emergency nurse should anticipate electrolyte abnormalities. Recognition of abnormalities and potential adverse effects is essential for effective treatment and prevention of complications.

REFERENCES

1. Beers MH, Porter RS, Jones TV et al: *The Merck manual of diagnosis and therapy*, ed 18, Whitehouse Station, NJ, 2006, Merck & Co, Inc.

2. Black JM, Hawks, JH: *Medical-surgical nursing: clinical management for positive outcomes*, ed 7, St. Louis, 2005, Saunders.

3. Chernecky C, Macklin D, Murphy-Ende K: *Fluids and electrolytes*, ed 2, St. Louis, 2006, Saunders.

4. Collins RD: *Illustrated manual of fluid and electrolytes disorders*, ed 2, Philadelphia, 1983, JB Lippincott.

5. Guyton AC, Hall JE: *Textbook of medical physiology*, ed 11, Philadelphia, 2006, Saunders.

6. Heitz U, Horne MM: *Fluid, electrolyte and acid-base balance*, ed 5, St. Louis, 2005, Elsevier Saunders.

7. Kasper DL, Fauci AS, Longo DL et al: *Harrison's principles of internal medicine*, ed 16, Chicago, 2005, McGraw-Hill.

8. Lewis SL, Heitkemper MM, Dirkson SR et al: *Medical-surgical nursing: assessment and management of clinical problems*, ed 7, St. Louis, 2007, Mosby.

9. Marx JA, Hockberger RS, Walls RM: *Rosen's emergency medicine: concepts and clinical practice*, ed 6, Philadelphia, 2006, Mosby.

10. Schaider JJ, Hayden SR, Wolfe RE et al: *Rosen's & Barkin's 5-minute emergency medicine consult*, ed 3, Philadelphia, 2007, Lippincott Williams & Wilkins.

CHAPTER 37

Endocrine Emergencies

Colette M. Morey

The endocrine system is an integrated complex of hormone-secreting glands. This system is instrumental in regulating metabolism, tissue function, growth and development, moods and emotions, and works to maintain homeostasis in response to physiologic stress.[8] Dysfunction of one endocrine gland can affect the physiology of the entire body. Without prompt assessment, identification, and management, endocrine disturbances may result in life-threatening consequences. The majority of endocrine emergencies encountered in the emergency department (ED) are related to diabetes. This chapter addresses selected disorders related to diabetes, pituitary, thyroid, and adrenal pathology, as well as alcoholic ketoacidosis, a metabolic emergency.

ENDOCRINE SYSTEM PHYSIOLOGY

The endocrine system consists of the hypothalamus, pituitary, thyroid, parathyroids, adrenals, pancreas, testes, and ovaries (Figure 37-1). Each gland produces and stores one or more hormones that have specific, unique functions. Table 37-1 identifies the hormones produced by the major endocrine glands, their target tissue, and their functions. Activities of the testes and ovaries are discussed in Chapters 35 and 43.

Hormone activity is the result of feedback loops, nerve stimulation, and intrinsic rhythms. Renal and liver function and external factors such as pain, stress, or fear also affect hormone release. Excessive amounts of circulating hormones inhibit hormone release, whereas low levels lead to increased hormone release. Neural stimulation triggers increased glandular activity and release of hormones. Intrinsic rhythms vary from hours to weeks and provide another method of hormone control.

Hypothalamus

The hypothalamus creates part of the walls and floor of the third ventricle. Various centers in the anterior and posterior hypothalamus control most endocrine functions and many emotional behaviors. Nerve tracts from the hypothalamus join the posterior pituitary, which lies just below. Posterior pituitary hormones are actually synthesized in the hypothalamus and then transferred along axons for storage in the posterior pituitary. The hypothalamus regulates anterior pituitary action by inhibiting or releasing certain hormones.

Pituitary

The pituitary gland, approximately 1 cm in all directions, lies within the sella turcica of the middle cranial fossa. Two physiologically distinct areas are found in the pituitary. The anterior pituitary contains secretory cells, whereas

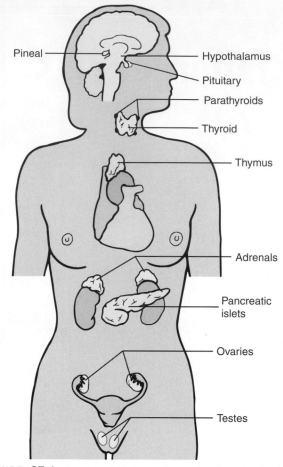

FIGURE **37-1.** Location of the major endocrine glands. Parathyroid glands actually lie on the posterior surface of the thyroid. (From Lewis SL, Heitkemper MM, Dirksen SR: *Medical-surgical nursing: assessment and management of clinical problems,* ed 7, St. Louis, 2007, Mosby.)

the posterior pituitary consists of neural cells that serve as a supporting structure for nerve fibers and nerve endings. Hormones secreted by the anterior pituitary include growth hormone, adrenocorticotropic hormone (ACTH), thyroid-stimulating hormone (TSH), prolactin, follicle-stimulating hormone, and luteinizing hormone. Antidiuretic hormone (ADH) and oxytocin are secreted by the posterior pituitary.

Thyroid

The thyroid gland consists of two lobes connected by an isthmus. This butterfly-shaped gland in the anterior neck below the cricoid cartilage partially surrounds the trachea. Thyroid hormone release is regulated through a complex feedback system between the hypothalamus and anterior pituitary. This main metabolic regulator contains follicular cells that secrete thyroxine (T_4) and triiodothyronine (T_3) in response to stimulation by the pituitary. Calcitonin originating in parafollicular cells in the thyroid affects calcium metabolism.

Parathyroids

The parathyroid glands are four or more small glands (the size and shape of a grain of rice) located on the posterior surface of the thyroid gland. The sole function of these glands is to maintain the body's calcium level within a very narrow range so that the nervous and muscular systems can function normally. When serum calcium levels drop, calcium-sensing receptors in the parathyroid gland are activated to release parathyroid hormone (PTH). PTH increases blood calcium levels by stimulating osteoclasts to break down bone and release calcium. It also increases gastrointestinal absorption of calcium by activating vitamin D and promotes calcium reabsorption by the kidneys.

Adrenals

The adrenal glands, located in the retroperitoneal area above the upper pole of each kidney, consist of an outer cortical layer and inner medullary layer. The adrenal cortex produces mineralocorticoids (e.g., aldosterone), glucocorticoids (e.g., cortisol), and androgens. Aldosterone is critical for maintaining internal fluid balance, whereas glucocorticoids are major players in the body's ability to resist stress. The adrenal medulla releases the catecholamines epinephrine and norepinephrine in response to sympathetic stimulation.

Pancreas

The pancreas is situated behind the stomach in the retroperitoneal space. The body of the pancreas extends horizontally across the abdominal wall with the head in the curve of the abdomen and the tail touching the spleen. Exocrine and endocrine cells are found in the pancreas. Acini are exocrine cells that release amylase, lipase, and other enzymes that aid in digestion. Three types of endocrine cells within the islet of Langerhans produce hormones that regulate serum glucose levels. Alpha cells secrete glucagon, beta cells produce insulin, and delta cells secrete somatostatin, which inhibits glucagon and insulin release.[5]

PATIENT ASSESSMENT

The endocrine system affects most, if not all, body systems. Complaints most commonly associated with endocrine disorders include fatigue and weakness, polyuria, polydipsia, weight changes, and mental status changes. The focused assessment should target the specific presenting complaint.

When a critically ill patient presents to the ED, an endocrine etiology should be considered as part of the differential diagnosis. Care of the patient begins with assessment and stabilization of the airway, breathing, and circulation (ABCs) as well as a neurologic assessment. The neurologic assessment includes evaluation of possible causes of altered consciousness such as trauma, blood glucose abnormalities, stroke, or toxins. Identification of a stressor or precipitating event may be elicited through patient history, family

Table 37-1. MAJOR ENDOCRINE GLANDS AND HORMONES

Hormones	Target Tissue	Functions
ANTERIOR PITUITARY (ADENOHYPOPHYSIS)		
Thyroid-stimulating hormone (TSH) or thyrotropin	Thyroid gland	Stimulates synthesis and release of thyroid hormones, growth and function of thyroid.
Adrenocorticotropic hormone (ACTH) or corticotrophin	Adrenal cortex	Fosters growth of adrenal cortex; stimulates secretion of glucocorticoids.
POSTERIOR PITUITARY (NEUROHYPOPHYSIS)		
Antidiuretic hormone (ADH) or vasopressin	Renal tubules, vascular smooth muscle	Promotes reabsorption of water. Raises blood pressure by inducing moderate vasoconstriction.
THYROID		
Thyroxine (T_4)	All body tissues	Precursor to T_3.
Triiodothyronine (T_3)	All body tissues	Regulates metabolic rate of all cells and processes of cell growth and tissue differentiation.
ADRENAL MEDULLA		
Epinephrine (adrenalin)	α- and β-adrenergic receptors	Increases heart rate and stroke volume, dilates pupils, constricts arterioles in the skin and digestive system, dilates arterioles in skeletal muscles. Relaxes bronchial smooth muscles. Triggers the release of glucose from energy stores.
Norepinephrine	α- and β-adrenergic receptors	Effects similar to epinephrine although longer acting. Also increased alertness and arousal.
ADRENAL CORTEX		
Corticosteroids (e.g., cortisol, hydrocortisone)	All body tissues	Maintains blood glucose, suppresses the immune response, and is released as part of the body's response to stress.
Mineralocorticoids (e.g., aldosterone)	Kidney	Regulates sodium and potassium balance and thus water balance.
PANCREAS		
Insulin (from beta cells)	General	Promotes movement of glucose out of blood and into cells.
Glucagon (from alpha cells)	General	Promotes movement of glucose from storage and into blood.

Modified from Lewis SL, Heitkemper MM, Dirksen SR: *Medical-surgical nursing: assessment and management of clinical problems,* ed 7, St. Louis, 2007, Mosby.

interviews, laboratory findings, radiographic analysis, or other diagnostic procedures.

SELECTED ENDOCRINE EMERGENCIES

The emergency nurse will encounter patients with varied severity of endocrine dysfunction. Selected conditions covered in this chapter include those situations that may lead to hemodynamic instability or altered neurologic function. Awareness of the potential for endocrine system abnormalities in every critical patient is extremely important for the ED nurse.

Diabetic Emergencies

Diabetes mellitus is a chronic condition characterized by hyperglycemia and disturbances of carbohydrate, fat, and protein metabolism. Two major types of diabetes mellitus exist: type 1, or insulin-dependent diabetes, is due to an absolute insulin deficiency; type 2, non–insulin-dependent diabetes mellitus or adult-onset diabetes, is characterized by impaired glucose secretion, peripheral insulin resistance, and increased hepatic glucose production. Type 2 is the most common type, accounting for approximately 90% of all diabetes in North America; obesity is a major risk factor for the development of this endocrine disorder.

Diabetic Ketoacidosis

Diabetic ketoacidosis (DKA) develops when a patient experiences relative or absolute depletion of circulating insulin. This potentially life-threatening condition may occur in previously undiagnosed patients, leading to the initial diagnosis of diabetes (particularly type 1). Infection, illness, pregnancy, or situational stressors can lead to gluconeogenesis, the manufacture of glucose from noncarbon substrates by the body. This creates a relative insulin deficiency. In some patients, excess circulating glucose secondary to poor dietary management can overwhelm an already stressed system. Absolute deficiency can occur in patients who fail to follow their prescribed insulin regimen or experience a stressor such as an illness and fail to take adequate insulin. The latter example demonstrates why diabetic education is critical.

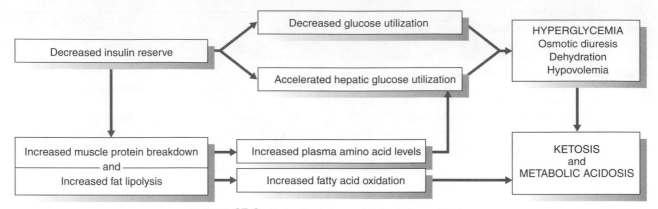

FIGURE **37-2.** Pathophysiology of diabetic ketoacidosis.

After prolonged insulin deficiency the patient can present with four acute problems: hyperglycemia, dehydration, electrolyte depletion, and metabolic acidosis (Figure 37-2). Stress causes release of counterregulatory hormones, which can lead to gluconeogenesis. Severe hyperglycemia increases serum osmolality and leads to osmotic diuresis, resulting in significant dehydration. Osmotic diuresis leads to urinary losses of water, sodium, potassium, magnesium, calcium, and phosphorus. The typical total body water loss in DKA is 6 L in adult patients.

It is thought that the hyperosmolarity further impairs insulin secretion and promotes insulin resistance. Without insulin, the newly liberated glucose cannot be used, further increasing serum blood glucose levels, urine glucose concentrations, and osmotic diuresis.[3] Fats and muscle proteins are metabolized for energy. The ensuing lipolysis causes a buildup of fatty acids, which overcomes the body's natural buffering system and leads to ketoacidosis.

DKA develops over a relatively short time, usually 2 to 3 days. The condition occurs most often in young adults and can result from infection, illness, stress, substance abuse, or failure to adhere to an insulin regimen. The patient describes a steady progression of symptoms, including polydipsia, polyuria, fatigue, and weakness. Patients with new-onset diabetes report recent weight loss. As ketoacidosis worsens, nausea, vomiting, decreased appetite, and abdominal cramping occur. The patient appears in moderate to severe distress with possible alteration in level of consciousness, confusion about recent events, or slow response to questions. Lethargy can progress to coma, and hyperthermia may be present.

Rapid, deep, Kussmaul respirations are present, and a fruity odor is usually noted on the breath. This acetone smell indicates worsening ketoacidosis. The cause of Kussmaul breathing is a respiratory compensation for a metabolic acidosis. Blood gas values from a patient with Kussmaul breathing will show a decreased PCO_2 level because of a forced increased respiration (blowing off the CO_2). The patient feels an involuntary urge to breathe rapidly and deeply. The skin is usually hot and dry, skin turgor is diminished, and mucous membranes are dry. Hypotension can result from severe dehydration. The most frequently seen cardiac rhythm is sinus tachycardia, but dysrhythmias related to

electrolyte disturbances also occur. This is a grave situation in the pregnant woman because of deleterious effects on the fetus. Early identification and aggressive interventions are critical to minimize effects on the fetus and the mother.

Initial laboratory studies should be obtained early and fluid therapy started on arrival to the ED. A serum glucose level higher than 300 mg/dL and normal or elevated potassium levels are usually present. Creatinine and blood urea nitrogen (BUN) levels may be elevated as a result of dehydration. Serum osmolality is greater than 310 mOsm/kg, and serum acetone titrations are positive. Serum ketone testing based on the measurement of β-hydroxybutyrate (BOHB or β-OHB, the main ketoacid causing acidosis) is recommended for diagnosis and monitoring. Mean BOHB levels in DKA are about 7 mmol/L, but can range from 4 to 42 mmol/L.[3] Urinalysis results include elevated levels of ketones and glucose. Blood gas results typically demonstrate normal arterial oxygen pressure (PaO_2), respiratory alkalosis, and metabolic acidosis. Infection can precipitate DKA, so blood cultures and a urine culture should be obtained when infection is suspected. After cultures are obtained, antibiotic therapy should begin. Radiographs may also be required to determine the primary site of infection.

Management in the ED should be aggressive. Treatment focuses on correction of hyperglycemia, dehydration, electrolyte imbalances, and metabolic acidosis. Close monitoring with frequent reassessment is essential to prevent complications. Serum glucose and potassium levels should be monitored every 1 to 2 hours, and pH should be monitored every 2 to 4 hours.[3] Oxygen therapy should be initiated for any signs of hemodynamic compromise or altered mental status.

Intravenous fluid replacement should start immediately with 1 to 2 L of normal saline over the first 1 to 2 hours of treatment for adults. In children the initial fluid bolus is weight based (5 to 20 mL/kg, dependent on the child's perfusion status); volume replacement is carefully titrated because of the high risk for cerebral edema in the pediatric population. The adult patient may require up to 8 to 10 L of fluid. Volume is gradually replaced after the initial fluid bolus because rapid infusion of a large volume increases the risk for development of cerebral edema. Close observation of intake and output is essential; placement of a urinary catheter ensures accurate output assessment. A continuous infusion of regular insulin is administered at 0.1 units/kg/hr to stop ketogenesis and achieve a steady decrease in serum glucose level of 50 to 75 mg/dL/hr; an initial intravenous (IV) bolus of 0.15 units/kg of regular insulin may be administered. The short duration of action for regular insulin allows better control of serum glucose levels. After serum glucose level reaches 250 to 300 mg/dL, fluids should be converted to 5% dextrose in normal saline (D_5NS) to provide fuel until the patient is able to eat. Resolution of a hyperglycemic emergency occurs when the serum glucose level is less than 200 mg/dL, serum bicarbonate level is greater than or equal to 18 mEq/L, and in DKA, the venous pH is greater than 7.3.[3]

Fluid replacement dilutes serum potassium and promotes diuresis. In addition, total body hypokalemia is exacerbated by metabolic acidosis, so potassium replacement should begin after the initial liter of IV fluids is infused, even when initial values are normal. Potassium levels frequently drop precipitously in the first few hours after treatment has been initiated because potassium moves back to the intracellular space along with the insulin and existing glucose. Serum potassium levels must be repeated every 1 to 2 hours during initial management. Cardiac monitoring is essential because dysrhythmias can develop with significant hypokalemia.

Acidosis generally corrects with insulin therapy. Insulin allows the cells to use available glucose for energy, leading to decreased proteinolysis and lipolysis, and the ketoacidosis resolves. Insulin infusion should be continued until the pH or serum bicarbonate level has normalized; IV fluids should be converted to D_5NS once the serum glucose level reaches 250 to 300 mg/dL to prevent hypoglycemia. Acidosis in DKA is not routinely treated with sodium bicarbonate because sodium bicarbonate administration can cause rebound alkalosis, which can worsen hypokalemia and increases the risk for development of cerebral edema.

Controlling nausea and vomiting not only improves patient comfort but prevents worsening dehydration. The patient may require analgesia to relieve abdominal pain, headaches, or other somatic complaints. Providing a quiet, calm environment can improve patient comfort. Stress reduction plays an important part in patient recovery. Thorough explanation of treatment, medications, and plan of care can alleviate stress related to hospitalization.

Potential complications include hypoglycemia, hypokalemia, dysrhythmias, and cerebral edema. Monitor capillary/serum glucose levels, electrocardiogram (ECG), laboratory values, vital signs, intake and output, and neurologic status carefully. If the serum glucose level falls rapidly, the resulting fluid shift can lead to cerebral edema, which is associated with a higher mortality rate. Cerebral edema remains the leading cause of death for children presenting in DKA.

Hyperosmolar Hyperglycemic State

Hyperosmolar hyperglycemic state (HHS), also known as hyperosmolar hyperglycemic nonketotic coma (HHNC), is a life-threatening emergency characterized by marked elevation of blood glucose level, hyperosmolarity, and little or no ketosis. HHS threatens type 2 (non–insulin-dependent) diabetic patients with mortality rates as high as 10% to 50%, although true mortality data are difficult to interpret due to the high incidence of comorbidities.[19] Delayed diagnosis in undiagnosed type 2 diabetes, alcoholics, and dialysis patients place these groups at the greatest risk.

With the increase in the prevalence of type 2 diabetes and the aging population, this condition is likely to be encountered more frequently in the future. The precipitating causes are numerous, with underlying infections, acute myocardial infarction, and stroke being the most common. Other causes include certain medications, medication and treatment noncompliance, undiagnosed diabetes, substance abuse, and coexisting disease. Physical findings include those associated with profound dehydration and various neurologic symptoms such as coma.

Typically, patients presenting with HHS are over 50 years of age and have undiagnosed diabetes or type 2 diabetes managed by diet and/or oral medications. In addition, they frequently are on medications that aggravate the problem, such as diuretics that cause mild dehydration.[19] Type 2 diabetic patients over 50 years typically present with other contributing health problems, so it is necessary to search for other underlying illness. When stressed with illness, surgery, or injury, the body responds with increased glucose levels. Type 2 diabetic patients produce enough insulin to avoid ketoacidosis but not enough to prevent profound hyperglycemia.

Increased serum glucose levels act as osmotic diuretics, leading to severe dehydration. Patients are unable to replace lost fluids, so their condition progressively worsens. Lack of sufficient circulating insulin causes the body to metabolize fat and muscle tissues, which increases circulating fatty acid and amino acid levels. The resulting hepatic gluconeogenesis compounds existing hyperglycemia. Underlying renal disease or decreased intravascular volume will decrease the glomerular filtration rate and cause the glucose level to increase. The loss of more water than sodium leads to hyperosmolarity. Insulin is present, but it is not sufficient to reduce blood glucose levels, particularly in the presence of insulin resistance.[19] Figure 37-3 illustrates the pathophysiology of HHS.

Onset of symptoms in HHS is much more insidious than with DKA, developing over days or even weeks. Subtlety of symptoms may account for delay in seeking treatment. The patient may notice vague abdominal pain, decreased appetite, polydipsia, and polyuria. As the disease progresses, neurologic symptoms such as headaches, blurred vision, and confusion develop. Changes in level of consciousness, seizures, or coma also occur. Tachycardia, dysrhythmias, and hypotension may also be present. Respirations may be increased but do not have the fruity smell associated with DKA. It is the decrease in mental status that usually brings the patient to the hospital.

Laboratory analysis includes complete blood count (CBC), electrolytes, urinalysis, and arterial blood gases.

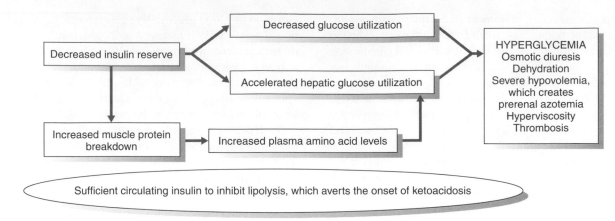

FIGURE **37-3.** Pathophysiology of hyperosmolar hyperglycemic nonketotic coma.

Typical laboratory findings in HHS include blood glucose levels greater than 600 mg/dL (33.3 mmol/L), serum osmolality greater than 320 mOsm/kg, pH levels greater than 7.30, and mild or absent ketonemia. Elevated white blood cell (WBC) count is present with infection. Serum sodium and potassium levels may be normal or elevated depending on the level of dehydration.

The treatment of HHS involves vigorous IV rehydration, correction of electrolyte imbalances, administration of IV insulin, and diagnosis and management of underlying illness and coexisting conditions. Due to the altered level of consciousness, oxygen therapy should be initiated immediately. Rapid IV fluid replacement is initiated with isotonic crystalloid solution. Continual assessment and reassessment are the keys to preventing complications associated with fluid therapy. Most patients are older than 50 years, so circulatory overload is a marked risk with rapid fluid therapy. Urinary catheter placement assists with monitoring of intake and output. Intravenous potassium may be indicated to prevent hypokalemia from hemodilution and insulin therapy. Continuous cardiac monitoring is essential due to the risk for dysrhythmias related to the potassium deficits. Once fluid replacement has been initiated, regular insulin should be administered as a continuous infusion of 0.1 unit/kg/hr; an initial bolus of 0.15 unit/kg regular insulin may be administered.

Serum glucose level should be lowered at a rate of 50 to 70 mg/dL/hr, because reductions greater than 100 mg/dL/hr may predispose the patient to cerebral edema from associated fluid shifts. Adequate fluids must be given before initiating insulin therapy because if insulin is administered before fluids, the water will move intracellularly, causing potential worsening of hypotension, vascular collapse, or death.[19]

After serum osmolality begins to normalize or the serum glucose level reaches 300 mg/dL, IV fluids are converted to D_5NS and insulin infusion decreased to 0.05 to 0.1 unit/kg/hr to maintain serum glucose level between 250 and 300 mg/dL until plasma osmolality is less than or equal to 315 mOsm/kg and the patient is mentally alert.

Patients with HHS are at particular risk for thrombus formation due to profound dehydration, hyperosmolarity, and immobility due to critical illness. Disseminated intravascular coagulation (DIC) can occur. Deep vein thrombosis prophylaxis should be considered.

Differentiation between HHS and DKA may be initially difficult; however, this should not alter the basic course of treatment. Management of ABCs is the top priority of emergency nursing care, and IV fluid therapy should begin immediately in both cases. Nursing actions are similar in both instances and include close observation of vital systems and laboratory values to prevent complications of therapy. Table 37-2 compares the clinical features of DKA and HHS.

Hypoglycemia

Hypoglycemia, a potentially life-threatening emergency commonly affecting patients with type 1 diabetes, is defined as a pathologic state characterized by a low serum glucose level. The precise level of glucose that is low enough to be considered hypoglycemia depends on the measurement method, the age of the person, presence or absence of symptoms, and the purpose of the definition. The debate continues as to what degree of hypoglycemia warrants medical evaluation or treatment or can cause harm.

Generally serum glucose levels below 60 mg/dL are indicative of hypoglycemia, although this value may vary based upon an individual's normal levels. How quickly the serum glucose decreases can influence the patient's symptoms; if glucose levels drop too quickly in relation to the body's compensatory ability, the patient may become symptomatic at levels of 60 to 80 mg/dL. Low serum glucose level is one of the more common causes of central nervous system (CNS) dysfunction seen in the ED.[2] The most dramatic effects of hypoglycemia are neurologic because glucose is the most important source of energy for the brain. The brain cannot synthesize glucose or store more than a few minutes' worth; it depends on a continuous supply from the circulatory system. Any unresponsive or neurologically altered patient should be promptly evaluated for hypoglycemia.

The most common cause of hypoglycemia is iatrogenic insulin effects in patients with type 1 diabetes. Other causes include pancreatic tumors, adrenal insufficiency, sepsis, and congenital metabolic disorders. In addition, several classes of

Table 37-2. COMPARISON OF DIABETIC KETOACIDOSIS (DKA) AND HYPERGLYCEMIC HYPEROSMOLAR STATE (HHS)		
Clinical Picture	**DKA**	**HHS**
Patient's age	Usually younger	Usually older adults
Type of diabetes mellitus	Type 1 (insulin-dependent)	Type 2 (non–insulin-dependent)
Duration of symptoms	Usually <2 days	Several days
Neurologic symptoms and signs	Rare	Very common
Glucose level	Usually <600 mg/dL	Usually >800 mg/dL
Ketone bodies	At least 4+ in a 1:1 dilution	<2+ in a 1:1 dilution
Serum sodium	Likely to be low or normal	Likely to be normal or high
Serum potassium	High, normal, or low	High, normal, or low
Serum bicarbonate	Low	Normal
Blood pH	Low, usually <7.3	Normal
Serum osmolality	Usually <350 mOsm/L	Usually >350 mOsm/L
Thrombosis	Very rare	Frequent
Mortality	3%-10%	20%-60%
Subsequent course	Ongoing insulin therapy usually required	Usually diet alone or oral agents

oral diabetes medications are associated with hypoglycemia; sulfonylureas and meglitinides are most frequently associated with hypoglycemia, whereas α-glucosidase inhibitors, biguanides, and thiazolidinediones alone do not normally cause hypoglycemia but can when used together with other diabetes medications. Factors that contribute to hypoglycemia include lack of dietary intake, increased physical stress, liver disease, changes in type of insulin or oral agents, pregnancy, alcohol ingestion, and certain drugs (e.g., nonsteroidal antiinflammatory drugs, phenytoin, thyroid hormones, and β-blockers).

Normally the body senses declining serum glucose levels and releases glucagon and epinephrine to stimulate release of glycogen by the liver. Glycogen functions as an alternate energy source; however, in acute hypoglycemia, glycogen stores cannot be broken down quickly enough to overcome the effects of insulin. Epinephrine release decreases utilization of existing glucose. Common symptoms of hypoglycemia, including shakiness, anxiety, palpitations, sweating, dry mouth, pallor, pupil dilation, and hunger, are attributed to catecholamine release. The known diabetic patient can usually recognize these symptoms and self-treat. β-Blocker therapy masks the sympathetic response, so these patients may not recognize onset of hypoglycemia.

As the brain becomes deprived of glucose, symptoms including abnormal mentation, irritability, confusion, difficulty speaking, ataxia, paresthesias, headaches, and stupor occur. The patient may or may not be able to self-treat or seek treatment at this point. Without treatment, neuroglycopenia can lead to seizures, coma, and even death. Patient and family education is essential. Often the family must initiate treatment after recognizing changes in the patient's behavior. Patients on insulin pumps are particularly vulnerable.

In the hospital setting, priorities include supporting the ABCs, ensuring patient safety, and initiating treatment. Treatment of the conscious patient consists of oral intake of 10 to 15 g of simple carbohydrates, usually in the form of glucose gel, juice, or hard candy, followed by a more complex carbohydrate snack or small meal. In the lethargic or unconscious patient, rapid administration of IV dextrose remains the treatment of choice (12.5 to 50 g of 50% dextrose for an adult). If IV access cannot be obtained, intramuscular glucagon 1 mg should be administered. Glucagon stimulates the liver to release glycogen, which is converted to glucose; patients must have adequate glycogen stores for this therapy to be effective. Because vomiting is common following the administration of glucagon, the patient should be positioned to minimize the risk for aspiration. If the patient has an insulin pump, the pump must be stopped immediately.

Laboratory study results obtained before glucose administration may provide helpful information, but administration of glucose should not be delayed to obtain laboratory samples. Severe neurologic deficits can result if the CNS is left without glucose. Once alert, the patient should be given a diet tray to provide complex carbohydrates to maintain an adequate glucose level. If the cause of the episode is identified, the patient may be discharged after a meal, observation, and confirmation that the glucose level has stabilized unless the patient is on oral antihyperglycemic agents that have a long half-life. Those patients will require further observation.

With the current focus on tight glycemic control and intensive insulin therapy, the risk for hypoglycemia is increased. Maintaining euglycemia decreases many of the macrovascular and microvascular complications associated with diabetes mellitus. Studies indicate that tight glycemic control results in a 42% reduction in heart disease, decreases the incidence of diabetic retinopathy by 76%, diabetic neuropathy by 69%, and the incidence of proteinuria by 34%.[7] Patients receiving intensive insulin therapy, however, have a threefold greater incidence of severe disabling hypoglycemia than those receiving conventional insulin therapy.[4] It is important to obtain a careful history of medication use, current illness, activity, etc., and the history of what led to this episode. This can be a key opportunity for patient teaching to prevent future episodes or to help the patient recognize and manage early signs of hypoglycemia.

Alcoholic Ketoacidosis

Alcoholic ketoacidosis (AKA) is an acute metabolic emergency that generally occurs 24 to 36 hours after a patient who has been ingesting large amounts of alcohol abruptly stops drinking. AKA is most common in adults with chronic alcohol abuse and a recent history of binge drinking, persistent vomiting, and decreased food intake; however, this disorder has been reported in less-experienced drinkers of all ages.[1] Although death is rare, illness often results from complications such as seizures, rhabdomyolysis, liver dysfunction, acute pancreatitis, heart failure, or systemic infection. AKA is characterized by elevated serum ketone levels and a high anion gap.[1] The anion gap $(Na^+ + K^+) - (Cl^- + HCO_3^-)$ is a calculation that represents unmeasured ions in serum plasma. The average anion gap for healthy adults is 6 mmol/L.

When dietary intake of carbohydrates is insufficient and hepatic glycogen stores are depleted by fasting, proteins and fats are broken down for fuel (gluconeogenesis), leading to production of ketones in the liver as an alternative source of energy. The body's response to starvation is a decrease in insulin activity and an increase in the production of counterregulatory hormones such as glucagon. Liver and pancreatic damage secondary to chronic alcohol consumption may further decrease glycogen stores and insulin levels. Inadequate glycogen leads to utilization of fat and muscle tissue for energy. Subsequent increased fatty acid production enhances an existing acidotic state.

Decreased insulin availability decreases glucose utilization, which also leads to increased fatty acid levels and acidosis. Actual alcohol metabolism decreases gluconeogenesis and compounds the altered metabolic state. Prolonged vomiting leads to dehydration. Circulating levels of epinephrine, cortisol, and growth hormones increase as a result of volume depletion, which further alters glucose utilization. As a result, the ketoacidotic cycle continues.

Patients present with abdominal pain, nausea, vomiting, and signs of alcohol withdrawal. Physical findings include tachypnea, tachycardia, mild to moderate abdominal tenderness, and some alteration in mental status, which may be mistakenly assumed to be due to alcohol intoxication rather than ketoacidosis. The skin may be cool and dry, and the patient may have a strong odor of ketones on the breath. Initial laboratory studies may show decreased pH, although serum pH levels can be misleading because patients with AKA often have a mixed acid-base disorder. In addition to metabolic acidosis due to ketone formation, a metabolic alkalosis can be present due to vomiting and volume depletion and a respiratory alkalosis can result from hyperventilation.

Other laboratory results may include a normal to slightly decreased potassium level, elevated liver function test results, and an elevated amylase level. Alcohol levels may be low or undetectable. Serum glucose levels can be low, normal, or slightly elevated, which may be useful in distinguishing AKA from DKA. Serum glucose levels are markedly elevated in cases of DKA. DKA should be ruled out when hyperglycemia is present. Hypomagnesemia, hypocalcemia, and hypokalemia are often present in chronic alcoholics.[1]

Management in the ED is focused on ABCs and correction of volume and glycogen depletion to restore metabolic functions. Once the diagnosis of AKA is established, the treatment is hydration with D_5NS. Carbohydrate and fluid replacement reverse the abnormalities that lead to AKA by increasing serum insulin levels and suppressing the release of glucagon and other counterregulatory hormones; exogenous insulin is rarely indicated to reverse the ketogenesis associated with AKA (life-threatening hypoglycemia can result from administering insulin to patients with depleted glycogen stores). As rehydration progresses and adequate renal function is established, electrolyte replacement should be considered. Potassium may be necessary because fluid therapy and shifting glucose molecules can lead to hypokalemia. Magnesium replacement may be indicated, because hypomagnesemia can increase the risk for seizures in alcohol withdrawal. Thiamine should be administered before or together with dextrose-containing fluids. CNS depletion of thiamine may result in Wernicke's encephalopathy, a syndrome characterized by ataxia, confusion and impairment of short-term memory; chronic thiamine deficiency may cause heart failure.

The patient with AKA requires close monitoring, seizure precautions, and supportive care. Frequent assessment of vital signs, intake and output, neurologic status, and electrolyte values is necessary to monitor effectiveness of therapy and to ensure an uncomplicated return to the patient's normal metabolic state.

Pituitary Disorders

Diabetes Insipidus

Diabetes insipidus (DI) is characterized by excretion of large volumes of dilute urine and can be life threatening if not properly diagnosed and managed. It can be caused by one of two different disturbances, inadequate or impaired secretion of ADH or impaired or insufficient renal response to ADH. Determining the type of disturbance is essential for effective treatment. Typically patients will present with extraordinary thirst despite copious water intake (up to 20 L/day), dry skin, and constipation. Patients are passing large amounts of dilute urine regardless of the body's hydration state.

Central diabetes insipidus results from any condition that impairs the secretion and release of ADH. Causes include damage to the hypothalamo-neurohypophyseal region as a result of head trauma, surgery, or tumors or may also be idiopathic or genetic.

In nephrogenic diabetes insipidus there is a sufficient amount of ADH, but the kidneys are unable to properly concentrate the urine. This may be genetic or acquired. Acquired forms are more common and are characterized by alterations in the structure or function of the kidney. Damage may be permanent or transient, caused by disease (the most common cause), drugs, or other conditions such as hypokalemia, hypercalcemia, pregnancy, and sickle cell anemia.[14]

Diagnosis is made by measurement of urine osmolality, which helps in determining whether polyuria is due to DI. A urine osmolality less than 200 mOsm/kg in the presence of polyuria characterizes DI. Determining if the pathologic condition is central or nephrogenic is essential; ADH replacement therapy is the treatment for central DI but will be ineffective in the treatment of nephrogenic DI.

The water deprivation test, although not required for the diagnosis of DI, is used to differentiate between central and nephrogenic DI. Cautious management is essential because the water deprivation test requires fluids to be withheld until the patient is sufficiently dehydrated to stimulate ADH secretion. Deprivation typically lasts 4 to 18 hours, with hourly measurements of body weight and urine osmolality until the patient experiences a 5% decrease in body weight or until two or three consecutive urine samples vary by less than 30 mOsm/kg. The serum ADH level is then measured, and the patient is given 5 units of ADH or 1 mcg of desmopressin. In central DI, urine osmolality will increase by more than 50% in response to ADH replacement, and in nephrogenic DI, the urine osmolality will increase by less than 50%.[14]

In central DI, sufficient quantities of water are essential to correct metabolic disturbances due to excessively dilute urine. Rapid volume correction should be avoided, however, because this can cause cerebral edema. Treatment consists of ADH replacement with medications such as desmopressin, chlorpropamide, or carbamazepine. Nephrogenic DI does not respond to ADH; therefore treatment includes correcting hypokalemia and hypercalcemia or discontinuing any drugs that may be the cause. In addition, thiazide diuretics can be used along with modest salt restriction to reduce the delivery of filtrate to the diluting portions of the nephron. This results in decreased sodium and chloride absorption in the distal tubule, which allows more sodium absorption and therefore more water absorption in the proximal tubule.[14]

Emergency management of the patient with DI includes close monitoring of fluid status, neurologic status, electrolyte levels, and resulting ECG rhythm or other systemic disturbances. Close monitoring of fluid intake, output, and urine osmolality, in addition to prompt distinction between central and nephrogenic DI, will determine the course of treatment.

Syndrome of Inappropriate Antidiuretic Hormone

The syndrome of inappropriate antidiuretic hormone (SIADH) occurs when the feedback system that regulates the ADH level fails, causing the pituitary gland to release excessive amounts of ADH. A patient with SIADH may present to the ED with dilutional hyponatremia, which can lead to seizures and death if left untreated. ADH is generated in the hypothalamus and stored in the pituitary gland. Any disease process that alters the hypothalamic secretion osmoreceptors or hypothalamic-pituitary-adrenal axis can precipitate SIADH. Thyroid and pituitary lesions, narcotics, tricyclic antidepressants, oral hypoglycemics, and carbamazepine also can precipitate SIADH. Other associated disorders include abscesses, pneumonia, tuberculosis, hypothyroid disorders, porphyria, and head injury, although the cause may be idiopathic.

Increased distal renal tubular permeability to water, resulting from ADH, decreases urine volume and returns water to the systemic circulation. Serum osmolality and circulating blood volume normally influence ADH release. Hypothalamic osmoreceptors sense an increased serum concentration and stimulate release of ADH. Serum concentration decreases when the kidneys respond with increased water reabsorption. As circulating volume expands, urinary output diminishes. The resulting hemodilution creates fluid overload with associated hyponatremia.

Subjective complaints include weakness, nausea, vomiting, diarrhea, abdominal and muscle cramps, sudden weight gain without edema, headache, and fatigue. The patient may note decreased urinary output despite regular oral intake; the greatest changes, however, may be in neurologic function. The patient appears confused and disoriented with seizures noted as hyponatremia worsens. Severe hyponatremia leads to fluid shifts, which can cause cerebral edema and hyponatremic encephalopathy.[10] Deep tendon reflexes are diminished.

Laboratory tests may reveal marked hyponatremia (serum sodium level less than 125 mEq/L) and low serum osmolality (less than 280 mOsm/kg). BUN and creatinine levels are low to normal, and renal function tests are usually normal. Urine osmolality, sodium, and specific gravity are increased; urine is hyperosmolar as compared to the plasma.

Management of SIADH is related to the severity of hyponatremia. Free water restriction is sufficient in mild cases.[10] Restrictions often start at 800 to 1000 mL/day; however, restrictions as severe as 500 mL/day may be required. The importance of accurate intake and output monitoring cannot be overemphasized. Acute, severe hyponatremia (less than 124 mmol/L) is often associated with neurologic symptoms such as seizures and should be treated urgently because of the high risk for cerebral edema and hyponatremic encephalopathy. The initial correction rate with hypertonic saline should not exceed 1 to 2 mmol/L/hr. Close monitoring is necessary for early identification of circulatory overload. Small amounts of loop diuretics increase urinary output and may prevent overload. Serial electrolyte evaluations help avoid complications in therapy and assist in monitoring therapy progress.

Administration of demeclocycline, 600 to 1200 mg/day, interferes with ADH action; however, this simply augments fluid restriction therapy. Ultimately, serum sodium and osmolality should improve. After the patient stabilizes, identification and treatment of the precipitating event become the next goals. Close observation and timely management ensure patient safety and prevent complications.

Thyroid Emergencies

Thyroid emergencies are rare but can be life threatening. The thyroid gland regulates the body's metabolic rate through the hypothalamic-pituitary-thyroid counterregulatory system. Thyroid gland activity depends on the hypothalamus secreting thyrotropin-releasing hormone (TRH), which is responsible for release of TSH by the anterior pituitary, which causes the release of T_4. Circulating T_4 is converted to T_3 in the peripheral system. The amount of TSH depends on the amount of TRH, which can be influenced by physical stressors such as surgery, infection, and extremely cold temperatures. Circulating levels of T_3 and T_4 also affect the amount of TRH released through negative feedback. If any part of this system malfunctions, the resulting hyperactivity or hypoactivity of the thyroid gland can lead to multisystem symptoms.

Hyperthyroidism

Hyperthyroidism can be caused by multiple disturbances. True hyperthyroidism is characterized by an overactive thyroid gland and excessive production of thyroid hormones. Graves' disease, an autoimmune disorder in which thyroid-stimulating immunoglobulins increase thyroid activity, is responsible for 60% to 80% of all cases of hyperthyroidism.[17] Tumors and thyroid nodules can also increase thyroid activity. An increased amount of circulating hormones without concurrent overactivity from the thyroid occurs in thyroiditis or ingestion of thyroid hormones (intentionally or unintentionally). Certain drugs, especially iodine and iodine-containing agents such as amiodarone and lithium, can induce hyperthyroidism.

Thyroid Storm

Thyroid storm is an acute, life-threatening complication of poorly managed hyperthyroidism or thyrotoxicosis (symptomatic hyperthyroidism). Rapid elevation in thyroid hormone levels results in a decompensated state of severe hypermetabolism, characterized by hyperthermia, agitation, tachydysrhythmias, and tremors. Neurologic symptoms may include delirium, syncope, or coma. Left untreated, mortality rates are around 90%[12]; exhaustion, cardiac failure, and death can occur within hours. Elevated hormone levels can occur in response to hospitalization, surgery, infection, emotional stressors, trauma, childbirth, sudden discontinuation of antithyroid medications, or overmanipulation of the thyroid.

Gathering a concise history regarding illnesses and current medications is important. The patient may have recently discontinued a medication or experienced a recent change in therapy. The patient commonly has a history of Graves' disease. Patients often report recent weight loss despite increased appetite and increased caloric intake. Complaints of abdominal pain are common.

The patient may be restless with a shortened attention span and appear to be having an anxiety attack. Tremors and manic behaviors are also common. In late stages the patient may have altered mental status progressing to coma. Hyperthermia may be extreme with temperatures reaching 105° to 106° F (40.5° to 41° C). Older adult patients may present with rapid, new-onset, atrial fibrillation. Tachycardia with rates as high as 200 to 300 beats/min increases the patient's risk for cardiac failure and arrest.[16] Pulmonary crackles secondary to cardiac failure may be heard.

The skin often progresses from warm and diaphoretic to hot and dry as dehydration worsens. Nausea, vomiting, and diarrhea are caused by increased gastric motility. Hepatic tenderness, jaundice, and thinning hair may occur. Goiter, an enlarged thyroid gland, develops as the condition progresses. Eyes become protuberant (exophthalmus), periorbital edema develops, and the patient has a staring gaze with heavy eyelids. Thyroid hormone levels may help differentiate the causative factor but are not readily available and make it difficult to differentiate between thyroid storm and thyrotoxicosis. If thyroid storm is suspected, rapid, aggressive therapy is essential to reduce hormone levels and preserve hemodynamic integrity.

Immediate goals for management of thyroid storm include inhibiting thyroid hormone synthesis and release, blocking peripheral thyroid hormone effects, and supportive care such as management of ABCs and control of hyperthermia and sympathomimetic symptoms. β-Blockers are given to inhibit adrenergic effects but should be used with caution in older patients and in patients with preexisting heart disease, chronic obstructive pulmonary disease, or asthma.

Propylthiouracil (PTU) and methimazole may be used to block further synthesis of thyroid hormone. Both are given orally or through a gastric tube. Onset of action is within 1 hour, but their full effect is not evident until 3 to 6 weeks. Iodides can be given to block the conversion of T_4 to T_3 and inhibit hormone release, but should be given at least 1 hour after antithyroid medications to slow release of stored thyroid hormone from the thyroid gland. If given sooner, iodine may actually be used to create new hormone. Patients with Graves' disease and thyroid crisis metabolize and use cortisol faster than normal, so administration of glucocorticoids has been shown to increase survival rates. Glucocorticoids prevent adrenal compromise and inhibit T_4 conversion to T_3.[16]

Increased body temperature raises metabolic demands, which increases the percentage of free T_4. Aspirin must be avoided because it can displace thyroid hormones from binding sites and worsen the situation. Cooling blankets are helpful for reduction of hyperthermia. Keep the patient from shivering because this increases the metabolic rate. Fluid replacement therapy replenishes fluids lost through hyperthermia, vomiting, and diarrhea. The patient's hemodynamic status and electrolyte levels determine the fluid of choice. Providing supplemental oxygen assists with increased multisystem oxygen demands.

After the patient stabilizes, close evaluation and assessment are necessary to identify the aggravating agent or illness. Laboratory analysis includes cultures, toxicology screens, thyroid functions, electrolyte levels, and CBC. Radiographs may be ordered to rule out infectious sources; head and neck computed tomography scans may be ordered to identify existing neoplasms or structural abnormalities. Antibiotic therapy may be started when infection is suspected as a causal agent.

Myxedema Coma

Myxedema coma is an extreme complication of hypothyroidism in which patients exhibit multiple organ dysfunction and progressive mental deterioration. Hypothyroidism is four times more common in women than in men, with 80% of the cases of myxedema coma occurring in females. Myxedema coma usually occurs in patients 60 years and older with more than 90% of cases occurring during the winter months. Mortality rates may be as high as 30% to 60 %. The factors associated with a poor prognosis include bradycardia, advanced age, and persistent hypothermia.[11]

Untreated hypothyroidism progresses over months to years before culminating in myxedema coma. All patients who develop myxedema coma have hypothyroidism.[11] Dysfunction may be related to autoimmune thyroiditis (e.g., Hashimoto's disease), ablation therapy (treatment for hyperthyroidism), iodine deficiency, tumor activity, or drug therapy. Secondary hypothyroidism stems from pituitary dysfunction. Alterations in pituitary function decrease TSH release, which lowers thyroid hormone secretion. Tertiary hypothyroidism occurs when the hypothalamus secretes inadequate amounts of TRH or TRH fails to reach the pituitary gland.

Medications such as lithium, amiodarone, β-blockers, anesthesia, and several anticonvulsants can precipitate myxedema coma. Other factors known to precipitate myxedema coma include burns, gastrointestinal hemorrhage, hypoglycemia, hypothermia, and infection.[11] In patients with a hypoactive thyroid, the entire metabolic system slows down. Fever, tachycardia, and diaphoresis are absent, so the crisis state may not be noticed initially. The patient may complain of pronounced fatigue, decreased activity tolerance, episodes of shortness of breath, and weight gain. Tongue swelling (macroglossia) may also occur. Patients may answer questions slowly and exhibit significant confusion. Altered mental status can progress to coma. "Myxedema madness" refers to associated psychiatric symptoms such as hallucinations, paranoia, depression, combativeness, and decreased concern for personal appearance.

Support of the ABCs is essential in patients with myxedema coma. The tongue may be thick and can obstruct the airway in a semiconscious or unconscious patient. Weak respiratory effort with decreased respiratory drive leads to alveolar hypoventilation and can predispose the patient to pulmonary infection. Alveolar hypoventilation also leads to hypercarbia, which can further confound an altered mental status. Obesity-related sleep apnea can further compromise the respiratory system. Respiratory failure is the usual cause of death.

Cardiac changes include decreased heart rate, decreased stroke volume, and decreased cardiac output. There may be widespread ST- and T-wave changes with prolonged QT intervals. Peripheral vasoconstriction is the body's attempt to conserve heat, so skin is cool and pale; body temperature is usually less than 96° F (35.5° C).

In myxedema coma renal blood flow, glomerular filtration rates, and sodium reabsorption decrease. Patients cannot excrete the usual volume of fluid; urine osmolality does not reflect the serum hypoosmolality. Generalized nonpitting edema may be observed. Occasionally hypoglycemia develops as a result of increased insulin sensitivity and decreased oral intake. Systemic metabolic slowing affects the

gastrointestinal tract, so constipation occurs. Oral medications may not be adequately absorbed because of decreased gastric motility.

Diagnostic tests reveal decreased WBC count, decreased hemoglobin and hematocrit (caused by low erythropoietin), and decreased thyroid levels. The creatine kinase (CK) and L-lactate dehydrogenase (LDH) levels may be elevated, secondary to increased muscle membrane permeability. Patients with myxedema coma may be misdiagnosed with myocardial infarction based on elevated CK levels in association with nonspecific ECG findings.[6]

Care focuses on thyroid hormone replacement along with stabilization and support of ABCs The patient may require mechanical ventilation to secure the airway, correct elevated carbon dioxide levels, and improve oxygenation. Hormone replacement is generally administered in the form of IV T_4. Large doses saturate empty receptor binding sites and replenish peripheral circulating hormone levels. T_3 does have a quicker onset of action, but increased mortality related to adverse cardiac effects has been associated with sole use of T_3. Some clinicians recommend a combination of T_4 and T_3 therapy; current guidelines, however, recommend hormone replacement with T_4.[9,15] After the patient can tolerate oral fluids, oral T_4 therapy may begin. Glucocorticoid administration may help prevent adrenal crisis in patients with compromised adrenal systems.[11]

Scans, radiographs, and further diagnostic tests are performed after the patient stabilizes. Severe systemic slowing exhibited in myxedema coma should not be underestimated. Slow warming is recommended because increased oxygen demands related to warming can add stress to an already overstressed system. Passive warming with blankets or heated, humidified mist is preferred. Supportive care includes analgesic administration, urinary catheter placement, and a gastric tube to decrease abdominal pressure and distention.

Adrenal Disorders

Acute Adrenal Insufficiency

Acute adrenal insufficiency, also known as adrenal crisis or addisonian crisis, is a rare occurrence with life-threatening potential characterized by depletion of adrenal glucocorticoids and mineralocorticoids. The crisis can occur in a person with Addison's disease or may be caused by sudden withdrawal of long-term steroid therapy, removal or injury of the adrenal glands, or destruction of the pituitary gland. Other risk factors include stress, trauma, surgery, or infection in a person with Addison's disease, or injury or trauma to the adrenal glands or the pituitary gland. Massive bilateral adrenal hemorrhage can occur under severe physiologic stress such as myocardial infarction, septic shock, or complicated pregnancy. Normally stress increases cortisol output from the adrenal system; therefore inability to meet these increased demands begins the sequence of events that leads to crisis.

When the adrenal system fails, the resulting decrease in cortisol and aldosterone levels leads to sodium and water loss from the kidneys and gastrointestinal tract. Water loss results in hypotension and hypovolemia, which can progress to cardiovascular collapse, coma, and death. As sodium decreases, serum potassium increases, leading to hyperkalemia and potentially fatal dysrhythmias. Gluconeogenesis, the normal hepatic response to stress, fails without sufficient levels of cortisol; therefore hypoglycemia can also occur in adrenal crisis. Decreased cortisol levels also alter activities of the adrenal medulla, which normally responds to stress through release of catecholamines to increase heart rate and serum glucose. Without a catecholamine response the severity of hypoglycemia and hypotension is magnified (Figure 37-4).

Diagnosing adrenal insufficiency can be difficult because symptoms often are insidious and nonspecific. An accurate history of prior illnesses (e.g., asthma with steroid therapy), recent medication changes, recent surgery, or injury helps determine precipitating factors. The patient may complain of headache, fatigue, weakness, weight loss, palpitations, and gastrointestinal symptoms such as nausea,

anorexia, abdominal pain, and chronic diarrhea. Signs and symptoms of adrenal crisis can include sudden pain in the abdomen, lower back, or legs; severe vomiting and diarrhea; high fever related to infection; dehydration; hypotension; and eventually loss of consciousness.

Physical findings are nonspecific and may include resting tachycardia, orthostatic hypotension, signs of dehydration such as dry mucous membranes, delayed capillary refill, poor skin turgor, and lethargy. Decreased cortisol levels cause the pituitary gland to increase secretion of ACTH and β-lipotropin, a substance that has melanocyte-stimulating activity, resulting in hyperpigmentation of skin and mucous membranes. Diffuse hyperpigmentation of the buccal mucosa and skin, especially over the elbows, knuckles, and axillary folds, is a sign of chronic primary adrenal insufficiency, but will not be present in all cases.[18]

Hyponatremia, hyperkalemia, hypoglycemia, and hypercalcemia are usually present. Hyperkalemia, the most sensitive of these conditions, is related to aldosterone deficiency. The ECG may reflect signs of hyperkalemia such as peaked

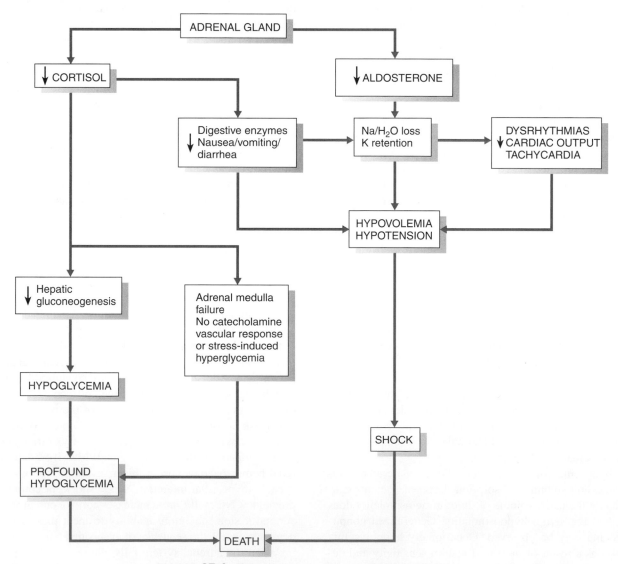

FIGURE 37-4. Pathophysiology of acute adrenal insufficiency.

T waves and a widening QRS. Decreased circulating volume also increases BUN. An ACTH challenge does help with diagnosis but is not useful in the emergency setting because treatment of the patient should not be delayed awaiting the test results. This challenge consists of obtaining a baseline serum cortisol level, administering synthetic ACTH, and then repeating the serum cortisol level 6 to 8 hours later. If the adrenal glands are functioning appropriately, the repeat cortisol level should be at least twice the baseline level.[20]

Maintenance of ABCs, replacement of glucocorticoids, and correction of fluid and electrolyte disturbances are cornerstones of care for the patient with adrenal crisis. Oxygen should be administered to meet increased oxygen demands caused by tachycardia. Hydrocortisone is the primary synthetic glucocorticoid given to stimulate gluconeogenesis, inhibit inflammatory response, and allow the body to increase its response to stress. Synthetic mineralocorticoids (e.g., fludrocortisone [Florinef]) are less commonly used because of the potential for excessive sodium retention.

Rapid IV fluid replacement assists in correcting volume deficit, which can be significant in adrenal crisis. A bedside glucose level should be obtained and hypoglycemia corrected if present. Hyperkalemia associated with adrenal crisis is usually mild and will resolve with IV fluids and replacement of glucocorticoid; however, the patient with clinical signs of hyperkalemia (muscle paralysis) or ECG changes (peaked T waves, widening QRS) should be treated appropriately (calcium, sodium bicarbonate, insulin, and 50% dextrose, etc.) Continuous cardiac monitoring is essential. Frequent reassessment of glucose and electrolyte levels is necessary to evaluate care and prevent complications. Observation of neurologic function, intake and output, and vital signs provides information on patient response to treatment.

Pheochromocytoma

A pheochromocytoma is a rare catecholamine-producing tumor derived from chromaffin cells in the adrenal medulla; the majority of these tumors are benign, secreting primarily norepinephrine. Clinical manifestations result from excessive (intermittent or continuous) catecholamine secretion. Patients characteristically present with severe hypertension accompanied by a triad of headache, palpitations, and diaphoresis. Visual disturbances (related to hypertensive retinopathy), fatigue, anxiety, pallor, tremors, fever, chest pain, abdominal pain, and mental status changes may also be noted. Life-threatening hypertension associated with pheochromocytoma can precipitate atrial and ventricular fibrillation, myocarditis, myocardial infarction, cardiomyopathy, pulmonary edema, stroke, and hypertensive encephalopathy. The diagnosis of pheochromocytoma may be suspected based on history and clinical findings. An abdominal computed tomography scan or magnetic resonance imaging may detect an adrenal mass. A 24-hour urine collection for catecholamines and metanephrines may be obtained.

Emergent care of the patient with pheochromocytoma entails controlling the effects of excessive catecholamine secretion. Intravenous α-blocking agents (phentolamine) or nitroprusside are commonly used to manage hypertensive crisis. The patient requires continuous cardiac monitoring to allow rapid detection and treatment of dysrhythmias. IV fluids are administered to maintain a normal circulating volume. Surgical resection of the tumor can reverse the clinical symptoms and may cure the hypertension.[13]

Cushing's Syndrome

Cushing's syndrome is caused by prolonged exposure to elevated levels of either endogenous or exogenous glucocorticoids. The majority of cases result from the administration of exogenous steroids. Patients affected with this disorder develop a characteristic cushingoid appearance due to increased adipose tissue in the face (moon facies), upper back at the base of the neck (buffalo hump), and above the clavicles.

Although Cushing's syndrome is not a medical emergency, exposure to excess glucocorticoids results in multiple medical problems, including hypertension, obesity, glucose intolerance, osteoporosis and fractures, impaired immune function, and impaired wound healing. These patients are at risk for developing adrenal crisis if steroids are abruptly stopped or dosage is not increased during an acute illness. The emergency nurse needs to be alert to the multisystem consequences of Cushing's syndrome when providing care for these patients in the ED.

SUMMARY

Endocrine emergencies can affect all body systems because of the diversity of hormones and their effects. Support of hemodynamic functions, identification of precipitating events, and detection of potential complications through frequent and thorough reassessment are essential for the survival of these patients.

REFERENCES

1. Adams S, Bontempo L: Alcoholic ketoacidosis. In Harwood-Nuss A, Wolfson A, editors: *The clinical practice of emergency medicine*, ed 3, Philadelphia, 2001, Lippincott Williams & Wilkins.
2. Bartlett D: Confusion, somnolence, seizures, tachycardia? Question drug induced hypoglycemia, *J Emerg Nurs* 31(2):206, 2005.
3. Brenner ZR: Management of hyperglycemic emergencies, *AACN Clin Issues* 17(1):50, 2006.
4. Briscoe VJ, Davis SN: Hypoglycemia in type 1 and type 2 diabetes: physiology, pathophysiology, and management, *Clin Diabetes* 24(3):115, 2006.
5. Carroll R: The metabolic system. In Black J, Hawks J, Keene A, editors: *Medical surgical nursing*, ed 6, Philadelphia, 2001, WB Saunders.
6. Citikowitz E: Myxedema coma or crisis, 2006, *eMedicine.* Retrieved July 11, 2008, from http://www.emedicine.com/med/topic1581.htm.

7. Clark W: Benefits of tight glycemic control: no end in sight, *Diabetes Self-Manag* 23(3):29, 2006.

8. Collier J, Longmore M: *Oxford handbook of clinical specialties*, ed 7, Oxford University Press, Oxford, UK 2006.

9. Cydulka R, Goldstein JR: Hypothyroidism. In Schaider J, Hayden SR, Wolfe R et al, editors: *Rosen and Barkin's 5-minute emergency medicine consult*, Philadelphia, 2006, Lippincott Williams & Wilkins.

10. Goh KP: Management of hyponatremia, *Am Fam Physician* 69(10):2387, 2004.

11. Guha B, Krishnaswanamy G, Peiris A: The diagnosis and management of hypothyroidism, *South Med J* 95(5):475, 2002.

12. Harris C: Recognizing thyroid storm in the neurologically impaired patient, *J Neurosci Nurs* 39(1):40, 2007.

13. Kudva YC, Sawka AM, Young WF: The laboratory diagnosis of adrenal pheochromocytoma: the Mayo Clinic experience, *J Clin Endocrinol Metab* 88(10):4533, 2003.

14. Makaryus AN, McFarlane SI: Diabetes insipidus: diagnosis and treatment of a complex disease, *Cleve Clin J Med* 73(1):65, 2006.

15. Perkins J: Hypothyroidism/myxedema coma. In Caterino JM, Kahan S, editors: *In a page emergency medicine,* Philadelphia, 2003, Lippincott Williams & Wilkins.

16. Ragland T, Urbanic R: Thyroid emergencies. In Harwood-Nuss A, Wolfson A, editors: *Clinical practice of emergency medicine*, ed 3, Philadelphia, 2001, Lippincott Williams & Wilkins.

17. Reid JR, Wheeler SF: Hyperthyroidism: diagnosis and treatment, *Am Fam Physician* 72(4):623, 2005.

18. Sabol VK: Addisonian crisis, *Am J Nurs* 101(7):24 AAA, 2001.

19. Stoner GD: Hyperosmolar hyperglycemic state, *Am Fam Physician* 71(9):1723, 2005.

20. Tintinalli JE: Adrenal insufficiency and adrenal crisis. In Tintinalli JE, Kelen G, Stapczynski J, editors: *Emergency medicine: a comprehensive study guide*, ed 6, New York, 2003, McGraw-Hill.

CHAPTER 38

Communicable Diseases

Sherri-Lynne Almeida

An infection is the detrimental colonization of a host organism by a foreign species. Three factors form the chain of infection: agent, host, and mode of transmission.[9] In an infection, the infecting organism seeks to use the host's resources to multiply (usually at the expense of the host). The infecting organism, or pathogen, interferes with the normal functioning of the host and can lead to chronic wounds, gangrene, loss of an infected limb, and even death. The host's response to infection is inflammation. A pathogen is usually considered a microscopic organism, though the definition is broader and includes bacteria, parasites, fungi, and viruses. The property of an infectious agent that determines the extent to which overt disease is produced or the power of an organism to produce disease is called pathogenicity. Some agents are highly pathogenic and routinely cause disease, whereas other agents cause disease only when normal host defenses are impaired.

A susceptible host is one who lacks effective anatomic and physiologic resistance to a pathogenic agent. Characteristics that influence susceptibility include nutritional and immunization status, hormonal influences, age, medical and medication history, underlying pathologic condition, and specific insult to the body such as trauma. The severity with which a pathogen causes disease in a specific host, the severity of the resulting diseases, the efficiency with which the organism is transmitted to or from the host, or a combination of these factors is known as the virulence of the pathogen.

Transmission of pathogens is essential to their ultimate survival. Major modes of transmission are contact (direct and indirect), airborne, and droplet. Direct transmission occurs when person-to-person contact occurs between an infected source and susceptible host with a receptive portal through which human or animal infection can enter. Examples of direct contact include biting, sexual intercourse, direct inoculation with contaminated blood (needlestick injury), or direct projection of droplet spray onto conjunctiva of the eye, nose, or mouth during sneezing, coughing, spitting, or vomiting. Indirect transmission occurs when susceptible hosts come in contact with an inanimate object contaminated with an infectious agent and the agent is transported and introduced into the host through a suitable portal of entry.

Vehicle-borne agents are contaminated, inanimate materials such as patient care equipment, soiled linen, surgical instruments, dressings, food, water, milk, and biologic products such as blood, serum, plasma, tissues, or organs. *Vector-borne* transmission occurs with injection of saliva during biting, regurgitation, or dermal exposure to feces or other material capable of penetrating nonintact skin. And finally, *airborne* transmission is defined as dissemination of microbial aerosols through a portal, usually the respiratory tract. Close contact with an infected source that is coughing or sneezing can transmit large infectious particles through the air. Factors that influence airborne transmission include ambient airflow, proximity, and spatial orientation to the infected person.

513

INFECTION PREVENTION IN THE ACUTE CARE SETTING

In the hospital environment, transmission of an infectious agent to a susceptible host occurs by contact and inhalation exposure. Nosocomial infections, also known as hospital-acquired infections, are infections acquired during hospital care that were not present or incubating at admission. Infections occurring more than 48 hours after admission are usually considered nosocomial.

Many factors contribute to the frequency of nosocomial infections: hospitalized patients are often immunocompromised, they undergo invasive examinations and treatments, and patient care practices and the hospital environment may facilitate the transmission of microorganisms among patients. The selective pressure of intense antibiotic use promotes antibiotic resistance. Although progress in the prevention of nosocomial infections has been made, changes in medical practice continually present new opportunities for development of infection.

Inappropriate or lack of hand washing is the most significant factor for development of nosocomial infections, and universal compliance with hand hygiene recommendations is poor. This is due to a variety of reasons, including lack of appropriate accessible equipment, high staff-to-patient ratios, allergies to hand-washing products, insufficient knowledge of staff about risks and procedures, and the duration of time recommended for washing.

When hands or other skin surfaces are contaminated with blood or other body substances, the area should be cleaned as soon as possible. Hands should be washed before and after every patient contact regardless of whether gloves are worn.

In addition to the protection of patients from infectious agents, clinical and nonclinical health care personnel need to protect themselves as well. Health care personnel are at risk for occupational exposure to bloodborne pathogens, including hepatitis B virus (HBV), hepatitis C virus (HCV), and human immunodeficiency virus (HIV). Exposures occur through needlesticks or cuts from other sharp instruments contaminated with an infected patient's blood or through contact of the eyes, nose, mouth, or skin with a patient's blood. Important factors that influence the overall risk for occupational exposure to bloodborne pathogens include the number of infected individuals in the patient population and the type and number of blood contacts.[1] Many needlesticks and other penetrating exposures can be prevented by using safer techniques (for example, not recapping needles by hand), disposing of used needles in appropriate sharps disposal containers, and using medical devices with safety features designed to prevent injuries. Using appropriate barriers such as gloves, eye and face protection, or gowns when contact with blood is expected can prevent many exposures to the eyes, nose, mouth, or skin.

Exposure to bloodborne pathogens is of concern in health care settings. The emergency nurse will encounter a number of communicable diseases, depending on where he or she

works and how mobile the patient population is. Most of the focus has been on HBV, HCV, and HIV, but any infectious agent presents a potential risk under the right circumstances. To control the spread of hepatitis A and E, enteric precautions should be implemented. Needlestick prevention and blood precautions will assist in the control of hepatitis B, C, and D.

DISEASES OF CONCERN
Hepatitis

Hepatitis is an acute or chronic viral infection of the liver that may be mild or life threatening. Acute viral hepatitis is caused by five agents, the hepatitis A, B, C, D, and E virus. Of the hepatitis viruses, only HBV, HCV, and hepatitis D (HDV) can cause chronic hepatitis.

Hepatitis A

Hepatitis A, one of the oldest diseases known to humankind, is a self-limited disease that results in fulminant hepatitis and death in only a small proportion of patients. However, it is a significant cause of morbidity and socioeconomic losses in many parts of the world.

Transmission of HAV is typically by the fecal-oral route.[7,10,12] Because HAV is abundantly excreted in feces and can survive in the environment for prolonged periods of time, it is typically acquired by ingestion of feces-contaminated food or water. Direct person-to-person spread is common under poor hygienic conditions.[7] Occasionally HAV is also acquired through sexual contact (anal-oral) and blood transfusions.[7] People who have never contracted HAV and who are not vaccinated against hepatitis A are at risk for infection. The risk factors for HAV infection are related to resistance of HAV to the environment, poor sanitation in large areas of the world, and abundant HAV shedding in feces.[7] In areas where HAV is highly endemic, most HAV infections occur during early childhood.

Nosocomial HAV transmission is rare. Outbreaks have occasionally been observed in neonatal intensive care units when an infant acquires the infection from transfused blood and subsequently transmits hepatitis A to other infants and staff.[10] Outbreaks of hepatitis A caused by transmission from adult patients to health care workers are typically associated with fecal incontinence, although the majority of hospitalized patients who have hepatitis A are admitted after onset of jaundice, when they are beyond the point of peak infectivity.[10] Data from serologic surveys of health care workers have not indicated an increased prevalence of HAV infection in these groups compared with that in control populations.

The course of hepatitis A may be extremely variable.[7] Patients with inapparent or subclinical hepatitis have neither symptoms nor jaundice. Children generally belong to this group. Asymptomatic cases can be recognized only by detecting biochemical or serologic alterations in the blood.[7] Patients may develop anicteric or icteric hepatitis and have symptoms ranging from mild and transient to severe and

Table 38-1.	CLINICAL PHASES OF HEPATITIS A
Incubation or preclinical period	Ranging from 10 to 50 days, during which the patient remains asymptomatic despite active replication of the virus. In this phase, transmissibility is of greatest concern.
Prodromal or preicteric phase	Ranging from several days to more than a week, characterized by the appearance of symptoms such as loss of appetite, fatigue, abdominal pain, nausea and vomiting, fever, diarrhea, dark urine, and pale stools.
Icteric phase	Jaundice develops at total bilirubin levels exceeding 20-40 mg/L. Patients often seek medical help at this stage of their illness. The icteric phase generally begins within 10 days of the initial symptoms. Fever usually improves after the first few days of jaundice. Viremia terminates shortly after hepatitis develops, although feces remain infectious for another 1-2 weeks. Extrahepatic manifestations of hepatitis A are unusual. Physical examination of the patient by percussion can help to determine the size of the liver and possibly reveal massive necrosis. The mortality rate is low (0.2% of icteric cases), and the disease ultimately resolves. Occasionally, extensive necrosis of the liver occurs during the first 6-8 weeks of illness. In this case, high fever, marked abdominal pain, vomiting, jaundice, and the development of hepatic encephalopathy associated with coma and seizures are the signs of fulminant hepatitis, leading to death in 70%-90% of the patients. In these cases mortality is highly correlated with increasing age, and survival is uncommon over 50 years of age. Among patients with chronic hepatitis B or C or underlying liver disease who are superinfected with HAV, the mortality rate increases considerably.
Convalescent period	When resolution of the disease is slow, but patient recovery uneventful and complete. Relapsing hepatitis occurs in 3%-20% of patients 4-15 weeks after the initial symptoms have resolved. Cholestatic hepatitis with high bilirubin levels persisting for months is also occasionally observed. Chronic sequelae with persistence of HAV infection for more than 12 months are not observed.

HAV, Hepatitis A virus.

prolonged, from which they either recover completely or develop fulminant hepatitis and die. The severity of the disease increases with age at time of infection.[7] The course of acute hepatitis A can be divided into four clinical phases identified in Table 38-1.

Hepatitis A cannot be differentiated from other types of viral hepatitis on the basis of clinical or epidemiologic features alone. Serologic testing to detect immunoglobulin M (IgM) antibody to the capsid proteins of HAV (IgM anti-HAV) is required to confirm a diagnosis of acute HAV infection. In the majority of persons, serum IgM anti-HAV becomes detectable 5 to 10 days before onset of symptoms.[8,11] IgG anti-HAV, which appears early in the course of infection, remains detectable for the person's lifetime and provides lifelong protection against the disease. In the majority of patients, IgM anti-HAV declines to undetectable levels less than 6 months after infection.[8,11]

Better hygienic and sanitary conditions and development of the hepatitis A vaccine have led to a decline in the overall incidence of hepatitis A in the United States over the past several decades. The vaccines containing HAV antigen that are currently licensed in the United States are the single-antigen vaccines HAVRIX (manufactured by GlaxoSmithKline) and VAQTA (manufactured by Merck & Co., Inc.) and the combination vaccine TWINRIX (containing both HAV and HBV antigens; manufactured by GlaxoSmithKline). All are inactivated vaccines. An inactive hepatitis A vaccine has been shown to be safe, immunogenic, and efficacious. Protection against clinical HAV may begin in some people 14 to 21 days after a single dose of vaccine; nearly all have protective antibodies by 30 days. Hepatitis A immunization is recommended for anyone who plans to travel repeatedly or reside for long periods in areas where people are at risk

for infection and for children living in communities with the highest rates of infection and disease. Individuals employed in hospitals or day care centers should also be immunized.

For proven cases of hepatitis A, enteric precautions are necessary during the first 2 weeks of illness but for no more than 1 week after onset of jaundice. Persons who have been recently exposed to HAV and who have not previously received hepatitis A vaccine should be administered a single dose of immune globulin (IG) (0.02 mL/kg) as soon as possible after exposure. Efficacy when administered more than 2 weeks after exposure has not been established. Persons who have been administered one dose of hepatitis A vaccine at greater than or equal to 1 month before exposure to HAV do not need IG. Hepatitis A vaccine and IG are not indicated for contacts if they do not fall into the following categories: close personal contacts, including household, sexual, or drug using; day care center attendees/workers if one or more cases of hepatitis A are identified; and common-source outbreak related to food handling.

The World Health Organization (WHO) has recommendations for the use of hepatitis A vaccine. In industrialized nations with low endemicity and high rates of disease in specific high-risk populations (men who have sex with men, injecting drug users, all susceptible persons traveling to or working in countries where HAV is endemic, persons who work with HAV-infected primates or in research laboratories), vaccination of these populations may be recommended.

Hepatitis B

HBV is a widely distributed pathogen that produces acute and chronic infection. Chronically infected people represent the major source of infection. Individuals have an increased risk for mortality and morbidity associated with chronic liver disease and primary hepatocellular carcinoma. HBV is a worldwide problem existing even in the most remote and isolated populations of the world. Prevalence of HBV infection varies widely. The disease is highly endemic in most of the developing world but is minimally endemic in developed countries. Of the 2 billion people who have been infected with HBV, more than 350 million have chronic (lifelong) infections. These chronically infected persons are at high risk for death from cirrhosis of the liver and liver cancer, diseases that kill about 1 million persons each year. Although the vaccine will not cure chronic hepatitis, it is 95% effective in preventing chronic infections from developing and is the first vaccine effective against a major human cancer. Despite vaccine availability, it is estimated that over 4 million new acute clinical cases occur each year.

Hepatitis B virus is transmitted by contact with blood or body fluids (saliva; cerebrospinal fluid; peritoneal, pleural, pericardial and synovial fluid; amniotic fluid; semen and vaginal secretions and any other body fluid containing blood; and unfixed tissues and organs) of an infected person. Transmission occurs by exposure to infected body fluids via the percutaneous or per mucosal route.

Worldwide, the major modes of HBV transmission include sexual or close household contact with an infected person, mother-to-infant transmission, the reuse of unsterilized needles and syringes, and nosocomial. Sexual transmission from infected men to women is about three times more efficient than that from women to men, and anal intercourse is associated with an increased risk for infection. The transmission of HBV in household occurs primarily from child to child. Perinatal transmission is common when the mother is hepatitis Be antigen (HBeAg)-positive. Intravenous (IV) drug users are at risk if they share syringes and needles contaminated with blood. In addition, hepatitis B virus is the major infectious occupational hazard of health care workers, despite the fact that most health care workers have received the hepatitis B vaccine.

The incubation period for HBV averages 60 to 80 days, with the norm 45 to180 days; however, the incubation period can range from 2 weeks to 6 to 9 months when hepatitis B surface antigen (HBsAg) appears. Extreme variation in the incubation period is related in part to the amount of virus in the inoculum, mode of transmission, alteration of viral pathogenicity by chemical or physical means, administration of a specific antibody, and unusual virus-host interactions.[7]

All people who are HBsAg-positive and HBeAg-positive are potentially infectious. Both antigens are detectable 1 to 3 weeks after exposure and 4 to 5 weeks before onset of jaundice. Infectivity of chronically infected individuals varies from highly infectious (HBeAg-positive) to sparingly infectious (anti–HBe-positive).[7]

Diagnosis of HBV is based on clinical, serologic, and epidemiologic findings. Detection of HBV infection serologic markers—HBsAg—confirms hepatitis B infection. Infection may present with a variety of symptomatology: acute illness with jaundice followed by recovery, subclinical infection followed by recovery, acute illness that progresses to chronic active hepatitis, subclinical infection followed by chronic active hepatitis, and fulminant disease.[7] Viral hepatitis is the most common infectious cause of jaundice. A short prodromal phase, varying from several days to more than a week, may precede onset of jaundice. Typical symptoms include anorexia, weakness, and fatigue. Nausea, vomiting, and diarrhea may also occur. Many patients complain of right upper quadrant abdominal pain. The preicteric phase may be characterized by fever (usually 103° F [39° C] or more), malaise, myalgia, and headache. Other symptoms are similar to serum sickness: arthritis, arthralgia, and urticaria or maculopapular rash.[7] The icteric phase begins with the appearance of dark urine resulting from bilirubinuria, followed by light or gray stools, and yellowish discoloration of mucous membranes, sclera, conjunctivae, and skin. Jaundice becomes apparent when total bilirubin levels exceed 2.0 to 3.0 mg/dL. Hepatic tenderness and hepatomegaly are also present.[7] Recovery begins with the disappearance of jaundice and other symptoms. HBsAg and HBeAg also disappear. The appearance of antibodies (anti-HBs and anti-HB) indicates the infection is subsiding. Liver failure may occur in 1% to 3% of patients with acute hepatitis B.[7] This potentially fatal disease is characterized by mental confusion, emotional instability, bleeding manifestations, and coma. The case fatality rate is about 1% higher in those over 40 years of age.

The most effective method of infection control against hepatitis B is the hepatitis B vaccine. Hepatitis B vaccine prevents hepatitis B disease and its serious consequences such as hepatocellular carcinoma (liver cancer). Hepatitis B vaccine has been available since 1982. The current vaccine used in the United State is a recombinant product derived from HBAg grown in yeast. Vaccines licensed in different parts of the world may have varying dosages and immunization schedules. In the United States the vaccine is primarily administered in three intramuscular (IM) doses. For infants, the first dose is administered at birth with subsequent doses at 1 to 2 and 6 to 18 months of age. In adults, the immunization schedule consists of three IM doses. After the first dose, subsequent doses are administered at 1 to 2 and 4 to 6 months. Current data show that vaccine-induced hepatitis B surface antibody (anti-HBs) levels may decline over time; however, immune memory (amnestic anti-HBs response) remains intact indefinitely following immunization. Therefore persons with declining antibody levels are still protected against clinical illness and chronic disease. Postvaccination testing for adequate antibody response is not necessary after routine vaccination of infants, children, adolescents, or adults. A combination of active and passive immunization is used for nonimmunized persons who have sustained a percutaneous or mucous membrane exposure to blood that might contain HBsAg. If the decision is made to provide postexposure prophylaxis, then a single dose of hepatitis B immune globulin (HBIG) (0.06 mL/kg) should be given as soon as possible, or at least within 24 hours of a high-risk needlestick, and the hepatitis B vaccine series should be started. If the vaccine cannot be given, a second dose of HBIG should be provided 1 month after the first.

WHO's hepatitis B prevention strategy is based on routine universal newborn or infant immunization. The current strategy in the United States includes screening of all pregnant women, providing HBIG and hepatitis B vaccine to infants of HBsAg- positive mothers, providing hepatitis B vaccine to susceptible household contacts, providing routine hepatitis B vaccine for all infants, and providing catch-up immunizations to unimmunized children and adolescents. In addition, there is also an effort to immunize adolescents and adults in defined risk groups.

Hepatitis C

HCV is transmitted parenterally. This infection has been found in every part of the world. The prevalence is directly related to poor parenteral practices in the health care setting and persons who share injection equipment. The WHO estimates that approximately 3% of the world's population is infected with the hepatitis C virus, 130 million of whom are chronic HCV carriers at risk for developing liver cirrhosis and/or liver cancer. WHO also estimates that 3 to 4 million persons are newly infected each year, 70% of whom will develop chronic hepatitis. HCV is responsible for 50% to 76% of all liver cancer cases and two thirds of all liver transplants in the developed world. The prevalence of HCV infection in some countries in Africa, the Eastern Mediterranean, Southeast Asia, and the Western Pacific (when prevalence data are available) is high compared to some countries in North America and Europe.

HCV is spread primarily by direct contact with human blood. Transmission through blood transfusions that are not screened for HCV infection; through the reuse of inadequately sterilized needles, syringes, or other medical equipment; or through needle sharing among drug users is well documented. Sexual and perinatal transmission may also occur, although less frequently. Other modes of transmission such as social, cultural, and behavioral practices using percutaneous procedures (e.g., ear and body piercing, circumcision, tattooing) can occur if inadequately sterilized equipment is used. HCV is not spread by sneezing, hugging, coughing, food or water, sharing eating utensils, or casual contact.

In both developed and developing countries, high-risk groups include injecting drug users, recipients of unscreened blood, hemophiliacs, dialysis patients, and persons with multiple sex partners who engage in unprotected sex.

In developed countries, it is estimated that 90% of persons with chronic HCV infection are current and former injecting drug users and those with a history of transfusion of unscreened blood or blood products.

In many developing countries, where unscreened blood and blood products are still being used, the major means of transmission are unsterilized injection equipment and unscreened blood transfusions. In addition, people who use traditional scarification and circumcision practices are at risk if they use or reuse unsterilized tools.

Health care workers frequently come into contact with blood, so there is increased risk for infection. However, prevalence of HCV infection is no greater among health care workers than among the general population.

The incubation period ranges from 2 weeks to 6 months with an average range at 6 to 9 weeks. The period of communicability may range from 1 or more weeks before the first onset of symptoms and may persist indefinitely. Peaks in virus concentration appear to correlate with peaks in serum alanine transaminase (ALT) activity.

Onset is usually insidious, with severity ranging from those without apparent disease to rare fulminating, fatal cases. Symptoms include anorexia, vague abdominal discomfort, nausea, and vomiting. Jaundice is seen less frequently than with the hepatitis B virus. The disease is usually less severe in the acute stage but chronicity is common, occurring more frequently than with hepatitis B in adults. Chronic infection may be symptomatic or asymptomatic. Persons with chronic hepatitis C may develop cirrhosis or hepatocellular carcinoma.

Diagnosis depends on detecting antibodies (anti-HCV) to HCV. Unfortunately, the antibody response in acute disease remains negative for 1 to 3 weeks after clinical onset and may never become positive in less than 20% of patients with acute, resolving disease. Assays of hepatitis C virus RNA by polymerase chain reaction (PCR) or other methods may be used for diagnosis, estimating progress, predicting interferon responsiveness, and monitoring therapy.

There is no vaccine against HCV. In the absence of a vaccine, all precautions to prevent infection must be taken, including screening and testing of blood and organ donors; virus inactivation of plasma-derived products; implementation and maintenance of infection control practices in health care settings, including appropriate sterilization of medical and dental equipment; promotion of behavior change among the general public and health care workers to reduce overuse of injections and to use safe injection practices; and risk reduction counseling for persons with high-risk drug and sexual practices.

Available data regarding prevention of HCV infection with IG indicate that IG is not effective for postexposure prophylaxis of hepatitis C.[3]

Hepatitis D

Hepatitis delta virus (HDV) is a defective virus that causes infection only in the presence of active HBV infection. HDV infection occurs as either coinfection with HBV or superinfection of an HBV carrier. Coinfection usually resolves, whereas superinfection frequently causes chronic HDV infection and chronic active hepatitis.

The prevalence of HDV varies widely, occurring epidemically and endemically in populations at high risk for acquiring HBV. Mode of transmission is thought to be similar to HBV, including exposure to blood and serous body fluids, needles, syringes, plasma derivatives, and sexual contact. Blood is potentially infectious during all phases of active HDV infection. Peak infectivity probably occurs before the onset of acute illness.

Onset is usually abrupt, with signs and symptoms resembling those of HBV infection. Symptoms may be severe and are always associated with a coexisting HBV infection. An HDV infection may be self-limiting or may progress to chronic hepatitis. Diagnosis is made by detection of total antibody to HDV (anti-HDV). ALT, alkaline phosphatase, and bilirubin levels are usually elevated.

General control measures against bloodborne pathogens apply. Prevention of HBV infection with hepatitis B vaccine prevents infection with HDV. However, hepatitis B immune globulin, IG, and hepatitis B vaccine do not protect HBV carriers from infection by HDV.

Hepatitis E

Hepatitis E virus (HEV) is the major causal agent of enterically transmitted non-A, non-B hepatitis worldwide. HEV infections account for more than 50% of acute sporadic hepatitis in some highly endemic areas.

Man is the natural host for HEV, and transmission occurs primarily by the fecal-oral route. Hepatitis E is a waterborne disease, and contaminated water or food supplies have been implicated in major outbreaks. Consumption of fecally contaminated drinking water has given rise to epidemics, and the ingestion of raw or uncooked shellfish has been the source of sporadic cases in endemic areas. Person-to-person transmission is uncommon.

The incubation period following exposure to HEV ranges from 3 to 8 weeks, with a mean of 40 days. The period of communicability is unknown. There are no chronic infections reported. Hepatitis E virus causes acute sporadic and epidemic viral hepatitis. Symptomatic HEV infection is most common in young adults 15 to 40 years of age.

Typical signs and symptoms of hepatitis include jaundice (yellow discoloration of the skin and sclera of the eyes, dark urine, and pale stools); anorexia (loss of appetite); an enlarged, tender liver (hepatomegaly); abdominal pain and tenderness; nausea and vomiting; and fever, although the disease may range in severity from subclinical to fulminant. Because cases of hepatitis E are not clinically distinguishable from other types of acute viral hepatitis, diagnosis is made by blood tests that detect elevated antibody levels of specific antibodies to hepatitis E.

There are no commercially available vaccines for the prevention of hepatitis E. Because almost all HEV infections are spread by the fecal-oral route, good personal hygiene, high-quality standards for public water supplies, and proper disposal of sanitary waste have resulted in a low prevalence of HEV infections in many well-developed societies.

Human Immune Deficiency Virus/Acquired Immunodeficiency Syndrome

Acquired immunodeficiency syndrome (AIDS) was first reported in 1981; however, isolated cases occurred in the United States and other areas of the world during the 1970s. Human immune deficiency virus (HIV) and AIDS have been recorded in virtually all countries among all races, ages, and social classes. At the end of 2003 an estimated 1,039,000 to 1,185,000 persons in the United States were living with HIV/AIDS, with 24% to 27% undiagnosed and unaware of their HIV infection.[4]

Worldwide, the Joint United Nations Programme on HIV/AIDS noted that in 2006, 4.3 million people were newly infected with HIV and 2.9 million people died of HIV-related illnesses.

The course of HIV disease is variable and dictated by the severity of the individual's immune deficiency and any resulting complications. The primary causative viral agent is the human immunodeficiency virus type 1 (HIV-1). In 1986 a second type of HIV, called HIV-2, was isolated from AIDS patients in West Africa. Both HIV-1 and HIV-2 have the same modes of transmission and are associated with similar opportunistic infections and AIDS. In persons infected with HIV-2, immunodeficiency seems to develop more slowly and to be milder. Compared with persons infected with HIV-1, those with HIV-2 are less infectious early in the course of infection. As the disease advances, HIV-2 infectiousness seems to increase; however, compared with HIV-1, the duration of this increased infectiousness is shorter. HIV-1 and HIV-2 also differ in geographic patterns of infection; the United States has few reported cases of HIV-2.

The primary mode of HIV transmission is person to person through unprotected intercourse; contact of abraded skin or mucosa with body secretions such as blood, cerebral spinal fluid (CSF), or semen; the use of HIV-contaminated needles and syringes; transfusion of infected blood or its components; and the transplantation of HIV-infected tissues or organs. HIV can also be transmitted from mother to child; 15% to 30% of infants born to HIV-infected mothers are infected through placental processes at birth.[6] Treatment of pregnant women has resulted in a marked reduction in infant infections. Breastfeeding by HIV-infected women can transmit infection to the infant, and this can account for up to half of mother-to-child HIV transmission.

Direct exposure of health care workers to HIV-infected blood through percutaneous exposure is associated with seroconversion in less than 0.5% of the cases.[6] The virus has been detected in saliva, tears, urine, and bronchial secretions; however, transmission after contact with these body fluids has not been reported.

The incubation period is variable. The most commonly used screening test for HIV, enzyme-linked immunosorbent assay, is highly sensitive and specific. When this test is reactive, an additional test such as the Western blot or indirect fluorescent antibody (IFA) test should be obtained. The time from infection to the development of detectable antibodies is generally 1 to 3 months; the time from HIV infection to diagnosis of AIDS has been noted to range from less than 1 year to 15 years or longer. The impact of highly active antiretroviral therapy has been shown to reduce the development of clinical AIDS in most industrialized nations. The only factor that has been associated with the progression from HIV infection to AIDS is the age of the patient at initial infection.

The period of communicability is unknown but is presumed to begin soon after onset of HIV infection and extend throughout life. Epidemiologic evidence suggests infectivity increases with increasing immune deficiency, clinical symptoms, and presence of other sexually transmitted diseases.

Table 38-2.	STAGES OF HIV DISEASE AND COMMON CLINICAL SYNDROMES				
Stages	**Constitutional**	**CNS**	**Gastrointestinal**	**Respiratory**	**Cutaneous**
Early disease (CD4 >500)	Bacterial pneumonia Tuberculosis				Rash Bacterial infections Kaposi's sarcoma lesions
Midstage disease (CD4 200-500)	Disseminated tuberculosis Sexually transmitted disease Anorectal infections		Thrush		Mucocutaneous candidiasis Oral hairy leukoplakia Herpes zoster Psoriasis Seborrheic dermatitis Atopic dermatitis
Late disease (CD4 75-200)	Disseminated tuberculosis Nontyphoid salmonella bacteremia Bartonellosis Fungal disease	Cryptococcal meningitis Herpes virus family Encephalitis *Toxoplasma* encephalitis *Cryptococcus* meningitis Herpes virus family Primary CNS lymphoma	*Candida* esophageal mucosal infection with oral lesions		More chronic skin infections that are refractory to therapy Eosinophilic folliculitis
Advanced disease (CD4 <75)	Disseminated *Mycobacterium avium* Systemic CMV infections	Primary CNS lymphoma Advanced AIDS dementia complex	*Candida* esophageal mucosal infection with oral lesions CMV and aphthous ulcers	*Pneumocystis jiroveci* pneumonia (PCP) Fungal pneumonia Kaposi's sarcoma–related pulmonary lesions	Unusual skin lesions Bacillary angiomatosis Molluscum contagiosum

AIDS, Acquired immunodeficiency virus; *CMV,* cytomegalovirus; *CNS,* central nervous system; *HIV,* human immunodeficiency virus.

Recent studies suggest infectiousness may be high during the initial period after infection.[1]

CD4 lymphocytes are the major cellular target for HIV. The CD4 count (Table 38-2) and the rate of decline have prognostic predictive value and are used to determine the need for antiretroviral therapy and for opportunistic infection prophylaxis. HIV infection can produce a variety of clinical syndromes. These syndromes correlate with the duration of the illness and severity of immunosuppression. More than a dozen opportunistic infections are considered AIDS infections, including several cancers, pulmonary and extrapulmonary tuberculosis (TB), recurrent pneumonia, wasting syndrome, neurologic disease (HIV dementia or sensory neuropathy), and invasive cervical cancer. AIDS is a severe, life-threatening clinical condition. This syndrome represents the late clinical stage of infection with HIV and is most often the result of progressive damage to the immune and other organ systems.

Currently there is not a vaccine to prevent HIV. Prevention of infection relies on controlling transmission of the virus. Control includes both prevention counseling and postexposure prophylaxis (PEP). Precautions to minimize the risk for transmission in the health care setting must be implemented. Prevention of occupational exposures should involve education

and reinforcement of the use of barrier precautions. In addition, the implementation of safety devices and the appropriate disposal of contaminated materials are essential.

Postexposure prophylaxis is complex but has become widely accepted after a high-risk occupational exposure. There are several factors to consider before recommending PEP: the nature of the exposure, whether the exposed worker might be pregnant, and the local occurrence of drug-resistant HIV strains (Box 38-1). Because of the complexity of selection of HIV PEP regimens, consultation with persons having expertise in antiretroviral therapy and HIV transmission is strongly recommended to adequately determine the need for PEP and most appropriate treatment regimen.[3] Resources for consultation are noted in Box 38-2.

Health care providers with occupational exposure to HIV should receive follow-up counseling, postexposure testing, and medical evaluation regardless of whether they receive PEP.

Methicillin-Resistant *Staphylococcus aureus*

Staphylococcus aureus bacteria are generally harmless unless they enter the body through a cut or other wound, and even then they often cause only minor skin problems in healthy

---

Box 38-1 SITUATIONS FOR WHICH EXPERT CONSULTATION FOR HIV POSTEXPOSURE PROPHYLAXIS (PEP) IS ADVISED

- Delayed (i.e., later than 24 to 36 hours) exposure report
  - Interval after which lack of benefit from PEP undefined
- Unknown source (e.g., needle in sharps disposal container or laundry)
  - Use of PEP to be decided on a case-by-case basis
  - Consider severity of exposure and epidemiologic likelihood of HIV exposure
  - Do not test needles or other sharp instruments for HIV
- Known or suspected pregnancy in the exposed person
  - Use of optimal PEP regimens not precluded
  - PEP not denied solely on basis of pregnancy
- Breastfeeding in the exposed person
  - Use of optimal PEP regimens not precluded
  - PEP not denied solely on basis of breastfeeding
- Resistance of the source virus to antiretroviral agents
  - Influence of drug resistance on transmission risk unknown

- If source person's virus is known or suspected to be resistant to one or more of the drugs considered for PEP, selection of drugs to which the source person's virus is unlikely to be resistant is recommended
  - Resistance testing of the source person's virus at the time of the exposure not recommended
  - Initiation of PEP not to be delayed while awaiting any results of resistance testing
- Toxicity of the initial PEP regimen
  - Adverse symptoms (e.g., nausea and diarrhea) common with PEP
  - Symptoms often manageable without changing PEP regimen by prescribing antimotility or antiemetic agents
  - In other situations, modifying the dose interval (i.e., taking drugs after meals or administering a lower dose of drug more frequently throughout the day, as recommended by the manufacturer) might help alleviate symptoms when they occur

From MMWR September 30, 2005, Vol 54, No. RR-9. Retrieved from http://www.cdc.gov/mmwr/PDF/rr/rr5409.pdf.
Updated US Public Health Service guidelines for the management of occupational exposures to HBV, HCV, and HIV and recommendations for postexposure prophylaxis, *MMWR Recomm Rep* 50(RR-11):1, 2001. Retrieved from http://www.cdc.gov/mmwr/preview/mmwrhtml/rr5011a1.htm.

Box 38-2 RESOURCES FOR CONSULTATION

Resources for consultation are available from the following sources:
- PEP line at http://www.ucsf.edu/hivcntr/Hotlines/PEPline; telephone 888-448-4911
- HIV Antiretroviral Pregnancy Registry at http://www.apregistry.com/index.htm
- FDA (for reporting unusual or severe toxicity to antiretroviral agents) at http://www.fda.gov/medwatch
- CDC (for reporting HIV infections in HCP and failures of PEP) at telephone 800-893-0485
- HIV/AIDS Treatment Information Service at http://aidsinfo.nih.gov

AIDS, Acquired immunodeficiency syndrome; *CDC,* Centers for Disease Control and Prevention; *FDA,* Food and Drug Administration; *HCP,* health care personnel; *HIV,* human immunodeficiency virus; *PEP,* postexposure prophylaxis.

people. Decades ago a strain of staphylococcus emerged in hospitals that was resistant to the broad-spectrum antibiotics commonly used to treat it and became known as methicillin-resistant *Staphylococcus aureus* (MRSA). It is resistant to antibiotics called β-lactams. β-Lactam antibiotics include methicillin and other more common antibiotics such as oxacillin, penicillin, and amoxicillin.

It is estimated that 25% to 30% of the United States population is colonized with *S. aureus* at any given time.[6] However, the number of MRSA-colonized people at any one time is not known.

Colonization is the presence of the bacteria on a person's body without observable clinical symptoms. When a person is colonized, bacteria live on the skin but cause no harm.

MRSA colonization can also occur in the nose, pharynx, axilla, rectum, and perineum.

Infection refers to the invasion of bacteria into tissue with growth of the organism. Infection may occur when the bacteria enter a break in the skin. *S. aureus* infections, including MRSA, generally start as small red bumps that resemble pimples, boils, or spider bites[6] but can quickly turn into deep, painful abscesses that require surgical draining. Sometimes the bacteria remain confined to the skin. But they can also burrow deep into the body, causing potentially life-threatening infections in bones, joints, heart valves, and lungs. MRSA infection can be fatal.

MRSA has become a prevalent nosocomial pathogen in the United States. *S. aureus* infections, including MRSA, occur most frequently among persons in hospitals and health care facilities (such as nursing homes and dialysis centers) who have weakened immune systems. Health care–associated MRSA (HA-MRSA) infections include surgical wound infections, urinary tract infections, bloodstream infections, and pneumonia.

In hospitals the most important reservoirs of HA-MRSA are infected or colonized patients. Although hospital personnel can serve as reservoirs for MRSA and may harbor the organism for many months, they have been more commonly identified as a link for transmission between colonized or infected patients.

It has been well documented that the primary route of transmission of MRSA is via the hands of health care workers, which may become contaminated by contact with colonized or infected patients; colonized or infected body sites of the personnel themselves; or devices, items, or environmental surfaces contaminated with body fluids containing MRSA.

The role played by the inanimate environment in transmission is uncertain. The ability of MRSA to contaminate a large variety of hospital items (e.g., chairs, bed frames, and mattresses) has been demonstrated in several studies. Studies have also shown that *S. aureus* has the potential to survive for long periods and is resistant to desiccation. Although there is no evidence demonstrating the direct transmission of MRSA from the environment to patients, there is evidence that contamination of the environment with MRSA is sufficient to contaminate the gloves of health care providers and thus lead to transmission to patients.

Doctors diagnose MRSA by checking a tissue sample or nasal secretions for signs of drug-resistant bacteria. In the hospital, patients may be tested for MRSA if they show signs of infection or if they are transferred into a hospital from another health care setting where MRSA is known to be present. Patients may also be tested if they have a previous history of MRSA.

Along with *S. aureus,* many significant infection-causing bacteria are becoming resistant to the most commonly prescribed antimicrobial treatments. Antimicrobial resistance occurs when bacteria change or adapt in a way that allows them to survive in the presence of antibiotics designed to kill them. In some cases bacteria become so resistant that no available antibiotics are effective against them. The leading causes of antibiotic resistance are the following:

- *Unnecessary antibiotic use in humans:* Like other resistant bacteria, MRSA is the result of decades of excessive and unnecessary antibiotic use. For years, antibiotics have been prescribed for viral infections that do not respond to these drugs, as well as for simple bacterial infections that normally clear on their own.
- *Antibiotics in food and water:* Prescription drugs are not the only source of antibiotics. In the United States, antibiotics can be found in cattle, pigs, and chickens. Antibiotics given in the proper doses to animals that are sick do not appear to produce resistant bacteria.
- *Germ mutation:* Even when antibiotics are used appropriately, they contribute to the rise of drug-resistant bacteria because they do not destroy every germ they target. Bacteria live on an evolutionary fast track, so germs that survive treatment with one antibiotic soon learn to resist others. And because bacteria mutate much more quickly than new drugs can be produced, some germs end up resistant to most available treatments.

At this time, treatment options still exist for HA-MRSA but are limited because HA-MRSA is resistant to many antibiotics. Vancomycin is one of the few antibiotics still effective against MRSA.

People infected with antibiotic-resistant organisms like MRSA are more likely to have longer and more expensive hospital stays and may be more likely to die as a result of the infection. When the drug of choice for treating an infection is not effective, treatment with second- or third-choice medicines may be less efficacious, more toxic, and more expensive.

According to the Centers for Disease Control and Prevention (CDC),[2] standard precautions and contact precautions

---

Box 38-3	**RISK FACTORS ASSOCIATED WITH MRSA**

- History of MRSA infection, colonization
- History of (within past 12 months) hospitalization, dialysis or renal failure, diabetes, surgery, long-term care residence, indwelling catheter or medical device
- Injection drug use, incarceration
- Close contact with someone known to be infected or colonized with MRSA
- High prevalence of MRSA in community or population
- Local risk factors: consult local public health department

MRSA, Methicillin-resistant *Staphylococcus aureus.*

---

should be used for all patients who present with open or draining skin or soft-tissue infections (SSTI) and all patients known to be infected with MRSA or at high risk (Box 38-3) for being infected with MRSA. The following conditions should apply:
- Examine patient in a private room.
- Wear gloves (clean nonsterile gloves are adequate) when providing care for patients; change gloves after having contact with infective material that may contain high concentrations of microorganisms (e.g., wound drainage or dressings). Remove gloves before leaving the patient's room, and wash hands immediately with an antimicrobial agent. After glove removal and hand washing, do not touch potentially contaminated environmental surfaces or items in the patient's room to avoid transfer of microorganisms to other patients and environments.
- Wear an isolation gown when providing care if there will be substantial contact with the patient's wound. This will protect skin and prevent soiling of clothes during procedures and patient-care activities that are likely to generate splashes or sprays of blood, body fluids, secretions, and excretions or cause soiling of clothing. Remove the gown before leaving the examination room.
- Wear a mask and eye protection or a face shield to protect mucous membranes of the eyes, nose, and mouth during procedures and patient-care activities that are likely to generate splashes or sprays of blood, body fluids, secretions, and excretions.
- Limit the movement and transport of the patient from the examination room to essential purposes only.
- Handle used patient-care equipment soiled with blood, body fluids, secretions, and excretions in a manner that prevents skin and mucous membrane exposures, contamination of clothing, and transfer of microorganisms to other patients and environments. Ensure that reusable equipment is not used for the care of another patient until it has been appropriately cleaned and reprocessed and that single-use items are properly discarded.
- Handle, transport, and process used linen soiled with blood, body fluids, secretions, and excretions in a manner that prevents skin and mucous membrane exposures, contamination of clothing, and transfer of microorganisms to other patients and environments. Any unused linen in the room should be discarded as if it were soiled.

- Ensure that patient-care items and potentially contaminated surfaces are cleaned and disinfected after use.
- Clean non-critical medical equipment surfaces with a detergent/disinfectant.
- Do not use alcohol to disinfect large environmental surfaces.
- Use barrier protective coverings as appropriate for noncritical surfaces that are (1) touched frequently with gloved hands during the delivery of patient care, (2) likely to become contaminated with blood or body substances, or (3) difficult to clean.
- Select Environmental Protection Agency (EPA)-registered disinfectants, if available, and use them in accordance with the manufacturer's instructions.
- Keep housekeeping surfaces (e.g., floors, walls, tabletops) visibly clean on a regular basis and clean up spills promptly.
- Use an EPA-registered hospital detergent/disinfectant designed for general housekeeping purposes in patient-care areas when uncertainty exists regarding the presence of multidrug-resistant organisms.

Tuberculosis

TB is caused by *Mycobacterium tuberculosis* and usually infects the lungs (pulmonary TB) or respiratory system. TB is a potentially life-threatening infection. If left untreated, TB can be fatal. Every year, TB kills nearly 2 million people worldwide. Prevalence of TB is not distributed evenly throughout the U.S. population. Some subgroups or individuals have a higher risk for TB because they are more likely than others in the general population to be exposed and infected or because their exposure is more likely to progress to active TB. The overall incidence of TB in the United States is quite low, but case rates are high among specific populations such as HIV-infected patients, the homeless, recent immigrants from countries that have a high prevalence of TB, intravenous drug users, inner-city dwellers, and minorities.

The number of new TB cases reported in the United States declined by 2.9% from 2004 to 2005, continuing a 13-year downward trend since the TB epidemic peaked in 1992, according to final data released by the CDC. A total of 14,097 TB cases were reported in 2005, an all-time low. Unfortunately, the incidence of TB is on the rise worldwide. The growing global TB epidemic could affect the declines made in the United States if TB defense systems are not maintained. In 2005 the proportion of total cases occurring in the foreign born was 55%, constituting a majority of cases for the fourth consecutive year.[5]

WHO estimates that the largest number of new TB cases in 2005 occurred in the South-East Asia Region, which accounted for 34% of incident cases globally. However, the estimated incidence rate in sub-Saharan Africa is nearly twice that of the South-East Asia Region, at nearly 350 cases per 100,000 population.

Until 50 years ago, there were no medications to cure TB. Now, strains that are resistant to a single drug have been documented in every country surveyed; what is more, strains of TB resistant to all major anti-TB drugs have emerged. Drug-resistant TB is caused by inconsistent or partial treatment, when patients do not take all their medications regularly for the required period because they start to feel better, because doctors and health care workers prescribe the wrong treatment regimens, or because the drug supply is unreliable. A particularly dangerous form of drug-resistant TB is multidrug-resistant TB (MDR-TB), which is defined as the disease caused by TB bacilli resistant to at least isoniazid and rifampicin (rifampin), the two most powerful anti-TB drugs available. Rates of MDR-TB are high in some countries, especially in the former Soviet Union, and threaten TB control efforts.

Although drug-resistant TB is generally treatable, it requires extensive chemotherapy (up to 2 years of treatment) with second-line anti-TB drugs that are more costly than first-line drugs and produce adverse drug reactions that are more severe, though manageable. The emergence of extensively drug-resistant (XDR) TB, particularly in settings where many TB patients are also infected with HIV, poses a serious threat to TB control and confirms the urgent need to strengthen basic TB control and apply the WHO guidelines for the management of drug-resistant TB.

TB spreads when a person is exposed to tubercle bacilli carried in airborne particles or droplet nuclei. The droplet nuclei are produced by people with pulmonary or respiratory tract TB during expiratory efforts such as coughing, singing, or sneezing. The nuclei are then inhaled into the pulmonary alveoli by a vulnerable contact, where they are taken up by the alveolar macrophages. Some macrophages are capable of killing the bacillus; others are not. The bacilli multiply within the cells and produce infection. Factors that influence the progression of infection to disease include the intensity of exposure, interval since infection, age, and other coexisting or comorbid diseases. Extrapulmonary TB develops when the bacillus travels to other organs by way of the bloodstream.

Although a person may harbor the TB bacteria, his or her immune system often can prevent the person from becoming sick. For that reason, doctors make a distinction between TB infection and active TB disease. TB infection, sometimes called latent TB, causes no symptoms and is not contagious. Latent infection may persist for a lifetime; however, risk for progression to TB disease is greatest within the first year or two. Active TB disease is defined as tissue involvement by the *M. tuberculosis* bacillus that progresses to produce clinical signs and symptoms. On average, illness develops in 3% to 5% of infected patients.

TB mainly affects the lungs, and coughing is often the only indication of infection initially. Signs and symptoms of active pulmonary TB include a cough lasting 3 or more weeks that may produce discolored or bloody sputum, unintended weight loss, fatigue, slight fever, night sweats, chills, loss of appetite, and pain with breathing or coughing (pleurisy).

The incubation period, the time from infection to demonstrable primary lesion or significant tuberculin reaction, is about 2 to 10 weeks. Theoretically, as long as viable tubercle bacilli are discharged in the sputum, the person may be infectious.

The degree of communicability is dependent on the number of bacilli discharged, virulence of the bacilli, adequacy of ventilation, exposure of bacilli to sun or ultraviolet (UV) light, and opportunities for aerosolization through coughing, sneezing, talking, or singing or during procedures.

Nosocomial transmission of TB has been associated with close contact with people who have infectious TB and performance of procedures such as bronchoscopy, endotracheal intubation, suctioning, open abscess irrigation, and autopsy. Sputum induction and aerosol treatments that induce coughing may also increase the potential for transmission

Diagnosis is confirmed by recovery of TB from a sputum sample, positive chest radiograph, and positive tuberculin skin test (purified protein derivative [PPD]). In some immunocompromised patients a PPD test result may be negative even though these patients are infected.

TB prevention and control programs should be established in all countries and health care settings. Triage guidelines should include identification of potential TB patients (Box 38-4). If a patient is diagnosed with active TB disease, the following therapeutic interventions should be considered: airborne precautions to prevent spread, administration of antituberculin drugs, and supportive care. For pulmonary TB, control of infectivity is best achieved through prompt, specific drug treatment, usually leading to sputum conversion in 4 to 8 weeks. Hospitalization is necessary for patients with severe disease requiring hospital level care and for those who are unable to care for themselves due to medical or social

circumstances. Negative-pressure ventilation rooms are recommended for isolation of these patients. Patients who have bacteriologically negative sputum, who do not cough, and are known to be on appropriate chemotherapy do not require isolation.

For patients with latent disease, preventive chemotherapy is recommended for persons who are or have been in contact with TB infection and TB disease has been ruled out. Treatment is also recommended for high-risk individuals.

In nonindustrialized countries the bacille Calmette-Guérin (BCG) vaccine is administered to prevent TB disease. BCG is used in many countries with a high prevalence of TB to prevent childhood tuberculous meningitis and miliary TB. However, BCG is not generally recommended for preventive use in the United States because of the low risk for infection with *M. tuberculosis,* the variable effectiveness of the vaccine against adult pulmonary TB, and the vaccine's potential interference with tuberculin skin test reactivity.

SUMMARY

Recognition of the potential for infectious disease is paramount in the care of any emergency department patient. With the prevalence of life-threatening infectious diseases, one must assume that any patient may be a potential source of infection and employ universal precautions whenever a potential for exposure exists. Careful attention to this matter reduces the spread of infection and contamination.

REFERENCES

1. Centers for Disease Control and Prevention: *Exposure to blood: what healthcare personnel need to know,* Atlanta, Ga, 2003, CDC.
2. Centers for Disease Control and Prevention: *Information about MRSA for healthcare personnel,* Atlanta, Ga, 2004, CDC.
3. Centers for Disease Control and Prevention: *Guidelines for the management of occupational exposures to hepatitis B, hepatitis C, and HIV and recommendations for postexposure prophylaxis,* Atlanta, Ga, 2005, CDC.
4. Centers for Disease Control and Prevention: *HIV/AIDS surveillance report: HIV infection and AIDS in the United States and dependent areas,* Atlanta, Ga, 2005, CDC.
5. Centers for Disease Control and Prevention: *Reported tuberculosis in the United States,* Atlanta, Ga, 2005, CDC.
6. Heymann DL, editor: *Control of communicable diseases in man,* ed 18, Washington, DC, 2004, The American Public Health Association.
7. Hollinger FB, Ticehurst JR: Hepatitis A virus. In Fields BN, Knipe DM, Howley PM, editors: *Fields virology,* ed 3, Philadelphia, 1996, Lippincott-Raven.
8. Liaw YF, Yang CY, Chu CM et al: Appearance and persistence of hepatitis A IgM antibody in acute clinical hepatitis A observed in an outbreak, *Infection* 14:156, 1986.

Box 38-4	**TRIAGE ASSESSMENT FOR POSSIBLE TUBERCULOSIS**

Historical and social information
- Recently moved from or traveled to a high-risk country
- Previous history of tuberculosis with no treatment or poor compliance with treatment regimen
- Resident of long-term care facility, nursing home, correctional institution, mental hospital, homeless shelter
- Close contact with an infected person
- Intravenous drug abuse or alcohol abuse
- Health care worker

Objective clinical information
- Weight loss, anorexia, malaise
- Cough worsening over weeks or months
- Productive cough with mucopurulent or blood-streaked sputum
- Night sweats, chills, low-grade fevers
- Malnourished
- Coinfection with human immunodeficiency virus
- Preexisting medical conditions e.g., diabetes mellitus, hematologic disorders, end-stage renal disease)
- Prolonged steroid or immunosuppressive therapy
- History of positive skin test or radiograph

9. Mandell G, Douglas R, Bennett J, editors: *Principles and practices of infectious diseases*, ed 3, New York, 1990, Churchill Livingstone.
10. Rosenblum LS, Villarino ME, Nainan OV et al: Hepatitis A outbreak in a neonatal intensive care unit: risk factors for transmission and evidence of prolonged viral excretion among preterm infants, *J Infect Dis* 164:476, 1991.
11. Stapleton JT: Host immune response to hepatitis A virus, *J Infect Dis* 171(suppl 1):S9, 1995.
12. Stapleton JT, Lemon SM: Hepatitis A and hepatitis E. In Hoeprich PD, Jordan MC, Ronald AR, editors: *Infectious diseases*, ed 5, Philadelphia, 1994, Lippincott Co.

CHAPTER 39

Influenza: Seasonal, Avian, and Pandemic

Sherri-Lynn Almeida

Historically, influenza has caused outbreaks of respiratory illness for centuries, including three pandemics (worldwide outbreaks of disease) in the twentieth century. There are three types of influenza viruses: A, B, and C. Influenza type A viruses have the potential to cause pandemics. Seasonal influenza outbreaks can be caused by either influenza type A or type B viruses. Influenza type C viruses cause mild illness in humans but do not cause epidemics or pandemics. Of the three types of influenza viruses, only type A is divided into subtypes. Subtype designations are based on the presence of two viral surface proteins (antigens): hemagglutinin (H) and neuraminidase (N). To date, 16 different hemagglutinin and 9 different neuraminidase surface proteins have been identified in influenza A viruses.[13] Subtypes are designated as the H protein type (1 to 16) solely or followed by the N protein type (1 to 9) (e.g., H5N1). Three different subtypes (i.e., H1N1, H2N2, and H3N2) caused pandemics in the twentieth century. Influenza A viruses vary in virulence, infectivity to specific hosts, modes of transmission, and the clinical presentation of infection.

Influenza viruses are normally highly species-specific, meaning that viruses infect an individual species and stay true to that species and only rarely spill over to cause infection in other species. Seasonal, avian, and pandemic influenza can occur in humans.[19]

Seasonal (or common) flu is a respiratory illness caused by influenza (A or B) viruses. Seasonal flu can be transmitted person to person. Most people have some immunity, and a vaccine is available.[3]

Avian (or bird) flu (AI) is caused by influenza viruses that occur naturally among wild birds. Low pathogenic AI is common in birds and causes few problems. Highly pathogenic H5N1 is deadly to domestic fowl, can be transmitted from birds to humans, and is deadly to humans. There is virtually no human immunity, and human vaccine availability is very limited.[2]

Pandemic flu is virulent human flu that causes a global outbreak, or pandemic, of serious illness. Because there is little natural immunity, the disease can spread easily from person to person and can sweep across the country and around the world in very short time.

PANDEMICS OF THE TWENTIETH CENTURY

During the past 100 years, three worldwide (pandemic) influenza outbreaks have occurred. Each differed from the others with respect to etiologic agents, epidemiology, and disease severity. The first was the "Spanish flu" (influenza A [H1N1]) of 1918. The origin of this pandemic has always been disputed and may never be resolved. It is estimated that approximately 20% to 40% of the world population became ill and over 20 million people died. Between September

1918 and April 1919 approximately 500,000 deaths from influenza occurred in the United States alone. Many people died very quickly. The Spanish flu was unique because the causative agent was very deadly. One of the most unusual aspects of the Spanish flu was its ability to kill young adults. The reasons for this remain uncertain. With the Spanish flu, mortality rates were high among healthy adults as well as the usual high-risk groups. The attack rate and mortality was highest among adults 20 to 50 years old. The severity of that virus has not been seen again.[6]

In February 1957 the Asian influenza, (influenza A [H2N2]) pandemic was first identified in the Far East. Immunity to this strain was rare in people less than 65 years of age, and a pandemic was predicted. In preparation, vaccine production began about 3 months after the first outbreaks occurred in China, and health officials increased surveillance for flu outbreaks. By June 1957, it had spread to the United States and subsequently caused approximately 70,000 deaths with the highest mortality among the older adult population. Infection rates were highest among school children, young adults, and pregnant women. By December 1957, the worst seemed to be over. However, during January and February 1958, there was another wave of illness among older adults. This is an example of the potential "second wave" of infections that can develop during a pandemic. The disease infects one group of people first, infections appear to decrease, and then infections increase in a different part of the population.[6]

The pandemic of 1957 provided the first opportunity to observe vaccination response in that large part of the population that had not previously been primed.

The third pandemic and the most recent, "Hong Kong flu" (influenza A [H3N2]), occurred in 1968. The first cases were detected in Hong Kong in early 1968. The pandemic, which was milder than 1957, is thought to have caused around 1 million deaths worldwide, and nearly 34,000 deaths in the United States. Those over the age of 65 were most likely to die. There could be several reasons why fewer people in the United States died as a result of this virus. First, the Hong Kong flu virus was similar in some ways to the Asian flu virus that circulated between 1957 and 1968. Earlier infections by the Asian flu virus might have provided some immunity against the Hong Kong flu virus that may have helped to reduce the severity of illness during the Hong Kong pandemic. Second, instead of peaking in September or October, as pandemic influenza had in the previous two pandemics, this pandemic did not gain momentum until near the school holidays in December. Because children were at home and did not infect one another at school, the rate of influenza illness among schoolchildren and their families declined. Third, improved medical care and antibiotics that are more effective for secondary bacterial infections were available for those who became ill. In the 1968 pandemic, vaccines became available 1 month after the outbreaks peaked in the United States.[6]

It is difficult to predict when the next influenza pandemic will occur or how severe it will be. Wherever and whenever a pandemic starts, everyone around the world is at risk. Countries might, through measures such as border closures and travel restrictions, delay arrival of the virus, but cannot stop it.

RECENT PANDEMIC FLU SCARES

In January 1976 an outbreak of respiratory disease was identified at Ft. Dix, New Jersey. On February 12 the Centers for Disease Control and Prevention (CDC) influenza laboratory notified the CDC director that a swine influenza virus strain (H1N1) had been isolated from patients that possessed hemagglutinin and neuraminidase subtypes that had not circulated for more than 50 years. Experience had led scientists to conclude that introduction of a new strain inevitably resulted in a pandemic. On March 24, 1976, President Ford met with representatives from the CDC, Food and Drug Administration (FDA), and National Institutes of Health (NIH), as well as other experts. There was a unanimous recommendation to initiate mass immunization. The first vaccine dose was given 7½ months after the virus was identified. Within 9½ months, 150 million doses of vaccine had been produced under a federal contract. The first vaccine was shipped to state health departments on September 22, 1976, and the first injections were given on October 1, 1976. Vaccination programs continued based on state plans and capacities, with some states aggressively implementing mass vaccinations and others implementing more limited programs. Overall, between October 1 and December 16, more than 40 million civilians were vaccinated. In November 1976 several cases of Guillain-Barré syndrome—a severe neurologic condition associated with paralysis that may include the respiratory muscles and may be fatal—were reported from Minnesota. On December 16, 1976, based on CDC's recommendation and after consultation with the president, the assistant secretary for health announced the suspension of the swine influenza vaccination program.[4]

In May 1977 influenza A(H1N1) viruses, isolated in northern China, spread rapidly and caused epidemic disease in children and young adults (less than 23 years of age) worldwide. The 1977 virus was similar to other influenza A(H1N1) viruses that had circulated before 1957. In 1957 the A(H1N1) virus was replaced by the new A(H2N2) viruses. Because of the timing of the appearance of these viruses, persons born before 1957 were likely to have been exposed to A(H1N1) viruses and to have developed immunity against A(H1N1) viruses. Therefore, when the A(H1N1) reappeared in 1977, many people over the age of 23 had some protection against the virus and it was primarily younger people who became ill from A(H1N1) infections. By January 1978 the virus had spread around the world, including the United States. Because illness occurred primarily in children, this event was not considered a true pandemic. Vaccine containing this virus was not produced in time for the 1977-1978 season; however, the virus was included in the 1978-1979 vaccine.[12]

Box 39-1 describes a more recent outbreak of influenza A(H1N1).

Box 39-1	SWINE FLU

In 2009 a swine influenza outbreak in Mexico resulted in a public health emergency in the United States. Swine flu virus (an influenza type A H1N1 virus) was first isolated from a pig in 1930. Before this outbreak there were limited reports of swine flu in humans. There were 12 U.S. human cases of swine flu reported to the Centers for Disease Control and Prevention between December 2005 through February 2009.

Swine flu is not typically transmitted to humans; however, there have been previous reports of swine flu outbreaks after direct contact with pigs. The symptoms of H1N1 virus infection is consistent with other influenza-like illnesses. People commonly report fever, general malaise, coughing, and decreased appetite. Runny nose, sore throat, nausea, vomiting, and diarrhea are also frequent presenting complaints. Management is aimed at supportive care; not a lot is known about the effectiveness of antiviral medications on the H1N1 swine flu virus. Disease transmission is believed to occur person to person through coughing or other droplet spread. Disease prevention is focused on good handwashing technique, use of a mask, and droplet precautions, as well as having those who believe they are infected with swine flu stay home.

From the Centers for Disease Control and Prevention: Swine flu. Retrieved April 30, 2009 from http://www.cdc.gov/h1n1flu/key_facts.htm.

AVIAN INFLUENZA A(H5N1) OUTBREAKS

Until 1997 the risk for avian flu was considered to be rare in humans. In 1997 at least a few hundred people became infected with the avian A(H5N1) flu virus in Hong Kong; 18 people were hospitalized, and 6 died. This virus was different because it moved directly from chickens to people, rather than having been altered by infecting pigs as an intermediate host. In addition, many of the most severe illnesses occurred in young adults similar to illnesses caused by the 1918 Spanish flu virus. To prevent the spread of this virus, approximately 1.5 million chickens were slaughtered in Hong Kong. The avian flu did not easily spread from one person to another, and after the poultry slaughter no new human infections were found. In 2001 Hong Kong reported an outbreak in its live bird markets of avian influenza type A(H5N1) that is highly pathogenic. As a preventive measure, 1.2 million susceptible birds were destroyed. The 2001 strain did not affect humans.[17]

Of all influenza viruses that circulate in birds, the H5N1 virus is of greatest present concern for human health for two main reasons. First, the H5N1 virus has caused the greatest number of human cases of very severe disease and the greatest number of deaths. It has crossed the species barrier to infect humans. Since 2003 the World Health Organization (WHO) has reported 319 human cases of avian influenza A(H5N1) with 192 deaths.[18] As more humans become infected with the H5N1 virus, transmissibility to humans improves.[15]

The virus can improve its transmissibility among humans via two principal mechanisms. The first is a reassortment event, in which genetic material is exchanged between human and avian viruses during co-infection of a human or pig. Reassortment could result in a fully transmissible pandemic virus, announced by a sudden surge of cases with explosive spread.[17]

The second mechanism is a more gradual process of adaptive mutation, whereby the capability of the virus to bind to human cells increases during subsequent infections of humans. Adaptive mutation, expressed initially as small clusters of human cases with some evidence of human-to-human transmission, would probably give the world some time to take defensive action, if detected sufficiently early.[17]

A second concern for human health is the risk that the H5N1 virus will develop the characteristics it needs to start an influenza pandemic. The virus has met all prerequisites for the start of a pandemic except one: the ability to spread efficiently and develop sustainability among humans. Although H5N1 is presently the virus of greatest concern, the possibility that other avian influenza viruses, known to infect humans, might cause a pandemic cannot be ruled out.[17]

Current available data indicate that close contact with dead or sick birds is the principal source of human infection with the H5N1 virus. Especially risky behaviors include the slaughtering, defeathering, butchering, and preparation for consumption of infected birds. At present, H5N1 avian influenza remains largely a disease of birds. Investigations of all the most recently confirmed human cases, in China, Indonesia, and Turkey, have identified direct contact with infected birds as the most likely source of exposure.[17]

Avian Influenza Clinical Signs and Symptoms

In many patients the disease caused by the H5N1 virus follows an unusually aggressive clinical course, with rapid deterioration and high fatality. Like most emerging disease, H5N1 influenza in humans is poorly understood. Clinical data from cases in 1997 and more recent outbreaks are beginning to provide a picture of the clinical features of disease, but much remains to be learned. However, the clinical picture could change given the propensity of this virus to mutate rapidly and unpredictably.[17]

The incubation period for H5N1 avian influenza may be longer than that for normal seasonal influenza, which is around 2 to 3 days. Current data for H5N1 infection indicate an incubation period ranging from 2 to 8 days and possibly as long as 17 days. However, the possibility of multiple exposures to the virus makes it difficult to define the incubation period precisely. WHO currently recommends that an incubation period of 7 days be used for field investigations and the monitoring of patient contacts.[17]

Initial symptoms include a high fever, usually with a temperature higher than 100.4° F (38° C) and influenza-like symptoms. Diarrhea, vomiting, abdominal pain, chest pain, and bleeding from the nose and gums have also been reported as early symptoms in some patients. Watery diarrhea without blood appears to be more common in H5N1 avian influenza than in normal seasonal influenza. The spectrum of clinical symptoms may, however, be broader, and not all confirmed patients have presented with respiratory symptoms. In two patients from southern Vietnam, the clinical diagnosis was acute encephalitis; neither patient had respiratory symptoms at presentation. In another case, from Thailand, the patient presented with fever and diarrhea, but no respiratory symptoms. All three patients had a recent history of direct exposure to infected poultry.[17]

One feature seen in many patients is the development of manifestations in the lower respiratory tract early in the illness. Many patients have symptoms in the lower respiratory tract when they first seek treatment. Based on present evidence, difficulty in breathing develops around 5 days after the first onset of symptoms. Respiratory distress, a hoarse voice, and a crackling sound when inhaling are common findings. Sputum production is variable and sometimes bloody. Most recently, blood-tinged respiratory secretions have been observed in patients in Turkey. Almost all patients develop pneumonia. During the Hong Kong outbreak, all severely ill patients had primary viral pneumonia, which did not respond to antibiotics. Limited data on patients in the current outbreak indicate the presence of a primary viral pneumonia in H5N1, usually without microbiologic evidence of bacterial suprainfection at presentation. Turkish clinicians also reported pneumonia as a consistent feature in severe cases; as elsewhere, these patients did not respond to treatment with antibiotics.[17]

In patients infected with the H5N1 virus, clinical deterioration is rapid. In Thailand, the time between onset of illness and the development of acute respiratory distress was around 6 days, with a range of 4 to 13 days. In severe cases in Turkey, clinicians observed respiratory failure 3 to 5 days after symptom onset. Another common feature is multiorgan dysfunction. Common laboratory abnormalities include leukopenia (mainly lymphopenia), mild-to-moderate thrombocytopenia, elevated aminotransferase levels, and some instances of disseminated intravascular coagulation.[17]

Prevention and Control of Avian Influenza: Antivirals and Vaccines

Limited evidence suggests that some antiviral drugs, notably oseltamivir (commercially known as Tamiflu), can reduce the duration of viral replication and improve prospects of survival, provided they are administered within 48 hours following symptom onset. However, before the outbreak in Turkey, most patients had not been detected and treated until late in the course of illness. For this reason, clinical data on the effectiveness of oseltamivir are limited. Moreover, oseltamivir and other antiviral drugs were developed for the treatment and prophylaxis of seasonal influenza, which is a less severe disease associated with less prolonged viral replication. Recommendations on the optimum dose and duration of treatment for H5N1 avian influenza, also in children, need to undergo urgent review, and this is being undertaken by WHO.[17]

In suspected cases, oseltamivir should be prescribed as soon as possible (ideally, within 48 hours following symptom onset) to maximize its therapeutic benefits. However, given the significant mortality currently associated with H5N1 infection and evidence of prolonged viral replication in this disease, administration of the drug should also be considered in patients presenting later in the course of illness.[17]

Recommended doses of oseltamivir for the treatment of influenza are contained in the product information at the manufacturer's Web site. The recommended dose of oseltamivir for the treatment of influenza, in adults and adolescents 13 years of age and older, is 150 mg per day, given as 75 mg twice a day for 5 days. Oseltamivir is not indicated for the treatment of children younger than 1 year of age.[17]

Because the duration of viral replication may be prolonged in cases of H5N1 infection, clinicians should consider increasing the duration of treatment to 7 to 10 days in patients who are not showing a clinical response. In cases of severe infection with the H5N1 virus, clinicians may need to consider increasing the recommended daily dose or the duration of treatment, recognizing that doses above 300 mg per day are associated with increased side effects. For all treated patients, consideration should be given to taking serial clinical samples for later assay to monitor changes in viral load, assess drug susceptibility, and assess drug levels. These samples should be taken only in the presence of appropriate measures for infection control.[17]

In severely ill H5N1 patients or in H5N1 patients with severe gastrointestinal symptoms, drug absorption may be impaired. This possibility should be considered when managing these patients.[17]

There currently is no commercially available vaccine to protect humans against the H5N1 virus that is being seen in Asia, Europe, and Africa. A vaccine specific to the virus strain causing the pandemic cannot be produced until a new pandemic influenza virus emerges and is identified.

The U.S. Department of Health and Human Services (HHS), through its National Institute of Allergy and Infectious Diseases, is addressing the problem in a number of ways. These include the development of prepandemic vaccines based on current lethal strains of H5N1 (the FDA has approved a vaccine based on an early strain of the H5N1 virus that is not commercially available, but is being added to the Strategic National Stockpile); collaboration with industry to increase the nation's vaccine production capacity; seeking ways to expand or extend the existing supply; and doing research in the development of new types of influenza vaccines.[11]

UNITED STATES AND GLOBAL PREPAREDNESS PLANNING

Although the timing of the next pandemic cannot be predicted, planning for a pandemic can be achieved through the integration of interventions to ensure a prompt and effective response. HHS and WHO have developed pandemic

---

Box 39-2 **WORLD HEALTH ORGANIZATION STAGES OF A PANDEMIC**

INTERPANDEMIC PERIOD

Phase 1: No new influenza virus subtypes have been detected in humans. An influenza virus subtype that has caused human infection may be present in animals. If present in animals, the risk[a] of human infection or disease is considered to be low.

Phase 2: No new influenza virus subtypes have been detected in humans. However, a circulating animal influenza virus subtype poses a substantial risk[a] of human disease.

PANDEMIC ALERT PERIOD

Phase 3: Human infection(s) with a new subtype, but no human-to-human spread, or at most rare instances of spread to a close contact.[b]

Phase 4: Small cluster(s) with limited human-to-human transmission but spread is highly localized, suggesting that the virus is not well adapted to humans.[b]

Phase 5: Larger cluster(s) but human-to-human spread still localized, suggesting that the virus is becoming increasingly better adapted to humans, but may not yet be fully transmissible (substantial pandemic risk).

PANDEMIC PERIOD

Phase 6: Pandemic: increased and sustained transmission in general population.[b]

---

[a]The distinction between *phase 1* and *phase 2* is based on the risk for human infection or disease resulting from circulating strains in animals. The distinction is based on various factors and their relative importance according to current scientific knowledge. Factors may include pathogenicity in animals and humans, occurrence in domesticated animals and livestock or only in wildlife, whether the virus is enzootic or epizootic, geographically localized or widespread, and/or other scientific parameters.

[b]The distinction between *phase 3*, *phase 4*, and *phase 5* is based on an assessment of the risk for a pandemic. Various factors and their relative importance according to current scientific knowledge may be considered. Factors may include rate of transmission, geographical location and spread, severity of illness, presence of genes from human strains (if derived from an animal strain), and/or other scientific parameters.

---

preparedness and response plans.[9,16] The HHS Pandemic Influenza Plan serves as a blueprint for all HHS pandemic influenza preparedness planning and response activities. The plan integrates changes made in the 2005 WHO classification of pandemic phases and expansion of international guidance and now is consistent with the National Response Plan (NRP), which is currently under review. The HHS Pandemic Influenza Plan has three parts. Part 1, the Strategic Plan, outlines federal plans and preparations for public health and medical support in the event of a pandemic. It identifies key roles of HHS and its agencies in a pandemic and provides planning assumptions for federal, state, and local governments and public health operations plans. Part 2, Public Health Guidance for State and Local Partners, provides detailed guidance to state and local health departments in 11 key areas. Parts 1 and 2 will be regularly updated and refined. These documents serve as tools for continued engagement with stakeholders, state, and local partners.

Part 3, which is currently under development, will consist of HHS Agencies' Operational Plans. Each HHS component will prepare, maintain, update, and exercise an operational plan that itemizes their specific roles and responsibilities in the event of a pandemic. These individual plans will also include detailed continuity of operations plans such as strategies for ensuring that critical everyday functions of each operating division are identified and maintained in the presence of the expected decreased staffing levels of a pandemic event. Recognizing that an influenza pandemic has the capacity to cause disruptions across all levels of governments and in all communities, pandemic influenza preparedness is a shared responsibility. The following list includes some of the additional plans that will be required to mitigate the impact of a pandemic and to ensure continuity of essential services: international and global planning; national strategy for pandemic influenza; state and local pandemic influenza plans; and corporate, infrastructure, and critical service provider plans.[9]

An influenza pandemic may require activation of the NRP if the first appearance of the disease in the United States occurs in one or a few isolated communities. The intent of the NRP is to reduce America's vulnerability to terrorism, major disasters, and other emergencies; to minimize the damage resulting from these emergencies; and to facilitate recovery. The NRP applies a functional approach that groups the capabilities of federal governmental departments and agencies and the American Red Cross into Emergency Support Functions to provide the planning, support, resources, program implementation, and emergency services that are most likely to be needed. The HHS will have primary responsibility for coordination of federal government assistance to state, local, and tribal resources.[9]

Stages of a Pandemic

WHO has identified three periods and six stages of a pandemic (Box 39-2).[16] To accomplish the public health goals for each phase, specific objectives and actions are divided into five categories: (1) planning and coordination, (2) situation monitoring and assessment, (3) prevention and containment, (4) health system response, and (5) communications. The WHO phases provide succinct statements about the global risk for a pandemic and provide benchmarks against which to measure global response capabilities. However, to describe the U.S. government's approach to the pandemic response, it is more useful to characterize the stages of an outbreak in terms of the immediate and specific threat a pandemic virus poses to the U.S. population.[14] The stages identified in Box 39-3 provide a framework for federal government actions.

In 2006 WHO issued a draft protocol for rapid response and containment of pandemic influenza. The protocol has three main parts. The first describes the steps needed to recognize the signal or triggering event. The second part describes the immediate actions that should follow recognition of the signal. The third part describes the actions that should be undertaken once the event has been verified, the overall situation has been assessed, and a decision has been made to launch the rapid-containment operation.[16]

Box 39-3	**FRAMEWORK FOR FEDERAL GOVERNMENT ACTIONS**

Stage 0: New domestic animal outbreak in at-risk country
Stage 1: Suspected human outbreak overseas
Stage 2: Confirmed human outbreak overseas
Stage 3: Widespread human outbreaks in multiple locations overseas
Stage 4: First human case in North America
Stage 5: Spread throughout United States
Stage 6: Recovery and preparation for subsequent waves

From World Health Organization. WHO Global Influenza Preparedness Plan. Available at: http://www.who.int/csr/resources/publications/influenza/GIP_2005_5Eweb.pdf. 2005. Accessed August 9, 2007.

Surveillance for Pandemic Influenza

Each country is responsible for surveillance of a novel influenza virus that has demonstrated the ability to be transmitted from person to person. When identified, WHO should be notified within 24 hours. According to WHO's rapid response and containment of pandemic influenza plan, they would then provide immediate recommendations to the affected country. The recommendations can vary based on the evidence to support the degree of the pandemic threat. WHO will coordinate international support and will work with the country to mobilize the necessary resources and initiate appropriate actions.

Pandemic influenza surveillance includes surveillance for actual influenza viruses (virologic surveillance) and surveillance for influenza-associated illnesses and deaths (disease surveillance). The goals of virologic surveillance are to rapidly detect the introduction and early cases of a pandemic influenza virus in the United States; to track the introduction of the virus into local areas; and to monitor changes in the pandemic virus, including development of antiviral resistance. The goals of disease surveillance are to serve as an early warning system to detect increases in influenza-like illness in the community; to monitor the pandemic's impact on health (e.g., by tracking outpatient visits, hospitalizations, and deaths); and to track trends in influenza disease activity and identify populations that are severely affected.[9]

Virologic and disease surveillance data—supplemented by data from outbreak investigations and special studies—can help decision makers identify effective control strategies and reevaluate recommended priority groups for vaccination and antiviral therapy. They can also facilitate efforts to mathematically model disease spread during a pandemic.[9]

Early detection is the key to the prevention of a pandemic influenza. The most important warning signal of a pandemic strain comes when clusters of patients with clinical symptoms of influenza, closely related in time and place, are detected. The clinical presentation and travel history of persons with influenza A(H5N1) or severe acute respiratory syndrome–coronavirus (SARS-CoV) infection may overlap. The CDC's interim recommendations for diagnostic

---

Box 39-4	**INTERIM RECOMMENDATIONS: ENHANCED U.S. SURVEILLANCE AND DIAGNOSTIC EVALUATION**

INFLUENZA A (H5N1) VIRUS INFECTIONS

Testing for influenza A(H5N1) is indicated for hospitalized patients with:

a. Radiographically confirmed pneumonia, acute respiratory distress syndrome (ARDS), or other severe respiratory illness for which an alternative diagnosis has not been established, **AND**

b. History of travel within 10 days of symptom onset to a country with documented H5N1 avian influenza in poultry and/or humans (for a listing of H5N1-affected countries, see the OIE Web site at http://www.oie.int/eng/en_index.htm and the WHO Web site at http://www.who.int/en/).

Testing for influenza A(H5N1) should be considered on a case-by-case basis in consultation with state and local health departments for hospitalized or ambulatory patients with:

a. Documented temperature of >38° C (>100.4° F), **AND**

b. One or more of the following: cough, sore throat, shortness of breath, **AND**

c. History of contact with domestic poultry (e.g., visited a poultry farm, household raising poultry, or bird market) or a known or suspected human case of influenza A(H5N1) in an H5N1-affected country within 10 days of symptom onset.

Adapted from http://www.hhs.gov/pandemicflu/plan/sup2.html#app2. Retrieved August 9, 2007.
OIE, World Organisation for Animal Health; *WHO*, World Health Organization.

evaluation for these agents in individuals who meet certain epidemiologic and clinical criteria are listed in Box 39-4.[1]

Prevention and Control in the Community

The three major goals of mitigating a community-wide epidemic through nonpharmaceutical interventions (NPIs) are (1) delay the exponential increase in incident cases and shift the epidemic curve to the right in order to "buy time" for production and distribution of a well-matched pandemic strain vaccine; (2) decrease the epidemic peak; and (3) reduce the total number of incident cases, causing a reduction in morbidity and mortality in the community. These three major goals of epidemic mitigation may all be accomplished by focusing on the single goal of saving lives by reducing transmission. NPIs may help reduce influenza transmission by reducing contact between sick persons and uninfected persons, thereby reducing the number of infected persons. Reducing the number of persons infected will also lessen the need for health care services and minimize the impact of a pandemic on the economy and society. The surge of need for medical care associated with a poorly mitigated severe pandemic can be only partially addressed by increasing capacity within hospitals and other care settings. Therefore reshaping the demand for health care services by using NPIs is an important component of the overall strategy for mitigating a severe pandemic.[8]

Pandemic mitigation strategies generally include (1) case containment measures, such as voluntary case isolation, voluntary quarantine of members of households with ill persons, and antiviral treatment/prophylaxis; (2) social-distancing measures, such as dismissal of students from classrooms and social distancing of adults in the community and at work; and (3) infection control measures, including hand hygiene and cough etiquette. Each of these interventions may be only partially effective in limiting transmission when implemented alone. To determine the usefulness of these partially effective measures alone and in combination, mathematical models were developed to assess these types of interventions within the context of contemporary social networks. The Models of Infectious Disease Agents Study (MIDAS), funded by the NIH, has been developing agent-based computer simulations of pandemic influenza outbreaks with various epidemic parameters, strategies for using medical countermeasures, and patterns of implementation of community-based interventions (case isolation, household quarantine, child and adult social distancing through school or workplace closure or restrictions, and restrictions on travel).[9] Mathematical modeling conducted by MIDAS participants demonstrates general consistency in outcome for NPIs and suggests the following within the context of the model assumptions.

Interventions implemented in combination, even with less-than-complete levels of public compliance, are effective in reducing transmission of pandemic influenza virus, particularly for lower values of $R0$ (i.e., reproductive number—the average number of infections resulting from a single case in a fully susceptible population without interventions). School closures and generic social distancing are important components of a community mitigation strategy because schools and workplaces are significant compartments for transmission. Simultaneous implementation of multiple tools that target different compartments for transmission is important in limiting transmission because removing one source of transmission may simply make other sources relatively more important.

Timely intervention may reduce the total number of persons infected with pandemic influenza. Each of the models generally suggest that a combination of targeted antiviral medications and NPIs can delay and flatten the epidemic peak, but the degree to which they reduce the overall size of the epidemic varies. Delay of the epidemic peak is critically important because it allows additional time for vaccine development and antiviral production. However, these models are not validated with empiric data and are subject to many limitations.[9]

Supporting evidence for the role of combinations of NPIs in limiting transmission can also be found in the preliminary results from several historical analyses.[9] One statistical model being developed, based on analysis of historical data for the use of various combinations of selected NPIs in U.S. cities during the 1918 pandemic, demonstrates a significant association between early implementation of these measures by cities and reductions in peak death rate.[5]

Taken together, these strands of evidence are consistent with the hypothesis that there may be benefit in limiting or slowing community transmission of a pandemic virus by the use of combinations of partially effective NPIs. At the present time this hypothesis remains unproven, and more work is needed before its validity can be established.

Appropriate matching of the intensity of intervention to the severity of a pandemic is important to maximize the available public health benefit that may result from using an early, targeted, and layered strategy while minimizing untoward secondary effects. To assist with prepandemic planning, the concept of a Pandemic Severity Index has been introduced. The index is based primarily on case fatality ratio 23% to 27% (i.e., the percentage of deaths out of the total reported cases), a measurement that is useful in estimating the severity of a pandemic on a population level and which may be available early in a pandemic for small clusters and outbreaks. Excess mortality rates may also be available early and may supplement and inform the determination of the Pandemic Severity Index.[7] Pandemic severity is described within five discrete categories of increasing severity (Category 1 to Category 5). Other epidemiologic features that are relevant in overall analysis of mitigation plans include total illness rate, age-specific illness and mortality rates, the reproductive number, intergeneration time, and incubation period. However, it is unlikely that estimates will be available for most of these parameters during the early stages of a pandemic; thus they are not as useful from a planning perspective.[8] The Pandemic Severity Index provides U.S. communities a tool for scenario-based contingency planning to guide prepandemic planning efforts.

Prevention and Control in Health Care Facilities

The CDC is revising its interim guidance for infection control precautions for avian influenza. The following interim recommendations are based on what are deemed optimal precautions for protecting individuals involved in the care of patients with highly pathogenic avian influenza from illness and for reducing the risk for viral reassortment (i.e., mixing of genes from human and avian viruses). The ability of low pathogenic avian influenza viruses to cause infection and serious disease is less well established, but appears to be lower than that of highly pathogenic viruses based on available information. Nonetheless, it is considered prudent to take all possible precautions to the extent feasible when caring for patients with known or possible avian influenza.

Rationale for Enhanced Precautions

Human influenza is thought to transmit primarily via large respiratory droplets. Standard precautions plus droplet precautions are recommended for the care of patients infected with human influenza. However, given the uncertainty about the exact modes by which avian influenza may first transmit between humans, additional precautions for health care workers involved in the care of patients with documented or suspected avian influenza may be prudent. The rationale for the use of additional precautions for avian influenza as compared with human influenza include the following: (1) the risk for serious disease and increased mortality from highly pathogenic avian influenza may be significantly higher than from infection by human influenza viruses; (2) each human infection represents an important opportunity for avian influenza to further adapt to humans and gain the ability to transmit more easily among people; and (3) although rare, human-to-human transmission of avian influenza may be associated with the possible emergence of a pandemic strain.

All patients who present to a health care setting with fever and respiratory symptoms should be managed according to the CDC's recommendations for respiratory hygiene and cough etiquette and questioned regarding their recent travel history.

Patients with a history of travel within 10 days to a country with avian influenza activity and who are hospitalized with a severe febrile respiratory illness, or are otherwise under evaluation for avian influenza, should be managed using isolation precautions identical to those recommended for patients with known SARS.[1] These precautions are discussed below.

Standard Precautions

Pay careful attention to hand hygiene before and after all patient contact or contact with items potentially contaminated with respiratory secretions.

Contact Precautions

Use gloves and gown for all patient contact.

Use dedicated equipment such as stethoscopes, disposable blood pressure cuffs, disposable thermometers, etc.

Eye Protection

Wear eye protection (e.g., goggles or face shields) when within 3 feet of the patient.

Airborne Precautions

Place the patient in an airborne isolation room (AIR). Such rooms should have monitored negative air pressure in relation to the corridor, with 6 to 12 air changes per hour (ACH), and air exhausted directly outside, or have recirculated air filtered by a high-efficiency particulate air (HEPA) filter. If an AIR is unavailable, contact the health care facility engineer to assist, or use portable HEPA filters (see CDC's Environmental Infection Control Guidelines) to augment the number of ACH.

Use a fit-tested respirator, at least as protective as a National Institute of Occupational Safety and Health–approved N-95 filtering face piece (i.e., disposable) respirator, when entering the room.

For additional information regarding these and other health care isolation precautions, see the CDC's Guidelines for Isolation Precautions: *Preventing Transmission of Infectious Agents in Healthcare Settings 2007.* These precautions should be continued for 14 days after onset of symptoms or until either an alternative diagnosis is established or diagnostic test results indicate that the patient is not infected with influenza A virus. Patients managed as outpatients or hospitalized patients discharged before 14 days with suspected avian influenza should be isolated in the home setting on the basis of principles outlined for the home isolation of SARS patients.[1]

In addition to the precautions noted above, the CDC recommends that health care workers involved in the care of patients with documented or suspected avian influenza should be vaccinated with the most recent seasonal human influenza vaccine. In addition to providing protection against the predominant circulating influenza strain, this measure is intended to reduce the likelihood of a health care worker's being coinfected with human and avian strains, where genetic rearrangement could take place, leading to the emergence of a potential pandemic strain.[1]

Although precautions and vaccinations are important to prevention, it is also vital that health care workers be vigilant for the development of fever, respiratory symptoms, and/or conjunctivitis (i.e., eye infections) for 1 week after last exposure to avian influenza–infected patients. Health care workers who become ill should seek medical care, and before arrival they should notify their health care provider that they may have been exposed to avian influenza. In addition, employees should notify occupational health and infection control personnel at their facility. With the exception of visiting a health care provider, health care workers who become ill should be advised to stay home until 24 hours after resolution of fever, unless an alternative diagnosis is established or diagnostic tests are negative for influenza A virus. While at home, ill persons should practice good respiratory hygiene and cough etiquette to lower the risk for transmission of the virus to others.[1]

IMPACT OF A PANDEMIC

A pandemic may come and go in waves, each of which can last for 6 to 8 weeks. An especially severe influenza pandemic could lead to high levels of illness, death, social disruption, and economic loss. Everyday life would be disrupted because so many people in so many places would become seriously ill at the same time. Impacts can range from school and business closings to the interruption of basic services such as public transportation and food delivery. A substantial percentage of the world's population would require some form of medical care. Health care facilities could be overwhelmed, creating a shortage of hospital staff, beds, ventilators, and other supplies. Surge capacity at nontraditional sites such as schools may need to be created to cope with demand. The need for vaccine is likely to outstrip supply, and the supply of antiviral drugs is also likely to be inadequate early in a pandemic.

Difficult decisions will need to be made regarding who gets antiviral drugs and vaccines. Death rates are determined by four factors: the number of people who become infected, the virulence of the virus, the underlying characteristics and vulnerability of the affected populations, and the availability and effectiveness of preventive measures.[1]

SUMMARY

According to WHO, there are 10 things we need to know about pandemic influenza.

• Pandemic influenza is different from avian influenza. Avian influenza refers to a large group of different influenza viruses that primarily affect birds. On rare occasions these bird viruses can infect other species, including pigs and humans. The vast majority of avian influenza viruses do not infect humans. An influenza pandemic happens when a new subtype emerges that has not previously circulated in humans. For this reason, avian H5N1 is a strain with pandemic potential, because it might ultimately adapt into a strain that is contagious among humans. Once this adaptation occurs, it will no longer be a bird virus—it will be a human influenza virus. Influenza pandemics are caused by new influenza viruses that have adapted to humans.

• Influenza pandemics are recurring events. An influenza pandemic is a rare but recurrent event. Three pandemics occurred in the previous century: "Spanish influenza" in 1918, "Asian influenza" in 1957, and "Hong Kong influenza" in 1968. The 1918 pandemic killed an estimated 40 to 50 million people worldwide. That pandemic, which was exceptional, is considered one of the deadliest disease events in human history. Subsequent pandemics were much milder, with an estimated 2 million deaths in 1957 and 1 million deaths in 1968. A pandemic occurs when a new influenza virus emerges and starts spreading as easily as normal influenza by coughing and sneezing. Because the virus is new, the human immune system will have no preexisting immunity. This makes it likely that people who contract pandemic influenza will experience more serious disease than that caused by normal influenza.

• The world may be on the brink of another pandemic. Health experts have been monitoring a new and extremely severe influenza virus—the H5N1 strain—for almost 8 years. The H5N1 strain first infected humans in Hong Kong in 1997, causing 18 cases, including 6 deaths. Since mid-2003, this virus has caused the largest and most severe outbreaks in poultry on record. In December 2003, infections in people exposed to sick birds were identified. Since then, over 100 human cases have been laboratory confirmed in four Asian countries (Cambodia, Indonesia, Thailand, and Vietnam), and more than half of these people have died. Most cases have occurred in previously healthy children and young adults. Fortunately, the virus does not jump easily from birds to humans or spread readily and sustainably among humans. Should H5N1 evolve to a form as contagious as normal influenza, a pandemic could begin.

• All countries will be affected. Once a fully contagious virus emerges, its global spread is considered inevitable. Countries might, through measures such as border closures and travel restrictions, delay arrival of the virus, but cannot stop it. The pandemics of the previous century encircled the globe in 6 to 9 months, even when most international travel was by ship. Given the speed and volume of international air travel today, the virus could spread more rapidly, possibly reaching all continents in less than 3 months.

• Widespread illness will occur. Because most people will have no immunity to the pandemic virus, infection and illness rates are expected to be higher than during seasonal epidemics of normal influenza. Current projections for the next pandemic estimate that a substantial percentage of the world's population will require some form of medical care. Few countries have the staff, facilities, equipment, and hospital beds needed to cope with large numbers of people who suddenly fall ill.

• Medical supplies will be inadequate. Supplies of vaccines and antiviral drugs—the two most important medical interventions for reducing illness and death during a pandemic—will be inadequate in all countries at the start of a pandemic and for many months thereafter. Inadequate supplies of vaccines are of particular concern, because vaccines are considered the first line of defense for protecting populations. Based on present trends, many developing countries will have no access to vaccines throughout the duration of a pandemic.

• Large numbers of deaths will occur. Historically, the number of deaths during a pandemic has varied greatly. Death rates are largely determined by four factors: the number of people who become infected, the virulence of the virus, the underlying characteristics and vulnerability of affected populations, and the effectiveness of preventive measures. Accurate predictions of mortality cannot be made before the pandemic virus emerges and begins to spread. All estimates of the number of deaths are purely speculative. WHO has used a relatively conservative estimate—from 2 million to 7.4 million deaths—because it provides a useful and plausible planning target. This estimate is based on the comparatively mild 1957 pandemic. Estimates based on a more virulent virus, closer to the one seen in 1918, have been made and are much higher. However, the 1918 pandemic was considered exceptional.

• Economic and social disruption will be great. High rates of illness and worker absenteeism are expected, and these will contribute to social and economic disruption. Past pandemics have spread globally in two and sometimes three waves. Not all parts of the world or of a single country are expected to be severely affected at the same time. Social and economic disruptions could be temporary, but may be amplified in today's closely interrelated and interdependent systems of trade and commerce. Social disruption may be greatest when rates of absenteeism impair essential services, such as power, transportation, and communications.

- Every country must be prepared. WHO has issued a series of recommended strategic actions for responding to the influenza pandemic threat. The actions are designed to provide different layers of defense that reflect the complexity of the evolving situation. Recommended actions are different for the present phase of pandemic alert, the emergence of a pandemic virus, and the declaration of a pandemic and its subsequent international spread.

- WHO will alert the world when the pandemic threat increases. WHO works closely with ministries of health and various public health organizations to support countries' surveillance of circulating influenza strains. A sensitive surveillance system that can detect emerging influenza strains is essential for the rapid detection of a pandemic virus. Six distinct phases have been defined to facilitate pandemic preparedness planning, with roles defined for governments, industry, and WHO. The present situation is categorized as phase 3: a virus new to humans is causing infections, but does not spread easily from one person to another.

Pandemic influenza will occur again sometime in the near future. Health care professionals should be aware of the facts as summarized above.

REFERENCES

1. Centers for Disease Control and Prevention: *Update on influenza A(H5N1) and SARS: interim recommendations for enhanced U.S. surveillance, testing, and infection control*, 2006. Retrieved August 10, 2007, from http://www.cdc.gov/flu/avian/professional/infect-control.htm.

2. Centers for Disease Control and Prevention: *Key facts about avian influenza (bird flu) and avian influenza A (H5N1) virus*, 2007. Retrieved August 8, 2007, from http://www.cdc.gov/flu/avian/gen-info/facts.htm.

3. Centers for Disease Control and Prevention: *Key facts about influenza and the influenza vaccine*, 2007. Retrieved August 8, 2007, from http://www.cdc.gov/flu/keyfacts.htm.

4. Gaydos JC, Top FH, Hodder RA et al: Swine influenza A outbreak, Fort Dix, New Jersey, *Emerg Infect Dis* 12(1):23, 2006. Retrieved August 8, 2007, from http://www.cdc.gov/ncidod/EID/vol12no01/05-0965.htm.

5. Institute of Medicine, Committee on Modeling Community Containment for Pandemic Influenza: *Modeling community containment for pandemic influenza: a letter report*, Washington, DC, 2006, The National Academies Press.

6. Kilbourne ED: Influenza pandemics of the 20th century, *Emerg Infect Dis* 12(1):9, 2006. Retrieved August 8, 2007, from http://www.cdc.gov/ncidod/EID/vol12no01/05-1254.htm.

7. Thompson WW, Comanor L, Shay DK: Epidemiology of seasonal influenza: use of surveillance data and statistical models to estimate the burden of disease, *J Infect Dis* 194(suppl 2):S82, 2006.

8. U.S. Department of Health and Human Services: *Community strategy for pandemic influenza mitigation*, 2007. Retrieved August 10, 2007, from http://www.pandemicflu.gov/plan/community/commitigation.html.

9. U.S. Department of Health and Human Services: *HHS pandemic influenza plan*, 2007. Retrieved August 10, 2007, from http://www.hhs.gov.pandemicflu/plan/#overview.

10. U.S. Department of Health and Human Services: *Understanding flu terms*, 2007. Retrieved August 8, 2007, from http://www.pandemicflu.gov/index.html.

11. U.S. Department of Health and Human Services: *Vaccination and treatment for H5N1 virus in humans*, 2007. Retrieved August 9, 2007, from http://www.pandemicflu.gov/vaccine/index.html. 2007.

12. U.S. Department of Health and Human Services, National Vaccine Program Office: *Pandemics and pandemic scares in the 20th century*, 2004. Retrieved August 8, 2007, from http://www.hhs.gov/nvpo/pandemics/flu3.htm.

13. U.S. Department of Labor, Occupational Safety and Health Administration: *Pandemic influenza preparedness and response guidance for healthcare workers and healthcare employers*, 2007. Retrieved February 12, 2009, from http://www.osha.gov/Publications/OSHA_pandemic_health.pdf.

14. U.S. Homeland Security Council: *National strategy for pandemic influenza implementation plan*, 2006. Retrieved August 10, 2007, from http://www.whitehouse.gov/homeland/nspi_implementation.pdf.

15. World Health Organization: *Ten things you need to know about pandemic influenza*, 2005. Retrieved August 9, 2007, from http://www.who/int/csr/disease/influenza/pandemic10things/en/index.html.

16. World Health Organization: WHO global influenza preparedness plan, 2005. Retrieved August 9, 2007, from http://www.who.int/csr/resources/publications/influenza/GIP_2005_5Eweb.pdf.

17. World Health Organization: *Avian influenza fact sheet*, 2006. Retrieved August 9, 2007, from http://www.who.int/mediacentre/factsheets/avian_influenza/en/index.html#history.

18. World Health Organization: *Confirmed human cases of avian influenza A(H5N1)*, 2007. Retrieved August 9, 2007, from http://www.who.int/csr/disease/avian_influenza/country/cases_table_2007_07_25/en/index.html.

19. Zinkovich L, Malvey D, Hamby E et al: Bioterror events: preemptive strategies for healthcare executives, *Hosp Top* 83(3):9, 2005.

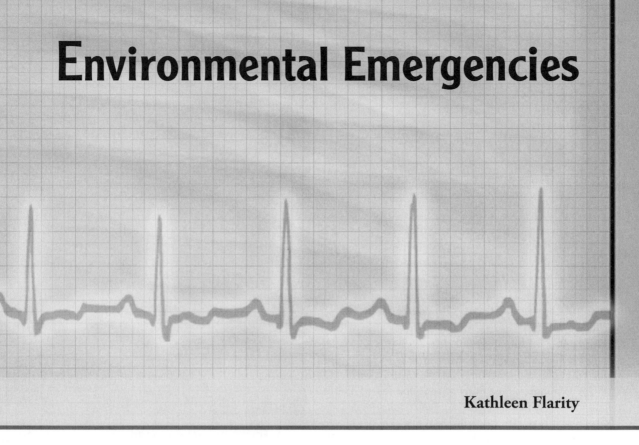

Kathleen Flarity

CHAPTER 40

Environmental Emergencies

O utdoor activities are extremely popular with individuals of all ages. Activities such as hiking, jogging, biking, swimming, and diving, however, place the individual at risk for illness and injury secondary to the weather, the activity, and various animals. Environmental hazards may be encountered during voluntary participation in an outdoor activity or involuntary exposure caused by confusion, mental illness, alcohol, or drugs. Specific environmental emergencies discussed in this chapter are related to heat and cold stress, water immersion, diving, carbon monoxide poisoning, bites, and stings.

HEAT-RELATED EMERGENCIES

Many cases of heat illness are reported annually in the United States. Only head injury, spinal cord injury, and heart failure are responsible for more deaths in athletes than heat illness.[23] Regardless of physical condition, anyone can suffer ill effects from heat stress if the exposure is intense or prolonged. The effects of environmental heat stress can be mild or severe, depending on the degree of heat and length of exposure. Emergencies related to heat stress range in severity from heat edema, heat cramps, and heat exhaustion to potentially life-threatening heat stroke.

Heat Edema

Heat edema occurs in nonacclimated individuals during prolonged periods of standing or sitting. Characteristic swelling of feet and ankles resolves in a few days. Treatment includes rest, elevation of the legs, and support hose. Heat edema is self-limiting and generally does not require further treatment.

Heat Cramps

Heat cramps are severe cramps (brief and intermittent) of specific muscles, usually in the shoulders, thighs, and abdominal wall. Associated symptoms include weakness, nausea, tachycardia, pallor, profuse diaphoresis, and cool moist skin. The person's core temperature may be normal or slightly elevated. Heat cramps usually develop suddenly when the victim is resting after exertion in a hot environment or one with high humidity. Salt depletion secondary to excessive perspiration in combination with excessive water consumption leads to muscle cramping. Increased water intake does not replace sodium losses caused by perspiration. Instead, water dilutes serum sodium, causing hyponatremia, the key factor in the development of heat cramps.[1]

Treatment includes removal of the person from the heat source, rest, and electrolyte replacement with oral or parenteral fluids. Discharge instructions should stress the importance of drinking commercially prepared electrolyte supplements (e.g., Gatorade, Powerade, All Sport) when working outdoors or participating in strenuous recreational activities during hot weather. Strenuous activity should be avoided for at least 12 hours after discharge.[1,22]

Heat Exhaustion

Heat exhaustion is a clinical syndrome caused by prolonged heat exposure, usually over hours or days. Excessive perspiration and inadequate fluid and electrolyte replacement lead to fluid loss, electrolyte depletion, and dehydration. Heat exhaustion occurs most often in individuals working in hot environments. Older adults and the very young are at greatest risk because they cannot or do not increase fluid intake sufficiently to compensate for increased fluid losses from sweating.[1,12,23]

Heat exhaustion is characterized by rapid onset (within minutes) of extreme thirst, general malaise, muscle cramping, headache, nausea, vomiting, anxiety, and tachycardia—ultimately leading to syncope and collapse. Associated dehydration may cause orthostatic hypotension and mild to severe temperature elevation (98.6° F to 105° F [37° C to 40.5° C]). Diaphoresis may or may not be present. Untreated, heat exhaustion can progress to heat stroke.

Initial treatment begins with moving the patient to a cool, quiet environment and removing constricting clothing. When significant hyperthermia is present, moist cloths placed on the patient reduce temperature by evaporation. Fluid and electrolyte replacement should be initiated. Oral replacement with a balanced commercial salt preparation can be used if the patient is not nauseated. Intravenous 0.9% saline solution should be used if the patient is nauseated or vomiting. Salt tablets are not recommended because of potential gastric irritation and hypernatremia. Monitor the patient's temperature during treatment. Hypotension may be corrected initially with a 300- to 500-mL bolus of 0.9% saline, with subsequent infusions correlated to clinical and laboratory findings. Patients with hypotension or a history of cardiac disease should be placed on a cardiac monitor because heat exhaustion can rapidly evolve into heat stroke. Admission should be considered for any patient who does not improve significantly after 3 to 4 hours of emergency treatment.[1,12,23]

Heat Stroke

Heat stroke is the least common but most emergent and life-threatening form of heat illness. Mortality as high as 70%[1] is directly related to the speed and effectiveness of diagnosis and treatment. Heat stroke is defined as an abnormal form of hyperthermia resulting from a failure of the body's physiologic systems to dissipate heat and cool down. Heat stroke is characterized by an elevated core temperature of 104°F (40° C) or greater. Environmental factors and the patient's ability to dissipate heat also affect the outcome of heat stroke.

Heat stroke occurs in one of two forms: classic heat stroke and exertional heat stroke. Classic heat stroke occurs during prolonged exposure to sustained high ambient temperatures and humidity. It commonly affects older adults, the chronically ill, and those who live in poorly ventilated homes without air conditioning. Children locked in cars on hot days are at great risk for developing heat stroke. Poor dissipation of environmental heat is the underlying cause of classic heat stroke. In contrast, those patients with exertional heat stroke are usually young and healthy, often athletes and military recruits. In these individuals heat production overcomes the internal heat dissipation mechanisms. Onset of heat stroke is usually sudden; however, older adults and patients in predisposing environments can develop heat exhaustion several hours before heat stroke develops (Box 40-1). Heat stroke may present with changes in neurologic function such as anxiety, confusion, hallucinations, loss of

| Box 40-1 | RISK FACTORS ASSOCIATED WITH HEAT STROKE |

AGE
Older adults
Infants

ENVIRONMENTAL CONDITIONS
High environmental temperatures
High relative humidity
Low wind

PREEXISTING ILLNESS
Cardiovascular disease
Dehydration
Autonomic neuropathies
Previous stroke/central nervous system lesions
Obesity
Diabetes
Cystic fibrosis
Low fitness
Skin disorders (e.g., large burn scars)

PRESCRIPTION DRUGS
Anticholinergics
Phenothiazines
Butyrophenones
Tricyclic antidepressants
Antihistamines
Antispasmodics
Diuretics
Antiparkinsonian drugs
β-Blockers

STREET DRUGS
Lysergic acid diethylamide (LSD)
Jimson weed
Amphetamines
Phencyclidine (PCP)
Alcohol

muscle coordination, combativeness, and coma. Direct thermal damage to the brain combined with decreased cerebral blood flow can lead to cerebral edema and hemorrhage. The brain, particularly the cerebellum, is extremely sensitive to thermal injury; therefore the range of neurologic symptoms is broad.[1,12,23]

Management of heat stroke is directed at reducing core temperature as rapidly as possible and treating subsequent complications. Heat stroke is often fatal despite rapid treatment. Maintenance of airway, breathing, and circulation (ABCs) is crucial for patient recovery. Establish an airway, and administer supplemental oxygen by the method most appropriate for the patient's level of consciousness. Fluid volume is not depleted in most victims of hyperthermia; therefore 1 to 2 L of 0.9% saline solution during the first 4 hours is usually adequate. Lactated Ringer's solution is not recommended because the liver may not be able to metabolize lactate. Hemodynamic monitoring is indicated until normal vital signs are restored. After the ABCs are secured, rapid, aggressive cooling becomes the next intervention.

Prehospital treatment starts with removing the patient from the external source of heat and removing all clothing. Aggressive ice- or cold-water cooling should be avoided in the field to prevent shivering and seizure activity, which will only increase the core body temperature. Spray the patient with tepid water while fanning the entire body to promote cooling by evaporation. Well-padded ice packs in vascular areas such as the groin, axilla, and neck are also useful. Ice water or cold water immersion is an effective method of rapidly lowering core body temperature; however, its use is one the of the more hotly debated topics in the heatstroke literature. In addition to being unpleasant for the patient and caregiver, access to the patient is limited. Ice water immersion can also cause shivering, which dramatically increases oxygen consumption and can increase body temperature. Intravenous chlorpromazine (Thorazine), 10 to 25 mg, may be used to prevent shivering during the cooling process. Massive peripheral vasoconstriction from ice water immersion can act as an insulator and prevent adequate cooling. After the patient is in the emergency department (ED), aggressive cooling measures such as ice water gastric and peritoneal lavage can also be used. Cooling blankets may be used; however, cooling from wet skin is 25 times more effective than cooling from dry skin

Cooling should be continued until the rectal temperature is 102° F (38.8° C) or less. Core temperature should be monitored frequently during the cooling phase to prevent inadvertent hypothermia. Aspirin and acetaminophen have not proved effective in reducing hyperthermia secondary to heat stroke. Corticosteroid therapy, usually with methylprednisolone, may be used to treat cerebral edema. Intracranial pressure monitoring may be helpful for some patients. To increase renal blood flow, intravenous mannitol, 0.2 g/kg over 3 to 5 minutes, is recommended in patients over 12 years of age whose urinary output is less than 50 mL/hr.

High-output cardiac failure may develop with heat stroke; therefore patients should be placed on a cardiac monitor.

Central venous pressure and pulmonary capillary wedge pressure monitoring may be considered in the critical phase to evaluate fluid status. Protecting the kidneys and liver from thermal and low-flow damage is critical. Myoglobinuria and poor renal perfusion put the kidneys at risk for renal failure; therefore urine should be carefully monitored for color, amount, pH, and myoglobin.[1,12,23]

COLD-RELATED EMERGENCIES

Approximately 700 fatalities occur annually in the United States from cold exposure.[6] In 2003 the majority of reported deaths from exposure to cold were male (67%), and 51% were older than 65 years of age.[6] Most deaths do not occur in the extreme northern areas but are reported in temperate regions, urban areas in poorly heated apartments, and among the homeless. Nicotine, alcohol intoxication, and major psychiatric disorders are also predisposing factors.[4]

Injuries related to cold exposure are localized or generalized. Localized cold emergencies include chilblains, immersion foot, and frostbite, whereas hypothermia is a generalized cold emergency. Cold-related emergencies occur with prolonged exposure to cold ambient temperatures, immersion in cold water, or as a result of factors such as alcohol. Ambient temperature is a product of air temperature and wind speed: the greater the wind speed, the lower the ambient temperature. Heat loss occurs 24 times more quickly with immersion in cold water.[12,19]

Chilblains

Chilblains are localized areas of itching and redness accompanied by recurrent edema to exposed or poorly insulated body parts such as the ears, fingers, and toes. Chilblains are usually seen in cool, damp climates with temperatures above freezing. Chilblains are probably a mild form of frostbite with gradual onset of symptoms. There is generally no pain; however, the patient may experience transient numbness and tingling. Initial pallor or redness of the nose, digits, or ears may evolve into plaques and small, superficial ulcerations over chronically exposed areas.

Prehospital treatment begins with removal to a warm area in conjunction with covering the affected area with a warm hand or placing fingers under the axilla.[19] Elevation of the affected area decreases edema, which increases circulation and allows gradual warming at room temperature. Never rub or massage injured tissue. Avoid direct heat application. Tissue damage is rarely seen with chilblains; however, the patient should be instructed to protect the area from injury and further environmental exposure and to watch for signs of secondary infection.[11,18]

Nonfreezing Cold Injury (Immersion Foot)

Nonfreezing cold injury, a syndrome also known as immersion foot or trench foot, results from damage to peripheral tissues from prolonged (hours to days) contact between a wet foot and cold temperature. This usually occurs when the patient is wearing a watertight boot that does not allow normal evaporative "breathing." This condition is commonly seen in hunters and soldiers on outdoor maneuvers. Feet initially are cold, damp, numb, and edematous but within 24 to 48 hours will appear warm. Vasodilation and hyperemia, which result from warming, cause intense burning and tingling. Prolonged and repeated exposure can lead to lymphangitis, cellulitis, thrombophlebitis, and liquefaction gangrene.

Therapeutic interventions include drying the feet and changing frequently into dry socks. After the patient is in a controlled environment, rewarm injured areas gradually by exposing them to air or soaking them in warm water (100° F to 105° F [37.7° C to 40.5° C]) before drying. Some clinicians recommend daily air-drying of the feet for 8 hours.[3] Immersion foot is reversible with timely treatment. Patients are usually hospitalized for observation and prevention of complications.

Frostbite

Frostbite, the most prevalent injury caused by extreme cold, occurs when ice crystals form in intracellular spaces as tissue freezes. These crystals enlarge and compress cells, causing membrane rupture, interruption of enzymatic activity, and altered metabolic processes. Histamine release increases capillary permeability, red cell aggregation, and microvascular occlusion.[1] Once frostbite occurs, damage is irreversible. Further exposure to extreme cold or trauma increases tissue damage and worsens the injury. The patient with frostbite may also have hypothermia. Treatment of hypothermia takes priority over management of frostbite. Frostbite can be superficial or deep, depending on the degree of the cold and the length of exposure. Estimation of the extent of injury may not be possible until several days after exposure.[6,12]

Superficial Frostbite

Superficial frostbite involves skin and subcutaneous tissue and is similar to a superficial burn. Fingertips, ears, nose, toes, and cheeks are the areas most commonly affected. Symptoms include tingling, numbness, burning sensation, and white, waxy color. Frozen skin feels cold and stiff. After the tissue thaws, the patient may feel a hot, stinging sensation. Affected areas become mottled and blisters develop within a few hours. Frostbite tissue is extremely sensitive to subsequent cold and heat exposure and therefore is susceptible to repeat frostbite or burn injury.

Injured tissue is friable, so recovery depends on very gentle handling. Do not rewarm if there is a chance of refreezing. Do not rub the affected area. Apply warm soaks (104° F to 110° F [40° C to 43.3° C]), and elevate the extremity. Place the patient on bed rest for several days until the full extent of the injury has been evaluated and normal circulation has returned. The patient's room should be warm; however, heavy blankets should be avoided because friction and weight on the affected area can lead to sloughing.[6,12]

Deep Frostbite

Deep frostbite occurs when the temperature of a limb is lowered. Deep frostbite usually involves muscles, bones, and tendons. The degree of frostbite depends on ambient temperature, wind chill factor, duration of exposure, whether the patient was wet while exposed or in direct contact with metal objects, and the type of clothing worn. Deep frostbite appears white or yellow-white and is hard, cool, and insensitive to touch.[1] The patient has a burning sensation followed by a feeling of warmth, then numbness. Blisters appear 1 to 7 days after injury. Edema of the entire extremity occurs and may persist for months (Figure 40-1). A gray-black mottling eventually progresses to gangrene (Figure 40-2).

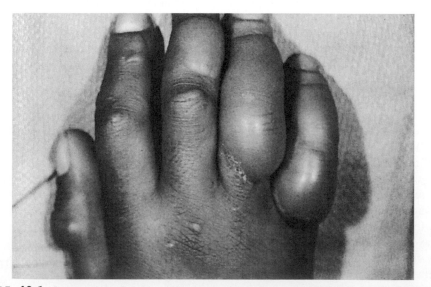

FIGURE **40-1.** Large, clear frostbite blisters on the right hand. (From Rosen P, Barkin RM, Hockberger RS et al, editors: *Emergency medicine: concepts and clinical practice,* ed 4, St. Louis, 1998, Mosby.)

Prehospital treatment includes transport with gentle handling and moderate elevation of the affected part.[3] Rewarming of the affected area is deferred until the patient reaches the ED. Do not rub the affected part with snow or ice. If the extremity has thawed, keep it immobile. Prevent heat loss by removing wet clothing, covering the patient with dry blankets, and removing the patient from the cold environment. If the patient is transported in a ground or air ambulance, warmed oxygen is recommended. Mylar or wool head coverings help prevent further heat loss.

Rapid rewarming under controlled conditions is the ideal treatment for maintaining tissue viability. Rewarming the patient with hypothermia and severe frostbite should occur with strict medical control. After the patient reaches the ED, obtain a baseline core temperature (rectal or esophageal), then immerse the affected area in warm (104° F to 110° F [40° C to 43.3° C]) water. Thawing frozen tissue is extremely painful, so liberal administration of parenteral narcotics is needed in severe cases. Warm all intravenous fluids before infusing them. Assess tetanus immunization status, and consider antibiotic therapy for deep infections. If hypothermia is not present, administer warm oral liquids. Cover the patient with warm blankets, but avoid friction and pressure on the affected area. Protect the thawed part with a large, soft, bulky dressing. Elevate the affected area to minimize edema. If severe vasoconstriction is present, escharotomy may be required. Final determination of the depth of injury may not be possible for several weeks; therefore amputation is not considered in the ED.

Hypothermia

Hypothermia can occur in many different situations, including cold ambient air, cold water immersion, or cold water submersion. Hypothermia can also occur as the result of a disease process (e.g., hypoglycemia), infusion of room temperature fluids, alcohol consumption, and ingestion of some medications. Hypothermia is defined as a core temperature below 95° F (35° C). Severe hypothermia is a core temperature less than 90° F (32.2° C). The American Heart Association has established 86° F (30° C) as the temperature for initiation of aggressive internal rewarming procedures.[17]

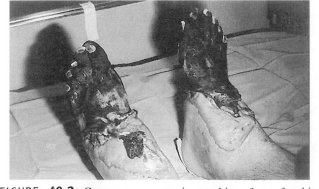

FIGURE **40-2.** Gangrenous necrosis resulting from frostbite injury. (From Auerbach P, editor: *Wilderness medicine*, ed 5, St. Louis, 2007, Mosby.)

The body's metabolic responses depend on a normal core temperature. As the core temperature drops, there is a progressive decrease in cellular activity and organ function. When the temperature drops by 18° F (10° C), the basal metabolic rate drops by two to three times the normal rate. The most obvious response is seen in the central nervous system (CNS). The patient becomes apathetic, weak, and easily fatigued, with impaired reasoning, coordination, and gait. The patient's speech is slow or slurred. Renal blood flow decreases, causing a decline in the glomerular filtration rate. Impaired water reabsorption leads to dehydration. Decreased respiratory rate and effort lead to carbon dioxide retention, hypoxia, and acidosis. Shivering consumes glucose stores, so the patient becomes hypoglycemic. Insulin levels fall, so available glucose decreases, forcing the body to metabolize fat for energy. Drug metabolism in the liver is sluggish, so medication effects may last longer.[8,17]

The cardiovascular system is also dramatically affected. Cold heart muscle is irritable and prone to dysrhythmias. The Osborne or J wave is a striking feature seen on electrocardiogram in approximately one third of hypothermic patients[32] (Figure 40-3). The J wave is described as a "humplike" deflection between the QRS complex and the early part of the ST segment. The most common dysrhythmias are atrial and ventricular fibrillation. The cold patient is in great danger of ventricular fibrillation when core temperature falls below 82° F (27.8° C). Ventricular fibrillation at these extremely cold temperatures does not respond to conventional treatment without prior rewarming. Defibrillation is limited to three shocks until core temperature is greater than 86° F (30° C).[10] Intravenous medications are also limited until the core temperature is greater than 86° F (30° C). Careful handling of hypothermic patients, especially when their temperatures reach the vulnerable mid-80s range, is imperative because even turning may cause ventricular fibrillation. Rewarming procedures are active or passive, based on external warming or internal warming.[17] Table 40-1 lists various procedures by category.

The goal in mild hypothermia (93.2° F to 96.8° F [34° C to 36° C]), in which the patient is still shivering, alert, and oriented, is to prevent further heat loss and rewarm the patient as rapidly as possible.[8,16,17] Passive external rewarming techniques such as moving the patient to a warm environment, replacing wet clothing with dry material, and wrapping with warm blankets may be effective. However, many patients require internal rewarming using warmed humidified oxygen. Giving the patient warmed, oral fluids that contain glucose or other sugars provides more heat through calories. Passive rewarming raises the temperature 1° F to 4° F (0.5° C to 2.0° C) per hour. Gradual rewarming minimizes the risk for active rewarming shock.

In moderate hypothermia (86° F to 93.2° F [30° C to 34° C]), rewarm truncal areas at 1° F (0.5° C) per hour using heating blankets such as Bair Hugger Therapy, radiant heating lamps, and hot water bottles. Monitor closely for marked vasodilatation and subsequent hypotension. American Heart Association guidelines recommend active

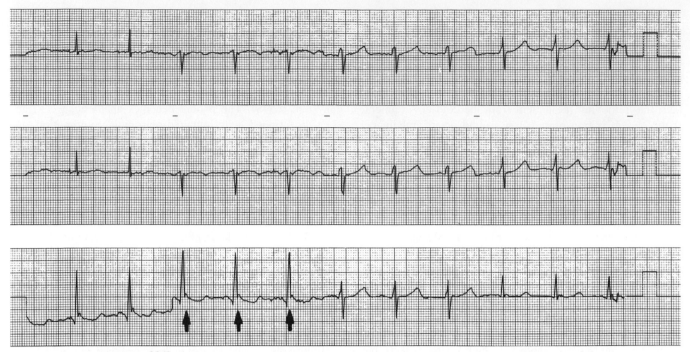

FIGURE **40-3.** Hypothermic J waves with QT prolongation. (From Rosen P, Barkin RM, Hockberger RS et al: *Emergency medicine: concepts and clinical practice,* ed 3, vol 1, St. Louis, 1992, Mosby.)

Table 40-1. **REWARMING TECHNIQUES**	
External Rewarming Procedures	**Internal Rewarming Procedures**
PASSIVE	**PASSIVE**
Move the patient to a warm area	Warmed humidified oxygen
Remove patient's wet clothing	Warmed intravenous fluids
Cover the patient with blankets	
ACTIVE	**ACTIVE**
Radiant heat lamps	Peritoneal lavage with KCL-free fluid
Heating blankets	Gastrointestinal irrigation
Bair Hugger warming blanket	Extracorporeal rewarming
Hot water bottles	Cardiopulmonary bypass
Heating pads	Hemodialysis
	Esophageal rewarming tubes
	Continuous arteriovenous rewarming (CAVR)

KCL, Potassium chloride.

internal rewarming when core temperature is less than 86° F (30° C) (see Table 40-1). Warmed humidified oxygen via endotracheal tube (108° F to 111° F [42.2° C to 43.8° C]), mechanically warmed intravenous fluid, peritoneal lavage, esophageal rewarming tubes, gastrointestinal irrigation, bladder irrigation, extracorporeal rewarming cardiopulmonary bypass, and hemodialysis may all be used.

In severe hypothermia (lower than 78.8° F [26° C]), active internal (core) rewarming in conjunction with active external rewarming procedures is essential to prevent rewarming shock. Rewarming shock can occur after rewarming is initiated. Cold peripheral blood returns to the central circulation, causing a continual drop in core temperature. Circulation of cold blood through the heart also increases ventricular irritability and leads to fibrillation. Rewarming may also cause peripheral vasodilatation, which can precipitate hypotension and cardiovascular collapse.

The continuous arteriovenous rewarming (CAVR) method, developed at the University of Washington, employs a modified bypass technique for rapid blood rewarming using a Level One fluid warmer normally used for trauma resuscitation. The treatment is preferred for patients with profound hypothermia. A spontaneous pulse is necessary because the patient's intrinsic blood pressure drives flow through the countercurrent module. (In true cardiothoracic bypass, an external pump is built into the machine.) The catheters are placed into a femoral artery and venous cordis, the blood is warmed as it flows through the countercurrent module. The CAVR method has rewarmed profoundly hypothermic patients five times more rapidly (39 minus versus 199 minutes) than standard methods and was demonstrated to decrease mortality rate.[13]

Successful rewarming depends on the patient's age, general condition before the hypothermic event, length of the patient's exposure, and careful handling by the ED team. To prevent hyperthermia secondary to aggressive rewarming, discontinue active rewarming when core temperature reaches 89.6° F to 93.2° F (32° C to 34° C).

SUBMERSION INCIDENTS

Each year in the United States more than 4,000 people die of drowning, with an additional 50,000 surviving submersion events annually.[7] The age distribution of victims is bimodal. One peak is for children less than 4 years of age (40% of all drowning victims); the other peak is for 15- to 25-year-olds.[31] Nearly 80% of teenagers who drown or suffer submersion injuries are male. Toddlers and young children are at risk because of their naturally inquisitive nature and inadequate supervision. Teenage boys are at risk because of risk-taking behavior during water-related activities, with alcohol as a contributing factor in more than 60% of teenage drownings.[7,20]

Submersion injury or near-drowning occurs when a patient initially survives suffocation while submerged in a liquid medium (Box 40-2). Drowning refers to death within 24 hours after a submersion event. Submersion can be intentional or unintentional. An estimated 59% of drownings in children younger than 1 year occur in bathtubs, and 56% are a result of child abuse. Because submersion victims rarely aspirate more than 3 to 4 mL/kg as a result of reflex laryngospasm, differentiating between saltwater and freshwater submersion is clinically insignificant.

Hypoxemia, laryngospasm, and fluid aspiration cause airway inflammation, obstruction, and collapse of the small airways. Pulmonary capillaries become leaky, resulting in pulmonary edema and acute respiratory distress syndrome (ARDS). Surfactant washout and inactivation contribute to the development of atelectasis and intrapulmonary shunting. Severity of neurologic outcome depends on the duration of submersion, temperature of the water, and the time elapsed before effective basic life support (BLS). Submersion greater than 5 minutes is generally associated with severe neurologic damage.

Complications associated with near-drowning are the direct result of the hypoxic event. Primary complications are pulmonary, cerebral, and cardiovascular, including pulmonary edema, pneumonitis, ARDS, anoxic encephalopathy, and cardiopulmonary arrest. Later complications include cerebral edema, disseminated intravascular coagulation (DIC), acute tubular necrosis, and renal failure. The most important part of treatment for a near-drowning victim is immediate resuscitation in the prehospital phase. If a submersion victim has appropriate airway and ventilation management, anoxic brain injury may be avoided.[7,11,16,26,27]

Secondary drowning can occur up to 72 hours after the initial insult; therefore every near-drowning victim should be taken to the hospital for observation, regardless of how he or she appears immediately after the event. Inflammatory reactions in the lung injure the alveolar-capillary membrane and alter surfactant function. Approximately 10% to 15% of deaths associated with drowning are due to secondary drowning. Near-drowning victims should be observed for at least 24 hours.[7,11,16]

Immersion in cold water can cause sudden death from cardiac dysrhythmias rather than drowning. Immersion syndrome occurs when cold water stimulates the vagus nerve, causing bradycardia or cardiac arrest. Many victims of cold water immersion have a good chance of survival without neurologic sequelae when resuscitation is initiated early.

Presenting symptoms with near-drowning vary with length of submersion, water temperature, quality of water, associated injuries, onset of BLS, and the patient's resuscitative response. Occasionally, near-drowning victims may be asymptomatic; however, most present with mild dyspnea, a deathlike appearance with blue or gray coloring, apnea or tachypnea, hypotension, heart rate as slow as 4 to 5 beats/min or pulselessness, cold skin, dilated pupils known as fish eyes, hypothermia, and vomiting.[33]

Field resuscitation of the near-drowning victim is crucial for survival. Performing immediate BLS procedures on the victim after removal from the water has been cited as a significant factor in survival, regardless of advanced life support availability. Initial resuscitation focuses on correcting hypoxia, associated acidosis, and hypotension as soon as possible. Box 40-3 highlights essential prehospital resuscitation. Establish a patent airway while initiating cervical spine protection (there is a high incidence of cervical spine injury in drowning victims). Additional interventions include applying a nonrebreather oxygen mask to patients with spontaneous respirations, initiating bag-mask ventilation or endotracheal intubation if indicated, ventilating with 100% oxygen to correct hypoxia and acidosis, and obtaining intravenous access.

All submersion victims require aggressive in-hospital resuscitation until all reasonable efforts prove futile and the patient is near normothermic. Resuscitation efforts emphasize stabilization of the ABCs and continued warming. Rewarming efforts should be aggressive if the victim's core temperature is below 86° F (30° C). The heart is resistant to drug therapy and electrical conversion when the core temperature is lower than 86° F (30° C); therefore early rewarming is essential to preventing ventricular fibrillation. The most

Box 40-3	ESSENTIAL GUIDELINES FOR NEAR-DROWNING MANAGEMENT

Determine duration of submersion.

Clear airway using cervical spine precautions, assess breathing, and provide rescue ventilations as soon as possible.

Assess circulation. If pulse is not palpated, begin chest compressions immediately. If advanced cardiac life support is available, proceed with gentle intubation.

Assess carefully for associated injuries when indicated by history and mechanism of injury.

Remove victim's wet clothing, and gently wrap him or her in dry blankets.

Do not attempt to warm victim if medical facility is less than 15 minutes away.

Initiate warming techniques (e.g., warm oxygen, warm intravenous fluids, or well-padded heat packs) if medical facility is more than 15 minutes away.

Transport the victim to a medical facility even if he or she recovers at the scene.

important factor in determining outcome is the patient's response to resuscitation as measured by serial neurologic examinations. Poor prognostic factors include a Glasgow Coma Scale score less than or equal to 5, prolonged submersion (more than 5 minutes), delay in initiating BLS procedures, pH less than 7.0, water temperatures of greater than 77° F (25° C), and asystole on arrival to the ED.[4,17]

DIVING EMERGENCIES

Over the past few decades self-contained underwater breathing apparatus (scuba) diving has enjoyed increased popularity. As equipment comfort and safety have improved, the recreational market has expanded significantly. Nearly 400,000 Americans achieve new scuba certification each year. There are thousands of commercial and military divers; however, most of the 5 million scuba divers in the United States are recreational divers.[1,2] As the number of divers increases, dive-related injuries increase. Most diving-related emergencies occur because the human body is not designed for the marine environment. Cold water, lack of available oxygen, and inability to run from hazards are intrinsic problems for which the diver must compensate. Diving accidents are increasing in all areas of the country, not just warm coastal resort areas. The most serious injuries are discussed in this section: arterial gas embolism, nitrogen narcosis, and decompression sickness.

Divers are exposed to pressure changes related to water. Water is denser than air, so pressure changes are greater under water. Even at relatively shallow depths, Boyle's law states that gas volume is inversely related to pressure at a constant temperature. For the diver, this means volume decreases and pressure increases as he or she descends. This principle is the mechanism behind all types of barotrauma, the most common medical problem that occurs with divers.

When a diver uses a scuba tank of pressurized air, lung volume remains constant at various depths. If the diver ascends but does not exhale, water pressure decreases and gas in the lungs expands, greatly increasing pressure in the lungs.[1,2,5]

Arterial Gas Embolism

Arterial gas embolism (AGE) is the most serious and dangerous of all diving emergencies, second only to drowning as cause of death among divers. As gas expands, lungs expand to the point of rupture, causing pneumothoraces. High-pressure air is forced into the circulatory system, producing air embolism. Exhaling during a controlled, slow ascent prevents air embolism. Divers risk injury when they ascend too rapidly or when they hold their breath during ascent.

AGE appears within seconds to minutes of ascent, usually less than 10 minutes from time of alveolar rupture. Complications of air embolism depend on the end point of air bubbles. If bubbles enter the coronary arteries, the patient may have signs of myocardial infarction, whereas an embolism entering the cerebral circulation causes neurologic symptoms. Other complications include blocked vascular flow to the spinal cord with subsequent spinal cord injury, altered blood coagulation leading to DIC, and hemoconcentration. The bubbles in AGE originate not from supersaturation of gases in the blood and tissue but from rupture of the alveoli due to the barotrauma of ascent. The bubbles enter the pulmonary vein and are carried to the heart and systemic circulation. The classic presentation is a sudden onset of unconsciousness within minutes of reaching the surface after a dive. Symptoms occur immediately, and the effects are devastating.[1,2,5,12]

Death is an immediate threat to the diver with AGE. The unconscious patient should be intubated immediately. Ensure proper ventilation with positive pressure ventilation and 100% oxygen. Perform needle thoracentesis for tension pneumothorax. Place the patient in the left lateral position to avoid cerebral embolism. If air transport is necessary, cabin altitude should not exceed 1000 feet. Definitive treatment is prompt and includes advanced life support measures, recompression, and hyperbaric oxygen therapy as quickly as possible.[1,2,12]

Nitrogen Narcosis

Solubility of any gas in a liquid is almost directly proportional to pressure of the liquid at a constant temperature (Henry's law). The composition of room air is 79% nitrogen. Nitrogen narcosis occurs when nitrogen becomes dissolved in solution because pressures are greater than normal. Symptoms begin to appear at depths of 100 feet or more and resolve with ascent. Experienced divers usually have fewer problems than novices, although nitrogen narcosis is a risk for all divers.

Dissolved nitrogen has neurodepressant effects similar to alcohol. The "martini" rule is used to evaluate effects of dives to different depths. Every 50 feet of descent is comparable to one martini. Initially the diver may exhibit impaired judgment, a feeling of alcohol intoxication, slowed motor response, loss of proprioception, and euphoria. Below 200 feet, nitrogen narcosis renders the diver unable to work; however, individual divers have varying tolerance levels for nitrogen narcosis. Loss of consciousness occurs at approximately 300 feet.

Nitrogen narcosis has no real metabolic significance. The risk lies with impairment of the diver's judgment. Jacques Cousteau aptly described this condition as "rapture of the deep." Divers become euphoric, silly, and unaware of the dangerous situation and the need to surface. Ascent to the surface causes symptoms to disappear completely, so no further therapy is required. Nitrogen narcosis can be avoided by limiting the depth of dives.[30]

Decompression Sickness

Decompression sickness, also called the bends, dysbarism, caisson disease, and diver's paralysis, is the most common form of diving emergency. Symptoms occur after rapid ascent. Speed of safe ascent is defined for each dive, depending on the depth-time relationship of the dive using standard U.S. Navy air decompression tables. According to Henry's law, gradual ascent allows the ambient pressure of nitrogen to reach an equilibrium that permits nitrogen to escape through respired air. Decompression sickness occurs during ascent and only when equilibrium cannot be established. Bubbles are squeezed into blood and tissues, obstructing flow and impairing tissue perfusion. Effects can be seen in almost every organ of the body.

Typically symptoms of decompression sickness begin within 30 minutes of ascent but may be delayed up to 36 hours. Some individuals (30%) exhibit symptoms before or on surfacing.[2] Nitrogen bubbles can develop in any tissue. The most significant mechanical effect is vascular occlusion in any tissue (e.g., supersaturation of lymphatic tissue with nitrogen causes lymphedema, cellular distention, membrane rupture). Physiologic effects are poor tissue perfusion and ischemia. Other symptoms characteristic of decompression sickness include cough, shortness of breath, and dyspnea (chokes); joint pain (bends); and neurologic symptoms such as fatigue, diplopia, headaches, dizziness, unconsciousness, paresthesias, and seizures.

Bends can occur at depths less than 33 feet, or 1 atmospheric pressure, if ascent is too rapid. Any joint pain within 24 to 48 hours of a dive should be treated as decompression sickness. Upper extremities are affected more often than lower extremities. A simple test for "joint bends" is inflation of a blood pressure cuff to 150 to 200 mm Hg or greater around the affected joint. Pain from the bends subsides as long as the cuff remains inflated. Initial treatment begins with high-flow oxygen (100%) via nonrebreather mask to improve oxygenation and eliminate nitrogen. Fluid replacement is performed with intravenous 0.9% saline or lactated Ringer's solution until urine output is 1 to 2 mL/kg/hr. Narcotic analgesics should be avoided because of their respiratory depressant

effect. Steroids are often recommended to reduce progression and reoccurrence. Aspirin (325 to 650 mg) is given prophylactically for its antiplatelet activity. Treat patients for symptomatic nausea, vomiting, or headache. Definitive treatment is immediate recompression in a chamber with hyperbaric oxygen therapy administered according to standardized protocols published by the U.S. Navy. The Navy dive treatment tables are very effective, especially when recompression is initiated early. The treatment selected is based on the severity of the patient's condition. The number of treatments is determined by physical examination and identifiable improvements from the baseline condition. When more information is required, 24-hour assistance is available through the national Divers Alert Network at Duke University at 919-684-8111, the local health department, or the nearest naval facility. Education and resource materials are available from the Divers Alert Network at 919-684-2948 (http://anesthesia.duhs.duke.edu/divisions/dan.html or http://www.diversalertnetwork.org/about/). The Undersea and Hyperbaric Medical Society, which publishes a directory listing all approved chambers in the United States and resources for international referral, can be contacted at 301-942-2980 or 410-257-6606 (http://www.uhms.org/).

Decompression sickness may be prevented by remaining within a safe range of depth and time during repeated dives and gradual ascent with delays at certain depths. This allows nitrogen absorption and can be accomplished with decompression tables to calculate rate of nitrogen absorption. The depth and length of each dive should be limited. The diver should carry a scuba identification card for at least 48 hours after a dive.[1,2,12]

Other Diving Problems
The Squeeze

The squeeze occurs when air is trapped in hollow chambers such as the ears, sinuses, pulmonary tree, gastrointestinal tract, teeth, and added air space such as the face mask or diving suit. Severe, sharp pain occurs when external pressure in these spaces exceeds internal pressure. The squeeze occurs if the diver descends to depths without exhalation. Pressure in the mask can cause pain, capillary rupture, skin ecchymosis, and conjunctival hemorrhage. Entrapped air in the external auditory canal from a tight-fitting diving hood causes ear squeeze on descent, resulting in pain, bleeding, hemorrhagic blebs, or tympanic membrane rupture. Middle-ear squeeze is caused by a blocked eustachian tube or paranasal sinus with inability to equalize pressure in these spaces. Diving should be avoided when these chambers are congested from colds or allergies. Gradual descents while diving allow pressures in air-filled chambers to equalize. If the symptoms are mild, decongestants are recommended. If the symptoms are moderate, a short course of oral steroids is often prescribed. If the tympanic membrane is ruptured, consider antibiotics for otitis media. A more serious but less common type of aural squeeze is inner-ear barotrauma. Structures of the inner ear may rupture with sudden pressure changes between the middle and inner ear. Permanent nerve damage and deafness can occur. Consultation with an otolaryngologist is recommended for the dive patient with tinnitus, vertigo, or deafness. Barodontalgia (dental barotrauma) occurs when air is trapped under a faulty filling as a result of pressure changes on descent. Abscesses and dental infections also can cause this syndrome.[1,2,12,30]

Treatment for all squeeze-related problems is gradual ascent to shallow depths to decrease pressure and maintenance of the ABCs. Symptomatic therapy with decongestants, both oral and nasal, is indicated for sinus squeeze. Pain control should be instituted with nonsteroidal antiinflammatory drugs.[1,2,12]

Barotrauma of Ascent

Barotrauma of ascent is the reverse of the squeeze. Although air-filled chambers may equalize during descent, air trapped in these spaces expands as atmospheric pressure decreases during ascent. If air cannot escape, barotrauma occurs. This condition is uncomfortable; however, no treatment is required because the condition subsides with time as the pressure gradually equalizes.

CARBON MONOXIDE POISONING

Carbon monoxide (CO) is a colorless, odorless, and tasteless gas. Most severe cases of CO intoxication are associated with inhalation of smoke from house fires; however, engine exhaust, improperly vented stoves, and faulty stoves or heating systems are also significant causes of unintentional poisoning. Poisoning occurs primarily during the winter, usually because of faulty heating systems. CO poisoning is the most frequent source of poisoning in the United States, with CO poisoning from engine exhaust a common means of suicide. Intentional and unintentional CO poisoning account for 3500 to 4000 deaths annually. Many victims die before transport to the hospital.[10]

The most significant effect of CO exposure is hypoxia. Toxicity is the result of the affinity of hemoglobin for CO, an altered oxygen-hemoglobin dissociation curve, and impaired cytochrome oxidase systems. Hemoglobin's affinity for CO is 200 times greater than for oxygen. Hemoglobin preferentially binds with CO, causing a decrease in oxygen-carrying capacity even when oxygen is available. Carboxyhemoglobin (COHb), formed when hemoglobin binds with CO, can be measured to determine severity of CO poisoning. COHb is measured in parts per million, with concentration indicated by percentage (Table 40-2). CO also binds with myoglobin at a rate 40 times greater than oxygen. Consequently, hypoxia occurs at the tissue level and in the oxygen transport system. Pulse oximetry is not reliable with carbon monoxide poisoning because it will indicate adequate saturation but does not differentiate CO from oxygen.

Generally oxygen diffuses from the blood into the tissues. The oxygen-hemoglobin dissociation curve describes this process. Any event that shifts the curve to the left or right affects cellular oxygenation. Hypoxia that results from a shift in the COHb dissociation curve is more significant than hypoxia that results from a simple reduction in functional hemoglobin. COHb shifts the oxygen curve to the right so that the partial pressure needed to unload oxygen from blood to the tissue is lower than in normal tissue. This makes it easier for more CO to bind with the hemoglobin.

Table 40-2. SIGNS AND SYMPTOMS OF CARBON MONOXIDE EXPOSURE

Exposure Level	Signs and Symptoms	Treatment
MILD		
10%-25% COHb when no cardiac or neurologic involvement	Throbbing headache, nausea, impaired function for complex tasks	Maintain airway; administer IV fluids; use cardiac monitor; ensure oxygen administration by tight-fitting mask for 4 hours or until COHb <5%
MODERATE		
20%-30% COHb; less if cardiac or neurologic involvement is present	Severe headache, irritability, weakness, visual problems, palpitations, loss of dexterity, nausea and vomiting, ECG abnormalities, confusion, and lethargy	Hyperbaric oxygen administration at 3 atm for 46 minutes; repeat in 6 hours if full CNS recovery does not occur; maintain airway; administer IV fluids; use cardiac monitor
SEVERE		
40%-50% COHb	Tachycardia, tachypnea, collapse, syncope	As above
LIFE-THREATENING		
50%-60% COHb	Coma, Cheyne-Stokes respirations, intermittent convulsions, cherry-red mucous membranes	As above
LETHAL		
Greater than 60% COHb	Cardiac and respiratory depression, likely cardiac arrest	CPR and as above

COHb, Carboxyhemoglobin; *CNS,* central nervous system; *CPR,* cardiopulmonary resuscitation; *ECG,* electrocardiogram; *IV,* intravenous.

CO also interferes with cytochrome oxidase systems. Cytochrome oxidase is an oxidizing enzyme found in mitochondria and important in cellular respiration. Decreased function of these systems impairs cellular respiration by displacing oxygen, particularly in high-rate metabolic organs (i.e., the brain and heart). Oxygen displacement is responsible for dysrhythmias and many CNS symptoms seen in CO poisoning.

Symptoms may initially be vague but worsen with increased exposure. Mild to moderate CO poisoning is often misdiagnosed as a viral illness or a benign headache. Variability of symptoms in individuals with identical exposure exists; the longer the time between exposure and presentation, the greater the variability. Children may have increased susceptibility to CO toxicity. A child's higher metabolic rate may cause syncope and lethargy at COHb levels of 25%. Specific signs and general management of CO poisoning are discussed in Table 40-2. The cornerstone for all treatment is high-flow oxygen to displace CO from hemoglobin. The half-life of CO is 5 to 6 hours on room air. Half-life is reduced to 1 hour with 100% oxygen and less than 20 minutes with hyperbaric oxygen therapy.

CO promotes dysrhythmias and myocardial ischemia. Alterations in the alveolar-capillary membrane may lead to pulmonary edema and hemorrhage. Neurologic deficits include seizures, cerebral edema, and coma. Renal failure can occur secondary to myoglobinuria. Patients with COHb levels greater than 25% or signs of cardiac ischemia or neurologic deficits should be admitted for observation and may be candidates for hyperbaric oxygen (HBO) therapy. HBO therapy is initiated to prevent life-threatening symptoms of cellular hypoxia and may prevent some of the delayed neurologic sequelae. If patients are discharged, instructions should include discussion of neurologic sequelae such as headache, loss of memory and concentration, irritability, personality changes, and excessive fatigue.

BITES AND STINGS

Specific environmental emergencies related to bites and stings include bites from snakes, animals, spiders, and ticks and stings from scorpions and hymenopterans (i.e., bees, wasps, hornets, and fire ants). Lethality is the result of poisonous venom and stings or secondary to anaphylaxis. Respiratory distress and anaphylactic shock are discussed in Chapters 30 and 32.

Snakebites

There are 3000 species of snakes in the world; of these, 375 species from five different families are venomous: Crotalidae, Elapidae, Viperidae, Colubridae, and Hydrophidae.[1,12,15] Two families of venomous snakes native to the United States are Crotalidae or pit vipers (rattlesnakes, copperheads, and cottonmouths) and Elapidae (coral snakes). Cobras and mambas belong to the Elapidae family but are not indigenous to the United States. It is estimated that as many as

2.5 million venomous snakebites occur internationally per year, and estimates of annual deaths from snakebites are as high as 125,000 worldwide.[1] Annually more than 45,000 snakebites occur in the United States. Envenomation occurs in only 8000 cases, and deaths from venomous snake bites account for 10 to 15 deaths each year.[1,2] Virtually all of the venomous bites in this country are from pit vipers (95%).[1,12,25,28] Pit vipers get their common name from a small "pit" between the eyes and nostrils that detects heat and allows the snake to sense prey at night. Venom is delivered through two fangs that the snake can retract at rest, but which spring into biting position rapidly. Figure 40-4 summarizes the differences between venomous and nonvenomous snakes.

Snakebite venom is a complex substance containing enzymes, glycoproteins, peptides, and other substances capable of causing tissue destruction—cardiotoxic, neurotoxic, hemotoxic, or any combination of these. Pit viper venom is primarily hemotoxic, whereas coral snake venom is primarily neurotoxic. In venomous creatures, all venom is designed to do the same thing: immobilize or kill the prey and begin the digestive process. Clinical presentations associated with envenomation are the result of digestive proteins, which break down muscles, break down cell barriers, destroy cell integrity, and trigger the coagulation cascade.

The amount of venom actually delivered by a pit viper bite varies. It is estimated that 20% to 30% of patients bitten by a snake, who actually have fang marks, have not received any venom at all. These are known as dry bites. The reason for this may be poor timing by the snake. Pit vipers have a very sophisticated mechanism that allows them to deliver venom at the exact instant their teeth are sunk into flesh. If the snake's timing is off, the venom may be squirted on the pant leg or released prematurely. A dry bite is defined as the absence of local, systemic, or coagulopathic effects. If there are no effects noted in 8 to 12 hours, the patient may be cleared for discharge. However, in some cases the venom effects may not become apparent for many hours after the bite.[1,12,25,28]

Signs and symptoms of snakebites depend on the circumstance of the bite, including the type and size of the snake, size and age of the patient, location and depth of the bite, number of bites, and amount of venom injected. Most snakebites occur in the lower extremities. Most bites occur around dawn or dusk during warm weather months.[1,2] The snake's teeth contain numerous microorganisms, so a bite can cause secondary infection. Major signs and symptoms are divided into local and systemic reactions. Local reactions include one or two fang marks, teeth marks, edema around the bite site 1 to 36 hours after the bite, pain at the site, petechiae, ecchymosis, loss of function of the limb, and possible necrosis 16 to 36 hours after the bite. Systemic reactions include nausea, vomiting, diaphoresis, syncope, and a metallic or rubber taste. The patient may develop paralysis; excessive salivation; difficulty speaking; visual disturbances; muscle twitching; paresthesia; epistaxis; blood in the stool, vomitus, or sputum; and ptosis. Neurologic symptoms include

CHARACTERISTICS

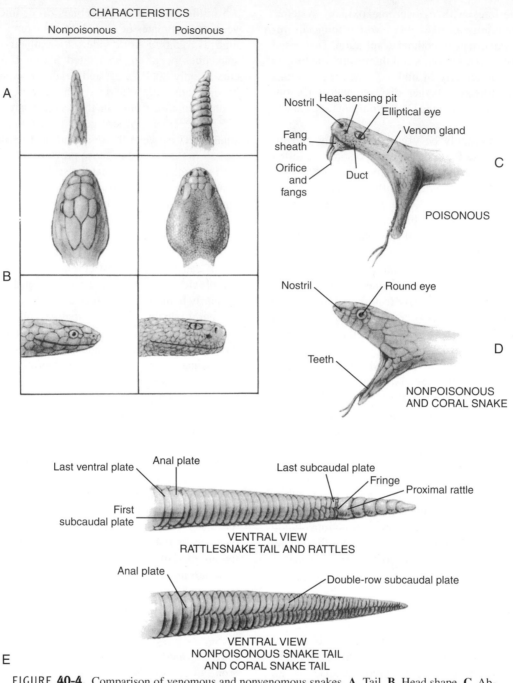

FIGURE **40-4.** Comparison of venomous and nonvenomous snakes. **A,** Tail. **B,** Head shape. **C,** Absence or presence of heat-sensing facial pit between the eye and the nostril. **D,** Absence or presence of well-developed venom glands, duct, and fangs. **E,** Belly scales leading up to the tail. (From Davis JH et al: *Surgery: a problem solving approach,* ed 2, vol 1, St. Louis, 1995, Mosby.)

constricted pupils and seizures. Life-threatening systemic reactions include severe hemorrhage, renal failure, and hypovolemic shock.

Initial assessment includes a history of the snakebite; for example, the size of the snake, location and depth of the injury, number of bites, and amount of venom injected (if known). Document the time of injury and all interventions before arrival in the ED. Stabilization of ABCs, keeping the patient calm and supine to minimize exertion, cardiac monitoring, and intravenous fluids should be initiated in the field when possible. Immobilize the limb at or below the level of the heart to reduce blood flow. Remove potentially constrictive jewelry or tight-fitting clothing. The following measures are not recommended treatment: incision, suction, tourniquets, electric shock, ice, and alcohol. Until recently the Sawyer Extractor pump was recommended, but various studies concluded it does not work for venomous snakebites and could potentiate the bite effects.[1,12] Mark the border of advancing edema with a pen every 15 minutes, so that an estimate of the severity of poisoning can be made by following the rate of progression. Venom sequestration techniques, such as applying a lymphatic or superficial venous constriction band or pressure immobilization, have been used effectively in Australia for field management of Elapid snake bites. One technique involves immediately wrapping the entire snake-bitten extremity with an elastic ACE wrap (as for a sprain). If used, it should not be removed until antivenin is available because of a potential bolus of venom release after removal.[1,12]

The initial management of hypotension or shock should include aggressive intravenous infusion of crystalloids (normal saline or lactated Ringer's). If organ perfusion remains inadequate after vigorous fluid infusion (2 L in adults), evidence supports a trial infusion of albumin, because of the rapid onset of increased vascular permeability after significant pit viper envenomation. Obtain a complete blood count; coagulation studies; electrolyte, blood urea nitrogen, creatinine, and creatinine phosphokinase levels; and blood type and crossmatch (coagulopathy). Clean the wound, and clearly mark and time the leading edges of envenomation every 15 minutes. Administer oral analgesics for pain or titrated does of intravenous opiates (e.g., morphine sulfate). Avoid aspirin and nonsteroidal antiinflammatory drugs because they may exacerbate coagulopathy. Administer tetanus prophylaxis if the patient's immunization history is incomplete or outdated. Plain radiographic films of the extremity may reveal retained teeth or fangs in the wound.

Suspect compartment syndrome if the extremity becomes increasingly tense secondary to edema and third-space fluid accumulation. Compartment pressures should be measured in this situation and an orthopedic consult obtained for possible fasciotomy to relieve pressure. Fasciotomy is usually indicated if compartment pressures remain persistently higher than 30 mm Hg despite appropriate use of antivenin.

Determine the severity of envenomation and need for antivenin. The general indication for antivenin treatment is the presence of progressive venom effects as indicated by worsening pain or swelling, a coagulopathy, or significant systemic effects such as hypotension or confusion. The main systemic effect of concern is hypotension. This typically reverses promptly with administration of antivenin, particularity if the patient is treated early. Neurologic and cardiac effects are also reversible with antivenin if treated early. The systemic manifestations include nausea, vomiting, paresthesia, and muscle fasciculations remote from the bite site. Local effects are manifest by progression of swelling up the extremity or toward the midline. A significant coagulation abnormality is also a relative indication for antivenom, particularity if it occurs within the first few hours after envenomation. Typical laboratory abnormalities include increased prothrombin time or international normalized ratio, decreased platelets, and hypofibrinogenemia, which improve with antivenin treatment.

Antivenin is most therapeutic when given within 4 to 6 hours of the bite and has limited value after 12 hours. Two antivenins for pit viper bites are currently available in the United States, Crotalidae Polyvalent Immune Fab (Ovine)

Table 40-3. ANTIVENIN CROTALIDAE POLYVALENT (ACP) DOSAGE REGIMEN

Signs and Symptoms	Degree of Envenomation	Dose
Fang marks; no local swelling or paresthesia	None	No skin test or antivenin required
Fang marks; local swelling of hands or feet; pain; no systemic responses	Minimal	3-5 vials*
Fang marks; progressive swelling beyond site of bite; mild systemic symptoms	Moderate	5-10 vials*
Multiple fang marks; progressive swelling, pain, and ecchymosis; marked systemic symptoms, hypotension, fasciculations, or clotting deficits	Severe	10-20 vials*

*Dilute antivenin in half-normal saline at a 1:4 ratio. Infuse within 2 hours. Repeat dose every 2 hours until symptoms subside. Children generally require 50% more antivenin.

(CroFab) (Protherics, Inc., Brentwood, Tennessee) and Antivenin (Crotalidae) Polyvalent (ACP) (Wyeth Laboratories, Marietta, Pennsylvania. Current research indicates that CroFab, available since 2000 and produced by injecting sheep with the venom, is more effective and safer to use than ACP, which is an equine-derived product. It appears that CroFab causes fewer acute anaphylactic reactions than ACP. (Fab) fragments with single antigen-binding sites are incapable of cross-linking immune complexes and stimulating the cascade of mediator release operant in anaphylaxis). Drawbacks to its use include significant cost and short half-life. In clinical trials the initial dosage of CroFab ranges from 4 to 12 vials, with repeated doses of 2 to 6 vials. No skin test or premedication is required for CroFab.[25,28]

ACP, an antivenin that has been used in the United States since 1954, is prepared in horse serum; therefore the patient should be questioned carefully about allergies to horse serum. Consider skin testing although controversial due to lack of efficacy. Monitor closely for systemic reactions such as urticaria, wheezing, or other symptoms of progressing anaphylaxis. Antivenin administration and dosing is guided by the clinical severity of envenomation. Table 40-3 provides a dosage regimen for ACP. Insufficient dosage is the most common cause of treatment failure. Administer antivenin until symptoms subside.

Lizard Bites

The iguana is a member of the family Iguanidae. The bite is generally nontoxic, causing pain without systemic reactions. Two venomous varieties, however, are the Gila monster (*Heloderma*) and the Mexican bearded lizard. Gila toxin is released in saliva. Symptoms may begin with pain and swelling, progressing to systemic symptoms of nausea, vomiting, weakness, hypotension, syncope, shock, and anaphylaxis. No antivenin is currently available for Gila toxin. Treatment includes wound care, tetanus prophylaxis, and analgesics. Meperidine enhances the effect of Gila toxin and should be avoided. Provide supportive care for systemic response.

Animal Bites

Estimates indicate that more than 5 million Americans are bitten by animals each year. Dogs and cats are involved in most of these bites.[1,12,22] Other animals involved in bites include rodents and other small mammals, such as ferrets and rabbits. Bites from more exotic animals (e.g., snakes, lizards, monkeys, farm animals) are rare. Dog and cat populations in the United States are estimated to exceed 50 million animals each. Many households in the United States include pets, and many children are bitten by family pets. Bites from both cats and dogs require careful management, and patients may experience long-term morbidity or may even die. Cat bites have a high incidence of infection (approximately 50%), and dog bites may cause severe injury to tissues. Treatment of animal bites includes cleaning the wound, tetanus prophylaxis, copious irrigation with saline solution, and analgesics as necessary. Careful wound excision may improve the cosmetic appearance of the scar and decrease the incidence of wound infection. Perform primary closure in certain wounds. Facial wounds rarely become infected because the face is well vascularized. Clean wounds also can be closed. Wounds on the hands or lower extremities should be left open. Patients who have a wound older than 6 hours are treated using delayed primary closure in lieu of primary closure. Consider rabies prophylaxis in certain circumstances (e.g., raccoon bites, bat bites, unprovoked attack by an unknown animal). Animal bites must be reported to health authorities based on local and state regulations.[1,12,15,21,24]

Dog Bites

Dog bites result in an estimated 340,000 ED visits annually throughout the United States. More than half of the bites seen by EDs occur at home. Dog bites account for 80% to 90% of all bites occurring to humans in the United States.[1,11,22] Most victims own the dogs that bite them, with children being the population at greatest risk. The most common sites of injury are the extremities. Dogs can produce crush injuries by the power of their jaws closing onto an extremity or other exposed body part. Bite injuries may result in damage to the face, hands, and feet, which may cause long-term scarring and loss of function. Dog bites are also responsible for the majority of reported deaths caused by nonvenomous animals.

Dog bite wounds may be simple punctures or major deforming lacerations, tears, avulsions, or soft-tissue crush injuries. Tissue necrosis may occur with a crush injury. The type of injury usually depends on the size of the dog and the body area where the wound is inflicted.

Treatment involves addressing ABCs immediately, especially in the event of facial and neck wounds. Wounds should be irrigated copiously with isotonic normal saline using a pressure irrigation set or an 18- to 20-gauge intravenous catheter. Use 100 to 200 mL of solution per inch of wound; however, heavily contaminated wounds may require more. Anticipate debridement of nonviable tissue. Puncture wounds are left open, whereas lacerations are loosely sutured. The extremity should be splinted and immobilized. Prophylactic antibiotic therapy is used with high-risk injuries such as hand and foot bites, puncture wounds, and wounds greater than 6 to 12 hours old. Report the incident to the local animal control or public health authorities. The dog should be quarantined for 10 days if immunization history is unknown or rabies is suspected. Consider tetanus prophylaxis.

Aftercare instructions for wound care should be given to the patient and family with careful explanation of signs and symptoms of infection. If a bite is not treated, infection, cellulitis, osteomyelitis, and residual neurovascular damage may occur. Puncture wounds have a higher rate of infection because of the depth of the wound. An estimated 5% of all dog bites become infected. Other complications include rabies. Fortunately, rabies is not a routine outcome of dog bites in the United States because of effective canine immunization programs.[1,11,21]

Cat Bites and Scratches

Although cats are found in nearly a third of U.S. households, cat bites are far less common than dog bites, accounting for 5% to 15% of all bites inflicted on humans in the United States each year.[1,12,21] There is little incidence of crush injury because cats' teeth are sharp, narrow, and long and the jaw lacks power. Cat bites do cause deep puncture wounds that can involve the victim's tendons and joint capsules. The tissue damage caused by cat bites is usually limited, but these wounds carry a high risk for infection. Whereas the infection rate for dog bite injuries is 15% to 20%, the infection rate for cat bites is 30% to 40%. Cats are hunters and often come in contact with bacteria-infected rodents, which contaminate their mouths with *Pasteurella multocida*. Consequently, rapid onset of infection can occur after the bite. Osteomyelitis, septic arthritis, and tenosynovitis have also been reported. Studies have shown that infections are polymicrobial. Antibiotic coverage for staphylococci and anaerobes is necessary. Treatment for cat bites is the same as for dog bites. Amoxicillin combined with a β-lactamase inhibitor is the oral antibiotic used most frequently. Patients who are allergic to penicillin and are tolerant of cephalosporins may be treated with ceftriaxone. Patients who are intolerant of cephalosporins may be treated with a combination of trimethoprim and sulfamethoxazole plus clindamycin. Prophylaxis also may be provided with erythromycin or a tetracycline. A 3- to 7-day course of antibiotic therapy commonly is used for prophylaxis. Cats also use their paws to groom themselves and may have considerable bacteria on their claws. Cat-scratch disease may cause lymphadenitis of the extremity days to weeks after the scratch. Because risk for infection is so great, thorough wound care instructions with clear instructions for follow-up are essential.[1,12,15]

Human Bites

There are approximately 70,000 human bites each year in the United States. Because the human mouth contains a multitude of potentially harmful microorganisms, human bites are more infectious than those of most other animals.

A human bite may cause a laceration, puncture, crush injury, soft-tissue tearing, or even amputation. The wounds are generally the consequence of a fight or sexual activity. Human bites are dangerous because of the organisms that may contaminate the bite wound, including *Staphylococcus aureus*, *Streptococcus,* and hepatitis virus. The most common sites for bites are the fingers, hands, ears, and tip of the nose. Boxer's fractures are often associated with an open wound over the knuckles that occurred when the fist impacted another person's teeth. Human bites have an increased risk for osteomyelitis, cellulitis, and septic arthritis. Treatment is similar to other bites, with the exception that the patient should always receive prophylactic antibiotics. If infection is already present, the patient is usually admitted for parenteral antibiotic therapy. Amoxicillin/clavulanate (Augmentin), 875 mg by mouth twice a day for 5 days, is the drug of choice for human bites caused by β-lactamase-producing strains of *S. aureus*. Human bites are reported to the local police in some states.[1,12,15]

Spider (Arachnid) Bites

All spiders inject venom when they bite. Most venom causes itching, stinging, swelling, or a combination of symptoms in a local area. Despite the vast number of arthropod bites and stings occurring on a daily basis, systemic reactions occur in only 4% of the population, with anaphylaxis in only 0.4%. In the United States, approximately four deaths per year are reported as a result of spider bites.[1,12,15] Tarantula bites usually cause only local reactions (i.e., slight pain and stinging). Black widow spider venom and brown recluse spider venom may cause systemic reactions and anaphylaxis.

Black Widow Spider Bites

The black widow, or hourglass, spider is the most dangerous species in the United States because of its potent venom. Spiders of the genus *Latrodectus* are worldwide in distribution. In the United States they are found in every state except Alaska. They are predominantly observed in southern and western states. Spiders of the *Latrodectus* genus are not aggressive, biting only when disturbed. Black widow spiders spin webs and await their prey. They can usually be found in their webs, which are often located near protected places, such as the undersides of stones and logs; in the angles of doors, windows, and shutters; and in littered areas such as city dumps, garages, barns, outhouses, and sheds. Often, these webs are found around outdoor toilet seats, resulting in bites on or near the genitalia. Adult females are recognizable by their shiny black body and the bright red hourglass

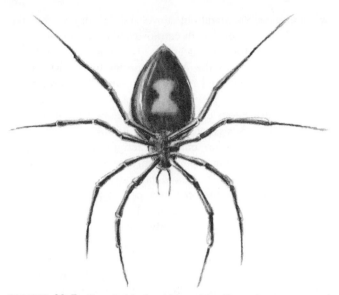

FIGURE **40-5.** Female black widow spider *(Latrodectus mactans)* with typical hourglass marking on the abdomen. (From Davis JH et al: *Surgery: a problem solving approach,* ed 2, vol 1, St. Louis, 1995, Mosby.)

marking on their abdomen (Figure 40-5). In the United States the incidence of envenomation from black widow spiders is unknown. In Texas 760 black widow spider bites were documented from 1998 to 2002, with an increased prevalence in western Texas. More than 13000 spider bites were reported to the American Association of Poison Control Centers in 1997, with no deaths; more than 1300 of the bites were described as moderate or severe. The reported death rate from documented bites occurs in less than 1% of reported cases.[1] Young children appear to be at highest risk for a lethal bite. The black widow spider's venom is neurotoxic. Initially a severe pain in local muscle groups occurs, which then spreads to regional muscle groups. Severe cramps and contraction of musculature may extend throughout the body. The abdominal pains are frequently most severe, mimicking appendicitis, colic, or food poisoning. Other symptoms include headache, restlessness, anxiety, fatigue, and insomnia.[1,12,14,15]

A local reaction begins within minutes, including pain out of proportion to the size of the bite. Two tiny red fang marks appear at the point of venom entry surrounded by a small papule. Because spiders rarely bite more than once, multiple bites tend to rule out spider envenomation. Systemic reactions develop within 1 hour and include nausea, vomiting, hypertension, hyperactive deep tendon reflexes, and elevated temperature. Patients may also have respiratory difficulty, headache, syncope, weakness, and chest and abdominal pain or spasms. Seizures and shock may also develop. Symptoms from envenomation peak 2 to 3 hours after onset but can last several days.

Reactions may be minor and require only local wound care; however, severe systemic responses also occur. The outcome, even in untreated cases of black widow bites, generally is favorable with supportive care. Symptoms usually subside in approximately 2 days, and most patients do not require hospitalization; however, the very young, the very old, and patients with cardiovascular disease are at an increased risk for complications.[1,15,22] Interventions begin with stabilization of the ABCs. Further treatment centers on alleviating pain and muscle cramping. The three main treatments are pain relievers such as narcotics, muscle relaxants, and intravenous calcium gluconate. A spider antivenin produced in horses is available for *Latrodectus* venom and appears efficacious no matter which *Latrodectus* species bit the victim. Patients appropriately treated with antivenin recover rapidly in 1 to 2 days, but fatigue, weakness, and other nonspecific symptoms may persist for 7 to 10 days. Because the possibility of anaphylaxis or serum sickness always exists, use antivenin only in those who are at high risk for severe complications. Premedication with diphenhydramine, methylprednisolone, ranitidine, and acetaminophen may help to decrease the possible allergic reaction to antivenin infusion. Apply ice to the bite area to slow action of the neurotoxin. Contact a poison control center for further consultation. With aggressive, supportive therapy, symptoms usually subside within 48 hours; however, hypertension and muscle spasms may recur for 12 to 24 hours.

Brown Recluse Spider Bites

The brown recluse spider, also know as the fiddleback or violin-back spider, is the most prevalent of the *Loxosceles* species in the United States. All *Loxosceles* species have the potential to inflict injury to varying degrees. Brown recluse spiders have a light-brown color with a dark-brown fiddleshaped mark that extends from the six white eyes down the back (Figure 40-6). These spiders are seen predominantly in the south central part of the United States; however, the brown recluse spider has been discovered as far north as Illinois and on both coasts. They prefer dark, dry, and undisturbed locations, such as the undersides of logs, boards, and rocks and inside barns and garages. Genital bites have been seen on patients using outhouses. Within homes they are found in attics, closets, and storage areas for bedding, clothing, and furniture. Both the male and female spider can envenomate. They are most active at night, from spring to fall. Bites are rare, even in houses heavily infested with brown recluse spiders; therefore a diagnosis of brown recluse spider bite is quite unlikely in areas that lack significant populations of *Loxosceles* spiders.

The venom of the brown recluse spider is cytotoxic and hemolytic. Bites of the recluse spider can cause a condition termed necrotic arachnidism, which begins with the development of an eschar at the bite site, followed by tissue necrosis and skin sloughing. Several groups of spiders have been linked to necrotic skin lesions, but recluse spiders cause most of these lesions. Although most recluse bites heal uneventfully, 10% have a protracted course, with the wound taking months to resolve completely. The bite typically is painless, and findings of a central papule and associated erythema may not be seen for 6 to 12 hours. Wounds destined for necrosis usually show signs of progression within 48 to 72 hours of the bite. Central blistering with a

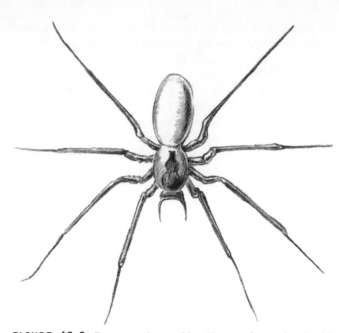

FIGURE 40-6. Brown recluse spider *(Loxosceles reclusa)* with typical dark violin-shaped marking on the cephalothorax. (From Davis JH et al: *Surgery: a problem solving approach,* ed 2, vol 1, St. Louis, 1995, Mosby.)

surrounding gray-to-purple discoloration of the skin may be seen at the bite site. A surrounding ring of blanched skin is itself surrounded by a large area of asymmetric erythema leading to the typical "red, white, and blue" sign of a brown recluse bite. At this stage of evolution, these bites may be associated with significant pain related to incipient necrosis of skin and subcutaneous tissues. The resultant eschar and ulceration may take months to resolve. Patients who are destined for a severe reaction usually develop key signs within 6 to 12 hours, such as bullae formation, cyanosis, and hyperesthesia. Areas with increased adipose tissue, such as the thighs, buttocks, and abdomen, are more likely to undergo severe necrosis than bites occurring at other sites. Methicillin-resistant *S. aureus* (MRSA) and cutaneous anthrax should also be considered in patients with these symptoms.[1,12,15]

Treatments for the bite of the brown recluse have been varied and controversial. Almost all brown recluse spider bites heal nicely in 2 to 3 months without medical treatment. The long-term medical outcome is excellent without treatment. Avoid performing surgery. When treatment is deemed appropriate, it should be conservative, using cold compresses, simple analgesics, elevation of an affected extremity, and cleansing of the bite site.[1,12,15]

If tissue breakdown occurs and/or the bite appears in an anatomic site that is difficult to keep clean, add prophylactic antibiotics (e.g., erythromycin, cephalosporin) to prevent the occurrence of a superimposed cellulitis; tetanus prophylaxis also is indicated. Dapsone has been shown to limit tissue destruction in some experimental models, but the results have been mixed and largely disappointing. A latency period of even a few hours before dapsone is started may negate any beneficial effects. Dapsone can cause hemolysis, especially in the setting of glucose-6-phosphate dehydrogenase (G6PD) deficiency. Intralesional steroids may do more harm than good and have not been of benefit. Systemic steroids may be involved in systemic brown recluse spider envenomation (loxoscelism) by preventing red blood cell hemolysis. Antivenin is not commercially available for *L. reclusa*. The only commercially available antivenin is for *Loxosceles laeta* in South America. In short, in most patients no systemic agent currently can be recommended to prevent necrosis. Prescribe systemic steroids only for patients with systemic loxoscelism.[1,12,15]

Necrotic skin lesions occur in 10% of patients with envenomation. Excision of a necrotic skin site may be advisable (especially for the rare large lesion) but only after 6 to 8 weeks of wound care, by which time an eschar has formed, adjacent tissues seem to have recovered, and normal healing is possible. Early surgery usually is inadvisable in the care of cutaneous loxoscelism. The practice of incising/lacerating the area of the bite to drain the venom is also not advised in light of the minute amount of venom injected. This surgery increases the amount of local inflammation, potentiates the venom's effects, usually increases morbidity, and is detrimental to the healing process by incurring an open wound that requires much more wound care than does the closed necrotic eschar.

Scorpion Stings

Scorpions are found primarily in the warm southwestern states and exotic pet shops across the country. Stings occur most often in the early evening and night hours. Scorpions appear to sting in self-defense; they are not by nature aggressive creatures. There are several kinds of scorpions, but only one is considered lethal—*Centruroides sculpturatus,* also known as "bark scorpions" because they dwell in tree bark. Ten percent of all calls to the Phoenix Poison Control Center are regarding scorpion stings.[1]

The tail of the scorpion contains a telson where venom is produced and stored. A stinger injects neurotoxic venom, which produces immediate local pain at the sting site, edema, discoloration, hyperesthesia, numbness, and agitation. Anxiety, restlessness, itching, speech disturbances, tachycardia, hypertension, and tachypnea occur with extensive envenomation. Systemic reactions include wheezing, respiratory stridor, profuse salivation, visual disturbances, ataxic gait, incontinence, muscle spasms of the jaw, nausea and vomiting, dysphagia, seizures, and anaphylaxis. Pain and numbness resolve without treatment in a few hours; however, systemic responses may last several days. Patients with severe envenomation may exhibit complicated neuromuscular and autonomic symptoms.

Most victims of scorpion envenomation, even those stung by potentially dangerous scorpions, demonstrate only local signs and symptoms and require only symptomatic outpatient treatment. However, it is prudent to observe them for several hours after the sting to ensure that progression to severe envenomation does not occur. Arizona experience has shown that progression of envenomation grade occurs rapidly, with a mean time of 14 minutes and a median time of less than 1 minute. Apply ice or cool compresses to relieve pain. For localized pain, many authorities recommend local anesthetics. Victims with significant systemic scorpion envenomation should receive supportive and symptomatic care in a monitored hospital setting. Treatment includes supporting the ABCs and fluid resuscitation as indicated secondary to fluid losses for vomiting, sweating, and increased insensible losses from hypothermia. Immobilize the extremity to slow venom absorption. Antihistamines are indicated for some patients. Scorpion antivenin is no longer available from the Antivenin Production Laboratories of Arizona State University. Specific antivenin for local species is available in other countries.[1]

Hymenopteran Stings (Bee, Wasp, Hornet, and Fire Ant)

Hymenopterans are an insect family found in temperate regions and include the honeybee, wasp, hornet, and fire ant. Stings are more common in the summer months. Hymenopteran venom varies among species and may be cytotoxic, hemolytic, allergenic, or vasoactive. Hymenopteran stings cause 40 to 150 deaths annually in the United States.[1]

Hymenopteran stings cause a variety of reactions, ranging from mild local reactions to anaphylactic shock depending on the type and amount of venom and the patient's sensitivity to the venom. Reactions can occur at the time of the sting and up to 48 hours later. Stings are usually cumulative. The greater the number of stings, the more severe the reaction. With the exception of the honeybee, most hymenopterans sting repeatedly. Fire ants have a painful sting that causes a wheal that expands to a large vesicle. The area then reddens and a pustule forms. When the pustule is reabsorbed, crusting and scar formation occur.

Symptoms vary from mild stinging or burning sensations, swelling, and itching to severe local reactions such as edema of the entire extremity. The patient may also have severe systemic reactions, including urticaria, pruritus, edema, bronchospasm, laryngeal edema, and hypotension.

Treatment begins with removal of the stinger as quickly as possible to prevent absorption of the venom. The stinger actively injects venom into the wound for 1 minute after the sting. Do not grasp or squeeze the stinger with tweezers because this squeezes out more venom. Scrape the stinger away using a dull object such as the side of a credit card or needle. Apply ice packs to the site. Further treatment is determined by severity of the reaction. If the reaction is mild, minimal medications are required—usually oral antihistamines will block the effects of some venom and of endogenously released histamine. If the reaction is severe, medications such as epinephrine, diphenhydramine, methylprednisolone, and famotidine may be required. Most stings resolve with no residual complaints.[1,12,15]

Tick Bites

Most tick bites are harmless; however, tick bites can cause Rocky Mountain spotted fever, Lyme borreliosis, and tick paralysis. Regardless of the species and subsequent illness, principal management consists of tick removal followed by supportive therapy.

Rocky Mountain Spotted Fever

Rocky Mountain spotted fever is caused by *Rickettsia rickettsii*. Occurring across the country, the disease is most prevalent in the south Atlantic and south central states. Most cases have been reported when ticks are most active, from April to September. Incubation period is 2 to 14 days. Major symptoms include fever, chills, malaise, myalgias, and headache. During the first 10 days the patient develops a pink, macular, or petechial rash over the palms, wrists, hands, soles, feet, and ankles. However, the rash may involve any part of the body. Treatment includes antibiotic therapy. Recovery occurs within 20 days. If untreated, mortality is between 8% and 25%.[1,16]

Lyme Disease

Lyme disease, the most widespread tickborne disease, is transmitted via the Ixodes tick and caused by the spirochete *Borrelia burgdorferi*. Incubation is 3 to 32 days. In 1992 more than 90% of reported cases occurred in the northeastern and Midwestern states.[14] Most cases occur in the spring and summer.

Within days of the tick bite, symptoms develop in three distinct stages. During the first stage, the patient experiences an expanding circular area of redness or rash (erythema migrans) at least 5 cm in diameter and flulike symptoms. This stage may last 2 months. First-line treatment recommendation is doxycycline for 14 to 21 days. However, the rash generally disappears without treatment. The second stage occurs days to weeks after the tick bite. Patients may exhibit neurologic, cardiac, and musculoskeletal complications such as meningitis, hepatitis, cranial neuropathies, atrioventricular blocks, cardiomyopathies, and arthralgia. Ceftriaxone is the most widely used agent in treating acute neurologic complications, third-degree heart block, and Lyme arthritis. Patients with first- and second-degree heart block are treated with doxycycline. The third and final stage may last months to years. In this stage the patient manifests primarily musculoskeletal and neurologic symptoms such as chronic arthritis and peripheral radiculoneuropathy. Lyme disease appears to respond to various medications; doxycycline, amoxicillin, or cefuroxime axetil are recommended for the early treatment of adult patients with early localized or early disseminated Lyme disease with erythema migrans but in the absence of neurologic or cardiac manifestations.[34] However, only 1% of untreated patients develop Lyme disease after a tick bite. Thus the Infectious Disease Society of America does not recommend or support the use of routine or selective prophylactic treatment.[35,36]

Tick Paralysis

Tick paralysis is a neurotoxic disease transmitted by a bite from a female *Dermacentor andersoni* (wood tick) or *Dermacentor variabilis* (dog tick). Incubation is 5 to 7 days. Most cases occur in the southeastern and northwestern United States. Tick paralysis is primarily an ascending motor paralysis occurring over 1 to 2 days. Symptoms include ataxia, lower extremity weakness progressing to upper extremities, paresthesia, decreased to absent reflexes, and eventual respiratory failure.

Treatment begins with tick removal. Gently grasp the tick with forceps at the point of entry and pull upward in a steady motion. After the tick is removed, cleanse the skin with soap and warm water. If you accidentally crush the tick, cleanse your skin with soap, warm water, and alcohol. Supportive care is necessary until symptoms resolve, usually within 48 to 72 hours.[1,12,15]

SUMMARY

Environmental emergencies cover a broad spectrum of diseases arising from a variety of environmental factors. These emergencies can occur in any geographic area and at any time of the year. Morbidity and mortality are directly related to the magnitude and duration of the exposure, regardless of the source. Prevention is the key to management of environmental emergencies. Those at greatest risk require information on protection against environmental dangers, use of good judgment, survival skills, and awareness of early signs and symptoms for specific emergencies.

REFERENCES

1. Auerbach PA: *Wilderness and environmental emergencies*, ed 5, St. Louis, 2007, Mosby.
2. Baratt DM, Harch PG, Van Meter K: Decompression illness in divers: a review of the literature, *Neurologist* 8:186, 2002.
3. Biem J, Koehncke N, Classen D et al: Out of cold: management of hypothermia and frostbite, *Can Med Assoc J* 168(3):305, 2003.
4. Bristow GK: Disturbances due to cold. In Rakel RE, editor: *Conn's current therapy 2000*, ed 52, Philadelphia, 2000, WB Saunders.
5. Carvalho MD, Shockley LW: Diving emergencies and dysbarism, In Rosen P, Barkin RM, Hockberger RS et al, editors: *Emergency medicine: concepts and clinical practice*, ed 6, St. Louis, 2007, Mosby.
6. Centers for Disease Control and Prevention: Hypothermia-related deaths: United States, 2003, *MMWR* 53(8):172, 2004.
7. Centers for Disease Control and Prevention: Nonfatal and fatal drowning in recreational water settings: United States, 2001-2002, *MMWR* 53(21):447, 2004.
8. Cochrane DA: Hypothermia: a cold influence on trauma, *Int J Trauma* 7(1):8, 2001.

9. CroFab website. CroFab Package insert http://www. savagelabs.com/Products/CroFab/Home/crofab_frame. htm accessed 2/12/09

10. Dart RC, McNally J. Efficacy, Safety, and Use of Snake Antivenoms in the United States [Abstract]. *Ann Emerg Med* 1(37):181, 2001.

11. Danzel DF; Frostbite. In Rosen P, Barkin RM, Hockberger RS et al, editors: *Emergency medicine: concepts and clinical practice*, ed 6, St Louis, 2007, Mosby.

12. Easley RB: Open air carbon monoxide poisoning in a child swimming behind a boat, *South Med J* 93(4):430, 2000.

13. Feldhaus KM: Submersion. In Marx JA, editor: *Rosen's emergency medicine: concepts and clinical practice*, ed 5, St Louis, 2002, Mosby.

14. Flarity K: Environmental emergencies. In Oman K, Koziol-McLain J, Scheetz L: *Emergency nursing secrets*, Philadelphia, 2007, Hanley & Belfus.

15. Gentilello LM, Cobean RA, Offner PJ et al: Continuous arteriovenous rewarming: rapid reversal of hypothermia in critically ill patients, *J Trauma* 32(3):316, 1992.

16. Goddard J: *Physician's guide to arthropods of medical importance*, ed 3, Boca Raton, Fla, 1999, CRC Press.

17. Greenberg MI, Henderickson RG, Silverberg, M: *Greenberg's text-atlas of emergency medicine*, Philadelphia, 2005, Lippincott.

18. Hanke BK, Schwartz GR, Gerace JE: Near drowning. In Schwartz GR, editor: *Principles and practice of emergency medicine*, ed 4, Baltimore, 1999, Williams & Wilkins.

19. Hazinski MF, Cummins RO, Field JM, editors: *2005 handbook of emergency cardiovascular care for healthcare providers*, Dallas, Tex, 2005, American Heart Association.

20. Johnson L: Hypothermia. In Schwartz GR, editor: *Principles and practice of emergency medicine*, ed 4, Baltimore, 1999, Williams & Wilkins.

21. Kazenbach TL, Dexter WW: Cold injury: protecting your patient from the dangers of hypothermia and frostbite, *Postgrad Med* 105:72, 1999.

22. Levy DT, Mallonee S, Miller TR et al: Alcohol involvement in burn, submersion, spinal cord, and brain injuries, *Med Sci Monit* 10(1):17, 2004.

23. Lewis LM, Levine MD, Dribben WH: Bites and stings. In Dale DC, Federman DD, editors: *Interdisciplinary medicine II*, WebMD, Scientific American Medicine, 2002.

24. Lugo-Amador NM, Rothenhaus T, Moyer P: Heat related illness, *Emerg Med Clin North Am* 22:315, 2004.

25. National Center for Injury Prevention and Control: *Water-related injuries,* Atlanta, 2007, Centers for Disease Control and Prevention. Retrieved August 5, 2007, from http://www.cdc.gov/ncipc/factsheets/drown.htm.

26. Newton E: Mammalian bites, In Schwartz GR, editor: *Principles and practice of emergency medicine*, ed 4, Baltimore, 1999, Williams & Wilkins.

27. Norris R: Snake envenomations, coral, 2005, *eMedicine,* http://www.emedicine.com/emerg/topic542.htm.

28. Orlowski JP, Szpilman D: Drowning, *Pediatr Clin North Am* 48(3):627, 2001.

29. Olshaker JS: Submersion, *Emerg Med Clin North Am* 22:357, 2004.

30. Otten EJ: Venomous animal injuries. In Rosen P, Barkin RM, Hockberger RS et al, editors: *Emergency medicine: concepts and clinical practice*, ed 6, St. Louis, 2007, Mosby.

31. Schwartz GR, Sipsey J, Hanke BK: Diving and altitude emergencies. In Schwartz GR, editor: *Principles and practice of emergency medicine*, ed 4, Baltimore, 1999, Williams & Wilkins.

32. Ulrich AS, Rathlev NK: Hypothermia and localized injuries, *Emerg Med Clin North Am* 22:281, 2004.

33. Van Mieghem C, Sabbe M, Knockaert D: The clinical values of the EKG in non-cardiac conditions, *Chest* 125:1561, 2004.

34. Vicarios S: Heat illness. In Rosen P, Barkin RM, Hockberger RS et al, editors: *Emergency medicine: concepts and clinical practice*, ed 6, St. Louis, 2007, Mosby.

35. Wormser GP, Dattwyler RJ, Shapiro ED et al: The clinical assessment, treatment, and prevention of Lyme disease, human granulocytic anaplasmosis, and babesiosis: clinical practice guidelines by the Infectious Diseases Society of America, *Clin Infect Dis* 43:1089, 2006.

36. Wormser GP, Nadelman RB, Dattwyler RJ: Practice guidelines for the treatment of Lyme disease, *Clin Infect Dis* 31:S1, 2000.

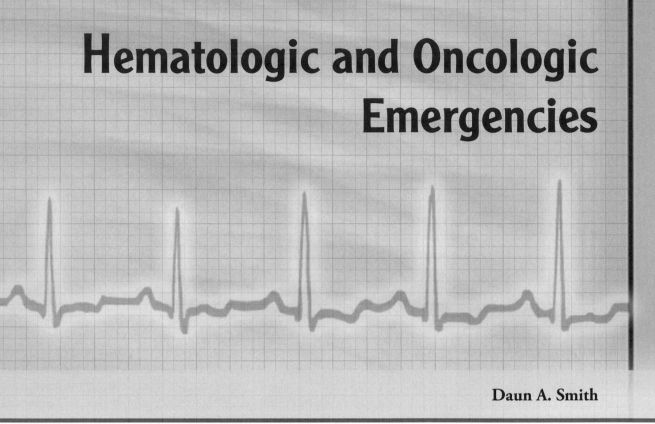

CHAPTER 41

Hematologic and Oncologic Emergencies

Daun A. Smith

The hematologic system (blood components and the organs that form them) plays a vital role in maintaining homeostasis of the whole body, affecting multiple cellular activities, including oxygen transport and delivery, hemostasis, and immune response. In turn, oncologic conditions and their treatments may have detrimental effects on the hematologic system. Patients with hematologic and oncologic disorders may present for emergency department (ED) care for an acute onset of a new condition, a sudden exacerbation of an existing disease, or with a therapy-related complication of their underlying disease. This chapter provides an overview of blood physiology, discusses general assessment of individuals with hematologic and oncologic emergencies, and describes specific hematologic and oncologic emergencies, including anemia, sickle cell disease (SCD), leukemia, thrombocytopenia, hemophilia, disseminated intravascular coagulation (DIC), fever and neutropenia, tumor lysis syndrome (TLS), syndrome of inappropriate antidiuretic hormone secretion (SIADH), superior vena cava syndrome, and spinal cord compression.

ANATOMY AND PHYSIOLOGY

Blood is a suspension of erythrocytes, leukocytes, platelets, and other particulate material in an aqueous colloid solution. This suspension provides a medium for exchange between fixed cells in the body and the external environment.

Nutrients such as oxygen and glucose are carried to each cell, whereas cellular wastes such as carbon dioxide and nitrogen are removed. Other essential functions include regulation of pH, temperature, and cellular water; prevention of fluid loss through coagulation; and protection against toxins and foreign microbes.

Plasma

Plasma is a clear, yellow fluid containing blood cells, electrolytes, gases, amino acids, glucose, fats, and nonprotein nitrogens such as urea, creatine, and uric acid.[11] These and other substances may be dissolved in the plasma or may bind with various plasma proteins for transport. Albumin, the primary plasma protein, maintains blood volume by providing colloid osmotic pressure, regulates pH and electrolyte balance, and transports substances, including many drugs. Other major plasma proteins include globulins and fibrinogen.

Erythrocytes

Adults have approximately 5 million erythrocytes or red blood cells (RBCs) per microliter of blood. The number of RBCs is slightly higher in men. Natives living at altitudes greater than 14,000 feet may have as many as 7 million/μL. The primary role of RBCs is transport of oxygen and carbon dioxide. Erythrocytes have no nucleus and cannot reproduce.

Their average life span is only 120 days, so new cells must be constantly produced.[5] The normal rate of hematopoiesis, or RBC production, is 2 million RBCs per second. Production occurs in the bone marrow but is regulated by the kidneys. When oxygen levels drop, the kidneys release erythropoietin, which stimulates RBC production by the bone marrow. Reticulocytes are erythrocyte precursors that mature within 24 to 48 hours of release into the circulation. Increased reticulocytes indicate increased bone marrow activity.

Erythrocytes are soft, pliable cells that change shape easily, thereby increasing the cell's oxygen-carrying capability by increasing surface area. The outer stroma of the cell contains antigens A, B, and Rh factor, whereas the inner stroma contains hemoglobin, the primary vehicle for oxygen transport. Hemoglobin molecules are so small they would leak across the blood vessel's endothelial membrane if left floating free in plasma. There are 300 different types of genetically determined hemoglobin (Hb). With the exception of normal fetal hemoglobin (Hb F), normal adult hemoglobin (Hb A), and sickle cell hemoglobin (Hb S), hemoglobins are identified by sequential letters of the alphabet. Abnormal hemoglobin molecules are produced in response to molecular abnormalities within blood. Tests such as hemoglobin electrophoresis are used to differentiate normal and abnormal hemoglobin. The most common hemoglobins are described in Table 41-1.

Red cell indices provide information about the size and weight of average red cells and are used to differentiate acute and chronic anemias. Mean corpuscular volume, mean corpuscular hemoglobin content, and mean corpuscular hemoglobin concentration values provide information on how well red cells function. Table 41-2 includes normal values for these indices as well as the other components of a complete blood count (CBC).

Erythrocyte sedimentation rate (ESR) measures the time required for erythrocytes in a whole blood specimen to settle to the bottom of a vertical tube. ESR is a product of red cell volume, surface area, density, aggregation, and surface charge.[2] Increased ESR occurs with widespread inflammation, red cell aggregation, pregnancy, and some malignancies, whereas polycythemia, SCD, and decreased plasma proteins are associated with decreased ESR.

Leukocytes

The body's primary defense against infection are leukocytes, or white blood cells (WBCs). Six types of leukocytes normally occur in the blood: neutrophils, eosinophils, basophils, monocytes, lymphocytes, and, occasionally, plasma cells (Table 41-3). The WBC count quantifies the total number of leukocytes in the circulation, whereas the differential count quantifies the percentage of each type. This count is based on 100 WBCs; therefore a differential count should always total 100%. The normal ratio of RBCs to WBCs is 700:1.

Table 41-1. TYPES OF HEMOGLOBIN (Hb)

Type	Significance
Hb A	Normal adult hemoglobin
Hb A$_{1c}$	Glycosylated hemoglobin
Hb A$_2$	β-Thalassemia, makes up 2% of hemoglobin in normal adults
Hb F	Fetal hemoglobin, thalassemia after 6 months
Hb C	Hemolytic anemia
Hb S	Sickle cell anemia
Hb M	Methemoglobinemia

Neutrophils

Neutrophils are the primary defense against bacterial infection. Bone marrow contains a reserve approximately 10 times greater than daily neutrophil production. About one half of all mature neutrophils adhere to vessel walls and are not measured by the traditional WBC count. The bone marrow reserve and the number of neutrophils on vessel walls allow for sudden increases in the circulating WBC count in response to stress or infection. After being released into the circulation, neutrophils live 4 to 8 hours. Immature neutrophils are called bands (also called stabs); mature neutrophils are called polymorphonuclear neutrophil leukocytes (PMNs or segs). An increased number of bands indicates acute infection.

Eosinophils

Eosinophils accumulate at the site of allergic reactions. Increases also occur during asthma attacks, drug reactions, and parasitic infections. Eosinophils decrease in response to stressors such as trauma, shock, or burns. Cell half-life is approximately 4½ to 5 hours after release into the circulation.

Basophils

Basophils contain histamine, heparin, bradykinin, serotonin, and lysosomal enzymes. During allergic reactions, basophils rupture and release these substances into surrounding tissue. This accounts for many of the typical manifestations of an allergic reaction. The number of basophils also increases in chronic inflammation and during times of stress.

Monocytes

Monocytes remain in the circulation less than 20 hours before moving into surrounding tissue to become macrophages. A macrophage acts as a "garbage collector," consuming bacteria and other debris in areas such as the spleen, lungs, and lymph nodes. Macrophages can live for months or even years. Monocytes are the body's second line of defense and are usually associated with chronic infection.

Lymphocytes

Lymphocytes play a major role in immunity against acquired infections. Their life span may be weeks, months, or years, depending on the body's needs. Two types of

Table 41-2. COMPONENTS OF COMPLETE BLOOD CELL COUNT

Component	Normal Values	Comments
White blood cell count	5000 to 10,000/mm^3	
Red blood cell count	Male: 4.6 to 6.2 million/mm^3	
	Female: 4.2 to 5.4 million/mm^3	
Hemoglobin level	Male: 14 to 18 g/dL	A conjugated protein responsible for oxygen and carbon
	Female: 12 to 16 g/dL	dioxide transport in the blood
Hematocrit	Male: 40% to 54%	Proportion of blood that consists of packed red blood cells;
	Female: 37% to 47%	expressed as a percentage by volume
Mean corpuscular volume	82 to 92 μm^3	Average volume of red blood cells in a sample
Mean corpuscular hemoglobin content	27 to 37 mcg	Average hemoglobin content of red blood cells in a sample
Mean corpuscular hemoglobin concentration	32% to 36%	Average hemoglobin content in 100 mL of blood
Platelets	150,000 to 400,000/μL	Platelets aid in hemostasis and maintenance of vascular integrity

Table 41-3. LEUKOCYTES: FUNCTIONS AND CHARACTERISTICS

Name	Percent of Total WBCs	Function	Circulatory Life Span
Neutrophils	62.0	Attack and destroy bacteria and viruses through phagocytosis	4-8 hr
Eosinophils	2.3	Attach to surface of parasites, then release substances that kill the organism; detoxify inflammatory substances that occur in allergic reactions	4-8 hr
Basophils	0.4	Prevent coagulation and speed fat removal from blood after a fatty meal	4-8 hr
Monocytes	5.3	Consume bacteria, viruses, necrotic tissue, and other foreign material	10-20 hr
Lymphocytes	30.0	Provide immunity against acquired infections; basis for antibody formation	2-3 hr
Plasma cells	—	Produce γ-globulin antibodies in response to specific antigens	Varies with need for antibodies

WBCs, White blood cells.

lymphocytes provide essential protection against bacteria and viruses: B-cell lymphocytes become antibodies and are responsible for humoral immunity; T-cell lymphocytes are responsible for cell-mediated immunity. At least three major types of T-cell lymphocytes have been identified: helper T cells, cytotoxic T cells, and suppressor T cells (Table 41-4). Lymphocyte increases are associated with viral infection.

Plasma Cells

Plasma cells produce γ-globulin (gamma globulin) antibodies in response to a specific antigen. Production continues until plasma cells die from exhaustion days or even weeks later.

Platelets

Platelets, or thrombocytes, provide hemostasis at the site of injury. These granular, disk-shaped fragments form when a parent cell breaks into thousands of cell fragments. The parent cell has no nucleus, so it cannot divide. Platelet life span is 9 to 12 days. Approximately one third of the body's platelets are stored in the spleen as a reserve. Clotting factors V, VIII, and IX are found on the platelet's surface. Platelets

Table 41-4. TYPES OF T-CELL LYMPHOCYTES

Name	Function
Helper T cells	Regulate immune functions by forming lymphokines or protein mediators such as interleukin and interferon; inactivated or destroyed by AIDS virus
Cytotoxic T cells	Also called killer T cells; capable of direct attack on microorganisms and on the body's own cells; role in destroying cancer cells and heart transplant cells
Suppressor T cells	Protect from attack by the person's own immune system; suppress helper and cytotoxic T-cell functions

AIDS, Acquired immunodeficiency syndrome.

provide hemostasis by clumping at the site of injury to form a platelet plug and seal bleeding capillaries. Substances such as ethanol and salicylates interfere with platelet aggregation

Table 41-5. COAGULATION FACTORS

Factor	Synonyms	Description/Function
I	Fibrinogen	Fibrin precursor
II	Prothrombin	Thrombin precursor
III	Tissue thromboplastin	Activates prothrombin
IV	Calcium	Essential for prothrombin activation and fibrin formation
V	Labile factor, proaccelerin	Accelerates conversion of prothrombin to thrombin
VII	Prothrombin conversion accelerator	Accelerates conversion of prothrombin to thrombin
VIII	Antihemophilic factor A (AHF)	Associated with factors IX, XI, and XII; essential for thromboplastin formation
IX	Christmas factor, antihemophilic factor B	Associated with factors VIII, XI, and XII; essential for thromboplastin formation
X	Thrombokinase factor, Stuart-Prower factor	Triggers prothrombin conversion; requires vitamin K
XI	Plasma thromboplastin antecedent, antihemophilic factor C	Formation of thromboplastin in association with factors VIII, IX, and XII
XII	Contact factor, Hageman factor	Activates factor XI in thromboplastin formation
XIII	Fibrin-stabilizing factor	Strengthens fibrin clot

by impairing their ability to clump. Decreased platelet aggregation leads to increased bleeding.

Hemostasis

Hemostasis refers to processes that prevent blood loss after vascular damage (i.e., vascular spasm, platelet aggregation, coagulation, and fibrinolysis). When vessel injury occurs, the initial response is reflex vasoconstriction. Arterioles contract, decreasing blood flow by decreasing vessel size and pressing endothelial surfaces together. Next, serotonin and histamine release cause immediate vasoconstriction and decrease blood flow to the injured area. Vasoconstriction is followed by platelet aggregation at the injury site. This temporary measure prevents bleeding by sealing capillaries.

Platelet aggregation is followed by clot formation, which requires activation of the coagulation cascade. The coagulation cascade is a complex network of 12 different clotting factors (Table 41-5). A defect of any clotting factor or an injury that overwhelms the entire system can cause failure of the coagulation cascade and lead to life- or limb-threatening hemorrhage. The cascade may be activated by intrinsic factors, such as damage to a vessel wall, or extrinsic factors, such as damage to surrounding tissue. Regardless of the method of activation, the end result of the coagulation cascade is formation of a clot—a protein mesh made of fibrin strands.

The final step in hemostasis is clot resolution via the fibrinolytic system. Clot resolution maintains blood in a fluid state by removing clots that are no longer needed. Without this system, circulation to affected areas may be permanently lost because of obstructed blood vessels.

PATIENT ASSESSMENT

The type and severity of hematologic or oncologic emergency depend on the individual's situation. Assessment is often complicated by vague complaints (e.g., fatigue, headache,

fever, syncope, dyspnea on exertion). Therefore it is important to observe the patient for clues to hematologic/oncologic problems, such as pale, jaundiced, or cyanotic skin. Ecchymosis, purpura, petechia, and ulcerations may be present. Evaluate skin for temperature, diaphoresis, warmth, coolness, texture, and turgor. Observe for joint deformity, edema, redness, limitation of movement, and difficulty or inability to ambulate. Obtain vital signs, noting pulse pressure; orthostatic blood pressure and pulse rate may be measured.

It is important to note new onset of fever, weakness, cough, rash, dyspnea, and increased or unusual bruising. Does the patient complain of spontaneous bleeding, such as epistaxis or menorrhagia? Are bleeding gums, hematemesis, melena, dark urine, or hemoptysis present? These symptoms suggest a hematologic/oncologic problem and indicate the need for more detailed evaluation.

Identify existing hematologic/oncologic diseases and family history of such disorders. Obtain medication history, including use of prescription and over-the-counter medications. It is also important to query the patient about herbals that may affect clotting. For example, evening primrose, garlic, and skull cap increase clotting time, whereas ginseng, cinnamon, and parsley decrease clotting time. Document allergies, exposure to toxic substances, and dietary history.

Complete Blood Cell Count

The CBC is used to determine the patient's hematologic status. Historically a CBC has been reported in two parts: the cell count and the differential count. The cell count is done by machine, with the differential count done manually. Electronic particle counters have made this process almost obsolete, providing an automated cell count and differential count; however, if the automated differential count reported is abnormal, a manual count is then done.

The cell count of the CBC provides normal values for leukocytes, erythrocytes, hemoglobin, and hematocrit (see Table 41-2). Normal CBC values vary with age and sex of the patient. The differential count provides information on red cell morphology and the percentage distribution of leukocytes.

SPECIFIC HEMATOLOGIC EMERGENCIES

Anemia

Anemia is a reduction in the total number of RBCs or a deficiency in the cells' ability to transport oxygen. Anemia may be acute or chronic. Severity depends on the patient's ability to compensate for RBC loss and provide essential oxygen to the cells. Oxygenation depends on blood flow and on hemoglobin's oxygen-carrying capacity and affinity for oxygen. A defect in any of these factors affects cellular oxygen.

Acute Anemia

Acute anemia is usually the result of blood loss. Causes include trauma, gastrointestinal hemorrhage, vaginal bleeding, and uterine rupture. Response to blood loss depends on the patient's age, physical condition, and rapidity of blood loss. Signs and symptoms include cool, clammy skin; tachycardia; decreased blood pressure; narrowing pulse pressure; tachypnea; postural hypotension; and decreased urinary output. Thirst and complaints of "feeling cold" are early clues to acute blood loss. A decreased level of consciousness may also occur.

Treatment begins with stabilization of the patient's airway, breathing, and circulation. Large-bore intravenous (IV) catheters and fluid resuscitation with normal saline or lactated Ringer's solution are used for volume replacement. Initial laboratory studies include CBC, type and crossmatch, prothrombin time (PT), partial thromboplastin time (PTT), international normalized ratio (INR), and serum electrolytes. Supplemental oxygen is indicated because these patients have lost a major source of oxygen delivery to the cells. Blood replacement therapy may be necessary in severe anemia.

Other causes of anemia include SCD, massive burns, DIC, toxins, infections, ABO incompatibility, transfusion reactions, carbon monoxide poisoning, and medications. Most chemotherapy agents adversely affect RBC production in some manner. SCD and DIC are discussed later in this chapter.

Chronic Anemia

Chronic anemia is not considered life threatening, has an insidious onset, and is often diagnosed before an ED visit. Patients complain of fatigue, headache, irritability, dizziness, and shortness of breath. Diagnosis is made by clinical assessment, history, and laboratory analysis, including a CBC with leukocyte differential, RBC indices, peripheral smear, and reticulocyte count. Patients are usually treated as outpatients unless they have acute shortness of breath, chest pain, severe dizziness, or altered level of consciousness.

Diminished RBC production occurs in iron deficiency anemia, thalassemia, lead poisoning, vitamin B_{12} deficiency, chronic liver and renal disease, and hypothyroidism.[9] Decreased bone marrow production causes aplastic anemia. Other causes of anemia include increased destruction of RBCs resulting from enzyme defects (e.g., glucose-6-phosphate dehydrogenase deficiency), cell membrane abnormalities, or abnormalities of the hemoglobin molecule (e.g., SCD).

Sickle Cell Disease

SCD is a genetically determined, inherited disorder that occurs in approximately 1 in 500 African Americans. Although SCD is primarily found in those of equatorial African descent, it also occurs in people of Mediterranean, Indian, Middle Eastern, Caribbean, and Central and South American lineage.[19] Forty-four states provide universal neonatal screening for SCD, and in the six remaining states, the screening is available on request.[19] RBCs contain Hb S, an abnormal hemoglobin that precipitates into long crystals when exposed to low oxygen concentrations, dehydration, infection, high altitudes, or strenuous exercise.[5] The resulting sickle shape of the cell gives the disorder its name. Sickle cell anemia is an autosomal recessive disorder. An individual who inherits one abnormal gene for sickle hemoglobin (Hb S) has sickle cell trait and may pass this gene on to his or her offspring. An individual with both genes for Hb S will have sickle cell disease. Hemoglobin electrophoresis shows a predominance of Hb S, variable amounts of Hb F, and no Hb A in the individual with sickle cell disease. In a person with sickle cell trait, Hb S and Hb A are both present.

As cells become hypoxic and sickling occurs, the cells are no longer flexible enough to pass through the smaller vessels and begin to clump in various parts of the body. The life span of RBCs that sickle is approximately 10 to 20 days compared to the normal 120-day life span of normal RBCs, leading to chronic anemia and a chronically elevated reticulocyte count. Ischemia resulting from vascular obstruction by clumps of sickled RBCs causes a painful sickle cell crisis, occurring most often in long bones, large joints, and the spine. It may be precipitated by exposure to cold, infection, or acidosis. Prolonged ischemia leads to local tissue necrosis. Treatment includes analgesia, oxygen, hydration, treatment of existing infections, local heat, and folic acid supplements.

Over the past few decades, early detection and early intervention have increased the life expectancy of the individual with sickle cell disease, but still many patients die before age 50.[5,19] Ongoing research into the disease may change this dismal outlook through use of stem cell transplants and other emerging treatment options. These patients develop hepatomegaly, hepatic infarctions, and jaundice. There is a high risk for pneumonia, meningitis, salmonellosis, osteomyelitis, pulmonary emboli, cor pulmonale, and chronic skin ulcers. Complications include recurrent sickle cell crisis, hemolytic anemia, transient aplastic crisis, cholelithiasis, cholecystitis, delayed sexual maturation, renal disease, bone disease, cardiac failure, and autosplenectomy. There is also a high incidence of spontaneous abortion, prenatal mortality, and maternal mortality.

Sickle cell crisis or vasoocclusive crisis is the most common painful complication of sickle cell disease and the main reason for seeking medical care in the ED. Acute episodes cause severe pain; however, providers are often reluctant to give patients adequate doses of narcotics.[5] Pain management in sickle cell disease should be individualized, and treatment should be driven by patient assessment. The ED nurse handling pain management also needs to remember that drug therapy should be adjusted for drug tolerance. Drug therapy should follow an analgesic ladder, using appropriate nonsteroidal antiinflammatory drugs and an opioid such as codeine or hydrocodone for mild-to-moderate pain.[5] Moderate-to-severe pain should be treated with an opioid such as morphine or hydromorphone.[5] Demerol (meperidine) is not advocated for pain control because Demerol's metabolite, normeperidine, may cause seizures and dysphoria with long-term use.[5]

Acute chest syndrome (ACS) is the second most common cause of hospitalization and the leading cause of mortality and morbidity in sickle cell disease.[14] Symptoms of acute chest syndrome include chest pain, dyspnea, cough, fever, wheezing, and hypoxemia, with pulmonary infiltrates that show up as a total white-out on chest x-ray film. ACS may rapidly progress to pulmonary failure, so immediate aggressive treatment is needed. This treatment includes broad-spectrum antibiotics, oxygen, analgesics, and close monitoring.[19]

Priapism may occur in males if sickling prevents exit of blood from the penis after normal erection. Treatment modalities include rehydration with oral and IV fluids, analgesics, anxiolytics, and possible intracavernosal aspiration of blood.[13]

Hydroxyurea (HU) is an effective therapy for adults with sickle cell disease, and recent studies have demonstrated that HU is safe and effective in children.[1] HU in children induces similar laboratory changes as seen in adults. HU stimulates Hb F production; however, its mechanism of action is not fully understood.

Leukemia

Leukemia is a malignant disorder of blood and blood-forming organs characterized by excessive, abnormal growth of leukocyte precursors in the bone marrow. An uncontrolled increase in immature leukocytes decreases production and function of normal leukocytes. Leukemia is classified as lymphogenous or myelogenous. Lymphogenous leukemias are caused by cancerous production of lymphoid cells, whereas myelogenous leukemias begin as the cancerous growth of myelogenous cells in the bone marrow. Both types may be acute or chronic. In the past, the terms reflected abruptness of onset and were used to predict survival time, but with the advances in therapy, the terms are presently used to reflect cell maturity, speed of onset, and aggressiveness of therapy needed.[9]

Acute lymphocytic leukemia (ALL) is most common in children less than 10 years of age, but also has another peak incidence after the age of 50 years. Newer therapies have increased the life expectancy for the childhood form. Presenting signs and symptoms are usually nonspecific and include fatigue, easy bruising, infections, and dyspnea. Diagnosis is made by the WBC count and confirmed by bone marrow examination. When the WBC counts rise above 50,000, the potential for leukostasis (a clumping or aggregation of WBCs) occurs. The two organs most affected by leukostasis are the brain and lungs, potentially precipitating stroke and pulmonary infarcts, respectively.

Chronic lymphocytic leukemia (CLL) is the most common leukemia seen above the age of 50 years. Signs and symptoms include spleen and liver enlargement, fatigue, easy bruising, infections, and weight loss. Leukostasis is rarely seen in CLL.[9]

Acute myelogenous leukemia (AML) is the most common type of acute leukemia and has its highest incidence in the population older than 60 years of age. It has an association with some genetic disorders, such as Down syndrome, Klinefelter's syndrome, and Fanconi's anemia. It has also been associated with radiation exposure and specific medications. Manifestations include fever, fatigue, bruising, and infections, and there is a higher risk for TLS and leukostasis.[9]

Chronic myelogenous leukemia (CML) is the least-common form and occurs most commonly in individuals over 40 years of age. Manifestations include weight loss, sweating, fatigue, and enlarged spleen. The Philadelphia chromosome is associated with CML. Patients with this form of leukemia are at risk for TLS and leukostasis.

Regardless of type, leukemic cells invade the spleen, lymph nodes, liver, and other vascular regions. Clinical manifestations include fatigue, fever, and weight loss. The patient may also complain of bone pain. Elevated uric acid levels, lymph node enlargement, hepatomegaly, and splenomegaly are usually present. Neurologic findings include headache, vomiting, papilledema, and blurred vision.

Treatment includes chemotherapy, immunotherapy, and bone marrow transplants. Blood transfusions, antibiotics, antifungal agents, and antiviral agents are also used. These patients are at significant risk for infection from their disease and their treatment; therefore it is critical that the patient be protected against exposure to potential infectious agents.

THROMBOCYTOPENIA

Normal platelet count is 150,000 to 450,000/μL. Thrombocytopenia is an abnormal decrease in circulating platelets; a platelet count less than 150,000/μL.[2] The platelet count is affected by menses, nutrition, and severe deficiencies in iron, folic acid, or vitamin B_{12}. Sepsis, tumors, medications (acetylsalicylic acid), and bleeding can also affect platelet count and platelet function.[9]

Thrombocytopenia may be secondary to congenital or acquired disorders such as decreased bone marrow production, increased splenic sequestration, or accelerated destruction of platelets.[6] Immune thrombocytopenic purpura (ITP), also known as idiopathic thrombocytopenic purpura, the most common form of thrombocytopenia, is an acquired disease in which increased platelet destruction is caused by immune autoreactive antibodies.[17]

Acute ITP usually occurs in children 1 to 3 weeks following a viral infection or a live-virus vaccination.[2] Acute ITP occurs equally in males and females, is self-limiting, and typically resolves spontaneously within 6 months. Peak incidence is between 2 and 4 years of age. Bruising and petechiae are considered universal presenting symptoms for acute ITP. Three to four percent may also present with purpura, epistaxis, mucous membrane bleeding, gastrointestinal bleeding, hematuria, and retinal bleeding. The diagnosis of ITP is usually based on patient history and confirmed with a platelet count. Treatment is generally unnecessary, but platelet transfusions, IV immunoglobulin, and splenectomy may be instituted for severe cases of spontaneous bleeding.

Chronic ITP most commonly affects individuals 20 to 50 years of age, with a higher incidence in women. Chronic ITP is an autoimmune disorder; platelet life span is shortened to a few hours. Early symptoms are vague and include ecchymoses, menorrhagia, mucous membrane bleeding, and epistaxis.

Chronic ITP is characterized by remissions and exacerbations with fluctuations in platelet counts. The decision to treat is based on the platelet count and on risk factors for bleeding (e.g., age, recent surgery, existing coagulation deficits).[2] A patient with a platelet count above 30,000/μL usually requires no treatment.[17] For patients with platelet counts below 30,000/μL and/or with additional risk factors, the first line of treatment is usually prednisone. Half of these patients will achieve a long-term beneficial effect. For patients unresponsive to steroids, IV immunoglobulin or anti-D immunoglobulin has a transient effectiveness in 85% of affected patients.[17] Second-line treatment involves splenectomy, with 75% achieving complete remission.[17] Treatments considered for refractory ITP include danazol, azathioprine (Imuran), cyclophosphamide (Cytoxan), vincristine, cyclosporin A, rituximab, and stem cell transplant.

Hemophilia

Hemophilia refers to a number of clotting disorders, including hemophilia A, hemophilia B, and von Willebrand's disease.[18] Hemophilia is an inherited, sex-linked disorder that occurs almost always in males. Females carry the disease and pass it on to their children. Severity ranges from mild to severe. The primary defect in hemophilia is absence or dysfunction of a specific clotting factor.

Hemophilia A, or classic hemophilia, is due to a factor VIII disorder. In the majority of patients with hemophilia A, factor VIII is not missing. It may even be present in excess quantities; however, available factor VIII does not function adequately. Disease severity is directly related to the functional activity of factor VIII.

Hemophilia B, or Christmas disease, occurs less often than hemophilia A. It is caused by the absence or functional deficiency of factor IX.

Von Willebrand's disease is usually less acute than hemophilia A or B and occurs in both sexes. The specific coagulation defect in this type of hemophilia is defective platelet adherence and decreased levels of factor VIII.

Hemophilia A and hemophilia B have similar clinical presentations. Patients with von Willebrand's disease exhibit less severe symptoms, with a lower incidence of bleeding into joints and deeper tissues. When a patient has hemophilia, even minor trauma can cause major bruises, visceral bleeding, and subdural hematomas. With the exception of lacerations or major trauma, one of the worst features of hemophilia is hemarthrosis—bleeding into a joint. Hemarthrosis usually begins in adolescence and involves primarily the knees, ankles, and elbows. Patients almost always come to the ED because of severe pain associated with hemarthrosis rather than actual bleeding. Improperly managed hemarthrosis can lead to arthritis and ultimately joint destruction. Platelet-mediated hemostasis does not depend on factor VIII or factor IX; therefore the affected extremity should be elevated whenever possible. Identification of the specific type of hemophilia is crucial because hemophilia A and hemophilia B present the same clinical picture but require treatment with different clotting factors. A bleeding history should be obtained from all patients with abnormal bleeding. A screening coagulation panel should also be considered.

Fresh frozen plasma (FFP) has been used to treat hemophilia A and von Willebrand's disease. Unfortunately, FFP contains relatively small amounts of factor VIII per unit of volume, so large quantities are required for successful treatment. Cryoprecipitate is rich in factor VIII per unit of volume; however, it has been associated with transmission of hepatitis and human immunodeficiency virus (HIV). Fortunately, recent product modifications have reduced this transmission risk and are also less expensive. Most individuals with hemophilia A are treated with replacement of factor VIII, either from pooled plasma or from a genetically engineered source. Antibody-purified factor IX is the treatment for hemophilia B patients with limited prior exposure to cryoprecipitate who are HIV-negative. Mild-to-moderate bleeding may be treated with FFP.

Disseminated Intravascular Coagulation

DIC is an acquired dysfunction of the clotting system that involves simultaneous clotting and bleeding. Conditions that can trigger DIC include infection (especially gram-negative sepsis), shock, severe trauma, neoplasms, and obstetric complications, such as pregnancy-induced hypertension, retained placenta, incomplete abortion, and amniotic fluid embolism.[8] In DIC, activation of the coagulation cascade leads to accelerated clotting, which triggers thrombosis as excessive fibrin is released in the circulation (especially thromboses in the small vessels). As coagulation continues at this accelerated rate, the fibrinolysis system also functions at an accelerated rate. Consequently, platelets, clotting factors, and fibrinogen are consumed faster than the body can replace them. As the system becomes overwhelmed, simultaneous hemorrhage and clotting occur.

Signs of DIC occur as the result of two mechanisms: thromboses that occur in the microcirculation from the over-function of the coagulation process and bleeding resulting from the consumption of platelets, fibrin and clotting factors. Thromboses-related signs include cyanosis; gangrene of fingers, toes, nose, and ears; bowel infarction; and renal failure.[6,8] Hemorrhagic signs include petechiae, purpura, bleeding from IV sites and surgical sites, epistaxis, altered level of consciousness, menorrhagia, hemoptysis, gastrointestinal bleeding, and hematuria. Other systemic signs may include cough, dyspnea, confusion, fever, and tachypnea. Diagnostic laboratory studies include PT, PTT, fibrinogen levels, platelet levels, fibrin split products, and fibrin degradation products (D-dimer).

DIC is frequently a life-threatening condition, and treatment should be initiated immediately. There are three components of treatment for DIC, which should be accomplished simultaneously: (1) to identify and treat or remove the trigger, (2) to maintain or restore tissue perfusion, and (3) to balance clot formation, clot breakdown, and clot prevention.[8]

The cornerstone of treatment in DIC is the recognition and treatment of the underlying cause. Many times, identifying the trigger of DIC may be difficult, but, knowing the trigger will help guide the treatment.

DIC both causes and is exacerbated by ischemia and necrosis, therefore adequate oxygenation and perfusion are essential in its treatment. Supplemental oxygen should be given to maintain oxygen saturation.[8] Volume replacement with IV fluids and packed RBCs may help restore intravascular volume. Vasopressors, such as dopamine, may be prescribed to maintain blood pressure and tissue perfusion. Achieving a balance in the coagulation process between clot formation, breakdown, and prevention is a difficult process. Replacement of the depleted clotting factors is one of the first orders of treatment and includes transfusions of FFP, packed RBCs, cryoprecipitate, and platelets. Packed RBCs will help to restore the oxygen-carrying capacity of the blood. FFP replaces clotting factors, while cryoprecipitate replaces fibrin. Platelet transfusions are used with caution because they may cause formation of antiplatelet antibodies.[8]

Heparin has been used to prevent the formation of new clots, but its use is controversial. It is contraindicated in some instances such as recent surgery, gastrointestinal bleeding, or central nervous system bleeding.[6] It has been used when there is evidence of organ damage or when loss of life or limb is imminent. Heparin has also been used with success in some obstetric-related cases of DIC, such as retained placenta and incomplete abortion.[8]

In 2001 the FDA approved the use of recombinant human activated protein C, which reduces the formation of thrombin and slows the clotting cascade. Activated protein C should not be used after recent strokes, spinal surgery, or in patients with brain cancer.[8]

Other therapies under investigation include antithrombin concentrate and protease inhibitors.

SPECIFIC ONCOLOGIC EMERGENCIES

Oncology-related emergencies are structural or metabolic problems that fall into three categories: cytopenias related to bone marrow suppression caused by disease process or treatment (anemia, neutropenia, and thrombocytopenia), electrolyte and fluid imbalances (hyperuricemia, TLS, and SIADH), and tumor-mediated compression of surrounding structures (superior vena cava syndrome and spinal cord compression). Structural emergencies are most often recognized by physical assessment, clinical findings, and imaging studies, whereas metabolic emergencies are confirmed by physical assessment, clinical findings, and laboratory values.

Fever and Neutropenia

Neutropenia is a condition in which the absolute neutrophil count is less than 1000 cells/mm^3 and indicates a moderate risk for infection. Neutropenia can be the result of a neoplastic process, medication/drug effects, or infection and is commonly associated with chemotherapy, radiation therapy, and bone marrow transplant.[14] The nadir (the period when neutrophil levels are at their lowest point) differs with each chemotherapeutic agent but usually occurs 10 to 14 days after the administration of chemotherapy. Many patients receive growth factors (e.g., filgrastim and pegfilgrastim) as a preventative measure to decrease the severity of neutropenia, although some patients may continue to progress to a severe state of neutropenia. The ED nurse should ask the patient if he or she is taking any of these growth factors.

Infection in patients with neutropenia often presents only as fever (febrile neutropenia). Sepsis is the leading cause of death in cancer patients, and in immunosuppressed patients, there may be few signs of infection/sepsis (fever, hypotension, site for infection focus). Development of an infection while the patient is neutropenic can result in death in hours.[14] Febrile neutropenia is defined as either a one-time temperature greater than or equal to 101 °F (38.3 °C) or a temperature of 100.4° F (38° C) for more than 1 hour.[14] Initial workup for febrile neutropenia should include two or more blood cultures from separate sites; complete blood count; electrolyte levels; kidney and liver function tests; chest x-ray examination; urinalysis; urine culture and sensitivity; and cultures of throat, stool, skin lesions, and vascular access devices.[3,14] Examination of cerebrospinal, pleural, or peritoneal fluids may also be indicated. Antibiotic therapy should be initiated immediately after cultures have been obtained. Initial antibiotic therapy should include one of the following: cefepime, ceftazidime, imipenem/cilastatin, meropenem, piperacillin/tazobactam.[14]

Admission should be to a private room, preferably with a positive-pressure airflow, and the patient should wear a mask when being transported throughout the hospital. Patients at higher risk for complications from febrile neutropenia are those who are older than 65 years of age, have comorbid chronic disease, have impaired renal or liver function, have been neutropenic for more than 1 week, or are status post stem cell or bone marrow transplantation.[12]

Tumor Lysis Syndrome

TLS occurs as the result of massive breakdown of tumor cells, either spontaneously or as a direct result of treatment (chemotherapy or radiation therapy). The destroyed cells release their intracellular contents (potassium and phosphorus are maintained at higher concentration levels within the cells) into the bloodstream,[4] leading to the following electrolyte imbalances: hyperkalemia, hyperphosphatemia, hypocalcemia, and hyperuricemia. The excess phosphorus in the blood binds with calcium, causing a reciprocal hypocalcemia. Nucleic acids are also released from the lysed cells and are broken down into uric acid, causing hyperuricemia.[4] The diagnosis of TLS is based on laboratory tests, patient history, and clinical manifestations.[16] Symptoms depend on the extent of the electrolyte imbalance and include fatigue, nausea, anorexia, muscle cramps, paresthesias, widened QRS, dysrhythmias, abdominal cramps, diarrhea, flank pain, and renal failure.[12,16] Hydration is the single most important intervention for TLS because it facilitates excretion of the excessive electrolytes. IV administration of sodium bicarbonate alkalinizes the urine to prevent renal failure from uric acid deposits in the kidneys.[12] Diuretics may be given to increase the excretion of uric acid and electrolytes. Allopurinol prevents the formation of uric acid. Hyperkalemia is managed by the administration of sodium polystyrene sulfonate (Kayexalate) to pull potassium into the gastrointestinal tract for excretion and by the IV administration of calcium chloride/calcium gluconate, sodium bicarbonate, hypertonic glucose, and insulin to move potassium from the serum into the intracellular spaces and/or nebulized administration of albuterol.[16] Phosphate-binding agents, such as aluminum hydroxide gel, help eliminate the hyperphosphatemia.[16]

Syndrome of Inappropriate Antidiuretic Hormone

Under usual circumstances, the pituitary gland produces and releases antidiuretic hormone (ADH) to manage increased serum osmolarity by reducing urine output. In certain types of cancers, especially small cell lung cancer, the tumors themselves release ADH, leading to an increase in fluid retention by the kidneys.[10] This causes a water intoxication with a dilutional hyponatremia (serum sodium level less than 129 mEq/L).[12] The excess fluid moves by osmosis into the cells causing cellular swelling.[10] Cerebral edema can be the most life-threatening sequela.

Symptoms of SIADH include headache, personality changes, mental status changes, irritability, lethargy, confusion, nausea, vomiting, anorexia, diarrhea, and muscle cramps.[10,16] As the hyponatremia becomes more severe, symptoms progress to seizure activity, papilledema, coma, and death.[16] Diagnosis is confirmed by laboratory tests: serum sodium levels, blood urea nitrogen, creatinine, urine osmolality.

Treatment includes fluid restrictions, cautious administration of hypertonic sodium chloride infusions, and diuretics.[10,16] Nursing care involves appropriate seizure precautions and monitoring.[16]

Superior Vena Cava Syndrome

Superior vena cava syndrome occurs when venous return from the head and arms is impeded by a mechanical obstruction.[3,7] This obstruction may arise from outside the vena cava as compression by a tumor or enlarged lymph node, or the obstruction may arise from within the superior vena cava by the formation of a thrombus caused by position of a venous access device. Advanced lung cancer accounts for approximately 75% of cases.[3,7] Most of the time, superior vena cava syndrome develops slowly, allowing collateral circulation to develop.[3] Symptoms are subtle and include gradual swelling of the face, neck, or arm, which is worse in the morning after sleeping in a supine position.[7] Other symptoms may include dyspnea, chest pain, and hoarseness. Symptoms accompanying a rapid onset of superior vena cava syndrome may include life-threatening manifestations such as cerebral edema (mental status changes, dizziness, visual changes) and airway obstruction from laryngeal swelling.

A definitive diagnosis of the cause and the type of tumor will direct the treatment regimen; therefore referral to an oncologist is of prime importance. Tumors that are drug sensitive will be treated with chemotherapy; others will be treated with radiation therapy. If the obstruction was caused by a thrombosis arising from a vascular access device, treatment modalities will include vascular catheter removal, fibrinolytic therapy, or anticoagulation.[3] Other supportive measures might include corticosteroids, oxygen therapy, and diuretics.[16] The patient should be placed in a semi-Fowler's position to facilitate breathing and to decrease facial and upper body swelling.

Spinal Cord Compression

The most frequent oncologic cause of spinal cord compression is vertebral body erosion from tumors, most commonly arising from breast, lung, and prostate cancer, and melanomas and lymphomas. Spinal cord compression affects 5% to 7% of all patients with cancer.[10] Symptomatic compression of the cord is an oncologic emergency because irreversible neurologic damage may occur in hours.[3] The most frequently reported symptom is back pain worsened by movement, coughing, sneezing, or by supine positioning. Many oncology patients have chronic back pain; therefore any new pain or a worsening or change in existing pain necessitates further assessment.[10,15] More specific symptoms depend on the location of the compression (most often thoracic) and may include lower extremity weakness progressing to paralysis, paresthesias, sensory losses, and loss of deep tendon reflexes, along with bowel and bladder dysfunction. Evidence of loss of neurologic function is an indication for emergent treatment to prevent further loss of function. Function that is lost is rarely regained. Diagnostic evaluation includes magnetic resonance imaging to rule out other causes of cord compression. Emergent treatment includes IV dexamethasone and radiation therapy.[3] Less emergent symptoms (pain without loss of neurologic function) may respond well to other treatment modalities such as chemotherapy or percutaneous vertebroplasty.[11] These patients need to be referred to their oncologist for timely intervention.

SUMMARY

Hematologic and oncologic emergencies cover an array of clinical conditions and represent a broad spectrum of patient acuity. Knowledge of the common disease processes and astute assessment skills enhance the ability of the emergency nurse to appropriately prioritize care to ensure optimal patient outcome.

REFERENCES

1. Anderson N: Hydroxyurea therapy: improving the lives of patients with sickle cell disease, *Pediatr Nurs* 32(6):541, 2006.
2. Brace L: Thrombocytopenia, *Clin Lab Sci* 20(1):38, 2007.
3. Brigden ML: Hematologic and oncologic emergencies, *Postgrad Med* 109(3):143, 2001.
4. Cope D: Tumor lysis syndrome, *Clin J Oncol Nurs* 8(4):415, 2004.
5. Dorman K: Managing the pain, *RN* 68(12):33, 2005.
6. Dressler DK: Coping with a coagulation crisis, *Nursing* 34(5):58, 2004.
7. Flounders J: Superior vena cava syndrome, *Oncol Nurs Forum* 30(4):E84, 2003.
8. Geiter H: Disseminated intravascular coagulopathy, *Dimens Crit Care Nurs* 22(3):108, 2003.
9. Hamilton GC, Janz TJ: Anemia, polycythemia, and white blood cell disorders, In Marx JA, editor: *Rosen's emergency medicine: concepts and clinical practice*, St. Louis, 2006, Mosby.
10. Held-Warmkessel J: Managing 3 critical cancer complications, *Nursing* 35(1):58, 2005.
11. Kim J, Mathis JM: Percutaneous vertebroplasty: rapid pain relief for vertebral compression fractures, *J Am Chiropract Assoc* 41(12):18, 2004.
12. Leon T, Pase M: Essential oncology facts for the float nurse, *Medsurg Nurs* 13(3):165, 2004.
13. Maples BL, Hageman TM: Treatment of priapism in pediatric patients with sickle cell disease, *Am J Health Syst Pharm* 61:355, 2004.
14. Marrs JA: Care of patients with neutropenia, *Clin J Oncol Nurs* 10(2):164, 2006.
15. Marrs JA: Nurse, my back hurts: understanding malignant spinal cord compression, *Clin J Oncol Nurs* 10(1):114, 2006.
16. Rokita S et al: Oncology: nursing management in cancer care, In Smeltzer SC, Bare BG, Hinkle JL et al, editors: *Brunner and Suddarth's textbook of medical-surgical nursing*, ed 11, Philadelphia, 2008, Lippincott Williams & Wilkins.
17. Stasi R, Provan D: Management of immune thrombocytopenia in adults, *Mayo Clin Proc* 79(4):504, 2004.
18. Thomas ML: Assessment and management of patients with hematologic disorders. In Smeltzer SC, Bare BG, Hinkle JL et al, editors: *Brunner and Suddarth's textbook of medical-surgical nursing*, ed 11, Philadelphia, 2008, Lippincott Williams & Wilkins.
19. Wilson RE, Krishnamurti L, Kamat D: Management of sickle cell disease in primary care, *Clin Pediatr* 42(6):753, 2003.

SUGGESTED READING

Flaherty AM: Spinal cord compression. In Yarbro CH, Frogge MH, Goodman M, editors: *Cancer nursing: principles and practice*, ed 6, Sudbury, Mass, 2005, Jones & Bartlett.

Gobel BH: Disseminated intravascular coagulation. In Yarbro CH, Frogge MH, Goodman M, editors: *Cancer nursing: principles and practice*, ed 6, Sudbury, Mass, 2005, Jones & Bartlett.

Hockett K: Oncologic emergencies, In Varricchio CG, editor: *A cancer source book for nurses*, ed 8, American Cancer Society, Sudbury Mass, 2004, Jones & Bartlett.

Hollis G, Crighton MH: Myelosuppression. In Varricchio CG, editor: *A cancer source book for nurses*, ed 8, American Cancer Society Sudbury Mass, 2004, Jones & Bartlett.

Keenan A: Syndrome of inappropriate antidiuretic hormone. In Yarbro CH, Frogge MH, Goodman M, editors: *Cancer nursing: principles and practice*, ed 6, Sudbury, Mass, 2005, Jones & Bartlett.

Lydon J: Tumor lysis syndrome. In Yarbro CH, Frogge MH, Goodman M, editors: *Cancer nursing: principles and practice*, ed 6, Sudbury, Mass, 2005, Jones & Bartlett.

Moore S: Superior vena cava syndrome, In Yarbro CH, Frogge MH, Goodman M, editors: *Cancer nursing: principles and practice*, ed 6, Sudbury, Mass, 2005, Jones & Bartlett.

CHAPTER 42

Toxicologic Emergencies

Patty Sturt

An estimated 5 million poisonings or drug overdoses occur annually in the United States.[25] Children account for approximately two thirds of all human toxic exposures reported to the American Association of Poison Control Centers.[3] Toxic agents are manufactured or naturally occurring chemicals that have deleterious effects on humans. Toxins can enter the body through ingestion, inhalation, injection, mucosal absorption, ocular exposure, or dermal contact. The quantity of toxin required to produce symptoms varies widely among substances. Exposure may be accidental or intentional and related to recreation or occupation.

Management of the poisoned patient may involve continuous respiratory and hemodynamic support, careful evaluation of toxicosis potential, interventions to reduce toxin absorption and promote excretion, and substance-specific therapy, including use of antidotes. An overview of assessment and management of the patient with a toxicologic emergency is followed by discussion of specific, common poisonings.

PATIENT MANAGEMENT

Determining the precise agent or agents involved in a toxicologic emergency can be challenging due to the vast number of potentially toxic substances. Poison control centers are an excellent resource for information on various drugs, potential toxicity, and patient management. Poison control centers, available nationwide through the telephone number

1-800-222-1222 and staffed by nurses and or pharmacists, provide professionals and the public with 24-hour telephone access to evidence-based treatment regimens. Many emergency departments (EDs) have rapid access to computer programs such as Micromedex that provide information on care of patients exposed to specific agents.

Symptoms of toxic exposures range from minor to severe and vary widely with the causative agent, dose, and extent of exposure. Toxins are capable of affecting every body system, and certain toxins produce predictable clinical signs and symptoms. Assess the patient carefully by obtaining a detailed history from the patient, family, or prehospital care providers. Consider the possibility of ingestion of or exposure to a toxic agent if the patient presents with a decreased level of consciousness without an identifiable cause. Table 42-1 describes essential assessment information related to toxic exposure.

Provision of meticulous supportive care, identification of patients requiring treatment with an antidote, and appropriate use of methods limiting poison absorption or increasing elimination remain the cornerstones of management[10] for patients with a toxicologic emergency.

General Interventions

Stabilization of airway, breathing, and circulation are the first priorities when caring for an individual with a toxicologic emergency. Protect the airway, ensure adequate oxygenation

Table 42-1. ESSENTIAL ASSESSMENT INFORMATION FOR TOXIC EXPOSURE

Item	Description
Substance	If possible, visually confirm substance(s) involved. Ask what medications the patient takes at home.
Time of exposure	Time since exposure influences both symptoms and treatment.
Acute or chronic	Acute exposures have different presenting symptoms and are managed differently than chronic exposures.
Amount of toxin	Determine the maximum quantity possible. Count pills in the bottle; confirm when the prescription was filled.
Signs and symptoms	Assess for symptoms in all systems. Toxins can affect every tissue in the body.
Prior treatment	Clarify any interventions provided by lay and prehospital personnel. Some home remedies can be detrimental.
Intentional or accidental	Poisoning is a popular form of suicide and suicidal gesture. Have there been previous suicide attempts? Does the patient have a history of depression or preexisting mental health problems? Was the poisoning recreational? Is this a possible homicide attempt?

and ventilation, and support the cardiovascular system while attempting to identify specific toxins involved. Significant exposures may require endotracheal intubation, mechanical ventilation, and vasoactive medications.

Substance-to-substance variations in toxicologic management exist; however, the need to ensure patient safety and provide emotional support is common to all poisonings. Knowledge of common toxidromes and interventions associated with each will assist the emergency nurse in the management of the patient with a toxicologic emergency.

Limit Absorption

Decontamination is a mechanism to limit or decrease absorption of the poison or toxic agent. Decontamination can be divided into gastrointestinal (GI) decontamination for ingestions and external decontamination for dermal or ocular injuries from a toxic agent. Specific interventions are determined by patient condition and the precise toxin involved.

GASTROINTESTINAL DECONTAMINATION.
GI decontamination refers to specific efforts used to inhibit absorption of drugs and poisons in the GI tract. There are five methods of GI decontamination: induced emesis, gastric lavage, activated charcoal, whole bowel irrigation, and binding agents.

Induced Emesis. Emesis may be induced with syrup of ipecac. It is prepared from the *Cephaelis* plant, which contains the alkaloids emetine and cephaeline. These emetics induce vomiting via gastric irritation and stimulation of the vomiting center in the brainstem. The use of syrup of

ipecac in the management of poisoned patients has declined. Several studies have found that use of syrup of ipecac has been associated with aspiration pneumonia, dehydration, a longer ED course, and more complications. In addition, no studies demonstrate that the use of ipecac in the treatment of acute poisoning changes or improves clinical outcomes.[4] The American Academy of Pediatrics no longer recommends home stocking of ipecac.

This agent has an unpredictable onset of action and intensity of effect. Violent, protracted vomiting after administration of ipecac predisposes the patient to fluid loss, acid-base abnormalities, electrolyte disturbances, and Mallory-Weiss tears and delays administration of activated charcoal and oral antidotes. Use of syrup of ipecac for hydrocarbon or caustic ingestion increases the incidence of oral, upper airway, and pulmonary injury.

Overall, the majority of clinical experts do not recommend the use of syrup of ipecac to induce vomiting for gastric decontamination in adult or pediatric patients.

Gastric Lavage. The benefit of using gastric lavage to decrease absorption is limited. Generally, gastric lavage is considered only when a patient has ingested a potentially life-threatening amount of poison and the procedure can be initiated within 60 minutes of exposure. Gastric lavage may propel gastric contents past the pylorus, moving the poison into the small intestine, where most of the ingested agent may be absorbed.[22] Some clinical trials indicate that gastric lavage does not improve patient outcomes and increases the risk for complications, such as hypoxia and aspiration, when compared to those treated without gastric lavage.[2]

Before initiating lavage, place the patient in a left lateral position to decrease risk for aspiration. Lavage should not be performed on patients who have ingested medications that may cause abrupt central nervous system (CNS) deterioration, such as tricyclic antidepressants (TCAs), unless the patient has been intubated. If the gag reflex is diminished, protect the airway with endotracheal intubation before lavage. Monitor for bradycardia secondary to vagal stimulation during tube placement. Lavage is not recommended for patients who have ingested a corrosive agent due to the increased risk for esophageal perforation. For adult patients with pill ingestion, insert a large-diameter (36 Fr to 40 Fr) orogastric tube with a bite block to prevent tube occlusion. Nasogastric tube aspiration may be effective in cases of liquid poisoning but is not adequate for ingestion of pills.

With mechanical suction or a catheter tip syringe, withdraw as much of the gastric contents as possible. To perform lavage, repeatedly instill and remove 200- to 300-mL aliquots of tepid tap water or normal saline until the return is clear; 2 to 5 L may be needed to achieve this goal.[11] For pediatric patients, administer 10 to 15 mL/kg in 50-mL boluses through a 24- to 28-Fr orogastric tube.

Activated Charcoal. Activated charcoal is the preferred means of GI decontamination for management of most toxic ingestions. Charcoal is "activated" by exposure to high temperatures that dramatically increase its surface area. This agent has an extensive network of interconnecting pores that are capable of binding and trapping chemicals within minutes of contact, thus preventing their absorption and toxicity. Binding prevents absorption into the bloodstream, allowing toxins to be eliminated in feces. Studies suggest that, used alone, activated charcoal administration is as effective as or even more effective than administration of activated charcoal after emesis or gastric lavage procedures.

Activated charcoal should be administered as soon as possible after the ingestion. Some clinical experts report it is most effective if administered within 60 minutes of the ingestion.[1,2] However, there is limited evidence to determine at what time frame activated charcoal is no longer beneficial. It may be effective for some agents beyond the 60-minute window, particularly for sustained-release preparations or anticholinergic medications.

Activated charcoal readily absorbs most poisons except heavy metals (e.g., lithium, iron) and alcohols (e.g., methanol, ethylene glycol). It is not recommended in patients who have ingested acidic or alkaline corrosives or who require endoscopy because charcoal will obstruct the view during the procedure. Substances poorly absorbed by charcoal include acids, alkali, cyanide, ethanol, fluoride, lead, mercury, mineral acids, organic solvents, and potassium. Contraindications to charcoal administration include bowel obstruction or bowel perforation. Adverse effects of activated charcoal include nausea, vomiting, GI obstruction, and pulmonary aspiration.

Activated charcoal is given orally or through a gastric tube in doses of 25 to 100 g (1 g/kg for children). The commercial product should be vigorously agitated before administration to resuspend all the activated charcoal. If the quantity of an ingested substance is known, give at least 10 times the ingested dose of toxin (by weight) to prevent desorption of the substance in the lower intestine. Administration of one or two follow-up doses at 1- to 2-hour intervals is common.

Activated charcoal is prepared as an aqueous solution with or without sorbitol. Sorbitol helps the toxins that are bound to the activated charcoal pass through the GI tract. Follow the recommendations of regional poison control centers for the type of activated charcoal to be used.

Binding Agents. Binding agents limit the bioavailability of certain poisons. Magnesium hydroxide has been found to be effective in reducing serum iron levels. Sodium polysterene sulfonate, often used to treat hyperkalemia, has been effective in limiting serum lithium levels. Other specific binding agents may not be as clinically applicable due to limited availability (e.g., cholestyramine, fuller's earth) Activated charcoal is often considered a binding agent because it limits absorption of many agents.

Whole Bowel Irrigation. Whole bowel irrigation is a method of GI decontamination that entails administering polyethylene glycol orally or through a gastric tube until the resulting rectal effluent is clear. Polyethylene is not absorbed and is less likely to produce a fluid or electrolyte imbalance. Whole bowel irrigation is used to treat large ingestions of drugs not absorbed by activated charcoal (such as lithium and iron), large ingestions of enteric-coated or sustained-release tablets, and patients who have ingested packages of illicit drugs (body packers).

The dose is usually 2 L/hr for adults and 500 mL/hr for children until the rectal effluent is clear. Contraindications to its use include bowel obstruction, paralytic ileus, or GI hemorrhage.

EXTERNAL DECONTAMINATION. External decontamination is the removal of a toxic substance from the skin or eyes to reduce the risk for absorption.

Dermal Decontamination. Skin decontamination is indicated for dermal exposure to any toxic substance. Remove contaminated clothing and jewelry as soon as possible, and rinse areas of contact for 10 to 15 minutes with copious amounts of water or saline. It is important to rinse the toxic agent from the hair, ears, nose, and skin folds. Dry substances should be brushed from the body before washing. Neutralizing agents should not be applied because the resulting chemical reaction produces heat and can increase local tissue damage. Depending on the substance and amount, both clothing and irrigation fluids may be considered hazardous waste. Individuals with toxic dermal exposures also represent a risk to others. Health care personnel should wear appropriate personal protective equipment (e.g., gloves, gowns, and goggles) to avoid secondary contamination.

Ocular Decontamination. Ocular decontamination involves vigorous eye irrigation with copious amounts of water or normal saline. Prolonged flushing may be necessary after exposure to caustic substances, particularly alkalis. An ophthalmologist should be consulted if ocular complaints persist after irrigation. Refer to Chapter 45 for discussion of eye irrigation and ocular burns.

Enhance Elimination

After initial efforts to limit absorption, enhancing elimination of absorbed toxins is the next priority in managing the poisoned patient. Techniques to enhance toxin elimination include repeat-dose activated charcoal, cathartic administration, forced diuresis, hemodialysis, charcoal hemoperfusion, and continuous hemofiltration.

REPEAT-DOSE ACTIVATED CHARCOAL. Repeat-dose activated charcoal is used in cases of theophylline, phenobarbital, dapsone, digoxin, and carbamazepine toxicity.[8] Even when parenterally administered, these agents may be effectively removed with activated charcoal in a process that is distinctly different from the agent's usual GI decontamination effect. Not only does charcoal bind toxins in the intestines and prevent absorption, it also facilitates elimination by decreasing serum concentrations of certain already absorbed poisons through a process of "gastrointestinal dialysis." This occurs as a result of the concentration gradient between charcoal in the gut and the toxin in the blood. Because of the intestine's tremendous blood supply, activated charcoal can draw select poisons from the circulation and bind them for elimination in feces, a process enhanced with repeated doses of charcoal.

CATHARTIC ADMINISTRATION. Cathartics, such as sorbitol and magnesium citrate, can be mixed with activated charcoal to increase elimination of ingested toxins by stimulating intestinal motility. Without concomitant use of a cathartic, charcoal may cause constipation, leaving both charcoal and toxins in the gut and creating the potential for toxin unbinding and systemic absorption. Cathartic use is contraindicated after corrosive ingestion and when vomiting, diarrhea, or ileus is present. Half the original cathartic dose may be repeated if there has been no charcoal stool within 6 to 8 hours. Multiple doses of cathartic agents should be avoided because the subsequent diarrhea has been associated with fatal electrolyte imbalances, particularly in children. Occasionally cathartics are used without activated charcoal to remove largely nontoxic materials or substances with poor affinity for charcoal, such as iron tablets or hydrocarbons. All cathartics should be used with caution in pediatric patients. Sorbitol is not recommended for infants because of the potential for fluid and electrolyte abnormalities.

HEMODIALYSIS, HEMOPERFUSION, AND HEMOFILTRATION. Hemodialysis, hemoperfusion, and hemofiltration not only remove toxins and their metabolites from the circulation, but also rapidly and effectively correct acid-base and electrolyte disturbances. Substances such as acetaminophen, alcohols, lithium, salicylates, and phenobarbital can be removed with dialysis. Because of requirements for vascular access, dialysis equipment, and skilled personnel, hemodialysis is generally reserved for poisonings associated with severe acidosis. Hemoperfusion is similar to hemodialysis, but it binds toxins as blood moves across a charcoal or resin filter rather than the traditional hemodialysis filter and dialysate. Hemoperfusion achieves greater clearance rates than hemodialysis and is particularly effective for severe cases of poisoning with paraquat, theophylline, phenytoin, and some sedative-hypnotic agents.[14] Continuous arteriovenous and venovenous hemofiltration have been suggested as alternatives to conventional hemodialysis when the need for rapid drug removal is less urgent. The role of these modalities in management of the acutely poisoned patient remains uncertain.

Substance-Specific Interventions

In addition to minimizing absorption and enhancing excretion, key interventions include antidote administration and urinary alkalinization.

Antidote Administration

Antidotes are available for specific drugs and poisons. If the ingested substance is unknown, determine if the signs and symptoms match with a specific classification of drugs. Table 42-2 lists antidotes and their indications.

Urinary Alkalinization

Urinary alkalinization can increase renal elimination of salicylates, phenobarbital, and chlorpropamide by changing them to a less-absorbable ionized form. Continuous infusions of sodium bicarbonate achieve desired urinary alkalinization.

Table 42-2. **RECOGNIZED ANTIDOTES**	
Antidote	**Indication**
Amyl nitrite	Cyanide
Atropine	Organophosphates
BAL/dimercaprol	Heavy metals
Calcium chloride/calcium gluconate	Calcium channel blockers
Deferoxamine	Iron
Ethylenediaminetetraacetic acid (EDTA)	Heavy metals
Ethanol	Ethylene glycol, methanol
Fab fragments	Digitalis
Flumazenil	Benzodiazepines
Fomepizole	Ethylene glycol, methanol
Glucagon	β-Blockers, calcium channel blockers
Insulin and glucose	Calcium channel blockers
Methylene blue	Nitrites
N-Acetylcysteine	Acetaminophen
Naloxone	Opiates
Octreotide	Sulfonylureas
Oxygen	Carbon monoxide
Penicillamine	Heavy metals
Physostigmine	Anticholinergics
Pralidoxime (2-PAM)	Organophosphates
Pyridoxine	Isoniazid
Sodium bicarbonate	Tricyclic antidepressants
Sodium nitrite	Cyanide
Sodium thiosulfate	Cyanide
Vitamin K	Warfarin

SPECIFIC TOXICOLOGIC EMERGENCIES

Patients may present with toxicity from a single agent or from ingestion of multiple agents. Caregivers should never assume the patient with a toxicologic emergency ingested only one pill or one type of pill. Specific toxicologic emergencies are reviewed in the following section.

Salicylates

Salicylates have analgesic, antiinflammatory, and antipyretic properties, making them frequent components of both prescription and nonprescription drugs. Aspirin (acetylsalicylic acid) is the most readily available salicylate. Oil of wintergreen (methyl salicylate) is a highly toxic, liquid form of salicylate used in products such as BenGay. Bismuth subsalicylate is an ingredient in Pepto-Bismol. The incidence of acute salicylate ingestion has dropped in the United States over the last two decades because of increased use of acetaminophen and ibuprofen. However, acute and chronic overdoses of salicylates continue to occur.

Clinical findings vary significantly with patient age, amount of salicylate consumed, and whether ingestion was chronic or acute. Acute salicylate ingestions can be divided into mild, moderate, and severe based on the dose ingested and the symptoms. Mild toxicity occurs with an ingested dose of greater than 150 mg/kg. Symptoms of mild toxicity include nausea, vomiting, dizziness, and tinnitus. Moderate toxicity occurs with an ingested dose of greater than 250 mg/kg, and symptoms include tachypnea, hyperpyrexia, sweating, dehydration, agitation, and ataxia. Severe toxicity is associated with an ingested dose of more than 500 mg/kg. Patients with severe toxicity (greater than 700 mg/dL) may exhibit hypotension, metabolic acidosis, renal failure, coma, and convulsion. Acidosis can lead to cardiac dysrhythmias and cardiac failure.

Chronic toxicity may occur with ingestion of more than 100 mg/kg/day for 2 or more days. Symptoms include lethargy, confusion, dehydration, hallucinations, pulmonary edema, elevated liver enzymes, and prolonged prothrombin time (PT). Direct GI irritation causes nausea, vomiting, and hematemesis. Patients may also exhibit hyperthermia, renal failure, tinnitus, and hypoglycemia.

Salicylates stimulate the respiratory center of the brainstem, resulting in hyperventilation and respiratory alkalosis. They also decrease adenosine triphosphate (ATP) production, which leads to metabolic acidosis. Metabolic acidosis decreases the renal elimination of salicylates and increases CNS toxicity. Children tend to present to the ED with metabolic acidosis whereas adults often present with respiratory alkalosis. Decreased platelet function can lead to petechiae. Hypoglycemia is more common in children.

Diagnostic studies include serial measurements of salicylate levels, arterial blood gases, electrolytes (particularly potassium), glucose, blood urea nitrogen (BUN), creatinine, platelets, PT, and urine pH. Obtain a serum salicylate level initially or at least within 4 hours after ingestion and then approximately every 4 hours until the concentration has peaked. Levels may not peak for 12 to 18 hours after ingestion of enteric-coated tablets.

Initial treatment consists of administration of activated charcoal. Repeat doses of activated charcoal should be administered at 2-hour intervals until serum levels start decreasing. Gastric lavage may be considered if patients present within 1 hour of ingestion of greater than 500 mg/kg. Urinary alkalinization is an effective method of increasing renal excretion of salicylates in patients who exhibit moderate toxicity.[21] This can be accomplished by adding 100 mEq of sodium bicarbonate to each liter of intravenous (IV) fluid and infusing at 200 to 300 mL/hr. Potassium may be added to the IV fluid to avoid potassium loss associated with alkaline diuresis. Hemodialysis is very effective for poisonings that do not respond to simpler measures and should be considered in patients with a salicylate level of more than 700 mg/dL who exhibit symptoms of severe toxicity that do not improve with treatment. Patients in significant metabolic acidosis may need 50 mL of 8.4% sodium bicarbonate IV push. Short-acting benzodiazepines should be used for emergency treatment of salicylate-induced seizures.

Table 42-3.	ACETAMINOPHEN TOXICITY	
Stage	**Time Frame**	**Symptoms**
I	0-24 hours	May be asymptomatic or experience lethargy, diaphoresis, mild gastric upset, including nausea, vomiting, and anorexia
II	24-48 hours	May have no complaints or develop liver failure, abnormal liver function tests, prolonged PTT, increasing bilirubin levels, right upper quadrant pain, hepatomegaly, oliguria
III	72-96 hours	Massive hepatic dysfunction, liver enzymes >100 times normal, hypoglycemia, jaundice, patient appears acutely ill, can progress to hepatic failure, encephalopathy, and death
IV	4 days to 2 weeks	If patient survives Stage III, enters recovery phase characterized by slow resolution of hepatic dysfunction

PTT, Partial thromboplastin time.

Acetaminophen

As with salicylates, acetaminophen is a common ingredient in many over-the-counter analgesics, antipyretics, and cold remedies. Acetaminophen overdoses are usually unintentional in the pediatric patient and intentional in adults. Although initial symptoms are mild, severe acetaminophen poisoning causes life-threatening hepatotoxicity.

Acetaminophen is rapidly absorbed from the gut and broken down by the liver, forming a toxic metabolite. In therapeutic doses, endogenous hepatic enzymes rapidly detoxify this intermediary product. However, toxic doses deplete these essential enzymes, damaging both the liver and kidneys as metabolites accumulate. An acute toxic dose of acetaminophen for children over the age of 6 years is 10 g or 200 mg/kg, and 7.5 g is considered an acute toxic dose in adults.[7] Higher levels are tolerated in pediatric patients without toxicity because of their ability to metabolize the drug better.

Serum acetaminophen levels of 200 mcg/mL or greater 4 hours post ingestion are considered toxic, and treatment should be initiated. Levels may continue to rise up to 4 hours after ingestion of a toxic amount. Individuals at risk for acetaminophen toxicity at lower doses include those with malnutrition, preexisting hepatic dysfunction, and those taking anticonvulsant medications such as phenytoin or carbamazepine.

Signs and symptoms of acetaminophen toxicity develop slowly and can be overlooked until significant damage has occurred. The clinical course of acetaminophen toxicity occurs in 4 phases. Table 42-3 describes the time frame and symptoms for each stage. Initial acetaminophen levels should be drawn 4 hours after ingestion. Plotting the

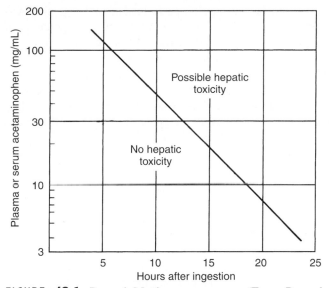

FIGURE **42-1.** Rumack-Matthew nomogram. (From Rumack BH, Matthew H: Acetaminophen poisoning and toxicity, *Pediatrics* 55:871, 1975.)

4-hour acetaminophen value on the Rumack-Matthew nomogram (Figure 42-1) determines whether the patient is at risk for potential hepatotoxicity. This nomogram is useful only for acute, single-dose poisonings not combined with other agents (such as opioids or anticholinergics) that delay absorption. Obtain liver function studies, PT, complete blood count, BUN, and creatinine levels on patients who present with clinical symptoms and those whose levels fall within the "possible hepatic toxicity" range on the nomogram.

Plot the patient's serum acetaminophen level on the nomogram. If a patient's 4-hour level remains below the identified level, no further treatment is required and serial acetaminophen levels are not indicated.[19] If the patient's serum acetaminophen level is above the potential risk line on the nomogram, antidotal treatment is indicated. N-Acetylcysteine is the antidote for acetaminophen and the preferred treatment for patients who have a hepatotoxic level. N-Acetylcysteine is available in an oral form (NAC, Mucomyst) and in an IV form (Acetadote). The oral and IV forms appear to be equally effective when administered within 8 to 10 hours of acetaminophen ingestion. N-Acetylcysteine is most useful when administered within 8 to 10 hours of ingestion but may be administered up to 24 hours after ingestion. N-Acetylcysteine works by replenishing the liver's supply of essential enzymes, allowing removal of acetaminophen metabolites.

Activated charcoal reduces acetaminophen absorption from the GI tract if administered within 2 hours of ingestion. Do not administer activated charcoal if more than 2 hours have elapsed since time of ingestion unless delayed absorption is suspected. Repeat or multiple doses of charcoal do not decrease serum acetaminophen concentration. Activated charcoal does not reduce the effectiveness of N-acetylcysteine. However, oral N-acetylcysteine has been shown in vitro to diminish the efficacy of activated charcoal to bind to acetaminophen.[24]

Because effective therapy depends on early initiation of oral N-acetylcysteine, it is important to treat nausea and vomiting with antiemetics such as prochlorperazine and metoclopramide. Ondansetron can be used if other antiemetics fail. All patients with a serum acetaminophen level that falls in the "possible hepatic toxicity" range should receive N-acetylcysteine. Patients in whom significant poisoning is suspected should begin N-acetylcysteine therapy on arrival without waiting for results of the serum acetaminophen level.[4]

The standard initial dose of oral N-acetylcysteine is 140 mg/kg, followed by half the calculated amount every 4 hours for 17 additional doses. Continue to treat if the patient remains symptomatic. Because of the foul taste and odor, N-acetylcysteine is usually given through a gastric tube or diluted in fruit juice or soft drinks. If the patient vomits within 1 hour of ingestion, the dose should be repeated.

Anaphylactic reactions with N-acetylcysteine are rare but have been reported to occur more frequently in patients receiving the IV form. Thus the oral form should be considered for patients with hypersensitivity reactions.[5] Administration of N-acetylcysteine in the United States generally occurs via the oral route unless the patient has refractory vomiting. Acetaminophen crosses the placenta and can cause fetal liver toxicity. N-Acetylcysteine can be used in pregnant patients.

Nonsteroidal Antiinflammatory Drugs

Ibuprofen is a common nonsteroidal antiinflammatory drug (NSAID). Ibuprofen ingestion of greater than 100 mg/kg is associated with GI symptoms, including abdominal pain, vomiting, and diarrhea. Very large ingestions may cause drowsiness, coma, acidosis, apnea, bradycardia, and renal failure. Patients presenting within 1 to 2 hours of an ingestion of greater than 100 mg/kg of ibuprofen or 10 tablets of any other NSAID should receive activated charcoal. Symptoms of gastric irritation can be treated with antacids, a mucosal protective agent, or a proton pump inhibitor.

Central Nervous System Stimulants

CNS stimulants are a loosely related group of legal and illegal drugs that act by simulating or mimicking the sympathetic branch of the autonomic nervous system. Illicit CNS stimulants include cocaine and methamphetamines. Street names for cocaine include crack, rock, coke, snow, and blow. Street names for methamphetamines include speed, meth, chalk, ice, crystal, crank, glass, and grit. Some CNS stimulants are available by prescription for the treatment of narcolepsy, obesity, and attention-deficit/hyperactivity disorder in children. Other CNS stimulants such as caffeine, phenylpropanolamine, and pseudoephedrine are common ingredients in over-the-counter diet pills, cold remedies, and alertness aids. Legitimate CNS stimulants are less potent and produce fewer euphoric or psychotic effects than their illegal counterparts; however, sufficient doses produce similar physiologic responses. CNS stimulants can be ingested, injected, inhaled, snorted, and absorbed rectally or vaginally.

Table 42-4.	CLINICAL EFFECTS OF CNS STIMULANTS
Degree of Intoxication	**Effects**
Mild	Insomnia, talkativeness, restlessness, garrulousness, agitation, aggression, tremor, hyperactivity
Moderate	Mydriasis, headache, nystagmus, hypertension, tachycardia, chest pain, dysrhythmias, hallucinations
Severe	Paranoia, shock, hyperthermia, rhabdomyolysis, acute tubular necrosis, acidosis, hyperkalemia, seizures, coma, myocardial infarction
Late	Chronic abusers may be exhausted after bingeing due to intense exertion and dopamine depletion; may sleep for hours; can be difficult to awaken but, when aroused, the patient is oriented

CNS, Central nervous system.

Although CNS stimulants are not all the same, their actions, side effects, and hazards are similar. Table 42-4 lists the effects of a stimulant based on the degree of intoxication. Street drugs, such as cocaine and amphetamines, are often diluted or "cut" with other CNS stimulants (e.g., caffeine, phenylpropanolamine, or phencyclidine hydrochloride [PCP]), making precise identification of specific agents difficult. CNS stimulants are rapidly absorbed from the gut, with onset of action minutes after injection or inhalation. These stimulants have relatively short half-lives and produce varying degrees of α-, β_1-, and β_2-adrenergic receptor innervation.

Patients present with a wide range of responses and symptoms related to the drug and quantity consumed (see Table 42-4). The patient may experience a sense of omnipotence, excitement, hyperalertness, hyperactivity, hypersexuality, anxiety, agitation, aggression, hallucinations, mania, or paranoia. Tachycardia, hypertension, cardiac dysrhythmias, hemorrhagic stroke, coronary artery spasms, and myocardial infarction can also occur. Neurologic effects include pupil dilation, tremors, restlessness, delirium, seizures, and coma. Stimulation of the GI tract produces nausea, vomiting, and diarrhea. Other effects include hyperthermia, rhabdomyolysis, piloerection (goose bumps), and coagulopathies.

The toxic dose is highly variable and depends on the agent or agents involved, route of entry, individual tolerance, and drug amount. Toxicologic screening of urine or blood provides a rapid qualitative test for common CNS stimulants; quantitative measures do not correlate well with clinical status. Initial care addresses airway, breathing, and circulatory issues; ongoing care is performed based on specific symptoms exhibited by the patient. Because of an increased metabolic rate, diaphoresis, and drug-induced diuresis, this population is frequently dehydrated. Adequate fluid volume is essential to minimize complications such as tachycardia, hyperthermia, and myoglobinuric renal failure.

Gastric lavage may be performed if oral ingestion was within an hour of arrival to the ED, there is no potential of airway compromise, and the risk for seizure is low. The treatment of choice is activated charcoal. Administer a single dose of activated charcoal as soon as possible. Gastric decontamination has no benefit when these drugs are inhaled, snorted, or injected. "Body packers" who have ingested cocaine-filled balloons or condoms may receive activated charcoal to absorb cocaine from the GI tract in case the containers rupture.

No specific measures are used to promote CNS stimulant elimination. Urinary acidification enhances excretion of some CNS agents but places patients at risk for rhabdomyolysis. Whole bowel irrigation has been used successfully to remove swallowed body-packed or body-stuffed drugs. Endoscopic or surgical removal may be necessary if packets rupture.

Treatment of CNS stimulant toxicosis is largely symptomatic. Symptoms can progress rapidly, mandating diligent observation. Continuous cardiac and blood pressure monitoring detect tachycardia, dysrhythmias, and hypertension. A 12-lead electrocardiogram (ECG) is indicated for patients with chest pain or shock. The risk for acute coronary syndrome is highest in the first hour, but the syndrome may occur 4 to 6 hours after cocaine use.[17] Cocaine-induced coronary artery vasospasm reduces myocardial oxygen supply when there is a greater myocardial oxygen demand. Cocaine-induced coronary artery vasospasm is more pronounced in smokers. Cocaine increases platelet activation and aggregation and produces vascular endothelial damage, which can lead to greater coronary artery damage in long-term users. Because of the potential for rapid development of severe hyperthermia, check body temperature frequently until symptoms subside.

The patient with a significant CNS stimulant overdose can be paranoid, incredibly strong, and anesthetized to pain. Prevent injury to the patient and others by sedating psychotic patients with benzodiazepines. Exclusive use of physical restraints can cause extreme agitation and intense muscle activity, contributing to hyperthermia and rhabdomyolysis. After the patient is under control, provide a minimal-stimulation environment.

CNS stimulants affect the sympathetic nervous system, so a β-blocker (e.g., propranolol, esmolol) may be used for treatment of significant overdoses, sometimes given in combination with a vasodilator. Intense muscle activity and increased metabolic rate can rapidly produce core temperatures greater than 104° F (40° C). Cool patients aggressively.

IV benzodiazepines are the agents of choice for treatment of actual or impending seizures. Adequate seizure control is essential because strenuous muscle use contributes significantly to hyperthermia.

Opiates

Originally derived from the opium poppy, opiates are among the oldest known analgesic agents, having been used for thousands of years. Today opium is refined into many different

Table 42-5.	EFFECTS OF NARCOTIC ABUSE AND TOXICITY
Etiology	**Potential Effects**
Narcotic	Pinpoint pupils, respiratory depression, mental changes, hypotension, visual hallucinations, analgesia, amnesia, sleep, coma
Lifestyle	Skin abscesses, cellulitis, endocarditis, septicemia, track marks, malnutrition, dental disease, hepatitis, human immunodeficiency virus infection, tuberculosis, pulmonary edema, fecal impaction, septic arthritis, frequent trauma
Withdrawal	Rhinorrhea, tearing, yawning, dilated pupils, abdominal pain, diarrhea, diaphoresis, nasal congestion, vomiting, headache, piloerection, chills, fever, joint pain, agitation, confusion, hyperactivity

drugs. Numerous synthetic opioids are also available. In the United States, single-agent and multidrug formula opiates can be legally obtained only by prescription. Narcotic toxicosis is often associated with IV abuse. Overdoses result from both pharmacologically prepared and "street drug" versions. Illicitly obtained opiates may be cut with caffeine, amphetamines, PCP, strychnine, lactose, or powdered sugar. Cointoxicants may be responsible for many of the patient's symptoms.

Although there are significant differences among opiate agents, all act on the CNS, producing variable degrees of sedation, euphoria, analgesia, and amnesia. Their psychic effects make opiates popular drugs of abuse. CNS depression sufficient to induce coma can occur with large drug doses or with relatively small amounts in novice users. Tolerance and dependence are common phenomena; addiction may follow chronic use. Table 42-5 lists potential effects of narcotic abuse and toxicity.

Opiates also act on the respiratory center in the brainstem, producing depression and apnea. These agents slow the GI system, making constipation a common side effect. Opiates such as paregoric and diphenoxylate hydrochloride with atropine (Lomotil) are prescribed specifically for this action. Signs and symptoms of opiate toxicity and abuse can be related to specific effects of the agent, substance abuse, lifestyle, or acute drug withdrawal.[13]

A qualitative toxicologic screen documents recent opiate use, but levels do not correlate with clinical presentation because of the number of substances available and the wide range of individual tolerance. Oral ingestions of opiates should be treated as soon as possible with activated charcoal, which effectively binds and reduces absorption into the circulation. Gastric emptying is not necessary if activated charcoal can be given promptly. Cathartic agents, in conjunction with charcoal, may be useful for enhancing drug elimination in opiate toxicity because of drug-induced intestinal hypomotility. However, they should be implemented only in patients with a secure airway.

Naloxone (Narcan) is the antidote for opiate poisoning or toxicity. Administer naloxone at 0.2-mg increments until the patient's respiratory status and level of consciousness improve. Naloxone may need to be redosed every 20 to 60 minutes in some patients. Naloxone can be administered intravenously, intramuscularly, subcutaneously, or intranasally. It antagonizes opiate receptor sites in the CNS, reversing opioid effects of respiratory depression and decreased level of consciousness. Doses of 4 mg or higher may be needed in cases of severe opiate toxicity. Full and sudden awakening is rarely desirable. Naloxone has a ½- to 2-hour duration of action, which may be less than that of the particular narcotic involved. Repeat doses or continuous IV naloxone infusions may be indicated and should be titrated to clinical response.

Benzodiazepines

Benzodiazepines are commonly prescribed anxiolytic and sedative-hypnotic agents. This class contains a large number of substances that vary widely in their indications, potency, and duration of effect. Fortunately, the level of toxicity associated with these drugs is generally mild. In overdose situations benzodiazepines ingested with other CNS depressants (e.g., ethanol, opiates, barbiturates) produce a more severe poisoning.

Benzodiazepines potentiate effects of the inhibitory neurotransmitter γ-aminobutyric acid (GABA), producing CNS depression. The toxic effects of benzodiazepines are an extension of their therapeutic effects, and a milligram-per-kilogram toxic dose has not been established.

Qualitative serum benzodiazepine levels confirm the presence of these agents. Quantitative levels are not particularly useful because of significant individual variability. Therefore interventions are dictated by the patient's clinical status rather than by serum drug levels.

The clinical features of benzodiazepine intoxication include slurred speech, incoordination, unsteady gait, drowsiness, lethargy, hypothermia, confusion, and coma. Profound coma suggests involvement of other CNS depressants. Significant circulatory compromise after isolated benzodiazepine ingestion is rare, so other causes should be considered.

Gastric emptying is of no additional value if activated charcoal can be given promptly. Administer a cathartic agent along with the charcoal to counteract GI hypomotility and enhance fecal drug elimination. Hemodialysis and charcoal hemoperfusion have little benefit in benzodiazepine overdose. Flumazenil (Romazicon) is the antidote for benzodiazepines. Flumazenil competes directly with benzodiazepines at their receptor sites. However, flumazenil administration can induce seizures in those with benzodiazepine addiction and in those with concomitant TCA overdose. Therefore, because benzodiazepine toxicosis is associated with a low morbidity and mortality, the decision to administer flumazenil must be considered carefully. The starting dose is 0.2 mg IV over 30 seconds. An interval of at least 30 seconds should pass before administering the next dose of 0.3 mg. Further doses of 0.5 mg may be administered every 60 seconds up to a total dose of 3 mg.

Tricyclic Antidepressants

There are a variety of TCA drugs available, including amitriptyline (Elavil), imipramine (Tofranil), and desipramine (Norpramin). The use of TCAs has decreased during the last decade because of the increase of selective serotonin reuptake inhibitors (SSRIs) for the management of depression. Along with depression, TCAs are used for patients with chronic pain, panic disorder, and obsessive-compulsive disorder. TCA overdoses are usually associated with suicidal intent.

TCAs inhibit the cardiac fast-sodium channels, α-adrenergic receptors, and histamine receptors. They are well absorbed from the GI tract and are difficult to remove from the body once absorbed. Toxicity may not be closely associated with a milligram-per-kilogram ingested dose. Generally an ingestion of greater than 10 mg/kg is likely to produce significant toxicity. Serum levels do not correlate well with clinical effects. A qualitative urine study is sufficient to confirm ingestion.

Because TCAs produce neurotoxicity, cardiotoxicity, and anticholinergic effects, signs and symptoms of TCA poisoning fall into three general categories. Neurotoxicity is characterized by lethargy, confusion, delirium, and hallucinations. CNS depression, coma, and seizures can occur. Profound CNS depression can lead to apnea and respiratory failure. Cardiac manifestations include hypotension and numerous ECG changes such as prolonged PR intervals, prolonged QRS intervals, prolonged QT intervals, ST- and T-wave abnormalities, conduction blocks, and tachycardia. Sinus tachycardia is a common rhythm seen in the early presentation of the patient. Ventricular tachycardia and fibrillation are more frequent in severe poisonings that are complicated by acidosis, hypotension, and extreme QRS prolongation. Polymorphic tachycardia (e.g., torsades de pointes) is not commonly associated with TCA overdose. TCA poisoning should be suspected in any patient with lethargy, coma, or seizures accompanied by QRS prolongation. A major cause of death from TCA poisoning is refractory hypotension due to decreased contractility and peripheral vasodilation.

Anticholinergic effects include mydriasis, flushed skin, dry mucous membranes, anxiety or psychosis, tachycardia, elevated body temperature, and urinary retention.

Respiratory arrest can occur quickly, and death from TCA toxicity may happen within a few hours of admission. Do not attempt to induce vomiting because CNS depression can develop rapidly. For large overdoses, protect the patient's airway with endotracheal intubation, then administer activated charcoal. Activated charcoal effectively binds TCAs, dramatically reducing their half-life. Gastric emptying is not recommended in the routine management of patients with TCA poisoning.[6] Because of TCA's anticholinergic effects, intestinal transit time is significantly lengthened; administering activated charcoal with sorbitol can increase drug

elimination and prevent GI obstruction. TCAs are highly tissue-bound, so hemodialysis is not effective.

Continuous cardiac monitoring is imperative for all significant TCA ingestions. Treat ventricular dysrhythmias with amiodarone or lidocaine. Do not administer procainamide (Pronestyl) or other type 1A antidysrhythmic agents. This class of antidysrhythmic has been associated with the development of QRS widening progressing to asystole. Serious conduction blocks may occur with acute TCA overdose; pharmacologic therapy is rarely helpful, and external pacing is usually the only effective intervention.

Systemic alkalinization with sodium bicarbonate is indicated in patients with QRS widening, ventricular dysrhythmias, and/or hypotension.[12] Sodium bicarbonate can narrow the QRS, improve systolic pressure, and control ventricular dysrhythmias. The increase in pH lowers free drug concentrations, making it less available to bind to sodium channels. Sodium bicarbonate is administered initially as a 1- to 2-mEq/kg bolus. Further doses are titrated to maintain a systemic pH of 7.5 to 7.55. This can be accomplished by the addition of sodium bicarbonate to IV fluids, guided by arterial blood gas values. Potassium chloride 10 to 20 mEq may be added to IV fluids to prevent hypokalemia secondary to sodium bicarbonate administration. Hypotension is initially managed with normal saline boluses; however, catecholamine vasopressors (e.g., norepinephrine, phenylephrine) are necessary for refractory hypotension. Treat seizures acutely with a short-acting benzodiazepine such as diazepam or lorazepam. Phenytoin is a sodium channel–blocking drug and should not be used to treat TCA-induced seizures.

Toxic Alcohols

In addition to ethanol, three other alcohols can cause severe poisoning. Toxic alcohols exist in many common household products not generally considered dangerous. Methanol, also known as "wood alcohol," is found in windshield wiper fluid, canned fuel (Sterno), and solvents such as paint removers. Isopropanol is a major component of rubbing alcohol, disinfectants, cleansers, and nail polish removers. Ethylene glycol is an odorless substance contained in antifreeze, detergents, paints, polishes, and coolants. Its sweet taste and fluorescent color are particularly appealing to children and pets. Toxic alcohol ingestions can be accidental, recreational, suicidal, or may occur in desperate alcoholics unable to obtain ethanol. In addition to oral ingestion, toxic alcohols may be inhaled or topically absorbed.

These alcohols are relatively nonpoisonous before hepatic conversion, by the enzyme alcohol dehydrogenase, to their toxic metabolites. The toxins—glycolaldehyde (ethylene glycol), formaldehyde and formic acid (methanol), and acetone (isopropanol)—produce widespread damage and metabolic dysfunction.

Clinical findings of alcohol intoxication include CNS and respiratory depression. Methanol toxicity causes nausea, vomiting, abdominal pain, blindness, and coma. The patient with isopropanol ingestion presents with acetone breath odor, vomiting, and possibly significant hypotension. Ethylene glycol causes seizures, ataxia, coma, nystagmus, cardiac conduction disturbances, and dysrhythmias. Profound acidosis, renal failure, and pulmonary edema may also occur.

Appropriate laboratory studies should be performed to detect the following predicted abnormalities. In methanol intoxication, pronounced metabolic acidosis results from accumulation of formic acid. Isopropanol poisoning causes elevated serum acetone levels with ketones present in blood and urine. Hyperglycemia may also occur. With significant ethylene glycol toxicity, both anion gap metabolic acidosis and a large osmolar gap are evident.

Gastric lavage may be used in severe cases to remove any alcohol remaining in the stomach. Because of the rapid absorption of alcohols, the effectiveness of gastric lavage and activated charcoal is limited. The lungs are responsible for eliminating a significant amount of toxic alcohols; therefore intubation and mechanical ventilation can be used to maximize respiratory excretion in severe poisoning. Hemodialysis both effectively removes toxic metabolites and reverses acidosis.[16]

Ethanol and each of the toxic alcohols rely on the enzyme alcohol dehydrogenase for metabolism; however, the liver preferentially metabolizes ethyl alcohol. Administration of IV ethanol (100 mg/kg/hr) saturates available alcohol dehydrogenase molecules and slows methanol and ethylene glycol degradation, preventing accumulation of toxic metabolites. Ethanol infusions must be continued during dialysis with the rate increased to maintain a serum ethanol level of 100 mg/dL. The antidote, fomepizole (Antizol), can be substituted for ethanol in the treatment of ethylene glycol and methanol poisoning.[15] Fomepizole is a competitive inhibitor of alcohol dehydrogenase and inhibits the metabolism of ethylene glycol and methanol to their respective toxic metabolites. Neither fomepizole nor ethanol is indicated for isopropanol toxicity.

Other treatable causes of altered level of consciousness such as hypoglycemia and opiate ingestion cannot be overlooked. Fifty percent dextrose in water ($D_{50}W$) is given to reverse hypoglycemia; however, thiamine should be given concurrently because it allows the brain to metabolize the glucose. Naloxone is used to reverse opiate toxicity.

Organophosphates

Organophosphates are major active ingredients in insecticides such as ant sprays, flea sprays, and insect sprays, powders, and liquids. Toxicity varies significantly among chemical formulations. Organophosphates can be ingested, inhaled, or absorbed topically. Mass poisoning occasionally occurs from ingestion of unwashed produce or airborne contamination during crop spraying. Several organophosphate nerve agents were developed in Germany during the 1940s with the intent for military warfare; however, they were not used. Tabun (GA), sarin (GB), and soman (GD) are three examples of such agents that fall in the organophosphate category.

The neurotransmitter acetylcholine is released into synaptic junctions in response to parasympathetic and sympathetic impulses. Acetylcholine plays a role in activation of specific smooth and skeletal muscles. Normally cholinesterase enzymes rapidly break down acetylcholine, halting its action until another stimulus is received. Organophosphates aggressively bind to cholinesterase molecules, inhibiting their effect and allowing acetylcholine to remain unopposed in the neural synapse. This leads to "overactivity" and specific signs and symptoms. Organophosphate-cholinesterase bonds do not spontaneously reverse. After 24 to 48 hours of continuous binding, cholinesterase molecules are destroyed. Complete regeneration of cholinesterase can take weeks or even months.

Clinical findings depend on the specific organophosphate and amount of poison involved. Most oral or respiratory exposures will produce signs and symptoms within 3 hours. Symptoms from toxic dermal exposures may be delayed up to 12 hours. A few lipophilic organophosphates such as dichlofenthion, fenthion, and malathion may not produce significant distress for 1 to 5 days. Acute toxicity from organophosphates presents with manifestations of cholinergic excess. Primary toxic effects involve the autonomic nervous system, neuromuscular junctions, and CNS. The dominant clinical features of cholinergic toxicity include bradycardia, miosis, lacrimation, salivation, increased respiratory secretions, bronchospasm, urination, emesis, and diarrhea. Other symptoms are based on the nicotinic effects and include fasciculations, muscle weakness, and paralysis. Delirium, coma, and seizures may occur. Respiratory arrest may occur because of paralysis of the respiratory muscles.

Dermal exposures necessitate removal of all clothing and jewelry, followed by copious soap and water skin cleansing. Contaminated irrigation fluid should be considered hazardous waste.[23]

Interventions are largely supportive. Severely poisoned patients with a markedly depressed mental status should receive 100% oxygen and intubation. Effective antidote therapy counteracts organophosphate effects, although recovery requires synthesis of new cholinesterase. Because organophosphates produce a cholinergic syndrome, anticholinergics are the treatment of choice. Immediate therapy includes administration of IV atropine titrated to the therapeutic end point of clearing of respiratory secretions and cessation of bronchospasms and bronchoconstriction. Atropine should be administered beginning at 2 to 5 mg IV for adults and 0.05 mg/kg IV for children. Cases of severe poisoning may necessitate up to 5 mg of atropine every 3 to 5 minutes. The presence of tachycardia is not a contraindication to atropine administration in the organophosphate-poisoned patient. Atropine does not treat neuromuscular dysfunctions such as muscle fasciculations and weakness. Pralidoxime (2-PAM) may decrease or inhibit the effects of organophosphates on nicotinic receptors. It should be administered once atropine therapy is initiated. The initial IV dose is 30 mg/kg (adults) and 25 to 50 mg/kg (children) administered slowly over 20 to 30 minutes and based on severity of symptoms.[9] An initial bolus is followed by additional boluses every 1 to 2 hours or by a continuous infusion of at least 8 mg/kg/hr in adults and 10 to 20 mg/kg/hr for children.[20] Seizures should be treated with diazepam. Phenytoin is not recommended for seizures induced by organophosphates.

The organophosphate-intoxicated individual is at significant risk for contaminating others. Perform resuscitation and decontamination in a well-ventilated, isolated area. All people coming into contact with the poisoned individual require full personal protective equipment, including gloves and goggles. The patient's clothing is considered contaminated. Vomitus, gastric lavage material, and stool must be handled with caution, followed by careful disposal, to avoid secondary contamination.

Heavy Metals

Heavy metals involved in poisoning include lead, mercury, zinc, arsenic, and cadmium. Because heavy metals are a by-product of the industrial age, all inhabitants of developed countries have measurable serum heavy metal levels. Intoxication by these agents is often chronic and subtle, making diagnosis difficult. For example, lead exposure may be related to daily use of glazed ceramic dinnerware or occasional ingestion of paint chips by a small child. Industrial exposure to button batteries, dental cement, marine paints, solder, and countless other products and manufacturing processes puts individuals at risk for heavy metal poisoning. Water pollution can cause mercury toxicity from seafood ingestion.

Absorption of these metals can occur through inhalation and ingestion. Chronic toxicities have a different presentation than acute poisonings. Exposure to an inorganic metal versus an organic metal salt also causes different effects. Heavy metal toxicosis is frequently associated with other poisons such as hydrocarbons (leaded gasoline), organophosphates (arsenic-containing pesticides), and carbon monoxide (mercury released in fuel burning). Without careful assessment and diagnostic evaluation, such polytoxicities can easily be missed.

Heavy metals have no known beneficial physiologic activity in humans and are not metabolized, so they accumulate in the tissues. The metals bind with reactive protein groups and enzymes, disrupting enzymatic function. Excretion from the body is slow, making the effects long term. Although symptoms vary with type of metal and extent of exposure, GI disturbances—ranging from nausea, vomiting, and diarrhea to GI hemorrhage—are frequently found. Central and peripheral nervous system effects include tremors, peripheral neuropathies, neuropsychiatric disturbances, and seizures. Acute inhalation produces chemical pneumonitis, pulmonary edema, and lung cancer.

Serum levels generally provide the best evaluation of heavy metal exposure, although urine and hair samples are sometimes tested. A plain film of the abdomen may show recently ingested metals in the GI tract. The need for therapeutic intervention is determined by extent of exposure and patient symptomatology. With certain chronic exposures, terminating contact with the offending agent or environment is all that is required. For very recent ingestions, standard gastric-emptying techniques can be employed; however, this is of no benefit for chronic ingestion or inhalation. Activated charcoal does not absorb metals.

Because heavy metals accumulate in tissues and are not metabolized, chelation therapy is the best means of eliminating these substances from the body. Chelating agents—administered orally, intramuscularly, or intravenously—bind to metals and facilitate excretion. Three chelating drugs are commonly used: dimercaprol, penicillamine, and ethylenediaminetetraacetic acid (EDTA). The particular agent selected and route of administration vary with the toxin involved. Dosage is dependent on patient size and symptom severity. Because of the highly individualized circumstances surrounding each exposure, consultation with poison control center personnel should be undertaken before administering any chelating drug. Other supportive measures are largely determined on a patient-by-patient basis as symptoms dictate. Fluid volume deficits, anemia, cardiopulmonary dysfunction, and renal failure require intervention as appropriate.

Iron

Iron overdose is one of the most common and severe poisonings in children younger than 6 years. Unlike heavy metals, iron plays an important physiologic role. Its therapeutic usefulness has made iron widely available in many over-the-counter formulations containing varying amounts of elemental iron. Iron toxicity begins with a direct corrosive effect on GI mucosa, leading to perforation, hemorrhage, and necrosis. After it is absorbed, iron initiates cellular toxicity by interfering with aerobic metabolism, causing lactic acidosis and producing free-radical injury.

Doses less than 20 mg/kg of elemental iron are generally asymptomatic. Ingestions between 20 and 40 mg/kg may produce self-limited vomiting, abdominal pain, and diarrhea. Doses higher than 40 mg/kg are considered serious, and doses greater than 60 mg/kg may be lethal.[18]

Classically the iron-poisoned patient passes through four clinical stages. In stage I, iron can produce GI corrosion. Symptoms of stage II range from nausea to massive hemorrhage. Patients who survive stage II may experience a latent period of apparent improvement over the next 12 hours. Stage III is signaled by abrupt onset of coma, shock, seizures, metabolic acidosis, coagulopathies, and hepatic failure. Survivors eventually enter stage IV, the recovery phase.

Diagnosis of iron ingestion is based on a history of exposure. Suggestive laboratory tests include elevated white blood cell count (greater than or equal to 15,000/mm^3 and hyperglycemia (greater than 150 mg/dL). Mild to moderate toxicity generally manifests with serum iron levels of 350 to 500 mcg/dL. Hepatotoxicity is observed at levels greater than 500 mcg/dL. Iron tablets may also be visible on abdominal radiographs.

If the acutely iron-toxic patient presents in hemorrhagic shock, early management focuses on basic stabilization. Gastric lavage may be considered if exposure was recent, tablets were chewed, or a liquid iron preparation was ingested. However, intact tablets are large and are unlikely to pass through a lavage tube. Activated charcoal does not absorb iron and is not recommended unless other drugs were ingested. Whole bowel irrigation is effective and can be considered. Massive ingestions may result in bezoar formation (i.e., a hard ball that develops in the stomach), requiring endoscopic or surgical removal.

Deferoxamine, the specific antidote for iron poisoning, is indicated in cases of serious intoxication.[1] This chelating agent is generally given intravenously by constant infusion at a rate of 15 mg/kg/hr. The chelated deferoxamine-iron complex is excreted in urine, usually producing a characteristic orange or pink-red color. Therapy may be stopped when urine color or serum iron levels return to normal or the patient's symptoms have resolved.

Calcium Channel and β-Blockers

Calcium channel blockers are used for the management of angina, hypertension, dysrhythmias, and migraine prophylaxis. Some of the common calcium channel blocker agents include verapamil, nifedipine, diltiazem, bepridil, and mibefradil. Calcium channel blockers are rapidly emerging as one of the most lethal prescription drug ingestions. Children can become symptomatic with as little as one tablet. Overdose by short-acting agents is characterized by rapid progression to cardiac arrest. Overdose from extended-release agents results in delayed onset of dysrhythmias, shock, cardiac collapse, and bowel ischemia. Calcium channel blockers result in peripheral vasodilation, decreased heart rate, decreased contractility, and decreased conduction. Significant bradycardia, hypotension, and heart blocks are classic symptoms of calcium channel blocker poisoning. Hyperglycemia may occur because calcium channel blockade inhibits insulin release. Serum drug levels may be obtained but often take hours to perform. Treatment must be instituted based on symptoms and history. A 12-lead ECG should be obtained and continuous cardiac monitoring implemented. Cardiac markers may help to differentiate drug-induced bradycardia from ischemic causes. Atropine may be tried if the patient has a hemodynamically unstable bradycardic rhythm; however, atropine is often not effective in calcium channel blocker toxicity. Transcutaneous pacing may be required for a hemodynamically unstable heart block. Dopamine at 5 to 10 mcg/kg/min may improve heart rate and contractility. Administer a fluid bolus of normal saline for hypotension if there is no evidence of decompensated heart failure. Administer 5 to 15 mg of glucagon IV if hypotension persists; glucagon is the accepted antidote for β-blockers. Glucagon competes for receptor sites and neutralizes the effects of β-blockers. Either calcium chloride or calcium gluconate (up to 4 g) may be administered for hypotension or heart block associated with acute or chronic calcium channel blocker toxicity. Calcium is essential for contractility; calcium channel blockers stop the movement of calcium, resulting in diminished perfusion. If performed within 1 to 2 hours of ingestion, gastric lavage may be helpful

for ingestion of extended-release formulas. Activated charcoal is recommended for calcium channel poisoning.

β-Adrenergic antagonists (β-blockers) are used in the treatment of hypertension, glaucoma, and various other disorders. They decrease cardiac rate and contractility. Recent data from the American Association of Poison Control Centers reported 2467 significant toxic ingestions.[26] Propranolol is considered the most toxic β-blocker. β-Blockers that are not sustained release are rapidly absorbed from the GI tract. The first critical signs of overdose may appear within 20 minutes but are more commonly observed within 1 to 2 hours. Bradycardia with hemodynamic compromise from hypotension is considered severe β-blocker toxicity and can lead to rapid clinical deterioration. Hypotension usually does not occur before the onset of bradycardia. β-Blockers may be associated with hypoglycemia, especially in patients with diabetes and in children. A 12-lead ECG and continuous cardiac monitoring are essential. Consider cardiac markers to rule out cardiac reasons for bradycardia and hemodynamic compromise. Administer a normal saline bolus in the hypotensive patient. Glucagon may enhance cardiac contractility and conduction; the initial IV bolus is 3 to 10 mg. Transcutaneous pacing may be needed in hemodynamically unstable bradycardic rhythms. Activated charcoal is indicated for the treatment of β-blocker poisoning.

Digitalis Glycosides

Digitalis glycosides are available in pharmaceutical preparations such as digoxin and digitoxin and can also be found in homes and yards in oleander, lily of the valley, rhododendron, and foxglove plants. At therapeutic and toxic doses, digitalis glycosides block the sodium-potassium-adenosine triphosphatase pump. With high serum concentrations, both vagal and sympathetic tone increase.

Clinical symptoms can be vague and difficult to diagnose, particularly with chronic overdoses in older adult patients. Findings include drowsiness, lethargy, and coma. Cardiac conduction disturbances (first-, second-, and third-degree heart block), ventricular dysrhythmias (premature ventricular contractions, ventricular tachycardia, and ventricular fibrillation), asystole, and profound hypotension also occur. (See Chapter 31 for discussion on management of various dysrhythmias.) Visual changes include the appearance of yellow or green halos around objects. The patient may experience anorexia, nausea, and vomiting, especially in cases of chronic poisoning. Elevated potassium levels are a prominent feature of cardiac glycoside poisoning, and hyperkalemia (greater than 5.5 mEq/L) must be treated aggressively.

Quantitative serum levels of digoxin or digitoxin can be useful for assessing an individual's degree of toxicity. Complete tissue distribution of cardiac glycosides requires at least 12 hours. Although serum levels are routinely drawn when toxicity is first suspected, samples collected before that time may not reflect a state of blood-tissue equilibrium. Because toxicosis can occur at various serum concentrations, symptomatology must guide therapy. Activated charcoal absorbs digitalis glycosides from the GI tract, decreasing systemic absorption. Multiple doses of activated charcoal have been suggested for the treatment of digoxin and digitoxin overdose, although limited clinical experience with this treatment has been reported.

High serum digitalis concentrations are an indication for antidote treatment. Digoxin immune Fab (Digibind), an ovine-derived antibody, attaches to digitalis glycosides and renders them inactive. Indications for Digibind are the presence of two or more of the following: life-threatening dysrhythmias, serum potassium levels higher than 5 mEq/L, or serum digoxin concentration greater than 10 ng/mL. The Digibind manufacturer also suggests administration if a single digitalis dose of more than 4 mg has been ingested by a child or more than 10 mg by an adult. An appropriate Digibind dosage is calculated based on a pharmacokinetic determination of total digoxin/digitoxin body load.[14]

Hydrocarbons

Hydrocarbons are found in petroleum, natural gas, coal, and bitumen. Exposure may be caused by inhalation, dermal contact, or ingestion. Accidental exposures are common in children younger than 5 years of age with access to kerosene, gasoline, or lighter fluid. Adults are usually poisoned as a result of occupational contact.

The effects of hydrocarbon toxicity can be divided into pulmonary aspiration and systemic absorption. The potential for pulmonary aspiration is inversely related to the substances' viscosity—the more viscous the hydrocarbon, the less toxic the substance. Aspiration of tiny amounts of low-viscosity hydrocarbons (gasoline, turpentine, lighter fluid, kerosene, petroleum, and ether) causes coughing and wheezing and can progress to a life-threatening chemical pneumonitis within hours. Systemic absorption occurs from ingestion, inhalation of hydrocarbon vapors, or dermal contact. Systemic manifestations of hydrocarbon toxicity vary widely by substance and time since exposure. Neurologic symptoms include confusion, headache, lethargy, ataxia, and coma. Hydrocarbons affect the heart's conduction system, causing complete heart block, asystole, and ventricular fibrillation. Nausea, vomiting, and GI bleeding have also been reported. Hepatic failure, renal failure, or hemolysis can occur days or even weeks after exposure. Dermal contact causes local irritation and chemical burns.

Exposure to high-viscosity substances (lubricating oil, petroleum jelly, grease, diesel oil, tar, and paraffin) with a low systemic toxicity potential, requires no treatment. Chemicals with a low potential for systemic problems, but with high risk for aspiration pneumonitis, only require observation for pulmonary embarrassment with appropriate respiratory support, should complications occur. Gastric suctioning and activated charcoal administration are indicated for recent ingestion of substances with low viscosity and high potential for systemic toxicity. A cuffed endotracheal tube must be inserted before gastric lavage to protect the patient from aspiration. Continuous cardiac and oxygen saturation monitoring are recommended. Remove clothing, and wash contaminated skin with copious amounts of soap and water. IV access should be established for emergency medications; however, fluids should be administered judiciously because of the potential for pulmonary edema development. Position the patient carefully to minimize risk for aspiration. Obtain a chest radiograph to rule out early pulmonary alterations. Do not administer steroids or prophylactic antibiotics. All symptomatic patients should be observed for 24 hours for pulmonary and cardiac problems. Patients who remain asymptomatic can be discharged after 4 to 6 hours.

Toxic Plants

Many plants found in the home and surrounding environment contain toxic substances. In fact, there are more than 100 species of toxic mushrooms alone. Some plants contain hallucinogenic, narcotic, or anticholinergic toxins, making them popular substances of abuse; others have neurotoxic or cardiotoxic effects. Many are simply GI irritants. Plants frequently associated with intentional or unintentional poisoning include poinsettia, jimsonweed, lily of the valley, and oleander. Consult poison control to determine needed interventions for toxic plant exposures.

SUMMARY

Toxicologic emergencies are a routine cause of ED visits. This chapter highlights some of the more frequently seen poisonings. Nursing diagnoses related to toxicologic emergencies may be found in the appendix at the back of the text. The initial focus of care in any intoxicated patient is always stabilization of cardiopulmonary or hemodynamic problems. Treatment priorities include limiting poison absorption, enhancing substance elimination, and providing toxin- and patient-specific supportive interventions. The reader is referred to a detailed toxicology text or the experts at a poison control center for further information on any of the toxicities discussed in this chapter.

REFERENCES

1. Alymara V, Bourantas D, Chaidos A: Effectiveness and safety of combined iron chelation therapy with deferoxamine and deferiprone, *Hematol J* 5(6):477, 2004.
2. American Academy of Clinical Toxicology and European Association of Poison Control Centers and Clinical Toxicologists: Position statement: gastric lavage, *J Toxicol Clinical Toxicol* 35:711, 1997.
3. Burns M: Activated charcoal as the sole intervention for treatment after childhood poisoning, *Curr Opin Pediatr* 12(2):166, 2000.
4. Burns MJ, Schartzstein RM: Decontamination of poisoned adults, *UpToDate,* 2008. Retrieved March 3, 2009, from http://www.uptodate.com/online/content/topic.do?topicKey=ad_tox/2200&selectedTitle=1~133&source=search_result.

5. Canter MZ: Comparison of oral and IV acetylcysteine in the treatment of acetaminophen poisoning, *Am J Health Syst Pharm* 63:1825, 2006.

6. Daragan PI, Coldbridge MG, Jones AL: The management of tricyclic antidepressant poisoning, *Toxicol Rev* 24(3):193, 2005.

7. Defendi GL: Toxicity: acetaminophen, *eMedicine.* Retrieved April 22, 2008, from http://www.emedicine.com/ped/topic7.htm.

8. Dorrington CL, Johnson DW, Brant R: The frequency of complications associated with MDAC, *Ann Emerg Med* 41(3):370, 2003.

9. Eddleston M, Szinicz L, Eyer P et al: Oximes in acute organophosphorous pesticide poisoning: a systematic review of clinical trials, *Q J Med* 95:275, 2002.

10. Greene SL, Daragan PI, Jones AL: Acute poisoning: understanding 90% cases in a nutshell, *Postgrad Med J* 81:204, 2005.

11. Heard K: Gastrointestinal decontamination, *Med Clin North Am* 89:1067, 2005.

12. Hutchison MD, Traub SJ: Tricyclic antidepressant intoxication, *UpToDate,* 2008. Retrieved March 4, 2009, from http://www.uptodate.com/online/content/topic.do?topicKey=ad_tox/10025&selectedTitle=6~133&source=search_result.

13. Karch S, Stephens B: Toxicology and pathology of deaths related to methadone, *West J Med* 172(1):11, 2000.

14. Kawasaki C, Nishi R, Uekihara S et al: Charcoal hemoperfusion in the treatment of phenytoin overdose, *Am J Kidney Dis* 35(2):323, 2000.

15. Lai MW, Klein-Schwartz W, Rodgers GC et al: 2005 Annual report of the American Association of Poison Control Centers' national poisoning and exposure database, *Clin Toxicol* (44):803, 2006.

16. Meyer R, Beard M, Ardagh M: Methanol poisoning, *NZ Med J* 113(102):11, 2000.

17. Mittleman MA, Mintzer D, Maclure M et al: Triggering of myocardial infarction by cocaine, *Circulation* 99:2739, 1999.

18. Morris C: Pediatric iron poisonings in the United States, *South Med J* 93(4):352, 2000.

19. Olson K, Acetaminophen: In Olsen K, editor: *Poisoning and drug overdose,* ed 3, Stamford, Conn, 1999, Appleton & Lange.

20. Pawar KS, Bhoite RR, Pillay CP et al: Continuous pralidoxime infusion versus repeated bolus injection to treat organophosphorous pesticide poisoning: a randomized control trial, *Lancet 368*:2136, 2006.

21. Proudfoot AT, Krenzelok EP, Val JA: Position paper on urine alkalinization, *J Toxicol Clin Toxicol* 42:19, 2004.

22. Saetta JP, March S, Gaunt ME et al: Gastric emptying procedures in the self-poisoned patient: are we forcing content beyond the pylorus? *J R Soc Med* 84:274, 1991.

23. Stacey R, Mofrey D, Payne S: Secondary contamination in organophosphate poisoning: analysis of an incident, *Q J Med* 97:75, 2004.

24. Tenebein PK, Sitar DS, Tenebein M: Interaction between *N*-acetylcysteine and activated charcoal: implications for the treatment of acetaminophen poisoning, *Pharmacotherapy* 21:1333, 2001.

25. Watson WA, Litovitz TL, Klein-Shwartz W et al: 2003 Annual report of the American Association of Poison Control Centers Toxic Exposure Surveillance System, *Am J Emerg MedL* 23:335, 2004.

26. Watson WA, Litovitz TL, Rodgers GC et al: 2004 Annual report of the American Association of Poison Control Centers, *Am J Emerg Med* 23(5):600, 2005.

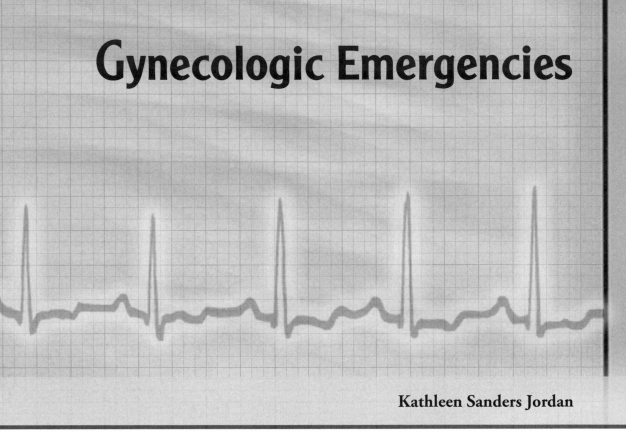

CHAPTER 43

Gynecologic Emergencies

Kathleen Sanders Jordan

Patients with gynecologic disorders are frequently seen in the emergency department (ED). Therefore the ED nurse must have a strong knowledge base of the normal anatomy and physiology of the female reproductive system in order to accurately assess and provide care for this patient population. Patients with gynecologic disorders may not seek care, or if they do, they may not disclose all of their concerns and symptoms. This could be due to a variety of reasons, including embarrassment or lack of knowledge regarding their own anatomy and physiology. Age, marital status, socioeconomic status, social support systems, and religious and cultural beliefs may also be key factors in preventing a female patient from seeking care or openly discussing problems related to the reproductive system.

ANATOMY AND PHYSIOLOGY

Gynecologic emergencies can affect any organ in the internal or external female reproductive system. The internal reproductive organs include the vagina, cervix, uterus, fallopian tubes, and ovaries. The external genitalia include the mons pubis, labia majora and minora, clitoris, vestibular glands, hymen, vaginal orifice, urethral orifice, and the ducts of Bartholin's and Skene's glands. The perineum is the triangular area between the posterior portion of the vestibule and the anus that supports portions of the urogenital and gastrointestinal tracts.

The ovaries, fallopian tubes, and uterus are located inside the peritoneal cavity. The ovaries are bilateral oval structures, located between the uterus and lateral pelvic wall. During childbearing years, each ovary is 2.5 to 5 cm long, 1.5 to 3 cm wide, and 0.6 to 1.5 cm thick. Size diminishes significantly after menopause. The number of ova present in the ovaries also decreases with age—from approximately 2 million at birth to 300,000 to 400,000 by puberty. During ovulation each ovary releases a single ovum that is transported down the fallopian tubes to the uterus. The fallopian tubes (approximately 10 cm long) transport the ovum to the uterus through smooth muscle contraction. These bilateral tubes are not contiguous with the ovaries; consequently, the ovum can migrate into the peritoneal cavity. This is the basic mechanism that leads to endometriosis and to ectopic pregnancy in the peritoneal space.

The uterus is a thick-walled organ shaped like an inverted pear. It is suspended in the anterior pelvis above the bladder and in front of the rectum. Length in nulliparous women is 6 to 8 cm. After pregnancy the uterus lengthens to 9 to 10 cm. A layer of peritoneum covers the superior portion of the uterus and forms the serous layer of the uterine wall. The middle layer of the uterine wall consists of smooth muscle with an inner mucous lining called the endometrium. The lower portion of the uterus is referred to as the cervix and provides entrance into the uterus. It is located in the vagina between the bladder on the anterior aspect and the rectum posteriorly. The top of the uterus is called the fundus.

Box 43-1 **INTERVIEW QUESTIONS FOR GYNECOLOGIC EMERGENCIES**

When was your last menstrual period? Was it normal?

How long does your period normally last?

Are you bleeding now? How much are you bleeding? How many pads or tampons have you used in the last hour? Are there any clots or tissue?

Is there a possibility you are pregnant?

How many pregnancies have you had? How many children do you have?

Do you normally have a vaginal discharge? Is there anything different about your discharge today?

Do you have any swelling, itching, redness, or pain?

Are you having other symptoms or problems?

Are you sexually active?

Do you have sex with men, women, or both?

In the past 2 months, how many partners have you had sex with?

What type of birth control do you use? Do you consistently use it?

Box 43-2 **TERMS USED TO DEFINE ABNORMAL UTERINE BLEEDING**

Amenorrhea—no menstruation

Oligomenorrhea—too few episodes of bleeding

Menorrhagia—too much blood loss

Metrorrhagia—too many episodes of bleeding

Menometrorrhagia—too much and too many episodes of bleeding

The female reproductive cycle consists of ovulation and menstruation, with each cycle determined by the level of female hormones. Changes in hormone levels prepare the endometrium for implantation of a fertilized ovum. If the ovum is not fertilized, the endometrium sheds the inner lining as menstrual flow. A normal menstrual cycle occurs every 21 to 45 days (average of 28 days for most females) with menstruation lasting from 2 to 7 days; an average of 35 to 150 mL of blood is lost with each cycle.

ASSESSMENT

An accurate history is critical to the assessment process. A patient's behavior during the assessment process may provide important clues as to the patient's feelings and attitudes regarding her illness. Pain and emotions related to one's reproductive organs and sexuality may cause a great deal of anxiety and fear for patients. It is important that the ED nurse create an environment to establish rapport and ensure confidentiality with each individual patient to facilitate the discussion of this sensitive material. Essential components of the history include chief complaint, pain assessment (i.e., provocation, quality, radiation, severity, and timing), presence of vaginal bleeding, presence of vaginal discharge, menstrual history, obstetric history, sexual history, medical/surgical history, medications and allergies. All female patients of reproductive age should be considered pregnant until pregnancy has been ruled out through a urine or serum pregnancy test. Box 43-1 summarizes essential interview questions for this patient population.

Patients with gynecologic emergencies can experience significant blood loss and hypovolemia. The physical examination must include a general survey consisting of the patient's general appearance; vital signs; skin color, moisture, and temperature; and cardiovascular and respiratory status. A focused assessment should include examination of the abdominal and genitourinary systems. The abdomen should be inspected, bowel sounds auscultated, and the entire abdomen palpated for areas of tenderness, masses, and signs of peritonitis. A complete pelvic examination should be performed, including assessment of the external genitalia, vagina, and bimanual examination of the uterus and ovaries; a speculum examination is commonly performed. Specimens should be obtained for sexually transmitted infection (STI) screening (e.g., chlamydial infection, gonorrhea, and trichomoniasis) and wet mount (i.e., normal saline and potassium hydroxide [KOH]).

Diagnostic tests indicated for the patient with a gynecologic emergency should include a urinalysis and urine or serum pregnancy test. A catheterized urine specimen should be obtained if the patient is bleeding from the vagina. Other laboratory tests that may be indicated include a complete blood count (CBC), prothrombin time (PT), activated partial thromboplastin time (aPTT), serum electrolyte levels, blood type and crossmatch, and C-reactive protein. Ultrasonography, abdominal and pelvic computed tomography (CT), and magnetic resonance imaging (MRI) may also be useful diagnostic tests for evaluating masses and abscesses.

SPECIFIC GYNECOLOGIC EMERGENCIES
Vaginal Bleeding/Dysfunctional Uterine Bleeding

Vaginal bleeding in the nonpregnant patient can be due to a variety of causes, including hormonal imbalance; vaginal, cervical, or uterine disorders; trauma; infection; malignancies; systemic disease; medications; or blood dyscrasias. Eating disorders, excessive weight loss, stress, and exercise can also cause abnormal vaginal bleeding or amenorrhea. More than 8 saturated pads per day or 12 tampons per day is considered excessive bleeding, although blood loss is difficult to estimate depending on the frequency of pad or tampon changes. Vaginal bleeding is abnormal in prepubertal females and necessitates a full diagnostic workup. Terms used to define abnormal uterine bleeding are listed in Box 43-2.

Dysfunctional uterine bleeding (DUB) is the most common cause of vaginal bleeding during a woman's reproductive years. The diagnosis of DUB is a diagnosis of exclusion and should only be made when other organic and structural causes for the abnormal bleeding have been ruled out.

Approximately 90% of DUB results from anovulation, which causes failure of the corpus luteum to develop. This leads to failure of normal progesterone secretion, resulting in continuous unopposed production of estrogen. Unopposed estrogen causes endometrial hyperplasia and irregular endometrial shedding, which can be excessive, prolonged, and life threatening.[13]

DUB may occur at any age; however, given the fact that most cases are due to anovulation, it is most common at the extremes of the reproductive years. Most cases in adolescent girls occur during the first 18 months after the onset of menstruation because of immaturity of their hypothalamic-pituitary axis.[7] In the perimenopausal period, DUB may be an early manifestation of ovarian failure. Vaginal bleeding in the postmenopausal patient should be considered a malignancy until this is ruled out.

Assessment of the nonpregnant patient with vaginal bleeding includes a detailed history followed by an abdominal and pelvic examination. The history should include the amount and duration of bleeding the patient has experienced. The patient with an established menstrual history should be asked to compare the number of pads used per day in a normal menstrual cycle to the number used at this time. The average tampon holds 5 mL of blood, the average pad 5 to 15 mL of blood. Additional information should be obtained regarding the presence or absence of pain; date of last normal menstrual period (LNMP), including duration and flow; menstrual regularity; obstetric history; contraceptive use; and sexual history. Additional information should be obtained regarding comorbidities and medications taken.

A physical examination should be conducted to assess volume status, hemodynamic stability, and extent of bleeding. Laboratory specimens should be obtained for urinalysis, urine or serum pregnancy test, and CBC. Other laboratory tests that may be indicated include PT, aPTT, liver function tests (in the presence of liver disease), and type and crossmatch. A pelvic or intravaginal ultrasound examination may be obtained to evaluate for structural abnormalities.

In the presence of hemodynamic instability, nursing interventions should be directed at immediate resuscitation and stabilization. If bleeding is severe and the patient is not responsive to initial fluid resuscitation, a 25-mg dose of intravenous (IV) conjugated estrogen (Premarin) should be administered. Repeat doses every 2 to 4 hours may be administered as needed. A course of oral estrogen therapy (Premarin) may also be prescribed for cessation of bleeding. Perimenopausal women may be treated with cyclic oral contraceptives 4 times per day for a period of 7 days to control and regulate bleeding.[12] A gynecology consultation should be obtained for all patients with hemodynamic instability while the patient is in the ED. Patients who are discharged should be given a referral to a gynecologist for further workup. All patients with anemia should be advised to take an iron supplement.

Pelvic Pain

Pelvic pain is a common presenting chief complaint in patients seeking care in the ED. Pain in the lower abdomen or pelvis may be due to a variety of causes. The uterus, cervix, and adnexa share the same visceral innervation as the lower ileum, sigmoid colon, and rectum. Therefore it may be difficult to distinguish pain originating in the gynecologic organs from pain originating in the gastrointestinal organs. Poorly localized visceral pain originates in organs and viscera innervated by autonomic nerves. This may be caused by distention of a hollow viscus (e.g., fallopian tube or bowel), distention of the capsule of a solid organ, or stretching of pelvic ligaments or adhesions. In contrast, pain that is well localized originates from somatic nerve irritation, such as irritation of the peritoneum caused by an inflamed organ (e.g., endometritis, appendicitis) or the presence of blood or purulent fluid (e.g., ruptured ectopic pregnancy or ovarian cyst).[6] Pelvic pain is classified as acute, chronic, or cyclic. Box 43-3 outlines the causes of pelvic pain originating from the reproductive organs. An accurate history and physical examination is crucial in this patient population because the condition causing the pain may be life threatening.

Dysmenorrhea

Pain with menstruation is a common gynecologic complaint, particularly in adolescents and young women. Primary dysmenorrhea is defined as pelvic pain during menstruation in the absence of other pelvic pathologic condition. It typically develops 1 to 3 years after menarche with an increasing incidence through the early to mid twenties as ovulatory cycles are established. Primary dysmenorrhea is the most common form of pain during menstruation. This problem may be

---

Box 43-3	**CAUSES OF PELVIC PAIN OF GYNECOLOGIC ORIGIN**

ACUTE PELVIC PAIN

Abortion (threatened or incomplete)
Ectopic pregnancy
Ovarian cyst
Ovarian torsion
Acute pelvic inflammatory disease
Tuboovarian abscess
Endometritis
Degenerating fibroid

CYCLIC PELVIC PAIN

Mittelschmerz
Endometriosis
Dysmenorrhea
Adenomyosis

CHRONIC PELVIC PAIN

Adhesions
Chronic pelvic inflammatory disease

significant, causing up to 10% of women to miss school or work days.[13] It is most severe in young, nulliparous women. Primary dysmenorrhea is characterized by crampy, low midline pain, which occurs secondary to progesterone-mediated uterine contractions and arteriolar vasospasm. The pain typically precedes menstrual flow by up to 24 hours and subsides after menses begins. There may be associated nausea, vomiting, back pain, headache, and irritability.[13]

Secondary dysmenorrhea is cyclic menstrual pain associated with a pelvic pathologic condition. This is most frequently caused by endometriosis or pelvic inflammatory disease (PID). Other causes include intrauterine devices, adhesions, and benign tumors of the uterus.

Management of primary dysmenorrhea includes the use of nonsteroidal antiinflammatory drugs (NSAIDs) to inhibit the synthesis of prostaglandins; narcotics should be avoided. To maximize pain relief, NSAIDs should be administered before the onset of menses. If NSAIDs fail to provide relief, cyclic oral contraceptives (COCs) should be started to inhibit ovulation, which will decrease the amount of menstrual pain and bleeding. If dysmenorrhea persists despite the use of COCs, a secondary cause of dysmenorrhea should be considered and an appropriate diagnostic workup should be pursued.[7] Sympathetic reassurance is helpful after other causes of acute pelvic pain have been ruled out. Gynecologic follow-up is indicated.

Endometriosis

Endometriosis is a common cause of cyclic pain in menstruating women. Endometrial tissue develops outside of the uterus, causing pain with menses. Organs involved may include the ovaries, posterior cul de sac, fallopian tubes, and uterosacral ligaments. Despite the abnormal location of endometrial tissue growth, the tissue sloughs and bleeds just as the uterine tissue does. As the disease progresses, pelvic adhesions may develop. Pain is cyclic or constant and may vary in character and intensity. It is generally worse just before or during menses. The character of the pain may range from midline pelvic cramping to severe diffuse pain.

Endometriosis may be strongly suspected, but it is not a diagnosis made in the ED. Diagnostic studies include a pregnancy test, CBC, and urinalysis. Laparoscopy is the standard modality used to definitively diagnose endometriosis. ED management focuses on pain control through the use of NSAIDs and possibly short-term narcotics. Further therapy depends on the severity of symptoms, stage of the disease, and desire for future fertility. Hormonal therapy may be used to mimic pseudopregnancy, chronic anovulation, and pseudomenopause.

Mittelschmerz

Pain with ovulation, referred to as mittelschmerz, is a transient, midcycle pelvic pain that occurs during or just after ovulation. The cause is increasing ovarian capsular pressure before the follicle erupts and leakage of prostaglandin-containing follicular fluid associated with ovulation. Mittelschmerz is characterized by sudden, sharp, and unilateral pelvic pain. Treatment includes antiprostaglandin therapy with NSAIDs for pain relief. Sympathetic reassurance is helpful after other causes of acute pelvic pain have been ruled out.

Ovarian Cyst

An ovarian cyst is a fluid-filled or semi–fluid-filled sac in an ovary that can develop at any time from the neonatal period to postmenopause. For most patients ovarian cysts cause no symptoms and are an incidental finding during ultrasonography performed for another reason. Follicle cysts of the ovary are the most common cystic structure found in healthy ovaries, and they develop during the first 2 weeks of the menstrual cycle. This type of cyst results from either failure of the mature follicle to rupture or failure of an immature follicle to undergo the normal maturation process. A follicular cyst may grow to a size of 8 to 10 cm, and stretching of the capsule is the cause of pelvic discomfort. Most of these cysts regress spontaneously over 1 to 3 months. Follicular cysts are thin walled and may rupture during sexual intercourse or strenuous exercise. The symptoms of a ruptured follicular cyst include sharp pelvic pain of sudden onset that resolves over a few days.

Corpus luteal cysts are much less common than ovarian cysts. These cysts develop during the latter half of the menstrual cycle during the luteal phase, and most regress at the end of the menstrual cycle. However, persistent corpus luteal cysts are blood filled and may rupture, producing sharp pelvic pain, intraperitoneal irritation, and bleeding, which may progress to anemia and hypovolemia. Bleeding from a ruptured corpus luteal cyst is usually self-limited but in rare cases may progress to hemorrhage and hypovolemic shock.[13]

Diagnostic studies include a pregnancy test, urinalysis, and CBC. Definitive diagnosis is made through pelvic ultrasonography and/or laparoscopy. Treatment of ruptured ovarian cysts is directed at pain control with NSAIDs and/or narcotics and treatment of complications, including hypovolemia and hemorrhage. Patients may need admission for observation and serial hematocrit determinations to monitor bleeding. Surgical intervention is usually not required except for the rare case of continued intraperitoneal hemorrhage.

Ovarian Torsion

Twisting of the ovary or fallopian tube is referred to as torsion. Most ovarian torsions result secondary to an ovarian cyst (most commonly dermoid cysts). The pain associated with this disorder is due to ischemia and is usually described as acute, severe, and unilateral. Pain may be intermittent or constant. Associated symptoms commonly include nausea and vomiting, low-grade fever, and leukocytosis. Diagnostic studies include a pregnancy test, CBC, and pelvic ultrasonography. Patients with torsion require hospital admission for surgical intervention. If untreated, an ovarian torsion can lead to infertility, infection, and eventual necrosis of the affected ovary or fallopian tube.

Vaginal Discharge and Vaginitis

Discharge from the vagina that is odorless and clear to milky in color is normal and the body's physiologic way of keeping the vagina healthy. A complex and intricate balance of microorganisms maintain the normal vaginal flora. Factors that can influence and alter the composition of the vaginal flora include age, stress, hormonal balance, sexual activity, contraceptives, hygiene products, antibiotics, and general health status.[10] Any change in the amount, color, odor, and/or associated symptoms of itching, burning, or irritation may indicate a change in this chemical balance in the vagina and lead to an infection. Vaginitis is common in postpubertal adolescents and adult women, but relatively uncommon in prepubertal females. The most common cause of vaginitis is bacterial vaginosis (40% to 50%), followed by *Candida albicans* (20% to 25%), and *Trichomonas vaginalis* (15% to 20%).[6]

Bacterial Vaginosis

Bacterial vaginosis (BV) occurs when the normal bacterial flora in the vagina is replaced with *Gardnerella vaginalis* and *Mycoplasma hominis*. BV is characterized by a vaginal discharge that is thin, homogeneous, malodorous, and white to gray in color. It is estimated that up to 50% of women with BV are asymptomatic. The Centers for Disease Control and Prevention (CDC) states that for this condition to be diagnosed three of the following signs and symptoms must be present: (1) a homogeneous, white, noninflammatory discharge that coats the vaginal walls; (2) the presence of clue cells on microscopic examination; (3) pH greater than 4.5; and (4) a fishy odor to the discharge after the addition of KOH (positive whiff test).[10] BV has also been associated with PID, endometritis, and vaginal cuff cellulitis after surgical procedures. Complications of BV in pregnancy include preterm labor and premature rupture of membranes. Metronidazole (Flagyl) and clindamycin are both effective for the treatment of BV. Both of these pharmacologic agents may be administered orally or intravaginally.

Candidiasis

Vaginal candidiasis is caused by vaginal colonization of the airborne fungi of the *Candida* species. Most commonly the organisms gain access to the vaginal lumen from the adjacent perianal area. Risk factors for the development of vaginal candidiasis include oral contraceptive use, intrauterine device (IUD) use, young age at first intercourse, increased frequency of intercourse, diabetes, human immunodeficiency virus (HIV) or other immunocompromised states, chronic antibiotic use, and pregnancy. Symptoms include pruritus (most common symptom); thick, odorless, white vaginal discharge (an appearance similar to cottage cheese, Figure 43-1); vulvar burning; dyspareunia; and vulvar dysuria. Erythema and swelling of the labia may be present with the vaginal discharge adhering to the walls of the vagina. Diagnosis is made microscopically by examining a wet mount sample of vaginal secretions for yeast buds and pseudohyphae. Treatment options include a 1-day treatment with oral fluconazole or the use of intravaginal azole preparations (fungistatic agents) with regimens ranging from 1 to 7 days.

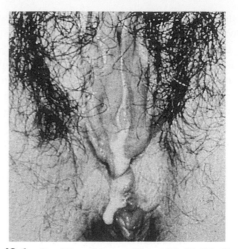

FIGURE **43-1.** *Candida albicans.* (From Zitelli BJ, Davis HW: *Atlas of pediatric physical diagnosis,* ed 4, St. Louis, 2002, Mosby.)

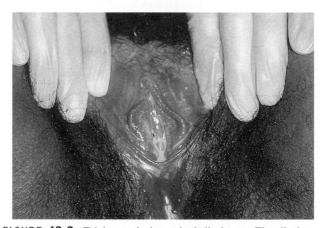

FIGURE **43-2.** Trichomoniasis vaginal discharge. The discharge is profuse and watery and appears purulent. (From Monahan FD, Neighbors M: *Medical-surgical nursing: foundations for clinical practice,* ed 2, Philadelphia, 1998, WB Saunders.)

Trichomoniasis

Trichomoniasis infection is caused by the protozoan *Trichomonas vaginalis*. Trichomoniasis is almost always an STI and is the most common nonviral STI in the world. It is estimated that 2 to 3 million American women contract the disease annually.[13] There is a high incidence of coinfection with gonorrhea in women with *T. vaginalis* infection. Risk factors include multiple sexual partners and increased frequency of sexual activity. Infection can range from an asymptomatic carrier state to severe, acute inflammatory disease. Symptoms commonly include a malodorous, copious frothy discharge (Figure 43-2) that is white to greenish-yellow; vulvovaginal soreness, fullness, and irritation; pruritus; dysuria; and dyspareunia. Gynecologic examination may reveal erythema of the cervix and upper portion of the vagina (strawberry cervix). Diagnosis is made microscopically through the examination of a wet mount sample for the presence of trichomonads. Diagnostic accuracy may be improved with a culture. The most effective treatment is metronidazole

(Flagyl) either in a single dose or a 7-day course. The single-dose treatment is preferable because of the lower cost, fewer side effects, and greater patient compliance.[4]

Pelvic Inflammatory Disease

Pelvic inflammatory disease is a term used to describe infection of the upper reproductive tract, including the endometrium, fallopian tubes, ovaries, pelvic peritoneum, and/or the pelvic connective tissue. PID may be acute, subacute, or chronic. The two most common organisms causing PID are *Neisseria gonorrhoeae* and *Chlamydia trachomatis,* which frequently coexist. Other aerobic and anaerobic organisms may also cause PID. Most cases of PID originate from STIs of the lower genital tract followed by an ascending infection to the upper tract. Another cause of PID is introduction of microorganisms through instrumentation such as endometrial biopsy, curettage, and hysteroscopy. Factors that facilitate the ascending migration of microorganisms include menses-related loss of the cervical barrier and hormonal changes reducing the bacteriostatic properties of the cervical mucus.[1] Risk factors for PID include multiple sexual partners, increased frequency of sexual activity, IUD use, history of other STIs, substance abuse, and frequent vaginal douching.

The most common symptom of PID is lower abdominal or pelvic pain that increases with movement—to limit this pain with walking, patients with PID characteristically shuffle (the "PID shuffle"). Other symptoms include abnormal vaginal discharge, vaginal bleeding, postcoital bleeding, dyspareunia, fever, malaise, nausea, and vomiting. Gynecologic examination usually reveals lower abdominal tenderness, mucopurulent cervicitis, cervical motion tenderness, and bilateral adnexal tenderness. Laboratory evaluation should include a pregnancy test, urinalysis, CBC, C-reactive protein and/or sedimentation rate, wet mount sample, and cervical culture and Gram stain. DNA probes for gonorrhea and chlamydial infection should also be included. An elevated white blood cell count and sedimentation rate and/or C-reactive protein support the diagnosis of PID. Imaging studies may include a pelvic sonogram, abdominal/pelvic CT scan, and/or MRI. Laparoscopy may also be performed for definitive diagnosis. Box 43-4 outlines the CDC diagnostic criteria for PID.

Complications of PID can include tuboovarian abscess, chronic pelvic pain, dyspareunia, infertility, and tubal adhesions and scarring, which increase the risk for ectopic pregnancy. The patient may also develop perihepatic inflammation, including right upper quadrant or pleuritic pain (Fitz-High-Curtis syndrome). The goals of treatment are to control pain, eliminate the acute infection, and prevent complications. Effective analgesia should be provided. Early initiation of empiric, broad-spectrum antibiotic therapy either on an outpatient or inpatient basis is critical to cover likely pathogens. Parenteral and oral therapy appear to have similar efficacy in achieving successful clinical outcomes in patients with mild to moderate PID. Refer to Box 43-5 for recommended treatment of PID. Hospital admission is suggested

---

Box 43-4 CDC CRITERIA FOR IDENTIFICATION OF PELVIC INFLAMMATORY DISEASE

Cervical motion tenderness OR uterine tenderness OR adnexal tenderness
Oral temperature >101° F (>38.3° C)
Abnormal cervical or vaginal mucopurulent discharge
Presence of abundant numbers of WBC on saline microscopy of vaginal secretions
Elevated erythrocyte sedimentation rate
Elevated C-reactive protein
Laboratory documentation of cervical infection with *Neisseria gonorrhoeae* or *Chlamydia trachomatis*

From Centers for Disease Control and Prevention: 2006 Guidelines for treatment of sexually transmitted disease, *MMWR* 55(RR-51):1, 2006.
CDC, Centers for Disease Control and Prevention; *WBC,* white blood cell.

Box 43-5 ANTIBIOTIC THERAPY FOR PELVIC INFLAMMATORY DISEASE

OUTPATIENT ANTIBIOTIC THERAPY

One of the following regimens is recommended.
Ceftriaxone 250 mg IM × 1 injection
  PLUS
Doxycycline 100 mg orally twice a day for 14 days
  WITH OR WITHOUT
Metronidazole 500 mg orally twice a day for 14 days
  OR
Cefoxitin 2 g IM and probenecid 1 g orally administered concurrently in a single dose
  PLUS
Doxycycline 100 mg orally twice a day for 14 days
  WITH OR WITHOUT
Metronidazole 500 mg orally twice a day for 14 days
  OR
Other parenteral third-generation cephalosporin
  PLUS
Doxycyclinc 100 mg orally twice a day for 14 days
  WITH OR WITHOUT
Metronidazole 500 mg orally twice a day for 14 days

INPATIENT ANTIBIOTIC THERAPY

Cefoxitin 2 g IV every 6 hours
  PLUS
Doxycycline 100 mg orally or IV every 12 hours

From Centers for Disease Control and Prevention: 2006 Guidelines for treatment of sexually transmitted disease, *MMWR* 55(RR-51):1, 2006.
IM, Intramuscular; *IV,* intravenous.

---

for patients who meet any of the following criteria: (1) surgical emergencies (appendicitis) cannot be excluded; (2) the patient is pregnant; (3) the patient does not respond clinically to oral antimicrobial therapy; (4) the patient is unable to follow or tolerate an outpatient oral regimen; (5) the patient

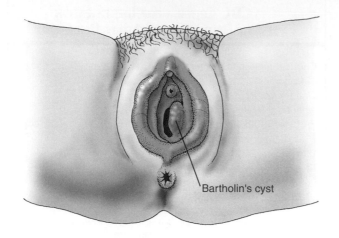

FIGURE **43-3.** Bartholin's cyst. (From Ignatavicius DD, Workman, ML, Mishler MA: *Medical-surgical nursing across the healthcare continuum,* ed 3, Philadelphia, 1999, WB Saunders.)

has severe illness, nausea and vomiting, or high fever; or (6) the patient has a tuboovarian abscess.[4]

Tuboovarian Abscess

A tuboovarian abscess (TOA) is a complication of PID and salpingitis with bacterial invasion into the disrupted capsule of the ovary. If the TOA ruptures, bacteria spills into the peritoneal space, which may lead to bacteremia and septic shock.[11] The patient with a TOA is ill appearing and presents with acute, severe pelvic pain. Associated symptoms include fever (which may be as high as 104° F [40°C]), nausea, vomiting, purulent vaginal discharge, and vaginal bleeding. Diagnostic studies include a pregnancy test, CBC, urinalysis, C-reactive protein, cervical culture, and Gram stain. DNA probes for gonorrhea and chlamydial infection should also be included. Imaging studies include pelvic ultrasonography, CT scan, or MRI. Treatment includes hospital admission, pain control, IV antibiotics, and surgical intervention for incision and drainage. Complications from TOA include chronic pelvic pain, pelvic adhesions, tubal factor infertility, and ectopic pregnancy.

Bartholin's Gland Abscess

The Bartholin's glands are located within the vestibule at the 5 and 7 o'clock positions. The glands secrete a clear viscous fluid that lubricates the vaginal vestibule. Under normal circumstances the glands cannot be palpated or visualized. Occasionally a Bartholin's gland forms a cyst or an abscess (Figure 43-3). A cyst develops when the duct of the gland becomes distended and gets occluded. A cyst is characterized by a small, painless lump. In the absence of infection, warm sitz baths are usually the only treatment required. An abscess is a primary infection of the gland with bacteria. Infection is generally the result of vaginal and fecal organisms (*Escherichia coli, G. vaginalis,* and other anaerobic bacteria);

however, STIs such as *N. gonorrhoeae* and *C. trachomatis* have also been cultured. The patient with an abscess complains of a progressive increase in unilateral pain, swelling, and redness of the labia. On physical examination there will be a labial mass that is erythematous, tender, and fluctuant on palpation. Treatment of a Bartholin's gland abscess is incision and drainage with placement of a Word catheter; a wound culture should be obtained. The Word catheter should remain in place for several weeks to prevent abscess recurrence. The patient should be advised to avoid sexual intercourse until the catheter has been removed. Other discharge instructions include sitz baths, pain control with NSAIDs or short-term narcotics, and gynecologic follow-up.[3]

Sexually Transmitted Infections

STIs are frequently encountered in the ED because the ED is used as initial entry into the health care system. The primary STIs include gonorrhea, chlamydial infection, trichomoniasis, syphilis, bacterial vaginosis, genital warts, genital herpes, hepatitis, and HIV infection. (See Chapter 38 for discussion of hepatitis and HIV.) The CDC estimates that 19 million new infections occur each year, almost half of them among young people ages 15 to 24.[4] STIs are associated with significant physiologic and psychologic morbidity. Complications associated with STIs include vaginitis, cervicitis, PID, infertility, urethritis, epididymitis, pharyngitis, proctitis, skin and mucous membrane lesions, and acquired immunodeficiency syndrome (AIDS) associated with the HIV virus (Table 43-1). Early diagnosis and treatment is critical in the prevention of the sequelae associated with STIs. Overall, prevention of STIs is possible; therefore primary prevention through health counseling should be a goal for all emergency care providers.

Genital Herpes

Genital herpes is most often caused by herpes simplex virus type 2 (HSV-2). However, it is estimated that 10% to 50% of infections are due to herpes simplex virus type 1 (HSV-1).[13] The virus is transmitted through microabrasions on mucosal surfaces during oral, vaginal, or rectal intercourse with an infected person. There may also be perinatal transmission of the herpes virus. Once the virus initially infects the mucosal surface, it enters the neurons, where it migrates to the ganglia. Viral replication occurs in the ganglia. Virus latency may be maintained in the ganglia, where it can undergo periods of reactivation and replication.

It is estimated that up to 1 million new cases occur each year with up to 50% of cases being asymptomatic. The incubation period for a primary infection is 2 to 12 days (average 4 days). If symptoms of the primary infection do develop, they are manifested by multiple, painful grouped vesicles or ulcerative and crusted external lesions on an erythematous base on the genitalia, buttocks, and/or thighs. The most common sites in females include the vulva and cervix and in males, the prepuce and glans penis (Figure 43-4). Systemic symptoms are common in primary infection

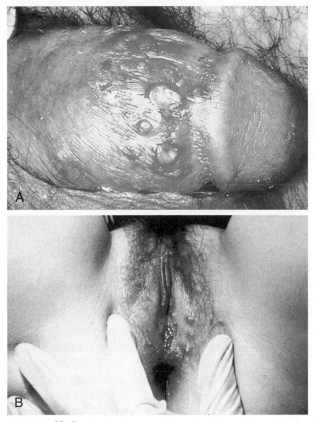

FIGURE 43-4. Genital herpes in a male (**A**) and in a female (**B**). (From Lewis SM, Collier IC, Heitkemper MM: *Medical-surgical nursing: assessment and management of clinical problems*, ed 4, St. Louis, 1996, Mosby.)

and include fever, malaise, headache, myalgias, regional lymphadenopathy, and dysuria. Females may also develop urinary retention secondary to severe dysuria. The primary illness lasts 10 to 20 days. It is estimated that 50% to 80% of patients will experience recurrent or reactivation eruptions 5 to 8 times per year because the virus remains latent.[9] These recurrent eruptions are not as severe as the primary infection, and systemic symptoms usually do not develop.

Definitive diagnosis of genital herpes is through viral culture. Treatment of this chronic illness is palliative and includes the use of antiviral therapy such as acyclovir, famciclovir, or valacyclovir. These drugs are reported to reduce both the severity and duration of symptoms in primary cases and may reduce recurrence. Once-daily suppressive therapy reduces the frequency of genital herpes recurrences in up to 80% of patients who have frequent recurrence (up to six per year). Analgesics and sitz baths may also be used to reduce pain. Recurrences often occur during times of stress; therefore rest, a balanced diet, and stress reduction are part of the treatment regimen. All patients should be counseled regarding the transmission of the virus. Sexual activity should be avoided during the 24-hour prodromal period and for the duration of the outbreak until the time at which all lesions are dry.

Table 43-1.	COMPLICATIONS CAUSED BY SEXUALLY TRANSMITTED ORGANISMS
Complication	**Causative Organisms**
Salpingitis, infertility, and ectopic pregnancy	*Neisseria gonorrhoeae* *Chlamydia trachomatis* *Mycoplasma hominis* *Ureaplasma urealyticum*
Reproductive loss (abortion/miscarriage)	*Neisseria gonorrhoeae* *Chlamydia trachomatis* Herpes simplex virus *Mycoplasma hominis* *Ureaplasma urealyticum* *Treponema pallidum*
Puerperal infection	*Neisseria gonorrhoeae* *Chlamydia trachomatis*
Perinatal infection	Hepatitis B virus Human immunodeficiency virus Human papillomavirus *Neisseria gonorrhoeae* *Chlamydia trachomatis* Herpes simplex virus *Treponema pallidum* Cytomegalovirus Group B streptococcus
Cancer of genital area	*Chlamydia trachomatis* Herpes simplex virus Human papillomavirus
Male urethritis	*Mycoplasma hominis* Herpes simplex virus *Neisseria gonorrhoeae* *Chlamydia trachomatis* *Ureaplasma urealyticum*
Vulvovaginitis	Herpes simplex virus *Trichomonas vaginalis* Bacteria causing vaginosis *Candida albicans*
Cervicitis	*Neisseria gonorrhoeae* *Chlamydia trachomatis* Herpes simplex virus
Proctitis	*Neisseria gonorrhoeae* *Chlamydia trachomatis* Herpes simplex virus *Campylobacter jejuni* *Shigella* species *Entamoeba histolytica*
Hepatitis	*Treponema pallidum* Hepatitis A, B, and C virus
Dermatitis	*Sarcoptes scabiei* *Phthirus pubis*
Genital ulceration or warts	*Chlamydia trachomatis* Herpes simplex virus Human papillomavirus *Treponema pallidum* *Haemophilus ducreyi* *Calymmatobacterium granulomatis*

From Ignatavicius DD, Workman ML: *Medical-surgical nursing: critical thinking for collaborative care*, ed 5, Philadelphia, 2006, WB Saunders.

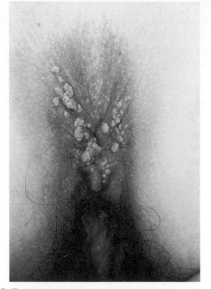

FIGURE **43-5.** Genital warts (condylomata acuminata). (From Black JM, Hawks JH: *Medical-surgical nursing: clinical management for positive outcomes,* ed 8, Philadelphia, 2009, WB Saunders.)

Genital Warts

Human papillomavirus (HPV) is the etiologic agent responsible for the development of genital warts (condylomata acuminata). Genital warts are considered to be the most common cause of STIs in the world. It is estimated that more than 24 million Americans are infected with HPV, and 50% of sexually active men and women will acquire HPV at some point in their lives. More than 100 strains of HPV have been isolated thus far, and more than 30 of the viruses are transmitted sexually. Many of these viruses have been associated with an increased neoplastic risk in both men and women; squamous cell cervical cancer is firmly linked to HPV.

The HPV virus invades the epidermal layer, penetrating skin and mucosal microabrasions in the genital and perineal area of males and females. A latency period of months to years may follow the initial virus transmission. Following the latency period, host cells become infected and genital warts develop. Warts are typically single or multiple papular eruptions of varying shapes, such as cauliflower or plaque-like. The color may vary from that of the skin to erythema or hyperpigmentation. The sites where warts are most commonly found include the vulva, perineum, cervix, penis, and perianal areas (Figure 43-5). Lesions may also be found in the mouth, pharynx, and larynx. The diagnosis of genital warts is established by appearance of the lesions without biopsy. The patient should be tested for other STIs.

There is no evidence that treatment of genital warts will eradicate the virus or reduce the risk for neoplasm. If left untreated, visible genital warts can undergo spontaneous resolution, increase in size and number, or remain unchanged. The goal of treatment is removal of symptomatic warts to induce wart-free periods. Treatment can be accomplished through cryotherapy, electrodessication, curettage, surgical excision, or carbon dioxide laser therapy. The patient may also use home medications such as imiquimod cream, podofilox gel or solution, or antiproliferative compounds. In June of 2006, Gardasil, a vaccine licensed by the Food and Drug Administration (FDA) to prevent cervical cancer and other diseases caused by HPV in females, was released. This vaccine is recommended to be administered to 11- to 12-year-old girls; it may be given in patients as young as 9 years. The vaccine is also recommended for 13- to 26-year-old females who have not yet received or completed the vaccine series. Gardasil is administered in three separate doses; the initial dose is followed by a second and third dose at 2 and 6 months after the first dose, respectively.[2,4] Emergency care providers are in an excellent position to educate patients regarding the importance of this vaccine.

Chancroid

The causative agent for chancroid is *Haemophilus ducreyi*, a gram-negative rod. It is a highly contagious disease that is most commonly found in third-world and developing countries. However, the incidence and prevalence in the United States is increasing. Coinfection with herpes or syphilis is found in 10% of patients with chancroid. An incubation period of 2 to 10 days is followed by the development of a papule or pustule that develops into a painful, shallow ulcer surrounded by an erythematous ring. The borders of the lesions are irregular, with a purulent exudate covering the base. Multiple lesions are common and may coalesce into a large ulceration. The lesions are most commonly found on the fourchette, the vestibule, the clitoris, and the labia. There may be associated dyspareunia, vaginal discharge, fever, or weakness. Painful inguinal lymphadenopathy, referred to as buboes, is found in up to 50% of patients.[7] Lymphadenopathy occurs within 1 to 2 weeks after the ulcer formation.

Cultures are insensitive and unreliable to confirm the diagnosis of chancroid. The World Health Organization (WHO) and the CDC suggest that a positive diagnosis be made if the patient has one or more painful ulcers without evidence of syphilis or HSV.[8] Serologic testing for syphilis, HIV, and other STIs should be performed with a retest in 3 months if the initial tests are negative. Chancroid is one of the STIs that may be associated with an increased risk for transmission of HIV. Treatment is with antibiotics: azithromycin 1 g by mouth (PO) in a single dose, ceftriaxone 250 mg intramuscular (IM), erythromycin 500 mg PO 4 times a day for 7 days, or ciprofloxacin 500 mg PO twice a day for 3 days. All patients should be counseled regarding safe sex practices and cautioned not to engage in sexual activity until the ulcers are healed.[8]

Syphilis

Syphilis is caused by the spirochete *Treponema pallidum*. The disease is almost always transmitted through direct contact with an infected lesion; however, perinatal and transfusion-related transmissions have occurred. The incidence of syphilis in the United States has increased, particularly among men who have sex with men. The spirochete penetrates abraded skin or intact mucous membranes easily and disseminates rapidly. There are numerous presentations of syphilis that can mimic several other infections; thus it is referred to as "the great imposter."

Syphilis is characterized by episodes of active disease and periods of latent infection. The disease occurs in three distinct phases: primary, secondary, and tertiary (latent). Primary syphilis is manifested by a single, painless genital ulcer, referred to as a chancre, which develops approximately 10 to 90 days after exposure. There is associated nontender inguinal adenopathy. The secondary phase of syphilis occurs 6 to 20 weeks after exposure. Secondary syphilis is manifested by a dull symmetric rash involving the palms and soles of the feet, fever and chills, lethargy, lymphadenopathy, patchy alopecia, loss of the lateral third of the eyebrow, and other nonspecific findings such as malaise, sore throat, and headache. The tertiary (latent) phase of syphilis develops years after the initial exposure and is manifested by neurologic findings, including meningitis, general paresis, progressive dementia, neuropathy, and tremulous extremities. Urinary incontinence may also occur. Cardiovascular complications of tertiary syphilis include aortic insufficiency and thoracic aneurysm. Figures 43-6 and 43-7 depict the clinical appearance of primary and secondary syphilis.

Early identification and antibiotic therapy are the keys to eradicating syphilis and the devastating complications associated with advanced disease. *T. pallidum* is too small to be visualized under a light microscope and cannot be cultivated in vivo; therefore diagnosis is made through serologic testing. The Venereal Disease Research Laboratories (VDRL) test and the rapid plasma reagent (RPR) test are the screening tests most commonly used. Confirmatory tests include the specific treponemal antibody tests, which are more specific. Refer to Table 43-2 for recommendations regarding the treatment of syphilis.

Chlamydia

Chlamydial genital infection is the most frequently reported STI in the United States. The causative organism is *C. trachomatis*. The prevalence is highest among persons 25 years of age or less, and within this young adult population 15- to 19-year-old adolescents are most frequently affected. An estimated 2.8 million Americans are infected with chlamydial infection each year.[4] Asymptomatic infection is common in both men and women, and therefore underreporting of this STI is substantial. Annual screening of all sexually active women age 25 years or younger is recommended, as is screening of older women who are at risk for contracting chlamydial infection. Risk factors include those who have a new sex partner or multiple sexual partners.

Chlamydial infection can be transmitted during vaginal, oral, or anal sexual contact with an infected person. In females the sequelae associated with chlamydial infection include cervicitis (most common), urethritis, bartholinitis, PID, and infertility. In males the complications that can result include epididymitis, prostatitis, and Reiter syndrome (arthritis, urethritis, and conjunctivitis). Chlamydial infection

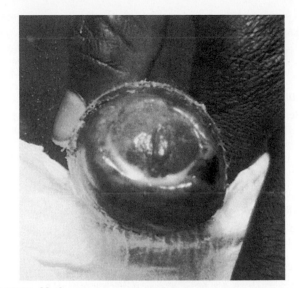

FIGURE **43-6.** Primary syphilis in the male. (From Greenberger NJ, Hinthorn DR: *History taking and physical examination: essentials and clinical correlates,* St. Louis, 1993, Mosby.)

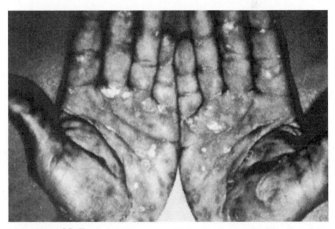

FIGURE **43-7.** Secondary syphilis. (From Goldstein BG, Goldstein AO: *Practical dermatology*, ed 2, St. Louis, 1997, Mosby.)

can also cause lymphogranuloma venereum, an uncommon STI that is characterized by unilateral, painful lymphadenitis. Chlamydial infection can also be transmitted to neonates passing through an infected birth canal with resulting conjunctivitis and/or neonatal pneumonia. Approximately 70% of women will be asymptomatic or have minimal symptoms such as dysuria, mild abdominal pain, or a vaginal discharge. Infected males may experience dysuria, urethral itching, and a thin mucopurulent discharge, although 50% of men are asymptomatic.

Diagnosis of chlamydial infection can be done through urine tests or vaginal/urethral swabs. Urine polymerase chain reaction (PCR), direct fluorescent antibody (DFA), nucleic acid amplification, and enzyme-linked immunoassay may all be used depending on the clinical site and test availability. The recommended treatment regimen for chlamydial infection is azithromycin 1 g in a single dose or doxycycline 100 mg PO twice a day for 7 days. Treatment regimens should be

Table 43-2. TREATMENT OF SYPHILIS

Primary, Secondary, or Early Latent	Late Latent, Unknown Duration, Tertiary (Excluding Neurosyphilis)	Neurosyphilis
ADULTS		
Benzathine penicillin G 2.4 million units IM in a single dose; or (in penicillin-allergic, nonpregnant patients) doxycycline 100 mg BID PO × 14 days; or tetracycline 500 mg QID PO × 14 days	Benzathine penicillin G 2.4 million units IM weekly × 3 weeks; or (in penicillin-allergic, nonpregnant patients) doxycycline 100 mg PO × 30 days; or tetracycline 500 mg QID PO × 30 days	Aqueous crystalline penicillin G 18-24 million units/day IV in 6 divided doses × 10-14 days; or procaine penicillin 600,000 units IM q day × 10-15 days and probenecid 500 mg PO QID × 10-14 days
CHILDREN		
Benzathine penicillin G 50,000 units/kg IM in a single dose up to 2.4 million units	Benzathine penicillin G 50,000 units/kg IM weekly up to 2.4 million units per dose × 3 weeks	Aqueous crystalline penicillin G 50,000 units/kg IV q 4-6 hr × 10-14 days

From Rosen P, Barkin RM, Hockberger RS et al: *Emergency medicine concepts and clinical practice,* ed 4, St. Louis, 1998, Mosby.
BID, Twice a day; *IM,* intramuscular; *IV,* intravenous; *PO,* by mouth; *QID,* four times a day.

effective against both *C. trachomatis* and *N. gonorrhoeae* because of the high frequency of concomitant infection.

Gonorrhea

Gonorrhea is the second most common STI in the United States. The causative organism is *N. gonorrhoeae,* a gram-negative diplococcus. In the United States an estimated 600,000 new cases occur each year. The greatest incidence of gonorrhea is found in the 15- to 19-year-old age-group, particularly among females.[4]

The organism causes infection at the site of acquisition and commonly results in mucopurulent cervicitis and urethritis. Three patterns of disease have been identified in females with gonorrhea: (1) asymptomatic carrier, (2) cervicitis, and (3) PID. Between 30% and 40% of females are asymptomatic. Gonococcal infection may involve the periurethral Skene's glands, labial Bartholin's glands, rectum, pharynx, and conjunctiva. Men are almost always symptomatic. In males the infection may involve the urethra, epididymis, and prostate gland. The infection may disseminate via the hematogenous route and lead to involvement of the joints, skin, meninges, and endocardium. Fever, chills, and a rash characterize disseminated gonococcal infections. Perinatal transmission may result in neonatal meningitis, sepsis, and ophthalmia neonatorum.

Diagnostic testing for *N. gonorrhea* can be done using endocervical, vaginal, male urethral, or urine specimens. Culture, nucleic acid hybridization tests, and nucleic acid amplification are available for diagnosis of gonorrhea. Patients infected with gonorrhea are frequently coinfected with *C. trachomatis;* therefore it is recommended that patients should be treated concurrently for chlamydial infection.

In many geographic areas and populations there has been an increasing resistance to quinolones for the treatment of gonorrhea. Quinolone-resistance has developed in parts of Europe, the Middle East, Asia, and the Pacific. In the United States quinolone resistance is becoming increasingly common. This has led to changes in the recommended treatment regimens. The current CDC recommendation for treatment of uncomplicated gonococcal infections of the cervix, urethra, and rectum is to administer ceftriaxone 125 mg IM or cefixime 400 mg PO in a single dose.[5]

SUMMARY

The patient with a gynecologic emergency presents challenging opportunities to the ED nurse. This patient population may have complex physiologic and psychosocial needs, particularly because a large proportion of this population are adolescents and young adults. In addition to meeting the physical needs of a patient, the ED nurse is afforded a great opportunity for patient teaching and counseling.

REFERENCES

1. Abel K, Aronson A: Ovarian cysts, last updated June 18, 2007, *eMedicine.* Retrieved April 24, 2008, from http://www.emedicine.com/emerg/topic352.htm.
2. Berman N: Preventing cervical cancer, *Adv Nurse Pract* 15(4):75, 2007.
3. Blumstein H: Bartholin gland disease, last updated May 24, 2005. *eMedicine.* Retrieved April 24, 2008, from http://www.emedicine.com/emerg/topic 54.htm.
4. Centers for Disease Control and Prevention: HPV vaccine questions and answers, 2006. Retrieved April 24, 2008, from http://www.cdc.gov/std/hpv/std act-HVP-vaccine.htm.
5. Centers for Disease Control and Prevention: Sexually transmitted disease treatment guidelines, *MMWR Morb Mortal Wkly Rep* 55(RR-11):1, 2006.
6. Centers for Disease Control and Prevention: Updated recommended treatment regimens for gonococcal infections and associated conditions—United States, April 2007, last updated June 5, 2007. Retrieved April 24, 2008, from http://www.cdc.gov/std/Treatment/2006/updated-regimens.htm.

7. Curran D, Gonzalez L, Suares T et al: Benign lesions of the ovaries, last updated August 19, 2007, *eMedicine*. Retrieved April 24, 2008, from http://www.emedicine.com/med/topic2358.htm.

8. Emans S, Laufer M, Goldstein D: *Pediatric and adolescent gynecology*, ed 5, Baltimore, 2004, Lippincott Williams & Wilkins.

9. Emergency Nurses Association: *Emergency nursing core curriculum*, ed 6, St. Louis, 2007, Saunders.

10. Gor H, Ching S, Nguyen P: Vaginitis, last updated August 21, 2006, *eMedicine*. Retrieved April 24, 2008, from http://www.emedicine.com/med/topic2358.htm.

11. Kliegman R, Marcdante K, Jenson H et al: *Nelson essentials of pediatrics*, ed 5, Philadelphia, 2006, Elsevier.

12. Mehta N, Silverberg M: Chancroid, last updated September 20, 2007, *eMedicine*. Retrieved April 24, 2008, from http://www.emedicine.com/emed/topic 95.htm.

13. Miller K, Ruiz D, Graves J: Update on the prevention and treatment of sexually transmitted diseases, *Am Fam Physician* 67(9):1915, 2003.

14. Owen M, Clenney T: Management of vaginitis, *Am Fam Physician* 70(11):2125, 2004.

15. Rosen P, Barkin R, Hayden S et al: *The 5 minute emergency medicine consult*, Philadelphia, 1999, Lippincott Williams & Wilkins.

16. Shepherd S, Gracia C, Meiner E et al: Salpingitis, last updated August 16, 2007, *eMedicine*. Retrieved April 24, 2008, from http://www.emedicine.com/med/topic2059.htm.

17. Tintinalli J, Kelen G, Stapczynski J: *Emergency medicine: a comprehensive study guide*, ed 6, New York, 2004, McGraw-Hill.

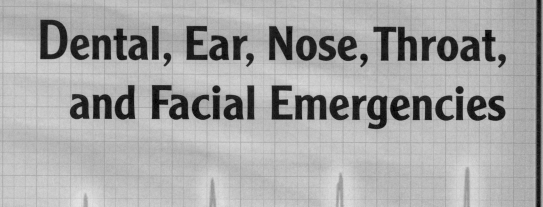

CHAPTER 44

Dental, Ear, Nose, Throat, and Facial Emergencies

Elizabeth Gaudet Nolan

Most emergencies of the face, mouth, ears, nose, and throat involve discomfort and pain. However, certain conditions can become life threatening if associated edema compromises the airway. Infectious processes in the mouth and face can spread to the brain, with potentially fatal systemic effects. Other concerns include loss of function and possible cosmetic deformities. This chapter describes conditions of the face, mouth, ears, nose, and throat that are frequently seen in the emergency department (ED). A brief review of anatomy is provided. Refer to Chapter 8 for a summary of patient assessment parameters for head, ears, eyes, nose, and throat.

ANATOMY

Structures of the mouth, nose, ears, throat, and face are intimately connected. Injury to one area can affect the others, just as infection from one site can spread to adjacent areas.

Mouth

Dentition consists of two main structures: the teeth and periodontium. Teeth comprise pulp, dentin, enamel, and root (Figure 44-1). The pulp, located at the center of the tooth, provides neurovascular supply and produces dentin. Dentin is a microtubular structure that overlays the pulp, provides hydration, and cushions teeth during mastication. Enamel,

which covers the crown, is the visible part of the tooth and the hardest substance in the body. The root anchors the tooth into alveolar tissue and bone. The periodontium is made up of gingiva and the attachment apparatus. Gingiva, or gums, is a mucous membrane with supporting fibrous tissue encircling the teeth and covering teeth not yet erupted. The attachment apparatus consists of the cementum, periodontal ligament, and alveolar bone.[1] In children, onset of primary and permanent teeth is important in determining management of injuries.[21] Normal primary dentition begins erupting at 6 months, with 20 teeth by age 3 years. Permanent dentition begins at 5 to 6 years with eruption of the first molar and is usually completed by age 16 to 18 for a total of 32 teeth.[1]

Ears

The ear is divided into three sections: external, middle, and inner ear (Figure 44-2). The external ear consists of the auricle (pinna), ear canal, and tympanic membrane (TM). The auricle is a cartilaginous appendage attached to each side of the head that collects and directs sound to sensory organs within the ear. The S-shaped ear canal is approximately 2.5 to 3.0 cm long in adults, terminating at the TM. Glands lining the canal secrete cerumen, a yellow, waxy material that lubricates and protects the ear.[8]

The TM, or eardrum, is a thin, translucent, pearly gray oval disk separating the external ear from the middle ear.

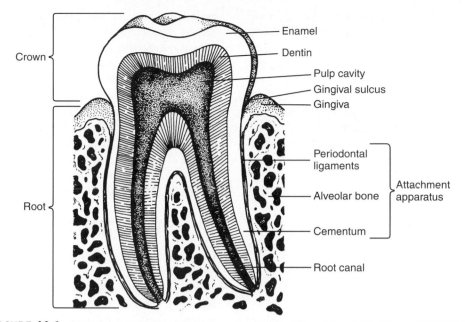

FIGURE 44-1. Dental anatomic unit and attachment apparatus. (From Marx J, Hockberger R, Walls R, editors: *Rosen's emergency medicine: concepts and clinical practice,* ed 6, St. Louis, 2006, Mosby.)

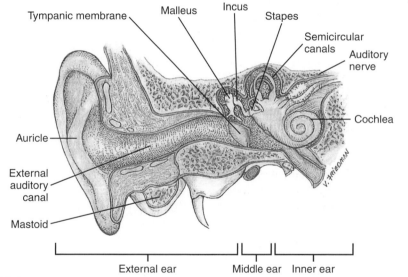

FIGURE 44-2. Ear structures. (From Potter PA, Perry AG: *Fundamentals of nursing,* ed 7, St. Louis, 2009, Mosby.)

It protects the middle ear and conducts sound vibrations to the ossicles.[3] On inspection with an otoscopic light, a cone of light at the anteroinferior aspect of the TM should normally be visible. Another landmark is the long process of the malleus (manubrium) pointing posterior and inferior and terminating in the center of the TM.

The middle ear, an air-filled cavity inside the temporal bone, consists of the ossicles, windows, and eustachian tube. Three tiny ear bones, or ossicles, are the malleus (hammer), incus (anvil), and stapes (stirrup), so named because of their appearance. Round and oval windows open into the inner ear, where sound vibrations enter. The eustachian tubes connect the middle ear with the nasopharynx, allowing passage of air to equalize pressure on either side of the TM.[11] They

also provide drainage for middle ear and inner ear secretions into the nasopharynx. The inner ear contains the bony labyrinth, which holds the sensory organs for equilibrium and hearing.[8]

Nose

Externally the nose is a triangular, mostly cartilaginous structure that warms, filters, and moistens inhaled air, provides a sense of smell, and is the primary passageway for inhaled air to the lungs. The upper third of the nose where the frontal and maxillary bones form the bridge is bony. Two nares at the base of the triangle allow air to enter and pass into the nasopharynx. The internal nose is formed by the palatine (hard palate) bones inferiorly and superiorly by the cribriform plate of the ethmoid bone. Branches of the olfactory nerve pass through the cribriform plate. The nasal cavity is separated by the septum, which forms two anterior vestibules. The septum is usually deviated slightly to one side. Lateral walls are formed by three parallel bony projections—the superior, middle, and inferior turbinates—that help increase surface area to warm inhaled air.[29]

Blood supply to the nose originates from the internal and external carotid arteries. The internal maxillary artery branch of the external carotid artery supplies the posterior nasal septum and lateral wall of the nose. As a branch of the internal carotid artery, the anterior ethmoidal artery supplies blood to the anterior septum at Kiesselbach's plexus in Little's area.[29] This area is also supplied by the septal branches on the sphenopalatine and superior labial arteries.

Throat

The throat, or pharynx, comprises the nasopharynx, oropharynx, and laryngopharynx. The nasopharynx is positioned behind the nasal cavities and extends to the plane of the soft palate. The pharyngeal tonsils, or adenoids, and eustachian tube openings are located in this area.[22] The oropharynx, a common passageway for both air and food, extends downward from the inferior soft palate to the level of the hyoid bone. The palatine tonsils, lymphoid tissue that filters microorganisms to protect the respiratory and gastrointestinal tracts, are found here. The laryngopharynx extends from the hyoid bone to the opening of the larynx anteriorly and esophagus, posteriorly.[24] The pharynx allows passage of air into the larynx. Pharyngeal constrictor muscles propel food or liquid into the esophagus. These muscles are also responsible for the cough and gag reflex, which are controlled by the cranial nerves. The larynx, or voice box, is a tubular, mostly cartilaginous structure that connects the trachea and pharynx; its main purpose is to allow air into the trachea. The epiglottis, a large, leaf-shaped piece of cartilage, lies on top of the larynx. This structure prevents aspiration by forming a lid over the glottis (the space between the vocal cords) so that liquids and food are routed into the esophagus and away from the trachea.[24] The larynx is also responsible for voice production via the vocal cords.

Face

The bony structures of the face are symmetric and consist of a single vomer and mandible and the following pairs of bones: maxillae, palatine, zygomatic, lacrimal, nasal, and inferior nasal conchae. The facial skull forms the shape of the face and provides attachment for muscles that move the jaw and control facial expressions. Cranial nerves V (trigeminal) and VII (facial) are responsible for facial innervation and movement, respectively. The paranasal sinuses are sterile, air-filled pockets situated behind and around the nose, which lighten the weight of the skull, provide resonance for speech, and move secretions into the nasopharynx

via ciliated mucous membranes.[8] Four pairs of sinuses are named for their craniofacial location. In children younger than 6 years, the sinuses are not fully developed.[29] The ethmoidal and frontal sinuses are fairly well developed between 6 and 7 years and mature along with the maxillary and sphenoidal sinuses during adolescence.[8]

The temporomandibular joint (TMJ) is the point where the mandible connects to the temporal bone of the skull; it can be palpated bilaterally just anterior to the tragus of the ear. The TMJ is a synovial joint that allows hinge action to open and close the jaws, gliding action for protrusion and retraction, and gliding for side-to-side movement of the lower jaw.[8]

DENTAL EMERGENCIES

Dental emergencies affect the teeth and gums. Specific emergencies involve infection, eruption of new teeth, or trauma. The most common emergencies seen in the ED are related to pain. Common causes of dental pain include dry socket, fractured teeth, periodontal disease, erupting teeth, maxillary sinusitis, and post root canal surgery.

Odontalgia

Dental caries are the most frequent cause of dental pain or odontalgia (Figure 44-3).[1] Too much sugar in the diet is largely responsible for decay. Dental caries are also caused by poor oral hygiene, which allows bacterial plaque to develop, which in turn form acids that break down and decalcify tooth enamel. Sodium fluoride, found in toothpaste, oral rinses, and public drinking water, helps stabilize the integrity of tooth enamel to prevent this breakdown. Affected teeth are usually tender to percussion and sensitive to heat, cold, or air.[19] If left untreated, decay progresses and invades dentin and pulp, eventually producing a hyperemic response. The pulp becomes inflamed, leading to pulpitis and finally pulpal necrosis. Occasionally pus leaks from the apex of the affected tooth as a periapical abscess forms.[3] Toothaches accompanied by facial or neck swelling should be assessed and promptly treated to prevent spread of infection. Clinical management includes antibiotics, topical anesthetics, nerve

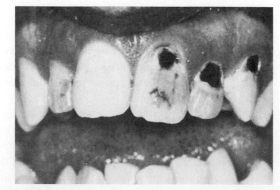

FIGURE **44-3.** Dental caries. (From Grundy JR, Jones JG: *A color atlas of clinical operative dentistry crowns and bridges,* ed 2, London, 1992, Wolfe Medical Publishing.)

blocks, and analgesics, including parenteral narcotics, as palliative treatment until the patient receives definitive care from the dentist.[2]

Tooth Eruption

Between 6 months and 3 years of age, children's primary teeth erupt, causing a variety of symptoms including pain, irritability, disrupted sleep, nasal discharge, and crying. Increased salivary gland production causes diarrhea, as well as significant drooling. Decreased fluid intake related to dental pain may cause dehydration and low-grade fever of 38.1° C (100.6° F). Care must be taken not to attribute significant fevers to this relatively benign process. Tonsillar or throat infections, thrush, other oral lesions, and respiratory emergencies such as epiglottitis (especially with excessive drooling) should be considered. In the second decade of life, third molars, or wisdom teeth, begin erupting, causing pain in adolescents and adults. Gingival inflammation secondary to wisdom tooth eruption may cause pericoronitis.

Topical anesthetics such as benzocaine are used sparingly to prevent sterile abscess formation. Acetaminophen is useful for analgesia in young children. To maintain hydration, Popsicles are usually well received and also provide pain relief. When there is minimal oral intake, a bolus of intravenous (IV) fluids may be necessary. In adults frequent saline irrigation may be used to remove debris from the affected tooth. Nonnarcotic analgesia is effective for pain relief in adult patients. Any consistent swelling or drainage from the eruption site requires referral to a dentist or oral surgeon.

Pericoronitis

If erupting molars become impacted or crowded, food and debris lodge under the pericoronal flap, causing gingival inflammation or pericoronitis. Pericoronitis is extremely painful, especially with opening and closing of the mouth. Earache on the affected side, sore throat, and fever may also occur.[2] Surrounding tissues appear red and inflamed with submandibular lymphadenopathy and trismus noted in some patients.

Warm saline or peroxide irrigation and mouth rinses are helpful in early stages of pericoronitis. When pus is present, incision and drainage may be necessary. Antibiotic therapy, usually penicillin or erythromycin, is indicated. Follow-up with an oral-maxillofacial surgeon within 24 to 48 hours for removal of the affected third molar is highly recommended.[1]

Fractured Tooth

The most frequently seen dental emergency in the ED is a chipped or broken tooth, usually anterior maxillary teeth. Trauma to dentition occurs as a result of sports activity, motor vehicle collisions, propulsive objects, falls, convulsive seizures, and physical assaults or abuse. With children, it should be noted that 50% of physical trauma in child abuse occurs in the head and neck region.[18] The emergency nurse should assess for concurrent head injury or maxillofacial trauma. Aspiration of a tooth or fragment or an embedded tooth should also be considered.

Management of fractures of the anterior teeth is determined by the relationship of the fracture to the pulp as well as patient age.[1] The Ellis classification system is used to describe location of tooth fractures. Class I fractures are the most common, involving only enamel. Injured areas appear chalky white. Cosmetic restoration is possible with dental referral within 24 to 48 hours. Class II fractures pass through the enamel and expose dentin. The fracture area appears ivory-yellow. Fractures are urgent for children because there is little dentin to protect pulp. Bacteria pass easily into pulp, causing an infection or abscess if exposed for longer than 6 hours.[21] Adults may be treated up to 24 hours later because the pulp is protected by a thicker layer of dentin, which reduces potential for infection. Place warm, moist cotton covered by dry gauze over the exposed area as needed for discomfort secondary to thermal sensitivity. Class III fractures are a dental emergency (Figure 44-4). Injury to the enamel, dentin, and pulp cause a pink or bloody tinge to the fractured area. Exposure of pulp also exposes the nerve, causing significant discomfort. Again, dry gauze can be used to minimize discomfort from thermal sensitivity. Some practitioners apply a layer of zinc oxide or calcium hydroxide to exposed dentin, which is then covered with dental foil.[17] The patient should be referred to a dentist with follow-up within 24 hours. Oral analgesics or a nerve block are usually effective for pain control. Tetanus immunizations should be administered as appropriate. Reassure the patient that cosmetic restoration is possible with enamel-bonding plastic materials.[2]

With facial trauma, assess the airway, breathing, and circulation (ABCs) before assessing the dental problem. History should include mechanism of injury, concomitant injuries, and tissue loss. Consider abuse in children, older adults, or disabled adults when the history does not correlate to the

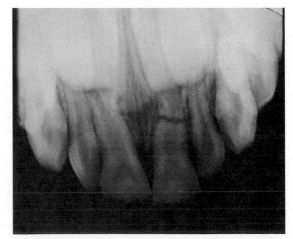

FIGURE **44-4.** This radiograph reveals a root fracture in the apical third of an upper primary incisor. This was suspected clinically because of tenderness and increased mobility. (From Zitelli B, Davis H: *Atlas of pediatric physical diagnosis,* ed 3, St. Louis, 1997, Mosby.)

injury. Assess for tooth pain, thermal sensitivity, stability of the tooth in the socket, and malocclusion. Complications of tooth fractures include infection (pulpitis), malocclusion, embedded tooth fragments, aspiration of tooth fragments, color change, or loss of affected teeth.

Tooth Avulsion

Tooth avulsion is a dental emergency. When a tooth has been torn from the socket, tissue hypoxia develops, followed by eventual necrosis of the pulp.[16] Reimplantation within 30 minutes greatly increases chances for reimplantation and healing. The periodontal ligament cells die if the tooth is out of the socket for more than 60 minutes. Determine the mechanism and time of injury immediately on arrival. Handle the avulsed tooth by the crown to avoid damage to attached periodontal ligament fragments. These fragments aid in healing of the reimplanted tooth.[21] Ideally the tooth should be rinsed and placed back in the socket as soon as possible. Immediate reimplantation is not always possible because of lack of patient cooperation, life-threatening injuries, or other factors at the scene of injury. In these cases the tooth should be transported in Hank's solution (pH-preserving fluid), milk, saline, or under the tongue of an alert patient. Use discretion with children, who may swallow or aspirate the tooth. Primary teeth (6 months to 6 years) are not reimplanted because fusion with the bone interferes with permanent tooth eruption and can cause cosmetic deformities.[1] If the tooth cannot be found, examine the oral cavity and face to ensure the tooth is not embedded in soft tissue. A chest x-ray examination is recommended to rule out tooth aspiration.

Symptoms include pain and bleeding at the site of the avulsion. Assess for concomitant head, neck, or maxillofacial injuries. Moist saline gauze may be applied to exposed oral tissues for comfort and to control bleeding. Administer analgesics and tetanus prophylaxis as indicated. Instruct the patient not to bite into anything with the affected tooth and to avoid hot or cold substances. Referral to a dentist or oral surgeon for definitive care is recommended.

Dental Abscess

Primary dental abscesses are periapical and periodontal. Periapical abscesses occur as an extension of pulpal necroses from a decayed tooth or traumatic injury. A pocket of plaque and food debris between the tooth and the gingiva causes localized swelling at the apex of the tooth, which leads to periodontal abscess formation.[18] Normally abscesses are confined; however, certain infectious processes can spread to facial planes of the head and neck.[1] The upper half of the face is affected with extension of infection from the maxillary teeth. Cellulitis in the lower half of the face and neck extends from the infection of the mandibular teeth.[1] With localized abscesses the patient may have severe pain unrelieved by analgesics, fever, malaise, foul breath odor, and slight facial swelling near the affected tooth. An extensive abscess causes facial and neck edema, trismus,

dysphagia, difficulty handling secretions, and potential airway obstruction.

Oral or parenteral narcotics, antipyretics, and antibiotics such as penicillin or erythromycin are recommended.[7] If abscess fluctuance is present, incision and drainage with culture and sensitivity of the exudate are required. The patient should be instructed to take medications as directed, use warm saline rinses, and follow up with an oral surgeon, dentist, or ear, nose, and throat (ENT) specialist within 24 to 48 hours for definitive care. Admission for further diagnostic studies and IV antibiotics may be necessary if the patient has abnormal vital signs or is unable to take oral medications.[18]

Gingivitis

Gingivitis, or inflammation of the gums, is usually caused by poor dental hygiene, allowing for the accumulation of food debris and plaque in crevices between the gums and teeth. This periodontal disease, along with periodontitis (loss of supporting bony structure of the teeth) affects approximately two thirds of young adults and 80% of middle-age and older adults. It is the most common cause of tooth loss today.[2] Gingivitis may also occur with vitamin C deficiency or in pregnancy and puberty because of changing hormone levels.[8] If inflammation continues, alveolar bone is lost, leading to periodontitis and eventual loss of teeth. Visual evidence of gingivitis includes red, swollen gum margins and possible bleeding. Pain unrelieved by over-the-counter analgesics, difficulty chewing, and low-grade fever also occur. Topical anesthetics, analgesics, and oral antibiotic therapy are indicated. Patient teaching regarding good oral hygiene, including brushing and flossing 3 to 4 times a day with peroxide and warm water rinses every hour, is extremely important to prevent extension of gingivitis.

Ludwig's Angina

Ludwig's angina is the spread of an existing, untreated dental infection or cellulitis into three mandibular spaces: submandibular, sublingual, and submental. Infection spreads downward from the jaw to the mediastinum and is characterized by bilateral, boardlike, brawny induration of involved tissues and elevation of the tongue. The inherent danger with Ludwig's angina is respiratory distress and airway obstruction.[18]

The patient develops significant swelling of the anterior and lateral neck. Swelling of the submandibular tissue displaces the tongue superiorly. Other symptoms include pain and tenderness, trismus, muffled voice, dysphagia, drooling, and fever or chills. Dyspnea and decreased oxygen pressure occur secondary to edematous tissues. The patient may be anxious or restless. Offer reassurance, check the patient frequently, and explain all procedures to ease fears.

Priorities in the ED include maintaining ABCs, pain relief, and IV antibiotics. Elevate the head of the bed to prevent aspiration of secretions. Administer supplemental oxygen in concert with continuous pulse oximetry monitoring.

Respiratory and mental status should be continuously monitored. Provide prescribed analgesics appropriate for the patient's degree of pain. Insert an IV catheter for IV fluids to prevent dehydration, to administer antibiotic therapy (usually high-dose penicillin), and as an access for emergency medications. Diagnostic procedures such as determination of arterial blood gas levels, complete blood count (CBC) with differential, erythrocyte sedimentation rate, culture and sensitivity of exudate, and soft tissue x-ray films, or computed tomography (CT) scan of the neck may be ordered.[18] Definitive care by an oral-maxillofacial surgeon includes determining site of the initial infection, surgical drainage of pus with removal of necrotic tissue, and continued antibiotic therapy.[1]

EAR EMERGENCIES

Ear emergencies commonly seen in the ED involve infection, pain, foreign body in the ear canal, or injury of the TM. Most ear emergencies require instillation of some type of otic drops (Figure 44-5).

Otitis

Otitis, or inflammation of the ear, may occur in any section of the ear. Symptoms vary with location; however, almost all cases of acute otitis cause significant discomfort.[18]

Otitis externa is inflammation of the external ear canal and auricle. Also known as swimmer's ear, this condition is seen most often during the summer. Factors that predispose the patient to otitis externa include swimming in contaminated water, exposure to chemical irritants, cleaning the ear canal with a foreign object, regular use of ear devices, and a perforated TM. The infectious agent is usually bacteria such as *Pseudomonas* species, *Proteus vulgaris,* streptococci, and *Staphylococcus aureus.* Symptoms include pain, swelling, redness, and purulent drainage of the auricle and ear canal (Figure 44-6). Pain is usually worsened by chewing or movement of the tragus or pinna. Regional cellulitis, partial

hearing loss, and lymphadenopathy may also be present. Basic treatment measures cure 90% of patients without complications.[27] Treatment includes keeping the ear dry; applying heat with a heating pad, heating lamp, or warm, moist compresses; and providing analgesics and antibiotics. Topical or otic antibiotics are used unless the patient has a persistent fever or regional cellulitis, in which case hospitalization and high-dose antibiotic therapy is needed.[27] Otitis externa usually resolves in 7 days but frequently recurs. Patients should be instructed to use earplugs for 2 to 4 weeks to protect the ear canal from water.

Otitis media (OM), or infection of the middle ear, occurs most often in children between 6 months and 3 years of age and is usually preceded by a viral upper respiratory infection (URI).[25] *Streptococcus pneumoniae* and *Haemophilus influenzae* are the most common causative organisms. Acute OM is characterized by rapid onset of ear pain, headache, tinnitus, hearing loss, and nausea or vomiting. Infants and young children may present with irritability, crying, rubbing or pulling the ears, restless sleep, and lethargy. Other symptoms such as fever, rhinitis, cough, otorrhea secondary to rupture of the TM, and conjunctivitis occur at any age.[25] Visualization of the TM, necessary for diagnosis, usually reveals a distorted light reflex and whitish-yellow opacity. Bulging may also occur as the infection progresses.[23] Redness of the TM is an inconsistent finding because it may be caused by crying or fever.[25] Sinusitis and purulent rhinitis frequently accompany otitis in children and infants.[28] Uncomplicated acute OM is treated with antibiotics, antipyretics, and analgesics such as acetaminophen or ibuprofen. Topical anesthetic otic solutions (e.g., Auralgan) for pain relief should be warmed before instilling. If not treated promptly, acute OM can cause serious complications such as ruptured TM, meningitis, acute mastoiditis, intracranial abscess, neck abscess, facial nerve damage, or permanent hearing loss.[25] Patients should complete the full course of antibiotic therapy and be reevaluated if there is no improvement in 48 to 72 hours.[27] Encourage parents to ensure children finish prescribed medications and to keep follow-up appointment. Children should be reevaluated

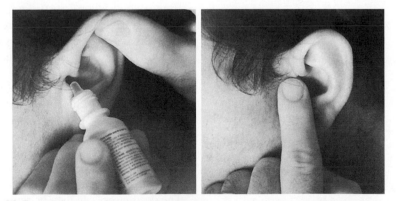

FIGURE **44-5.** Ear drop instillation. Turn the head to the side so that the affected ear faces upward. The orifice is exposed, and the drops of medicine are directed toward the internal wall of the canal. The pinna is pulled up and back in a person older than 3 years of age and down and back in a younger child. The tragus is then pushed against the ear canal to ensure that the drops stay in the canal. (From Potter PA, Perry AG: *Fundamentals of nursing,* ed 7, St. Louis, 2009, Mosby.)

in 14 to 21 days to confirm the infection has been eradicated or to determine if middle ear effusion (serous OM) persists. Chronic or persistent pediatric OM may require prophylactic antibiotics or referral to an otolaryngologist for myringotomy tube placement if intractable pain is present.

Labyrinthitis, or inflammation of the inner ear, is rare. Causes include acute febrile illness and chronic OM. The inner ear is the body's center of balance. The patient usually develops severe vertigo with nausea and vomiting, but without tinnitus and hearing loss. Vertigo usually lasts 3 to 5 days but may persist for weeks. Treatment includes bed rest, meclizine (Antivert) to control vertigo, and fluids for dehydration secondary to vomiting. Antibiotics are indicated for purulent labyrinthitis.

Ruptured Tympanic Membrane

A ruptured TM is most often the painful result of a bacterial infection—acute or chronic OM. Trauma such as skull fracture, foreign body insertion (e.g., cotton swabs, hairpins), explosions, or blows to the ear also rupture the TM. Children, especially those with chronic ear infections, are most often victims of this disorder. Symptoms include pain, bloody or purulent discharge, hearing loss, vertigo, and fever. Or the patient may be pain free because pain and pressure are relieved with rupture. In trauma-related TM rupture, ear drainage should be checked for the presence of cerebrospinal fluid, which is indicative of basilar skull fracture. Otoscopic examination reveals the TM as slit-shaped or irregular. X-ray examination of the skull, temporal bone, and cervical spine may be indicated with trauma. Hearing loss may be present in the affected ear, so speak slowly and clearly toward the unaffected ear while facing the patient. Large perforations require myringoplasty. If the middle ear is also involved, a tympanoplasty is performed.[3] More than 90% of perforations heal spontaneously.[23]

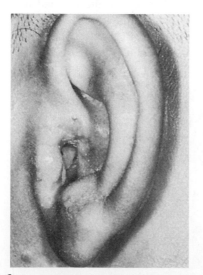

FIGURE **44-6.** Acute external otitis. Note swelling of the ear canal and lymphadenopathy in front of the tragus. (From Schuller D, Schleuning A, and II Schleuning J II, editors: *Deweese and Saunders' otolaryngology: head and neck surgery,* ed 8, St. Louis, 1994, Mosby.)

Management includes antibiotics, analgesics, and antipyretics. Carefully clean the ear canal of blood or debris with gentle suction, and obtain a culture and sensitivity of drainage. Irrigation is contraindicated with TM rupture. Instillation of antibiotic ear drops is generally not necessary.[23] The patient should be instructed to keep water out of the ears because this provides an environment conducive to bacterial or fungal growth. A piece of cotton lightly coated with petroleum jelly and placed in the affected ear helps repel water. The patient should follow up with an otolaryngologist for definitive care.

Foreign Body

Cerumen is the most common obstructive material seen in children's ears, often caused by cotton swabs pushing wax and cotton fibers deeper into the ear canal. Therefore remind parents to put "nothing smaller than an elbow into the ear." Cerumen is a yellow-brown, waxy material that obstructs view of the TM and must be removed. Adults, especially older patients, are also prone to impacted cerumen. In long-term care residents the estimated incidence of cerumen impaction is almost 40%. Use of hearing aids is a contributing factor because of increased cerumen production and obstruction of natural outflow from the ear.

The patient who presents with a foreign body in the ear is most often a child under 5 years of age. Beads, small stones, beans, corn, and dry cereal are common culprits. Parents, often unaware of the foreign body, bring the child to the ED with an earache or purulent, foul-smelling ear discharge. Older children and adults may complain of decreased hearing and fullness in the affected ear. Insects, including roaches, can fly or crawl into the ear and become trapped, moving and buzzing in the ear, causing great distress and anxiety for the patient. Children with insects in the ear may be extremely frightened.

Before attempting removal of impacted cerumen or a foreign body, evaluate for a history of ruptured TM or current infection. Explain the procedure to the patient in terms that are appropriate for his or her age. Cooperation is elicited from a child whose trust is not violated. Conscious sedation or restraints may be required in difficult situations.[23] Methods for foreign body removal include suctioning, irrigation, or use of special tools under direction visualization. A good light source such as an operating otoscope or head lamp is imperative for these procedures. To best expose the ear canal, pull the auricle up and back for adults, down and back for children. Vegetables or other soft materials that may absorb water should not be irrigated. Subsequent swelling caused by water absorption makes removal more difficult. Live insects can be killed by placing a few drops of mineral oil in the ear or by filling the ear canal with 2% lidocaine. The dead insect can then be removed with direct instrumentation.[12] If removal is difficult, referral to an ENT specialist within 24 hours is recommended.

Irrigation, often the safest and most effective method for removal of impacted cerumen, is contraindicated with a history of TM rupture, infection, a soft or vegetable-like foreign body, or in children younger than age 5. Any solutions for the ear should be warmed to 98.6° F (37° C) before instillation to prevent inner ear stimulation, which may cause dizziness, nausea, and vomiting. Suggested guidelines for ear irrigation are illustrated in Figure 44-7.

Other methods of foreign body removal include use of an ear curette, right-angle hook, Frazier suction catheter, soft flexible catheter with funnel-shaped tip, and alligator forceps. Surfactant ear drops (i.e., Cerumenex, glycerin and peroxide) may soften cerumen for easier removal. If an impacted foreign body cannot be removed, refer the patient to an ENT specialist within 24 hours. Emergent referral is necessary with severe pain or presence of a caustic foreign body substance. Antibiotics may be prescribed to prevent or treat an existing infection. Complications include hearing loss, TM rupture, and acute OM or otitis externa from injury during attempted foreign body removal or from retained foreign body material.

NASAL EMERGENCIES

Nasal emergencies involve infection, hemorrhage, or a foreign body. Most problems are minor such as infection or nasal fracture. However, life-threatening hemorrhage can also occur.

Rhinitis

Rhinitis is inflammation of nasal mucosa that usually accompanies the common cold. Acute rhinitis, the most prevalent disease among all age-groups, is spread by droplet contact.[8] Upper respiratory viruses such as rhinovirus, adenovirus, or influenza virus are the most common causative organisms. Symptoms include copious, mucopurulent nasal secretions; red and swollen nasal mucosa; mild fever; and decreased sense of smell. Allergic rhinitis (hay fever) may be perennial or seasonal—caused by pollens, grasses, trees, or flowers. Perennial allergic rhinitis is a chronic condition caused by environmental factors such as dust, animal dander, mold, and foods. Perennial rhinitis is characterized by nasal mucosa that appears pale to bluish and swollen, tearing, periorbital edema, and thin, watery nasal discharge.

The single most effective treatment for all forms of rhinitis is warm saline irrigation; however, not all patients are willing to continue this treatment on their own.[20] Systemic or topical antihistamines are used to shrink swollen nasal tissues. Instruct the patient in effective use of nasal sprays. It is recommended to spray each nostril and lie supine for 2 minutes and then repeat procedure. The first dose shrinks the nasal mucosa, allowing the second dose to reach the upper turbinates and sinus ostia.[3] Using nasal sprays just before bedtime may enhance relief.[19] Analgesics and

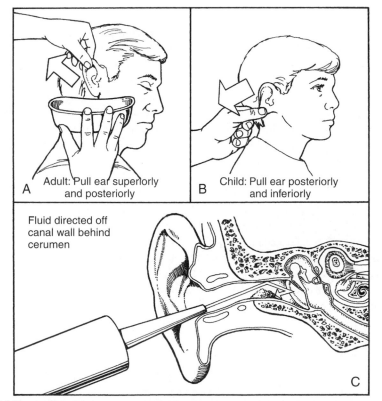

FIGURE **44-7.** Ear irrigation. **A,** The external auditory canal in the adult can best be exposed by pulling the earlobe upward and backward. **B,** The same exposure can be achieved in the child by gently pulling the auricle of the ear downward and backward. **C,** An enlarged diagram showing the direction of irrigating fluid against the side of the canal. NOTE: This is more effective in dislodging cerumen than if the flow of solution were directed straight into the canal.

antipyretics are administered as necessary. The patient should be instructed to drink plenty of clear fluids, humidify the home environment, avoid allergens, and rest. Complications associated with rhinitis include serous OM, nasal polyps, sinusitis, and exacerbation of asthma. Excessive use of topical medications and nose blowing may cause epistaxis.[20]

Epistaxis

Epistaxis, or nosebleed, is seen frequently in the ED. Causes include infection, trauma, local irritants, foreign bodies, anticoagulant drug therapy, hypertension, congenital or disease-induced coagulation disorders, and tumors. However, the most common cause is nose picking. Bleeding may occur anteriorly or posteriorly. Anterior bleeding is usually acute and almost always originates at Kiesselbach's plexus in Little's area, a highly vascularized area of the nose. Posterior epistaxis is usually chronic and common in older adults. Bleeding is more profuse, involving posterior branches of the sphenopalatine artery. Hypertension as the cause of epistaxis may be undetected if blood loss lowers blood pressure to normal.[20] In mild cases bleeding may stop spontaneously within minutes or by simply pinching the nares. Bleeding may be profuse and continuous with a potential for hypovolemia, requiring aggressive management.

The patient usually presents clutching bloody tissues or towels to the nose and can be extremely anxious. A calm, reassuring systematic approach by the emergency nurse helps ease anxiety and allows efficient management. Obtain a quick history, including duration, frequency, and amount of bleeding; recent trauma or surgery; nausea or vomiting; recreational drug use; and pertinent medical history. All staff caring for this patient should observe universal precautions including gloves, goggles, mask, and gown, because potential for blood splashing is high.

Maintain the patient in an upright seated position with the head tilted downward and nostrils pinched. Assess ABCs, and initiate appropriate interventions such as suction, IV access, cardiac monitor, and oxygen saturation monitor. Obtain CBC, prothrombin time, partial thromboplastin time, and type and crossmatch as ordered. The bleeding site is determined after clearing the nose of clots by having the patient blow the nose or with suction using an 8 Fr or 10 Fr Frazier catheter. A nasal speculum is required to visualize the posterior nasal cavity. Treatment of anterior epistaxis begins with identification of the bleeding site followed by application of topical vasoconstrictors (i.e., 2% to 5% cocaine hydrochloride, Neo-Synephrine), direct pressure for 5 to 10 minutes, chemical (silver nitrate) or electrical cautery, and packing if necessary.[19] Nasal packing may be done with standard petrolatum-iodoform gauze or newer commercial products such as the Merocel nasal sponge or Gelfoam, which eventually dissolve and do not require removal. Coat packing material with antibiotic ointment before insertion to help prevent sinusitis and toxic shock.[20] Anterior nasal packing is left in place 24 to 72 hours. The patient should follow up with an otolaryngologist or return to the ED immediately for persistent bleeding or dislodged nasal packing.[6]

With posterior epistaxis, bleeding is much more difficult to control. Direct pressure is ineffective, and packing often difficult. A posterior nasal pack should be inserted in anyone with posterior nasal hemorrhage.[19] Devices such as a Merocel nasal sponge, Nasostat epistaxis balloon, or 12 Fr to 16 Fr urinary catheter with the distal tip cut off can be used for posterior packing. These devices should be removed in 2 to 3 days. Posterior nasal packing predisposes the patient to respiratory obstruction, so admission is necessary for airway monitoring, sedation, antibiotic therapy, and humidified oxygen. Surgical ligation of vessels may be required for control of severe posterior epistaxis.[20] Antihypertensive agents may be needed for patients whose blood pressure remains elevated.

Complications of anterior and posterior epistaxis include hypoxia, dislodged nasal packing, airway occlusion, hypovolemia, severe discomfort, sinusitis, toxic shock, cardiac dysrhythmias, and respiratory or cardiac arrest. With severe blood loss, blood transfusion may be necessary. Posterior epistaxis is often associated with significant atherosclerosis and can precipitate myocardial or cerebral infarction.[20]

Foreign Body

A foreign body in the nose usually occurs in children and is often discovered when a purulent nasal discharge is noticed.[4] Usually self-inserted, foreign bodies in the nose may also occur with trauma. Nasal cavities are easily expanded, so unusual, large, or multiple retained foreign bodies are possible. The patient may present with pain and fullness from a recently placed foreign body or with purulent, foul-smelling nasal discharge, recurrent epistaxis, sinus pain, fever, and edematous nasal mucosa.[7] Care should be taken to prevent damage to the highly vascular nasal septum and mucosa during removal of a nasal foreign body. Children may require conscious sedation or a papoose board for restraint. Ask the cooperative patient to occlude the unobstructed nostril, close the mouth, and make a forceful nasal exhalation at least 15 times.[15] If unsuccessful, apply a topical anesthetic agent and place the patient in Trendelenburg's position. The object is then removed with hooked probe or forceps.[4] Balloon catheters, stick and glue, suction catheter tip, and positive pressure ventilation may prove helpful.[4] Extreme care must be taken not to dislodge or drive the foreign body deeper into the nasopharynx because aspiration may occur.[10] Complications such as epistaxis, septal hematoma, septal perforation, or inability to remove the foreign body should be referred to an otolaryngologist. (Refer to Chapter 27 for discussion of septal hematoma and nasal trauma.)

THROAT EMERGENCIES

Throat emergencies represent a threat to the patient's airway. The emergency nurse should evaluate the patient's ABCs carefully and monitor for significant changes in breathing and mentation. (Refer to Chapter 47 for assessment and management of epiglottitis.)

Pharyngitis

Pharyngitis, inflammation of the pharynx, often accompanies the common cold. Symptoms include bright red throat, swollen tonsils, white or yellow exudate on tonsils and pharynx, swollen uvula, and enlarged, tender cervical and tonsillar nodes.[22] The patient may complain of sore throat, fever, dysphagia, and halitosis (foul breath odor). Treatment for pharyngitis depends on underlying pathologic condition.[3] A throat culture and sensitivity should be obtained to distinguish bacterial or viral cause. Many EDs use a rapid strep test to screen for streptococcal infections. Most sore throats in adults are viral and do not warrant antibiotics.[14] For bacterial pharyngitis (i.e., streptococcal pharyngitis), treatment consists of antibiotics, antipyretics, and analgesics. Encourage the patient to gargle frequently with warm saline. Stress the importance of bed rest, increased fluid intake, and completing the full course of antibiotics. Tonsillectomy, or removal of tonsils, may be necessary in severe cases. Complications include retropharyngeal abscess, glomerular nephritis, and acute rheumatic fever and toxic shock syndrome.[9]

Laryngitis

Acute laryngitis, inflammation of the vocal cords, may accompany URI or can exist alone. Causes of acute laryngitis include overuse, allergies, irritants, and viral or bacterial infections.[5] Tension in the vocal cords determines the amount of vibration produced when air flows upward through the glottis. Anything that alters this tension affects the ability to speak. The patient presents with partial or complete voice loss, with or without URI symptoms. Dyspnea or stridor should be evaluated and treated immediately as potential airway obstruction. Throat culture and CBC are the usual diagnostic procedures. Treatment includes voice rest, steam inhalations to thin secretions and improve moisture, increased fluid intake, and topical anesthetic throat lozenges. Patient teaching should emphasize preventive therapy, avoiding airway irritants such as cigarette smoke and loud or excessive use of the voice.[5] In the presence of infection administer antibiotics and instruct the patient to complete the entire course. Aspirin is contraindicated for analgesia because of its anticoagulant properties, which increase the risk of vocal cord hemorrhage and subsequent scarring and changes in voice quality. Complications of laryngitis are aspiration pneumonia, decreased cough reflex, and airway compromise or obstruction.

Tonsillitis

Tonsillitis refers to inflammation of the palatine tonsils. Tonsils are lymphatic tissue that filters bacteria and other microorganisms to prevent infection in the body.[26] Culture for streptococcus bacteria may be taken because it is the most common and most dangerous form of tonsillitis.[26] Viruses are also a leading cause of this contagious, airborne infection. Symptoms are similar to pharyngitis and may include a feeling of fullness in the throat, malaise, otalgia (ear pain), and tenderness in the jaw or throat.[26] The patient may have difficulty speaking or swallowing. The tonsils may be covered by a white or yellow exudate and the patient can have foul breath. Rapid strep test, throat culture and sensitivity, CBC, monospot test, and chest radiograph may be ordered. As with pharyngitis, warm saline gargles, topical anesthetic lozenges, analgesics, antipyretics, and antibiotics (usually penicillin or erythromycin) are indicated. Surgery is recommended for recurrent streptococcal infections unresponsive to antibiotic therapy or tonsillar hypertrophy that predisposes the patient to respiratory obstruction or dysphagia. Retropharyngeal and peritonsillar abscess, glomerular nephritis, and rheumatic fever with subsequent cardiovascular disorders are potential complications of tonsillitis.[26]

Peritonsillar Abscess

Untreated acute or chronic suppurative tonsillitis may evolve into a peritonsillar abscess caused by a perforated tonsillar capsule and extension of the infection into deep soft tissue.[13] Usual causative organisms are species of *Streptococcus* (aerobic) and *Prevotella* or *Peptostreptococcus* (anaerobic.)[13] The abscess is usually unilateral with dysphagia, drooling, hot potato/muffled voice, painful swallowing, trismus, and anxiety present.[8] Fever, malaise, and dehydration are usually seen. Treat dehydration with fluid resuscitation; administer antipyretics and analgesics as needed. Tonsillectomy may be required to prevent recurrence of the abscess. Patients can be managed on an outpatient basis unless they show signs of sepsis, airway compromise, or complications.[13]

In mild cases, needle aspiration relieves trismus and painful swallowing; therefore the patient is discharged on oral antibiotics with ENT specialist follow-up.[13] Ice packs to the neck help decrease pain and edema. Encourage oral hygiene; however, gargling should be avoided because this may cause inadvertent rupture of the abscess.

In more severe cases with airway compromise, surgical incision and drainage or needle aspiration is followed by IV antibiotic therapy. Stability of the ABCs is a priority. Provide oxygen, monitor arterial oxygen saturation levels and respirations, and keep the head of the bed elevated 80 to 90 degrees. Patients with an airway compromise will need immediate endotracheal intubation. If unable to intubate, then cricothyroidectomy or a tracheotomy may need to be performed. Dangerous sequelae associated with peritonsillar abscess include aspiration, airway obstruction, parapharyngeal abscess, dehydration, glomerulonephritis, and subacute bacterial endocarditis. Fortunately complications can be avoided with aggressive antibiotic treatment (penicillin based or erythromycin.)

FACIAL EMERGENCIES

Facial emergencies affect structures of the face such as the nerves, bones, and sinuses. These emergencies may be secondary to infection or other disease processes.

Sinusitis

Acute sinusitis, inflammation of mucous membranes in any of the paranasal sinuses, generally occurs as a result of blockage and backup of secretions. The cause is usually attributed to URI or allergic rhinitis. Other causes include foreign bodies, trauma, dental disorders, inhalation of irritants (e.g., cigarette smoke, cocaine use), deviated nasal septum, polyps, and tumors. Secretions are retained in the sinus cavity as a result of altered ciliary activity and obstruction of the sinus ostia.[10] Negative pressure and air-fluid levels result from fluid accumulation and reabsorption of air in the sinus. Fluid accumulation forms a medium for bacteria to grow and multiply, resulting in bacterial sinusitis. *H. influenzae* and *S. pneumoniae* are common causative organisms.[29]

Chronic sinusitis is a result of unresolved acute sinusitis of more than 3 weeks' duration.[29]

In chronic sinusitis the mucous membrane becomes permanently thickened from prolonged or repeated inflammation or infection. The patient with sinusitis complains of dull, achy pain over the affected sinus. In adults, frontal sinusitis with periorbital and forehead pain that worsens when bending over is common. Ethmoidal sinusitis, common in children, causes pain at the bridge of the nose and behind the eyes. Fever, decreased appetite, and nausea may also be present. Ethmoidal sinusitis is especially serious in children because of the tendency for the infection to extend toward the retroorbital area and central nervous system.[19] The patient has tenderness to palpation over the involved sinus; swollen, erythematous mucosa with purulent nasal discharge; and diminished transillumination. Radiographic studies are not always conclusive or reliable in diagnosis of sinusitis. Findings that are most reliable include sinus opacity, air-fluid level, or 6 mm of mucosal thickening. Absence of radiographic evidence does not exclude the diagnosis of sinusitis.[19] Other diagnostic methods include CT scan, sinus endoscopy, and sinus cultures of the ostia via needle aspiration.

Over-the-counter nasal decongestant sprays (e.g., Afrin or Neo-Synephrine) may provide immediate relief; however, topical decongestants should not be used for more than 3 days because of a dangerous rebound effect.[3] Isotonic saline nose drops may also help. Encourage increased fluid intake and use of a humidifier in the home. Warm, moist compresses to the sinus areas promote drainage and comfort. Administer antibiotics and analgesics as prescribed. Instruct the patient to avoid environmental irritants and avoid bending over because this increases sinus pressure and pain. If the condition worsens despite antibiotic therapy for 3 to 5 days, the patient should return to the ED immediately or see an ENT specialist. Complications of undertreated acute sinusitis are chronic sinusitis, orbital or periorbital cellulitis or abscess, cavernous sinus thrombosis, sepsis, brain abscess, meningitis, and osteomyelitis of the frontal bone.

Temporomandibular Joint Dislocation

TMJ dislocation refers to anterior and superior bilateral displacement of the jaw. Unilateral dislocation rarely occurs. Jaw muscles attempt to close the mandible, but the resulting spasm prevents condyles from returning to normal position in the mandibular fossae.[1] TMJ dislocation usually occurs when opening the mouth too wide, as in yawning or laughing. Trauma or dystonic reaction to drugs may also be responsible. The patient usually presents with the chin protruding, the mouth open, drooling, and pain related to muscle spasms. The patient cannot close the mouth, talk, or swallow and may be extremely anxious.[3] Diagnostics include prereduction and postreduction radiographs. Muscle relaxants may be administered to reduce muscle spasm and relax the patient.

To reduce the dislocation, seat the patient facing the emergency physician. The physician places the thumbs intraorally onto the lower molar ridge and applies a downward and backward pressure to return the condyle to the normal position.[1] The physician should pad the thumbs with a thick layer of gauze because the strong masseter muscles of the jaw contract with great force with reduction of the TMJ. Postreduction pain is rare and is minimal when present. Nonsteroidal antiinflammatory drugs and muscle relaxants may be helpful.[1] Instruct the patient to avoid stress on the TMJ by consuming a soft diet for 3 to 4 days. Because patients with one episode of TMJ dislocation are predisposed to further dislocations, referral to an otolaryngologist is recommended.[4]

SUMMARY

Emergencies of the mouth, face, nose, and ears are a routine part of emergency nursing. Most are not life threatening. However, the ability to discern problems that represent a potential threat to the patient's life is a requisite skill for the emergency nurse.

REFERENCES

1. Amsterdam JT: Oral medicine. In Marx J, Hockberger R, Walls R, editors: *Rosen's emergency medicine: concepts and clinical practice*, ed 6, Philadelphia, 2006, Mosby.
2. Beaudreau RW: Oral and dental emergencies. In Tintinalli JE, Kelsen GD, Stapczynski JS, editors: *Emergency medicine: a comprehensive study guide*, ed 6, New York, 2004, McGraw-Hill.
3. Black JM, Matassarin-Jacobs E: *Medical-surgical nursing: a psychophysiologic approach*, ed 6, Philadelphia, 2000, WB Saunders.
4. Cox RJ: Foreign bodies, nose, 2000, updated October 6, 2005, *eMedicine*. Retrieved January 13, 2008, from http://www.emedicine.com/emerg/topic186.htm.
5. Demetroulakos JL: Laryngitis, updated July 25, 2007, *MedicinePlus medical encyclopedia*. Retrieved January 13, 2008, from http://www.nlm.nih.gov/medicineplus/ency/article/001385.htm.
6. Evans J, Rothenhaus T: Epistaxis, updated July 19, 2005, *eMedicine*. Retrieved January 13, 2008, from http://www.emedicine.com/emerg/topic806.htm.
7. Ignatavicius DD, Workman ML, Mishler MA: *Medical-surgical nursing: across the healthcare continuum*, ed 3, Philadelphia, 1999, WB Saunders.

8. Jarvis C: *Physical examination and health assessment*, ed 5, Philadelphia, 2007, WB Saunders.
9. Kazzi AA, Will J: Pharyngitis, updated April 21, 2005, *eMedicine*. Retrieved January 13, 2008, from http://www.emedicine.com/emerg/topic419.htm.
10. Kennedy E: Sinusitis, updated August 8, 2007, *eMedicine*. Retrieved January 13, 2008, from http://www.emedicine.com/emerg/topic536.htm.
11. Leonard CH: *Gray's pocket anatomy*, New York, 1984, Crown.
12. Mantooth R: Foreign body ear, updated March 13, 2007, *eMedicine*. Retrieved January 13, 2008, from http://www.emedicine.com/emerg/topic185.htm.
13. Mehta N, Silverberg M: Peritonsillar abscess, updated November 4, 2008, *eMedicine*. Retrieved January 13, 2008, from http://www.emedicine.com/emerg/topic417.htm.
14. Melio F: Upper respiratory tract infections. In Marx J, Hockberger R, Walls R, editors: *Rosen's emergency medicine: concepts and clinical practice*, ed 6, Philadelphia, 2006, Mosby.
15. Peacock WF: Face and jaw emergencies. In Tintinalli JE, Kelen GD, Stapczynski JS, editors: *Emergency medicine: a comprehensive study guide*, ed 6, New York, 2004, McGraw-Hill.
16. Peng L, Kazzi AA: Dental, avulsed tooth, updated November 8, 2007, *eMedicine*. Retrieved January 13, 2008, from http://www.emedicine.com/emerg/topic125.htm.
17. Peng L, Kazzi AA: Dental, fractured tooth, updated September 27, 2007, *eMedicine*. Retrieved January 13, 2008, from http://www.emedicine.com/emerg/topic127.htm.
18. Peng L, Kazzi AA: Dental infections, updated September 26, 2007, *eMedicine*. Retrieved January 13, 2008, from http://www.emedicine.com/emerg/topic128.htm.
19. Pfaff JA, Moore GP: Otolaryngology. In Marx J, Hockberger R, Walls R, editors: *Rosen's emergency medicine: concepts and clinical practice*, ed 6, Philadelphia, 2006, Mosby.
20. Pons PT: Nasal foreign bodies. In Rosen P, Barkin RM, Hockberger RS et al, editors: *Emergency medicine: concepts and clinical practice*, ed 5, St. Louis, 2002, Mosby.
21. Rahman WM, O'Connor TJ: Facial trauma. In Barkin RM, editor: *Pediatric emergency medicine: concepts and clinical practice*, ed 2, St. Louis, 1997, Mosby.
22. Shores CG: Infections and disorders of the neck and upper airway. In Tintinalli JE, Kelen GD, Stapczynski JS, editors: *Emergency medicine: a comprehensive study guide*, ed 6, New York, 2004, McGraw-Hill.
23. Tintinalli A, Lucchesi M: Common disorders of the external, middle, and inner ear. In Tintinalli JE, Kelen GD, Stapczynski JS, editors: *Emergency medicine: a comprehensive study guide*, ed 6, New York, 2004, McGraw-Hill.
24. Tortora G, Derrickson BH: *Principles of anatomy and physiology*, ed 11, New York, 2005, Harper & Row.
25. Uphold CR, Graham MV: *Clinical guidelines in family practice*, ed 4, Gainesville, Fla, 2003, Barmarrae Books.
26. Uppaluri R: Tonsillitis, updated January 30, 2007, *MedicinePlus medical encyclopedia*. Retrieved January 13, 2008, from http://www.nlm.nih.gov/medicineplus/ency/article/001043.htm.
27. Walsh M, Cook K: Otitis externa, updated July 26, 2007, *eMedicine*. Retrieved January 13, 2008, from http://www.emedicine.com/emerg/topic350.htm.
28. Walsh M, Cook K: Otitis media, updated July 16, 2008, *eMedicine*. Retrieved January 13, 2008, from http://www.emedicine.com/emerg/topic351.htm.
29. Waters TA, Peacock WF IV: Nasal emergencies and sinusitis. In Tintinalli JE, Kelen GD, Stapczynski JS, editors: *Emergency medicine: a comprehensive study guide*, ed 6, New York, 2004, Mosby.

CHAPTER 45

Ocular Emergencies

Darcy Egging

Emergency nurses care for patients with eye problems on a regular basis; however, true ocular emergencies are not an everyday occurrence. The ability to identify those conditions that represent a threat to the patient's vision is essential. This chapter provides a brief description of anatomy, ocular assessment, and common ocular emergencies encountered in the emergency department (ED).

According to the National Hospital Ambulatory Medical Care Survey: 2004 Emergency Department Summary, approximately 3.6 million individuals present to the ED annually with complaints related to the eyes or ears. This number is approximately 11% of all ED visits. Of the 3.6 million visits, 1.6 million are for traumatic eye injuries according to the 2004 report.[28] The typical ocular emergencies treated in the ED include corneal or conjunctival foreign body, conjunctivitis, and corneal abrasion. These conditions do not cause significant morbidity; however, the patient does experience discomfort and disruption of routine. True ocular emergencies, those conditions with potential for vision loss, include chemical burns, angle-closure glaucoma, globe rupture, and retinal artery occlusion.

ANATOMY AND PHYSIOLOGY

The eyes are the windows to the world. Vision is often considered the most important of the five senses. Basic understanding of ocular structures facilitates assessment and treatment of ocular problems. Figure 45-1 illustrates these ocular structures. The eyes are protected by the surrounding bony structures, eyelids, and sclera. Lacrimal glands secrete tears, which continuously bathe the eye to decrease friction and remove minor irritants. Meibomian and Zeis glands are sebaceous glands that line the eyelid margins and prevent tears from evaporating and running out of the conjunctival sacs.

Light enters the eye through the cornea, passes through the lens, and is reflected off the retina. The amount of light entering the posterior chamber is controlled by the iris as it expands and contracts to open and close the pupil. Six oculomotor muscles control movement of the eye itself.

PATIENT ASSESSMENT

Assessment of the patient with an ocular problem begins with triage and continues into the treatment area. A potential threat to vision should be triaged as emergent, whereas a patient with a reddened eye and no potential for loss of vision could be triaged as nonurgent if no other problems exist.

After a brief assessment to ensure that the airway, breathing, and circulation (ABCs) are stable, the patient is evaluated to identify potential threats to vision. Focused assessment includes determination of precipitating events, duration of symptoms, and identification of anything that worsens or improves symptoms. When the patient verbalizes discomfort, description

602

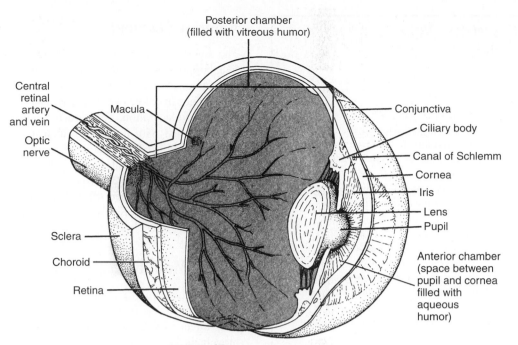

FIGURE **45-1.** Anatomy of the eye.

of the discomfort helps clarify the patient's problem. Does the patient describe itching, burning, or the sensation of something in the eye? Determine the degree of pain and where the pain occurs. Clarify reported visual changes to determine if the loss is partial or complete, and in one or both eyes. Biocular changes suggest a neurologic condition rather than an ocular condition, whereas the presence of floaters suggests retinal tear.

When the patient has a history of trauma, determine the mechanism of injury and when it occurred. If the injury occurred as a result of a motor vehicle crash, did the air bag deploy? Injuries associated with air-bag deployment include orbital fractures, retinal detachment, hyphema, and globe rupture; an increased incidence of globe rupture and hyphema has been noted in older adults.[40] The alkaline powder in air bags can also cause significant eye irritation.[46] Question the patient regarding use of protective eyewear, glasses, or contact lenses. Evaluate medical history, including ocular history, use of corrective lenses, ocular medications, past ocular surgery, and disease such as diabetes. Tetanus status should be determined if signs of ocular trauma are noted.

The primary elements of the ocular examination for all patients are visual acuity and evaluation of external features, pupils, anterior segment, and extraocular movement (EOM).[1,20] The physician may perform a slit-lamp examination, intraocular pressure (IOP) measurement, and direct ophthalmoscope examination.

Visual Acuity

Visual acuity is a "vital sign" for patients with an ocular concern. This simple test is done on all patients presenting with any type of eye or vision complaint.[1,20,24] Physical examination begins with visual acuity unless the patient has sustained ocular exposure to a chemical. In these situations irrigation takes priority over determination of visual acuity.[1,2,4,24,30] Measure visual acuity both with and without the patient wearing corrective lenses. When corrective lenses are not available, the pinhole test can be used for measurement of visual acuity. This is accomplished by punching a hole in a note card with an 18-gauge needle. Looking through a pinhole usually corrects any refractory error to at least 20/30.[29,31] Test the affected eye first, then the unaffected eye, and finally both eyes. The Snellen chart is the standard method for determination of visual acuity. For the examination, have the patient stand 20 feet from the chart and cover the eye without applying pressure to the orbit. Alternative techniques for visual acuity when a Snellen chart is not available are using a pocket vision screener held 14 inches from the nose or having the patient read a newspaper and record the distance at which the paper must be held for the patient to read. If the patient is unable to read, hold fingers up, record the distance at which the patient can see your fingers, then ask the patient how many fingers you are holding up. If the patient cannot see fingers moving; record the distance at which the patient perceives hand motion. If unable to see hand motion, is the patient able to perceive light? Table 45-1 describes documentation of visual acuity for the Snellen chart and alternative techniques for reporting visual acuity. For people who are illiterate or do not speak English, there is an E chart where the patient indicates the direction of the letter *E*. The Allen card of objects is used for children. Be sure to name the objects before the test so that they are identified correctly. The patient with a corneal abrasion or foreign body may have difficulty with photophobia, pain, and tearing. Placing a drop of topical anesthetic in the affected eye may assist in accomplishing an accurate visual acuity in these patients.[25]

Table 45-1.	EXAMPLES OF VISUAL ACUITY EXAMINATION
20/20	Standing at 20 feet, patient can read what the normal eye can read at 20 feet.
20/20 2	Standing at 20 feet, patient can read what the normal eye can read at 20 feet; however, missed two letters.
20/200	At 20 feet, patient can read what the normal eye can read at 200 feet. Patient is considered legally blind if reading is obtained while wearing glasses or contact lenses.
10/200	When the patient cannot read letters on the Snellen chart, have patient stand half the distance to the chart. Record findings at the distance the patient is standing from the chart over the smallest line he or she can read.
CF/3 ft	Patient can count fingers at a maximum distance of 3 feet.
HM/4	Patient can see hand motion at a maximum distance of 4 feet.
LP/position	Patient can perceive light and determine the direction from which it is coming.
LP/no position	Patient can perceive light but is unable to tell the direction from which it is coming.
NLP	Patient is unable to perceive light.

External Features

External examination of ocular complaints begins by inspecting the patient. Observe for bruising, lacerations, lesions, and other differences between the eyes. Assess eyelids, lashes, and how the eyes rest in the socket. Examine the conjunctiva and sclera for abnormal color.

Pupil Examination

Pupil examination includes assessment of shape, size, and reactivity. Testing should be performed in a dimly lit examination room. Pupils are normally round, black, and equal in size. Variations may indicate a potentially serious problem or may reflect a normal physiologic variation. Up to 20% to 25%[13] of the population have unequal pupils (physiologic anisocoria) as a normal finding.[7] Physiologic anisocoria is a normal finding when the difference in pupils is 1 mm or less and both pupils react briskly to light.[41] An oval pupil may be caused by a tumor or retinal detachment. A pupil that is the shape of a teardrop suggests a ruptured globe, with the teardrop pointing to the rupture site.[24] Pupil size is measured in millimeters. Assess and document the change in size that occurs in each pupil in response to direct and consensual light stimulation. Normally both pupils constrict equally when a strong light is directed at one eye (direct response in eye to which light is directed and consensual response of the other eye).[24]

Anterior Segment

The anterior segment is composed of the sclera, conjunctiva, cornea, anterior chamber, iris, lens, and ciliary body.[20] The conjunctiva or the white of the eye should be inspected for changes in color, swelling (chemosis), discharge, foreign bodies, and laceration. The cornea should be clear. The cornea is stained with fluorescein to inspect for the presence of any abrasions. The anterior chamber is inspected for hyphema (blood in the anterior chamber) or hypopyon (pus in the anterior chamber). To inspect the anterior chamber, hold a light tangential or at a 90-degree angle to the eye. A slit lamp is used to perform an adequate assessment of the anterior chamber.[20,25]

Ocular Motility

Evaluate the patient's ability to move the eyes through six cardinal positions of gaze by asking the patient to follow your finger as you move it through these positions. Ocular movement is controlled by the cranial nerves that regulate the oculomotor muscles. Figure 45-2 shows these positions of gaze and identifies the specific oculomotor muscles and cranial nerves involved. Impaired ocular movement may occur with an entrapped muscle secondary to a blowout fracture, muscular injury, orbital cellulitis, or underlying central nervous system problem. Evaluation of ocular motility in children requires patience and creativity. Hold toys, keys, or lights in different areas so that the child glances in that direction. Children become easily bored with the same object, so a general rule of thumb is to use a different toy for each position.[24,29]

Other Examinations

Other techniques used to evaluate ocular function include fluorescein staining, measurement of IOP, and funduscopic examination. Fluorescein is used to determine if the corneal epithelium is intact. Before staining, the patient should remove his or her contact lenses. Explain the procedure to the patient. Moisten end of a sterile fluorescein strip with normal saline solution. Pull down on the lower lid and touch the moistened fluorescein strip to the inner canthus of the lower lid. Ask the patient to blink several times before examining the patient with a cobalt blue light; disruptions of the corneal epithelium appear as a bright yellow spot. Following fluorescein application, flush the eye with normal saline and instruct the patient not to insert contact lenses for at least 3 to 5 hours.[34]

IOP is measured with a Schiøtz tonometer (Figure 45-3) or a Tono-Pen. This procedure is contraindicated in patients with possible globe rupture. The Tono-Pen is a handheld instrument that has gained popularity because of its ease of use and decreased incidence of contamination; the tip is covered with a sterile cover that is discarded after each patient. Regardless of technique, the cornea must be anesthetized before measurement. Normal IOP is 10 to 21 mm Hg. A low

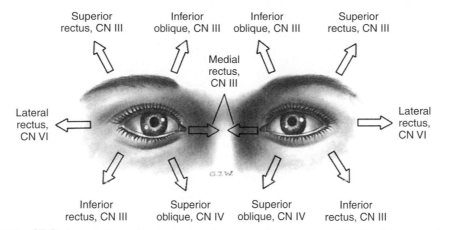

FIGURE **45-2.** Innervation and movement of extraocular muscles. *CN,* Cranial nerve. (From Thompson JM, McFarland GK, Hirsch JE et al: *Mosby's clinical nursing,* ed 5, St. Louis, 2002, Mosby.)

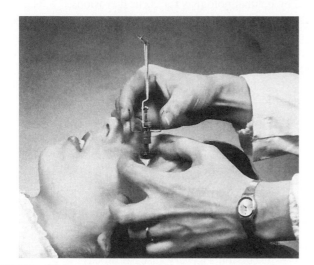

FIGURE **45-3.** Measurement of ocular tension with Schiøtz tonometer. (From Newell FW: *Ophthalmology: principles and concepts,* ed 8, St. Louis, 1996, Mosby.)

reading indicates decreased IOP, whereas a high reading indicates increased IOP. Any obstruction to aqueous outflow, such as glaucoma, can result in an elevated IOP.[25,29,34]

Direct ophthalmoscopy, or funduscopic evaluation, is used to evaluate the posterior chamber of the eye using a light beam directed through the pupil.[20] Mydriatic drops may be administered to dilate the pupil and make visualization of the disc, retinal artery, and macula easier; however, they are contraindicated in patients who have sustained a head injury.[25] Ophthalmoscopes provide different shapes and colored light beams to assist in detecting various abnormalities.

PATIENT MANAGEMENT

General management of ocular emergencies includes removal of contact lens, instillation of ocular medication, irrigation, and eye patching.

Figure 45-4 illustrates removal of hard contacts; Figure 45-5 illustrates soft contact removal.

Eye drops and ophthalmic ointments are used to decrease pain, provide antibiotic therapy, change pupil size, reduce allergic reactions in the eye, and cleanse the eye. Topical ophthalmic medications are prepared under sterile conditions and distributed in single-dose containers. Container caps are color coded by the medication's effect on the pupil. For example, a red cap indicates a mydriatic (pupil dilating) medication, green for a pupil constrictor (miotic); white is for a topical anesthetic, blue an irrigating or lubricating agent, and a yellow cap denotes medications that decrease aqueous humor production.

Instilling eye drops or ointments requires attention to detail to prevent contamination and minimize systemic effects of the medication. Before instilling eye drops or ointments, explain the procedure to the patient, and place the patient in the supine position. Instruct the patient not to roll his or her eyes because this can worsen injury, particularly when anesthetic drops have been used; topical anesthetics may be used to facilitate the examination but should not be prescribed for continuous use because these agents retard epithelial healing. Instillation of eye drops and ointments are relatively easy procedures to master; in both instances have the patient gaze upward because this will help to ensure that the patient does not blink at an inopportune time. Pull the lower eyelid downward and instill the medication in the conjunctival sac. Monitor patients carefully following instillation of eye drops; systemic effects secondary to eye drops may occur. These systemic effects can be minimized by instructing patients to apply pressure to the medial canthus for several minutes after medication instillation to close the nasolacrimal duct. If more than one type of drop is ordered, wait several minutes between applications to allow maximal exposure for each drop.

Irrigation is used to remove chemicals, small foreign bodies, and other substances. Isotonic saline or lactated Ringer's are the fluids of choice for ocular irrigation.[25,32,38] Dextrose solutions should not be used because they are sticky and irritate the eye. Irrigation is contraindicated in the patient with a possible ruptured globe. There is no documented literature on the correct length of tubing to be used; however,

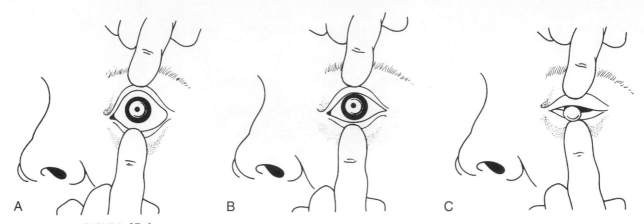

FIGURE 45-4. Technique for removing hard corneal contact lens from eye. **A,** Spread eyelids apart. **B,** Push lids toward center of eye under contact lens. **C,** Remove lens.

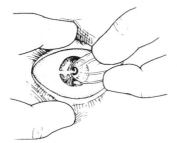

FIGURE 45-5. Soft contact lens removal. Lift lens off cornea.

the shorter the tubing, the faster the flow. Before irrigating the eye, make sure the outer aspects of the eye are cleansed so that additional debris does not inadvertently contaminate the eye and cause further problems. When using intravenous tubing to irrigate, gently separate the eyelids and have the patient look around while the irrigant is flowing. Sweep from the inner to the outer canthus. Occasionally allow the patient to blink for comfort. A Morgan Lens can also be used for irrigation. In the case of a chemical exposure, a baseline pH measurement of the eye should be obtained by placing pH paper in the conjunctival sac before irrigation is initiated. Irrigation is continued until the pH of the tear film is neutral (normal conjunctival pH is 7.1). As a rule of thumb, for acidic chemical exposure 1 L of fluid will be necessary, whereas exposure to an alkali will require a minimum of 2 L of fluid.[25,32]

Eye patching is performed to minimize ocular stimulation by reducing movement and limiting light exposure. A common intervention in the past, this procedure is currently not being used for routine management of uncomplicated corneal injuries because evidence does not support its use.[25] A Cochrane review of the literature shows that patching of a simple corneal abrasion does not increase healing time nor does it decrease pain.[36] Patching of both eyes simulates total blindness; patching one eye alters depth perception. Eye patches should not be used when there is an increased risk for a *Pseudomonas* organism infection, for example, in the contact lens wearer. Although not widely available in the ED, a collagen shield that is similar to a contact lens is being

used by ophthalmologists for corneal erosions.[25,33] The correct method of patching the eye includes asking the patient to gently close both eyes and placing a folded eye pad over the affected eye followed by an unfolded eye pad. The eye pad is taped obliquely, ensuring that the entire eye patch is covered. Ask the patient if he or she can blink under the pad: if the patient is able to blink, the patch has not been applied correctly. When the patient is discharged with an eye patch, discharge instructions must include discussion of altered vision and the hazards of driving or using machinery. Eye patches should not be applied for more than a 24-hour period; therefore follow-up is essential.[33]

SPECIFIC OCULAR EMERGENCIES

Injury or disease may cause ocular emergencies. Comprehensive discussion of every disease process is beyond the scope of this text; however, situations encountered most often by the emergency nurse are discussed.

Trauma

General principles pertaining to ocular examination are essentially the same for the patient with an eye injury; however, the patient's ABCs should be evaluated and stabilized before interventions for the ocular problem. Ocular injury often occurs in conjunction with head and facial trauma; therefore these patients should be carefully evaluated for an associated eye injury. Check for contact lenses in the unconscious patient, and remove them as soon as possible. Do not instill eye drops before evaluation of ocular injury. Severe pain associated with ocular trauma can be minimized without medication by patching both eyes. When the patient cannot blink, protect the cornea from drying with ophthalmic ointment or artificial tears. The eyes may be taped shut when ointment is used.

Obtain pertinent details of history, including mechanism of injury, time of injury, energy source, material involved when there is ocular penetration, and use of protective eyewear. If the foreign material is organic, there is increased risk for infection, whereas metallic materials cause vitreous and ocular reactions.

Blunt Trauma

Blunt trauma to the eye may be caused by a motor vehicle collision, assault with various weapons, or a fall. The most commonly seen ocular injury is periorbital contusion or a black eye. This injury is usually benign, but the patient should be assessed for more serious injury, such as a hyphema or basilar skull fracture. Symptoms usually include ecchymosis of the lids, which can make it very difficult to visualize the globe. If the globe appears intact, rule out orbital fracture and hyphema. If no obvious associated problems are identified, therapeutic interventions such as ice, head elevation, and reassurance are initiated. Resolution of noncomplicated periorbital ecchymosis usually occurs within 2 to 3 weeks.[29]

ORBITAL FRACTURES. Orbital fractures involve the orbital floor and the orbital rim. A fracture of the orbital floor, sometimes called a blowout fracture, is serious and usually results from direct blunt trauma to the eye. A blowout fracture occurs when direct trauma increases IOP to the point where the orbital floor fractures. Orbital contents may herniate into the maxillary or ethmoid sinuses and trap the inferior rectus muscle in the defect. A blowout fracture is diagnosed by history and observation of periorbital ecchymosis, subconjunctival hemorrhage, periorbital edema, enophthalmos (sunken eye), an upward gaze, and a complaint of diplopia.[24] The latter three conditions occur when the inferior rectus and oblique muscles are trapped in the fracture. Computed tomography (CT) scan is most often used for the diagnosis of orbital fractures; facial radiographs are rarely used. Magnetic resonance imaging (MRI) is not generally used in acute orbital trauma and is contraindicated if there is a possibility of a metallic foreign body. CT or MRI is more helpful in identification of entrapment than plain radiographs.[24,29]

Orbital fractures are not considered an ocular emergency unless visual impairment or globe injury is present. Surgical intervention is usually delayed until swelling resolves in 7 to 10 days. Patients without eye injury or entrapment may be referred to an ophthalmologist and treated conservatively. Patients who have fractures involving the sinuses should receive a prescription of antibiotics. Discharge instructions should include ice and cautions against Valsalva maneuvers, sneezing, and nose blowing (activities that increase IOP).[24,29,42]

HYPHEMA. Hyphema refers to bleeding into the anterior chamber of the eye, usually secondary to blunt trauma (Figure 45-6). It occurs when blood vessels of the iris rupture and leak into the clear aqueous fluid of the anterior chamber.[43] Hyphema size varies from microscopic to total involvement of the anterior chamber. The term "eight-ball hyphema" describes a total hyphema that has begun to clot.[18] A large clot can obstruct aqueous outflow and lead to secondary glaucoma. Any patient with a hyphema requires evaluation by an ophthalmologist.

Symptoms of hyphema include pain, photophobia, and blurred vision. Blood in the anterior chamber may be easily seen in patients with lighter-colored eyes but may be extremely difficult to see in dark-eyed patients. Suspect

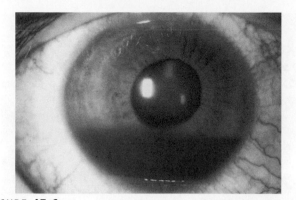

FIGURE **45-6.** Traumatic hyphema. (From Abrams D: *Ophthalmology in medicine: an illustrated clinical guide,* St. Louis, 1990, Mosby.)

concurrent head injury if the patient has an altered level of consciousness. Patients with bleeding disorders, anticoagulant therapy, kidney disease, liver disease, or sickle cell disease have an increased risk for complications; therefore these patients should be monitored carefully for increased bleeding. The most common complication of hyphema is rebleeding, which occurs in 30% of patients, usually within 2 to 5 days, but can occur up to 14 days after the initial injury.[18,29,39] Other complications include corneal blood staining, secondary glaucoma, loss of vision, and loss of the eye.

Management of hyphema is variable and controversial, particularly relative to activity. The controversy regards whether the patient should be allowed quiet activity or placed on strict bed rest. Regardless of the decision, when the patient is in bed, the head of the bed should be elevated 30 to 45 degrees. There is also disagreement regarding hospitalization and eye patching. Some clinicians advocate leaving the eye uncovered while the patient is awake, allowing visual changes to be recognized. Conservative therapy should be considered for those patients at risk for complications, children and older adults. Hospitalization should be considered when noncompliance with treatment is an issue. Pharmacologic management includes β-blockers to control elevated IOP, mydriatic agents to increase patient comfort, steroids to decrease inflammation in the anterior chamber, and an antifibrinolytic agent to delay clot dissolution and decrease the rate of rebleed. Analgesics may also be used; however, aspirin and nonsteroidal antiinflammatory medications should be avoided. Antiemetics may be used to decrease the risk for vomiting if the patient is nauseated because vomiting increases IOP. Regardless of the above information, it is imperative that all patients with a hyphema be referred to an ophthalmologist for follow-up.[18,29,39]

SUBCONJUNCTIVAL HEMORRHAGE. Subconjunctival hemorrhage is a harmless ocular condition that can frighten patients by its appearance. It is usually caused by trivial trauma such as a cough, sneeze, or the Valsalva maneuver. This condition is caused when a small blood vessel underneath the conjunctiva ruptures and bleeds (Figure 45-7). The symptoms include a painless, bright red flat patch on the sclera. Most patients usually discover a subconjunctival

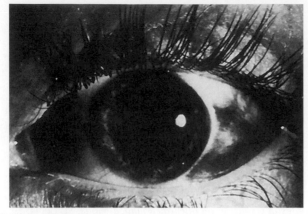

FIGURE 45-7. Subconjunctival hemorrhage. (From Stein HA, Slatt BJ, Stein RM: *The ophthalmic assistant,* ed 7, St. Louis, 2000, Mosby.)

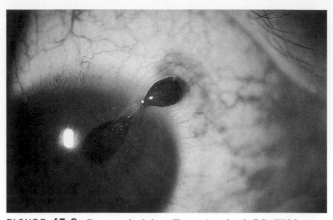

FIGURE 45-8. Ruptured globe. (From Auerbach PS: *Wilderness medicine,* ed 5, St. Louis, 2007, Mosby; courtesy Steve Chaflin, MD, University of Texas Health Science Center, San Antonio, Tex.)

hemorrhage as a surprise when looking in the mirror. Although a subconjunctival hemorrhage is benign, there is a need to differentiate it from a bloody chemosis, which can be indicative of scleral rupture, conjunctivitis, iritis, or coagulopathy. No treatment is required for a subconjunctival hemorrhage; blood will usually reabsorb in 2 to 3 weeks.[19,29,45]

Penetrating Trauma

Penetrating injury to the eye may occur during work or play and is often associated with lack of protective eyewear. Injury may affect surface structures such as the cornea or involve damage to the globe.

PERIORBITAL WOUNDS. Periorbital wounds involve injury to the eyelids and surrounding periorbital tissue. Tissues lie in close proximity to the globe, so wounds should be examined carefully for globe penetration. Depending on mechanism of trauma, careful examination for foreign bodies should be part of the examination. Therapeutic interventions for lacerations include wound care and early closure with careful approximation of wound edges before edema develops. For major lacerations or injuries with missing tissue, a plastic surgeon is recommended. An ophthalmologist may be consulted to rule out ocular damage. The eyelid has an excellent blood supply, so trauma to the eyelid has a low incidence of infection; antibiotic treatment is rarely required.[29,41,44]

GLOBE RUPTURE. Globe rupture is a major ocular emergency that results from blunt or penetrating trauma. Rupture occurs at a point of weakness in the ocular structures, usually insertion of the extraocular muscles or the corneoscleral junction (limbus). Penetrating injuries to the globe are caused by perforation with a sharp object such as a knife, stick, or other projectile object. Blunt forces cause globe rupture secondary to an abrupt rise in IOP.

Signs and symptoms of globe rupture include an unusually deep or shallow anterior chamber, altered light perception, hyphema, and occasionally vitreous hemorrhage (Figure 45-8). The pupil assumes a teardrop shape with the tip pointing to the perforation. In addition, the patient may experience eye pain with nausea. When globe rupture is suspected, further eye manipulation should be avoided. If an impaled object is present, do not remove it. Secure the object, and patch the opposite eye to decrease eye movement and prevent further damage. Detailed examination is not performed until the ophthalmologist arrives; during this time a CT scan maybe ordered. General anesthesia may be necessary to perform an adequate examination. Eye drops should not be used when globe rupture is suspected. Aggressive pain management is crucial to prevent or decrease expulsion of intraocular contents. If the patient is nauseated, antiemetics should be given. Tetanus immunization should be updated. While waiting for the ophthalmologist, a Fox Shield or other protective device should be placed over the affected eye. The unaffected eye should be patched as well to minimize consensual movement. Keep the patient NPO (nothing by mouth), and prepare for surgery.[22,24,29]

Superficial Trauma

CORNEAL ABRASION. Corneal abrasions are a common injury seen in the ED. The cornea is damaged when a foreign body such as a contact lens scratches, abrades, or denudes the epithelium. Damage to the cornea exposes superficial corneal nerves, causing tearing, eyelid spasms, and pain. The patient will usually complain of a foreign body sensation, photophobia, and acute onset of pain.

Instillation of a drop of topical anesthesia will assist in obtaining a visual acuity. It will also alleviate the sensation of a foreign body and decrease pain. The upper eyelid should be inverted to ensure that no foreign body is found. Diagnosis is made with fluorescein staining and examination with a cobalt light and a slit-lamp examination. If the abrasion is large, cycloplegics may be prescribed to decrease ciliary spasms; however, there is no supporting evidence for this treatment.[3] Topical antibiotics are usually prescribed to prevent secondary infection. Additional medications that may be given are topical nonsteroidal agents and analgesics. Patching is no longer recommended as standard management of this injury; patching should never be done if the patient wears contact lenses. The injury should be reevaluated in 24 hours.[1,27,29,45]

CORNEAL LACERATIONS. Corneal lacerations present similarly to corneal abrasions; they may be small or large. Small lacerations are treated as corneal abrasions, or a corneal band aid maybe applied. Larger corneal lacerations may require surgery to preserve the integrity of intraocular contents. Corneal lacerations are identified by the Seidel test. The Seidel test uses fluorescein to detect the laceration; it will appear as a stream of dye on the cornea.[25] An ophthalmology consult is indicated for these patients.[21]

Foreign Body

CONJUNCTIVAL/CORNEAL FOREIGN BODY. The most common foreign body is a small particle of dust. The patient usually presents with photophobia, excessive tearing, or pain, especially when opening or closing the eye. Foreign bodies and corneal abrasions feel similar to the patient. With a foreign body, the first step is to locate the object. Local anesthesia may be required to examine the eye adequately. Good lighting and a magnification source are essential to locate and safely remove a foreign body from the eye.

With a suspected foreign body in the conjunctiva and cornea, determine identity of the foreign body (what the patient believes is in the eye). A history of high-speed projectiles should increase the index of suspicion for an intraocular foreign body. Organic foreign bodies have a higher incidence of infection, whereas metallic objects leave a rust ring unless the object is removed within 12 hours. Inert foreign bodies do not cause infection but have a greater risk for penetration.

Therapeutic intervention includes inverting the upper eyelid with a cotton-tipped swab, irrigating with normal saline solution, and gently removing the foreign body with a moistened cotton-tipped swab. Never use a dry cotton-tipped swab on the cornea because it may create a large corneal defect. If the foreign body adheres to the cornea, a topical anesthetic is applied, and then a 25- to 27-gauge needle is used at a tangential angle to remove the object. Larger embedded objects are referred to the ophthalmologist for removal or follow-up. After the foreign body is removed, the cornea should be carefully examined for other objects, rust ring, or corneal abrasion. Ocular burr drills are also used to remove rust rings and may be used to free foreign bodies stuck to the cornea. Treat subsequent corneal abrasions. If the patient has a rust ring, an ophthalmologic referral should be arranged so that the patient is seen within the next 24 hours.[16,29]

INTRAOCULAR FOREIGN BODY. Intraocular foreign bodies are usually small and easily overlooked. Metal fragments and other small projectiles enter the eye at high speed and come to rest within the posterior chamber. The entry site may be small and difficult to locate. A high index of suspicion is required to prompt a vigorous evaluation for this type of injury. Many patients experience only slight discomfort. Visual acuity may be significantly decreased or may be normal. The pupil may assume the shape of a cat's eye, which may indicate a ruptured globe.

An intraocular foreign body is an ocular emergency. Early therapeutic intervention is essential to preserve vision. The amount of damage to the eye depends on size, shape, and composition of the foreign body. All foreign bodies in the eye are considered contaminated, so the patient is treated with antibiotics and tetanus prophylaxis as appropriate. A CT scan is the best way to locate an intraocular foreign body. Surgery is indicated for most patients to prevent further damage to the eye secondary to hemorrhage, infection, or detached retina.[24,29]

Ocular Burns

Ocular burns pose an immediate threat to the patient's vision. Burns to the eye may result from a chemical, heat source such as a curling iron, or radiation. Regardless of cause, these injuries cause significant discomfort.

CHEMICAL TRAUMA. A chemical burn is the most urgent of all ocular emergencies. Chemical burns from acids, alkalis, or petroleum-based products occur at home and work. These substances, particularly alkalis, have a devastating effect on the eye. Acid burns cause immediate damage to the cornea by denaturing the tissue, so the cornea appears white and opaque. No further damage occurs after the initial impact because the acid is neutralized on contact. Alkalis such as concrete, lye, and drain cleaners also cause the cornea to opacify; however, alkalis continue to penetrate and damage the cornea until the substance is removed.[24,25]

Chemical burns are the only ocular emergency in which visual acuity is temporarily postponed. Copious irrigation should be initiated as soon as possible, preferably before the patient arrives in the ED. With alkaline burns, irrigation should continue until ocular pH reaches approximately 7.5 to 8. Irrigation for a minimum of 30 minutes with 2 L of fluid is the norm. The pH should be measured periodically during and after the initial irrigation. With severe cases, irrigation for 2 to 4 hours may be necessary. After pH reaches the desired level, the eyelid should be inverted, and then the cul-de-sac swabbed and irrigated to remove any remaining particles. Patients should receive topical antibiotics, cycloplegic agents, and steroids. Parenteral or oral narcotic analgesia is also recommended. Administer tetanus as appropriate. Obtain ophthalmologic consult for all ocular burns.[8,25,29]

THERMAL BURNS. Thermal burns affect the eyelids but rarely involve the globe because of reflex lid closure. Thermal burns are treated similarly to other burns that occur on the body. If the lids are damaged so they do not close adequately, special attention must be given to ensure that the globe is not injured. Burns to the eyelids may cause lid contracture, which is disfiguring and affects vision. Therapeutic interventions include analgesia, sedation, eye irrigation, antibiotics, cycloplegics, and bilateral eye patches.[24]

RADIATION BURNS. Radiation burns may be ultraviolet or infrared. Severity of the burn depends on wavelength and degree of exposure. Ultraviolet burns occur in welders, snow skiers, ice climbers, people who read on the beach, and those who use sun lamps. Ultraviolet radiation is absorbed by the cornea and produces keratitis, conjunctivitis,

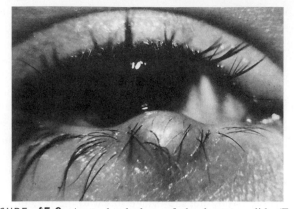

FIGURE **45-9.** Acute hordeolum of the lower eyelid. (From Newell FW: *Ophthalmology: principles and concepts,* ed 8, St. Louis, 1996, Mosby.)

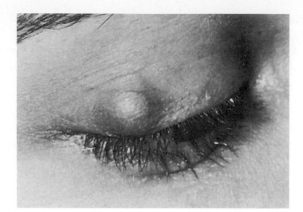

FIGURE **45-10.** Chronic chalazion of meibomian gland of the upper eyelid. (From Newell FW: *Ophthalmology: principles and concepts,* ed 8, St. Louis, 1996, Mosby.)

or both. Pain, tearing, photophobia, and a foreign body sensation usually begin 8 to 12 hours after exposure. Ultraviolet burns are considered the most painful of all ocular burns. Visual acuity is usually decreased. Therapeutic interventions include topical antibiotics, cycloplegics to reduce ciliary spasm, systemic analgesics, topical antibiotic ointment, and light avoidance (e.g., sunglasses or patching). The cornea usually heals within 24 hours without residual scarring. Slit-lamp examination with fluorescein staining reveals superficial punctate keratitis that looks like small microdots on the corneal surface.[24,29]

Infrared burns are more serious than radiation burns but uncommon, due primarily to use of protective eyewear. In the past, infrared injuries were associated with eclipses and atomic bomb detonation. In recent years, however, the laser has been implicated in causing infrared burns. Class IV lasers are the most dangerous to vision and are used in surgery, cutting, and drilling. The typical laser pointer is a Class II laser, classified as a low-power laser. Eye damage can be caused even with a Class II laser if someone is staring at the light.[26] Infrared injuries usually do not produce pain but can result in permanent loss of vision. A thorough examination is required to assess the degree of visual changes with referral to an ophthalmologist.

Medical Problems Involving the Eye

Many ocular problems that present to the ED are not related to trauma. Problems may be a minor annoyance or represent a significant threat to the patient's vision. The most common medical conditions seen in the ED are described in the following section.

Infections

LID INFECTIONS

Hordeolum. Hordeolum, or an external sty, is an infection of an eyelash oil gland of Zeis or Moll. The patient develops a small external abscess, pain, redness, and swelling (Figure 45-9). Therapeutic intervention includes application of warm compresses 4 times per day until the abscess comes

to a point. A hordeolum may rupture spontaneously; if unresponsive to a few weeks of conservative therapy, the patient should be referred to an ophthalmologist for consideration of incision and drainage. Ophthalmic antibiotic ointment should be applied every 4 hours. The patient should be instructed not to squeeze the abscess because this can spread infection and worsen the condition.[17,29]

Chalazion. A chalazion is an internal hordeolum caused by chronic granulomatous inflammation of the meibomian gland (Figure 45-10). The patient usually presents with several weeks of painless, localized swelling. A chalazion is differentiated from a hordeolum by the absence of acute inflammation. Treatment in the early stages includes topical antibiotic ointment; incision and drainage is indicated when the chalazion affects vision.[15,29]

Blepharitis. Blepharitis is an acute or chronic inflammation of the lid margin; the cause is multifactorial. Symptoms include burning, stinging, and itching of the lids, as well as conjunctival irritation. The eye appears rimmed with red, and scales may appear on the lashes. There are no specific diagnostic tests; however, a culture of the lids may be performed to determine if the condition is caused by a staphylococcal infection. Treatment consists of removing the crusts and cleaning lid margins twice daily with a mild shampoo, warm compresses, and use of artificial tears; severe blepharitis is treated with an antibiotic ophthalmic ointment.[1,14]

CORNEAL INFECTIONS

Keratitis. Keratitis is a generic term for inflammation of the cornea. The cornea becomes light sensitive, red, and painful, with profuse tearing. A corneal ulcer, bacteria, or fungus may cause keratitis. Risk factors for keratitis include ultraviolet light exposure and corneal injury secondary to contact lens use (*Acanthamoeba* keratitis), viral infections, and blepharitis. The typical presentation is conjunctivitis, pain, photophobia, mucopurulent discharge, and decreased vision. Pus in the anterior chamber (hypopyon) may also be present. Culture and sensitivity should be obtained to determine the specific cause of the infection. Therapeutic interventions include warm compresses, broad-spectrum antibiotics, and possibly fungal drops. A topical cycloplegic agent may be used to control pain. The eye should not be patched because of the risk for *Pseudomonas* organism infection. Referral to an ophthalmologist within 24 hours is required to prevent further complications.[1,29]

Viral Keratoconjunctivitis. Viral keratoconjunctivitis is an acute conjunctivitis and keratitis usually caused by adenovirus. The patient complains of redness to the eye, tearing, and pain.[1,20] Photophobia usually begins several days later. Eyelids and conjunctiva become swollen. In adults this condition is confined to the eye; however, children may have fever, pharyngitis, and diarrhea. Therapeutic intervention is usually symptomatic. Topical antibiotics may be started while awaiting culture results. This type of infection spreads easily; therefore it is critical to stress scrupulous hand washing to the patient. All instruments used on the patient should be sterilized.

HERPES SIMPLEX. Herpes simplex infection can affect the eyelids, conjunctiva, and the cornea. Symptoms include watery discharge, burning, and a foreign body sensation. Skin involvement includes vesicular lesions; the conjunctiva appears inflamed. Fluorescein staining reveals a corneal dendrite. Outbreaks on the lids and conjunctiva can be treated with oral and topical antiviral agents. Ophthalmology referral in 2 to 3 days is recommended.[1,20,29]

HERPES ZOSTER OPHTHALMICUS. Herpes zoster ophthalmicus represents shingles in the ophthalmic division of the trigeminal nerve. Patients will often have prodromal signs of fever, fatigue, and malaise before the eruption of vesicles along the affected dermatome appearing as a unilateral rash over the forehead, upper eyelid, and nose. Patients will often have significant pain and scalp tenderness on half the forehead. If the tip of the nose is involved, ocular involvement is more likely (Hutchinson's sign). Standard management includes local wound care, analgesics, and antiviral therapy; topical steroids may be indicated for ocular involvement, and antibiotics may be required for secondary bacterial infection of the lesions. Administration of antivirals, specifically within 72 hours of vesicular eruption, has been demonstrated to decrease complications. At times hospitalization may be necessary for intravenous acyclovir, especially if any intracranial symptoms are present or if the patient is immunocompromised.[1,10,29]

Long-term complications include permanent loss of sight and postherpetic neuralgia.

CONJUNCTIVITIS. Conjunctivitis, or pink eye, is a frequent problem seen in the ED. Conjunctivitis has many etiologic factors: bacterial, viral, or allergic.

Bacterial conjunctivitis usually presents with a yellow-green purulent discharge. Patients will usually complain that eyes are matted shut in the morning. This infection can involve one or both eyes. It is important to ask the patient if he or she been exposed to someone with pink eye. Infections can be caused by *Streptococcus pneumoniae, Staphylococcus aureus,* and *Moraxella* and *Haemophilus* organisms.[1,11,35] Signs and symptoms of bacterial infection include purulent discharge, reddened eye, and swollen eyelid associated with

tenderness; symptoms are usually unilateral. Treatment usually consists of a topical ocular antibiotic for 5 to 7 days. For contact lens wearers, a fluoroquinolone or aminoglycoside is prescribed to cover a *Pseudomonal* organism infection. Warm soaks are used to keep the lids and lashes free of debris.[35]

Bacterial and viral conjunctivitis are both contagious. Detailed aftercare instructions should include how to prevent the disease from spreading. Teaching should include discussion of cross-contamination through eye makeup, pillows, washcloths, and towels. Children should be kept out of school until the discharge subsides. Appropriate hand-washing techniques should also be reviewed.[1,35]

Conjunctivitis secondary to *Neisseria gonorrhoeae* causes copious purulent discharge with extremely red and swollen conjunctiva. The clue to this type of conjunctivitis is the amount of discharge; it has been described as "a waterfall of pus."[1] Gonococcal conjunctivitis is usually seen in sexually active adolescents and in newborns. Diagnosis is made on the presence of purulent discharge from the eyes; genital discharge may also be noted. A positive culture confirms the diagnosis by showing gram-negative diplococci.[1] Therapeutic intervention is ceftriaxone 125 mg intramuscularly or intravenously. There is controversy on the optimal dosage; however, based on Centers for Disease Control and Prevention guidelines, 125 mg intramuscularly is recommended.[47] Immediate referral to an ophthalmologist is essential, because this condition left untreated can result in permanent visual impairment. Other potential contacts, including sexual contacts, should be treated.[37]

Viral conjunctivitis is usually caused by an adenovirus. Viral infections are highly contagious and may accompany an upper respiratory infection. Onset is usually abrupt and unilateral (rapidly progressing to bilateral) and at times resembles a cold. Eye drainage is usually clear, and the conjunctiva is reddened. Treatment consists of cool compresses and artificial tears; decongestant or antihistamine eye drops may be used. A topical antibiotic may be prescribed if the diagnosis is uncertain; however, evidence does not support this management.[1] Detailed aftercare instructions should include how to prevent the disease from spreading.[29]

Allergic conjunctivitis is usually caused by an allergen that causes the eye to tear and the lids to itch. Treatment may consist of eye drops containing antihistamines, decongestants, and/or nonsteroidal agents; cool compresses; and systemic antihistamines.[29]

UVEITIS/IRITIS. Uveitis/iritis is an inflammation of the uveal tract, including the iris, ciliary body, and choroid. Uveal inflammation usually affects the anterior portion of the uveal tract and is categorized as iritis. Uveitis can be caused by inflammation, infection, or trauma. Symptoms include decreased vision, photophobia, pain with direct and consensual light reflex, reddened eye, and excessive tearing. Anterior uveitis and iritis need an ophthalmic referral. Initial treatment includes cycloplegics and topical steroids. This decreases photophobia and inflammation.[1,20]

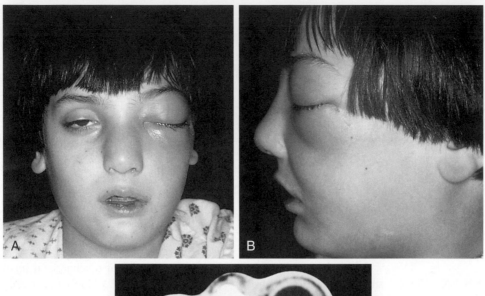

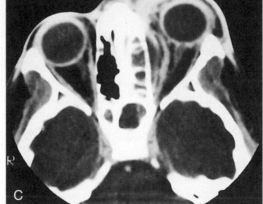

FIGURE 45-11. Orbital cellulitis. **A** and **B,** This child had a fever, severe toxicity, and marked lethargy. He experienced intense orbital and retroorbital pain, and showed a limited range of ocular motion. **C,** This computed tomography scan shows preseptal swelling, proptosis, and lateral displacement of the globe and orbital contents by a subperiosteal abscess. (From Zitelli B, Davis H: *Atlas of pediatric physical diagnosis,* ed 4, St. Louis, 2002, Mosby.)

ORBITAL CELLULITIS. Orbital cellulitis (Figure 45-11), an infection deep into the orbital septum, can be a life-threatening infection. Usual causes are *S. pneumoniae, S. aureus,* and *Haemophilus influenzae.* There is usually an associated sinus infection. Symptoms include pain, fever, and impaired EOM. Impaired EOM is a crucial clue to differentiating between periorbital cellulitis and orbital cellulitis. With periorbital cellulitis there is no impairment of the extraocular muscles. Decreased visual acuity is a late finding. A CT scan of the orbits and sinuses, blood cultures, and admission to the hospital is required. The patient is given intravenous antibiotics. Immediate ophthalmologic referral is required.[1]

Orbital cellulitis may progress to a life-threatening condition called cavernous sinus thrombosis. This is an infection that has spread from an infected sinus to the orbital area. Signs and symptoms include chills, headache, lethargy, nausea, pain, and decreased vision. The patient may also have fever, vomiting, and other signs of systemic involvement.[6,29]

Retinal Emergencies

CENTRAL RETINAL ARTERY OCCLUSION. Central retinal artery occlusion (CRO) produces sudden, painless blindness and is usually limited to one eye. This is a true ocular emergency. Retinal circulation must be reestablished within 60 to 90 minutes to prevent permanent loss of vision. Occasionally, before total occlusion occurs, the patient may experience transient episodes of blindness called amaurosis fugax. This can be equated to a transient ischemia attack of the retinal artery. Patients usually describe the episode as a shade coming down over the eye. Causes of CRO include embolus (carotid and cardiac), thrombosis, hypertension, giant cell arteritis, or simple angiospasm (rare) associated with a migraine or atrial fibrillation. Hence the patient will need to be thoroughly evaluated to rule out other systemic problems. To prevent permanent damage, retinal perfusion needs to be reestablished as rapidly as possible. Interventions include vasodilation techniques (having the patient breathe into a paper bag), ocular massage, and administration of

IOP-lowering drugs, none of which have been shown to be extremely beneficial.[1,12,20]

RETINAL DETACHMENT. Retinal detachment occurs when the retina tears and allows vitreous humor to seep between the retina and the choroid. Normal function of the retina is to perceive light and send an impulse to the optic nerve. When the retina is torn, loss of blood and oxygen supply renders the retina unable to perceive light. With retinal detachment, the patient complains of "flashing lights," "floaters," and a "veil" or curtain effect in the visual field. The prognosis is excellent if treated early. Diagnostic workup may include CT, MRI, or ultrasonography. Based on the medical evidence, ophthalmic ultrasonography appears to be the superior testing method.[20] Ophthalmologic consultation for immediate referral is necessary for definitive treatment (laser repair or scleral buckling).[1,9,20,29]

Glaucoma

Glaucoma is the second most common cause of blindness in the United States. Glaucoma occurs when aqueous humor cannot escape from the anterior chamber, causing volume to increase and IOP to rise. Normally, aqueous humor leaves the anterior chamber and enters the vascular system via Schlemm's canal at the junction of the iris and cornea. With glaucoma, increased anterior chamber pressure decreases circulation to the retina and increases pressure on the optic nerve. If left untreated, these high pressures eventually cause blindness.

Glaucoma is classified as primary or secondary and open angle or closed angle. Secondary glaucoma is associated with some type of underlying ocular or systemic condition, whereas with primary glaucoma there is no underlying or known cause. Closed-angle glaucoma is caused when the anterior chamber angle is narrowed; open-angle glaucoma has a normal anterior chamber angle. Primary open-angle glaucoma is the most common form of glaucoma. The most concerning type of glaucoma is primary angle-closure glaucoma (PACG).

ACUTE ANGLE-CLOSURE GLAUCOMA. The prevalence of PACG increases with age and is more common in women. There is a higher incidence of acute angle-closure glaucoma in Asians and Eskimos.[23] PACG is estimated to be the cause of 46% of all cases of irreversible blindness worldwide.[5] Acute angle-closure glaucoma occurs with blockage of the anterior chamber angle near the root of the iris (Figure 45-12). The patient presents with severe eye pain, a fixed and slightly dilated pupil, hard globe, foggy-appearing cornea, severe headache, complaints of halos around lights, diminished peripheral vision, and nausea and vomiting.[23] IOP greater than 60 to 70 mm Hg damages the corneal endothelium, lens, iris, optical nerve, and retina. Diagnosis may be difficult because symptoms can mimic cardiovascular or gastrointestinal processes. Therapeutic intervention focuses on decreasing IOP as quickly as possible by decreasing production and increasing removal of aqueous humor. Treatment includes topical miotics (e.g., pilocarpine 2%), β-blockers (e.g., timolol 0.5%), and carbonic anhydrase inhibitors (e.g., acetazolamide, Diamox). Antiemetics and narcotics may be

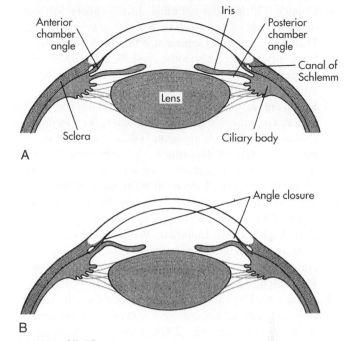

FIGURE **45-12.** Comparison of normal angle of eye (**A**) with closed angle in angle-closure glaucoma (**B**).

useful. Ophthalmologic consultation for definitive treatment is required.[1,23,27,29]

Summary

Most ocular emergencies do not represent a threat to the patient's life; however, these conditions represent a great threat to the patient's well-being. Once lost, vision cannot be replaced. The emergency nurse should assess the patients who present with various ocular problems and identify those patients with actual or potential threats to vision. Early recognition of true ocular emergencies is essential for preservation of sight.

REFERENCES

1. Alteveer JG, McCans K: The red eye, the swollen eye, and acute vision loss: handling non-traumatic eye disorders in the ED, *Emerg Med Pract* 4(6):1, 2002.
2. Blais BR: *Eye*, 2004, updated August 17, 2007, National Guideline Clearinghouse. Retrieved July 12, 2008, from http://www.guideline.gov.
3. Carley F, Carley S: Towards evidence based emergency medicine: best BETs from the Manchester Royal Infirmary—mydriatics in corneal abrasion, *Emerg Med J* 18:270, 2001.
4. Chech A I: Ocular burns, 2006, *eMedicine*. Retrieved July 12, 2008, from http://www.emedicine.com/emger/topic736.htm.
5. Coleman AL, Law SK: *Primary angle-closure glaucoma,* July 2007. Retrieved July 12, 2008, from http://www.medscape.com/viewprogram/ 7394_pnt.

6. Conners GP: Orbital cellulitis. In Greenberg MI, editor: *Greenberg's text-atlas of emergency medicine*, Philadelphia, 2005, Lippincott Williams & Wilkins.

7. Eggenberger ER: Anisocoria, June 29, 2007, *eMedicine*. Retrieved July 12, 2008, from http://www.emedicine. com/oph/topic160.htm.

8. Eisenberg J: Ocular alkali injury. In Greenberg MI, editor: *Greenberg's text-atlas of emergency medicine*, Philadelphia, 2005, Lippincott Williams & Wilkins.

9. Fintak D: Retinal detachment. In Greenberg MI, editor: *Greenberg's text-atlas of emergency medicine*, Philadelphia, 2005, Lippincott Williams & Wilkins.

10. Gejer W: Herpes zoster ophthalmicus. In Greenberg MI, editor: *Greenberg's text-atlas of emergency medicine*, Philadelphia, 2005, Lippincott Williams & Wilkins.

11. Gorton N: Bacterial conjunctivitis. In Greenberg MI, editor: *Greenberg's text-atlas of emergency medicine*, Philadelphia, 2005, Lippincott Williams & Wilkins.

12. Gorton N: Central retinal artery occlusion. In Greenberg MI, editor: *Greenberg's text-atlas of emergency medicine*, Philadelphia, 2005, Lippincott Williams & Wilkins.

13. Greenberg M: Anisocoria. In Greenberg MI, editor: *Greenberg's text-atlas of emergency medicine*, Philadelphia, 2005, Lippincott Williams & Wilkins.

14. Greenberg M: Blepharitis. In Greenberg MI, editor: *Greenberg's text-atlas of emergency medicine*, Philadelphia, 2005, Lippincott Williams & Wilkins.

15. Greenberg M: Chalazion. In Greenberg MI, editor: *Greenberg's text-atlas of emergency medicine*, Philadelphia, 2005, Lippincott Williams & Wilkins.

16. Greenberg M: Corneal/Conjunctival foreign body. In Greenberg MI, editor: *Greenberg's text-atlas of emergency medicine*, Philadelphia, 2005, Lippincott Williams & Wilkins.

17. Greenberg M: Hordeolum. In Greenberg MI, editor: *Greenberg's text-atlas of emergency medicine*, Philadelphia, 2005, Lippincott Williams & Wilkins.

18. Greenberg M: Hyphema. In Greenberg MI, editor: *Greenberg's text-atlas of emergency medicine*, Philadelphia, 2005, Lippincott Williams & Wilkins.

19. Greenberg M: Subconjunctival hemorrhage. In Greenberg MI, editor: *Greenberg's text-atlas of emergency medicine*, Philadelphia, 2005, Lippincott Williams & Wilkins.

20. Guluma K: An evidence-based approach to abnormal vision, *Emerg Med Pract* 9(9):1, 2007.

21. Haroz R: Corneal laceration. In Greenberg MI, editor: *Greenberg's text-atlas of emergency medicine*, Philadelphia, 2005, Lippincott Williams & Wilkins.

22. Horowitz M: Ruptured globe. In Greenberg MI, editor: *Greenberg's text-atlas of emergency medicine*, Philadelphia, 2005, Lippincott Williams & Wilkins.

23. Jackson J, Carr LW, Fisch BM et al: *Optometric clinical practice guideline: care of the patient with primary angle closure glaucoma*, St. Louis, 2001, American Optometric Association.

24. Kim G, Witt M: Ocular trauma: an evidence-based approach to evaluation and management in the ED, *Pediatr Emerg Med Pract* 3(11):1, 2006.

25. Knoop KJ, Dennis WR, Hedges JR: Ophthalmologic procedures. In Roberts JR, Hedges JR, editors: *Clinical procedures in emergency medicine*, ed 4, Philadelphia, 2004, WB Saunders.

26. *Laser safety*. Retrieved July 12, 2008, from http://www. microscopyu.com/articles/fluorescence/lasersafety. html.

27. Mazzeo AS: Corneal abrasion. In Greenberg MI, editor: *Greenberg's text-atlas of emergency medicine*, Philadelphia, 2005, Lippincott Williams & Wilkins.

28. McCaig LF, Nawar EW: *National hospital ambulatory medical care survey: 2004 emergency department summary*, Washington, DC, 2006, U.S. Department of Health and Human Services, No. 372.

29. Mitchell JD: Ocular emergencies. In Tintinalli JE, Kelen GD, Stapczynski JS, editors: *Emergency medicine: a comprehensive study guide*, ed 6, New York, 2004, McGraw-Hill.

30. Nervi SJ: Chemical burns, June 20, 2006, *eMedicine*. Retrieved July 12, 2008, from http://www.emedicine. com/ped/topic2735.thm.

31. Quigley MT: Assessing visual acuity, In Proehl JA, editor: *Emergency nursing procedures*, ed 3, St. Louis, 2004, WB Saunders.

32. Quigley MT: Eye irrigation. In Proehl JA, editor: *Emergency nursing procedures*, ed 3, St. Louis, 2004, WB Saunders.

33. Quigley MT: Eye patching. In Proehl JA, editor: *Emergency nursing procedures*, ed 3, St. Louis, 2004, WB Saunders.

34. Quigley MT: Tonometry. In Proehl JA, editor: *Emergency nursing procedures*, ed 3, St. Louis, 2004, Saunders.

35. Quinn CJ, Matthews DE, Noyes RF, et al: *Optometric clinical practice guideline: care of the patient with conjunctivitis*, ed 2, St. Louis 2002, American Optometric Association.

36. Rabiu TA: Patching for corneal abrasion, *Cochran Database Syst Rev* 2006(2):CD004764, DOI:10.1002/ 14651858.CD004764.pub2.

37. Roemer B: Gonococcal conjunctivitis. In Greenberg MI, editor: *Greenberg's text-atlas of emergency medicine*, Philadelphia, 2005, Lippincott Williams & Wilkins.

38. Saidinejad M, Burns MD: Ocular irrigant alternatives in pediatric emergency medicine, *Pediatr Emerg Care* 21(1):23, 2005.

39. Sheppard JD: Hyphema, November 3, 2006, *eMedicine*. Retrieved July 12, 2008, from http://www.emedicine. com/oph/topic765.htm.

40. Stitzel JD, Hansen GA, Herring IP et al: Blunt trauma and the aging eye, *Arch Ophthalmol* 123(6):789, 2005.

41. Trobe JD, Hackel RE: Managing common ophthalmic problems, In Trobe JD, Hackel RE, editors: *Field guide to the eyes*, Philadelphia, 2002, Lippincott Williams & Wilkins.

42. Trobe JD, Hackel RE: Orbital wall fracture. In Trobe JD, Hackel RE, editors: *Field guide to the eyes*, Philadelphia, 2002, Lippincott Williams & Wilkins.

43. Trobe JD, Hackel RE: Traumatic hyphema. In Trobe JD, Hackel RE, editors: *Field guide to the eyes*, Philadelphia, 2002, Lippincott Williams & Wilkins.

44. Trott AT: Special anatomic sites. In Trott AT, editor: *Wounds and laceration emergency care and closure*, ed 3, Philadelphia, 2005, Mosby.

45. Uphold CR, Graham MV: Corneal abrasion. In Uphold CR, Graham MV, editors: *Clinical guidelines in family practice*, ed 4, Gainesville, Fla, 2003, Barmarrae Books Inc.

46. Wallis LA, Greaves I: Injuries associated with airbag deployment, *Emerg Med J* 19:490, 2002, http://www.emjonline.com.

47. Workowski KA, Berman SM: Sexually transmitted diseases treatment guidelines, 2006. *MMWR Recomm Rep* 55(RR-11):1, 2006.

UNIT VI

Special Patient Populations

CHAPTER 46

Obstetric Emergencies

Donna L. Mason

mergency departments (EDs) handle obstetric emergencies throughout all stages of pregnancy. The goal for obstetric emergencies is to stabilize the mother and ultimately prevent any harm to the unborn child or children. Management of obstetric emergencies requires acute assessment skills to identify life-threatening conditions and rapid intervention to prevent adverse outcomes for mother and baby. This chapter describes changes in pathophysiology related to pregnancy, assessment of the pregnant patient, and management of emergencies commonly associated with pregnancy. Refer to Chapter 29 for discussion of obstetric trauma.

ANATOMY AND PHYSIOLOGY

The female reproductive system consists of the fallopian tubes, ovaries, uterus, vagina, and external genitalia. The cervical os, or opening to the uterus, is located within the vagina. The vagina serves as the exit route for menstrual blood flow, entry point for sperm, and the birth canal. Physiologic activity of the reproductive system is cyclic. Each month the uterus prepares for implantation of a fertilized egg through proliferation of the uterine endometrium. Eggs are stored in the ovaries and released in a cyclic pattern. If the egg is not fertilized, the uterine lining sloughs and is shed as menstrual blood flow. If the egg is fertilized, it begins to reproduce and replicate. The embryo is formed, transported through the

fallopian tube, and embedded in the uterine wall to continue its growth.

As the pregnancy progresses, it is characterized by an increasing embryo size and development of various sexual organs. Uterine size increases from about 50 g to about 1100 g.[4] Concurrently, breast size doubles and the vagina enlarges. Total weight gain during pregnancy is about 25 pounds. Other body systems affected by pregnancy include the cardiovascular, respiratory, gastrointestinal, and genitourinary systems (Table 46-1).

PATIENT ASSESSMENT

Many EDs will provide pregnancy-related care for patients; however, some provide care only for complaints not related to the pregnancy (e.g., colds, flu, sprains, strains, fractures, and lacerations). Each pregnant patient should be carefully assessed and referred to other specialty care as needed (Box 46-1).

Regardless of gestational age, the priorities for assessments for a woman with an obstetric emergency are airway, breathing, and circulation (ABCs). The age of fetal viability is considered 24 weeks' gestation, and though there has been an increased rate of survivability before 24 weeks' gestation, complications to the preterm infant are greater. Management of obstetric emergencies after onset of fetal viability involves two patients, mother and fetus.

Table 46-1.	PHYSIOLOGIC CHANGES RELATED TO PREGNANCY
Body System	**Changes**
Cardiovascular	Cardiac output increases 30%-40% by week 27.
	Placental blood flow is 625-650 mL/min.
	Blood volume increases by 30%.
	Heart rate increases throughout pregnancy.
Respiratory	Respiratory rate increases.
	Oxygen consumption increases by 20%.
	Minute volume increases by 50%.
	Arterial pCO_2 decreases secondary to hyperventilation.
Urinary	Rate of urine formation increases slightly.
	Sodium, chloride, and water reabsorption increases as much as 50%.
	Glomerular filtration rate increases about 50%.
Gastrointestinal	Smooth muscle relaxes, which increases gastric emptying time.
	Intestines are relocated to the upper abdomen.
Other	Anemia develops because of increased iron requirements by mother and fetus.

pCO_2, Pressure of carbon dioxide.

Box 46-1	ASSESSMENT GUIDELINES FOR THE PREGNANT PATIENT

Last normal menstrual period
Birth control method
Gravida, parity, and abortion history
Bleeding, discharge, or tissue present
Nausea or vomiting
Urinary symptoms
Abdominal pain—location, duration, description
Estimated date of confinement
Prenatal care
Problems with present or previous pregnancies
Medications and allergies
Maternal medical and surgical history
Blood type and Rh factor if known

See Chapter 47 for discussion of neonatal resuscitation. After assessment of the patient's ABCs, the next priority is determination of gestational age and evaluation for impending delivery. Specific emergencies are divided into those associated with the first, second, and third trimester and the postpartum period.

FIRST-TRIMESTER EMERGENCIES

First-trimester emergencies involve only one patient—the mother. Mortality is usually related to blood loss. Other issues relate to loss of pregnancy and potential loss of fertility.

Ectopic Pregnancy

Ectopic pregnancies often result from scarring caused by a past infection in the fallopian tubes, surgery on the fallopian tubes, or a previous ectopic pregnancy. Up to 50% of women who have ectopic pregnancies have a past history of inflammation of the fallopian tubes (salpingitis) or pelvic inflammatory disease (PID).[6]

Ectopic pregnancy occurs when the fertilized ovum implants anywhere other than the endometrium, such as in the fallopian tube, ovary, or abdominal cavity. Ninety-five percent of all ectopic pregnancies occur in one of the fallopian tubes, with the most common site for implantation being the ampulla followed by the isthmus (Figure 46-1). The ovum begins to grow but may rupture, usually after the twelfth week of pregnancy. Ectopic pregnancy is one of the major causes of maternal death, usually from hemorrhage.

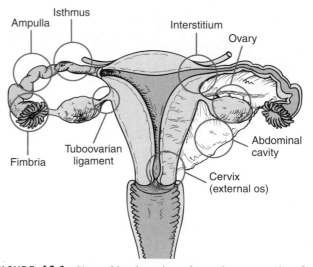

FIGURE 46-1. Sites of implantation of ectopic pregnancies. Order of frequency of occurrence is ampulla, isthmus, interstitium, fimbria, tuboovarian ligament, ovary, abdominal cavity, and cervix (external os). (From Lewis SL, Heitkemper MM, Dirksen SR et al: *Medical-surgical nursing: assessment and management of clinical problems,* ed 7, St. Louis, 2007, Mosby.)

On assessment the patient gives a history of being pregnant, usually about 12 weeks. However, 15% of patients with ectopic pregnancy are symptomatic before the first missed period. Complaints include pelvic pain or vaginal bleeding. Pain, if present, may be mild to severe. If the ectopic pregnancy is leaking or has ruptured, the diaphragm may become irritated from blood in the peritoneum, causing referred pain to the shoulder (Kehr's sign).

A pregnancy test should be obtained on all women presenting with pelvic pain and vaginal bleeding or spotting. A pelvic examination is done to evaluate the cervical os and identify the amount and source of bleeding. Bimanual pelvic examination defines uterine size and allows for palpation of masses outside the uterus.

If an ectopic pregnancy is suspected, intravenous (IV) access should be established with a large-bore IV catheter in anticipation of potential life-threatening hemorrhage. Quantitative serum β-human chorionic gonadotropin (β-hCG) level, complete blood count (CBC), and type and screen should be obtained. An ultrasound scan is done to identify an ectopic pregnancy.

Treatment for ectopic pregnancy includes nonoperative and operative interventions. For selected cases, ectopic pregnancy can be medically managed as an alternative to surgery. Methotrexate, a folic acid antagonist that prevents further duplication of fetal cells, is administered intramuscularly, and the patient is followed as an outpatient with serial β-hCG tests. Occasionally β-hCG levels do not fall, so additional methotrexate injections may be necessary. Operative interventions are indicated when the ectopic pregnancy has ruptured, the patient is in shock, or nonoperative interventions are unsuccessful or not appropriate.

In addition to assessment and intervention for physiologic needs, the emergency nurse must recognize the need for emotional support for the patient and the family. The patient may fear for her life and her future childbearing ability, feel concern because the pregnancy is not normal, or experience personal guilt related to the pregnancy.

Abortion

Abortion is defined as any interruption in pregnancy that occurs before the fetus is viable. Fetal viability is usually between 20 and 24 weeks' gestation or fetal weight of 500 g. This can occur spontaneously as a miscarriage or be artificially induced by chemical, surgical, or other means.[2]

Abortion is the number one cause of vaginal bleeding in women of childbearing years, with an estimated 10% to 15% of all pregnancies resulting in spontaneous abortion.[3] This is one of the differential diagnoses for any woman of childbearing years with vaginal bleeding. Table 46-2 summarizes the types of abortion. Causes of abortion include infection, injury, and an incompetent cervix.

The patient presents to the ED complaining of vaginal bleeding with abdominal pain frequently noted. A missed period may or may not be reported. Gynecologic history should be elicited from the patient, including amount of bleeding. Ask the patient how many pads or tampons she has used in the past hour; a general rule of thumb is a saturated pad or tampon equals 5 to 15 mL of blood loss.

Obtain a urine pregnancy test or serum β-hCG level. Palpate the patient's abdomen for pain or tenderness, which may indicate ectopic pregnancy. A pelvic examination determines the source of bleeding, visualizes any products of conception, and determines dilatation of the cervical os. Observe for vaginal discharge. A bimanual examination is performed to determine the size of the uterus and other reproductive organs, and palpation is performed to determine tenderness. Consider ultrasonography to exclude ectopic pregnancy.

Therapeutic interventions depend on the type of abortion. Fifty percent of threatened abortions result in complete or incomplete abortion within a few hours. A patient with a threatened abortion should be observed closely for changes

Table 46-2. TYPES OF ABORTION

Type	Signs and Symptoms
Threatened	Vaginal bleeding
	Mild abdominal cramping
	Closed or slightly open os
Inevitable	Heavy vaginal bleeding
	Severe abdominal cramping
	Open os
Incomplete	Heavy vaginal bleeding
	Abdominal cramping
	Some products of conception retained
Complete	Slight vaginal bleeding
	No abdominal cramping
	All products of conception passed
Missed	Usually no maternal symptoms
	Discrepancy in fetal size when compared to dates
Septic	Severe abdominal pain
	High temperature
	Malodorous vaginal discharge

in hemodynamic status. Document the amount of blood loss. If the patient exhibits signs of shock, replace blood loss with fluids or blood. Provide emotional support to the patient, significant other, and family.

If the abortion is inevitable or incomplete, obtain blood for CBC, Rh type, and type and screen. Start at least one IV line with a large-bore catheter, and administer fluids (normal saline or lactated Ringer's solution). Prepare for suction curettage, which may be performed in the operating room, labor and delivery area, or in some cases, the ED.

If the patient will be discharged, aftercare instructions should include information on bed rest and instructions to return to the ED or call the primary caregiver for increased vaginal bleeding, increasing abdominal pain, passage of tissue, fever, or chills. The patient should also be told to avoid douching and intercourse while on bed rest because these can increase vaginal bleeding, worsen cramping, or cause infection if the cervical os begins to open. The patient should be instructed to follow up with the appropriate referral caregiver. RhoGAM should be given within 72 hours if the mother is Rh negative.

ANTEPARTUM EMERGENCIES

Emergencies that occur during the last months of pregnancy threaten the mother and the fetus. Neurologic sequelae such as seizures and anoxic brain damage are also possible.

Pregnancy-Induced Hypertension

The term *pregnancy-induced hypertension* (PIH) refers to toxemia of pregnancy and includes preeclampsia and eclampsia. This condition usually occurs in the last few months of pregnancy (after 20 weeks' gestation) and can appear up to 2 weeks after delivery. Actual etiology is unknown, though the syndrome occurs most often in women who have a family history of preeclampsia, are primigravida, or are younger than 20 years or older than 40 years of age. There is also increased risk if there is a history of chronic vascular disease, renal disease, diabetes, multiple fetuses, or hydatidiform mole. PIH can cause maternal morbidity and mortality with high fetal mortality.

PIH is characterized by hypertension, proteinuria, and edema. Systolic blood pressure is greater than 140 mm Hg, or there is an increase of 30 mm Hg over the nonpregnant level. An increase of 15 mm Hg of the diastolic over baseline or diastolic blood pressure of 90 mm Hg or more is classified as hypertension.[2] Hypertension leads to vasospasm and hemolysis and affects several organ systems.

Blood pressure elevation is the paramount symptom of preeclampsia, and readings are compared to prenatal or early pregnancy blood pressure measurements. Proteinuria is a late sign and is an indicator of severity of the disease. Edema is the least reliable sign because of the normal frequency of occurrence during pregnancy. However, sudden onset of facial edema with weight gain is a significant indicator of preeclampsia (Table 46-3). Pulmonary edema may also be present. Subjective signs of preeclampsia may include visual changes, headaches, epigastric pain, and decreased urination. Preeclampsia left untreated may progress to eclampsia. In eclampsia the patient presents with seizures or coma. This situation is an immediate threat to the mother and fetus.

Treatment includes oxygen, IV access, and fetal monitoring. The woman is placed in the left lateral recumbent position,

so the gravid uterus does not cause aortocaval compression. Pharmacologic therapy to control hypertension is usually initiated when diastolic blood pressure is higher than 90 to 100 mm Hg. Magnesium sulfate is the drug of choice to prevent seizures. Continuous monitoring, including blood pressure, pulse, and respirations every 15 to 30 minutes, is essential to identify changes in the patient's condition due to PIH and magnesium toxicity. Signs of magnesium toxicity include absent deep tendon reflexes, respirations less than 12 per minute, urine output less than 30 mL/hr or 120 mL/4 hr, and signs of fetal distress. If magnesium toxicity occurs, the patient is given calcium gluconate 1 g IV. Lorazepam can be used to control seizures, although magnesium may also be considered. Fetal monitoring is essential. Any drop in fetal heart rate or deceleration of heart rate during contractions indicates the need for immediate emergency cesarean section. Delivery does not always resolve preeclampsia. Symptoms of concern up to 6 weeks following delivery include headache, elevated blood pressure, vision changes, oliguria, and decreased platelets. These patients should receive a high priority for care.

HELLP Syndrome

The HELLP syndrome is a potentially life-threatening form of preeclampsia that occurs when the patient develops multiple organ damage. *H*emolysis, *E*levated *L*iver enzymes, and *L*ow *P*latelets (HELLP) affects up to 12% of women with

Table 46-3.   CHARACTERISTICS OF MILD VERSUS SEVERE PREECLAMPSIA

Characteristics	Mild Preeclampsia	Severe Preeclampsia
Blood pressure	Greater than 140/90 mm Hg but less than 160/110 mm Hg 30 mm Hg systolic rise; or 15 mm Hg diastolic rise over baseline readings of early pregnancy (Readings are obtained after rest in a sitting position two times at least 6 hr apart)	Blood pressure greater than 160/110 mm Hg
Proteinuria (albuminuria)	300 mg/L/24 hr or two separate random daytime specimens 6 hr apart (true clean catch) of 1+, 2+	5 g or more per 24 hr, 3+, 4+ in true clean-catch or catheterized specimen
Edema	Weight gain of more than 3 lbs (1.4 kg) per week or 6 lbs (2.72 kg) per month—any sudden weight gain is suspicious Minimal or marked edema 1+, 2+ of lower extremities	Weight gain advances at accelerated rate Edema more pronounced, especially of hands, face 3+, 4+ (as condition worsens, edema of lungs, brain, and other organs)
Urine output	Not below 500 mL/24 hr	Oliguria less than 500 mL/24 hr
Neurologic signs and symptoms	Absent or only occasional headaches, blurred vision, or spots before eyes Normal peripheral reflexes	More persistent headaches, blurred vision, and spots before eyes—retinal arteriole spasms on ophthalmic examination Hyperactive knee jerk and other tendon reflexes +3, +4 with clonus Irritability, tinnitus
Other organ involvement		Liver involvement causing epigastric or right upper quadrant abdominal pain, nausea, vomiting (often said to precede convulsion/ coma or onset of eclampsia) Pulmonary edema manifested by respiratory distress, rales, cyanosis

From Novak JC, Broom BL: *Ingalls and Salerno's maternal and child health nursing,* ed 9, St. Louis, 1999, Mosby.

preeclampsia-eclampsia syndrome.[2] Unlike preeclampsia, which usually affects primigravidas, HELLP syndrome is more common among the multigravida population. HELLP syndrome, characterized by complaints of epigastric or right upper quadrant pain, can imitate a variety of nonobstetric medical problems. Serious medical and surgical pathologic conditions must be ruled out (Box 46-2).

Clinically the woman develops respiratory distress, usually secondary to an inadequate amount of hemoglobin available to carry oxygen to the cells. Hypotension and tachycardia often are seen because of blood loss from significant coagulopathies. Supportive care for the mother takes precedence, and emergent cesarean section may also need to be performed. Intubation, ventilatory support, fluid resuscitation, and administration of blood may need to occur to stabilize the mother before emergent cesarean section. Delivery often reverses many of the physiologic sequelae associated with this syndrome. In rare occasions this syndrome can occur after delivery; therefore the emergency nurse needs to be alert for physiologic presentation in the postpartum patient that could represent this syndrome.

Box 46-2 **DIFFERENTIAL DIAGNOSES OF HELLP SYNDROME**

Autoimmune thrombocytopenia purpura
Chronic renal failure
Pyelonephritis
Cholecystitis
Gastroenteritis
Hepatitis
Pancreatitis
Thrombotic thrombocytopenia purpura
Hemolytic-uremic syndrome
Acute fatty liver of pregnancy

From Pearlman M, Tintinalli J: *Emergency care of the woman*, New York, 1998, McGraw-Hill.
HELLP, Hemolysis, elevated liver enzymes, and low platelets.

THIRD-TRIMESTER EMERGENCIES

Fetal viability and the mother's survival are the primary focus for emergencies during the third trimester. Hemorrhage can be obvious or occult, so the emergency nurse must be alert to changes in the mother and fetus.

Placenta Previa

Previa means in front of, so placenta previa occurs when the placenta presents before the fetus. Placenta previa is caused by implantation and development of the placenta in the lower uterine segment rather than normal implantation in the upper uterine wall. Implanting in the lower segment of the uterus puts the placenta in the zone of effacement and dilation, which causes the placenta to partially or completely cover the internal cervical os. Three types of placenta previa are defined in relation to how much of the os is covered (Figure 46-2):

• Complete—the placenta completely covers the os.
• Partial—the placenta partially covers the os.
• Marginal or low implantation—the placenta is adjacent to but does not extend beyond the margin of the os.

Approximately 1 in every 250 pregnancies results in placenta previa at term. The condition is much more common in early pregnancy. However, because the uterus grows during pregnancy, the majority of early placenta previa cases resolve without treatment by the time of delivery.[2] Seventy-five percent of placenta previa cases occur in multiparous women. Multiparity with advancing age and a rapid succession of pregnancies are believed to be predisposing factors for placenta previa.

Hemorrhage, the first and most commonly seen sign of placenta previa, is not accompanied by contractions, so there is usually no associated pain. Because the cervix begins to dilate and efface in the eighth month, maternal vessels can tear even when the patient is asleep. Bleeding may cease spontaneously or continue, depending on the size of torn vessels. After two or three hemorrhages, labor usually begins. Associated membrane rupture can lead to infection.

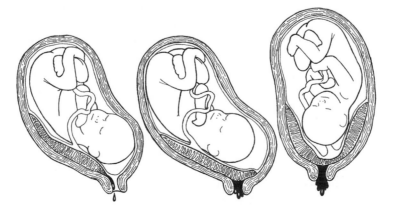

Marginal implantation   Partial implantation   Complete implantation

FIGURE **46-2.** Placenta previa. (Modified from *AJN/Mosby nursing boards review for NCLEX-RN,* ed 10, St. Louis, 1997, Mosby.)

Premature labor and an abnormal presenting part can further complicate delivery. In total placenta previa, bleeding occurs earlier and is more profuse. Suspect placenta previa when painless uterine bleeding occurs in the last half of the pregnancy.

Diagnostic studies include ultrasonography to determine the specific position of the placenta. A CBC, type and crossmatch for several units of blood, and clotting studies should be immediately obtained. Establish a large-bore IV line, administer a crystalloid solution such as lactated Ringer's solution, and transfer the patient to labor and delivery for monitoring and if indicated, immediate cesarean section. Pelvic examination is contraindicated because of potential perforation of the placenta and catastrophic hemorrhage.

Assessment of vital signs should always include assessment of fetal heart rate. If fetal heart tones are not heard, this finding should be reported immediately. A normal fetal heart rate is 120 to 160 beats/min. Stay with the patient, and encourage her to talk. Provide necessary assistance for her husband or significant other with admitting procedures and contacting other family members.

Abruptio Placentae

Abruptio placentae, or separation of the placenta from the uterine wall, accounts for approximately 30% of episodes of bleeding in late pregnancy. In addition, small subclinical or marginal separations may be undetected until the placenta is examined at delivery. In nontraumatic abruptions, spontaneous hemorrhage occurs. Placental hemorrhage may be an acute problem or an occult problem throughout the later stages of pregnancy. It is associated with maternal hypertension and is commonly associated with increasing maternal age, increased parity, smoking, and cocaine use.[3]

Partial separation causes occult or frank hemorrhage. Frank hemorrhage is always an emergency because of blood loss and associated hypotension and hypoxia; however, the more dangerous of the two is occult hemorrhage.

Abruptio placentae should be considered in any woman in the third trimester who presents to the ED with vaginal bleeding and abdominal pain or contractions. This is an emergency requiring immediate intervention.

Maternal assessment with vital signs and fetal heart rate are essential. At least one IV line should be started with a large-bore IV catheter and crystalloid solution. A CBC and type and crossmatch should be sent to the laboratory immediately. Fetal monitoring is essential. The patient should be sent to labor and delivery for monitoring and if indicated, immediate cesarean section.

DELIVERY

With decreasing access to a dwindling number of obstetricians, the probability of deliveries occurring in prehospital care settings and the ED is high. If a patient in labor arrives in the ED and time permits, rapid obstetric examination should be performed and a brief obstetric history obtained. An in-depth, rapid maternal assessment should be completed. And, remember that when the mother says, "The baby is coming," she is always right.

The first stage of labor is the time from onset of regular contractions until complete cervical dilation. This is generally the longest of the three stages of labor. The second stage of labor is the time from full cervical dilation until delivery of the baby. The mother may have the urge to push in this stage. The average time for stage two is 20 minutes to 1 hour. The third stage of labor is from delivery of the baby until delivery of the placenta. This stage usually lasts from 5 to 15 minutes. In cases where the placenta fails to detach from the uterine wall, it may be necessary to manually remove the placenta.

When a woman in labor arrives at the ED, if time permits, a brief physical examination should be performed. First check fetal heart tones; normal fetal heart tones are 120 to 160 beats/min. Prolonged bradycardia or tachycardia may indicate fetal distress. If this occurs, place the mother on her left side and give supplemental high-flow oxygen. Arrange for immediate obstetric consultation for possible emergency delivery by cesarean section.

After it has been determined that the fetus is in no distress, examine the mother's abdomen and measure uterine height. A full-term fetus elevates the uterus to the level of the xiphoid. Palpate contractions as they occur. Help the mother to relax between contractions. The emergency nurse involved in a delivery should remember that the mother does most of the work. Some of the roles of the nurse are to provide psychologic support, "coach" the mother, and ensure that the infant, once delivered, is breathing adequately, has a good pulse, and is kept warm.

If crowning is not present, a manual vaginal examination using sterile technique is performed to determine dilation, effacement, and station of the fetus. If fluid is present, identify if it is amniotic fluid by determining acidity of the fluid. Amniotic fluid is neutral, whereas normal vaginal secretions are acidic. If the test is equivocal because of the presence of blood, assume the membranes have ruptured and that amniotic fluid is present.

A rapid decision should be made as to whether delivery is imminent and the baby will be delivered in the ED or if time permits transport of the mother to labor and delivery. If there is any indication that the mother will deliver imminently (i.e., crowning), keep her in the ED for delivery.

If an emergent delivery is imminent, place the mother on a stretcher and obtain equipment necessary for delivery of the fetus. Sterile disposable delivery kits usually have most equipment necessary for an emergent delivery. Do not place equipment between the mother's legs; place it on a surface beside the stretcher. Minimum essential equipment includes cord clamps, scissors, towels, and bulb syringe.

After donning appropriate attire, cover one hand with a sterile towel or a 4 × 4 inch dressing. Apply gentle pressure to the infant's head as it crowns to prevent explosive delivery and possible tearing of the perineum. When the head is delivered, quickly suction the infant's mouth and then the nose to prevent aspiration. At this point, check for the umbilical cord around the infant's neck. If the cord is found and is loose, carefully slip it over the infant's head. If it is tight, clamp it in two places and cut the cord. After the head is delivered and has rotated, hold it gently in both hands. Apply gentle downward pressure to assist with delivery of the anterior shoulder and gentle upward traction to assist with delivery of the posterior shoulder. Carefully support the infant's head. After the shoulders are delivered, delivery of the rest of the infant's body usually occurs quite rapidly (Figure 46-3).

Keep the infant in a head-dependent position at the level of the introitus to prevent aspiration. Once again, suction the mouth and then the nose. If spontaneous breathing or crying does not occur, gently rub the infant's back with a towel to stimulate breathing.

If not already done, clamp the umbilical cord in two places at least 6 inches from the umbilicus. The cord can be

cut as soon as it is convenient, usually when it has stopped pulsating.

Place the infant in a warmed environment. Assess ABCs. If necessary, open the infant's airway with a slight chin lift, being careful not to overextend the neck. If breathing is absent or the heart rate is less than 60 beats/min despite 30 seconds of assisted ventilation, begin resuscitation measures following current American Heart Association guidelines for neonatal resuscitation.[1] For additional information on neonatal resuscitation, see Chapter 47.

Determine the infant's Apgar score at delivery, and repeat 5 minutes after delivery (Table 46-4). The Apgar score is a system used to predict health outcomes by scoring and totaling five key factors. Each factor is scored from 0 to 2. Zero is a poor response or absence of the factor being measured, 1 indicates some response, and 2 indicates a normal finding. A total score of 10 is possible, with 7 to 10 considered very good. A score of

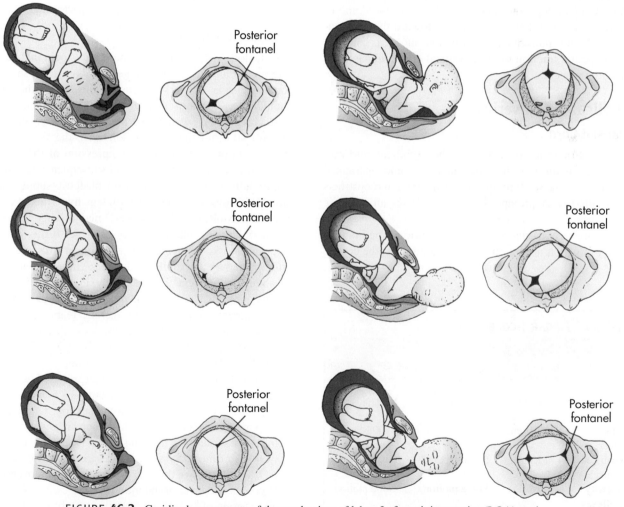

FIGURE 46-3. Caridinal movements of the mechanism of labor. Left occipitoanterior (LOA) position. **A,** Engagement and descent. **B,** Flexion. **C,** Internal rotation to occipitoanterior position (OA). **D,** Extension. **E,** External rotation begining (restitution). **F,** External rotation. (From Lowdermilk DL, Perry SE: *Maternity and women's health care,* ed 9. St. Louis, 2007, Mosby.)

4 to 6 indicates a moderately depressed infant, whereas a score of 0 to 3 indicates a severely depressed infant.

After ensuring health of the infant and its continued warmth, place the infant on the mother's abdomen and encourage the mother to breastfeed the infant if appropriate. Be sure to cover the mother and baby to keep the baby warm. Sucking stimulates the uterus to contract, reassures the mother the infant is fine, and helps to keep the infant warm. Put an identification band on the infant's wrist and ankle.

After delivery of the infant, the third stage of labor begins. At this point, unclamp the cord and obtain laboratory specimens from the cord for determinations of hematocrit and hemoglobin levels, blood type, Rh factor, and bilirubin level and reclamp the cord. Palpate the uterus through the abdominal wall. Prepare for delivery of the placenta; this usually occurs 5 to 10 minutes after the infant is born. A sudden gush of blood occurs when the placenta separates from the uterine wall; the uterus rises into the abdomen and the umbilical cord protruding from the vagina lengthens. Do not pull on the umbilical cord; this could cause uterine inversion.

When the placenta has separated, apply slight traction to the umbilical cord and place your hand on the dome of the uterus, pressing downward slightly toward the suprapubic area. As the placenta enters the vaginal area, continue applying gentle traction to the umbilical cord and carefully remove the placenta.

Complicated Deliveries

Prolapsed Cord

A prolapsed umbilica occurs when the umbilical cord precedes the fetus through the birth canal, becomes entrapped when the fetus passes through the birth canal, and obstructs fetal circulation. A prolapsed cord constitutes an obstetric emergency.

There are three variations of this condition. The first is a situation in which uterine membranes are intact; the cord is compressed by fetal parts but is not visible externally. This variation should be suspected when there are signs of fetal distress, most prominently bradycardia. This variation is actually called "cord presentation" rather than true prolapse.

In the second variation the cord may not be visible but can be felt in the vagina or cervix. In the third and most extreme variation, the umbilical cord actually protrudes from the vagina.

Cord compression can be determined in two ways. First, on examination the cord is felt as the presenting part. However, cord compression is usually identified when the fetus suddenly develops distress, which is noted on the fetal monitor as a decreasing fetal heart rate or decelerations.

Therapeutic intervention is aimed at relieving pressure on the cord and minimizing fetal anoxia. Either elevate the mother's hips, or place the mother in the knee-chest position with the bed in Trendelenburg's position. Instruct her to not push because this may cause further compression of the cord.[5,8] Administer oxygen via nonrebreather mask at 100%. An exposed cord dries out, so cover it with saline-moistened sterile gauze. If the cervix is completely dilated, forceps may be used to rapidly deliver the baby. If the cervix is not fully dilated, emergency cesarean section is performed.

Shoulder Dystocia

Risk factors associated with shoulder dystocia include large infants, prolonged second stage of labor, and use of high forceps during delivery. Whatever the cause, the infant's shoulder has difficulty passing through the pelvis. Shoulder dystocia is an emergency that presents in fewer than 2% of deliveries.[7] After the head is delivered, the shoulders cannot pass through the pelvis. Compression of the shoulders can lead to cord compression and subsequent fetal distress. Rapid delivery is critical! Call for obstetric support if possible. Positioning the mother with legs hyperflexed over the abdomen (McRoberts' maneuver)[5] may disengage the anterior shoulder and make delivery possible. If this maneuver does not work, application of suprapubic pressure will be attempted to try and facilitate delivery.[6] Infant complications of shoulder dystocia include asphyxia, traumatic brachial plexus injuries, fractured clavicle or humerus, and Erb's palsy. Maternal complications include tears to the cervix, vagina, perineum, or rectum.

Breech Delivery

With breech delivery, the head—the largest fetal body part—is delivered last. A woman whose fetus is a breech presentation is often scheduled for cesarean section. Unfortunately, in the emergency setting when a woman arrives in labor with delivery imminent and the fetus is in a breech position, there may not be time to arrange for cesarean section. Delivery must be completed in the ED, especially if the fetus has been delivered to the level of the umbilicus.

Categories of breech presentation are frank breech, full or complete breech, and footling breech. Frank breech is the most common variation, occurring when fetal legs are extended across the abdomen toward the shoulders and the

Table 46-4. **APGAR SCORE**			
	Score		
Factor	**0**	**1**	**2**
A Appearance (color)	Blue	Blue limbs, pink body	Pink
P Pulse (heart rate)	Absent	<100 beats/min	>100 beats/min
G Grimace (muscle tone)	Limp	Some flexion	Good flexion
A Activity (reflexes irritable)	Absent	Some motion	Good motion
R Respiratory effort	Absent	Weak cry	Strong cry

buttocks are presenting. Full (or complete) breech is reversal of the usual cephalic presentation. The head, knees, and hips are flexed, but the buttocks are presenting. Footling breech is when one or both feet present.

With any breech presentation, call for obstetric support if possible. It is usually best to allow the fetus to deliver spontaneously to the level of the umbilicus. If the fetus is in a frank breech presentation, the legs may require extraction after the buttocks are delivered. After the umbilicus is visualized, gently extract a generous amount of umbilical cord. Rotate the fetus to align shoulders in an anterior-posterior position. Place gentle traction on the fetus until the axilla are seen. Pull upward gently on the feet to allow delivery of the posterior shoulder. Carefully extract the posterior arm, then gently pull downward on the feet to deliver the anterior shoulder. Rotate the buttocks to the mother's front. Using a Mauriceau maneuver, rest the fetus on your arm, and then place your index and middle finger in the fetus's mouth, gently flexing the head. Do not apply traction with this hand. Grasp the fetus at the base of the neck and tip of the shoulders with your other hand and apply gentle traction. If assistance is available, have the other person apply firm, steady pressure to the top of the fundus toward the suprapubic area. The neonate should then be suctioned and the cord clamped.

Meconium Aspiration Syndrome

Meconium aspiration syndrome occurs when meconium enters fetal lungs during delivery. Relaxation of the anal sphincter in utero caused by fetal hypoxia leads to meconium staining of amniotic fluid. Staining is seen most often in postterm deliveries. Meconium staining of amniotic fluid can be an emergency for the fetus, but delivery must be adapted to address potential fetal respiratory distress. The 2005 American Heart Association recommendations no longer advise routine intrapartum oropharyngeal and nasopharyngeal suctioning for infants born to mothers with meconium-stained amniotic fluid. Previously the recommendation was that meconium-stained infants have endotracheal intubation performed immediately following birth and that suction be applied to the endotracheal tube as it is withdrawn. There has been no benefit found in performing this procedure in infants who are born vigorous (strong respiratory effort, good muscle tone, and heart rate greater than 100 beats/min). For meconium-stained infants who are not born vigorous, endotracheal suctioning with a meconium aspirator should be performed immediately after birth.[1]

Multiple Fetuses

With delivery of twins or other multiple births, there are additional concerns. Often multiple-birth neonates are premature or have a host of other problems. The initial and most important objective is to ensure safe delivery of all fetuses. The best advice is to take one fetus at a time, as they come. The first may present vertex or breech. Follow the previous information for various presentations. The second fetus usually has membranes intact. If the second fetus is in the headfirst position, you may rupture the membranes and allow the mother to deliver the fetus by pushing when she has a contraction. If the second fetus is breech, deliver the feet, and then rupture the membranes. Both neonates should be suctioned as they are delivered. Both cords should be clamped and both neonates should receive identification bands. Multiples increase the risk for complications; if at all possible there should be two teams available in the event neonatal resuscitation is required.

Amniotic Fluid Embolism

Amniotic fluid embolism is a catastrophic event with high maternal mortality because amniotic fluid leaks into the mother's venous circulation during labor or delivery. This embolus of squamous epithelial cells, lanugo, and vasoactive chemicals travels to the pulmonary circulation, causing sudden, severe obstruction and respiratory arrest, which is usually followed quickly by cardiac arrest.

Amniotic fluid emboli are seen most commonly with placenta previa, abruptio placentae, precipitate labor in the multiparous woman, and intrauterine fetal death. Amniotic fluid emboli occur in about 1 of every 100,000 deliveries. The mother may initially demonstrate profound hypotension, tachycardia, tachypnea, cyanosis, and hypoxia followed by cardiopulmonary arrest. Coagulopathies can also occur.

Therapeutic interventions must be rapid and aggressive. Administer oxygen at high-flow via a nonrebreather mask. Rapid endotracheal intubation and mechanical ventilation with positive end-expiratory pressure is required for many patients. Crystalloid solutions and blood products should be administered. Fresh frozen plasma may be infused for identified coagulopathies.

POSTPARTUM EMERGENCIES
Postpartum Hemorrhage

Postpartum hemorrhage, defined as 500 mL or more of blood, is the most common complication of labor and delivery. Bleeding can occur immediately (within 24 hours) after delivery or be delayed (24 hours to 6 weeks). The main causes of postpartum bleeding are uterine atony, which can cause subinvolution; a decreased or absent decrease in size of the uterus; retained products of conception, such as pieces of the placenta or membranes; and vaginal or cervical tears incurred during delivery. Subinvolution usually occurs 7 to 14 days after delivery when thrombi detach from placental-attachment sites and those sites begin to bleed. If involution does not occur, the gravid uterus will not return to the nonpregnant state and life-threatening hemorrhage can occur. Retention of membranes or placental fragments can also cause sudden hemorrhage because they interfere with the involutional process. The emergency nurse should also be aware of a condition known as placenta accreta. When the placenta fails to separate from the uterine wall after delivery because it has grown into the uterine muscle itself, postpartum bleeding results and immediate surgery is indicated. Cervical tears and vaginal lacerations can also cause postpartum hemorrhage.

When assessing the patient with postpartum bleeding, survey the patient's general condition. Note the presence or absence of pain, skin color, posture, gait, motor activity, and facial expression. The following information should be elicited when obtaining history of the problem.

- Quantity, character, and duration of bleeding. How does it compare with the patient's normal menstrual period? How many pads has she used in the past hour? During the past 24 hours? How does it compare with the number she normally requires during a period?
- Menstrual history. When was the date of her last period?
- Does she have pain? What is the nature of the pain—dull, achy, cramping, constant, or radiating? Where is the pain? How long has she had it? Was onset gradual or sudden?
- Is there any history of trauma?
- When did she deliver? Has she ever had any infections of the reproductive system? Has she had previous episodes of bleeding?

Continued assessment should include vital signs, palpation of the uterine fundus for firmness, and evaluation of vaginal bleeding. If the fundus is boggy and relaxed, gently massage it until firm. Check the pad the patient is wearing to objectively evaluate the amount of bleeding. Note presence or absence of clots or odor. Examine and save any clots or tissue that the patient may have brought with her for laboratory examination. If bleeding is profuse, establish two IV lines with large-bore catheters for administration of warmed crystalloids and blood. If respirations are labored, administer oxygen. Obtain a CBC, sedimentation rate, and type and crossmatch.

While collecting data and stabilizing the patient, prepare for a vaginal examination. Explain each procedure, and reassure the patient by allowing her to express her feelings.

Postpartum bleeding generally responds to administration of IV oxytocin (Pitocin), bed rest, and fundal massage. If bleeding continues, prepare the patient for operative evaluation of bleeding. Treatment of retained products of conception includes removal of the offending piece by dilation and curettage and a thorough exploration of the uterus after the patient is under general anesthesia. Suturing of vaginal lacerations can be performed in the ED. However, with the possibility of damage at the cervix, suturing is best performed after general anesthesia. A complete pelvic examination can also be performed after anesthesia.

Disseminated Intravascular Coagulation

Disseminated intravascular coagulation is characterized by acceleration and hyperactivity of clotting mechanisms in pregnancy. This condition of simultaneous bleeding and clotting is seen most often in severe cases of abruptio placentae in the form of hypofibrinogenemia but can also occur after excessive blood loss, amniotic fluid embolus, or fetal death in utero. In this hypercoagulable state, clotting factors are consumed before the liver has time to replace them.

See Chapter 41 for additional discussion of disseminated intravascular coagulation.

Postpartum Infection

Vaginal lacerations, cervical tears, episiotomy sites, placental implant sites, and retained tissue can become host sites for infection. Patients develop fever and abdominal or pelvic pain and occasionally have foul-smelling lochia. Therapeutic interventions include culture of drainage and administration of antibiotics as indicated. In rare cases the postpartum patient may become septic and require fluid resuscitation and stabilization.

OTHER EMERGENCIES
Molar Pregnancy (Hydatidiform Mole)

Molar pregnancy occurs when trophoblast villi grow very rapidly and then die. If an embryo is formed, it dies very early. As trophoblast cells degenerate, they fill with a jelly-like fluid. The cells become vesicles that look like grapes filled with fluid. Bleeding occurs early in the second trimester as these vesicles enlarge and rupture. There is a definite association between hydatidiform mole and choriocarcinoma (a rapidly growing carcinoma), so early diagnosis is critical.

In the United States, molar pregnancy occurs in 1 in 1000 pregnancies. It is seen more frequently in women of poor socioeconomic status who lack protein in their diet, mothers younger than 18 years or older than 35 years, and women of Asian background.

Because the trophoblast secretes hCG and grows very rapidly, the uterus grows larger than expected for the due date. At about 16 weeks' gestation, the woman develops vaginal bleeding. Bleeding may be mixed with clear fluid as the vesicles begin to rupture. The patient will have a positive pregnancy test with enlarging uterus; however, fetal heart tones cannot be auscultated. A viable fetus is not evident on pelvic ultrasonography.

Intervention for molar pregnancy is removal of the mole. The patient should be prepared for suction dilation and curettage. The patient and family need much emotional support. They now know this is an abnormal pregnancy (without a fetus) and must also worry about the possibility of a tumor.

SUMMARY

The emergency nurse uses the nursing process to assess and prioritize care for women with obstetric complaints. Through this process, the emergency nurse can identify life-threatening problems and intervene quickly. The ability to do this while providing emotional support for the mother and family is the hallmark of emergency care for the obstetric patient in the ED. Knowledge of common obstetric emergencies will promote optimal outcomes for the infant and mother.

REFERENCES

1. American Heart Association: Guidelines 2005 for cardiopulmonary resuscitation and emergency cardiovascular care, *Circulation* 102(suppl I):I-1, 2005.
2. Cunningham GF, Leveno KL, Bloom SL et al: *Williams obstetrics*, ed 22, Columbus, OH, 2007, McGraw-Hill.
3. Gorrie TM, McKinney ES, Murray SS: *Foundations of maternal-newborn nursing*, ed 4, Philadelphia, 2006, WB Saunders.
4. Guyton AC, Hall GE: *Textbook of medical physiology*, Philadelphia, 2006, Elsevier.
5. Jarvis C: *Physical examination and health assessment*, ed 4, Philadelphia, 2004, WB Saunders.
6. Mallon WK, Henderson S: Labor and delivery, In Marx JA, Hockberger RS, Walls RM, editors: *Rosen's emergency medicine: concepts and clinical practice*, ed 6, Philadelphia, 2006, Mosby.
7. Marx JA, editor: *Emergency medicine: concepts and clinical practice*, ed 6, St. Louis, 2006, Mosby.
8. Novak JC, Broom BL: *Ingalls and Salerno's maternal and child health nursing*, ed 9, St. Louis, 1999, Mosby.
9. Stacey JF, Proehl JA: Emergency childbirth, In Proehl JA, editor: *Emergency nursing procedures*, ed 4, St. Louis, 2009, Saunders.
10. Wright M, Grant HP: How competent are you and your staff with shoulder dystocia? *AWHONN Lifelines* 3(1):35, 1999.

CHAPTER 47

Pediatric Emergencies

S ick children present distinctive challenges to many health care professionals. Assessment and treatment of children is unique because of the developmental, anatomic, and physiologic differences between adults and children. Understanding and appreciating these differences is the foundation for developing a working knowledge of pediatrics. Once a health care professional is able to separate normal from abnormal behaviors and assessment findings, care and treatment of children becomes much easier. However, being able to quickly recognize a sick child is an acquired skill that takes time and practice to develop. The caregiver who is not accustomed to caring primarily for children may also feel confused or overwhelmed when assessing and caring for patients that require a different communication style than what they may be accustomed to using. A child's fear and anxiety of being ill and in a hospital, as well as the parent's fear and anxiety, can at times make simple communication a challenge.

In most cases, when a child is sick, the parents or guardian should be encouraged to stay with their child during all phases of the visit. Fear and uncertainty surrounding the child's condition, coupled with a loss of control of the situation, add to the stress that both the parent and child may be experiencing. Begin the assessment as soon as the child enters the emergency department (ED); approaching the child slowly while interviewing the parent is the best way to start the interaction with the child. Positive, caring interactions with the

child and parent help alleviate the stress and facilitate assessment of the child. Calling the child by name, making direct eye contact, using simple understandable terms, and offering choices when appropriate are all basic guidelines that can be used with patients and families of all ages.

Most emergency nurses, regardless of practice area, will encounter a sick child at some point in their career. The ability to intervene in critical situations requires a strong foundation of knowledge and assessment skills. This chapter provides an overview of pediatric assessment and common pediatric emergencies. Pediatric trauma and child abuse are discussed in Chapters 28 and 48, respectively.

TRIAGE

Pediatric patients, defined by the Centers for Disease Control and Prevention (CDC) as individuals less than 15 years of age, account for approximately 21% of annual ED visits nationally.[11] The triage nurse needs to have outstanding assessment, communication, and organization skills. The emergency nurse who becomes skilled at triage will also develop a "sixth sense" for identifying the "sick" infant or child.

A sick child in the ED can make nurses who are unfamiliar with children uneasy, just as an adult with chest pain can generate alarm in a pediatric nurse. Triage of a child does not require familiarity with every childhood disease, medication, and neurologic reflex or a horde of specialized equipment.

Pediatric triage does require understanding of concepts related to pediatric emergencies, including the following:

- Anatomic, physiologic, and developmental differences between children and adults
- Recognition of conditions leading to pediatric arrest (hypoxia and shock) and appropriate interventions
- Effective communication with parents
- "Rules" of pediatric triage

Children are a challenge to evaluate when compared with adults for several reasons. Children often have nonspecific symptoms, such as fever, and communication can be difficult. In the younger infant, because of limited vocabulary and verbal skills, the nurse must depend on the parent and subtle clues from the child for history. A child's response to illness or injury depends on his or her current developmental stage. Toddlers cling to parents, whereas adolescents are independent. Children compensate physiologically for longer periods in the face of illness; therefore they may not be outwardly symptomatic despite the presence of a life-threatening condition. Normal vital signs do not always indicate stability in the pediatric patient.

Special Pediatric Considerations

Some of the most significant differences between children and adults are found in the respiratory and circulatory systems. One of the most obvious anatomic differences is that infants and young children have larger tongues in proportion to the size of their mouths. This means that the tongue can easily obstruct the airway; proper positioning is often all that is necessary to provide airway patency. Because of the smaller diameter of their airway structures, children have increased airway resistance compared to an adult; small amounts of mucus or swelling exacerbate this difference and can easily obstruct the airway. Infants less than 4 months of age are obligatory nose breathers; any process that obstructs the nose can lead to respiratory distress. Cartilage of a child's larynx is softer than in an adult. The cricoid cartilage is the narrowest portion of the larynx, providing a natural seal for endotracheal tubes.[13] The sternum and ribs of the pediatric patient are cartilaginous, the chest wall is soft, and intercostal muscles are poorly developed, leading easily to fatigue. All of these factors contribute to a more inefficient respiratory system and the cause of frequent respiratory distress.

There are some specific differences in the cardiovascular system of the pediatric patient that have clinical significance. Infants and children have a higher cardiac output than adults (200 mL/kg/min versus 100 mL/kg/min).[5] Cardiac output is the volume of blood ejected by the heart each minute; it is defined by the following equation: heart rate × stroke volume = cardiac output. A higher cardiac output is required because the pediatric patient has a higher oxygen demand as a result of a higher metabolic rate and greater oxygen consumption (6 to 8 mL/kg/min compared to 3 to 4 mL/kg/min in adults). In pediatric patients the myocardial fibers are shorter and less elastic, which means the myocardium has poorer compliance and less ability to adjust stroke volume

in an altered cardiac output state. This is why heart rate is such an important and sensitive indicator of cardiac output in pediatric patients.[13]

Children have a greater percentage of total body water than adults (80 mL/kg versus 70 mL/kg in adults) and are more susceptible to volume depletion with even small loses that are not replaced. This is why children are at a greater risk for dehydration than adults. However, part of the challenge with pediatrics is that children can maintain an adequate cardiac output for long periods of time by compensating for fluid loss with an increased heart rate (tachycardia) and peripheral vasoconstriction.[13] Because of their strong compensatory mechanisms, 25% to 30% of circulating volume may be lost before a decrease in systolic blood pressure (SBP) occurs, indicating the child has progressed to a decompensated shock state.[13] By the time the shock state is recognized the child may already be in critical condition.

Neonates, term infants from birth to 28 days of age, and particularly preterm neonates, possess unique physiologic characteristics and should be assessed and treated very carefully. The thermoregulatory system is very immature in the neonatal period, and thus keeping newborns warm without overheating them can be a challenge. There can be serious consequences of hypothermia, as well as hyperthermia. Hypoglycemia, apnea, metabolic acidosis, and poor feeding can result from cold stress. Warm stress can also lead to poor feeding, lethargy, hypotonia, and hypotension. Simply taking care to not leave the newborn undressed or unwrapped for long periods of time during the ED visit is a simple way to avert problems. Other methods that may be used to keep the newborn warm include the use of warmed intravenous (IV) fluids, covering the head of the newborn, use of an overhead radiant warmer, or even the use of warm blankets. An effortless way to ensure thermoregulation of the newborn in the ED is to maintain a higher temperature in the room where the newborn will be examined. As a rule of thumb, if an adult in short sleeves is feeling warm, the room temperature should be about right for the newborn. However, as mentioned, overheating can become an issue for the newborn as well, so it is important not to overdo the heating methods. Temperature monitoring should not be overlooked. The neonatal immune system is also immature; therefore a fever of 100.4° F (38° C) is considered significant for a newborn. The inability to localize infections makes the neonate even harder to assess for infectious processes because they have fewer signs and symptoms.[10] Newborns, young infants, and children have limited glycogen stores and are vulnerable to hypoglycemia when stressed by an illness, injury, or cold stress.

Rules of Pediatric Triage

The following unofficial rules of pediatric triage may assist triage nurses in evaluating children.

1. Parents know their children better than you do—listen to them. Parents' history can give clues to the cause of an illness or injury and help triage nurses determine urgency.

2. Remember airway, breathing, and circulation (ABCs)—children are different. Do not always focus on the obvious; a subtle, more serious problem can be overlooked.

3. Some children can talk, walk, and still be in shock; do not depend solely on the child's appearance. Consider history and vital signs, but do not allow normal vital signs to give you a false sense of security.

4. Never tell parents their child cannot be evaluated in the ED, no matter what the chief complaint.

Pediatric Triage Evaluation

Depending on the facility, the triage assessment may be brief, limited to determining chief complaint and looking at the child, or it may be more comprehensive and include obtaining vital signs and providing treatment such as antipyretics, splinting, or ice packs. Whatever triage protocols or pathways exist, the first and most important aspect is prompt assessment with observation. This first assessment is sometimes referred to as the "across-the-room assessment," or the "looks good–looks bad" assessment using the Pediatric Assessment Triangle (PAT).[10] The PAT uses three physiologic parameters that reflect severity of illness or injury: the child's general appearance, work of breathing, and circulation to skin (Figure 47-1). General appearance refers to the child's tone, interactiveness, consolability, look/gaze, and speech/cry. Work of breathing is evaluated by signs such as airway sounds, positioning, retractions, and flaring. Circulation to the skin is obtained by assessing skin color (pink, pale, gray, dusky, cyanotic). The parameters can be assessed in any order.[10] With experience and practice a triage nurse can look at a room of children and quickly sort out who needs to be triaged first.

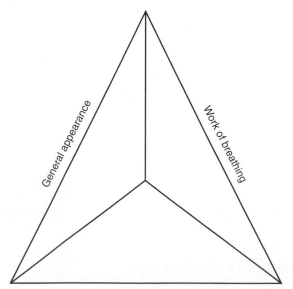

FIGURE **47-1.** Pediatric Assessment Triangle. (From Emergency Nurses Association: *Emergency nursing pediatric course provider manual,* ed 3, Hawkins HS, editor, Des Plaines, Ill, 2004, The Association.)

Primary Assessment

Primary assessment consists of evaluation of the ABCs and neurologic status of the child. ABCs may be the only part of the assessment performed in triage if the child has an emergent condition. The primary survey includes assessment of level of consciousness; respiratory effort, rate, and quality; skin color, temperature, and capillary refill; and pulse rate and quality.[13]

Secondary Assessment

Secondary assessment consists of vital signs and head-to-toe survey. During triage, secondary assessment is usually limited to evaluating the area of chief complaint or focused examination. The rest of the examination is performed later in a treatment area. When performing a secondary assessment on a child, do not focus only on the obvious injury. Do not forget to take into account the patient's chronic condition(s) or any significant past medical history when determining how high risk the patient may be (e.g., fever in the immunosuppressed patient or headache and vomiting in the patient with a ventriculoperitoneal [VP] shunt in place). Communicate your findings to other health care team members, and document your assessment.

History

Obtaining a standardized history of the child's illness is an important part of the pediatric assessment. If the triage nurse identifies a life-threatening condition during the PAT assessment, the standardized history can be obtained by the patient's primary nurse. In infants less than 1 year of age, and especially with neonates, history may be vague, nonspecific, and limited by the parents' ability to communicate their concern for their child. Past medical history is also important in determining if the child has a prior condition that may affect assessment (e.g., congenital heart disease, chronic respiratory condition, prematurity). The CIAMPEDS mnemonic is a standardized tool that describes components of basic pediatric history (Table 47-1).

Vital Signs

Obtaining accurate vital sign measurements on children is one of the more challenging aspects of pediatric assessment. Temperature, pulse rate, respiratory rate, blood pressure, weight, and pain scores should be obtained on every patient. (See Chapter 12 for further discussion on pain assessment.) Vital signs vary with age (Table 47-2); therefore alterations from normal must be viewed in light of the child's history and other symptoms.[13] Infants localize infections poorly because of their immature immune system; therefore any child younger than 3 months of age should be evaluated for possible bacterial infection when the child has fever greater than 100.4° F (38.0° C). Temperatures less than 96.8° F (36.5° C) in this age-group can be a sign of infection as well.

Weight can be obtained at triage, but whether at triage or in the patient care area, it needs to be measured near the

Table 47-1. COMPONENTS OF BASIC PEDIATRIC ASSESSMENT (CIAMPEDS)[5,10]

C	Chief complaint	Reason for the child's ED visit and duration of complaint (e.g., fever lasting 2 days).
I	Immunizations	Evaluation of the child's current immunization status:
		• The completion of all scheduled immunizations for the child's age must be evaluated. The most current immunization recommendations are published by the American Academy of Pediatrics.
		• If the child has not received immunization because of religion or cultural beliefs, document this information.
	Isolation	Evaluation of the child's exposure to communicable diseases (influenza, chickenpox, shingles, mumps, measles, whooping cough, tuberculosis):
		• A child with active disease or who is potentially infectious, based on a history of exposure and the disease incubation period, must be placed in respiratory isolation on arrival in the ED.
		• Immunosuppressed or immunocompromised children can develop active disease even when previously immune. These children must also be protected from inadvertent exposure to viral and bacterial illness while in the ED and placed in *protective* or *reverse isolation.*
		• Other exposures that may be evaluated include exposure to meningitis (with or without evidence of purpura), pneumonia, and scabies.
A	Allergies	Evaluation of the child's previous allergic or hypersensitivity reactions:
		• Document reactions to medications, foods, products (e.g., latex), and environmental allergens. The type of reaction must also be documented.
M	Medications	Evaluation of the child's current medication regimen, including prescription and over-the-counter medications:
		• Dose administered.
		• Time of last dose.
		• Duration of medication use.
P	Past medical history	A review of the child's health status, including prior illnesses, injuries, hospitalizations, surgeries, and chronic physical and psychiatric illnesses. Use of alcohol, tobacco, drugs, or other substances of abuse must be evaluated, as appropriate:
		• The medical history of an infant must include the prenatal and birth history:
		• Complications during pregnancy or delivery.
		• Number of days infant remained in hospital post birth.
		• Infant's birth weight.
		• The medical history of the menarcheal female includes the date and description of last menstrual period.
	Parent's/caregiver's impression of the child's condition	• Identification of the child's primary caregiver.
		• Consider cultural differences that may affect the caregiver's impressions.
		• Evaluation of the caregiver's concerns and observations of the child's condition. Especially significant in evaluating the special needs child.
E	Events surrounding the illness or injury	Evaluation of the onset of the illness or circumstances and mechanism of injury:
		• Illness:
		• Length of illness, including date and day of onset and sequence of symptoms.
		• Exposure to others with similar symptoms.
		• Treatment provided before ED visit.
		• Examination by primary care provider.
		• Injury:
		• Time and date injury occurred.
		• M: Mechanism of injury, including the use of protective devices such as seat belts and helmets.
		• I: Injuries suspected.
		• V: Vital signs in prehospital environment.
		• T: Treatment by prehospital providers.
		• Description of circumstances leading to injury.
		• Witnessed or unwitnessed.
D	Diet	Assessment of the child's recent oral intake and changes in eating patterns related to the illness or injury:
		• Changes in eating patterns or fluid intake.
		• Time of last meal and last fluid intake.
		• Regular diet: Breast milk, type of formula, solid foods, diet for age, developmental level, and cultural differences.
		• Special diet or diet restrictions

(Continued)

Table 47-1. COMPONENTS OF BASIC PEDIATRIC ASSESSMENT (CIAMPEDS)[5,10] — CONT'D

	Diapers	Assessment of the child's urine and stool output: • Frequency of urination over last 24 hours (number of wet diapers); changes in frequency. • Time of last void. • Changes in odor or color of urine. • Last bowel movement; color and consistency of stool. • Change in frequency of bowel movements.
S	Symptoms associated with the illness or injury	Identification of symptoms and progression of symptoms since the onset of the illness or injury event.

ED, Emergency department.

Table 47-2. NORMAL VITAL SIGNS BY AGE

Age	Heart Rate (beats/min)	Respiratory Rate (breaths/min)	Systolic Blood Pressure (mm Hg)	Weight (kg)
Preterm	120-180	55-65	40-60	2
Term newborn	90-170	40-60	52-92	3
1 month	110-180	30-50	60-104	4
6 months	110-180	25-35	65-125	7
1 year	80-160	20-30	70-118	10
2 years	80-130	20-30	73-117	12
4 years	80-120	20-30	65-117	16
6 years	75-115	18-24	76-116	20
8 years	70-110	18-22	76-119	25
10 years	70-110	16-20	82-122	30
12 years	60-110	16-20	84-128	40
14 years	60-105	16-20	85-136	50

Modified from Barken RM, Rosen P: *Emergency pediatrics,* ed 6, St. Louis, 2003, Mosby.

beginning of the ED visit. Weight is important for calculating medication doses for pediatric patients, and it is in the best interest and safety of the child to have an accurate weight. A length-based resuscitation tape (e.g., Broselow tape) may be used in those situations in which a measured weight cannot be readily obtained. Recording the child's weight in kilograms reduces the chance of error in medication calculations. Birth weight should be documented for infants younger than 8 weeks of age.

Pulse and respirations can be measured consecutively while the nurse is evaluating airway and breathing. An apical pulse can be obtained with the stethoscope on the child's chest, and a full minute of respirations can also be counted while the stethoscope is on the chest. Temperatures may be obtained by a variety of routes, including oral, tympanic, temporal artery, axillary, or rectal. The method chosen will depend on the age of the child, medical history of the child, institutional preference, and the needed reliability of the measurement. When an accurate temperature is required to make a treatment decision, a measurement strategy that approaches core temperature is desired—rectal temperature is considered the gold standard.

Obtaining a blood pressure can be a bit more difficult in the younger child. Beginning with the correct size cuff is the first priority. The cuff must cover two thirds of the area being used.[15] A cuff that is too small gives a false high reading, whereas an oversized cuff gives a false low reading. Having a wide variety of cuff sizes is very important when caring for pediatric patients. Using the lower extremity on younger infants and toddlers while distracting them during the procedure is often an alternative way to obtain an accurate blood pressure reading. Manual methods of obtaining blood pressures by auscultation, palpation, or by use of a Doppler are skills that often need to be employed when caring for the pediatric patient.[8,13] This is especially true with the critically ill or injured child, but these methods, when practiced, can be easier and faster when used on all children. Noninvasive blood pressure (NIBP) monitor limitations may be due to very low blood pressures that the NIBP is unable to detect accurately.[8] In the pediatric patient, if a low blood pressure is obtained from a NIBP, a manual blood pressure should be obtained to verify.[8] Also if a NIBP is unable to obtain a blood pressure and the child has signs and symptoms suggestive of shock, a manual blood pressure must be attempted. It is not acceptable to document "unable to obtain" simply because the NIBP will not record a blood pressure.

Children With Special Needs

As a result of improvements in health care and technology, children with many different congenital conditions and survivors of life-threatening illness or injury are living to adulthood.[10] Children with special health care needs may present to all levels and types of EDs for treatment related to their underlying disorder or for childhood conditions unrelated to their particular condition. These children can be a challenge to assess and care for, but the same basic principles used for all pediatric patients should be used for this group as well. There are, however, some important points to keep in mind. A basic assessment can be difficult, because cardiopulmonary and neurologic status may be abnormal at baseline. When this is the case, parents or other frequent caregivers are the best source of information about baseline status. Asking the parent or caregiver about vital signs and past medical history specifics is an integral part of the history and assessment. Do not assume you know what the risk factors are for a particular patient or particular congenital condition because often these children are unique.[10] Preexisting problems in many different organ systems can complicate assessment findings and may make it difficult to determine an acute problem. Children with special health care needs may also have less cardiopulmonary reserve than an average pediatric patient. They may not compensate for illness in the same way and can deteriorate more rapidly than most children.[10] The health care provider needs to stay objective when interpreting the assessment findings. Clearly communicating any concerns with the parent and other health care providers on the team is vital.

RESPIRATORY EMERGENCIES

Recognition of respiratory distress and failure in the pediatric patient is crucial because unrecognized or undertreated respiratory compromise is almost always the precursor to cardiac arrest in children.[5,13] A child having difficulty breathing can display a variety of symptoms. Upper airway conditions can cause the child to be apprehensive, restless, stridorous, and exhibit intercostal and sternal retractions. Sudden onset of respiratory distress may suggest foreign body obstruction or laryngeal spasms. Airway obstruction in children results from a myriad of causes, including congenital anomalies, peritonsillar abscess, laryngeal obstruction, drug intoxication, and foreign bodies such as coins or toy parts.

Gradual onset of respiratory distress with coughing and an increased work of breathing that could include wheezing, retractions, hypoxia, and nasal flaring is more suggestive of a lower airway problem.[1] Viruses cause 80% to 90% of childhood respiratory infections with respiratory syncytial virus (RSV), rhinovirus, parainfluenza, influenza, and adenovirus the most common ones in the pediatric population. An individual virus can cause several different patterns of illness (e.g., RSV can cause bronchiolitis, croup, pneumonia, or the common cold).

Assessment

When a child first arrives in the ED with any respiratory problem, rapid assessment should be completed using a systematic approach with the least-intrusive methods first. Observe the child quickly to obtain vital information on respiratory effort and level of consciousness. Inspect the child's bare chest for structural abnormalities, symmetry of movement, and use of accessory muscles. Note the child's position. A child in respiratory distress finds a position of comfort with the body leaning slightly forward and the head in the "sniffing" position, as if smelling a flower; this position allows maximum airway opening.

Respiratory Rate and Pattern

The young child's respiratory muscles are not well developed, so the diaphragm plays a critical role in breathing. Chest auscultation and observation of rise and fall of the abdomen are the best methods for assessing respiratory rate in patients younger than 2 years. Respiratory rates are often irregular in small children, so the rate should be carefully assessed for 1 full minute.

Normal respiratory rates vary by age. A neonate has a normal respiratory rate from 40 to 60 breaths/min, which slows as the child gets older. With respiratory distress the child's respiratory rate initially increases. A resting respiratory rate greater than 60 breaths/min is a sign of respiratory distress in a child, regardless of age. As respiratory distress progresses to failure, the child becomes more acidotic, mental status changes occur, and respiratory rate slows. Bradypnea is an ominous sign in a pediatric patient.

Work of Breathing

Children in respiratory distress exhibit increased work of breathing as evidenced by the use of accessory muscles for breathing. As work of breathing increases, intercostal, substernal, and supraclavicular retractions are observed.

Inspiration is an active process in which muscles expand the chest. Exhalation is passive, relying on elastic recoil of the lungs and chest wall. Under normal circumstances these two processes are balanced with expiration roughly the same length as inspiration (inspiration/expiration ratio 1:1). When air passages are narrowed by inflammation or obstruction, time required for inhalation may remain the same with an increase in effort; however, exhalation takes substantially longer than inspiration (inspiration/expiration ratio 1:2 or 1:3).

Alertness, general responsiveness to the environment, and consolability are important observations for assessing mental status with children. Inconsolability is often a sign of hypoxia; however, a restless child who becomes progressively quieter should be carefully assessed to make certain improved oxygenation rather than respiratory failure or exhaustion is causing the restlessness to abate.

Quality of Breathing

Quality of breathing includes depth and sound of breathing. A child's chest should expand symmetrically; therefore asymmetry or inadequate expansion indicates serious problems such as pneumothorax or hemothorax, foreign body obstruction, or flail chest. To auscultate a child's chest, place the stethoscope at the anterior axillary line level with the second intercostal space on either side. This helps identify the location of any abnormal breath sounds. The small size of a child's chest and thinness of the chest wall allow sounds from one side to resonate throughout the thorax (and even into the abdomen). Therefore listening to the anterior and posterior aspects of the chest may not be as useful for pediatric assessment as it is for an adult.

Breath Sounds

Various disorders produce adventitious sounds that are not normally heard over the chest. Stridor is suggestive of an upper airway obstruction. Stridor is usually heard in the inspiratory phase of respiration as the child works to get air past the obstruction. Stridor will be high-pitched in croup, anaphylaxis, and foreign body aspiration. Sounds heard in the expiratory phase suggest lower airway disorders. Crackles result from passage of air through moisture or fluid. Wheezes are produced as air passes through airways narrowed by exudates, inflammation, or spasm. Bilateral wheezing suggests asthma or bronchiolitis, whereas unilateral wheezing suggests foreign body aspiration. Decreased or unequal breath sounds may be suggestive of an airway obstruction, pneumothorax, pleural effusion, or pneumonia.

Grunting is caused by early closure of the glottis during exhalation with active chest wall contraction. It is a forced expiration that creates positive end-expiratory pressure (PEEP) and prevents airway collapse. Grunting is seen in diseases with diminished lung compliance such as pulmonary edema; it also occurs as a result of pain.

Monitoring

The child with a respiratory problem should be monitored carefully for changes in level of consciousness, work of breathing, and level of fatigue.

Blood gas analysis gives the clearest picture of the patient's respiratory status. For pediatric patients, a venous or capillary gas sample is easier to obtain than an arterial sample and can provide helpful information on ventilatory and acid-base status. Pulse oximetry is a useful, noninvasive means of continuously measuring the oxygen saturation of hemoglobin in the capillaries and correlates well with arterial blood gas (ABG) measurement. An oxygen saturation of 90% to 93% is the lowest acceptable range in children living at sea level. At higher elevations, saturations that fall into the 88% to 89% range are considered normal. Pulse oximetry's major limitation is that carbon dioxide and acid-base balance are not evaluated. Many pulse oximeters rely on analysis of hemoglobin color and may not be useful when extremity perfusion is diminished from trauma, cold ambient temperature, or vasopressors or when the number of erythrocytes is decreased, as in anemia. It can be challenging to effectively apply and monitor an infant or small child on a pulse oximeter.

There are several types of probes that can be used, depending on the type of oximeter available. The adhesive type of pediatric or neonatal probe is generally the most useful probe to use with the younger age-group. Common sites of application include the fingers, toes, earlobes, and the bridge of the nose; in infants, flexible probes work through the palm, foot, penis, or arm.[7] Placing the probe on the foot or great toe and then reapplying the child's sock to limit artifact and lessen the chance the child will remove it can be a very successful approach. In EDs across the country it is becoming more common to see capnography used not only in the intubated patient but in the spontaneously breathing patient as well. In the spontaneously breathing patient it can be used to determine adequacy of ventilation for patients with asthma, patients undergoing procedural sedation, or unconscious patients.[9]

Airway Obstruction by Foreign Body

Small children spend a good deal of time exploring their world. Small objects hold a special fascination for children and are likely to end up in their mouths. Foreign body aspiration can occur at any age but is most commonly seen in children younger than 3 years of age. A child brought to the ED with sudden onset of respiratory distress should be evaluated for foreign body aspiration if no other cause is apparent. Initially a foreign body obstruction produces choking, gagging, wheezing, or coughing. If the object becomes lodged in the larynx, the child cannot speak or breathe. If an object is aspirated into the lower airways, there may be an initial episode of choking/gagging followed by an interval of hours, days, or even weeks when the child is without symptoms. Secondary symptoms are related to the anatomic area in which the object is lodged and usually caused by a persistent respiratory infection.

Foreign body obstruction that completely occludes the airway is an acute emergency. Initial treatment is immediate removal of the object using back slaps and chest thrusts for infants less than 1 year of age. For children 1 year or older, abdominal thrusts should be used. Blind finger sweeps are not recommended to relieve upper airway obstruction; however, any visible foreign objects should be removed. Immediate cricothyrotomy or tracheostomy must be performed to open the airway if it remains obstructed. If ventilation appears adequate, allow the child to assume whatever position is most comfortable. Unless the object is observed high in the upper airway, its exact location must be determined by radiograph. Bronchoscopy may be necessary for removal. A swallowed object is allowed to pass normally through the gastrointestinal tract, unless it is long and sharp. Those objects present significant danger of intestinal perforation. Nickel-cadmium batteries must be removed because of the potential for toxic leakage.

Asthma

Asthma is the most common chronic illness in childhood, affecting 5% to 10% of all American children. This chronic lung disease is characterized by hyperreactivity of the airway, bronchospasm, widespread inflammatory changes, and mucous plugging. Wheezing, the most obvious sign of asthma, may range from mild to severe and is accompanied by tachycardia, retractions, and anxiety. Expiration may be prolonged because of narrowed airways. Obtaining a thorough history may be useful in trying to determine the cause and severity of the attack. Repeated asthma attacks are a dangerous sign because of increasing fatigue and potential complications. Recent hospitalization is likely to be an indication of a seriously ill child.

When assessing a child with asthma, evaluate respiratory rate, quality, and effort to determine the degree of respiratory distress; peak flow measurement should be obtained in older children. The child may require supplemental oxygen if saturation on room air is low and tachypnea and tachycardia are present.

Treatment of a child in the ED with moderate to severe distress involves nebulized or metered-dose inhaled β_2-agonist agents (e.g., albuterol and levalbuterol). Nebulized treatments are usually given every 20 minutes for three doses; nebulized anticholinergic agents such as ipratropium (Atrovent) may be added to potentiate the effects of the β_2-agonists. Oral systemic corticosteroids are given to suppress and reverse airway inflammation. Adequate hydration for children with asthma is important. They are prone to fluid loss during hyperventilation because of decreased intake due to an increased work of breathing. IV fluids may be necessary for some patients.

Bronchiolitis

Bronchiolitis, a viral infection commonly found in infants younger than 24 months of age, can be a life-threatening illness in high-risk children. Those at high risk include the very young (0 to 3 months of age), premature infants, and children with heart or lung disease or chromosomal abnormalities. The viral infection causes an inflammatory process that produces edema in the bronchial mucosa with resultant expiratory obstruction and air trapping. The virus also causes necrosis of the epithelial cells in the upper airways, which produces thick copious mucus. Bronchiolitis has a broad spectrum of severity. Determination of when the respiratory distress began helps predict the course of the illness because the critical period of bronchiolitis usually occurs during the first 24 to 72 hours after onset of respiratory distress. History typically includes symptoms of a cold, cough, and copious amounts of thick nasal drainage for a few days before onset of respiratory distress. High-risk infants can present with apnea and be very ill in appearance compared to the older child. Hospitalization is necessary for high-risk infants younger than 2 months of age and those with an apneic episode.

RSV, the most common causative organism of bronchiolitis, is a highly contagious respiratory pathogen transmitted by direct contact with infected respiratory secretions or contaminated objects. The virus enters the body by contact of contaminated hands with the nose, eye, or other mucous membranes. Aerosol spread occurs but is less common. Care includes appropriate isolation precautions.

Treatment of bronchiolitis is controversial; bronchodilators and corticosteroids are commonly used, but the efficacy of these treatments has not consistently been shown in studies.[3] Nasal suctioning, oxygen therapy, and adequate hydration along with other appropriate supportive care measures are the mainstays of treatment.

Carbon Monoxide Poisoning

Carbon monoxide (CO) is a colorless, odorless gas resulting from incomplete burning of organic substances, such as gasoline, coal products, tobacco, and building materials. Injury and death occur when CO interferes with or inhibits cellular respiration. CO has a higher affinity for hemoglobin than does oxygen, so when CO enters the bloodstream, it readily combines with hemoglobin to form carboxyhemoglobin, decreasing the amount of oxygen available to be released to the cells. Tissue hypoxia can reach dangerous levels before oxygen is available to meet tissue needs.

Unintentional poisoning is often the result of fumes from heaters or smoke from structural fires. Signs and symptoms of CO poisoning are the result of tissue hypoxia. Severity varies with the level of carboxyhemoglobin. Mild symptoms include irritability, headache, visual disturbances, and nausea, whereas more severe cases cause confusion, hallucinations, ataxia, and coma. Bright cherry-red lips and skin, described as classic signs of poisoning, occur less often than pallor and cyanosis. Pulse oximetry will not be accurate in CO poisoning; a reading within normal limits may be present even though tissues are hypoxic because the pulse oximeter cannot differentiate hemoglobin saturated with CO from hemoglobin saturated with oxygen.

Primary treatment is administration of 100% oxygen with a nonrebreather mask or bag-valve mask. Efforts should be made to reduce the child's metabolic demand for oxygen by keeping the child quiet and calm. Severe cases may require intubation or hyperbaric oxygen therapy. Children with suspected or known inhalation of CO should be admitted for close observation and oxygen therapy. Because CO has a half-life of approximately 2 hours, oxygen therapy is needed for a prolonged period.

Croup

Croup, or laryngotracheobronchitis, is viral inflammation of the subglottic area, including the trachea and bronchi. Croup occurs most frequently in infants and children 6 months to 3 years of age but may occur in older children. It is slightly more prevalent in boys. Croup is seen most frequently in cooler months.

The inflammatory process of viral croup produces edema of the trachea and surrounding structures. Edematous airways secrete tenacious mucus, which leads to problematic removal of secretions. The child's effort to inspire air through edematous structures produces the characteristic stridor of croup.

History usually includes an upper respiratory infection for a few days followed by nocturnal onset of the characteristic "barking" cough. The child may have a hoarse voice or cry. Nursing assessment should be performed carefully to keep the child calm. The stress of crying increases the work of breathing, so both stridor and retractions markedly increase. Assessment should focus on cardiorespiratory status, hydration, anxiety, and fatigue level as well as parental anxiety.

Nursing interventions for croup focus on relieving anxiety and reducing work of breathing. The child should be kept as comfortable as possible (e.g., sitting on parent's lap); painful interventions should be minimized. Heart rate, respiratory rate, and work of breathing should be monitored. Cool mist therapy has been the mainstay of ED treatment, though little evidence supports its clinical efficacy.[12,13] Corticosteroids are administered to reduce airway inflammation and swelling. Dexamethasone has the same efficacy if administered intravenously, intramuscularly, or orally. Nebulized racemic epinephrine is used in severe cases to reduce mucosal edema and laryngospasm. Children should be monitored for at least 2 to 3 hours after racemic epinephrine is administered because the medication's effect may not be sustained, producing a "rebound" effect. Soft-tissue radiograph of the neck may be indicated to rule out epiglottitis; croup is associated with tracheal narrowing, a "steeple sign" on neck films.

The decision for hospital admission depends on the patient's degree of respiratory distress, ability to maintain adequate hydration, ability to rest, and the degree of parental apprehension.

Epiglottitis

Epiglottitis, or supraglottic laryngitis, is the most emergent acute bacterial upper airway obstruction of childhood. This condition produces a rapid onset of inflammatory edema of the epiglottis. Because most pediatric cases are caused by *Haemophilus influenzae* type B, the incidence of epiglottitis has significantly declined since the *H. influenzae* type B conjugate vaccine became available. A child with epiglottitis typically presents in an anxious state, with respiratory distress, drooling because of difficulty swallowing, and sitting forward with the neck extended (tripod position) to maximize airway patency. The child may have audible respiratory sounds and appears flushed and toxic with a high temperature. The epiglottis becomes swollen and cherry red and can cause total airway obstruction if manipulated during examination.

The child should be allowed to assume a position that maximizes his or her respiratory effort. Initially, no attempts should be made to perform invasive procedures or look down the patient's pharynx unless absolutely necessary. Most patients with severe respiratory distress from epiglottitis go directly to the operating room for intubation or tracheostomy. Hospital admission is always required for known or suspected epiglottitis. IV fluids are necessary until oral fluids can be swallowed. IV administration of antibiotics is preferred; however, IV access, fluids, and antibiotics should be deferred until the patient's airway is secured and protected.

Peritonsillar and Retropharyngeal Abscess

Other diseases with signs and symptoms similar to epiglottitis include peritonsillar abscess and retropharyngeal abscess. A peritonsillar abscess, on rare occasions, can compromise a child's airway. Retropharyngeal abscesses have a less abrupt onset than epiglottitis but also pose a substantial risk to airway patency. A child with a peritonsillar or retropharyngeal abscess requires the caregiver to frequently assess and support respiratory and circulatory function. Retropharyngeal abscesses require drainage in the operating room, whereas a peritonsillar abscess may be drained in the ED if there is danger of airway compromise. Both conditions are treated with IV antibiotics.

Pertussis

Pertussis, or whooping cough, is an acute respiratory infection caused by *Bordetella pertussis*. Whooping cough usually occurs in children younger than 4 years of age who have not been immunized. Highly contagious, whooping cough is particularly threatening to young infants, resulting in higher morbidity and mortality rates. Incidence is highest in the spring and summer.

Pertussis is usually indistinguishable from a common cold until the paroxysmal stage. During this stage the child has a fever and whooping type of spasmodic cough that can lead to hypoxia, gagging, vomiting, and exhaustion. Petechiae above the nipple line, ear infection, atelectasis, pneumothorax, and vomiting may also be present. Hernias may appear suddenly as a result of exertion during coughing.

Excitement and crying tend to worsen the coughing paroxysms, so care should be taken to keep the child as calm as possible. Airway clearance is important in management of pertussis and may require gentle suctioning. Humidified oxygen should be used, the child should be isolated from other patients, and antibiotic therapy should be initiated as soon as possible. Hospitalization is recommended for those infants who exhibit respiratory distress and have a significant oxygen desaturation associated with coughing paroxysms. Infants may also require IV fluids for dehydration secondary to inability to feed caused by coughing.

Pneumonia

Pneumonia, inflammation of the pulmonary parenchyma, is common throughout childhood but occurs more frequently in infancy and early childhood. Clinically, pneumonia may occur as a primary disease or complication of other illnesses.

Viruses cause the majority of pneumonias in children, although bacterial pneumonia, usually caused by group B streptococci and gram-negative bacilli, is more likely to occur in the first weeks of life. Whether viral or bacterial, pathogens reach the lung and cause an inflammatory response that leads to accumulation of fluid in the lungs, tachypnea, cough, and fever. Bacterial pneumonia tends to have an abrupt onset with high fever, 101.3° to 105.8° F (38.5° to 41° C). In viral pneumonia, fever is usually lower than 102.2° F (39° C). With bacterial pneumonia there is an increase in the number of granulocytes and bands on the white cell differential count.

Treatment varies with the child's age, suspected causative agent, severity of symptoms, and immune status of the child. Infants younger than 2 months usually require a complete septic workup and hospitalization for IV antibiotic treatment. Children with minimal distress and who are tolerating oral fluids well can usually be treated at home with oral antibiotic therapy.

Pneumothorax

A pneumothorax is a collection of air in the pleural space caused by the rupture of an alveolar bleb on the surface of the pleura and results in the partial collapse of one or both lungs. A pneumothorax may occur spontaneously or secondary to obstruction, trauma, cancer, or tuberculosis. A history of a previous spontaneous pneumothorax increases the likelihood of recurrence.

Symptoms depend on how much air escapes into the pleural space. Small amounts may be asymptomatic. A large amount of air prevents full expansion of the affected lung, causing tachypnea, dyspnea, grunting, hypoxia, and cyanosis. Most respiratory problems cause retraction of chest wall musculature; however, a pneumothorax may cause bulging of these muscles, especially intercostal muscles over the affected area. Bilateral breath sounds are usually heard in infants and small children with a pneumothorax because their thin chest wall allows breath sounds to be readily transmitted from one area to another.

Hospital admission is almost always recommended. Oxygen administration and bed rest are used in mild cases. Children with more than 40% pneumothorax usually require a chest tube with closed drainage and suction to evacuate air from the pleural space and reexpand the lung. The child must be continually assessed for development of a tension pneumothorax, which is a life-threatening problem. If a tension pneumothorax is suspected, a needle thoracentesis must immediately be done. Prepare for a chest tube insertion following the needle thoracentesis.

CARDIOVASCULAR EMERGENCIES

Causes of cardiovascular emergencies in the pediatric population differ from those in adults, but the three basic categories of cardiovascular compromise are the same: inadequate heart function (rhythm disturbances, heart failure, congenital heart disease), inadequate volume for circulation (dehydration, burns, trauma), and inadequate fluid distribution (distributive shock states such as sepsis and anaphylaxis).

Most pediatric cardiac arrests are related to respiratory arrest rather than primary cardiac arrest.[1] Supporting the child's respiratory efforts and intervening early can prevent potential cardiac problems.

Assessment

Blood volume in a child is 80 mL/kg, with total blood volume much less than in an adult. Loss of 1 cup (8 oz or 240 mL) of blood in a 10-kg child is equivalent to blood loss of 1 quart (32 oz or 960 mL) in an adult. With infants and children, the immature sympathetic innervation of the ventricles and the shorter and less elastic myocardial fibers keep the stroke volume at a relatively fixed rate.[14] A child responds to the need for increased cardiac output with an increased heart rate. Tachycardia may initially increase cardiac output during periods of distress; however, prolonged tachycardia causes cardiac decompensation and decreases cardiac output. Close attention to heart rate, skin perfusion, and mental status is the key to early recognition of compensated shock. Capillary refill time is also recommended as a sensitive indicator of perfusion in the pediatric patient. Use of this parameter has not been studied extensively; however, normal capillary refill time is about 2 seconds. More than 3 seconds may indicate poor perfusion in a normothermic child.

Cardiovascular assessment should identify shock or conditions that could lead to shock that require intervention by the emergency nurse. A history of illness or injury is important in interpreting signs and symptoms. Observing the child plays a major role. Important elements to assess include the following:

- *Skin color:* Pallor and mottling may indicate decreased perfusion caused by diminished cardiac output.
- *Capillary refill:* A delay of 3 seconds or more is abnormal.
- *Level of consciousness:* Decreased perfusion to the brain may cause restlessness, confusion, or lethargy.
- *Skin turgor:* Estimates the state of hydration and, to a lesser extent, nutrition of the child. To assess, grasp the skin on the back of the hand, lower arm, or abdomen between two fingers so the child's skin is tented up. Hold the skin for a few seconds then release. Skin with normal turgor snaps rapidly back to its normal position. Skin with decreased turgor remains elevated and returns slowly to its normal position (tenting). This is a late sign of moderate to severe dehydration.
- *Mucous membranes:* Membranes should be moist. Dry, cracked, parched lips suggest moderate to severe dehydration.
- *Anterior fontanel:* A bulging fontanel may indicate increased intracranial pressure, whereas a sunken fontanel suggests dehydration. The anterior fontanel generally closes by 9 to 18 months of age.

- *Peripheral pulse quality:* Decreased perfusion to extremities results in weak peripheral pulses. Inappropriate distribution of fluids, as in a distributive shock state (sepsis and anaphylactic) causes bounding pulses.
- *Vital signs:* Temperature, pulse rate, respiration rate, and blood pressure. Normal vital sign parameters for the pediatric patient are listed in Table 47-2.

Vital signs should be documented as part of the baseline assessment. Children in early shock may have a normal SBP because of their strong compensatory mechanisms (tachycardia and vasoconstriction). Trending pulse pressure (systolic pressure minus diastolic pressure) provides valuable clues to perfusion status: a narrowing pulse pressure indicates further vasoconstriction; a widening pulse pressure indicates increasing vasodilation. Declining SBP is a sign of a decompensated shock state warranting immediate intervention. A child can lose a significant amount of circulating volume before hypotension ensues. SBP can be estimated using the following formula:

$$\text{Normal systolic pressure} = 80 + (\text{age in years} \times 2)$$

$$\text{Minimal acceptable systolic pressure} = 70 + (\text{age in years} \times 2)$$

Inadequate Heart Function

Rhythm Disturbances

Children generally have young, strong hearts, so rhythm disturbances are seldom primary events. Dysrhythmias usually result from hypoxia or metabolic disturbances. Because of increased survival rates, pediatric patients with rhythm disturbances from congenital cardiac problems are seen with increasing frequency in the ED. The most common congenital problems causing rhythm disturbances are transposition of the great vessels and congenital mitral stenosis. Acquired cardiac diseases such as cardiomyopathies, rheumatic heart disease, and viral myocarditis may also cause rhythm disturbances.

Abnormal rhythms in pediatric patients are often divided into three categories: fast, slow, and absent (Table 47-3). Sinus tachycardia and supraventricular tachycardia (SVT) are two major rhythm disturbances found in children. Sinus tachycardia is caused by a variety of factors, including fever, anxiety, pain, and hypovolemia. The rate of sinus tachycardia is 140 to 220 beats/min. Treatment of sinus tachycardia is focused on the underlying cause; for example, if the child is febrile, control the fever and then reassess the heart rate. SVT is caused by a reentry mechanism and is characterized by a nonvarying heart rate higher than 220 beats/min in infants and greater than 180 beats/min in children. Infants often present with symptoms of poor feeding, rapid breathing, pale skin color, or fussiness. SVT can be initially well tolerated; however, it will ultimately lead to congestive heart failure if left untreated. Stable SVT may respond to vagal maneuvers: an example of a vagal maneuver

appropriate for an infant would be putting a bag of ice water over the forehead, eyes, and bridge of the nose (not obstructing the airway).[14] An example of a vagal maneuver for an older child would be to have the child blow through an obstructed straw.[14] Adenosine should be considered if there is no response to the vagal maneuvers. Bradycardia is an ominous sign in a pediatric patient. Sinus bradycardia is frequently caused by hypoxia and should be treated aggressively with ventilation and oxygenation. A child with a heart rate less than 60 beats/min with signs of poor perfusion requires immediate cardiac compressions.[5,14] Junctional and idioventricular rhythms are usually terminal rhythms. Absent, disorganized, and nonperfusing rhythms require cardiopulmonary resuscitation and advanced life support procedures.

Heart Failure

Congenital heart disease accounts for the majority of children seen in the ED with heart failure (HF). Preload, afterload, and myocardial contractility are major factors in determining the amount of blood pumped through the vascular system. When the heart is not able to pump effectively because of chronic disease, rhythm disturbance, pressure on the heart, or excessive fluid volume, the fluid backs up in the system, causing signs of overload such as pulmonary edema, jugular vein distention, and enlarged liver.

Signs of HF include tachycardia, tachypnea, cough, wheezes, pulmonary crackles, cyanosis, pallor, poor appetite, and failure to thrive. Many times infants with HF have a very rapid respiratory rate (60 to 100 breaths/min) but do not appear in distress. Lack of distress is evidence of the infant's ability to compensate. Observe for presence and degree of other indicators of respiratory effort such as nasal flaring, intercostal retractions, head bobbing, and expiratory grunting.

Primary treatment of HF is aimed at improving myocardial contractility and decreasing cardiac workload by using pharmacologic agents. These agents include inotropic drugs (dobutamine, milrinone, digoxin) that improve myocardial contractility, diuretics (furosemide) to reduce preload, and afterload-reducing agents (sodium nitroprusside, captopril) to reduce ventricular afterload.

Inadequate Volume

The major medical cause of hypovolemia in children is dehydration. A child who has been sick for even a short time with vomiting and diarrhea is at risk, as is a child who has been ill for several days with fever and decreased fluid intake. When output exceeds intake over time, dehydration becomes clinically significant and electrolyte imbalances occur; electrolyte disturbances cause more nausea and vomiting, starting a downward spiral that can be reversed only with medical intervention. The degree of dehydration is categorized as a percentage of lost body weight (mild—5%, moderate—10%, severe—15%). When 5% or more of the child's body mass (weight) is lost, skin and mucous membranes appear dry. It

Table 47-3. Rhythm Disturbances in Children

Rhythm	Cause	Characteristics	Treatment
FAST RHYTHMS			
Sinus tachycardia	Fever, anxiety, pain, hypovolemia	Rapid sinus rhythm; rate 140-220 beats/min	Treat underlying cause.
Supraventricular tachycardia	Reentry mechanism	Paroxysmal sinus rhythm; P waves often undetectable; rate >220 beats/min (infant), rate >180 beats/min (child)	*Stable:* Vagal maneuvers. Consider adenosine if no response. Adenosine 0.1 mg/kg IV bolus (maximum initial dose: 6 mg). May double and repeat dose once (maximum second dose: 12 mg). If no response consider: Alternative medications (e.g., amiodarone, procainamide). Cardioversion 0.5-1 J/kg. *Unstable:* Cardioversion 0.5-1 J/kg; if not effective, increase to 2 J/kg. Sedate if possible, but do not delay cardioversion. May attempt adenosine if this does not delay cardioversion.
Ventricular tachycardia	Structural disease, hypoxia, acidosis, electrolyte imbalance, toxic ingestion (e.g., tricyclic antidepressants)	Rate ≥120 beats/min; wide QRS; no P waves	*Pulse and stable:* Amiodarone 5 mg/kg IV (max 300 mg) over 20-60 min or procainamide 15 mg/kg IV over 30-60 min or lidocaine 1 mg/kg IV bolus. Consider sedation, and cardiovert at 0.5-1 J/kg. *Pulse but unstable:* Cardioversion 0.5-1 J/kg; if not effective, increase to 2 J/kg. Sedate if possible, but do not delay cardioversion. *Pulseless:* Defibrillation at 2 J/kg, high-quality BLS for 2 minutes; if no response, repeat defibrillation using 4 J/kg followed by high-quality BLS for 2 minutes; repeat as needed. Epinephrine IV/IO: 0.01 mg/kg (1:10,000: 0.1 mL/kg) as soon as vascular access obtained. ET: 0.1 mg/kg (1:1,000: 0.1 mL/kg). Repeat dose every 3 to 5 minutes. Consider antidysrhythmics: Amiodarone 5 mg/kg (max 300 mg) IV/IO. Lidocaine 1 mg/kg IV/IO. Magnesium 25-50 mg/kg IV/IO if torsades de pointes.
SLOW RHYTHMS			
Sinus bradycardia	Hypoxemia, hypotension, acidosis	Sinus rhythm; slow rate (<80 beats/min in infants, <60 beats/min in children)	Ventilation, oxygenation, cardiac compressions for heart rate <60 beats/min with signs of poor perfusion. Epinephrine (1:10,000), 0.01 mg/kg IV/IO. Repeat every 3-5 minutes. If increased vagal tone or primary AV block: Atropine, 0.02 mg/kg IV; may repeat. (Minimum dose 0.1 mg; maximal total dose for child: 1 mg.) Consider cardiac pacing.
Junctional rhythm, heart blocks	Hypoxemia, hypotension, acidosis	Rare in children; slow rate; P waves may or may not be present	Ventilation, oxygenation, cardiac compressions for heart rate <60 beat/min with signs of poor perfusion. Atropine, 0.02 mg/kg IV; may repeat. (Minimum dose 0.1 mg; maximal total dose for child: 1 mg.) Epinephrine (1:10,000) 0.1 mL/kg IV. Consider cardiac pacing.

Table 47-3.	RHYTHM DISTURBANCES IN CHILDREN—CONT'D		
Rhythm	**Cause**	**Characteristics**	**Treatment**
ABSENT/DISORGANIZED/NONPERFUSING RHYTHMS			
Asystole/PEA	Hypoxia, hypovolemia, acidosis, hypo/hyperkalemia, hypoglycemia, hypothermia, toxins, cardiac tamponade, tension pneumothorax, thrombosis (coronary or pulmonary), trauma	Asystole: Flat line on ECG; absent pulse; absent respirations PEA: Pulselessness, with organized electrical activity on ECG	BLS, identify/treat underlying cause. Epinephrine IV/IO 0.01 mg/kg (1:10,000): 0.1 mL/kg; ET; 0.1 mg/kg (1:1,000: 0.1 mL/kg). Repeat every 3 to 5 minutes.
Ventricular fibrillation	Rare in infants and children; hypoxia, hypovolemia, acidosis, hypo/hyperkalemia, hypoglycemia, hypothermia, toxins, cardiac tamponade, tension pneumothorax, thrombosis (coronary or pulmonary), trauma	No identifiable P, QRS, or T waves; wavy line on ECG	Defibrillation at 2 J/kg, highquality BLS for 2 minutes; if no response, repeat defibrillation using 4 J/kg followed by high-quality BLS for 2 minutes; repeat as needed. Epinephrine IV/IO: 0.01 mg/kg (1:10,000: 0.1 mL/kg) as soon as vascular access obtained. ET: 0.1 mg/kg (1:1,000: 0.1 mL/kg). Repeat dose every 3 to 5 minutes. Consider antidysrhythmics: Amiodarone 5 mg/kg (max 300 mg) IV/IO. Lidocaine 1 mg/kg IV/IO. Magnesium 25-50 mg/kg IV/IO if torsades de pointes.

BLS, Basic life support (ventilations and compressions); *ECG,* electrocardiogram; *ET,* endotracheal tube; *IO,* intraosseous; *IV,* intravenous; *PEA,* pulseless electrical activity.

is often helpful to ask the parent about intake and output—the number of bottles the child has taken and the number of stools or wet diapers per day for small children (six to eight wet diapers per day is considered normal). Mild dehydration is commonly treated with oral rehydration. Parents may be instructed to give the child small amounts of an oral electrolyte solution at frequent intervals (a teaspoonful at a time). Changes in mental status, skin perfusion, heart rate, pulse quality, urinary output, and blood pressure occur in moderate and severe dehydration; eyes appear sunken and infants exhibit a sunken anterior fontanel. Unless fluid volume is replaced and balance between intake and output restored, the condition will progress to hypovolemic shock.

Increasing heart rate, mottled cool skin, decreasing mental status, narrowing pulse pressure, and extremely prolonged capillary refill time suggest that the child's perfusion status is worsening. Resuscitation requires ensuring adequate ventilation and oxygenation, rapid bolusing with 20 mL/kg of crystalloid solution, and repeated fluid boluses until improvement is seen.[14] If vascular access cannot be rapidly obtained, intraosseous (IO) access should be attempted, and in some cases of severe decompensated shock IO access should be the initial access. IO access can be performed safely on children of all ages.[10] IO access is a quick, safe, and dependable route for administering fluids, medications, and blood products.

Diagnostic tests may include complete blood count (CBC); determination of electrolytes, glucose, and blood urea nitrogen (BUN) values; and urinalysis. The decision to admit is based on the child's condition after evaluation and management and the ability to tolerate oral feeding.

Inadequate Fluid Distribution

Septic Shock

Sepsis, or septicemia, is a profound, life-threatening bacterial infection in the bloodstream. Septic shock occurs in patients with septicemia when inadequate tissue perfusion occurs in the wake of massive vasodilation. The massive vasodilation causes a relative hypovolemia in the intravascular space, which is why pediatric septic shock frequently responds well to early aggressive fluid resuscitation. The clinical diagnosis of septic shock is made in children with a suspected infection, manifested by hyperthermia or hypothermia, who exhibit other signs of decreased perfusion. Septic shock may be manifest as a warm shock or a cold shock state. Tachycardia and decreased mental status are seen in both shock states. Warm shock may occur initially characterized by a flushed ruddy appearance, bounding peripheral pulses, and flash capillary refill; cold shock is associated with mottled cool extremities, diminished peripheral pulses, and capillary refill greater than 3 seconds.[2,6]

The ABCs should be rapidly assessed and supported. The nurse must keep in mind that hypotension is a late sign of shock in infants and young children, and when present, it indicates decompensated severe shock. Skin should be inspected for petechiae or purpuric lesions which would be "red flag" skin signs of septic shock caused by meningococcemia.

Management in the ED focuses on preservation of vital functions. Adequate ventilation and oxygenation are the first priority. Administer supplemental oxygen, and assist with breathing if ventilation is inadequate. Maintaining normal perfusion is a priority. Vascular access should be quickly obtained, and rapid fluid boluses of 20 mL/kg should be repeatedly administered with the goal of attaining normal perfusion.[2,6] The average fluid requirement to obtain normal perfusion is 40 to 60 mL/kg in the first hour. This can vary depending of the severity of the presentation.[2] Isotonic crystalloids such as normal saline are given for volume replacement. After the diagnosis of sepsis or septic shock is made, IV antibiotic therapy should be instituted immediately. Ideally, all cultures (blood, urine, others) are collected before antibiotic administration. The antibiotics administered vary with the child's age and the presumed source of infection. After culture results are available, antibiotic therapy can be more specific. Sympathomimetic and inotropic drugs such as epinephrine and dopamine may be used to increase heart rate and cardiac output in patients with poor myocardial function and systemic perfusion despite adequate oxygenation and fluid resuscitation. Serum glucose level should be carefully monitored. In younger infants and children, limited glycogen stores in the liver place the child at risk for hypoglycemia. A child is considered hypoglycemic if his or her blood glucose level is less than 60 mg/dL in a child or less than 40 mg/dL in a neonate. The child is admitted, usually to the intensive care unit, for continued IV fluid replacement, antibiotics, and monitoring.

Anaphylaxis

Anaphylaxis is a serious allergic reaction with a rapid onset and the potential to cause death.[16]

This severe, potentially fatal, multisystemic response occurs after exposure to an allergy-causing substance (allergen). Anaphylaxis is highly likely when at least *one* of following three clinical criteria is present:

1. Acute onset (minutes to several hours) of illness with involvement of skin and/or mucosal tissue (hives, itching, flushing, swollen lips) and at least one of the following:
   - Respiratory compromise (e.g., difficulty breathing, wheeze, stridor, hypoxemia)
   - Reduced SBP or associated symptoms of end-organ hypoperfusion (e.g., syncope, incontinence, hypotonia)
2. Two or more of the following that occur rapidly after exposure to a *likely* allergen for that patient (onset of minutes to several hours):
   - Skin and/or mucosal involvement (e.g., hives; itching; flushing; swollen lips, tongue, or uvula)
   - Respiratory compromise
   - Reduced SBP or associated symptoms of end-organ hypoperfusion
   - Persistent gastrointestinal symptoms
3. Reduced SBP after exposure to *known* allergen for that patient (onset of minutes to several hours):
   - Infants 1 month to 1 year: less than 70 mm Hg
   - Children 1 year up to 10 years: less than (70 mm Hg + [2 × age in years])
   - Children 11 years or older and adults: less than 90 mm Hg or greater than 30% decrease from patient's baseline

Recovery from anaphylactic reactions depends on rapid recognition and institution of treatment. The goal of treatment is to provide ventilation, restore adequate circulation, and prevent further exposure by identifying and removing the cause. Establishing an airway is the first concern. The child should be placed on high-flow oxygen, cardiac monitoring should be initiated, and vital signs should be assessed. Epinephrine intramuscularly, 1:1000 solution: 0.01 mg/kg (0.01 mL/kg), maximum 0.3 mg (0.3 mL), should be given immediately and repeated every 5 to 15 minutes as necessary.[1,17]

Fluids are given to restore volume. The amount of fluid given should be determined by the clinical situation. Children with anaphylaxis should be hospitalized and monitored for at least 24 hours because of the risk for a biphasic reaction.

Second-line treatments, such as antihistamines and steroids, are slower acting than epinephrine and have little effect on acute blood pressure changes. They are helpful for symptomatic relief of itching, angioedema, or hives and are commonly administered in the ED setting.

Sickle Cell Disease

Sickle cell disease (SCD) is an inherited hemoglobinopathy characterized by the presence of hemoglobin S. In SCD, red blood cells that are normally round assume an irregular sickle shape when deoxygenated. These sickled cells clump together, occluding small blood vessels and causing tissue ischemia. Sickling is precipitated by multiple factors, including infection, dehydration, fatigue, cold exposure, and stress.

There are three major categories of sickle cell crisis. Vasoocclusive crises occur when small vessels in bone, soft tissue, and organs (e.g., liver, spleen, brain, lungs, penis) are occluded, causing ischemia, pain, and swelling. The first presentation of vasoocclusive crisis, usually after 2 or 3 months of age, is manifested by warmth and swelling of one or both hands or feet. Older children have pain in affected organs, visual disturbances, respiratory distress, and priapism. Management is primarily focused on correcting the precipitating cause, if identified, supporting hydration and oxygenation as needed, and pain management.

Aplastic crisis is characterized by impaired red blood cell production in the bone marrow. Aplastic crisis worsens the anemia of SCD and leads to high-output congestive heart failure. The diagnosis of aplastic crisis is made on the basis of CBC and reticulocyte count results. Management is focused on restoring depleted blood components.

Sequestration crisis is the most fulminant manifestation of SCD. It is less common than other crises but can be rapidly fatal. Incidence is greater in young children, several months to 6 years of age. Blood suddenly pools in the spleen and other visceral organs, causing severe anemia and hypovolemic shock. Emergent management is focused on restoration of circulating blood volume.

Acute chest syndrome (ACS) is a major cause of morbidity and mortality for children with SCD. There is a higher incidence of ACS during the winter months, and the peak incidence occurs in patients 2 to 4 years of age. The specific cause of ACS is not easily determined. Triggers such as a vasoocclusive crisis, infection, asthma, or postoperative complication have all been implicated. Regardless of the cause, deoxygenation occurs and sickling of the red cells is triggered, resulting in occlusion, ischemia, and vessel injury within the pulmonary vasculature.[19] Signs and symptoms include pleuritic chest pain, cough, dyspnea, fever, tachypnea, hypoxia, and pleural effusions.

Because of the need for close monitoring, specialists care for most patients with SCD. However, a first crisis or severe crisis may lead to treatment in the ED. Medical management is usually directed at supportive, symptomatic treatment. The main objectives are pain management, oxygenation, hydration with oral or IV solutions, electrolyte replacement, rest, blood replacement as needed, and antibiotics as required. The administration of narcotics should be anticipated for pain control because SCD is a chronic painful disease.

NEUROLOGIC EMERGENCIES

Head trauma is the most common cause of neurologic emergency in children; however, seizures, shunt malfunction, and rarely, brain tumors and congenital vascular malformations can also affect mental status in the pediatric population. Infectious processes such as meningitis and sepsis are another cause for neurologic changes in children. Refer to Chapter 28 for discussion of pediatric trauma.

Assessment

When a child has an altered mental status, it is important to remember the first priority is airway and ventilation. Neurologic assessment of pediatric patients presents special challenges, especially for the nonverbal child. When parents say their child is "not acting normal," this should be taken seriously. Early signs and symptoms of increased intracranial pressure include altered mental status, restlessness, inconsolability, headache, and vomiting. Constricted or dilated pupils and decorticate (abnormal flexion) or decerebrate (abnormal extension) posturing are late signs of increased intracranial pressure.

Numerous methods of assessing neurologic function in children have been proposed, including pediatric adaptations of the Glasgow Coma Scale (see Table 28-3). The simplest and probably the most useful in the emergency setting is the mnemonic AVPU:
- **A** *A*lert
- **V** responds to *V*erbal stimuli
- **P** responds to *P*ainful stimuli
- **U** *U*nresponsive

Serial assessment with this mnemonic, together with a description of the patient's behavior, is the clearest means for documenting changes. An accurate history from parents is also helpful. When a child presents with an altered mental status, ask about trauma, previous medical problems, ingestions, headache, and signs and symptoms of infection. An altered level of consciousness in any child needs to be recognized as an emergent condition.

Treatment for children who arrive in the ED with an altered level of consciousness includes assessment of ABCs along with assessment for injury or illnesses. The child must be evaluated for signs and symptoms of increased intracranial pressure to prevent secondary central nervous system injury. Laboratory studies may be ordered to detect toxins or electrolyte abnormalities; diagnostic imaging may be ordered to rule out injury or other pathologic processes as the precipitator of the child's change in mental status.

Seizures

Seizures are involuntary movements or alteration in sensation, behavior, or consciousness caused by abnormal electrical activity in the brain. In young children seizures associated with fever are one of the most common neurologic disorders of childhood, affecting 3% to 5% of children. Most febrile seizures occur after 6 months of age and usually before 3 years, with increased frequency in children younger than 18 months.

The cause of febrile seizures is still uncertain. In most children, height and rapidity of temperature elevation or rapidity of the temperature drop seem to be important factors; however, seizures usually occur during temperature fluctuations rather than after prolonged elevation. Febrile seizures may accompany upper respiratory infection, gastrointestinal infection, or ear infection. Between 25% and 30% of children with simple febrile seizures have a recurrence with subsequent infections.[5]

Treatment for febrile seizures consists of ensuring the child's safety during the seizure, controlling the seizure, and reducing the temperature. Parents also need reassurance of the generally benign nature of febrile seizures.

Other seizure disorders have numerous and varied causes. Seizure disorders are idiopathic if the cause is unknown and organic or symptomatic if the cause is identifiable. Epilepsy is the diagnosis when seizures are recurrent with no apparent cause for the seizures. Seizure patients may exhibit a wide range of behaviors, from lip smacking and staring to violent muscular contractions or sudden loss of consciousness; urinary and bowel incontinence may also occur. Status epilepticus occurs when seizure activity is prolonged (greater than 30 minutes) or the patient has sequential seizures without regaining consciousness between each seizure. Airway management, prevention of injury, and cessation of seizure activity with drug therapy are indicated for management of seizures. Whether the patient is admitted to the hospital or discharged home depends on the patient's history, laboratory findings, and physical findings.

Status Epilepticus

Prolonged continuous seizure activity, or status epilepticus, may be a manifestation of anoxia, infection, trauma, ingestion, or metabolic disorder. In about half the children with status epilepticus, the cause is not identified. Sustained seizure activity can potentially produce cerebral anoxia and possible ischemic brain damage, so airway maintenance, oxygenation, and rapid termination of convulsive activity are priorities.

Ensure the child's safety. If the child is in severe respiratory distress or stops breathing, bag-mask device ventilation should be used until intubation is possible. An IV or IO catheter should be inserted for administration of fluids and medication. Anticonvulsant medications (e.g., benzodiazepines) may be administered rectally, intranasally, or intramuscularly until seizure activity abates and vascular access can be established. Common laboratory tests include CBC; determination of electrolytes, glucose, calcium, magnesium, BUN, and anticonvulsant drug levels; urinalysis; and toxicology screen.

GASTROINTESTINAL AND GENITOURINARY EMERGENCIES
Gastroenteritis

Innumerable children are brought to the ED with complaints of nausea, vomiting, diarrhea, and poor feeding. Gastroenteritis is an inflammation of the gastrointestinal tract caused by bacterial, viral, or parasitic agents. Viral diarrhea is the most common infection, with rotavirus being the most common cause. Morbidity results from dehydration and electrolyte imbalances. Diagnostic tests may include CBC; measurement of electrolyte, glucose, and BUN levels; urinalysis; and stool cultures. Gastroenteritis associated with signs of severe dehydration/hypovolemic shock is treated with 20 mL/kg boluses of IV crystalloid solutions. Fluids boluses of 20 mL/kg should be repeated until perfusion improves. Patients whose laboratory analyses are within normal limits, those who are only mildly dehydrated, and those who are able to take fluids by mouth are generally discharged to home after rehydration. Parents are instructed to give the child small amounts of clear liquids at frequent intervals (a teaspoonful at a time). Oral rehydration fluids are preferred; apple juice should be avoided because it is hyperosmolar and may worsen diarrhea. The traditional strategy of treating diarrhea with oral rehydration therapy followed by food restriction with bowel rest (e.g., the BRAT diet—bananas, rice, applesauce, and tea and toast) is being challenged by evidence supporting prompt refeeding without a restrictive diet.[5] Parents should be instructed to return to their physician or the ED if the child does not improve within 24 hours, abdominal pain increases, or the child is acting strangely in any way.

Abdominal Pain

Other illnesses that can cause gastrointestinal upset or abdominal pain are infection with bacterial agents and parasites; surgical emergencies such as appendicitis, strangulated hernia, intussusception, testicular torsion, or bowel obstruction; urinary tract infection (UTI); and toxic ingestion. For the most part, ED treatment of the stable patient with abdominal pain focuses on assessing the patient, including history and vital signs, deciding whether the patient can be discharged or requires hospitalization, and determining if the problem needs medical or surgical intervention. If the child has abdominal pain, an acute abdominal condition must be ruled out, so the child should not be allowed to drink any fluid until evaluation is complete. In general, the possibility of a surgical abdomen should be considered for any patient with abdominal pain associated with palpation or movement. Basic diagnostic tests include a CBC and urinalysis; imaging studies of the chest, abdomen, or pelvis may be needed. Adolescent female patients should be asked about pregnancy, and a menstrual history should be obtained. Assume that any female of childbearing age could be pregnant and obtain a pregnancy test to rule out gestation as the potential cause of abdominal pain.

Appendicitis

Appendicitis is inflammation of the vermiform appendix or blind sac of the cecum. It is the most common condition requiring surgical intervention during childhood. Primarily an acute condition, appendicitis can progress to perforation and peritonitis without appropriate treatment. Signs and symptoms of appendicitis vary greatly but commonly include pain that begins in the periumbilical region and migrates to the right lower quadrant, rebound tenderness, nausea, and vomiting. Appendicitis in the nonverbal child often presents very late; the appendix may be ruptured and the peritoneum contaminated by the time symptoms are recognized and the child goes to surgery. The most important diagnostic tests are a white blood cell count with differential and urinalysis. With appendicitis, total white blood cell count is usually 15,000 to 20,000 cells/mL with bands present. Fever is usually present, varying from 99.5° F to 101.3° F (37.5° to 38.5° C). If the temperature is greater than 102.2° F (39° C), viral illness or perforation is likely. Imaging studies (e.g., abdominal computed tomography or ultrasonography) may be obtained if diagnosis is uncertain. Definitive treatment for appendicitis is surgical removal of the appendix, or appendectomy. The child should have no oral intake, and fluid and electrolyte imbalances should be corrected before the child goes to surgery. Prophylactic antibiotics may be started before surgery for patients with evidence of perforation.

Incarcerated Hernia

A hernia is a protrusion of a portion of an organ through an abdominal opening. Classic presentation is an asymptomatic bulge that becomes more prominent with crying, defecation, coughing, or laughing.[5] Danger from herniation arises when the intestine protruding through the opening is constricted to the extent that circulation is impaired. Hernias can often be manually reduced in the ED. Giving pain medication, placing the patient in Trendelenburg's position, and applying ice to the area may assist in this process. Surgical intervention is eventually required for most patients.

Intussusception

Intussusception occurs when a proximal portion of the intestine telescopes into a more distal portion of intestine. This generally occurs in infancy, most often between ages

3 months and 1 year. Telescoping prevents passage of intestinal contents, including fecal material, beyond the defect. Stools passed in this disorder contain primarily blood and mucus, resulting in the "currant jelly" stools characteristic of intussusception. The child may have intermittent spasmodic type of pain. Occasionally a sausage-shaped mass can be palpated in the abdomen.

In most cases initial treatment is nonsurgical hydrostatic reduction by barium enema concurrent with diagnostic testing. If this does not reduce the obstruction, surgical intervention is necessary.

Pyloric Stenosis

Pyloric stenosis results from hypertrophy of the circular muscle of the pylorus causing constriction and obstruction of the gastric outlet. Although it is has been reported in infants from birth to 5 months, it most commonly occurs at 3 to 4 weeks of life; projectile, nonbilious vomiting after feeding is common. The infant is persistently hungry and easily re-fed. Weight loss, constipation, and dehydration result from the continuing emesis. An olive-shaped mass may be palpable in the right upper quadrant, and peristaltic waves may be visualized across the abdomen. This condition is diagnosed by history, physical examination, and abdominal ultrasonography. Management consists of correcting dehydration with IV fluid, inserting a gastric tube to decompress the stomach, and preparing the infant and family for a surgical pyloromyotomy.

Testicular Torsion

A prepubertal male with sudden onset of severe scrotal pain radiating to the abdomen may have testicular torsion. Twisting of spermatic vessels causes ischemia, swelling, and a high-lying testis. Patients may complain of nausea and vomiting. Scrotal edema is present, and blood pressure may be elevated because of pain and anxiety. Fever is rarely present. Diagnosis can often be made clinically, but Doppler ultrasound flow studies may also be used. Testicular torsion is a surgical emergency. Testicular salvage is approximately 80% to 100% if detorsion is accomplished within 6 hours; salvage is less than 20% with more than 12 hours of torsion, and after 24 hours the rate of salvage approaches 0%. If the torsion has been present less than 3 or 4 hours, manual reduction by the ED physician or urologist may be possible. If surgery is indicated, make sure the patient has no oral intake and administer analgesics as ordered. Patients with suspected testicular torsion should receive a higher triage priority because of increased potential for functional recovery with early resolution of the problem.

Urinary Tract Infections

UTIs are a major concern in children. About 3% to 5% of all girls and 1% of boys will have a symptomatic UTI before puberty.[10] Neonatal UTIs usually result from a bacteremia, whereas infants and children become infected from bacteria that travel up the urethra to the bladder. The presence of a possible UTI should be considered in all febrile infants, even if there is another source of infection identified. The gold standard for obtaining a urine specimen in a child with a suspected UTI is a catheterized sample, not a bagged collection. Urinary reflux can move bacteria up into the kidneys and lead to abnormal renal function and pyelonephritis if left undetected.

ENDOCRINE EMERGENCIES
Diabetic Ketoacidosis

Diabetic ketoacidosis (DKA) is a life-threatening medical emergency characterized by hyperglycemia, dehydration, metabolic acidosis, and ketonemia or ketonuria resulting from an absolute or relative insulin deficiency. DKA is more common in young children and adolescents with type 1 diabetes mellitus than in adults and remains the most common cause of death in diabetic children. DKA is the most common presentation of diabetes in children under 4 years of age; overall, 20% to 40% of children newly diagnosed with type 1 diabetes present for medical care in DKA.[18] Early symptoms of hyperglycemia, including polyuria, polydipsia, polyphagia, weight loss, and fatigue, are often subtle and are easily missed in infants or preschool children. As hyperglycemia progresses, nausea, vomiting, lethargy, altered mental status, deep rapid breathing (i.e., Kussmaul respirations), acetone odor to the breath, and abdominal pain are commonly identified, signaling the onset of DKA. In children with known type 1 diabetes, infection and noncompliance with insulin regimen are the most common precipitators of DKA. Diagnosis of this disorder is based on the result of blood gas analysis, blood glucose level, and serum and/or urine ketones.

Once the child's ABCs have been supported, management of the patient in DKA should focus on the correction of metabolic acidosis. Systematic interventions are implemented to restore fluid volume, stop ketogenesis, correct electrolyte disturbances, and avoid complications (cerebral edema, hypoglycemia, and hypokalemia). Cerebral edema is the most frequent, serious complication of pediatric DKA; children less than 5 years of age and patients previously undiagnosed with type 1 diabetes are at high risk for developing this potentially devastating complication.

The current recommendations for the management of pediatric DKA are as follows. Initially, a bolus of 5 to 20 mL/kg of 0.9% saline or other isotonic fluid is administered and repeated as necessary to restore hemodynamic stability. Subsequently, the remaining fluid deficit should be replaced over a 36- to 48-hour period. Gradual correction of fluid status is advised to minimize the risk for developing cerebral edema. Insulin should be administered by continuous infusion at a rate of 0.1 unit/kg/hr until ketosis/acidosis is resolved. This low dose of insulin usually decreases serum glucose concentration by 50 to 75 mg/dL/hr. The insulin drip should be continued until the metabolic acidosis has resolved (pH greater than or equal to 7.3, bicarbonate greater than or equal to

18 mEq/L). Serum glucose concentrations generally decrease to the normal range before ketosis and acidosis have resolved. To prevent hypoglycemia during insulin infusion, dextrose-containing fluids should be added when the serum glucose falls below 250 to 300 mg/dL. Serum glucose levels should be checked every hour until stabilized.

Initial serum potassium levels may be low, normal, or high. Potassium levels drop as acidosis is corrected, and replacement therapy should be initiated once adequate renal function has been ensured, generally after the child's first void. Potassium is typically administered at a concentration of 30 to 40 mEq/L of fluid. Potassium may be administered as potassium chloride and potassium phosphate or potassium acetate. Ongoing monitoring should include serial evaluation of vital signs, neurologic checks, intake and output, and laboratory samples (e.g., glucose, pH, electrolytes).

INFECTIOUS DISEASE EMERGENCIES

Children with upper respiratory infections such as colds, sore throats, sinusitis, and ear infections are often brought to the ED. For the most part they are rapidly discharged and followed by their private physicians. Some of the more serious infectious diseases are described in this section.

AIDS

Infants and children with acquired immunodeficiency syndrome (AIDS) or those infected with the human immunodeficiency virus (HIV) present to the ED with numerous physical problems requiring both physiologic and psychologic support. In the pediatric population, three age-groups are primarily affected. These are children exposed in utero to an infected mother, children who received blood products infected with the virus, and adolescents infected through high-risk behaviors. The majority of children with AIDS are younger than 2 years of age and constitute a small percentage of the total AIDS population. Most children with AIDS have recurrent bacterial and fungal infections, chronic diarrhea, chronic anemia, renal disease, cardiomyopathy, neurologic deterioration, or general failure to thrive.

Treatment is primarily supportive, aimed at prevention of infections and complications, early recognition of complications, and support of optimal general health.

Tuberculosis

Tuberculosis (TB) is caused by *Mycobacterium tuberculosis,* and the source of infection in most situations is a member of the household. It is a disease controlled in most developed countries that still remains a health hazard and leading cause of death in many parts of the world. A steady increase in new cases has occurred during the past several years, attributed in part to the influx of foreign-born people and recognition of the disease in the native-born population.

Clinical manifestations of TB are extremely variable. Fever, malaise, anorexia, weight loss, or cough may be present. Coinfection with HIV is also common. Most children with pulmonary TB have noninfectious disease; therefore they seldom require isolation. Hospitalization is seldom necessary because most children can be managed at home. Antimicrobial agents cure most cases of TB, with the limiting factor being patient compliance with drug administration. Drug therapy usually lasts 6 to 9 months. Historically, TB has been regarded with fear of infection, so it is important to clarify any misconceptions parents may have regarding this disease.

Bacteremia

The effects of bacterial invasion of the bloodstream may range from relatively mild symptoms of infection (bacteremia) to overwhelming, life-threatening infection (sepsis or septic shock). Bacteremia and septic shock represent the two extremes on a continuum of severity rather than disparate entities.

Bacteremia may occur in association with meningitis, cellulitis, or UTI. It may also occur without localized findings (occult bacteremia). Bacteremia is most common in children younger than 2 years of age and may be difficult to detect in the child less than 2 months of age. Any child younger than 2 years of age should be suspected of bacteremia when there is fever and documented infection (white blood cell count greater than 15,000 cells/mL) without an observable focus of infection. Bacteremia may be especially difficult to detect in young infants because they do not always respond to infection with fever. Bacteremia should be suspected when a child has fever with malaise, poor feeding, irritability, or is not playful or easily consoled. The diagnostic workup commonly includes CBC, blood cultures, urinalysis, urine culture, and lumbar puncture if indicated. Broad-spectrum antibiotics are initially administered.

If the patient is discharged, careful attention should be given to the parent's ability to understand and appreciate the importance of the diagnosis and the need to continue antimicrobial therapy as prescribed. The child should be reevaluated within 24 to 48 hours. Bacteremia can progress to sepsis if the patient is not adequately treated.

Meningitis

Meningitis, acute inflammation of the meninges, is a common cause of death and disability in children. Annual incidence of meningitis is 1 case per 2000 children with a peak in children 2 months to 5 years of age.[10] Causative organisms are often bacterial, but viral meningitis also occurs. With bacterial meningitis, organisms can enter the bloodstream through focal infection or by routes such as open wounds, skull fractures, and surgical procedures. The infection spreads through the subarachnoid space, causing swelling and pain. Recognition and treatment are essential to prevent death and residual damage.

Increased intracranial pressure is a major concern in meningitis. As inflammation increases, expansion within the rigid skull causes direct pressure on the brain. Narrow passageways to the ventricles are occluded, and cerebrospinal fluid outflow is obstructed, producing altered sensorium.

Many children diagnosed with meningitis present with headache, nausea, vomiting, or poor feeding. Most children have an elevated temperature; however, infants may have normal temperature or even hypothermia. A classic sign of meningitis is nuchal rigidity, which is rarely seen in infancy. Common signs and symptoms of increased intracranial pressure may be evident, including inconsolability, restlessness, altered mental status, and seizures. A bulging fontanel is a late sign. A severely ill child may be in respiratory distress, exhibit cyanosis, and have a rash or petechiae.

In the late stages, meningitis requires aggressive intervention, including airway management, control of increased intracranial pressure, IV medication (e.g., vasopressors, mannitol, diuretics, antibiotics), and admission to the intensive care unit. Definitive diagnosis requires a lumbar puncture and laboratory analysis of cerebrospinal fluid for protein, glucose, cell count, and Gram stain.

Meningococcemia

Meningococcemia, caused by invasion of the bloodstream with *Neisseria meningitidis,* can occur with or without meningitis. The child with meningococcemia has fever, headache, and rash (usually maculopapular rash), petechiae, and purpuric lesions. Figure 47-2 illustrates the cutaneous effects of meningococcemia. Meningococcemia can be rapidly fatal. Shock and disseminated intravascular coagulation occur very quickly; therefore rapid assessment and intervention are critical. Aggressive resuscitation, including advanced airway management, fluid bolusing, antibiotics, and vasopressors, should be anticipated. Diagnostic tests may include

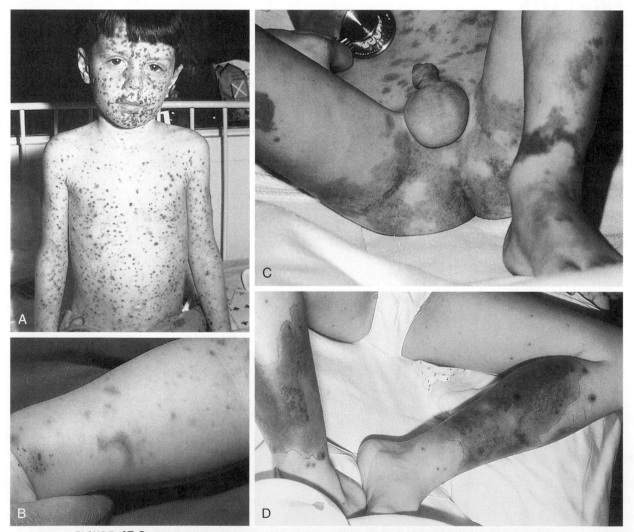

FIGURE **47-2.** Meningococcemia. **A,** This child manifests the generalized purpuric and petechial rash characteristic of acute meningococcemia. **B,** Petechiae are more apparent in this close-up of an infant. Gram stain of petechial scrapings may reveal organisms. **C** and **D,** Purpura may progress to form areas of frank cutaneous necrosis, especially in patients with disseminated intravascular coagulation. (From Zitelli B, Davis H: *Atlas of pediatric physical diagnosis,* ed 5, St. Louis, 2007, Mosby.)

CBC, electrolytes, glucose, clotting studies, blood cultures, urinalysis and urine culture, and lumbar puncture. Isolation with droplet precautions should be initiated immediately upon suspicion of meningococcemia to protect caregivers from exposure to this life-threatening illness.

Encephalitis

Acute encephalitis, or inflammation of brain parenchyma, may be caused by direct viral invasion or may follow an infection such as measles. Symptoms and treatment of encephalopathy vary by cause. Associated symptoms include but are not limited to headache, fever, altered sensorium, and nuchal rigidity. Supportive measures, including fluid restriction and monitoring electrolyte levels, may be all that are required for acute encephalitis. However, herpes encephalitis is a life-threatening disease requiring aggressive intervention.

One type of encephalitis, Reye's syndrome, is rarely seen today. This illness is associated with fatty infiltration of the liver and develops a few days after a mild viral illness. Cause is unknown, but genetic predisposition and use of aspirin during viral illness have been proposed.

Kawasaki Disease

Kawasaki disease is an acute systemic vasculitis occurring mainly in children under the age of 5 years. The acute disease is self-limiting; however, without treatment, one in five children can develop cardiac sequelae (aneurysms of the coronary arteries). Kawasaki disease is the leading cause of acquired heart disease in children in the United States. The etiology remains a mystery, and diagnosis can be a challenge. The classic criteria for diagnosis include high fever for at least 5 days and a minimum of four of the five following clinical findings: (1) bilateral nonpurulent conjunctival redness and irritation; (2) irritation and inflammation of the mouth, lips, and throat; (3) redness and swelling of hands and feet (peeling of fingers and toes); (4) erythematous rash, primarily involving the trunk; (5) cervical lymphadenopathy.

Treatment is focused on prevention of complications. High-dose γ-globulin (2 g/kg) has been useful in reducing the risk for coronary artery disease. High doses of aspirin, 30 to 100 mg/kg per 24 hours, are often given simultaneously. Beyond these two medications, treatment is largely supportive. IV fluids should be given to correct dehydration.

Lyme Disease

Lyme disease is a systemic, tick-borne illness. A skin lesion, known as erythema chronicum migrans, is present in a majority of cases. Lyme disease, caused by the spirochete *Borrelia burgdorferi,* is carried by a tick that lives primarily on white-tailed deer and white-footed field mice. The multisystem nature and slow evolution of the illness make diagnosis difficult. In a child with suspected Lyme disease, a history of tick bite or being in a wooded area is important. The small

size of the tick may prevent the patient from realizing its presence. General malaise, aching, sore throat, or fever may cause the patient to seek treatment.

Antibiotic therapy varies, depending on clinical presentation and progression of the disease. Early Lyme disease is treated with oral doxycycline, amoxicillin, or erythromycin. More serious symptoms such as Lyme carditis, neurologic manifestations, or Lyme arthritis require IV therapy with ceftriaxone or penicillin G. Prevention of the disease involves awareness and taking precautions before and after being in areas where the ticks reside. Parents should check the child's entire body after being in a wooded area.

Skin Rashes

Children are often brought to the ED with a concern of a rash. In fact, rashes are quite a common pediatric complaint. Most rashes, such as neonatal acne, diaper dermatitis, and viral exanthema, are not life threatening. Other diseases have long-term consequences and should be taken seriously. Some infectious diseases that present with a skin rash are shown in Table 47-4.

OTHER CONDITIONS
Cellulitis

An injury that breaks the skin barrier, such as an insect bite, abrasion, laceration, or surgical procedure, may allow entry of organisms that cause cellulitis (e.g., *Staphylococcus aureus,* group A streptococci). An inflammatory response causes edema and swelling of the affected area, usually without fever. Most patients are treated on an outpatient basis. Children younger than 3 years old with facial cellulitis are more likely to have bacteremia and require IV antimicrobial therapy.

Community-acquired methicillin-resistant *Staphylococcus aureus* (CA-MRSA) infection is becoming a more common concern, especially in children with skin and soft tissue infections. When children are placed on antibiotics for soft tissue cellulitis on an outpatient basis, close follow-up to ensure clearance of the infection is vital.

Hair Tourniquets

Hair tourniquet syndrome is a relatively common finding in infants. The infant usually presents with excessive crying, or the parent or caretaker notices redness of the extremity. It is an emergency because failure to promptly remove the hair acting as a tourniquet can lead to serious infection or even amputation.

This syndrome usually affects the toes, fingers, or external genitalia with the third toe and third finger the most commonly involved areas. Hair is more commonly associated with toes (Figure 47-3) and external genitalia, whereas threads are more often found around fingers.

Treatment includes removal with fine scissors and forceps. If unable to remove, some physicians have used depilatory agents to dissolve the hair and material. In rare

Table 47-4. INFECTIONS WITH SKIN RASHES

Characteristic	Measles (Rubeola)	Chickenpox (Varicella)	Scarlet fever	Roseola (Exanthema Subitum)	Petechial Rash (From Meningitis)
Incubation	10-11 days	10-20 days	2-4 days	10-15 days	None
Signs and symptoms	3-5 days of fever, cough, coryza, toxic appearance, conjunctivitis; Koplik's spots (mucosal lesions) appear 2 days before rash	Fever and cough, simultaneously with rash; headache; malaise	Fever for 1-2 days, sore throat, strawberry tongue, vomiting, chills, malaise	Rapid onset of high fever lasting 3-4 days in otherwise well child	May be sudden onset or preceded by fever and malaise; if sudden onset and accompanied by fever, may indicate sepsis
Exanthem (rash)	Reddish brown; begins on face, spreads downward; confluent high on body, discrete lesions in lower portions; lasts 7-10 days	Vesicles appearing in crops; trunk, scalp, face, extremities; lesions in all stages of development	Punctate, sandpaper texture; blanches on pressure; appears first in flexor areas; rash lasts 7 days	Appears discrete, rose-colored; appears after fever; begins on chest and spreads to face	Reddish purple vascular, *nonblanching* rash
Complications	Pneumonia, encephalitis, otitis media	Pneumonia, encephalitis, Reye's syndrome	Rheumatic heart disease	None	Sepsis, septic shock, long-term sequelae from increased intracranial pressure

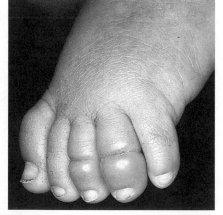

FIGURE **47-3.** Hair tourniquet. The mild erythema and edema of the third and fourth toes are the result of constriction by hairs that accidentally became wrapped around them. (From Zitelli B, Davis H: *Atlas of pediatric physical diagnosis,* ed 5, St. Louis, 2007, Mosby.)

incidents, surgery may be required if the hair/thread is very deep. Usually there is no sequela after removal.

Impetigo

Impetigo is a skin infection caused by group A streptococci. It is typically found in children younger than 6 years of age. The patient has skin lesions that ooze serous fluid and honey-colored crust when dry. Most cases of impetigo can be treated on an outpatient basis with oral or intramuscular antibiotics.

Scabies

Scabies is caused by the itch mite *Sarcoptes scabiei.* The major symptom of scabies is severe itching. Infestation results in eruption of wheals, papules, vesicles, and often visible threadlike burrows. Scabies is transmitted by direct contact. Topical application of lindane or crotamiton is the treatment for children older than 1 year. Oral antihistamines may be required to control itching. All bedding and clothing should be removed and washed.

FAMILY PRESENCE

The Emergency Nurses Association, American Association of Critical Care Nurses, and American Heart Association are among the growing number of professional organizations that support the option of family presence during invasive procedures and resuscitation. Family presence can be looked at as a natural extension of family-centered care, which is a fundamental part of pediatric emergency care. Well thought-out planning needs to be a crucial component of any family presence guidelines used in the emergency care setting. Some of the key points to consider for a family presence guideline include the following[14]:

• Discuss the plan with all resuscitation team members in advance.

- One team member must be assigned to stay with the family to clarify information and answer questions.
- Have a specific space for the family member to be in during the resuscitation, and if possible, facilitate the opportunity for the family to touch their child.
- Resuscitation team members must be aware of the family presence and communicate in a sensitive way.

SUMMARY

Children seen in the ED can cause great anxiety for health care providers, especially those who are not accustomed to caring for children on a regular basis. Developing skill in pediatric triage, assessment, and care requires the emergency nurse to develop a system that is comfortable, systematic, thorough, and adaptable to the age of the child. Acquiring the habit of beginning a pediatric assessment as soon as the child enters the ED is good practice. Focus on the child, not the parent, yet realize the important role the parent has to play, especially with a nonverbal child. Appreciate the differences physically, physiologically, and developmentally between adults and children, and be mindful of the differences with each child you assess. Take special care when obtaining and interpreting vital signs in pediatric patients because abnormal vital signs may be the first clues you detect that tell you your patient is "sick," is not responding to interventions, or is decompensating. Showing concern and offering support for the family, including the family in the child's care whenever possible, and giving thorough, clear discharge instructions lay the groundwork for ongoing care of the child after the emergency is over.

REFERENCES

1. Anchor J, Settipane RA: Appropriate use of epinephrine in anaphylaxis, *Am J Emerg Med* 22(6):488, 2004.
2. Carcillo JA, Fields AI; Task Force Committee Members: Clinical practice guidelines for hemodynamic support of pediatric and neonatal patients in septic shock, *Crit Care Med* 30(6):1365, 2002.
3. Corneli H, Zorc J, Mahajan P et al: A multicenter, randomized, controlled trial of dexamethasone for bronchiolitis, *JAMA* 351(4):331, 2007.
4. Duro D, Duggan C: The BRAT diet for acute diarrhea in children: should it be used? *Pract Gastroenterol* 31(6):60, 2007.
5. Emergency Nurses Association: *Emergency nursing pediatric course provider manual,* ed 3, Hawkins HS, editor, Des Plaines, Ill, 2004, The Association.
6. Goldstein B, Girior B, Randolph A et al: International pediatric sepsis consensus conference: definitions for sepsis and organ dysfunction in pediatrics, *Pediatr Crit Care Med* 6(1):2, 2005.
7. Grap MJ: Pulse oximetry, *Crit Care Nurse* 22(3):69, 2002.
8. Hazinski M: Cardiovascular disorders. In Hazinski M, editor: *Nursing care of the critically ill child,* ed 2, St. Louis, 1999, Mosby.
9. Lightdale JR, Goldmann DA, Feldman HA et al: Microstream Capnograph improves patient monitoring during moderate sedation: a randomized controlled study, *Pediatrics* 117(6):1170, 2006.
10. Martin S, Morfin M: Shock. In Bernardo L, Thomas D, editors: *Core curriculum for pediatric emergency nursing,* Boston, 2003, Jones & Bartlett.
11. McCaig LA, Nawar EW: National hospital ambulatory medical care survey: 2004 emergency department summary, *Adv Data* 372:1, 2006.
12. Molodow RE, Defendi GL, Muniz A: Croup, last updated September 19, 2007, *eMedicine,* http://www.emedicine.com/PED/topic510htm.
13. Neto GM, Kentab O, Klassen TP et al: A randomized controlled trial of mist in the acute treatment of moderate croup, *Acad Emerg Med* 9(9):873, 2001.
14. Ralston M, Hazinski M, Zaritsky A et al, editiors: *Textbook of pediatric advanced life support,* Chicago, 2006, American Academy of Pediatrics and American Heart Association.
15. Rutkowski EM: Vital signs: blood pressure. In Bowden V, Smith Greenberg C, editors: *Pediatric nursing procedures,* ed 2, Philadelphia 2007, Lippincott Williams & Wilkins.
16. Sampson HA et al: Second symposium on the definition and management of anaphylaxis: summary report—second National Institute of Allergy and Infectious Disease/Food Allergy and Anaphylaxis Network symposium, *J Allergy Clin Immunol* 117(2):391, 2006.
17. Simons F, Roberts J, Gu Z et al: Epinephrine absorption in children with a history of anaphylaxis, *J Allergy Clin Immunol* 101:33, 1998.
18. Steinmann RA: Pediatric diabetic ketoacidosis, *Am J Nurs* 107(3):72CC, 2007.
19. Vichinsky EP, Neumayr LD, Earles AN et al: Causes and outcomes of the acute chest syndrome in sickle sell disease, National Acute Chest Syndrome Study Group, *N Engl J Med* 342(25):1855, 2000.

CHAPTER 48

Child Abuse and Neglect

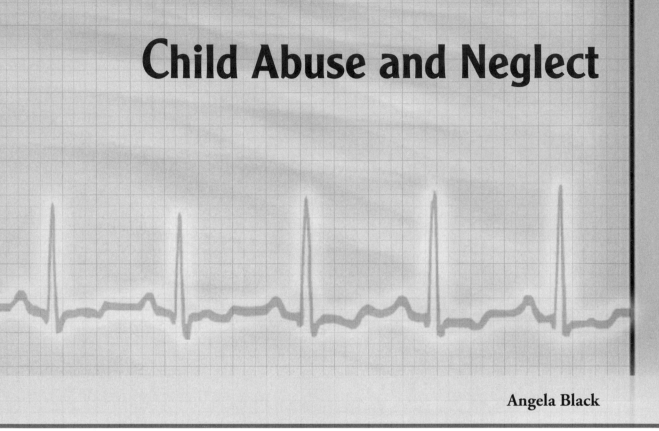

Angela Black

Child abuse and neglect affect children of all ages, ethnicities, genders, and socioeconomic groups. Approximately 1460 children died as a result of abuse in 2005 alone.[19] This figure may be conservative due to potential inaccurate determination of the manner and the cause of death. Several researchers suggest that deaths related to maltreatment are underreported by as much as 60%.[8,13,17] These tragic figures represent the death of approximately four children in the United States each day. Younger children experience the highest rate of fatalities: children under the age of 4 years account for three quarters (76.6%) of children killed as a result of child maltreatment.[19]

In Chicago a 35-year-old mother kicks and throws her 16-month-old baby out a window because he will not stop crying; an Alabama couple shackles their twin daughters above the knees and locks them in a room to live in their own excrement; a Detroit drug addict sells her son to settle a $1000 crack cocaine debt; a trusted priest is sentenced to more than 30 years for sexually abusing children during his reign as youth leader; in California a teenage girl is abducted from her home and later found raped, beaten, and dead; a 4-year-old is beaten to death by her father while a neighbor reports she had to walk to another part of the house and turn up the television volume to drown out the child's screams; a 3-year-old raped by a trusted family friend is left infected with *Neisseria gonorrhoeae* and human immunodeficiency virus (HIV); and in South Carolina, the drowning of two young boys at the hand of their mother horrifies the nation. Children are the future of our communities, and they must be protected; yet they are not able to protect themselves. Child abuse and neglect are a burden to society in many ways. Abused children are more likely to develop alcoholism, abuse drugs, and suffer from depression. Tragically, abused children often grow up to be abusive adults. There is also a significant financial burden. Annual direct costs related to child abuse exceed $24 billion, whereas annual indirect costs approach $70 billion.[20] Direct costs include hospitalization, the child welfare system, and the judicial system; indirect costs encompass special education, juvenile delinquency, and adult criminality.

In 2005 approximately 3.3 million incidents of suspected child abuse and neglect, involving approximately 6 million children, were reported to child protection services.[19] Reports of violence against children have almost tripled since 1976. The most common pattern of abuse is neglect, usually perpetrated by the female parent, whereas physical and sexual abuse is most often inflicted by a male acting alone.[20]

More often than not, abused children present to the emergency department (ED) without a declaration of abuse or neglect. This, along with a false presentation of the history surrounding the child's injury or illness, or a caregiver's intentional withholding of information, leads to difficulty in identifying child maltreatment. A detailed history and

Box 48-1	INDICATORS OF CHILD ABUSE OR NEGLECT
Child	**Caregiver**
Extreme change in behavior (regressive, passive, or overly aggressive)	No explanation or changing explanation for the child's injury
Flat affect	Explanation of injury does not match clinical findings
Does not cry during painful procedures	Delay in seeking health care
Appears malnourished, unkempt	Uncooperative or hostile toward health care team
Sudden drop in school performance	Inappropriate response to the seriousness of the child's condition
Sexual behavior toward adults or other children	

Box 48-2	POTENTIAL INDICATORS OF CHILD NEGLECT
Behavioral Findings	**Physical Findings**
Begs or steals food	Height and weight significantly below normal for age level
Falls asleep in school, lethargic	Inappropriate clothing for weather
Poor school attendance, frequent tardiness	Poor hygiene, including lice, body odor, scaly skin
Chronic hunger	
Dull, apathetic appearance	Child abandoned and left with inadequate supervision
Runs away from home	Untreated illness or injury
Reports no caregiver in the home	Lack of safe, warm, and sanitary shelter
Assumes adult responsibilities	Lack of necessary medical and dental care

From *For kids sake: a child abuse prevention and reporting kit,* rev ed, Oklahoma City, 1992, Oklahoma State Department of Health.

thorough physical assessment are essential when identifying these small victims of maltreatment. The historical data and physical findings must be compared and evaluated to determine congruency. The interactions among the child, caregivers, and staff are also important to evaluate. Some behaviors that could indicate that the child is suffering from abuse or neglect are reviewed in Box 48-1.

NEGLECT

The lack of visible bruises or broken bones belies the fact that ongoing child neglect is a silent, serious attack on children that can leave lasting mental and physical problems. Currently 62.8% of all abuse cases involve neglect, and 42% of the deaths in 2005 were attributed to neglect.[19] Neglect, defined as intentional or unintentional omission of needed care and support, may appear to the emergency nurse as a child who is unkempt, left unattended, not dressed appropriately for the weather, malnourished, or diagnosed with "failure to thrive." Identification of neglect must recognize parental attempts to provide essentials despite limited resources. Failure to provide adequate physical protection, nutrition, or health care is generally considered neglect, but neglect can also include lack of human contact and love. Recognizing neglect is often difficult in the ED because of limited, one-time contact with most patients. However, the emergency nurse should be alert for behaviors that suggest neglect (Box 48-2). Figure 48-1 depicts a case of neglect.

Neglect can be physical, medical, educational, or emotional. Physical neglect accounts for the majority of child maltreatment in the United States. Physical neglect includes cases such as child abandonment, inadequate supervision, and failing to adequately provide for the child's safety and physical and emotional needs. This type of neglect can lead to failure to thrive, malnutrition, serious illness,

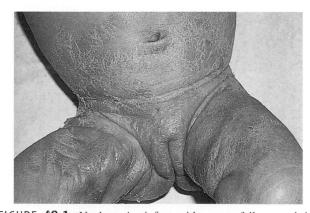

FIGURE **48-1.** Neglect. An infant with severe failure to thrive has a badly neglected case of irritant diaper dermatitis. (From Zitelli BJ, Davis HW: *Atlas of pediatric physical diagnosis,* ed 4, St. Louis, 2002, Mosby.)

physical harm from injuries due to lack of supervision, and a lifetime of low self-esteem.[16] Medical neglect is the failure to provide appropriate health care for a child such as immunizations, recommended surgery, or other interventions necessary for a serious health problem. In some cases a parent may withhold traditional medical care because of religious beliefs. These cases generally do not fall under the definition of medical neglect; however, some states will intervene through the court system and force medical treatment for the child to save the child's life or prevent life-threatening injury. Medical neglect can lead to poor overall health and compounded medical issues.[16] Educational neglect occurs when a child is allowed to engage in chronic absenteeism or is of mandatory school age but not enrolled in school or receiving needed special educational training.

This can ultimately lead to inability to acquire necessary basic skills, dropping out of school, and continual disruptive behaviors.[16] Finally, emotional neglect is difficult to recognize and diagnose because of the lack of physical evidence. Emotional neglect is often typified by child behaviors such as depression, habit disorders (sucking, biting, rocking, enuresis), or conduct and learning disorders such as antisocial behaviors (e.g., cruelty). Emotional neglect includes actions such as chronic or extreme spousal abuse in the child's presence, failure to provide needed psychologic care, belittling and withholding of affection. This can lead to poor self-image, alcohol or drug abuse, destructive behavior, and even suicide.[16]

Failure to Thrive

Failure to thrive is defined as a condition in children younger than age 5 years whose growth persistently and significantly deviates from norms for age and sex based on national growth charts. Measurements for height, weight, and head circumference are plotted against normal childhood growth patterns. Failure-to-thrive children generally fall below average in all three areas. Actual weight less than 70% of predicted weight for length requires urgent attention.[5] The cause of failure to thrive may be organic, which is caused by a medical condition (e.g., *Giardia* organism infection, celiac disease, lead poisoning, malabsorption) or inorganic, caused by psychosocial issues.

Psychosocial causes are often linked to and reported as child neglect. Maladaptive parenting practices, chronic family illnesses, parental depression, and substance abuse among caregivers are recognized causes. Failure to thrive does not necessarily imply abuse or neglect but does require aggressive treatment and follow-up by appropriate health care professionals. Untreated, failure to thrive can lead to developmental and behavioral difficulties secondary to nutritional deprivation of the nervous system and other systems. A multidisciplinary approach in treating failure to thrive has the best opportunity for success. Family assessment, nutritional counseling, medical intervention, and family support are needed to correct failure to thrive.

The medical evaluation for suspected neglect and failure to thrive should include a thorough history, physical examination, feeding observation, and a home visit by a health care provider. The history should review the child's family history, including genetic conditions, growth histories, endocrine disorders, caregivers' knowledge of normal growth and development, family functioning, eating patterns, types of food available in the home, and family stressors.[5] The physical examination should include past and present growth parameters, including head circumference using appropriate growth charts. Along with a general examination, a careful neurologic examination and observation of the child's developmental skills and interactive behaviors with parents is necessary. Laboratory and radiologic studies are frequently unnecessary, and the yield of

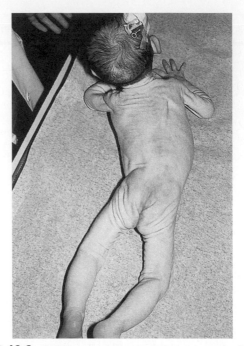

FIGURE **48-2.** Psychologic failure to thrive as a result of neglect. **A,** This 4½-month-old infant was brought to the emergency department because of congestion, where she was found to be below her birth weight and to be suffering from severe developmental delay. Note the marked loss of subcutaneous tissue manifested by the wrinkled skin folds over her buttocks, shoulders, and upper arms. (From Zitelli BJ, Davis HW: *Atlas of pediatric physical diagnosis,* ed 4, St. Louis, 2002, Mosby.)

positive laboratory data is less than 1%.[5] Figure 48-2 illustrates a case of failure to thrive.

PHYSICAL ABUSE

Physical abuse is intentional injury to a child younger than age 18 years by a parent or caregiver. Of the four types of child maltreatment, physical abuse is second to neglect, accounting for approximately 17% of all abuse cases.[19] In 2004, 152,250 children were confirmed victims of physical abuse in the United States.[6] It is estimated that the rate of physical abuse in children with disabilities is 2.1 times greater than for children without disabilities. Despite these statistics, physical abuse remains underreported for several reasons, including individual and community variations in what is considered abuse, inadequate knowledge among professionals in recognition of abusive injuries, and unwillingness to report suspected abuse.[6] Child abuse is typically a pattern of behavior repeated over time, but it can also be a single attack. The condition is characterized by injury, torture, maiming, or use of unreasonable force. Abuse may result from harsh discipline or severe punishment. Box 48-3 identifies behavioral and physical indicators found in physical abuse. Children rarely tell anyone about physical abuse because of feelings of shame or confusion. They may also fear breaking up their family, isolation, or threats from the abuser.[1]

Box 48-3	PHYSICAL ABUSE FINDINGS
Behavioral Findings	**Physical Findings**
Requests or feels deserving of punishment	Unexplained bruises or welts found most frequently, usually on face, torso, buttocks, back, or thighs; can reflect shape of object used (e.g., electric cord, hand, belt buckle); may be in various stages of healing
Afraid to go home, or requests to stay in school or daycare	
Overly shy, tends to avoid physical contact with adults, especially parents	Unexplained burns often on palms, soles of feet, buttocks, or back; can reflect pattern of cigarette burn, electrical appliance, or rope burn
Displays behavioral extremes (withdrawal or aggressiveness)	
Cries excessively or sits and stares	Unexplained fractures or dislocations involving skull, ribs, and bones around joints; may include multiple fractures or spiral fractures
Reports injury by parent or caretaker	
Gives unbelievable explanations for injuries	Other unexplained injuries such as lacerations, abrasions, human bite, or pinch marks; loss of hair or bald patches; retinal hemorrhages; abdominal injuries
Clings to health care worker rather than parent	

Modified from *For kids sake: a child abuse prevention and reporting kit,* rev ed, Oklahoma City, 1992, Oklahoma State Department of Health.

Skin Injuries

In contrast to unintentional injuries, inflicted injuries tend to occur on surfaces other than bony prominences such as the head, trunk, upper arms, buttocks, and backs of the thighs. Location, size, and shape of bruises, lacerations, burns, or bites should be documented in the medical record accompanied by high-quality photographs.[6] Measurement of skin injuries will help in determining the mechanism of injury, as well as the object used to inflict the injury. Bite marks should be carefully measured and photographed if possible. Referral to professionals that can gather specific forensic information is ideal. Causes of burn injuries may be chemical, thermal, or electrical. The history and continuity of the burn pattern may indicate a greater probability of inflicted trauma. Unintentional scalds commonly involve hot liquids that are pulled or splashed onto the child's head, torso, and upper extremities. Inflicted injuries will be sharply demarcated with few or no splash marks.

Cranial Injuries

Head trauma is the leading cause of death for victims of child abuse.[6] Inflicted injuries tend to occur in younger children. Abuse should be suspected in infants with a history of a minor head trauma, such as a short fall off a sofa, presenting with multiple, complex, or occipital skull fractures. A funduscopic examination for retinal hemorrhages should be performed in any infant who is a suspected victim of physical abuse. Retinal hemorrhages occur in approximately 85% of infants who are subjected to abusive shaking with or without impact.[6]

Skeletal Injuries

Skeletal fractures are common in childhood, leading to difficulty determining whether a fracture is unintentional or inflicted. Fractures that are particularly suspicious for abuse include multiple fractures in different stages of healing, long-bone fractures including metaphyseal fractures, spiral/oblique fractures, and bilateral or symmetric fractures. If a fracture is suspected, the skin should be carefully assessed for grab marks; however, the absence of bruising does not exclude an abusive mechanism of injury. Rib fractures in infants are usually caused by forceful squeezing of the chest. Posterior or lateral rib fractures or multiple rib fractures are especially predictive of abusive trauma.[6]

Specific Abuse Patterns

Children can experience a multitude of insults and injuries at the hands of primary caregivers or other adults. Two patterns seen with increasing frequency are shaken baby syndrome (SBS) and Munchausen syndrome by proxy (MSP) (also referred to as factitious disorder by proxy).

SBS occurs when infants are shaken vigorously. Approximately 1500 cases of SBS occur each year in the United States; however, the true number of cases is unknown due to misdiagnosis and underreporting.[14] According to the American Academy of Pediatrics, SBS is a violent form of abuse that occurs in infants younger than 2 years but can involve children as old as 5 years.[2,15] Acceleration-deceleration of the head creates a triad of injuries: subdural hemorrhage (Figure 48-3), retinal hemorrhage (Figure 48-4), and altered level of consciousness. There are often no external signs of trauma. Babies shaken into unconsciousness are often put to bed in hopes the injuries will resolve; therefore the window for therapeutic intervention is lost. The spectrum of symptoms may vary from vomiting and irritability in mild shakings to unconsciousness, convulsions, and even death in severe shakings. A funduscopic examination of the pupils should be performed to look for retinal hemorrhages. Pupil dilation may be required in some patients. A computed tomography scan should be obtained to identify brain hemorrhages. Magnetic resonance imaging, when available, is extremely helpful for detection of subdural hematoma. A skeletal survey should be obtained to rule out fractures, especially in the area of the ribs. The diagnosis of SBS is made following a thorough history of the circumstances of the injury(s), pattern of injury, and social context in which they occur. Recent legal and medical controversies over SBS have led to questions regarding its diagnosis and even its existence. The controversies concern the precise cause of

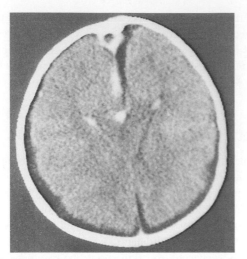

FIGURE **48-3.** Subdural hematoma secondary to shaken baby syndrome. (From Zitelli BJ, Davis HW: *Atlas of pediatric physical diagnosis,* ed 4, St. Louis, 2002, Mosby. Courtesy the Division of Neuroradiology, University Health Center of Pittsburgh.)

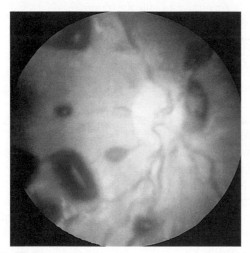

FIGURE **48-4.** Retinal hemorrhages secondary to shaken baby syndrome. (From Zitelli BJ, Davis HW: *Atlas of pediatric physical diagnosis,* ed 4, St. Louis, 2002, Mosby. Courtesy Dr. Stephen Ludwig, Children's Hospital of Philadelphia.)

brain injury and the retinal and subdural hemorrhages, the degree of force required, and whether impact in addition to acceleration-deceleration forces is needed.

MSP is a complex condition in which a parent, usually the mother, knowingly keeps a child ill or fabricates an illness for secondary gain or attention through the child's illness. The child is subjected to illnesses perpetuated by caregivers who may administer emetics, laxatives, or other drugs, introduce pathogens, or otherwise contribute to a child's illness. Commonly seen signs and symptoms of MSP include apnea, seizures, vomiting, diarrhea, simulated or actual hemorrhage, bacteremia, rash, and fever.[9] The history provided is often sophisticated and elaborate. The parent often demands extensive medical evaluations and appears very concerned for the child. The child's history may also include the parent's seeking health care at multiple locations and from multiple

physicians. Often undetected by health care professionals, MSP can lead to emotional problems, chronic disabilities, and death.

One difficulty in identifying abuse is the number of conditions that mimic physical abuse. Physiologic or pathologic causes for physical findings should always be considered.[7]

- Sudden infant death syndrome can appear as child abuse because of pooling of blood, mottling, and other discoloration associated with death. The definitive cause of death should be determined by a complete autopsy with appropriate ancillary studies, a review of clinical findings, and a scene investigation.
- Disorders such as erythema multiforme, Henoch-Schönlein purpura, leukemia, Wiskott-Aldrich syndrome, hemophilia, and idiopathic thrombocytopenic purpura can cause bruising or lesions resembling burns.
- Mongolian spots are benign bluish gray birthmarks found predominantly in African Americans, Hispanic Americans, Asians, Latinos, Native Americans, or anyone with dark pigmentation. Mongolian spots are usually located over the sacral area and buttocks but may also be located on the legs, shoulders, upper arms, and face.
- Multiple petechiae and purpuric lesions of the face can occur when vigorous crying, retching, or coughing increases vena caval pressure. Unlike intentional choking, there are no marks around the neck.
- Bullous impetigo may appear as an infected wound or burn. This condition may reflect neglect if caregivers are apathetic about care of lesions.
- Glutaricaciduria type 1, a rare disorder of amino acid metabolism, can cause subdural hematomas and retinal hemorrhages after minimal trauma.
- Cultural or ethnic practices such as coining or cupping are used to treat pain, fever, or poor appetite. Coining—rubbing a coin over bony prominences—causes a striated "pseudoburn." Cupping (warming a cup, spoon, or shot glass in oil and then placing it on the neck, back, or ribs) can result in a petechial or purpuric rash over the affected area.
- Osteogenesis imperfecta, or "brittle bone disease," is an inherited disease characterized by abnormal collagen synthesis that can result in multiple fractures with minimal trauma and causes a tendency to bleed easily.

Interviewing Caregivers

When maltreatment is suspected, the caregiver should be carefully interviewed to obtain as much information as possible. If there is more than one caregiver present, be sure to interview them separately. Make every effort to establish rapport, conveying genuine concern and understanding. A nonjudgmental approach is essential. Judgmental attitudes hinder communication and limit information. Tactfully determine issues of concern to the caretaker. The person may feel desperate and inadequate. Use reflective statements, such as "You sound really frustrated right now." Do not agree or condone, merely listen and reflect, using critical listening skills. Any statements made by the caregiver regarding the injury should be documented accurately and verbatim.

Parents often feel intense neediness and helplessness about their inability to meet their own needs, so a child who is needy, demanding, or misbehaves proves extremely stressful. Parents may also feel intensely negative about themselves and dwell on their own worthlessness, helplessness, and incompetence. Support the caregiver, but do not convey pity. Emphasize anything positive; for example, that the parent sought help. Reinforce the decision to seek help; normal behavior is to withdraw without seeking help. Help parents draw on personal strengths. Helplessness and worthlessness are self-destructive, so effort should be made to draw parents away from negative feelings. Parents may be agitated, embarrassed, or tearful, so work to make them feel valued as individuals.

Parents are often distressed because of isolation and lack of a social network. Discuss places for support such as church, family, and friends. Talk about stressors the person is experiencing, including economic worries, unemployment, poverty, illness, divorce, and single-parenting concerns.

Allegations of Abuse

Allegations of child abuse sometimes arise during separation, divorce, and child custody proceedings. Perceptions exist that false allegations are made during divorce or custody proceedings in an attempt to place one parent in a "favored" position for child custody. Although false accusations are sometimes made, all allegations of abuse or neglect during divorce proceedings deserve serious consideration because of the increased risk for abuse during this time. A higher index of suspicion for abuse and neglect is required with divorcing families because families are experiencing increased stress and are dysfunctional as a result of the divorce process. Separation of parents increases the opportunity for sexual and physical victimization but can also provide an opportunity for a child to disclose that abuse has taken place if the abuser is out of the home. Risk for extrafamilial abuse is higher because of changes in caregivers or presence of a nonbiologic caregiver in the home.

Reporting Abuse

When suspicion of intentional trauma, neglect, or sexual abuse is raised, appropriate agencies must be notified immediately. Each state defines child abuse and neglect differently; however, the ultimate goal, regardless of geographic location, is prevention of further injury through prompt intervention. It is estimated that child abuse may recur up to 35% of the time without appropriate detection or intervention.[6] If child endangerment is a concern, the child should be taken into protective custody. State statutes regarding protective custody vary, so become familiar with local requirements. Such statutes now exist in all 50 states. These statutes designate specific individuals as mandated reporters (e.g., law enforcement, physicians, health care professionals, and educators) who must report suspected child abuse and neglect.

State reporting laws grant immunity for good-faith reporting. In most states liability exists only if the reporter knows the allegations are false or the individual acted with malicious purpose.

The health care team should inform the parents or caregivers when an inflicted injury is suspected. Avoid inflammatory statements when relaying information to caregivers; instead, relay the team's concern for the child and his or her safety. When child protection services and/or the police are contacted, simply state the team's legal responsibility to report suspicions.

Treatment

Care of injury is the primary medical concern. After immediate physical needs are resolved, further assessment is then initiated. Query the child and caregivers, avoiding judgments of possible perpetrators or reasons the injury occurred. Health care providers must remember that investigation of child abuse allegations is the responsibility of police or the appropriate division of family services. Emergency nurses who suspect child abuse or neglect must report specific concerns and the reasons for those concerns.

Reassure the child and caregiver that you are there to help. Establish trust, allay fears, and lay groundwork for expression of concerns. Give the child some degree of control by providing choices. "Which color gown do you want—blue or green?" "May I listen to your heart, or do you want to listen to it first?" Be clear, and explain what you are doing. Be honest; if something will hurt, say so.

Obtain a detailed history, paying close attention to the sequence of events. Is the history consistent with the child's age and nature of injury? Interview the child and parent(s) separately if the child is old enough to talk. Is the parent at high risk for abusing—isolated, abused as a child, low self-esteem? Is the child at high risk for abuse—difficult child, difficult developmental age, premature infant? Is the family experiencing a crisis—financial, social? Are other children at home at risk for abuse? Is alcohol or drug abuse present? Box 48-4 discusses several risk factors for child maltreatment. A combination of individual, societal, and relational factors contribute to the risk for child maltreatment. Certain individual characteristics in both the child and caregiver have been found to increase the risk for a child being maltreated. It is important to remember that risk factors are contributing factors, not a direct cause of abuse. The presence of risk factors should also not be used as indicators of abuse but rather provide guidance in developing prevention strategies as well as treatment plans.[6]

Physical Examination

Identify and document all injuries, old and new, comparing historical information to clinical evidence. Measure, draw, and describe location, color, induration, and scarring. Assess for limited range of motion, which may indicate old fractures. Look for patterned injuries such as cigarette burns, strap marks (Figure 48-5), electric cord marks (Figure 48-6),

Box 48-4	RISK FACTORS FOR CHILD MALTREATMENT[9]	
Child	**Caregiver**	**Community**
Prematurity	Childhood history of abuse	Social isolation
Prenatal drug exposure	Acute or chronic stressors	Domestic violence
Product of unwanted pregnancy	Lack of parenting knowledge	Community violence
		Unemployment
Developmental or physical disability	Rigid or unrealistic expectations	Homelessness
		Frequent relocations
Chronic illness	Alcohol or substance abuse	
Difficulty with milestones (e.g., walking, toilet training)	Low self-esteem	

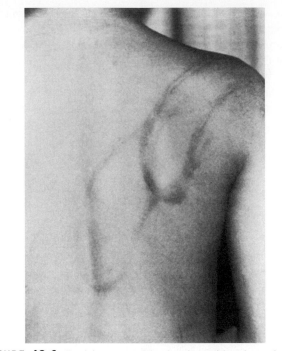

FIGURE **48-6.** Bruising caused by beating with a looped cord. (From Rosen PR, Barkin RM, Hockberger RS et al: *Emergency medicine: concepts and clinical practice*, ed 4, St. Louis, 1998, Mosby. Courtesy J. Brummitt, MD, Alberta Children's Hospital.)

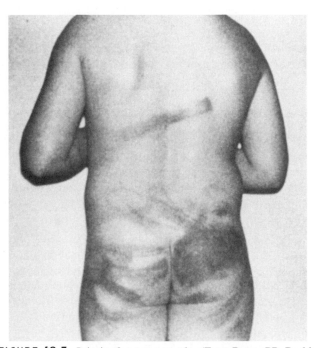

FIGURE **48-5.** Injuries from strap marks. (From Rosen PR, Barkin RM, Hockberger RS et al: *Emergency medicine: concepts and clinical practice*, ed 4, St. Louis, 1998, Mosby. Courtesy J. Brummitt, MD, Alberta Children's Hospital.)

or spiral femur fractures in a nonambulatory child. Examine for imprint marks (Figure 48-7), bruising on the buttocks (Figure 48-8), and inflicted scald burns (Figure 48-9). Downturned marks at the corners of the mouth occur when the child has been gagged.[11] Measure height, weight, and head circumference, and compare the measurements to standard growth charts. Assess developmental level of function. An ocular and funduscopic examination is required to identify retinal hemorrhages. Skeletal surveys are obtained on children younger than 2 years to rule out existing or healed fractures. Prothrombin time, partial thromboplastin time, factor XIII, fibrinogen level, platelet count, and bleeding time results are recommended to rule out an existing blood dyscrasia.

SEXUAL ABUSE

In 2002 more than 88,000 children were confirmed victims of sexual abuse in the United States.[4] Child sexual abuse, involvement of children in sexual activities that violate social taboos, is usually done for gratification or profit of a significantly older person. Children do not understand these acts and are not able to give informed consent. Types of sexual abuse include, but are not limited to, fondling, digital manipulation, exhibitionism, pornography, and actual or attempted oral, vaginal, or anal intercourse. Unfortunately, the definition of child sexual abuse varies from state to state and there is no national reporting system, so determination of actual incidence and prevalence rates is difficult.

The primary portal of entry into the health care system for children with sexual abuse is the ED. One study showed 46% of children with suspected sexual abuse were first evaluated in the ED. Without appropriate intervention there is a 50% chance of further abuse and a 10% chance for death. Physicians historically hesitate to become involved because they lack confidence in the medical examination, fear testifying in court, and are uncomfortable handling social problems that accompany a diagnosis of sexual abuse. However, legal

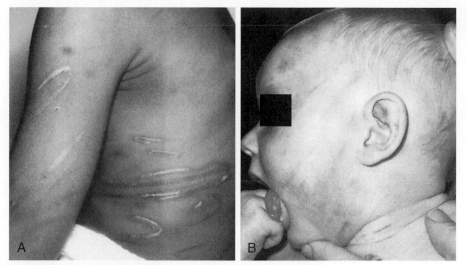

FIGURE **48-7.** Imprint marks reflecting the weapons used to inflict them. **A,** Hypopigmented and hyperpigmented scars that were the result of beatings with a looped electrical cord. **B,** The characteristic pattern of parallel lines that results from blows with a belt. (From Zitelli BJ, Davis HW: *Atlas of pediatric physical diagnosis,* ed 4, St. Louis, 2002, Mosby.)

and social systems depend heavily on medical examination to provide evidence that can withstand intense scrutiny when used to protect children from further abuse and prosecute the offender. Consequently, emergency care professionals must recognize sexual abuse and be skilled in examinations with medical and forensic strength. Knowledge of normal and abnormal sexual behaviors, physical signs of sexual abuse, appropriate diagnostic tests for sexually transmitted diseases, and medical conditions confused with sexual abuse is useful in the evaluation of such children.[4] Screening and treatment protocols specifically addressing child sexual abuse are recommended for all EDs.

Clinical Presentation

Most children are brought to the ED by their mothers for evaluation of complaints directly related to the anogenital region such as discharge, bleeding, pain, swelling, dysuria, or difficulty stooling and nonspecific symptoms such as headache, abdominal pain, or fatigue. Patients may present with sexually transmitted diseases such as genital herpes (Figure 48-10) and genital warts (Figure 48-11). Behavioral symptoms such as excessive masturbation, depression, inappropriate sexual expression (verbal or physical), suicidal gestures, delinquency, fearfulness, anxiety, decline in school performance, sleep disturbances, or drug and alcohol abuse may also be identified. It is estimated that 12% to 25% of girls and 8% to 10% of boys are sexually victimized by 18 years of age.[4] Children may be sexually abused by family members or nonfamily members with the majority of perpetrators being male. Adolescents are perpetrators in at least 20% of reported cases.[4] Male victims abused by males may be reluctant to report sexual abuse because of fear of being labeled a homosexual. In most cases, abuse has been ongoing for many years before it is reported to the authorities.

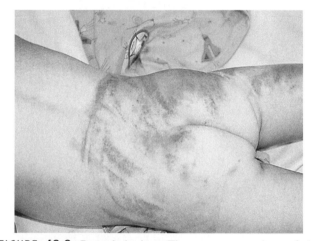

FIGURE **48-8.** Buttock bruises. The severe contusions of the buttocks and lower back seen in this child were inflicted by hand, hairbrush, and belt. (From Zitelli BJ, Davis HW: *Atlas of pediatric physical diagnosis,* ed 4, St. Louis, 2002, Mosby.)

Urgency for medical evaluation depends on timing of the last abuse episode and presenting symptoms. Immediate examination is required if abuse occurred within 72 hours or there is bleeding, pain, or discharge. Evidence may still be present, so specimens for a forensic evidence collection kit are collected for law enforcement officials. Body swabs collected in children more than 24 hours after a sexual assault are unlikely to yield forensic evidence; however, nearly two thirds of forensic evidence may be recovered from the linen or clothing worn during the assault.[4] The physical examination of sexually abused children should not result in additional physical or emotional trauma. The examination should also be explained to the child before it is performed. If more than 72 hours has passed and no acute injuries are present, an emergency examination is usually not necessary.

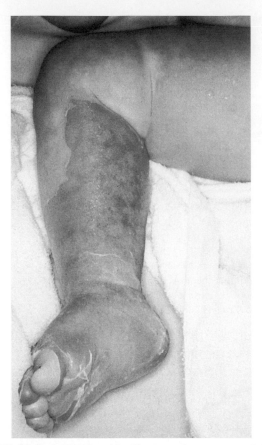

FIGURE **48-9.** Inflicted scalds. Close-up of severe second-degree burns of the foot and lower leg. (From Zitelli BJ, Davis HW: *Atlas of pediatric physical diagnosis,* ed 4, St. Louis, 2002, Mosby.)

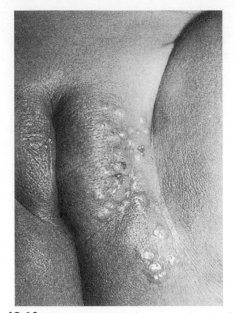

FIGURE **48-10.** Herpes genitalis in a prepubertal girl. (From Barkin RM: *Pediatric emergency medicine: concepts and clinical practice,* ed 2, St. Louis, 1997, Mosby. Courtesy N. Esterly, MD.)

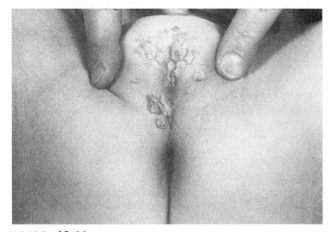

FIGURE **48-11.** Condyloma acuminata in a prepubertal girl. (From Barkin RM: *Pediatric emergency medicine: concepts and clinical practice,* ed 2, St. Louis, 1997, Mosby. Courtesy N. Esterly, MD.)

Rather, a well-coordinated evaluation and examination can be scheduled with an advocacy center through child protective services if this service is available. This option is only appropriate if the child is in a safe and protective environment and the health care team is assured that the caregiver will in fact follow through with this arrangement. A general physical examination should be performed before patient discharge to ensure that no acute problems exist.

Emergency personnel should ascertain safety of the child and of the home environment and treat current conditions (e.g., pelvic inflammatory disease, sexually transmitted infections [STIs]). Prophylaxis against pregnancy should be given for the pubescent female. Other responsibilities include emotional support, reporting suspected abuse to child protection authorities (including law enforcement), and involving the hospital-based child protection team or medical social worker.[13]

The most important component of sexual abuse evaluation is obtaining the patient history.[2] The diagnosis of sexual abuse often can be made on the basis of a child's history. Physical findings or behavioral indicators rarely stand alone; they are most valuable in supporting the history given by the child.[13] Physical findings are often absent even when penetration is involved. Many types of sexual abuse leave no physical evidence, and mucosal injuries often heal rapidly

and completely.[4] The type and extent of interview are contingent on many factors. If a multidisciplinary forensic interviewing team is available, emergency health care providers should collect just enough information to complete the medical examination and make recommendations. When a team is not available, a social worker may be helpful in coordinating care. History taking requires a quiet, child-friendly environment. A health care professional should begin by interviewing the adult who accompanied the child—without the child present. A careful, comprehensive medical history should document previous traumas to the anogenital area and attempt to gain an understanding of the adult's perception and emotional response to what has occurred.

Table 48-1. SECONDARY SEX CHARACTERISTICS (TANNER STAGES)

BREAST DEVELOPMENT

Stage I	Preadolescent; elevation of papilla only
Stage II	Breast and papilla elevated as small mound; areolar diameter increased
Stage III	Breast and areola enlarged; no contour separation
Stage IV	Areola and papilla form secondary mound
Stage V	Mature; nipple projects; areolar part of general breast contour

NOTE: Stages IV and V may not be distinct in some patients.

GENITAL DEVELOPMENT (MALE)

Stage I	Penis, testes, and scrotum preadolescent
Stage II	Enlargement of scrotum and testes, texture alteration; scrotal sac reddens; penis usually does not enlarge
Stage III	Further growth of testes and scrotum; penis enlarges and becomes longer
Stage IV	Continued growth of testes and scrotum; scrotum becomes darker; penis becomes longer; glans and breadth increase in size
Stage V	Genitalia adult in size and shape

PUBIC HAIR (MALE AND FEMALE)

Stage I	None; preadolescent
Stage II	Sparse growth of long, slightly pigmented downy hair, straight or only slightly curled, chiefly at base of penis or along labia
Stage III	Considerably darker, coarser and more curled; hair spreads sparsely over junction of pubes
Stage IV	Hair resembles adult in type; distribution still considerably smaller than in adult. No spread to medial surface of thighs
Stage V	Adult in quantity and type with distribution of the horizontal pattern
Stage VI	Spread up linea alba: "male escutcheon"

Modified from Tanner JM: *Growth at adolescence,* ed 2, 1962, Blackwell Scientific Publications.

Although children may not exhibit external trauma, a mental health emergency may develop because the victim and family are in a state of crisis.[13] Ideally the child and caregivers should be interviewed separately. Obtaining a child's statement requires an interviewer who is sensitive, nonjudgmental, nonthreatening, and trained in forensic interviewing of children. Interviewers must respond to the child's developmental and cognitive level and ask questions accordingly, using the child's terminology for body parts. The interviewer should avoid asking leading questions or showing strong emotions such as shock and disbelief and maintain a "tell me more" or "and then what happened" approach.[4] Allow time for the child to ask questions. General questions should include inquiries about the caregiver, where the child lives, sleeping arrangements, school habits, friends, names for body parts, and primary care provider. Focus on specific questions by addressing hurtful touches, pain, bleeding, or other "ouches."[13] Health care professionals should not be overzealous; however, interviewers should attempt to determine what abuse occurred, who was involved, when the last abuse occurred, and where it occurred. If the child becomes uncomfortable at any time, stop the interview. Children should not be further traumatized in an attempt to collect history. Always close the interview with praise for the child and reassurance that he or she has done nothing wrong and is not at fault for someone else's actions.

Physical Examination

Health care providers must be confident in their ability to correctly identify anatomy and detect acute injuries, nonspecific findings, scars, and healed tissue of genital trauma.[11] Physical findings in the female genital area are communicated using the face of a clock. The clitoris is always at 12 o'clock with the posterior fourchette at 6 o'clock. The area of the anus closest to the posterior fourchette is always at 12 o'clock. Tanner staging determines a child's outward sexual development and helps communicate level of sexual maturity (Table 48-1).

Preparing the child for medical evaluation is extremely important (Table 48-2). Give the child lots of decisions to make, such as what color of gown to wear, who he or she wants in the examination room, and if he or she wants to sit on the right or left side of the table. Always tell the truth, and promise only what you can control. While the child is fully clothed, explain the purpose of the examination. Most experts in the field use a colposcope, which allows magnification of the genital area up to 25 times, serves as an excellent light source, and is capable of photographing physical evidence. A colposcope can be frightening to a small child and should be fully explained before use. Demonstrate the colposcope, saline, and culture swabs. Use this time to assess the developmental, behavioral, and emotional status of

Table 48-2.	Preparing the Child for Medical Examination
Questions/Concerns	Helpful Responses
Do you know why you're here today?	To make sure your body is okay. We are going to look in your eyes, ears, nose, throat, mouth, where you go pee-pee (private area), and your skin all over. (Justify why they must undress.)
What is that big machine?	That is called a colposcope or big flashlight. It helps us see little bitsy things. The camera lets us take pictures. Do you think you could take some pictures for us? (Let child use long shutter cord to take pictures.)
Explain culture collection	We all have germs on our hands. They are also all over your body. I'm going to use a "bug-collector" (Dacron swab) to see if we can catch some germs, and if we do, let's feed them this chocolate bug food (modified Thayer-Martin culture medium for *Neisseria gonorrhoeae*) and give them some orange bug drink (*Chlamydia* culture medium).

the child. Allow the child as much control as possible. Let the child take pictures or hold swabs.

When the child appears comfortable, begin with a general head-to-toe examination to deemphasize the anogenital examination and look for other medical conditions. In males, the penis, testes, and scrotum are examined in the standing position. Look for urethral discharge, bleeding, swelling, bruising, or bite marks. Females are placed in the supine frog-leg position on a pelvic table, flat examination table, or mother's lap. With legs open, identify external genitalia and assess Tanner stage of development. Assess for ecchymoses, bleeding, lacerations, or abrasion. Use gloved hands to grasp the labia majora with thumb and forefinger, and apply gentle traction in a lateral, downward, and outward motion (toward the examiner). Gentle traction can best be explained as "opening double doors so we can look where you go pee-pee and make sure everything is okay." A normal hymen can exist in many shapes and forms: crescentic, annular, septate, redundant, cribriform, or rarely imperforate. If the hymen does not visualize well, saline solution may be squirted on the hymen, and then a moist Dacron swab is used to tease the hymenal edge up for better view. If the edge is still difficult to visualize, place the child in the knee-chest position. The knee-chest position is often the position in which abuse occurs and may be very uncomfortable for the child. The knee-chest position uses gravity to help redundant hymenal tissue fall downward for inspection. Assess for loss of tissue, lesions, transections, tears, notches, or bumps. Look for discharge or signs of foreign body. Speculum and digital examination is not recommended for the prepubertal child unless there is vaginal bleeding, laceration requiring suturing, or strong suspicion of a foreign body. The child should be sedated or placed under anesthesia if such examination is required. In rare circumstances in which the child is unable to cooperate and the examination must be performed because of the likelihood of trauma, infection, and/or the need to collect forensic evidence, an examination under sedation should be considered.

Conditions that may be mistaken for sexual abuse include unintentional trauma such as a straddle injury, urethral prolapse, congenital malformations, hemangioma,

inflammatory bowel disease such as Crohn's disease, and perianal streptococcal infection.

Multiple studies have shown that a high percentage of children with documented sexual abuse have no physical findings.[4] For example, oral-genital contact and fondling do not cause physical trauma. The anus is designed to allow large objects to easily pass with care and lubrication, so signs of abuse may not be evident. Physical findings are usually nonspecific and require a good history to determine significance. Legal and social systems are often unwilling to protect children unless evidence of physical trauma exists.

Anorectal examination is performed with the child in a lateral decubitus position. Observe for rugae symmetry of verge tissue. Gently separate the buttocks and inspect for tears, fissures, bruising, abrasions, and sphincter tone. Holding traction can prevent blood flow from the anus, resulting in venous pooling, which can be mistaken for bruising.

Explain actions with a soft, reassuring voice throughout the examination to keep children informed and to decrease anxiety. Remind children that they are in charge, so if anything hurts, the examiner will stop and together they will decide a different way to do things. When the examination is over, reassure them that their "bottom is okay," and then give them a chance to ask questions.

Specimen Collection

For prepubertal females, use saline-moistened Dacron swabs to obtain cultures from the vagina, pharynx, and rectum for *N. gonorrhoeae* and the endocervix and rectum for *Chlamydia trachomatis*. Obtain wet preparation, potassium oxide (KOH) slide, and Gram stain for vaginal discharge and viral cultures if herpes is suspected. If there is a history of penile-genital contact, obtain a serum pregnancy test.

In males, culture the urethra, rectum, and pharynx for *N. gonorrhoeae,* and the rectum and urethra (if there is a discharge) for *C. trachomatis*. Obtain a Gram stain of any discharge from male or female victims of acute assault and in those situations in which the perpetrator has a high risk for STIs. Obtain hepatitis B surface antigen,

Venereal Disease Research Laboratory (VDRL) or rapid plasma reagin test (repeat in 12 weeks), and HIV antibody test (repeat in 6 months).

Documentation

Child protection services rely heavily on the medical record; however, many child protective service workers admit they cannot read the writing, understand the terminology, or discern the significance of findings or lack of findings in these records. Health care providers have a responsibility to disseminate information in an understandable manner to law enforcement, child protective service workers, and the judicial system. Document findings accurately and precisely. Use quotation marks, draw pictures, and write clearly and legibly. Not only does this help law enforcement and child protective services, it also provides you a reference if you are called to testify in the case. Often these cases do not go to court for years, and health care professionals often have to rely on their documentation rather than memory alone. Avoid statements such as "hymen intact" or "has not been sexually abused" because these statements are ambiguous, and children with normal examinations may have been sexually abused.

EMOTIONAL ABUSE

As with other forms of child maltreatment, the true incidence of emotional abuse is unknown. The U.S. Department of Health and Human Services estimates that 7.1% of child abuse victims experienced emotional abuse in 2005. However, emotional abuse is almost always found with every form of child maltreatment.[17] Emotional abuse is defined as a repeated pattern of damaging interactions between caregiver(s) and child that becomes typical of the relationship.[3] Psychologic maltreatment of children occurs when a person conveys to a child that he or she is worthless, flawed, unloved, or unwanted.[3] This can be defined as acts or the lack of acts that cause or could possibly cause serious cognitive, behavioral, emotional, or mental disorders. Caregivers that use extreme measures of discipline such as locking a child in a closet or less severe acts such as habitual belittling or scapegoating are sufficient to warrant child protection intervention. Verbal abuse is one of the most common forms of emotional abuse.[10]

OTHER ISSUES RELATED TO CHILD ABUSE AND NEGLECT
Multidisciplinary Teams and Sexual Assault Nurse Examiners

Child abuse and neglect issues are complex and require the expertise of many professionals. Many hospitals and communities have adopted a multidisciplinary approach, using a core team with a health care provider (physician or nurse practitioner), social worker, and team coordinator. A con-

sulting team may include a child psychiatrist, developmental specialist, psychologist, public health coordinator, adult psychiatrist, and attorney. Professionals who can offer opinions on a case-by-case basis include family physicians, public health nurses, child protection workers, police officers, mental health therapists, guardians ad litem, foster parents, county attorneys, and teachers.

A cooperative approach has decreased the incidence of reabuse, serious injury, and child death and consistently ensured that hospitals fulfill the legal mandate to report suspected abuse. Consistent use of trained experts increases case findings and reporting within the community while focusing treatment on the entire family. A team approach also provides expert collection of forensic evidence and court testimony, ensures continuing education across disciplines, and decreases burnout for professionals in this field. An interdisciplinary approach appears to be extremely successful but does have drawbacks, such as high salaries and communication. Without effective communication among team members, there is a chance for conflict; however, strong direction and coordination can overcome these and other obstacles.

Sexual Assault Nurse Examiners

A sexual assault nurse examiner (SANE) is a registered nurse (RN) who has advanced education and clinical preparation in forensic examination of sexual assault victims.[21] The SANE program began in 1977 in Minneapolis and has now grown to more than 116 programs nationwide. The primary mission of a SANE program is to "meet the needs of the sexual assault victim by providing immediate, compassionate, culturally sensitive and comprehensive forensic evaluation and treatment by trained, professional nurse experts within the parameters of the individual's State Nurse Act, the SANE Standards of the International Association of Forensic Nurses, and the individual agency policies."[20] The SANE is responsible for performing the entire sexual assault evidentiary examination. This includes the perineal examination, collection of forensic evidence, STI prevention, pregnancy risk evaluation and interception, crisis intervention, and referrals for follow-up care.[18] SANE programs are enhancing evidence collection for more effective investigations and better prosecutions, particularly in nonstranger sexual assault cases.[21]

Testifying for Child Abuse and Neglect Cases

Health care providers are often the first professionals who become aware of child maltreatment; therefore the quality of documentation is critical to future prosecutorial decisions. The medical record and the health care professional who examined the child will almost certainly be involved if the case goes to court. Consequently, effective communication skills are essential for charting, obtaining history, handling parents, and interacting with investigators and attorneys. Physician testimony is not considered hearsay, so physicians are allowed to testify as to what the child told them during a medical examination.

If you do receive a subpoena and have never testified, contact the attorney. Find out what is expected from your testimony, and discuss what you can and cannot say. If you are called as a material witness, there is an expectation to "tell what you observed." An "expert" witness is required to prepare and support expert knowledge with current scientific literature.

Child Death Review Teams

The past 10 years have seen an increased focus on child deaths resulting from abuse and neglect. The National Center on Child Abuse and Neglect found a 49% increase in reports of child death since 1985.[12] In 2005 an estimated 1460 child fatalities from abuse were reported with a rate of nearly 2 deaths per 100,000 children in the United States.[19] In general, fatality rates decrease as children get older. Children vulnerable to serious or fatal abuse are those least visible to the community, educational programs, and protective services. Although many feel that perpetrators are those not related to the victim, approximately 77% of child fatalities occur at the hand of one or more parents.[19] Neglect accounted for approximately half of fatalities with combinations of maltreatment, physical abuse, and medical neglect accounting for the rest.

Child death review teams grew from an effort to determine how and why children were dying. In 1983 a tiny infant was beaten and eventually starved to death. A Los Angeles deputy sheriff mapped more than 52 contacts with 10 agencies. Investigations of drug abuse, domestic violence, reports of suspicious injuries, and drunken brawls were conducted; however, no agency knew the other was involved, and no one saw a need to remove the infant. From that meeting, a small group of professionals began to meet, share records, and make team decisions. Teams stood together, faced judges returning children to abusive settings, and started asking questions about siblings. Michael Durfee, a child psychiatrist, pressed for child death review teams across the country. Because of Durfee's efforts, most states have designated teams to review child deaths.

The death of a child in an ED is usually unexpected and sudden. Health care providers need to be sensitive to the family's needs while trying to obtain a history and conduct an examination to determine cause of death. After the death has been called, provide the family an opportunity to view and hold the child. Every ED should have written policies and procedures accompanied by checklists (Box 48-5) that should be followed in the event of a child's death. The medical examiner and child's primary medical caregiver should be notified of the death. Autopsies should be required on suspicious, obscure, or otherwise unexplained deaths.[7] Community resources should be offered for grief counseling. Hospital resources such as critical incident stress debriefings should be made available to all caregivers who have been emotionally stressed by a child's death.[1]

Box 48-5 CHECKLIST FOR CHILD DEATH IN THE EMERGENCY DEPARTMENT

Obtain a complete history (medical, family, social)
Describe the circumstances of death (especially when SIDS is suspected):
  Position in which the child was put to sleep
  Type of bed and bedding
  Did child sleep alone or cosleep?
  What and when child last ate
  Position in which child was found and by whom
  Clothing child was wearing
  Temperature of room
Core temperature upon arrival at ED
Perform a complete physical examination (head to toe, including eyes, skin, and genitalia)
Photograph any bruises or wounds if present
Review prior medical records
Skeletal survey
Laboratory tests such as cultures, drug screen, and routine blood studies
Grief support for family and ED staff
Autopsy (documentation of circumstances and laboratory specimens should accompany body to morgue)

SIDS, Sudden infant death syndrome; *ED,* emergency department.

Prevention

Prevention of child abuse and neglect is extremely difficult. It is essential that health care providers be able to recognize children and families at risk for child maltreatment. Precursors to physical maltreatment include excessive parental physical discipline, failure to provide basic necessities such as food and a safe home, and unobtainable goals set by parents. Programs for prevention of child abuse and neglect typically focus on physical abuse, centering on the parent, parenting skills, and damaging practices. Pilot programs such as home visiting and increased public awareness have decreased physical abuse of children in some areas. Changing attitudes and modifying behaviors require at least 6 to 12 months. To successfully reduce physical abuse and neglect within diverse populations, preventive services should begin before or shortly after birth of the first child—through support of effective child-rearing skills. Prevention efforts should tie the child's developmental level to parent enhancement education. Parents must observe and be able to model desired parental behaviors. Child safety can depend on the parent's ability to take advantage of social programs and obtain assistance as needed. All prevention programs must recognize and accept cultural differences.

Current sexual abuse prevention focuses on the child.[17] The child is given permission to say "no." Classroom education teaches "good touches" and "bad touches" and who the child should tell if someone tries to hurt him or her. But what if the abuser is the child's mom or dad? Sexual abuse is convoluted; secrecy is a large component of manipulation. Effective prevention programs should stress community involvement, self-confidence, and the child's cognitive abilities.

SUMMARY

Child abuse and neglect are complex, life-threatening situations. Medical professionals who work with children must speak out for abused children. No one agency or discipline can be solely responsible for protection of children. The community, law enforcement, child protection workers, mental health counselors, legislators, educators, health care providers, and the judicial system must work together to remove barriers to identification, treatment, and prevention of child abuse and neglect.

REFERENCES

1. American Academy of Pediatrics: Care of children in emergency department: guidelines for preparedness, *Pediatrics* 107(4):777, 2001.
2. American Academy of Pediatrics: Shaken baby syndrome: rotational cranial injuries (policy statement), *Pediatrics* 108(1):206, 2001.
3. American Academy of Pediatrics: The psychological maltreatment of children—technical report, *Pediatrics* 109(4):1, 2002.
4. American Academy of Pediatrics: The evaluation of sexual abuse in children, *Pediatrics* 116(2):506, 2005.
5. American Academy of Pediatrics: Failure to thrive as a manifestation of child neglect, *Pediatrics* 116(5):1234, 2005.
6. American Academy of Pediatrics: Evaluation of suspected child physical abuse, *Pediatrics* 119(6):1232, 2007.
7. American Academy of Pediatrics: Committees on Child Abuse and Neglect and Community Health Services: Investigation and review of unexpected infant and child deaths, *Pediatrics* 99(104):1158, 1998.
8. Bonner BL, Crowe SM, Logue MD: Fatal child neglect, In Dubowitz H: *Neglected children: research, practice, and policy*, Thousand Oaks, Calif, 1999, Sage.
9. Emergency Nurses Association: *Emergency nursing pediatric course provider manual*, ed 3, Des Plaines, Ill, 2004, The Association.
10. Emergency Nurses Association: *Emergency nursing core curriculum*, ed 6, Des Plaines, Ill, 2007, The Association.
11. Giardino AP, Finkel MA, Giardino E, et al: *A practical guide to the evaluation of sexual abuse in the prepubertal child*, Newberry Park, Calif, 1992, Sage.
12. Herman-Giddens ME, Brown G, Verbiest S et al: Underascertainment of child mortality in the United States, *JAMA* 282(5):463, 1999.
13. Monteleone JA, Brodeur AE: *Child maltreatment: a clinical guide and reference*, St. Louis, 1994, GW Medical Publishing.
14. The National Shaken Baby Coalition: *Facts about SBS*. Retrieved August 21, 2007, from http://www.shakenbabycoalition.org/facts.htm.
15. Peddle N, Wang C: *Current trends in child abuse prevention, reporting, and fatalities: the 1999 fifty state survey*, 2002, National Center on Child Abuse Prevention Research. Retrieved February 21, 2002, from http://www.preventchildabuse.org.
16. Prevent Child Abuse America: *Neglect*. Retrieved August 23, 2007, from http://preventchildabuse.com/neglect.htm.
17. Prevent Child Abuse America: *Total estimated cost of child abuse and neglect in the United States*. Retrieved February 21, 2002, from http://www.preventchildabuse.org.
18. U.S. Department of Health and Human Services: *Child maltreatment 1998: reports from the state to the national child abuse and neglect data system*, Washington DC, 2000, U.S. Government Printing Office.
19. U.S. Department of Health and Human Services: *Child maltreatment 2005: annual report*, Washington, DC. Retrieved August 9, 2007, from http://www.acf.hhs.gov.
20. U.S. Department of Health and Human Services: Office for Victims of Crime: *Sexual assault nurse examiner development and operation guide*, Washington, DC, 2000, U.S. Government Printing Office.
21. U.S. Department of Justice: *Sexual assault nurse examiner (SANE) programs: improving the community response to sexual assault victims*. Retrieved August 23, 2007, from http://www.ojp.usdoj.gov/ovc/publications/bulletins/sane_4_2001/welcome.html.

CHAPTER 49

Intimate Partner Violence

Mary Jagim

Although recognizing, assessing, and intervening with victims of intimate partner violence in the emergency department (ED) can be challenging, the emergency nurse has an opportunity to affect the victim's outcome. Intimate partner violence (IPV) is defined as "a pattern of assaultive and coercive behaviors including inflicted physical injury, psychological abuse, sexual assault, progressive social isolation, stalking, deprivation, intimidation and threats. These behaviors are perpetrated by someone who is, was, or wishes to be involved in an intimate dating relationship with an adult or adolescent, and are aimed at establishing control by one partner over the other."[19]

INCIDENCE

IPV occurs in adolescents and adults, in all social and cultural groups, among lesbian and gay, heterosexual, and transgendered couples, and in married and unmarried relationships. The most prevalent incidence of IPV is among women. The National Crime Victimization Survey found that 85% of IPV victims were women.[3] Nearly 5.3 million incidents of IPV occur each year among U.S. women ages 18 and older, and 3.2 million occur among men.[3] Approximately 1.5 million women and more the 800,000 men have been victims of sexual or physical assault by an intimate partner. National studies have shown that 29% of women and 22% of men

have experienced physical, sexual, or psychologic IPV during their lifetime.[4]

IPV impacts women of all ages. In a study of older adult women age 65 and older, 18% reported that they had suffered sexual or physical abuse by intimate partners at some point in their lives, and 22% said they been victims of nonphysical abuse, including being threatened, called names, or having their behavior controlled by a partner.[1]

Higher incidence of risk for IPV exists for women of certain racial, ethnic, and socioeconomic groups. The ethnic groups most at risk are Native American/Alaskan Native women and men, African American women, and Hispanic women.[21] Also, young women and those below the poverty line are disproportionately victims of IPV.[21]

Pregnant women also note a higher incidence of IPV. A review of 13 studies found the prevalence of IPV ranging from 0.9% to 20.1%. One study, using a three-question screening tool, revealed a 17% prevalence of physical or sexual abuse during pregnancy with 60% of abused pregnant women reporting two or more occurrences. Common sites of physical abuse in pregnancy include the face, head, breasts, and abdomen. IPV may be a contributing risk factor for low birth weight and delays in prenatal care.[20]

IPV results in nearly 2 million injuries and 1200 deaths nationwide every year. At least 42% of women and 20% of men who were physically assaulted since age 18 sustained injuries during their most recent victimization. Most of the injuries were minor such as scratches, bruises, and welts. More severe physical consequences of IPV are dependent upon the severity and frequency of abuse.[3]

Alcohol and drug abuse are comorbidity factors to IPV. Sixty to seventy percent of violent men assault their partners while drunk. Another 13% to 20% of violent men assault their partners while on drugs. Overall, the presence of an alcohol or drug problem increases the risk for severe violence by 70% to 158%.[11]

The economic impact of IPV is notable. IPV costs exceed $8.3 billion, which includes $460 million for sexual assault, $6.2 billion for physical assault, $461 million for stalking, and $1.2 billion in value of lost lives. In addition, victims of severe IPV lose nearly 8 million days of paid work annually.[3]

RISK FACTORS

Associated risk factors identified as contributing to a greater likelihood of being a victim of IPV include but are not limited to the following:

- Prior history of IPV
- Witnessing or experiencing violence as a child
- Low self-esteem
- Low academic achievement
- High-risk sexual behavior
- Heavy alcohol and drug use
  The following are relationship factors:
- Couples with income, education, or job status disparities
- Dominance and control of the relationship by the male
  Community and societal factors include the following:
- Poverty and associated factors
- Low social capital; lack of institutions, relationships, and norms that shape the quality and quantity of a community's social interactions
- Weak community sanctions against IPV
- Traditional gender norms (e.g., belief that women should stay at home and not enter workforce, should be submissive)[3]

Rural Victims

Victims of IPV who reside in rural areas may have an additional risk factor related to increased availability of weapons. Rural victims of IPV may also have greater challenges in seeking help. There are often geographic isolation, very traditional gender roles, poverty, shortage of health providers, lack of public transportation systems, and decreased access to resources and other opportunities. In small communities where everyone knows everyone, seeking confidential assistance may be nearly impossible.[15] Victims may have limited ability to go to another location to seek assistance. In some cases the abuser could be a local person of authority.

CYCLE OF VIOLENCE

The central functions of intimate partner violence are intimidation and control. Control is accomplished by the perpetrator through physical, sexual, and emotional abuse; social

isolation; and financial dependency. Several theories exist as to the development of a batterer. One of the primary explanations centers on borderline personality organization. Borderline personality organization is characterized by intense and unstable interpersonal relationships coupled with intense anger, impulsivity, and fear of abandonment. It is thought that early attachment difficulties, primarily surrounding parental rejection, later develop into an excessive dependency and abandonment anxiety with their adult partner. Other contributing factors may be an exposure to physical or sexual abuse, either as a direct victim or a witness to interfamilial conflict. Batterers come to see violence as necessary, normal, and good. They often have traditional sex role expectations about acceptable behavior in women.[11]

The cycle of intimate partner violence is repeated by the batterer until it is disrupted. The cycle consists of three phases:

Phase one: increased tension, anger, blaming
Phase two: battering, use of objects as weapons, sexual abuse, verbal threats and abuse
Phase three: calm state, apology (most difficult time for the victim to leave)[22,24]

Impact on the Victim

Battering can have a physical, emotional, and psychologic impact on the victim. As a result, the victim may exhibit depression, antisocial behavior, suicidal behavior in females, anxiety, low self-esteem, inability to trust men, and a fear of intimacy.

Due to the social isolation batterers often impose, victims are isolated from social networks such as family or friends, have restricted access to services, and may experience strained relationships with health care providers and employers.

Women experiencing IPV are more likely to display negative health behaviors that present further health risks. Some noted behaviors are engaging in high-risk sexual behavior such as unprotected sex or multiple partners, using or abusing harmful substances such as alcohol or drugs, and unhealthy diet-related behaviors such as vomiting after eating or overeating.[3]

Impact on Children

The long-lasting ramifications of IPV on children are difficult to measure. Children who may become injured include those who witness IPV incidents between their parents. There is also a positive correlation between IPV and child maltreatment. One study found that children of abused mothers were 57 times more likely to have been harmed because of IPV incidents between their parents, compared with children of nonabused mothers.[3] Children whose lives are touched by IPV may have resultant low self-esteem, depression, ineffective coping, higher levels of aggression, oppositional behavior, fear, anxiety, withdrawal, and poor peer and other social relationships. Also noted are lower cognitive functioning, poor school performance, lack of conflict resolution skills, limited problem-solving skills, proviolence attitudes, and belief in rigid gender stereotypes and male privilege.[2]

Why Do Women Stay?

Understanding why a woman chooses to stay in a violent relationship is probably the most challenging aspect of providing care for the victims of IPV. It would seem obvious that the solution to the violence is to just "get out." But for the victim of IPV, this is often the solution that seems most out of reach or inconceivable. As awful as their world is, it is the world they know versus the unknown should they choose to leave. Women feel they are the "victim" and feel a loss of control over their lives. They often believe that if they just love their abuser enough and behave appropriately, things will change. Many have a negative self-concept, and they doubt they can manage on their own. These victims may be afraid they will be unable to financially support themselves or their children and that they will be stigmatized. There may also be cultural factors that shape what is considered acceptable and unacceptable behaviors.[12] Victims may be justifiably afraid of retaliation. The greatest risk for homicide often occurs when the victim has decided to leave or just after the victim has left.[2] The emergency nurse needs to repeatedly ask the questions and assist victims with knowing what options exist until they are ready to take action.

Treatment of Batterers

Legal interventions, such as being arrested and/or prosecuted, are often the primary impetus for batterers to receive treatment. Treatment of batterers is focused on prevention and decreased recidivism. Interventions are tailored to a specific type of batterer based on psychologic factors, risk assessment, or substance abuse history.[13] The effectiveness of batterer treatment programs remains in question because of variable results.[14]

ROLE OF THE EMERGENCY NURSE

The primary role of the health care provider in caring for potential victims of IPV is to ensure care and recognition of injuries, offer victims the chance to tell their story, and initiate interventions and referrals to assist victims in planning for safety. Forty-four percent of women murdered by their intimate partner had visited an ED within 2 years of the homicide. Of these women, 93% had at least one injury visit.[3] The greatest number of ED visits tends to occur during the month of the assault.[16] The chance of being screened or identified with intimate partner violence increases with repeated visits.

Screening

The Joint Commission established its initial standards regarding victims of abuse in 1990.[6] The standards identified the importance of identifying, assessing, intervening,

and initiating a referral for victims of abuse. The requirement to screen for abuse was integrated into routine care of all patients. In addition, they noted that it is necessary to collect information and evidentiary materials for potential future actions as part of a legal process for victims of reported abuse or neglect.[6] A 2004 recommendation by the U.S. Preventive Services Task Force[23] noted that there is insufficient evidence to recommend for or against routine screening of women for intimate partner violence; the belief and support of many professional organizations remains that screening in the ED is beneficial to victims.[10] The rationale behind ED screening is that it is the access point for all populations, particularly the underserved; the ED is generally a secure environment; and it affords the opportunity for greater anonymity in an environment where there is no ongoing health care relationship.[8,17] The ED visit may be the only "window of opportunity" to assess and provide assistance to victims of intimate partner violence. With the evidence that clinician inquiry is the strongest determinate of intimate partner violence disclosure, the Emergency Nurses Association recommends "routine assessment of risk factors for both the victim and perpetrator."[7] However, clinically documented compliance with universal screening remains low, as does the provision of appropriate counseling and intervention services.[5] In order for universal screening to be most effective, appropriate assessment, intervention, and referral practices must also be in place.

The Partner Violence Screen is a brief screening instrument designed for use in EDs or other urgent care settings. This screening tool includes the following questions:

1. Have you been kicked, hit, punched, or otherwise hurt by someone in the past year? If so, by whom?
2. Do you feel safe in your current relationship?
3. Is there a partner from a previous relationship who is making you feel unsafe now?[9]

The first question is nearly as sensitive and specific as the combination of the three questions.[9] In the busy ED setting the first question may be asked at triage if privacy is possible. Positive answers on the initial screen itself can be explored after the patient is in the treatment area away from the partner. Escorting the patient to the bathroom for a urine sample provides an ideal opportunity to ask the patient about potential abuse.

Patient Presentation

The emergency nurse must have a high index of suspicion and be alert for physical and behavioral clues. The majority (72%)[16] of patients who visit the ED as a result of IPV will present with medical complaints such as abdominal pain, back pain, pelvic pain, urinary tract infections, headaches, anxiety, substance abuse, sexually transmitted diseases, or symptoms of posttraumatic stress disorder. If victims of IPV do present with trauma-related injuries, the injuries often appear inconsistent with the story, and evidence of old injuries may also be present.[12] The most common sites of injuries are the head, face, neck, and areas usually covered by clothing, such as the chest, breasts, and abdomen. Maxillofacial trauma is also common, including eye and ear trauma, hearing loss, soft tissue injuries, and fractures of the mandible, nasal bones, orbits, zygoma, and maxilla.[25] Patient behaviors that may indicate possible abuse are concerns about confidentiality, comments regarding their carelessness or stupidity in getting hurt, fear of their partner leaving them in the ED, and appearing anxious to leave or to get their partner out of the room. Abusive partners who are present with the victims may stay very close during the assessment and interview of a patient or even respond to questions for their partner. The abuser may also be very aggressive and demanding toward staff.[25]

Evidence Collection

Evidence should be collected that may be required for prosecution, including sexual assault kits or photographs of injuries. Collaborate with law enforcement regarding evidence collection and maintaining appropriate chain of custody. Consider testing for pregnancy or sexually transmitted diseases if appropriate.

Safety Planning and Referrals

When a patient responds positively to any of the screening questions, further assessment needs to occur to assess the incidence of violence and identify safety concerns. The emergency nurse assesses for safety of the patient by asking questions such as the following:

- Are you afraid to go home?
- Have there been threats of homicide or suicide?
- Are there weapons present in the home?
- Can you stay with family or friends?
- Do you need access to a shelter?
- Do you want police intervention?

Initial crisis management begins immediately. Arrangements should be made to provide for advocacy services and follow-up appointments for primary care. It is ideal if a social worker or advocate can come to the ED to meet with the victim and assist in developing an initial action plan for securing the victim's safety. Information regarding available shelters and other community resources should be provided. The patient should be given resources such as a phone number he or she can call 24 hours a day to get help (National Domestic Violence Hotline: 800-799-SAFE, pamphlets or cards with phone numbers). Be aware that patients may refuse cards or phone numbers because it may not be safe to bring home material that deals with IPV. If the patient will not take any material, give the number of the ED or the name of a local IPV organization to him or her to look up in the phone book.

Reassure the patient that he or she is not to blame for the battering. Many patients believe they have done something to incite the violence or are sure they can prevent further violence if they simply behave in the appropriate manner.

This is a false assumption, however; the pattern of abuse will continue until an outside intervention stops it. Reinforce that even risk factors such as high-risk sexual activity do not make the victim responsible for the batterer's actions.

Documentation and Reporting

Documentation is a crucial step in the care of the victim of IPV. Documentation should include the responses to all screening and safety questions and incidents surrounding the injury or other physical complaints using the patient's own words in quotations. Include accurate descriptions of all injuries, using a body map to mark location and size and support these with instant photographs. Documentation serves multiple purposes, including the following:

- Alerting other health care providers of ongoing domestic violence in a patient's life
- Serving as objective documentation that injuries not consistent with accidental origin have been observed
- Assisting those who monitor quality of care to determine the rate of screening that is occurring
- Contributing data to hospital and clinic policy decisions so that scarce resources are allocated to the problems that patients are most typically presenting[12]

To summarize these key elements in caring for the victim of IPV, in 1992 the Massachusetts Medical Society developed the acronym RADAR:

- **R**emember to routinely ask patients about intimate partner violence
- **A**sk them directly, using specific questions
- **D**ocument assessment and injuries
- **A**ssess victim safety
- **R**eview possible options with the victim, and provide referrals

Forensic nurse examiners, already available in many EDs, are an excellent resource to assess and document injury related to IPV. Forensic nurse examiners routinely work with law enforcement, clinicians, advocacy agencies, and community services as part of a multidisciplinary team. They are well versed in principles of forensic evidence collection, photo-documentation, and legal testimony. A 2003 pilot study examining ED use demonstrated that 85% of IPV victims chose to work with law enforcement with a subsequent 90% conviction rate when a forensic nurse examiner was involved in their care. These victims also had fewer ED visits in the year after forensic nursing services were used than in the year before.[18]

Emergency nurses must be familiar with the mandatory reporting laws of their state. Most states require that health care providers report when they treat patients who have been shot, stabbed, or injured. Some states have laws that specifically address IPV. The Family Violence Prevention Fund provides a listing and evaluation of mandatory reporting laws for all states, which can be found at http://www.endabuse.org/health/mandatoryreporting.

SUMMARY

As emergency nurses, we may feel great frustration in caring for victims of IPV, especially when victims choose to remain in a violent relationship or place themselves at risk. Although the process is often slow, many women do leave their abusive partners. Our role is not to judge but rather to provide the treatment needed, assess patients' current situation for safety risks, and convey to victims the knowledge that they have options and resources to make a change should they so choose. We can be an essential part of a process that supports the patient's autonomy, offers hope, and empowers the patient to eventually take action to stop the cycle of violence. For information on additional resources, see Box 49-1 for a summary of national resources.

REFERENCES

1. Bonomi AE, Anderson ML, Reid RJ: Intimate partner violence in older women, *Gerontologist* 47(1):34, 2007.
2. Campbell JC, Lewandowski LA: Mental and physical health effects of intimate partner violence on women and children, *Psychiatr Clin North Am* 20(2):353, 1997.
3. Centers for Disease Control and Prevention: *Intimate partner violence: overview,* Atlanta, 2007, CDC, National Center for Injury Prevention and Control. Retrieved September 3, 2007, from http://www.cdc.gov/ncipc/factsheets/ipvoverview.htm.
4. Coker AL, Davis KE, Arias I et al: Physical and mental health effects of intimate partner violence for men and women, *Am J Prev Med* 23(4):260, 2002.
5. Datner EM, Omalley M, Schears RM et al: Universal screening for interpersonal violence: inability to prove universal screening improves provision of services, *Eur J Emerg Med* 11:35, 2004.
6. Dienemann J, Trautman D, Shahan JB et al: Developing a domestic violence program in an inner-city academic health center emergency department: the first 3 years, *J Emerg Nurs* 25(2):110, 1999.
7. Emergency Nurses Association: *Intimate partner and family violence, maltreatment, and neglect position statement,* Des Plaines, Ill, 2006, Emergency Nurses Association. Retrieved September 3, 2007, from http://www.ena.org/about/position/.
8. Family Violence Prevention Fund: *National consensus guidelines on identifying and responding to domestic violence victimization in health care settings,* 2004. Retrieved September 3, 2007, from http://fvpfstore.stores.yahoo.net/natconguidon.html.
9. Feldhaus KM, Koziol-McLain J, Amsbury H, et al: Accuracy of 3 brief screening questions for detecting partner violence in the emergency department, *JAMA* 277(17):1357, 1997.
10. Glass N, Dearwater S, Campbell J: Intimate partner violence screening and intervention: data from eleven Pennsylvania and California Community Hospital Emergency Departments, *J Emerg Nurs* 27(2):141, 2001.
11. Gortner ET, Gollan JK, Jacobson NS: Psychological aspects of perpetrators of domestic violence and their relationships with the victims, *Psychiatr Clin North Am* 20(2):337, 1997.
12. Griffin MP, Koss MP: Clinical screening and intervention in cases of partner violence, *Online J Issues Nurs* 7(1), 2002. Retrieved September 3, 2007, from http://www.nursingworld.org/ojin.
13. Healey K, Smith C, O'Sullivan C: *Batterer intervention: program approaches and criminal justice strategies,* Washington, DC, 1998, U.S. Department of Justice, Office of Justice Programs, National Institute of Justice. Retrieved September 3, 2007, from http://www.ncjrs.gov/pdffiles/168638.pdf.
14. Jackson S, Feder L, Forde D et al: *Batterer intervention programs: where do we go from here?* 2003, U.S. Department of Justice, Office of Justice Programs, National Institute of Justice. Retrieved September 3, 2007, from http://www.ncjrs.gov/pdffiles1/nij/195079.pdf.
15. Johnson R: *Rural health response to domestic violence: policy and practice issues,* Publication No. 99–0545(P), Washington, DC, August 30, 2000, Federal Office of Rural Health Policy, Health Resources and Services Administration, U.S. Department of Health and Human Services. Retrieved March 15, 2007, from http://ruralhealth.hrsa.gov/pub/domviol.htm.
16. Kothari CL, Rhodes KV: Missed opportunities: emergency department visits by police-identified victims of intimate partner violence, *Ann Emerg Med* 47(2):190, 2006.
17. Koziol-McLain J, Campbell JC: Universal screening and mandatory reporting: an update on two important issues for victims/survivors of intimate partner violence, *J Emerg Nurs* 27(6):602, 2001.
18. Markowitz JR, Steer S, Garland M: Hospital-based intervention for intimate partner violence victims: a forensic nursing model, *J Emerg Nurs* 31(2):166, 2005.

19. National Health Resource Center on Domestic Violence: *A call to action: the nursing role in routine assessment for intimate partner violence,* Family Violence Prevention Fund. Retrieved September 3, 2007, from http://fvpfstore.stores.yahoo.net/nursingfolio.html.

20. Shah AJ, Kilcline BA: Trauma in pregnancy, *Emerg Med Clin North Am* 21(3):615, 2003.

21. Tjaden P, Thoennes N: *Extent, nature, and consequences of intimate partner violence: findings from the National Violence Against Women Survey,* Publication No. NCJ 181867, Washington, DC, 2000, U.S. Department of Justice. Retrieved September 3, 2007, from http://www.ojp.usdoj.gov/nij/pubs-sum/181867.htm.

22. University of Virginia Women's Center: *The cycle of violence in abusive relationships.* Retrieved September 3, 2007, from http://womenscenter.virginia.edu/sdvs/domestic/cycle.htm.

23. U.S. Preventive Services Task Force: Screening for family and intimate partner violence: recommendation statement, *Ann Intern Med* 140:382, 2004.

24. Walker L: *Dynamics of domestic violence—the cycle of violence.* Retrieved September 3, 2007, from http://www.enddomesticviolence.com/include/content/filehyperlink/holder/The%20Cycle%20of%20Violence.doc.

25. Warshaw C, Ganley AL: *Improving the health care response to domestic violence: a resource manual for health care providers,* 1998, Family Violence Prevention Fund. Retrieved September 3, 2007, from http://endabuse.org/programs/display.php3?DocID=238.

CHAPTER 50

Elder Abuse and Neglect

Nancy Stephens Donatelli

Elder abuse and neglect take different forms; however, the common denominator is harm or threatened harm to the health or welfare of the older adult.[6] Abuse and neglect have increased steadily as the number of older adults requiring dependent care has increased. The emergency nurse needs to cultivate a sensitivity and heightened consciousness of the scope of this problem and its risk factors, and approach the suspicion of elder abuse in the same manner that suspected child abuse is addressed.

DEFINING ELDER ABUSE AND NEGLECT

According to the American Medical Association, older adult abuse is defined as "actions or the omission of actions that result in harm or threatened harm to the health or welfare of the elderly."[7] Neglect is defined as the deliberate refusal to meet basic needs. Seven primary categories of elder mistreatment have been identified: physical abuse, neglect, self-neglect, psychologic or emotional abuse, abandonment, violation of personal rights, and financial abuse.[6]

SCOPE OF THE PROBLEM

The life span of the average American is increasing, whereas the U.S. birth rate has declined. More people require care, but fewer people are available to provide care. Consequently, the literature suggests that the number of older adult abuse incidents will increase over the next 30 years because people are living longer, which increases the need for long-term care; the baby-boomer generation is entering the age-group of 60 plus; there is an increased demand on caregivers; and there is an increased legal obligation to report suspected abuse.

Obtaining a clear, accurate picture of demographics surrounding elder abuse is difficult. Significant shame and embarrassment are associated with this problem, so abused individuals may keep the problem hidden within the family to decrease further embarrassment. Study findings confirm commonly held theories that officially reported cases of abuse are only the "tip of a much larger iceberg." For every case of abuse and neglect that is reported to authorities, experts estimate that there may be as many as five cases that have not been reported.[6]

The best national data report that a total of 565,747 older adults, age 60 and over, experienced abuse, neglect, or self-neglect in domestic settings in 2004.[10] According to these estimates, between 1 and 2 million Americans age 65 or older have been mistreated by someone they depend upon for care or protection.[8] It occurs among men and women of all racial, ethnic, and socioeconomic groups. Most neglect is due to ignorance, lack of resources, or the frailty of the caregiver. Individuals age 80 and older are abused and neglected two to three times more often than those of other ages. This is attributed to the fact that they tend to have more health problems and are living longer, which increases stress on the caregiver.

Older women are far more likely than men to suffer from abuse or neglect, probably because they make up a larger proportion of the senior population. In 2003, two out of three (67.7%) elder abuse victims were women.[7] The more dependent the person, the more likely he or she is to be abused. In descending order of frequency, substantiated types of maltreatment were self-neglect (37.2%), caregiver neglect (20.4%), financial exploitation (14.7%), emotional/psychologic/verbal abuse (14.8%), physical abuse (10.7%), sexual abuse (1%), other (1.2%).[7] As for the perpetrator of the abuse, 62% of the time it is a family member; 52% are men, with spouses representing 30% of the total. Most often the abuser is 36 to 50 years of age; race is white about three fourths of the time, and less than one fifth of abusers were black.[6]

An area of elder maltreatment that is quickly coming to the forefront is known as "gray murders." The expectancy that an older adult will die is such a fact of life that details concerning the death are often not questioned. Homicide related to elder abuse has long been overlooked. Since 1960 the rate of homicide in those 65 years of age or older has increased.[3] According to police veteran, Joseph Soos, "Gray murders might be among the most overlooked violent crimes in America."[2]

ORIGIN OF THE PROBLEM

Four main theories may explain elder abuse: role theory, transgenerational theory, psychopathology theory, and stressed-caregiver theory.

Role Theory

As the parent ages and becomes more childlike, the child must assume a parental role. The elder who once helped the child must now take orders from that child. The psychologic impact of this role reversal is significant for both generations. When role conflicts are present, the potential for abuse increases substantially. Many family caregivers find themselves "sandwiched" between the need to provide care for their own children while providing care for their older parent(s) or spouse's parent(s), a situation creating additional stress and role conflicts.

Transgenerational Theory

The underlying philosophy of transgenerational theory is that violence is a learned behavior. If a child grows up in a family in which aggressive behavior is a part of life, the child exhibits similar behavior. If the parent abused the child, then the child, as the caregiver, abuses the parent in retribution.

Psychopathology Theory

Altered impulse control caused by psychologic problems such as mental illness or drug or alcohol dependence places the elder at greater risk for abuse. The typical abuser is a middle-age, white woman who lives with the victim, is an alcohol or drug addict, and has long-term financial problems and high stress levels. The abuser perceives the victim as the source of this stress.

Stressed-Caregiver Theory

This is one area in which the nurse providing long-term care for older adults can abuse their charge as easily as can the family caregiver. Caregivers under stress have limited amounts of internal resources. Stress associated with the health care environment and stress in the individual's personal and family life may lead the caregiver to express stress through maltreatment of older adults.

PRIMARY CATEGORIES OF MALTREATMENT AND ASSOCIATED CLINICAL FINDINGS

Physical abuse is an act of violence that results in bodily harm or mental distress, including pain, injury, and physical confinement. Injuries result from slapping, shoving, hitting, beating, pushing, kicking, incorrect positioning, pinching, burning, biting, overmedicating or undermedicating, or improper use of restraints. Signs of physical abuse include bruises or grip marks around the arms or neck, lacerations, fractures, and rope marks or welts on the wrists and/or ankles.

The possibility of sexual abuse, unwanted sexual activity forced on a person by another through coercion or threats, must also be considered. Signs include unexplained genital or anal bleeding, bruised breasts, and sexually transmitted infections.

Neglect is the deliberate refusal to meet an individual's basic needs, including activities such as withholding assistance vital to performance of activities of daily living, behavior that causes mental anguish, and lack of compliance with medication administration and treatment regimens. Signs of neglect include dehydration, malnutrition, decubitus ulcers, and poor personal hygiene.

Self-neglect encompasses behaviors of an older adult that threaten his or her own health or safety. Victims are usually depressed, confused, or extremely frail. Excluded are situations in which a mentally competent older adult makes a conscious and voluntary decision to engage in acts that threaten his or her health or safety.

Psychologic or emotional abuse includes verbal aggression, intimidation, and humiliation; threats to deprive the elder of property or services, placement in a nursing home, or removal of financial support; unreasonable demands; deliberately ignoring the person; isolating the elder from family, friends, or activities; and failure to provide companionship. Findings suggestive of psychologic abuse include elders that are uncommunicative and unresponsive; unreasonably fearful or suspicious; lack interest in social contacts; have chronic physical or psychiatric health problems; or exhibit emotional pain, distress, and evasiveness.

Violation of personal rights is the deprivation of inalienable rights (i.e., personal liberty, personal property, free speech, privacy, voting).

Abandonment is the desertion of an older adult by an individual who has physical custody or otherwise has assumed responsibility for providing care for an elder or by a person with physical custody of an elder.

Financial abuse is the unauthorized use of money or goods for personal gain. Inappropriate conduct includes misuse of funds, petty theft, material exploitation, coercion of the elder to sign contracts, failure to pay bills, or declaration of the elder as incompetent in order to confiscate property. This type of exploitation is not unique to family caregivers—it can also be perpetrated by individuals or corporations who take advantage of seniors through confusing or misleading mail or telephone offers (e.g., elders who have multiple magazine subscriptions or who get checks in the mail not realizing that their signature on the check is a contract for a service they did not solicit or a loan with an extremely high interest rate).

RISK FACTORS FOR MALTREATMENT

Risk factors can be divided into four broad categories: economic, caregiver related, social, and physical. An example of an economic situation might be the stress of living in cramped conditions with associated financial problems. Caregiver factors may be inexperience of the caregiver in dealing with complex needs of the frail, ill older adult; caregiver mental illness; and stress resulting from the "sandwich generation," when the addition of an older adult to the household brings sudden, unwanted, and unexpected dependency to the caregiver who has young children in the home. The greater the dependency on the caregiver, the greater the risk for abuse. Social factors may be seen in a role reversal in which the parent abused the child and now the child abuses the parent. Physical factors may include advanced age of the caregiver or the older adult and alcohol or drug abuse in the older adult or the caregiver.

RECOGNIZING CLUES OF MALTREATMENT

Clues to abuse may be detected during the review of the patient's medical history, during the physical assessment, and/or by the patient's psychologic status.

History taking may show a pattern of "health care shopping," a series of missed appointments, or excessive concern with health care costs by the older adult or the caregiver. The elder person's history should be obtained from several sources whenever possible.

Physical clues may be evidenced as previously unexplained injuries, the presence of old and new bruises, weight gain or loss, or poor personal hygiene. Alopecia secondary to repeated pulling and tugging of the person's hair or positioning of the head in one position for a long period of time is another significant finding.[5] Blows to the eyes can cause dislocation of the lens, subconjunctival hemorrhage, or retinal detachment. Whiplash injuries are seen after repeated, violent shaking. Consider the possibility of sexual abuse if there is difficulty walking or sitting. This may be a subtle sign, whereas bruises or lacerations of the inner thighs or genitalia are more overt findings. Pain or itching in the genital area may indicate a sexually transmitted infection. Multiple decubitus ulcers without interventions suggest neglect. Be alert to the implication that "old people always get bed sores." Photographs of bruises, lacerations, and other injuries should be obtained to document type and extent of injuries.

Psychologic clues of maltreatment manifest as extreme mood changes, withdrawn or agitated behavior, depression, fearfulness, insomnia or excessive sleeping, and ambivalent feelings toward family and/or caregivers. The older adult may not be given the opportunity to speak for himself or herself; the caregiver may exhibit an attitude of indifference or anger toward the older adult. The caregiver may blame the patient for his or her condition (e.g., incontinence is viewed as a deliberate act and not a result of physical dysfunction).

Forensic and medical specialists investigating possible elder abuse may have discovered a new screening clue: how healthy is the household pet? "If a pet shows signs of mistreatment, we need to be worried about the person." The caregiver may threaten or mistreat a pet to silence its owner, or a person may want to leave a relationship but is afraid of leaving the animal behind. "If someone seems really worried about their pet, it can be a clue something's not right," according to Jane Raymond of the Wisconsin Department of Health and Family Services.[4]

ASKING THE RIGHT QUESTIONS

The Elder Assessment Instrument (EAI)[5] is a 41-item Likert scale that has been referenced in the literature since 1984. The various sections of this instrument review signs, symptoms, and subjective complaints suggestive of elder abuse, neglect, exploitation, and abandonment. There is no score; instead it serves as a screening tool that heightens the clinician's awareness of potential elder abuse and maltreatment.

When screening for elder abuse, the patient and suspected abuser should be interviewed separately. Begin with general questions about the patient's perception of safety in the home:
- Do you feel safe where you live?
- Do you need help taking care of yourself?
- Who prepares your meals?
- Who handles your checkbook?
- How many people are living in your home?

More specific questions about maltreatment might include the following:
- Do you have frequent disagreements with your caregiver?
- When you disagree, what happens?

- Are you ever physically hurt or confined to your room?
- Do you ever have to wait long periods for food or your medicine?
- Has anyone ever failed to answer your request for help?

When talking with the suspected abuser, empathy and an understanding approach go a long way in obtaining information about the patient's care environment. Try to identify specific issues that may present problems resulting from the patient's diagnosis. For example, close monitoring for skin breakdown in a patient with dementia and frequent episodes of incontinence is a challenge. In talking with this patient's caregiver you might say, "Caring for your father in this stage of his dementia must be a real challenge at times. Do you ever feel overwhelmed with the responsibility? How do you deal with it?" It is essential to avoid confrontation in this phase of the assessment.

INTERVENTIONS IN ABUSE AND NEGLECT

Access is a major issue in assessment and intervention for alleged abuse or neglect of older adults. The competent elder has the right to make his or her own personal care decisions. The elder may choose to stay in the abusive situation despite all efforts to effect a change; this does not negate the emergency nurse's responsibility to report the suspected maltreatment. Victims of abuse often have both positive and negative feelings toward their abusers. Such ambivalence makes separation from the abuser difficult for the abuse victim.

The Older Americans Act of 1965 and its 1987 and 2000 amendments require each state to identify agencies involved in recognizing and treating abused, neglected, and exploited elders and to determine the need for appropriate services. Although all 50 states have adult protection legislation, mandatory reporting laws vary from state to state. Emergency nurses should be familiar with the reporting requirements for their specific state. The Older Americans Act Amendment of 2000 provided, for the first time, critical and much-needed support for families caring for elderly loved ones who are ill or disabled. This legislation included programs for respite care for family members struggling to care for older relatives at home and other needed services. The Older Americans Act Amendment of 2006, the most recent reauthorization legislation, further defines and expands these responsibilities and services.[9]

The primary goal of intervention is to protect the patient from immediate and future harm. A secondary and equally important goal of intervention is to break the cycle of maltreatment. The well-being of the abused individual must be considered concurrently with the coping ability of the abuser.

With regard to intervention, family-mediated elder abuse is divided into two broad categories.[1] First are cases in which the elder has physical or mental impairment and is dependent on the family for daily care needs. The second group comprises individuals with minimal needs or care needs overshadowed by pathologic behavior of the caregiver. Potential intervention strategies for both categories include referrals to community agencies for continual monitoring of the situation, support services to decrease caregiver stress, close health care follow-up to prevent switching to another health care provider, reports to adult protective services with removal of the individual from a harmful environment, or use of 24-hour supervision through a home care agency.

Care needs of elders in the home increase over time; however, resources of the family in terms of psychosocial and financial reserves do not always increase at the same rate. Intervention requires a multidisciplinary team approach. Such a team is able to assess aspects of the situation such as physical injury, mental status, competency, financial irregularities, legality, treatment, assistance, protection, or prosecution. When there is a high degree of suspicion for elder abuse, consult social services or the responsible agency in your area. When appropriate, contact a home care agency to make an initial home assessment. In acute situations the elder may require shelter or protective care.

Unfortunately, prosecuting elder abuse cases often proves challenging. Difficulties arise from diminished mental capacity of the victim, physical health of the victim, cooperation by the victim, proving undue influences, and witness intimidation.[8]

SUMMARY

The American population is living longer. As baby boomers enter their senior years, there are more and more elders with mounting health problems who require assistance to perform simple activities of daily living. Caregivers are frequently balancing demands of a young family, career, and aging parents.

As children, we are taught to honor our mothers and fathers and to respect and care for older adults. The notion of frail older adults facing a life of fear and pain caused by someone they love and trust is beyond our comprehension. Likewise, understanding the frustration, fear, and sadness of the person who has gone from being a child cared for and nurtured by a parent to being the adult caring for that parent as one would a small child is also difficult to accept. For health care professionals to successfully diagnose and treat elder abuse, a nonjudgmental, open, and caring attitude toward all those involved is essential.

REFERENCES

1. All AC: A literature review: assessment and intervention in elder abuse, *J Gerontol Nurse* 20(7):25-32, 1994.
2. Cheshes J: Gray murders, *Modern Maturity* 45(2):56, 2002.
3. Falzon AL, Davis GG: A 15 year retrospective review of homicide in the elderly, *J Forensic Sci* 43(2):371, 1998.
4. Kardim R: Pets may hold clues to elder abuse, *AARP Bulletin*, November 2004.

5. National Center on Elder Abuse: *Elder mistreatment, abuse, neglect and exploitation in an aging America*, 2003. Retrieved August 20, 2007, from http://ncea@nasua.org.

6. National Center on Elder Abuse: *Frequently asked questions*. Retrieved September 5, 2007, from http://www.elderabusecenter.org.

7. Teaster PB, Otto JM: Abuse of adults aged 60+: 2004 survey of adult protective services, *Fact Sheet*, National Center on Elder Abuse, February 2006. Retrieved August 20, 2007, from http://www.nationalcenteronelderabuse.org.

8. Top 5 most difficult aspects of prosecuting elder abuse cases, *National Center on Elder Abuse Newsletter* 6(3), 2003. Retrieved September 5, 2007, from http://www.elderabusecenter.org/pdf/newsletter/newsletter031217.pdf.

9. US Dept of Health and Human Services, Administration on Aging: *Older Americans Act of 2006 Information and Resources*. Retrieved March 16, 2009, from http://www.aoa.gov/oaa2006/Main_Site/oaa/oaa.aspx.

CHAPTER 51

Behavioral Health Emergencies

Lynne Gagnon

Psychiatric emergencies are presenting in Emergency Departments (EDs) at an alarming rate. Centers for Disease Control and Prevention (CDC) data indicate that 30% of all cases treated in EDs are psychiatric in nature. These emergencies take many forms in the ED. These patients may arrive with severe dysfunction of behavior, mood, thinking, or perception that represents a significant threat to life, daily living, or psychologic integrity. Severity is related to the patient's ability to function and adapt but also depends on the person's support systems. Working with this type of patient requires patience, understanding, and flexibility. Comprehensive discussion of psychiatric emergencies is beyond the scope of this chapter. Therefore material presented herein focuses on those conditions seen more often in the ED—anxiety, panic disorder, depression, suicidal ideation, schizophrenia, and substance abuse with co-occurring illness. Anorexia nervosa and bulimia are also discussed.

Initial assessment for all psychiatric disorders should include vital signs, medical history, visual examination, urine toxicology screen, cognitive examination, pregnancy test for fertile women, and a cursory medical examination for medical clearance. Goals of interventions for psychiatric emergencies are to mitigate the risk to the patient and to staff. Calming the patient without sedation is most desirable.

AGITATION

Agitation is demonstrated by abnormal and excessive verbal, physically aggressive, or purposeless motor behaviors, heightened arousal, or other symptoms that cause clinically significant disruption of patient's ability to function. Initial history is important in trying to establish triggers that precipitated the event.

Treatment should include management of the agitation by deescalation, or if necessary, with physical or chemical restraint. Medications used to treat agitation are listed in Table 51-1. Plan of care would include psychiatric assessment for any underlying disorder and follow-up with appropriate services.

Restraints

Restraints should be used in the ED to manage aggression, or any patient with a behavioral emergency, only when all other less-restrictive means have been exhausted. In 2007 the Centers for Medicare and Medicaid Services (CMS) revised the conditions of participation for all acute hospitals and now require that the patient rights explicitly include the "right to be free of restraint." The CMS definition of restraint is "any means to restrict movement of a patient." In this revision the restraint application training and management

Table 51-1. **MEDICATIONS USED TO TREAT AGITATION**

Generic Name	Brand Name	Indications
Olanzapine	Zyprexa	Calming but not sedating
Risperidone	Risperdal	Mood stabilizer
Haloperidol	Haldol	Second line for agitation
Ziprasidone	Geodon	Second line for agitation

required in behavioral health units is required for all acute hospitals. Demonstration of annual physical restraint training is now mandated, and specifics related to restraint use and patient management must be described. Any hospital death of a patient in restraints or who has been in restraint within the past 24 hours must be reported as a sentinel event and reported directly to the regional offices of CMS. States that also provide requirements for hospital licensing may have additional requirements related to restraint use. Use of a sitter in the ED may also be considered "restraint" and is subject to CMS rules as well. Reasons for restraints or seclusion should be documented and include immediate threat to life and failure of less-restrictive methods. Orders must be time specific: "restraint is needed" or "restraint is needed for duration of visit" is not an acceptable order. Once a patient is in restraints, safety and well-being must be assessed every 15 minutes and documented.

ANOREXIA NERVOSA

Anorexia nervosa is an eating disorder characterized by severe weight loss to the point of significant physiologic consequences. Diagnostic criteria include the following:

- Intense fear of obesity despite slenderness
- Overwhelming body-image perception of being fat
- Weight loss of at least 25% from baseline or failure to gain weight appropriately (resulting in weight 25% less than would be expected from the patient's previous growth curve)
- Absence of other physical illnesses to explain weight loss or altered body-image perception
- At least 3 weeks of secondary amenorrhea or primary amenorrhea in a prepubescent adolescent.[13]

Associated physical characteristics include excessive physical activity, denial of hunger in the face of starvation, academic success, asexual behavior, and history of extreme weight loss methods (e.g., diuretics, laxatives, amphetamines, emetics). Psychiatric characteristics include excessive dependency needs, developmental immaturity, behavior favoring isolation, obsessive-compulsive behavior, and constriction of affect. Patients with anorexia nervosa generally fall into two categories—those with extreme food restriction and those with food binge and purge behavior.

Anorexia nervosa is thought to result from psychologic, biologic, and societal stresses involving sexual development at puberty. There is a high incidence of premorbid anxiety disorder in prepubescent patients who subsequently develop anorexia nervosa. The patient's altered body image results in a perception of fatness. Attempts to correct this misperception through food restriction or progressive purging lead to progressive starvation. Modern preoccupation with slenderness and beauty is thought to contribute greatly to the mindset of slenderness in girls and young women.

Anorexia malnutrition causes protein deficiency and disrupts multiple organ systems. Other nutritional deficiencies, including hypoglycemia, severe loss of fat stores, and multiple vitamin deficiencies, follow.

Cardiovascular effects of anorexia include atrial and ventricular tachydysrhythmias, bradycardia, orthostatic hypotension, and shock. Renal aberrations lead to decreased glomerular filtration rate, elevated blood urea nitrogen, edema, metabolic acidosis, hypokalemia, and hypochloremic alkalosis resulting from vomiting. Gastrointestinal findings include constipation, delayed gastric emptying, gastric dilation and rupture, dental enamel erosion, esophagitis, and Mallory-Weiss tears. Bone marrow suppression leading to platelet, erythrocyte, and leukocyte abnormalities have been reported.

Anorexia nervosa occurs in approximately 1 of 100 adolescent females and is most frequently found in middle- and upper-class families. Recent studies suggest there is no increased incidence in anorexia nervosa over the last four decades. There does appear to be a familial component to the disease.

Suspect anorexia in patients presenting with extreme weight loss and history of food refusal, amenorrhea, dehydration in an otherwise healthy individual, flat affect, or near-catatonic behavior. Patients may be depressed, so the risk for suicide should be carefully assessed. Obtain a mental health history because there is a strong association with depression and substance abuse.

Assessment

The most striking physical attribute in patients with moderate to severe anorexia is their cachectic appearance. Physical examination may reveal hypothermia, peripheral edema, and thinning hair.[9] Behaviorally, these patients have a flat affect and display psychomotor alterations. Physical and behavioral symptoms also occur in other conditions, so it is important to rule out potentially treatable causes.

A complete blood count (CBC) may reveal normocytic, normochromic anemia resulting from bone marrow suppression from starvation. Serum chemistry determinations often indicate varying degrees of hypokalemia from laxative abuse. In addition, dehydration can cause significant electrolyte abnormalities, including hyponatremia. Hypocalcemia from dietary deficiency of calcium and associated protein deficiency also occur. β-Human chorionic gonadotropin can determine whether pregnancy is the cause of vomiting and electrolyte abnormalities. Urinalysis is used to rule out urinary tract infections, dehydration, or renal acidosis. Positive fecal occult blood suggests esophagitis, gastritis, or repetitive colonic trauma from laxative abuse and a bleeding disorder or severe protein malnutrition. Serum erythrocyte sedimentation rate and thyroid function tests are unlikely to alter ED management but may be ordered to rule out inflammatory or endocrine pathologic processes.

An electrocardiogram (ECG) should be obtained because anorexia can precipitate several heart rhythm disturbances. Recognized ECG changes include nonspecific ST- and T-wave abnormalities, atrial or ventricular tachydysrhythmias, idioventricular conduction delay, heart block, nodal rhythms, ventricular escape, premature ventricular contractions, and prolonged QTc interval. These abnormalities are attributable to starvation, ipecac toxicity, and electrolyte and neuroendocrine abnormalities.

Rib fractures from repetitive vomiting in the presence of hypocalcemia do occur, so a chest x-ray examination should be obtained. Cardiomegaly from ipecac toxicity or malnutrition has been noted in many patients. Electrolyte disturbances or malnutrition can lead to development of an ileus, so abdominal x-ray films are often obtained.

Treatment

Care in the ED may include rehydration, correction of electrolyte abnormalities, and appropriate referral for continuing medical and psychiatric treatment.[12] Consultations with psychiatry and adolescent medicine specialists are recommended for inpatient care and to facilitate outpatient follow-up care.

No specific medications have been shown to alleviate the disordered body image characteristic of anorexia. For nutritional therapy, forced feedings with total parenteral nutrition or tube feedings may be used to replace nutrients, stabilize nutrient deficiency syndromes, and alter mood when the patient becomes nutritionally replenished.

ANXIETY

Anxiety is a complex feeling of apprehension, fear, and worry often accompanied by pulmonary, cardiac, and other physical sensations.[2] Anxiety is a normal response to threatening situations. Patients experiencing severe anxiety present in the ED with panic disorders, phobic disorders, obsessive-compulsive disorders, acute distress, posttraumatic stress disorder, anxiety due to medication conditions, and anxiety due to substance abuse. Anxiety disorders are the most common of all psychiatric disorders and can result in functional as well as emotional impairment.

A heightened physiologic response and elevated catecholamine levels play an important role in the normal physiologic response of the body to stress and anxiety. It has been hypothesized that disturbances in the cerebral cortex play a pathologic role in anxiety. The data specifically cite the limbic system (hypothalamus, septum, hippocampus, amygdala, cingulate), other neural bodies (thalamus, locus caeruleus, medial raphe nuclei, dental or interpositus nuclei of the cerebellum), and connections between these structures.[2]

Three neurotransmitters are associated with anxiety—norepinephrine, γ-aminobutyric acid (GABA), and serotonin.[2] The efficacy of benzodiazepines in treating anxiety has implicated GABA in the pathophysiology of anxiety disorders. Drugs that affect norepinephrine such as tricyclic antidepressants and monoamine oxidase inhibitors are efficacious in treatment of several anxiety disorders.[23]

Assessment

Anxiety in its most severe form can be quite debilitating. The condition is categorized as mild, moderate, severe, or panic disorder. Organic illness, medications, drug abuse, and obvious psychotic causes of an anxious state must be ruled out and documented before treatment of anxiety. Patients require ED treatment for anxiety when they are in such an acutely anxious state that they pose a danger to themselves and others. A thorough medical and psychiatric history is critical. Documentation should include any changes in behavior and somatic symptoms such as headaches, dizziness, disorientation, confusion, and syncope. Family and significant others are reliable sources of history for the patient with acute anxiety. Previous psychiatric illnesses and any current medical problems should be documented. Identify any agents that can cause anxiety (e.g., caffeine, nicotine, prescribed drugs, over-the-counter medications, illicit drugs, alcohol). Thorough physical assessment is required to identify potential life-threatening illnesses. The clinician should focus on signs and symptoms of anxiety; however, organic causes should be eliminated first. Diagnostic studies are used to rule out physical causes of anxiety such as metabolic disorders. Needle marks indicate illicit drug involvement, whereas hepatomegaly, ascites, and spider angioma suggest alcohol abuse.

A patient with anxiety may present as a classic panic attack, which is characterized by sudden onset of fear and a sense of impending doom with at least four of the following symptoms—palpitations, diaphoresis, tremulousness, shortness of breath, chest pain, dizziness, nausea, abdominal discomfort, fear of injury or going crazy, derealization (perception of altered reality), and depersonalization (perception that one's body is surreal). Evaluation of mental status can be especially helpful in distinguishing functional disorders from organic disorders. Assessment should include the following:

- Level of consciousness
- Affect
- Behavioral observation
- Speech pattern
- Level of attention
- Language comprehension
- Memory, calculation, and judgment

Anxiety states are associated with increased prevalence of other physical illnesses. Avoid falsely attributing somatic symptoms of anxiety to other medical conditions.

Laboratory tests to rule out physical illness include a CBC with differential, serum chemistry profile, pregnancy test, and serum or urine screens for drugs. Specific serum endocrine panels are also available to diagnose illnesses such as hyperthyroidism. Cardiopulmonary disorders such as pneumonia, congestive heart failure, and pneumothorax can be ruled out through physical assessment and a chest x-ray examination. An ECG can identify tachydysrhythmias and myocardial infarction as the cause of palpitations and other symptoms.

While remaining vigilant for life-threatening illness, emergency nurses should reassure patients suffering from anxiety. Place the patient in a calm, quiet room for formal evaluation. Rhythmic breathing, imagery techniques, and hypnotic suggestion have been used for patients with anxiety.

Treatment

Acute anxiety has been effectively treated with the passage of time, social support, and a short course of fast-acting anxiolytics, preferably a benzodiazepine (Table 51-2).[20] In chronic anxiety psychotherapy anxiolytics are the recommended course. Chronic anxiety often requires a comprehensive approach using psychotherapy, counseling, and a wider spectrum of anxiolytics (e.g., benzodiazepines, buspirone, antidepressants). Short-acting benzodiazepines in parenteral form are most useful for acute treatment. Benzodiazepines should be prescribed only in motivated and cooperative individuals with reliable follow-up arrangements. β-Blockers do not reduce intrinsic anxiety but may be beneficial in treatment of associated tachycardia. Buspirone may be initiated in the ED after consultation with a psychiatrist or the patient's primary care physician. Antidepressants have well-known pharmacologic profiles and could be useful in the patient with concomitant depression and anxiety.[23] They have demonstrated benefit as adjunct agents in the treatment of generalized anxiety disorder. Antidepressants have been relegated to long-term outpatient use for other chronic anxiety disorders.

Anxiety disorders are often chronic illnesses and require follow-up psychiatric intervention for successful treatment. Any patient with anxiety who presents with suicidal ideation, homicidal ideation, or acute psychosis requires emergent psychiatric consultation.[15] Some studies report the failure

rate for diagnosing anxiety disorders as high as 50%.[28] This can result in overuse of health care resources and increased morbidity and mortality rates for anxiety disorders and comorbid medical conditions. Listening to the patient and allowing expression of concern makes the patient feel safe.

BULIMIA

Bulimia nervosa is an eating disorder characterized by eating binges followed by self-induced vomiting, laxative or diuretic abuse, prolonged fasting, or excessive exercise.[3] The patient with binge eating exhibits the following characteristics:

* Eating, in a discrete period of time (e.g., within any 2-hour period), an amount of food that is definitely larger than most people would eat during a similar period of time under similar circumstances
* A perceived lack of control over eating during the episode (i.e., a feeling that one cannot stop eating or cannot control what or how much one is eating)

Some patients with anorexia nervosa also manifest bulimia; however, patients with bulimia have a normal weight or are overweight. Recurrent inappropriate compensatory behavior is used to prevent weight gain (e.g., self-induced vomiting; misuse of laxatives, diuretics, enemas, or other medication; fasting; excessive exercise). Binge eating and inappropriate compensatory behaviors occur at least twice a week for 3 months on average.[6] Self-evaluation is unduly influenced by body shape and weight.

Bulimia nervosa is categorized as purging type when the person regularly engages in self-induced vomiting or misuse of laxatives, diuretics, or enemas. If other inappropriate compensatory behaviors, such as fasting or excessive exercise, are used without self-induced vomiting or misuse of laxatives, diuretics, or enemas, the diagnosis is bulimia nervosa, nonpurging type. Individuals who binge eat without regular use of characteristic inappropriate compensatory behaviors of bulimia nervosa are included under the category of eating disorders not otherwise specified.

It has been reported that 5% to 35% of women ages 13 to 20 years have a history of bulimia.[4] Other investigators have reported the prevalence of bulimia as 1.5% in young girls, whereas partial syndromes or mild variants of the disorder occur in 5% to 10% of young women.[4] Symptoms of bulimia, such as isolated episodes of binge eating and purging, have been reported in up to 40% of college women. Anorexia and bulimia nervosa may be increasing in incidence, although increased reporting of cases resulting from greater medical and public awareness of the disorders over the past two decades cannot be discounted.[12]

Bulimia nervosa is a chronic disorder with a waxing and waning course.[9] Mortality rates are not known. Comorbid conditions associated with bulimia nervosa include affective disorders, personality disorders, anxiety disorders, substance abuse, and adverse events related to aggression or poor impulse control.[21,25]

The vast majority (90% to 95%) of patients with bulimia nervosa are women. Eating disorders also occur frequently

Table 51-2. **ANTIANXIETY MEDICATIONS**		
Generic Name	**Brand Name**	**Drug Class**
Alprazolam	Xanax	Benzodiazepine
Chlordiazepoxide	Librium	Benzodiazepine
Clonazepam	Klonopin	Benzodiazepine
Diazepam	Valium	Benzodiazepine
Lorazepam	Ativan	Benzodiazepine
Oxazepam*	Serax	Benzodiazepine
Hydroxyzine hydrochloride	Atarax	Antihistamine
Hydroxyzine	Vistaril	Antihistamine

*May be addictive. Sudden withdrawals may cause convulsions.

among men who participate in sports with a weight requirement (e.g., wrestling) or in whom low body fat is important (bodybuilders).[4] As in anorexia, a morbid fear of obesity is the overriding psychologic preoccupation in bulimia nervosa. Bulimia, however, is more frequent in people with a history of obesity. The common behavior of dieting may be related to the development of bulimia. Bulimia may occur after an episode of anorexia nervosa or substance abuse. Self-loathing and disgust with the body are even more severe in bulimia than in anorexia nervosa.

Binges may occur habitually or may be triggered sporadically by unpleasant feelings of anger, anxiety, or depression. Food deprivation (i.e., dieting) also plays a role in inducing bingeing. Guilt and dysphoria are common feelings after binges; however, some patients find these binges themselves soothing.

Binges are typically followed by efforts to prevent weight gain. Generally patients attempt to prevent weight gain by self-induced vomiting; however, ingestion of ipecac syrup is occasionally used to prevent weight gain. Laxative or diuretic misuse is also common, although these substances almost exclusively produce fluid loss rather than calorie loss. Individuals may display extreme caloric restriction between episodes, exhibit wide fluctuations in weight, or become obese.

Although the act of self-induced vomiting may occur only occasionally and may be of little consequence, a chronic pattern may develop, leading to poor overall health, decreased muscle strength, dental erosion, serious electrolyte abnormalities, cardiac arrhythmias, or death. Electrolyte abnormalities resulting from vomiting may be compounded by those from laxative-induced diarrhea or diuretic use. Chronic laxative (phenolphthalein) overdose has been reported. Menstrual irregularities may be caused by weight fluctuations, nutritional deficiency, or emotional stress.[6]

Deaths related to bulimia are thought to result from cardiac arrhythmias. Gastric or esophageal rupture, Mallory-Weiss tear, pneumomediastinum, and postbinge pancreatitis have resulted from gorging and vomiting and may be life threatening.[14] Diet pills can cause hypertension and cerebral hemorrhage when taken in excess. Ipecac-related deaths have been reported, probably resulting from emetine cardiotoxicity in conjunction with electrolyte imbalances.[14]

Assessment

Common complaints include muscle weakness, cramps, dizziness, carpopedal spasm, hematemesis, abdominal pain, chest pain, heartburn, sore throat, or menstrual irregularity. Unrecognized bulimia nervosa has been associated with perioperative cardiac dysrhythmias.[25] Patients are characteristically young and female. Males with bulimia often have a history of participation in sports with weight requirements.[3] Patients may admit to use of diuretics for edema but often deny self-induced vomiting or laxative use. Caffeine, pseudoephedrine, phenylpropanolamine (now off the market), ginseng, thyroid replacement preparations, ma huang, and other "cleansing" or "dieter's" herbs may be used in an attempt to increase metabolic rate and calorie loss. Many "natural" or herbal remedies thought to be completely safe actually contain substances that increase blood pressure or promote electrolyte imbalance.

Vital signs may be normal. Tachycardia and hypotension, when present, suggest volume depletion, whereas hypertension should raise the suspicion of stimulant use. Physical examination may reveal signs of dehydration and erosion of tooth enamel with or without frank caries. A callus resulting from repetitive contact with the upper teeth during self-induced vomiting may be found on the dorsal surface of the index and long finger of the patient's dominant hand. Alopecia, hypertrichosis, and nail fragility are other common skin findings.[9]

Weight is frequently normal or above normal with the remainder of the physical examination usually normal. Specific complications, however, may be found on examination of the abdomen (e.g., epigastric tenderness, guaiac-positive stools), chest (e.g., Hamman crunch resulting from air in the mediastinal space from an esophageal tear), or extremities (e.g., edema). These symptoms can be found with other conditions, so care should be taken to rule these out.

Research is ongoing regarding the potential role of other chemical mediators in the pathogenesis of eating disorders. Significantly higher rates of sexual assault and aggravated assault among women with bulimia nervosa support the hypothesis that victimization may contribute to development or maintenance of the disease.

Obtain electrolyte measurements even in patients with normal weight. Hypokalemia, hypomagnesemia, and metabolic alkalosis secondary to compulsive vomiting are confirmatory for bulimia. Sodium and chloride levels may be decreased. In patients who abuse laxatives but are not vomiting, hypokalemia is associated with metabolic acidosis, whereas hypocalcemia is caused by loss of bicarbonate and calcium in diarrheal stool. Diuretic abuse can decrease serum sodium and potassium levels and increase uric acid and calcium levels.

Urinary findings vary with the degree of vomiting or laxative-induced diarrhea, diuretic use, and volume status. Findings also depend on whether the condition is acute or chronic. If abdominal pain is present, serum lipase and amylase measurements are used to screen for pancreatitis. Gastric rupture should be ruled out with an upright chest x-ray film. Pneumomediastinum secondary to esophageal rupture may also be evident. If hematemesis or melena has been reported, placement of a nasogastric tube may be indicated. A pregnancy test should be obtained in all female patients of childbearing age.

Treatment

Emergency nurses should anticipate and be prepared to intervene for the complications of bulimia, including volume depletion, electrolyte abnormalities, esophagitis, Mallory-Weiss tear, esophageal or gastric rupture, pancreatitis, arrhythmias, or adverse effects of medication (e.g., ipecac, appetite suppressants). Associated illnesses, including depression, anxiety disorders, and substance abuse, put patients at risk for other illness and injury. Directly question patients regarding suicidal ideation.

For patients unable to halt the dangerous sequence of dieting, bingeing, and purging, admission may be necessary to break the cycle. Psychiatric hospitalization may be necessary for patients with severe depression and suicidal ideation, weight loss greater than 30% over 3 months, failure to maintain outpatient weight contract, or family crisis. Medical admission is warranted for patients with significant metabolic disturbance or other physical complication of bingeing or purging, such as Mallory-Weiss tear, esophageal rupture, or pancreatitis.

Treatment usually combines individual psychotherapy with a cognitive-behavioral approach, group or family therapy, and pharmacotherapy.[11] The pharmacotherapy of bulimia nervosa is based on two models—seizure disorder and affective disorder. Medications include thiamine, multivitamins, and magnesium. Antidepressants have been reported to reduce binge eating, vomiting, and depression.[12] They may improve eating habits, although their impact on body dissatisfaction remains unclear. There are a number of potential complications associated with bulimia.

Patients should be educated about the risks of using diet pills, amphetamines, and energy pills and diet teas that claim to be natural. These often contain herbal forms of caffeine and ephedrine and have been associated with hypertension, cerebrovascular accident, and death. Phenylpropanolamine, the most common ingredient in both over-the-counter diet pills and decongestants, has been taken off the market because of the fear of severe hypertension leading to stroke and other serious pathologic processes (especially in females).

Patients with serious eating disorders often mistrust health care professionals, whom they see as being interested only in refeeding them or making them lose their will so they become fat. Education about body weight regulation and the effects of starvation, vomiting, and laxatives on bodily functions may be helpful. Discussion of issues of self-esteem is important, especially how basing self-worth entirely on body size leads to forcing oneself to be something that is not natural.

DEPRESSION

Depression is a potentially life-threatening mood disorder that afflicts up to 10% of the population.[8,17] This holistic disorder affects the body, feelings, thoughts, and behaviors. Considerable pain and suffering significantly affect the individual's ability to function. It is important to note that depression also adversely affects significant others, sometimes destroying family relationships or work dynamics between the patient and others. The economic cost of depressive illness is estimated in the tens of billions of dollars each year in the United States alone.[27] The human cost cannot be overestimated. As many as two thirds of the people suffering from depression do not realize they have a treatable illness and therefore do not seek treatment.

Mortality of depression is measurable and is the direct result of suicide, the eleventh leading cause of death in the United States.[3] Almost all those who kill themselves intentionally have a diagnosable mental disorder with or without substance abuse.[10] Ironically, substance abuse is often the result of attempted self-treatment for symptoms of depression. The majority of suicide attempts are expressions of extreme distress, not bids for attention.[18] Lifetime risk is an estimated 5% to 12% for men and 10% to 25% for women.

The condition may be due to biologic, physiologic, genetic, or psychosocial factors. Medications (prescription, over-the-counter, recreational, and herbals) should also be considered. Serotonin and norepinephrine are the primary neurotransmitters involved, although dopamine has also been related to depression. A family history of depression is common. Bipolar disorder has a prominent depressive phase but is a different clinical entity from depression.

An ED presentation of major depressive disorder will include symptoms that disrupt one's personal and social functioning. These patients *must* be assessed for suicidality. Any treatment that initiates antidepressant medications should also require a follow-up appointment because it can take up to 2 weeks for these medications to have a noticeable effect. Antidepressant medications are listed in Table 51-3.

Assessment

Depression is often difficult to diagnose because it can manifest in many different forms. To establish the diagnosis of major depression, a patient must express at least one primary symptom and at least five secondary symptoms. Such disturbances must be present almost daily for at least 2 weeks; however, symptoms can last for months or years. The individual may experience significant personality changes during this period, making it difficult for others to feel charitable toward the sufferer. Some symptoms are so disabling they interfere with the ability to function from day to day. In severe cases patients may be unable to eat or leave their beds. Episodes may occur only once in a lifetime, may be recurrent, or may

Table 51-3. ANTIDEPRESSANTS

Generic Name	Brand Name	Indications
Amitriptyline*	Elavil	Typical
Imipramine*	Tofranil	Typical
Doxepin*	Sinequan	Typical
Fluoxetine	Prozac	Atypical
Citalopram	Celexa	Atypical
Fluvoxamine	Luvox	Atypical
Sertraline	Zoloft	Atypical
Trazodone	Desyrel	Atypical
Venlafaxine	Effexor	Atypical
Bupropion	Wellbutrin	Other
Mirtazapine	Remeron	Other
Nefazodone	Serzone	Other

*These medications can be cardiotoxic—need baseline electrocardiogram.

be chronic and long-standing. Occasionally symptoms are precipitated by life crises or other illnesses, whereas at other times depression can occur at random. Clinical depression often occurs concurrently with other medical illnesses and worsens the prognosis for these illnesses.

In addition to depression, alcohol and substance abuse, impulsiveness, and certain familial factors are highly associated with risk for suicide.[10] Familial factors include history of mental illness or substance abuse, suicide, family violence of any type, and separation or divorce. Other risk factors include prior suicide attempts, presence of a firearm in the home, incarceration, and exposure to suicidal behavior of family members, peers, celebrities, or even highly publicized fictional characters.

A standard tool such as the Beck Scale, IS THE PATH WORN, or SADD PERSONS scale should be used as part of the initial assessment.[19]

The emergency nurse's responsibility when caring for a patient with depression is to maintain a high index of suspicion for the diagnosis, especially in populations at risk for suicide. Primary at-risk populations include young adults and older adults; however, depression and suicide can occur in any age-group, including children.[13] Depression should be suspected as an underlying factor in drug overdose (including alcohol), self-inflicted injury, or intentionally inflicted injury when the assailant is known to the victim. In any such patient, screening for diagnostic symptoms of major depression and suicide is essential.[24]

When a patient has contemplated or attempted suicide, the patient should be carefully assessed to determine the presence of suicidal ideation and accessible means and plans.[18] Psychiatric evaluation should occur only after this screening evaluation is complete and all acute medical complications are addressed.

Treatment

Depression is a clinical diagnosis; however, symptoms associated with depression may be the result of medications, metabolic disorders, and other nutritional abnormalities. Assessment and treatment of the person with depression should rule out various treatment conditions. Laboratory tests are primarily used to rule out other diagnoses such as renal failure, hypoglycemia, and drug toxicity. Additional diagnostic studies include computed tomography (CT), magnetic resonance imaging (MRI), and electroencephalogram to rule out organic brain syndrome or other central nervous system (CNS) problems. Inpatient care is recommended when there is significant concern for the patient's safety.

PANIC DISORDERS

Understanding panic disorder (PD) is important for emergency nurses because patients with PD frequently present to the ED with various somatic complaints. As many as 70% of PD patients are unrecognized.[1] These patients have a fourfold higher risk for alcohol abuse and eighteenfold higher risk for

suicide than the general population. Some studies do suggest panic disorder itself is not a risk factor for suicide in the absence of other risks such as affective disorders, substance abuse, eating disorders, and personality disorders. Serious medical problems—such as asthma—cardiac dysrhythmia, or metabolic disturbances—such as hypoglycemia, hypoxia, and thyroid storm—can mimic panic attack. After exclusion of somatic disease and other psychiatric disorders, confirmation of the diagnosis with a brief mental status screening examination and initiation of appropriate treatment and referral is time- and cost-effective in patients with high rates of medical resource use.

PD appears to be a genetically inherited neurochemical dysfunction that involves autonomic imbalance, increased adenosine receptor function, increased cortisol, diminished benzodiazepine receptor function, and disturbances in serotonin, norepinephrine, GABA, dopamine, cholecystokinin, and interleukin-1-β. Some theorize that PD may represent a state of chronic hyperventilation and carbon dioxide (CO_2) receptor hypersensitivity.

Positron emission tomography (PET) scanning has demonstrated increased flow in the right parahippocampal region of panicky patients. MRI has demonstrated smaller temporal lobe volume despite normal hippocampal volume in these patients. In experimental settings symptoms can be elicited in panic subjects by hyperventilation, inhalation of CO_2, caffeine consumption, or intravenous infusions of sodium lactate, cholecystokinin, isoproterenol, or flumazenil.

Other conditions found in the patient with PD include depression, obsessive-compulsive disorder, specific phobias, social phobia, agoraphobia (fear of being unsafe in public settings), irritable bowel syndrome, migraine, mitral valve prolapse, and alcohol and drug abuse. Lower oxygen consumption and exercise tolerance than the general population has been identified in patients with PD.

Symptoms of PD create a significant hindrance in lifestyle for many patients. Those with agoraphobia may be unable to travel alone, be in crowds, malls, or on public transportation. Unemployment, depression, substance abuse, and suicide are also common. Studies have found PD present in 30% of patients with chest pain and normal angiograms, 5% to 40% of asthmatics, 15% of headache patients, 20% of epilepsy patients, 8% to 15% of patients in alcohol treatment programs, and 10% of patients in primary care settings.[7]

Panic attacks may be triggered by injury, surgery, illness, interpersonal conflict, or personal loss. Use of stimulants such as caffeine, decongestants, cocaine, and sympathomimetics (e.g., amphetamine) can precipitate panic attacks in susceptible individuals.[7] Bouts of panic can also occur in certain settings, such as stores and public transportation, especially in patients with agoraphobia.

Assessment

Patients in the throes of a panic attack complain of sudden onset of fear or discomfort, typically peaking in 10 minutes. Attacks are associated with a constellation of systemic symptoms.

During an acute episode patients have the urge to flee or escape—they experience a strong sense of impending doom as though they are dying from a heart attack or suffocation. Severe personality disorganization may be present. Other symptoms include headache, cold hands, diarrhea, insomnia, fatigue, intrusive thoughts, and ruminations. Patients with PD have recurring episodes of panic with fear of recurrent attacks causing significant behavioral changes (avoiding situations or locations) and worry about implications of the attack or its consequences (e.g., losing control, going crazy, dying).

Assessment should include precipitating events, suicidal ideation or plan, phobias, agoraphobia, obsessive-compulsive behavior, and involvement of alcohol, illicit drugs, and medications with stimulatory effects (e.g., caffeine). Determination of a family history of panic or other psychiatric illness is indicated.

Patients with PD may manifest any one of several physical symptoms. They appear anxious and may have cool, clammy skin. Heart rate and respiratory rate are usually elevated; however, blood pressure and temperature are usually normal. Hyperventilation may be difficult to detect by observing breathing because respiratory rate and tidal volume may appear normal.

Room air pulse oximetry values are normal to high normal; however, arterial blood gas analysis is indicated to rule out the presence of acid-base abnormalities. Hypoxemia with hypocapnia or a widened A-a gradient should raise the possibility of pulmonary embolus in the patient who appears to be having a panic attack. Laboratory studies that may be helpful in excluding other medical disorders include serum electrolytes to exclude hypokalemia and acidosis; serum glucose to exclude hypoglycemia; cardiac markers in patients suspected of acute coronary syndromes; hemoglobin in patients with near-syncope; thyroid-stimulating hormone in patients suspected of hyperthyroidism; and urine toxicology screen for amphetamines, cocaine, and phencyclidine in patients suspected of intoxication.[22]

Chest x-ray films are useful in excluding various causes of dyspnea. An ECG should be inspected for signs of ventricular preexcitation (short PR and delta wave) and long QT interval in patients with palpitations and for ischemia, infarction, or pericarditis patterns in patients with chest pain—conditions that share symptoms with or may precipitate a panic attack.

Treatment

Patients presenting to the ED that appear anxious but also complain of chest pain, dyspnea, palpitations, or near-syncope should be treated as they clinically present. Place the patient on oxygen, and monitor pulse oximetry, ECG, and frequent vital signs. PD patients require frequent reassurance and explanation; many may benefit from social service intervention after more serious organic causes of symptoms are ruled out. A major component of therapy involves education that the symptoms are neither from a serious medical condition nor from mental deficiency, but rather from a chemical imbalance in the fight-or-flight response.

The ED staff should listen, remain empathic, and be non-argumentative with these patients. Statements such as "It's nothing serious" and "It's related to stress" can be misinterpreted as implying lack of understanding and concern. Intravenous medication (e.g., Ativan, 0.5 mg intravenously [IV] every 20 minutes) may be necessary in PD patients who, as a result of subsequent poor impulse control, pose a risk to themselves or to those around them.[5] PD patients are best served by referral to a qualified mental health professional who can establish constructive rapport with the patient and follow his or her needs on a long-term basis before beginning anxiolytic medications.

Aside from IV medications required to treat acute anxiety states in the ED, the use of pharmacotherapy for panic disorder patients should, in most instances, be deferred to the psychiatrist following the patient long-term. Benzodiazepines are optimal for ED and outpatient abortive therapy because of their immediate antipanic effects.[28] Coexisting disorders may influence medication choice (e.g., monoamine oxidase inhibitors [MAOIs], clonazepam, and selective serotonin reuptake inhibitors [SSRIs] for social phobia; SSRIs or clomipramine [Anafranil] for obsessive-compulsive disorder; tricyclic antidepressants [TCAs] for depression).[5] Institution of treatment for PD in the ED is appropriate in a very limited subset of PD patients. Those who are very motivated, cooperative, and possess an understanding of the psychologic nature of their disorder and whose symptoms are elicited as a response to temporary stress are good candidates. In such cases pharmacotherapy with an oral benzodiazepine for no longer than 1 week may be appropriate.

Inpatient treatment is necessary in patients with suicidal ideation and a suicide plan, serious alcohol or sedative withdrawal symptoms, or when potential medical disorders warrant admission (e.g., unstable angina, acute myocardial ischemia). Follow-up with a chemical dependence treatment specialist should be arranged when indicated. All discharged PD patients should be referred to a psychiatrist, psychologist, or other mental health professional.

SCHIZOPHRENIA

Insanity, psychosis, madness . . . regardless of how it is labeled, schizophrenia is a chronic psychotic disorder with onset typically in adolescence or young adulthood. Schizophrenia results in fluctuating, gradually deteriorating, or relatively unstable disturbances in thinking, behavior, and perception. These disturbances include the presence of both positive and negative symptoms. Positive symptoms include delusions, hallucinations, and disorganized speech and behavior; negative symptoms include poverty of speech, flattened affect, and social withdrawal.

Current diagnostic requirements are met if the syndrome continues for at least 6 months with at least 1 month in which active symptoms are present and these symptoms result in significant impairment of occupational and social functioning. Other schizophrenia-related disorders have a milder, less global, or more transient course but share strong familial association with schizophrenia.

Persons with schizophrenia occupy up to 25% of all hospital psychiatric beds at any given time.[8] The condition is devastating, with a profound effect on family and the patient's social and occupational life. Premature death may result from poor health maintenance, substance abuse, poverty, and homelessness. Onset of symptoms is insidious in about half of all patients. The prodromal phase can begin years before the full-blown syndrome. It is characterized by losses of previously achieved functioning in home, society, and occupation (e.g., poor school or work performance, deterioration of hygiene and appearance, decreasing emotional connections with others, behaviors considered odd for this individual).

Gradual onset predicts a more severe and chronic illness course, whereas abrupt onset of hallucinations and delusional, bizarre, or disorganized thinking in previously functioning patients can lead to better intermediate and long-term outcome. Such patients arrive in the ED in a psychotic crisis requiring acute management, often without having been previously diagnosed with a psychiatric illness. They present diagnostic dilemmas regarding organic versus psychiatric etiology and primary psychotic versus affective disorder that may be further complicated by the presence of alcohol or drug intoxication.

Because of the variability of symptom expression and diagnostic requirements of chronicity, the diagnosis of schizophrenia in the ED should be provisional at best. As a diagnosis by exclusion, schizophrenia must be distinguished from the numerous psychiatric and organic disorders that also lead to psychotic behaviors.

Assessment

The most common causes for severe mental status changes in the ED are organic, not psychiatric. They include medications, drug intoxication, drug withdrawal syndromes, and general medical illnesses causing delirium.[15] The presence of an affective disorder (e.g., major depression, bipolar disorder, schizoaffective disorder) must be excluded. Conditions that can be mistaken for schizophrenia have very different prognoses and therapies. In addition, an organic cause (e.g., drug intoxication, medical illness) must be ruled out. Commonly problems with antipsychotic medications are the chief complaint. Medical illness can cause or complicate a psychotic process. Obtain a complete medication history; many commonly prescribed medicines can cause psychotic reactions.

Psychiatric and organic illness can coexist and interact at the same time in the same patient. Acute psychiatric symptoms and difficulty obtaining a reliable history can mask serious organic illness. History obtained in the ED may relate to a complication of treatment (medication side effects) or crisis arising from socioeconomic factors secondary to schizophrenia, such as poverty, homelessness, social isolation, and failure of support systems.

Information should be elicited about the actual or potential likelihood for acts of violence. Acutely psychotic patients presenting to the ED place other patients and staff in danger. A paranoid schizophrenic, in response to delusions and command hallucinations, can be extremely dangerous and unpredictable. Identify threats made to others, expressions of suicidal intent, and possession of weapons at home or on the person.

The schizophrenic patient may be wildly agitated, combative, withdrawn, or severely catatonic. Conversely, they may appear rational, cooperative, and well controlled. Blunting of affect may be noted, or the person may be subtly odd, unkempt, or grossly bizarre in manner, dress, or affect. Physical examination with attention to vital signs, pupillary findings, hydration status, and mental status should be performed. Diagnostic evaluation is required when organic cause or drug intoxication may be related to mental status changes.

Pay particular attention to fever (tachycardia can be a sign of neuroleptic malignant syndrome), heat stroke (antipsychotics inhibit sweating), and other medical illness. Look for dystonia, akathisia, tremor, and muscle rigidity. Tardive dyskinesia is a common, often irreversible sequela of long-term (and sometimes brief) antipsychotic use. The condition is characterized by uncontrollable tongue thrusting, lip smacking, and facial grimacing. Mental status is usually normal with sensorium clear and the person oriented to person, place, and time. Assess attention, language, memory, constructions, and executive functions.

Treatment

There are no specific laboratory findings diagnostic of schizophrenia; however, some studies may be necessary to rule out organic causes for psychosis or to uncover complications of schizophrenia and its treatment. Blood levels of certain psychiatric drugs, specifically lithium and mood-stabilizing antiseizure medications, can confirm compliance or indicate toxicity. Serum alcohol and toxicology tests can be useful when substance abuse is suspected. A fingerstick glucose test is a rapid, inexpensive method of ruling out a diabetic emergency masquerading as an exacerbation of a psychotic illness. Similarly, oxygen saturation can disclose hypoxia as a potential cause of behavioral or CNS disturbances. Electrolyte levels may reveal hyponatremia secondary to water intoxication (psychogenic polydipsia), which is common in undertreated or refractory schizophrenia.

A CT scan and an MRI scan can disclose abnormalities of brain structure and function in the schizophrenic patient. Although they are of interest for research, such studies have very narrow clinical relevance.

Evolving from the efficacy of modern antipsychotic medications and the subsequent widespread budget cutting of psychiatric services over the past two decades, deinstitutionalization of the schizophrenic patient has had a major impact on emergency nursing. The schizophrenic patient is now a frequent visitor to the ED, with problems ranging from disease exacerbation, medication noncompliance, or side effects to medical and socioeconomic crises arising from substance abuse, poverty, homelessness, and failed support systems.

Care for the schizophrenic patient in the ED may be limited to diagnosis and treatment of an urgent or nonurgent medical complaint. In some patients brief medical evaluation before psychiatric, crisis intervention, or social service consultation is adequate. For others, evaluation and treatment of a psychiatric drug adverse reaction is necessary. Physical and chemical restraint is indicated when the patient represents an immediate threat to self or others and alternatives have failed.

Crisis liaison teams, typically made up of clinical social workers, psychologists, or psychiatric nurses, are available in many EDs 24 hours a day through the hospital or local psychiatric agencies. Psychiatry consultation should be used as soon as organic processes are ruled out to correctly diagnose or safely treat a severely disturbed schizophrenic patient.

Antipsychotic medications (previously referred to as neuroleptics or major tranquilizers) have revolutionized the treatment of and prognosis for schizophrenia (Table 51-4). These agents block dopamine receptors in the brain, whereas newer atypical agents also affect serotonin transmission. The newer agents (e.g., risperidone, clozapine, olanzapine, quetiapine) are less likely to produce dystonia and tardive dyskinesia and more likely to improve negative symptoms. However, with the possible exception of clozapine, they are no more effective than traditional agents (e.g., haloperidol, fluphenazine) in the treatment-resistant patient. Benzodiazepines also have a role in schizophrenia, especially for emergency care of the acutely psychotic patient. Anticholinergic medications are used to counteract dystonic and parkinsonian side effects (extrapyramidal symptoms [EPS]) of antipsychotics, particularly higher-potency agents that are less sedating but more likely to produce EPS.

Schizophrenia is a chronic and disabling illness. Fewer than 20% of patients recover fully from a single psychotic episode; a few have little or no recovery from the first episode and persist with chronic, pervasive psychotic illness. Approximately 60% will recover sufficiently to lead functional lives, but only 50% of those will be employed. Approximately 30% remain severely and permanently handicapped, with 10% being chronically hospitalized. Rapid and aggressive medication therapy of acute psychotic episodes is correlated with better overall prognosis.

SUBSTANCE ABUSE

ED visits involving nonmedical use of pharmaceuticals, such as pain killers, narcotic analgesics, benzodiazepines, and muscle relaxants, usually involve multiple drugs as well as alcohol. These drugs are easy to obtain, and they are viewed as "safer" than street drugs.[16] Of particular note is the increase in Vicodin, OxyContin, and methadone overdoses being reported across the country.

The Drug Abuse Warning Network (DAWN) reported in 2005 that there were 1.4 million ED visits associated with misuse or abuse. Substance abusers are at high risk for suicide, homicide, and overdose.

Assessment

History of patient's past use, and/or what did he or she take just before coming to the ED?
Has the patient been treated for substance abuse previously?
Any history of blackouts or seizures?
Any history of withdrawal symptoms or overdoses?
Any family history of drug or alcohol problems?
Does the patient have any coexisting physical conditions?
What is the patient's current medical status?
What is the patient's current mental status?
Any history of physical or sexual abuse?
Any history of violence toward self or others?

Treatment

Immediate medical treatment of withdrawal or overdose symptoms should be undertaken to avert any life-threatening problems. Are there any physical complications related to drug abuse (acquired immunodeficiency syndrome [AIDS], abscesses, hepatitis)? Once necessary medical interventions have been completed and the patient is stable, the focus of treatment should be on appropriate follow-up.

SUICIDE ASSESSMENT

People at risk for suicide present with a variety of complaints: mental disorders, substance abuse, physical abuse, chronic illness, or recent losses.

The Joint Commission reports inpatient suicide is the number one reported sentinel event. Suicide is the eighth leading cause of death of all ages. The Joint Commission revised their national patient safety goals in 2007 to require identification and assessment of patients at risk for suicide. This is applicable to all behavioral health units and EDs.[26]

Table 51-4. ANTIPSYCHOTICS

Generic Name	Brand Name	Indications
Chlorpromazine*†	Thorazine	Typical
Thioridazine*†	Mellaril	Typical
Haloperidol*†	Haldol	Typical
Clozapine*†	Clozaril	Atypical
Olanzapine*†	Zyprexa	Atypical
Quetiapine*†	Seroquel	Atypical
Risperidone*†	Risperdal	Atypical

*Antiparkinsonian medications (Artane, Cogentin, amantadine, Benadryl) may be used to decrease side effects of antipsychotic medications.
†Neuroleptic malignant syndrome is a potentially life-threatening adverse effect that can occur with anyone taking antipsychotics. Symptoms include fever, muscle rigidity, and altered consciousness. The patient may also demonstrate decreased blood pressure, appetite, and urine output; and increased white blood cell count, sweating, and pulse rate.

Assessment

Risk factors associated with suicide include being male, white, over 65, widowed or divorced; living alone; and having current life stressors, access to firearms, family history of suicide or previous attempt, and history of mental illness. Symptoms include, but are not limited to, depression, hopelessness, insomnia, anxiety, panic attacks, and impaired concentration.

EDs are encouraged to implement an assessment tool such as the SADD PERSONS scale to provide a consistent approach to the assessment of these patients. These tools are not a definitive prediction of suicide but can provide some suggestions for a course of treatment based on scoring.

Assessment is critical in determining imminent risk to the patient. Essential elements of the assessment require a complete history, including current ideation, intent, and plan; history of previous attempts; family history of suicide; history of mental illness and any current treatment; history of alcohol or substance abuse; current medical problems; recent life stressors; and any history of aggression or violence. It is also important to determine if the patient has social supports, such as family or friends.

Treatment

Treatment should include a plan for keeping the patient safe. If the patient is discharged, there should be plans for immediate follow-up. "Contracting" with the patient for safety is usually part of the plan of care when the patient is in the ED. Those patients with a plan for suicide should be admitted until appropriate safety measures can be implemented. Patients may need to be watched or closely supervised while in the ED.

SUMMARY

Psychosocial conditions found in the ED are varied and challenging. Regardless of presenting symptoms it is important for the emergency nurse to treat the patient with empathy and respect while protecting the patient and others from harm. Recent decreases in federal and state funding for mental health services are a harbinger for increases in the number of patients presenting to the ED.

REFERENCES

1. Ballenger JC, Davidson JR, Lecrubier Y et al: Consensus statement on panic disorder from the International Consensus Group on Depression and Anxiety, *J Clin Psychiatry* 59(8 suppl):47, 1998.
2. Brawman-Mintzer O, Lydiard RB: Biological basis of generalized anxiety disorder, *J Clin Psychiatry* 58 (3 suppl):16, 1997.
3. Centers for Disease Control and Prevention: *Web-Based Injury Statistics Query and Reporting Systems (WISQARS)*, 2005, National Center for Injury Prevention and Control, http://www.cdc.gov/ncipc/wisqars/default.htm.
4. Corcos M, Flament MF, Giraud MJ: Early psychopathological signs in bulimia nervosa: a retrospective comparison of the period of puberty in bulimic and control girls, *Eur Child Adolesc Psychiatry* 9(2):115, 2000.
5. den Boer JA: Pharmacotherapy of panic disorder: differential efficacy from a clinical viewpoint, *J Clin Psychiatry* 59(8 suppl):30, 1998.
6. Fairburn CG, Cooper Z, Doll HA: The natural course of bulimia nervosa and binge eating disorder in young women, *Arch Gen Psychiatry* 57(7):659, 2000.
7. Fleet RP, Marchand A, Dupuis G et al: Comparing emergency department and psychiatric setting patients with panic disorder, *Psychosomatics* 39(6):512, 1998.
8. Gagnon L: Psychiatric/Psychosocial emergencies. In ENA: *Emergency nursing core curriculum*, ed 6, Philadelphia, 2007, WB Saunders.
9. Glorio R, Allevato M, DePablo A: Prevalence of cutaneous manifestations in 200 patients with eating disorders, *Int J Dermatol* 39(5):348, 2000.
10. Harwitz D, Ravizza L: Suicide and depression, *Emerg Med Clin North Am* 18(2):263, 2000.
11. Jacobs D, editor: *The Harvard Medical School guide to suicide assessment and intervention*, San Francisco, 2000, Jossey-Bass Publishers.
12. Jacobs D: A resource guide for implementing the Joint Commission on Accreditation of Healthcare Organizations 2007 patient safety goals on suicide, *Screening for Mental Health*, 2006.
13. Knesper D: *Guide to suicide assessment*, 2003, Department of Psychiatry University of Michigan.
14. Kreipe RE, Birndorf SA: Eating disorders in adolescents and young adults, *Med Clin North Am* 84(4):1027, 2000.
15. Lagomasino I, Daly R, Stoudemire A: Medical assessment of patients presenting with psychiatric symptoms in the emergency setting, *Psychiatr Clin North Am* 22(4):819, 1999.
16. Maxwell JC: Trends in the abuse of prescription drugs, Austin, Tex, 2006, The Gulf Coast Addiction Technology Transfer Center.
17. Mental health emergencies, *Emergency medicine*, 2001, eMedicine. Retrieved February 21, 2002, from http://www.emedicine.com.
18. Muzina D: Suicide intervention: how to recognize risk, focus on patient safety. Retrieved November 13, 2007, from http://www.currentpsychiatry.com.
19. Patterson WM, Henry HD, Bird J, Patterson GA et al: Evaluation of suicidal patients: the SAD PERSONS scale, *Psychosomatics* 24:343, 1983.
20. Rickels K, Schweizer E: The clinical presentation of generalized anxiety in primary-care settings: practical concepts of classification and management, *J Clin Psychiatry* 58(11 suppl):4, 1997.
21. Ringskog S: Somatic complications in anorexia and bulimia nervosa, *Lakartidningen* 96(8):882, 1999.
22. Roy-Byrne P, Stein M, Bystrisky A et al: Pharmacotherapy of panic disorder: proposed guidelines for the family physician, *J Am Board Fam Pract* 11(4):282, 1998.

23. Schatzberg AF: New indications for antidepressants, *J Clin Psychiatry* 61(11 suppl):9, 2000.

24. Suicidal patients: assessing and managing patients presenting with suicidal attempts or ideation, *Emergency medicine practice*, 2004, http://empractice.net.

25. Suri R, Poist ES, Hager WD: Unrecognized bulimia nervosa: a potential cause of perioperative cardiac dysrhythmias, *Can J Anaesth* 46(11):1048, 1999.

26. The Joint Commission: 2008 *National patient safety goals*, http://www.jointcommission.org/NR/rdonlyres/82B717D8-B16A-4442-AD00-CE3188C2F00A/0/08_HAP_NPSGs_Master.pdf.

27. Varcarolis E, Carson V: Shoemaker: *Foundations of psychiatric mental health nursing: a clinical approach*, ed 5, 2006, Saunders.

28. Zun LS: Panic disorder: diagnosis and treatment in emergency medicine, *Ann Emerg Med* 30(1):92, 1997.

CHAPTER 52

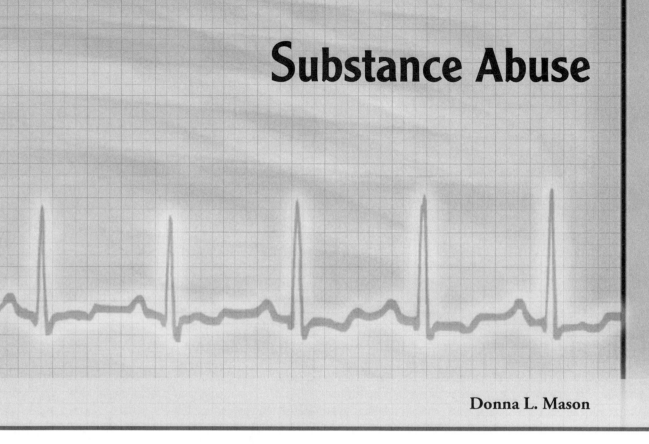

Substance Abuse

Donna L. Mason

S ubstance abuse refers to the inappropriate use of prescription drugs or use of illicit substances and continues to be a significant problem in the United States.[9] It occurs among persons of all socioeconomic groups and ages, including children, older adults, pregnant women, incarcerated persons, and health care workers. The reasons for abuse are multifactorial and can include experimentation, recreational use, and self-medication for serious underlying disease.

A 2006 report identified that more than 20 million persons over 12 years of age in the United States had abused substances within the previous month. The scope of the problem includes the following statistics: 31% of America's homeless suffer from substance abuse or alcoholism; in 2006 workplace substance abuse affected 8.8% of those employed full-time and 9.4% of those employed half time. Of unemployed adults 18 years of age or older, 18.5% were current (past month) illicit drug users.[11] Marijuana remains the most commonly abused substance; in 2006 there were 14.8 million current users. During the same period, rates of current use of other substances by persons over the age of 12 years were 2.4 million using cocaine, 1 million using hallucinogens, 7 million misusing prescription psychotherapeutic drugs, and 731,000 using methamphetamines.[10] The patient with substance abuse is at increased risk for poor health outcomes and can pose a unique challenge to the emergency nurse.

Regardless of legal status, abused substances generally fall into five categories: cannabis, depressants, hallucinogens, narcotics, and stimulants. For the purposes of this chapter, specific information is presented on alcohol, tobacco, cocaine, designer drugs, and heroin. The reader is encouraged to seek other sources for a more comprehensive discussion of prescription drug abuse.

ADDICTION

Researchers have discovered evidence that some alcoholics are genetically predisposed to alcoholism; however, scientists have not been able to determine if drug abusers have a similar genetic predisposition. Some drug abusers say they feel normal after substance abuse rather than euphoric. This may indicate that drug abuse has a biologic basis in certain individuals.

Drug addiction is a biologically based disease that alters the pleasure center and other aspects of the brain via the neurotransmitter dopamine. Dopamine connects neurons through the dendrite synaptic junction to a receptor site. When a neurotransmitter couples with a receptor, like a key fitting into a lock, the biochemical process in that neuron is activated. This process, called chemical neurotransmission, allows a receptor neuron to connect with other neurons. Heroin mimics the effects of this natural neurotransmitter (dopamine), whereas substances such

689

as lysergic acid diethylamide (LSD) block receptors and prevent natural transmission. Cocaine interferes with the process of neurotransmission by preventing release of dopamine. Phencyclidine (PCP) interferes with the way messages proceed from the surface receptors into the cell interior.

The biologic basis for addiction is the repeated process of altering chemical neurotransmission. Repeated use of these drugs can and will affect the brain on a permanent basis. Addiction begins when the pleasure circuit is repeatedly stimulated. The pleasure circuit is activated in a variety of ways, depending on the drug of choice. Heroin activates the opiate receptors, whereas cocaine allows dopamine to accumulate in the synapses, where it is released. Increasing amounts of dopamine at the synapses lead to euphoria.

Drugs exert a powerful control on behavior because of these physiologic effects. If you do something pleasurable, the message received reinforces the behavior responsible for the pleasure. Understanding this process makes it easier to understand addiction.

SPECIFIC SUBSTANCES

Emergencies related to substance abuse may be acute or chronic. The patient may come to the emergency department (ED) with an injury secondary to substance abuse, acute withdrawal symptoms, severe drug intoxication, or seeking help for addiction. This chapter focuses on addiction rather than acute drug intoxication. Refer to Chapter 42 for information on other toxicologic emergencies.

Cannabis

Cannabis is often used interchangeably for marijuana but also refers to other forms of the plant such as sinsemilla, *Cannabis indica* (hashish), and hash oil. Any form of cannabis should be recognized as possessing mind-altering or psychoactive properties.[13]

Marijuana

Marijuana is the most commonly used illegal substance. However, ED visits due to marijuana use alone are rare. Some states have legalized its use for certain conditions (e.g., decrease chemotherapy side effects, glaucoma). Marijuana is a mixture of dried, shredded leaves and other parts of the *Cannabis sativa* plant. Marijuana is most often smoked as a cigarette (commonly referred to as a joint) or in some type of smoking device such as a bong. Marijuana may be used in combination with another drug, such as crack cocaine, and has been mixed into food such as brownies or brewed into a drink.

The main active chemical in marijuana is delta-9-tetrahydrocannabinol (THC). The effects of THC include altered perception, an inability to problem solve, difficulty thinking rationally, loss of coordination, anxiety, and tachycardia. The only treatment, if needed, is supportive until the effects wear off.

Depressants

There are many depressant agents that are misused and abused. In the past, barbiturates (e.g., Seconal, pentobarbital) have been frequently abused depressants. Ketamine, also called vitamin K,[1] is one of the more commonly abused depressant class drugs and is second to ecstasy as a drug of choice at raves. Alcohol is also a depressant and will be covered in more depth later in the chapter.

Ketamine

Ketamine is a rapid-acting, dissociative anesthetic that provides hypnotic, analgesic, and amnesic effects with minimal respiratory depression.[10] When given as an intramuscular injection, the onset of action is 6 minutes. The person appears to be in a coma with the eyes open. The first priority in the management of adverse effects of ketamine ingestion is protecting the airway because muscle tone is lost when an overdose of this drug occurs. Ketamine may also be considered a club drug because of its use at raves.[9]

Hallucinogens
Lysergic Acid Diethylamide

LSD, a hallucinogen developed in 1938, has recently become popular again in the adolescent and young adult population.[4] It comes as a tablet or liquid that is sold on squares of blotter paper. Effects are primarily sensory and emotional. Colors, sounds, and smells are greatly intensified. The user may hear or feel colors and all sounds. The effects can be erratic and combined with hallucinations that can be pleasurable or terrifying. Psychosis has been reported. Physical effects can include dilated pupils, hyperthermia, tachycardia, elevated blood pressure, loss of appetite, sweating, and tremors. Many users of LSD can have flashbacks, which are a recurrence of certain parts of a previous LSD experience. Flashbacks most commonly occur with chronic users but can happen to any LSD user.

Phencyclidine

PCP is a hallucinogen that alters reality, touch, hearing, smell, taste, and visual perceptions. These effects may lead to serious bodily injury to the user. Chronic and long-term use can cause permanent changes in cognitive ability, memory, and fine motor function. Pregnant women who use PCP often deliver babies with visual, auditory, and motor disturbances.

The patient under the influence of PCP may be extremely violent with an increased risk for harm to self and others. Decrease stimulation for these patients, and monitor carefully for escalating violence.

Club Drugs

Club drugs (also called designer drugs), often used by teenagers and young adults at clubs, bars, and parties, including all-night dance parties (raves) attended by teenagers, are often a combination of stimulant and hallucinogen.[6,10] Rave parties are typically held in large open areas such as empty warehouses or open fields, are advertised by word of mouth, and attract adolescents and young adults. Liberal use of drugs has caused concern and scrutiny of raves. Club drugs include ecstasy (3,4-methylenedioxymethamphetamine [MDMA]), γ-hydroxybutyrate (GHB), flunitrazepam (Rohypnol), and ketamine (Table 52-1).[4,6,8] Not all rave attendees use drugs, but many illicit drugs are available. Alcohol is usually absent because it is believed to cause aggression and violence. GHB and Rohypnol have been used to "spike drinks," and all of the club drugs have been used to facilitate sexual assault. Victims may present to the ED reporting suspected assault, loss of memory, and little or no alcohol intake.

Ecstasy

Ecstasy is a synthetic amphetamine derivative that was originally developed as an appetite suppressant in 1914.[4,6,10] Ecstasy produces both stimulant and hallucinogenic effects and is potentially life threatening.[6,8] As with other street drugs, ecstasy is a combination of other illicit drugs with numerous recipes used to produce it. A newer variation called herbal ecstasy is composed of ephedrine or pseudo-ephedrine and caffeine from the kola nut. Ecstasy comes as a tablet, powder, or capsule and in virtually any color. The drug is primarily taken orally or snorted but can also be injected or taken rectally. Imprints may or may not be present. The butterfly is the universal symbol for ecstasy and appears on drug paraphernalia used at raves. These include cigarettes and other products that do not actually contain ecstasy.

Ecstasy is one of several drugs used to facilitate sexual assault, also called "date-rape drugs." In combination with alcohol, these drugs increase feelings of sexual arousal. This heightened sense of sexuality, coupled with short-term narrow cognitive focus, increases the likelihood that sexual assault will occur. Patients crave touch and experience a heightened sensuality, giving rise to many of the names for ecstasy such as "love" and the "hug drug." Other effects include hyperthermia, hypertension, tachycardia, and ataxia. An ecstasy high can last up to 24 hours.

Use of ecstasy in adolescents is of significant concern: there continues to be a high rate of ecstasy abuse, which may be due to availability of the drug, as well as its intoxicating effects. All-night raves are where many users are introduced to this drug. Another factor that may contribute to increased use is the duration of the effects.

Gamma-Hydroxybutyrate

GHB, thought to function like a neurotransmitter, is structurally related to γ-aminobutyric acid (GABA) and glutamic acid and has been the subject of investigation since 1960. GHB is a naturally occurring metabolite of GABA that produces a biphasic dopamine response and triggers release of an opiate-like substance that affects sleep cycles, temperature regulation, cerebral glucose metabolism, blood flow, and memory and emotional control, and it crosses the blood-brain barrier.[8] In low doses GHB can cause drowsiness, dizziness, nausea, and visual disturbances. In larger doses it can cause seizures, respiratory depression, unconsciousness, and coma. There is no antidote for GHB overdose; treatment is restricted to nonspecific supportive care, which includes ventilatory support and atropine for persistent bradycardia. Upon presentation to the ED, patients often require intubation and ventilation, but the central nervous system/respiratory depression usually resolves suddenly and rapidly within a few hours.

Inhalants

Use of inhalants is more likely to occur in younger adolescents, and they are the substances of first use for many. There are thousands of inhalants available, including solvents, glues, paints, gasoline, and aerosols.[1,7,9] Inhalants are cheap, usually free if found at home, easily available, and readily used. Huffing refers to direct inhalation or inhaling deeply from a chemical-soaked cloth within a paper bag. Inhalants can have immediate and extremely deleterious consequences, including death. Short-term symptoms include palpitations, delirium, respiratory distress, dizziness, and headaches. Frostbite injury to the roof of the mouth has been noted with use of some substances. Prolonged use can lead to irreversible brain damage, muscle weakness, nosebleeds,

Table 52-1. DRUGS ASSOCIATED WITH RAVES			
Drug	**Street Name[1]**	**Clinical Features**	**Toxicities**
Ecstasy (MDMA)	E, X, XTC, love	Heightened perception and sensual awareness, mydriasis, bruxism, jaw tension, and ataxia; sympathomimetic	Dysrhythmias, hyperthermia, rhabdomyolysis, DIC, hyponatremia, seizures, death
Ketamine	Kit-kat, special K, vitamin K	Nystagmus, increased tone, purposeful movements, amnesia, and hallucinations; sympathomimetic	Loss of consciousness, respiratory depression, catatonia, highly addictive
GHB	G, liquid grievous bodily harm, Georgia home boy	Agitation, nystagmus, ataxia, sedation, amnesia, hypotonia, vomiting, and muscle spasm	Seizures, apnea, sudden reversible coma with abrupt awakening and violence, bradycardia

DIC, Disseminated intravascular coagulation; *GHB*, γ-hydroxybutyrate; *MDMA*, 3,4-methylenedioxymethamphetamine.

sensory disturbances, arrhythmias, kidney and liver damage, cognitive problems, and violent behavior.[7] Boys and girls are at equal risk for use of inhalants.[9,11]

Narcotics

Heroin

Heroin is an opiate that affects the pleasure center. In 2006 there were 91,000 first-time users of heroin,[11] and the rates did not change significantly from 2005 to 2006.[10] Use of intravenous heroin (or other intravenous drug use) increases the risk for human immunodeficiency virus (HIV), hepatitis, skin abscesses/soft tissue infections, phlebitis, and bacterial endocarditis. Heroin may be intentionally used with cocaine to enhance the rush or high (speedball). The heroin dealer may also cut the heroin with other substances such as strychnine or PCP.

Heroin use can lead to physical dependence, and any attempt to stop using the drug will cause severe, painful withdrawal symptoms, including watery eyes, runny nose, yawning, loss of appetite, tremors, panic, chills, sweating, nausea, muscle cramps, and insomnia. Elevated blood pressure, pulse, respiratory rate, and temperature occur as withdrawal progresses. Heroin causes shallow breathing, pinpoint pupils, nausea, panic, insomnia, and a need for increasingly higher doses of the drug to achieve a high or to prevent withdrawal.

The heroin addict may present to the ED in acute withdrawal, after an overdose, or with problems related to intravenous drug injection. The patient in acute withdrawal is treated symptomatically with antianxiety agents, antihypertensive agents, and in some cases, administration of methadone. Acute heroin intoxication is treated with administration of naloxone, ventilatory support, and intravenous fluids when appropriate. Naloxone administration can precipitate severe withdrawal in some patients, so careful monitoring is essential.

Stimulants

Cocaine

Cocaine is a strong stimulant that can be snorted, smoked, or injected. Approximately 35.3 million Americans 12 years of age and older had tried cocaine by 2006,[11,12] 6.1 million had used some form of cocaine in the past year, and 2.4 million admitted using it in the past month.[11] Crack, the smokable form of cocaine, was introduced to the drug scene in 1986. The "high" is 10 times more powerful than that caused by snorting the drug. The associated rush or euphoria lasts only 5 to 10 minutes, which encourages more frequent use, so greater dependency develops. Many individuals addicted to cocaine say they continued to use in an attempt to experience the rush of their first time.

Injecting cocaine and other drugs carries the added risk for contracting HIV. Effects of cocaine on the cardiovascular system include chest pain, myocarditis, cardiomyopathy, endocarditis, ventricular arrhythmias, aortic dissection, hypertension, and cerebrovascular accident. Acute coronary syndrome (ACS) is the most commonly reported cardiovascular consequence of cocaine use. Other effects of cocaine are excitation, increased alertness, increased heart rate, increased blood pressure, loss of appetite, insomnia, dilated pupils, runny nose, and nasal congestion. In some situations cocaine can trigger paranoia. Cocaine may lead to seizures, cardiac and respiratory arrest, and even stroke. Long-term snorting of cocaine causes mucous membranes of the nose to disintegrate, and heavy use can actually cause the nasal septum to collapse. Despite views to the contrary, cocaine does not improve performance. Use can lead to loss of concentration, irritability, loss of memory, loss of energy, anxiety, and a loss of interest in sex.

Cocaine is also an issue in pregnancy. Literature supports the fact that cocaine, as with other drugs, can increase the risk for prematurity, stillbirth, low birth weight, central nervous system damage, and uterine rupture. Concomitant use of alcohol increases these risks and contributes to long-term developmental problems. Table 52-2 summarizes effects of maternal cocaine use on mothers and fetuses or babies.

It is not uncommon for a substance abuser to use more than one drug. Polysubstance abuse creates additional problems and often jeopardizes the health of the user. The most frequently used substance in association with cocaine or crack is alcohol; however, barbiturates, marijuana, and tranquilizers are often taken with or immediately after cocaine or crack. Combining cocaine or crack with heroin, called "speedballing," can be deadly. Reports from the National Institute on Drug Abuse indicate increasing use of cocaine or crack with a hallucinogenic drug such as PCP, also called a "space ball." Another combination that is extremely deadly is freebasing, which is the process of converting street cocaine to pure form by removing some of the cutting agents. The result is a more powerful drug that reaches the brain in seconds. The high occurs rapidly, but the euphoria disappears quickly, so the user has a craving to freebase again and again.

Life-threatening emergencies related to cocaine include chest pain, ACS, seizures, severe hypertension, and stroke. Management of these life-threatening emergencies is no different in the patient who uses cocaine than in other patients with these problems. Recognition of cocaine as a causative agent is not essential to managing these patients in the ED; however, long-term management must address the issue of substance abuse. Other cocaine-related problems include agitation, paranoia, and epistaxis. There is an increased risk for injury to self and others with these patients. Decrease stimulation, and monitor the patient carefully.

Methamphetamine

Methamphetamine is an addictive stimulant that can be injected, snorted, smoked, or ingested orally. Users experience a brief intense "rush" when the drug is used. Methamphetamine is a central nervous system stimulant that causes increased activity and decreased appetite. The drug has limited medical uses for the treatment of narcolepsy, attention deficit disorders, and obesity.[14]

Table 52-2. EFFECTS OF MATERNAL COCAINE USE ON MOTHERS AND FETUSES OR BABIES		
System	**Effects on Mother**	**Effects on Fetus or Baby**
Neurologic	Seizures	Increased irritability
	Neural damage*	Increased startle response
	Insomnia	Difficult to console
		Tremors
		Jittery
Ocular	Retinal crystals causing flashes of light called snow lights	Eye defects*
Respiratory	Shortness of breath	Increased respiratory rate
	Lung damage, if smoked	Abnormal ventilatory patterns
	Nasal membrane burns and lesions	Increased risk for sudden infant death syndrome*
	Respiratory paralysis in overdose	
Cardiovascular	Acute hypertension	Intrauterine growth retardation
	Angina	Tachycardia
	Arrhythmias	Cerebral artery injury/infarction*
	Tachycardia	Acute hypertension*
	Palpitations	
	Cerebral artery injury or cerebrovascular accident	
	Cardiac failure	
Gastrointestinal	Sore throat	Diarrhea
	Hoarseness	Poor tolerance for oral feeding
	Anorexia leading to weight loss and malnutrition	Prune-belly syndrome*
Renal		Hydronephrosis*
Reproductive	Increased uterine contractility	Cryptorchidism*
	Abruptio placentae	
	Spontaneous abortion	
	Premature labor	
	Stillbirth	

*Suspected but not established.

Methamphetamine is easily produced in "meth labs" using ingredients that were previously easily available. Increased illegal manufacturing of methamphetamine has resulted in a controlled substance restriction of many over-the-counter medications containing pseudoephedrine and other similar agents. Methamphetamine is made by a process called "cooking." Cooking methamphetamine is dangerous because the chemicals used are volatile and the by-products are extremely toxic. Meth labs are dangerous to anyone who comes into contact with the lab setting. Persons exposed to a meth lab may require decontamination, and special precautions may need to be taken for young children.

The current incidence of methamphetamine use was estimated at 731,000 current users 12 years of age and older. Lifetime (ever having used) use of methamphetamine was approximately 5.8% of the United States population above age 12 in 2006.[11]

ALCOHOLISM

Over 50% of the American population has a drink of alcohol at least once a month, which represents about 125 million people. Heavy drinking is defined as five or more drinks on 5 or more days of the week and is reported by 17 million Americans; another 57 million persons report binge drinking.[11] Twenty-three million people needed treatment for alcohol or other substance abuse in 2006.[11] In 2005, crashes involving drunk drivers accounted for 39% of all traffic deaths. This translates to one death every 31 minutes; nonfatal crashes occurred every 2 minutes.[5]

Comorbidities of substance abuse and mental illness exacerbate symptoms and often lead to treatment noncompliance, greater depression, and the likelihood of suicide, incarceration, family friction, and increased use and cost of public and hospital services.

Alcoholism is defined as a primary or chronic disease with genetic, psychosocial, and environmental factors influencing development and manifestation. The disease is often progressive and fatal and is characterized by impaired control over drinking, preoccupation with alcohol despite adverse consequences, and distortions in thinking, most notably denial.

Alcohol consumption affects all organs and systems of the body but the most significant effect is on the central nervous system. Alcohol depresses inhibitory control mechanisms, which has a major effect on neurotransmitters of the brain. Alcohol intake results in diminished judgment and impulsiveness that leads to risky and reckless behaviors. Excessive intake can cause severe impairment, respiratory compromise, blackouts, unconsciousness, and death.

Alcohol Screening, Brief Intervention, and Referral to Treatment (SBIRT) has been successfully implemented by emergency nurses. Every patient whom you suspect has been drinking or who responds positively to drinking alcohol when questioned should be screened by the CAGE test and asked the questions in Box 52-1. The CAGE test is an easy and effective way to determine if someone has a drinking problem (Box 52-2). The test has a 70% sensitivity and a 90% specificity. At-risk drinking is defined as one or more positive answers on the CAGE and for men greater than 14 drinks per week or more than 4 drinks per occasion; for females or those over the age of 65, greater than 7 drinks per week or more than 3 drinks per occasion. Those identified as being at-risk drinkers need to receive appropriate counseling or referral information based on screening answers.

Effects of Ethanol on Body Systems

Cardiovascular System

Alcohol initially depresses myocardial contractility and causes peripheral vasodilatation, resulting in a mild drop in blood pressure and a compensatory increase in heart rate and cardiac output. An increase of three or more drinks per day can result in hypertension and dysrhythmias.

Central Nervous System

After a few drinks, rapid eye movement sleep is affected, resulting in a faster than normal alternation between sleep stages and a deficiency in deep sleep. Peripheral neuropathy is noted in 5% to 15% of cases as a result of thiamine deficiency. Two syndromes, Wernicke's encephalopathy and Korsakoff's psychosis, are caused by thiamine deficiency. Clinical findings in Wernicke's encephalopathy are mental status changes, ocular dysfunction, and ataxic gait. Korsakoff's psychosis presents with profound anterograde amnesia. Alcoholics can show severe cognitive problems and impairment in recent and remote memory for weeks to months. Wernicke's encephalopathy is characterized by lesions in several parts of the brain causing double vision, involuntary and rapid eye movements, lack of muscular coordination, and decreased mental function. Almost every psychiatric syndrome can be seen during heavy drinking or subsequent withdrawal.

Gastrointestinal System

Acute alcohol intake can cause inflammation of the esophagus (esophagitis) and the stomach (gastritis). Gastritis is the most frequent cause of gastrointestinal bleeding in heavy drinkers. Violent vomiting can result in a Mallory-Weiss tear. Most gastrointestinal symptoms are reversible; however, two complications of chronic alcoholism, esophageal varices secondary to cirrhosis-induced portal hypertension and atrophy of gastric cells, may be irreversible.[5]

Alcoholics commonly develop acute or chronic pancreatitis. Glyconeogenesis is impaired, lactate production increases, and there is an increase in fat accumulation within liver cells resulting from decreased oxidation of fatty acids in the citric cycle. With repeated exposure to alcohol, more severe changes in the liver function are likely to occur. Hepatitis and cirrhosis are due to repeated exposure to alcohol.

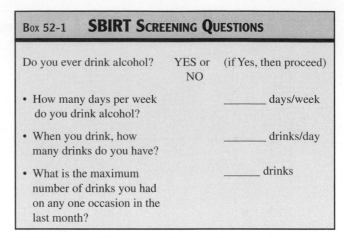

Box 52-1	**SBIRT** SCREENING QUESTIONS	
Do you ever drink alcohol?	YES or NO	(if Yes, then proceed)
• How many days per week do you drink alcohol?		_____ days/week
• When you drink, how many drinks do you have?		_____ drinks/day
• What is the maximum number of drinks you had on any one occasion in the last month?		_____ drinks

SBIRT, Screening, Brief Intervention, and Referral to Treatment.

Box 52-2	**CAGE** SCREENING
C: Have you ever felt the need to **C**ut down on your drinking?	
A: Have you ever felt **A**nnoyed by criticism of your drinking?	
G: Have you ever felt **G**uilty about your drinking?	
E: Have you ever felt the need for an **E**ye-opener in the morning?	

Jaundice, bruising, spider angiomata, and hepatomegaly are common findings in people who abuse alcohol.

Genitourinary System

Initially, modest intake of alcohol can increase sexual drive in men and simultaneously decrease erectile function. However, men with chronic alcoholism exhibit testicular atrophy that is irreversible, with concomitant loss of sperm cells.

In women with chronic alcoholism, amenorrhea, decreased ovarian size, infertility, and spontaneous abortions have been reported. Alcohol abuse during pregnancy is responsible for fetal alcohol syndrome.

Hematopoietic System

Anemia is a common finding in the person with severe alcoholism. Mild thrombocytopenia and an elevated mean corpuscular volume are also seen in alcoholics. Alcohol affects platelets and their ability to clump or stick to each other. Consequently, these patients may bleed more easily and longer from even minor cuts.

Skin

Findings seen in people who abuse alcohol include distal extremity hair loss, facial telangiectases, rosacea, seborrheic dermatitis, skin atrophy, and superficial infections.

Other Effects of Ethanol

Chronic intake and abuse of alcohol cause various nutritional deficiencies, increased risk for fractures resulting from alterations in calcium metabolism, modest but reversible

Box 52-3	SYMPTOMS OF ALCOHOL WITHDRAWL

Restlessness, irritability, anxiety, agitation
Anorexia, nausea, vomiting
Tremor, elevated heart rate, increased blood pressure
Insomnia, intense dreaming, nightmares
Impaired concentration, memory, judgment
Increased sensitivity to sounds, alteration in tactile sensations
Delirium—disorientation to time, place, and situation
Hallucinations—auditory, visual, or tactile
Delusion—usually paranoid
Grand mal seizures
Elevated temperature

decrease in thyroxine (T_4), and a marked decrease in triiodothyronine (T_3).

FETAL ALCOHOL SYNDROME. Infants who are exposed to prenatal alcohol are at risk for development of fetal alcohol syndrome disorders. These disorders include physical, psychologic, behavioral, and cognitive effects over the individual's lifetime. Fetal alcohol syndrome is characterized by abnormal facial features, growth abnormalities, and disorders of the central nervous syndrome. The clinical presentation of these infants varies dependent on the amount of alcohol they were exposed to during pregnancy.

ALCOHOL AND AGING. Decreased lean body mass related to aging affects distribution of alcohol; therefore older adults have an increased peak alcohol concentration with any given dose of alcohol. Drug absorption is affected by delayed gastric emptying and fluctuation in drug clearance; therefore drugs with narrow therapeutic indexes, such as warfarin or anticonvulsants, can produce hazardous consequences. Alcohol intake can affect adherence to treatment, and medication regimens may be entirely abandoned.

Alcohol Withdrawal

Individuals with severe alcoholism experience withdrawal when their serum ethanol drops below the patient's normal level. Symptoms may be mild during the early hours of withdrawal and can progress to full-blown delirium tremens within days. Box 52-3 highlights symptoms of alcohol withdrawal. It is important to note that symptoms occur when there is a drop below the person's normal level, not necessarily when there is no alcohol in the person's system. Withdrawal scoring is commonly being done in EDs and other acute care settings to provide an opportunity for pharmacologic interventions before full-blown delirium tremors.

In younger alcoholics, tremors usually begin 8 to 12 hours after the last drink and peak in 24 to 36 hours. In older alcoholics it is not unusual to see the effects of withdrawal delayed, with symptoms starting several days after cessation. Confusion rather than tremor is often the predominant clinical sign. Hallucinations in older adults are usually tactile; delirium tremens is a late manifestation of withdrawal that occurs 2 to 10 days after cessation of drinking.

Acute treatment of alcohol withdrawal includes a safe environment and treatment of nutritional and electrolyte deficiencies. Benzodiazepines have proven effective and are the drugs of choice because of their rapid onset and their short- and long-term effects. Lorazepam is preferred for individuals with liver dysfunction because it does not depend on hepatic metabolism for clearance. The literature supports use of long-term benzodiazepines; however, there is controversy in use of short- and long-term benzodiazepines. Antipsychotic medications such as thioridazine or haloperidol are sometimes used; however, they must be prescribed with care because they can lower the seizure threshold.

TOBACCO

Tobacco use includes cigarettes, pipes, cigars, and smokeless tobacco. Despite extensive education, tobacco use remains prevalent in the United States with an incidence of almost 73 million current users of tobacco in 2006.[2,3] In addition to the previously mentioned substances of abuse, many individuals abuse tobacco, steroids, and some natural stimulants available in health food stores. It is beyond the scope of this text to describe all potential substances of abuse; however, the use of tobacco does warrant brief discussion.

Tobacco abuse is related to a multitude of health care problems, including cardiovascular disease, lung cancer, bronchitis, and many more. Ironically, tobacco abuse is also common in the health care community. The emergency nurse should recognize the broad effects of tobacco abuse and provide pertinent education to the patient and family. The addictive component of tobacco products is nicotine. There are many commercial products available to assist with nicotine withdrawal for those interested in cessation of tobacco use.

NURSING CONSIDERATIONS

Emergency nurses should continue to educate themselves and others about the effects of substance abuse. Drug abuse knows no social boundaries; therefore emergency nurses should be meticulous in assessment of patients seen in the ED. Obtain a detailed history, and observe the patient for behaviors or physical symptoms that indicate drug use or abuse. Table 52-3 summarizes the effects of the most common illegal drugs. If you suspect the patient is abusing drugs, report your findings to the physician managing the patient's care so that appropriate testing or screening can be initiated. Obtain a urine specimen to screen for drugs of abuse for patients who present with unusual or erratic behavior. Ensure a safe environment for the patient, visitors, and personnel working in the ED.

The potential for violence increases in individuals under the influence of drugs. Increased injury severity and increased length of hospital stay occur in the presence of drug abuse. Patients often present for treatment of injuries associated with high-risk behavior such as assaults, penetrating trauma, blunt trauma, and sexually transmitted diseases rather than the drug abuse. Treat potentially life-threatening

Table 52-3. ILLEGAL DRUGS AND THEIR EFFECTS[1]				
Drugs	**Street Name**	**Signs of Use**	**Overdose**	**Route Taken**
Cocaine/Crack cocaine	Coke Crack Snow Dust Blow Girl Rock Freebase rocks	Excitation Increased alertness Increased heart rate Increased blood pressure Insomnia Runny nose Nasal congestion Dilated pupils	Agitation Increase in body temperature Hallucinations Seizures Possible death	Snorted Smoked (freebased) Injected
Amphetamines/ Methampheta- mines	Crank Ice Meth Speed Crystal Ecstasy	Excitation Increased alertness Increased heart rate Increased blood pressure Insomnia Runny nose Nasal congestion Dilated pupils	Agitation Increase in body temperature Hallucinations Seizures Possible death	Swallowed Snorted Smoked Injected
Heroin	Smack Stuff Horse Dope Boy	Excitation Drowsiness Respiratory depression Constricted pupils Nausea	Respiratory depression Seizures Coma Clammy skin Possible death	Injected Smoked Snorted

Phencyclidine	PCP
	Angel dust
	Hog
	Loveboat
		Illusions and hallucinations
		Poor perception of time and
		  distance
			Psychosis
			Longer, more intense "trip"
			  episodes
			"Awake" coma
			Bizarre behavior
			Violence
			Possible death
				Oral
				Injected
				Snorted
				Smoked

Lysergic acid diethylamide	LSD
	Acid
	Mickey Mouse
	Paper acid
	Blotter acid
	Green/Red dragon
		Illusions and hallucinations
		Poor perception of time and
		  distance
			Psychosis
			Longer, more intense "trip"
			  episodes
			Violence
			Possible death
				Oral

Marijuana	Weed Grass Pot THC Acapulco gold Joint Roach	Difficulty concentrating Euphoria Short-term memory loss Dilated pupils Loss of depth perception Disciplinary problems Increased appetite Disoriented	Fatigue Paranoia Possible psychosis	Oral Smoked

injuries, and then evaluate the patient for drug-related problems. Patients with acute signs and symptoms of abuse need medical intervention for the effects of the drug taken. Consultation or referral to a drug treatment center is indicated for substance abuse treatment after the patient is medically cleared.

SUMMARY

Substance abuse remains a significant challenge for emergency care providers and law enforcement officials. Continued misuse of both legal and illegal substances can compromise schools, the workplace, and our society. Increases in violence and crime have been strongly correlated with substance abuse, resulting in significant health concerns. Prevention of substance abuse is essential. The emergency nurse must be knowledgeable of licit and illicit drug abuse warning signs. Caring for this population is challenging and consumes many emergency care resources. Evidence has shown that regulatory and statutory mandates are essential to affecting substance abuse. The emergency nurse needs to be prepared to care for, advocate for, and educate patients with substance abuse illnesses and injuries.

REFERENCES

1. Addiction Science Network: *Illicit drug index: common street names of various drugs.* Retrieved February 3, 2008, from http://www.addictionscience.net/ASNdrugs. htm#StimulantClass.

2. Centers for Disease Control and Prevention: Cigarette smoking among adults—United States, 2006, *MMWR Morb Mortal Wkly Rep* 56(44), 2007. Retrieved February 17, 2008, from http://www.cdc.gov/tobacco/data_ statistics/Factsheets/adult_cig_smoking.htm.

3. Centers for Disease Control and Prevention: *Health effects of smoking among young people.* Retrieved February 17, 2008, from http://www.cdc.gov/tobacco/data_ statistics/Factsheets/youth_tobacco.htm.

4. National Clearinghouse for Alcohol and Drug Information: *Drugs of abuse.* Retrieved February 17, 2008, from http://www.drugabuse.gov/drugpages.html.

5. National Highway Traffic Safety Administration, U.S. Department of Transportation: Traffic safety facts 2005: alcohol, Washington, DC, 2006, The Administration. Retrieved February 17, 2008, from http://www-nrd.nht-sa.dot.gov/pdf/nrd-30/NCSA/TSF2005/AlcoholTSF05. pdf.

6. National Institute on Drug Abuse: *Drugs of abuse: ectasy.* Retrieved February 17, 2008, from http://www. drugabuse.gov/infofacts/ecstasy.html.

7. National Institute on Drug Abuse: *Drugs of abuse: inhalants.* Retrieved February 17, 2008, from http://www. nida.nih.gov/DrugPages/Inhalants.html.

8. National Institute on Drug Abuse: *NIDA InfoFacts: Rohypnol and GHB.* Retrieved February 17, 2008, from http://www.nida.nih.gov/infofacts/RohypnolGHB.html

9. National Institute on Drug Abuse: *Epidemiologic trends in drug abuse,* Bethesda, MD, 2007, U.S. Department of Health and Human Services National Institutes of Health.

10. National Institute on Drug Abuse, Research Report Series: *Hallucinogens and dissociative drugs.* Retrieved February 17, 2008, from http://www.drugabuse.gov/ResearchReports/Hallucinogens/Hallucinogens.html.

11. National Institute on Drug Abuse, Research Report Series: *Methamphetamine.* Retrieved February 17, 2008, from http://www.drugabuse.gov/ResearchReports/Methamph/Methamph.html.

12. National Institute on Drug Abuse, Research Report Series: *NIDA InfoFacts: crack and cocaine.* Retrieved February 17, 2008, from http://www.nida.nih.gov/infofacts/cocaine.html.

13. Office of National Drug Control Policy: *Drug facts.* Retrieved February 3, 2008, from http://www.whitehousedrugpolicy.gov/drugfact/index.html.

14. Substance Abuse and Mental Health Services Administration: *Results from the 2006 national survey on drug use and health: national findings,* Office of Applied Studies, NSDUH Series H-32, DHHS Publication No. SMA 07-4293, Rockville, Md, 2007, DHHS.

CHAPTER 53

Sexual Assault

Anita Ruiz-Contreras

S exual assault can be defined as any type of sexual contact or behavior that occurs without the explicit consent of the recipient, including such activities as forced sexual intercourse, sodomy, child molestation, incest, fondling, and attempted rape.[18] Sexual assault is one of the most feared and least understood crimes. Of all the choices made in our lives, the most intimate choices are sexual. In a sexual assault, choice is taken away. Sexual assault is not a crime of passion. The perpetrator does not attack because of overwhelming lust. It is not the victim's clothing or his or her perceived seductive behavior that causes the assault. The perpetrator's sexual gratification is a myth.

In a classic study of more than 600 sex offenders, Amir[1] was one of the first to describe rape as a crime of power and control. Groth[11] interviewed more than 500 sexual "aggressors" and found power and anger described as motivating factors. Sex is used by the rapist as a tool to control and humiliate the victim.

Sexual assault is not defined by gender, social level, ethnic origin, religious affiliation, or cultural lines.[9] Anyone, male, female, young or old, can be a victim of sexual assault. Prostitutes who normally charge for sexual services can be raped. A wife, a husband, a boyfriend, or a girlfriend can be raped. One in six women describe being sexually assaulted in their lifetime.[15] Sixty percent of women are acquainted with their assailant.[17] Many victims, possibly as high as 61%, do not report the crime.[7]

There are many factors that contribute to victims not reporting sexual assault. There is a perceived shame that the victim should have been able to prevent the event. There is concern about what others will say or think about the victim. In most states, health care professionals are mandated reporters and should speak honestly about this requirement. The patient has the right to report or not report as he or she sees fit.

Male sexual assault may be one of the most underreported of all groups. Myths surrounding male sexual assault include beliefs that these assaults only happen in prison or that homosexuality is a causative factor. Lipscomb et al,[9] in a study of 99 adult male victims of sexual assault, found no statistically significant difference between incarcerated and not incarcerated victims. All people are potential victims regardless of sexual orientation. Men are raped for the same reason women are raped: power, control, and humiliation. The male survivor needs the same level of compassion and recognition as any other patient who has been sexually assaulted.

SEXUAL ASSAULT PATIENTS ARE SURVIVORS

The term *survivor* has been used to identify patients who have been sexually assaulted. The patient who has experienced sexual assault has lived through a life-threatening,

698

life-altering event. Use of the term *victim* may denote a person who is helpless and who feels hopeless. The term *survivor* has more of a positive, empowering connotation. Use of *survivor* as an identifying term can be helpful when counseling patients. However, there are some professionals working in the area of sexual assault treatment who do not use the term *survivor* because it is felt that it may minimize or take away from addressing the devastation of the actual event. In determining the terms to be used, the health care professional must consider the impact of his or her choice of words on the individual presenting for care.

MYTHS AND MISCONCEPTIONS

Common myths such as "victims are women wearing suggestive clothing" or "a woman cannot be raped by an acquaintance" have long ago been dispelled. Regrettably, other myths remain prevalent. The media often portray women as secretly wanting to be raped, which is the so-called rape fantasy. When an individual fantasizes, he or she selects the players, the setting, and the sexual acts. In sexual assault all choice is taken away. This myth confuses sex and rape. Sex becomes the tool used by the rapist to degrade and humiliate the victim. Emergency nurses can use their knowledge regarding myths and misconceptions when counseling patients and families to dispel these beliefs and help begin the process of healing.

The patient may arrive with expectations about the hospital and the staff that are based on misconceptions; law enforcement officers and emergency nurses may also have long-held beliefs based on misconception. It is important for health care professionals to examine their own attitudes regarding survivors of sexual assault.[10] Myths and misconceptions surrounding sexual assault harm the patient and hamper development of a trusting relationship with the emergency nurse.

RAPE-TRAUMA SYNDROME

In a landmark study of 94 rape victims, Burgess and Holmstrom[3] first identified rape-trauma syndrome, a cluster of symptoms experienced by survivors of sexual assault. Symptoms include somatic, behavioral, and psychologic reactions. The framework of rape-trauma syndrome includes recognition of the long-term reorganization a survivor goes through when recovering from the assault. Reorganization may take weeks or even years. There is recognition of differences in lifestyle choices made by individuals, in which lifestyles are not judged but seen as normal for that person.

Rape-trauma syndrome is an approved nursing diagnosis and can be used to plan nursing care. The initial hospital experience can have a major effect on the acute phase of the sexual assault survivor's recovery. When interacting with the sexual assault victim, it is essential for the emergency nurse to develop a trusting relationship. As with any patient, a calm, confident approach facilitates this process. Listen to the patient, and explain what will happen during the examination. Show concern for the patient's experience. Specific questions that require the patient to relive the assault are not needed. Determining the presence of physical trauma that requires immediate treatment is the initial priority. The extent of emotional injury cannot be estimated. Each person's response to a sexual assault is different. Individuals may laugh, cry, tell a joke, or become catatonic. Patients may blame themselves for fighting back or for not fighting back. Inform the patients that their actions helped get them through the ordeal, regardless of what action was taken. Patients may believe they caused the rape by accepting the ride or opening the door. Remind these patients that they did not cause the assault. Patients need to hear that they have the right to decide what to do with their own bodies and that no one has the right to hurt them.

THE SEXUAL ASSAULT SURVIVOR IN THE EMERGENCY DEPARTMENT

Evaluation of the sexual assault survivor in the emergency department (ED) requires planning, development of specific policies and procedures, and staff education. The goal is to provide sensitive, individualized care for each person in a manner that ensures adherence to legal and regulatory requirements. Staff should be knowledgeable about state laws and regulations regarding sexual assault. A standard documentation form or protocol may be required by local or state policy. For example, the California State Medical Protocol for the Examination and Treatment of Sexual Assault Victims must be used by all California hospitals and health care practitioners who perform examinations on survivors of sexual assault.[4] If hospitals do not wish to comply, they must develop a referral protocol with a hospital that does comply. For each case, a standard documentation form is used with copies for law enforcement, the criminalistics laboratory, and the hospital. The protocol outlines the steps of examination, including evidence collection, laboratory testing, medications, and follow-up care.

Sexual Assault Response Teams

For more than 20 years, specialized teams of nonphysician medical providers have been responsible for performing sexual assault medical and legal examinations.[2] The teams are identified as sexual assault response teams (SARTs) or suspected abuse response teams and consist of a nurse examiner, rape crisis advocate, and law enforcement personnel. Nurses with specialized training are identified as sexual assault/abuse nurse examiners (SANEs) or sexual assault forensic examiners (SAFEs). Some programs have started with the registered nurse serving as a patient care coordinator. This nurse assists the physician with the examination and follow-up. At the same time the nurse is learning how to perform examinations on his or her own. Other programs begin with adult patients and then progress to evidentiary examinations of pediatric patients as well.[16] The SANEs are usually on call and respond when a sexual assault victim arrives at an identified hospital/clinic. The SART programs train registered nurses to obtain patient histories, conduct evidentiary examinations, provide sexually transmitted infection (STI) prophylaxis, offer pregnancy prevention medication, and ensure follow-up care. The proliferation of these programs across the United States is evidence of their need and effectiveness. Most programs hold monthly case review meetings to ensure that all staff are kept up-to-date and there is consistent adherence to protocols. SANE personnel become the medical and legal experts in the field of sexual assault. The National Institute of Justice found that SART programs enhanced the quality of health care for women, improved the quality of forensic evidence, and increased the ability of law enforcement to collect information, file charges, and convict the assailant.[16] The International Association of Forensic Nurses reports that there are over 500 functioning sexual assault treatment programs (499 of these are in the United States—approximately 80% in hospitals with the remaining programs being community-based) (International Association of Forensic Nurses, personal communication, K. Day, March 9, 2009).

Development of a specialized team is the ideal; however, hospitals without specialized programs can treat sexual assault victims effectively. Individual hospitals can train all ED nurses or an identified number of nurses to care for sexual assault survivors during their work hours. Identified personnel may conduct the complete evidentiary examination independently or in conjunction with a physician. The nurse acts as a patient care coordinator, ensuring adherence to established protocols and procedures.

The Examination Begins

Sexual assault survivors should receive an emergent triage priority, only behind patients experiencing acute life-threatening events. The patient should be immediately placed in a safe, secure room. A medical screening examination should be performed to rule out an emergency medical condition. One nurse should be instructed to remain with the patient throughout the ED visit to provide continuity and decrease repetition of data collection. The patient should be allowed a support person such as a family member, friend, or representative from a rape crisis center. Asking "Whom can I call for you?" allows the patient to think of a name, whereas asking "Is there someone I can call for you?" is often followed by a "No" answer. Rape crisis advocates are an integral part of any sexual assault treatment program. If available, a rape crisis advocate should be part of the SART and be called to the hospital whenever the patient arrives. Law enforcement personnel should not be in the examination room during the examination.

Consent

Consent for medical treatment as well as evidentiary examination and photographs should be obtained. The nurse should ensure that the patient is well informed and understands the examination process. In obtaining consent for forensic evaluation, the nurse begins to develop a therapeutic relationship with the patient. The examination of a sexual assault survivor has been called "another rape." The goal of the hospital or clinic experience is to cause as little additional stress as possible. All interactions should be handled with sensitivity and understanding. Every effort should be made to ensure that the patient has the opportunity to make informed choices about medical care. Patients must be informed if the hospital is required to notify law enforcement. The hospital may be required to report; however, the patient has the right to decide whether he or she wishes to speak with law enforcement. It has been found that women assaulted by a partner are significantly less likely to report sexual assault to police or seek medical care.[8] Patients should be informed of the nurse's and the hospital's mandatory reporting responsibility. The patient may wish to speak to an advocate before talking to hospital staff or the law enforcement officer. Law enforcement officers today are well prepared to deal sensitively with survivors of sexual assault. The patient must understand that the evidence collected will be used for prosecution of the accused rapist if a report is made. Many patients are not ready to file a report with law enforcement, even with treatment in the ED. One study of 337 sexual assault victims found only 62% were certain they wanted to file such a report.[12]

History

A standard form should be used to gather the patient's history. This history helps the nurse determine the type of evidence collection required. Examinations performed within 72 hours of the assault are more likely to yield evidence of assault[8]; however, this time frame should not negate performing examinations on individuals assaulted beyond the 72-hour time frame. Evidence of sexual assault has been found after as many as 5 to 6 days.[5] When questioning the patient, the patient does not need to describe the assault in specific minute-by-minute detail. Questions should be asked in a manner understood by the patient, translating medical terms into everyday language. History taking may be delayed when the patient's emotional response to questioning makes it impossible to ascertain the information. Documentation should be completed legibly and clearly. If this case is called to court, the nurse may be asked to discuss what was written in the record. The nurse must be able to understand what he or she wrote months or even years after it was written. The nurse should write in such a manner that the information can be easily read and explained to the jury.

Potential use of various drugs (e.g., Rohypnol, γ-hydroxybutyrate [GHB], ketamine) should be assessed while obtaining other historical data. This data helps the SANE or other examiner determine the need for drug screening. Assaults committed using these agents are referred to as drug-facilitated sexual assaults. These drugs are used to incapacitate a victim in order to perpetrate a sexual assault. Blood and first-void urine specimens are collected as quickly as possible because of the short half-life of these types of drugs. Signs and symptoms commonly found in patients who have experienced a drug-facilitated sexual assault include the following[13]:

- A history of being out drinking, having just one or two drinks (too few to account for the extreme level of intoxication), suddenly feeling "very drunk" or "disoriented," or being told he or she suddenly appeared drunk or drowsy with impaired motor skills, judgment, or amnesia.
- Reports from witnesses or from the victim that he or she acted "intoxicated" approximately 15 minutes after drinking a beverage that he or she accepted from someone or after drinking a beverage that was left unattended.
- The victim remembers very little of the incident other than flashes of memory, sometimes referred to as "cameo appearances," in which he or she remembers "waking up" or "coming to" but being unable to move, then losing consciousness once again. Cameo appearances are often associated with a loud noise or pain.
- The victim awakens hours later and finds himself or herself undressed or partially dressed, possibly in bed with a person he or she may or may not know, or the victim awakens with vaginal or rectal soreness, indicating sexual contact may have occurred without consent.
- Clothing is not worn as he or she normally wears it (e.g., underwear inside out).
- Possible nausea and vomiting upon awakening (not always, because this reaction is drug specific).
- History of being at a party, possibly a rave, or being with "friends" and taking "Roofies," "R-2," "Special K," "Ecstasy," etc.

Physical Examination and Evidence Collection

Collection of laboratory specimens should be accomplished early to allow for pregnancy test results. A negative pregnancy test is needed to administer medication for prevention of pregnancy. The patient's clothing is collected and placed in paper rather than plastic bags for evaluation at the local crime laboratory. Paper bags better serve to maintain the evidence for trial evaluation. Paper does not facilitate mold growth or provide for the static electricity lifting of trace evidence as plastic bags do. A head-to-toe physical assessment is completed to assess for all injuries. Documentation of any injuries should include color and size of injuries such as bruises, abrasions, lacerations, or avulsions. Use of body figures on the documentation tool can assist in recording this data. A Wood's lamp or other ultraviolet light is used to identify fluorescent areas on the patient's skin. Semen may appear as orange or blue-green on the skin. The fluorescent area should be swabbed with a moistened cotton-tipped applicator. A control swab should then be taken from an area of the body adjacent to where the swab was taken. Caution should be taken when reporting Wood's lamp findings because other materials such as lint also fluoresce. Oral swabs are taken for evidence of semen and as a reference sample. Reference samples include saliva, blood, semen, pubic hair, and body hair. The criminalistics laboratory results of these reference samples are compared to specimens from potential suspects.

For the female patient the pelvic examination begins with a gross visual examination. The external genitalia are examined for signs of injury or foreign materials. Injuries should be described by size, appearance, and location.

Photographs are then used to detect and document genital trauma.[6] Colposcopic photographs have become standard as part of the pelvic or genital evaluation. The colposcope provides binocular vision, magnifies the area by 5 to 30 times, and can take photographs.[10] Lenahan found that the colposcope improved detection of genital trauma when compared with gross visualization alone.[6] Documentation should indicate if the injury is apparent without use of the colposcope. Pubic hair is combed and collected to allow for microscopic evaluation of foreign hairs by the criminalistics laboratory. A representative number of the patient's pubic hairs are cut close to the skin for comparison. During the pelvic examination, swabs and slides are taken from the vaginal pool. Historically, baseline testing for chlamydia and gonorrhea has also been performed. Recently, some established programs have stopped performing these tests routinely because each patient is offered prophylactic antibiotic treatment.

Rectal examination includes anoscopy (if indicated), colposcopy, swabs, slides, and baseline testing for STIs (as indicated by local policy). The perianal area should be cleansed after taking vaginal/penile specimens to avoid contamination from vaginal or perianal drainage.[8] All swabs and slides must be labeled to identify the patient and the source along with the time, date, location of collection, and the name of the person collecting the evidence. After collection, swabs or slides should be placed in a drying box with cool airflow. If a facility does not have a dryer, measures should be taken to ensure that all swabs and slides are dry before packaging; drying swabs and slides also prevents deterioration of evidence. Testing of swabs and slides is done by a criminalistics laboratory in the hope of linking evidence to potential suspects. Current methods of deoxyribonucleic acid (DNA) typing allow detection of semen donor type beyond the 72-hour time frame. Special care must be taken by the nurse to prevent any contamination of evidence collected. All pieces of evidence are placed in separate containers or paper bags. All equipment that comes in contact with evidence must be clean. The nurse should limit handling of evidence and take care not to leave any of his or her own DNA on the evidence. This can be facilitated by using gloves, hair covering, masks, and gowns and by avoiding talking directly over collected, unsealed evidence. See Chapter 16 for more details of the forensic evaluation.

Chain of Custody

To maintain the integrity of evidence collected, the nurse must be able to verify the whereabouts of all evidence. A chart can be used to indicate that evidence was taken from the patient by the nurse and then given to the law enforcement officer. All transfers of evidence must be logged to show that evidence was transferred from one person to another, with each transfer dated and timed. The best practice is to keep transfers of evidence to a minimum. If a drying box is used, it should have a lock that is closed and opened only by the nurse.

After Examination

A shower and clean clothing should be available for the patient after the sexual assault examination. Ideally the hospital maintains a closet with clean, new or used clothing. If desired by the patient, medication should be provided for prevention of pregnancy and STIs (Box 53-1). The Centers for Disease Control and Prevention (CDC) currently recommends prophylactic treatment for trichomoniasis, bacterial vaginosis, gonorrhea and chlamydial infections.[5]

Consent for pregnancy prevention should be obtained after a negative pregnancy test result and after the patient is informed of associated risks. A specific postcoital consent form should be completed before administration of the medication. Prophylaxis for HIV and Hepatitis B should be considered.[5] SART programs in California, New York, and Vancouver (British Columbia) do offer the option of HIV and hepatitis B prophylaxis to all patients.[14] HIV seroconversion has occurred when the only known risk factor was sexual assault, although the frequency is low.[5] Providers might also consider administration of an antiemetic medication when pregnancy prophylaxis is given.[5] The CDC recommendations, along with local medical authority, should be consulted to ensure an effective medication regimen.

Follow-up Care

Patients should be rechecked in 10 days to 2 weeks. Referral to a gynecologist or nearby clinic is essential. Cultures for chlamydia and gonorrhea can be obtained at this time. At the follow-up appointment, timelines for HIV testing can be discussed. Many established specialized teams include

---

Box 53-1	**MEDICATION PROPHYLAXIS IN SEXUAL ASSAULT**

PROPHYLACTIC TREATMENT OF SEXUALLY TRANSMITTED INFECTION (TRICHOMONIASIS, BACTERIAL VAGINOSIS, GONORRHEA, CHLAMYDIA)

Ceftriaxone 125 mg IM in a single dose
PLUS
Metronidazole 2 g orally in a single dose
PLUS
Azithromycin 1 g orally in a single dose
OR
Doxycycline 100 mg orally twice a day for 7 days

PREGNANCY PROPHYLAXIS (GIVE ONLY AFTER OBTAINING NEGATIVE PREGNANCY TEST)

Ovral 2 tablets orally and 2 tablets in 12 hours

Modified from Centers for Disease Control and Prevention: *Sexually transmitted diseases: treatment guidelines,* 2006. Retrieved November 11, 2007, http://www.cdc.gov/std/treatment/2006/sexual-asssault.htm.

---

follow-up care as part of their overall program. A rape crisis advocate available at the time of the follow-up examination can assess the patient's need for counseling.

LEGAL ASPECTS

Should the criminal case go to court, the nurse may be called as a witness to describe what he or she did and saw. In some situations the nurse will be qualified by the judge as an expert witness. The expert witness is allowed to give opinion testimony and offer conclusions regarding his or her findings. Each encounter with a sexual assault patient has the potential for becoming a court case. In court the nurse is not there to represent one side or the other. The nurse may receive a subpoena from the district attorney's office or a defense attorney representing the accused. In preparation for court the nurse should review the patient's medical record. The nurse should also have a professional curriculum vitae that can be reviewed by both attorneys. The nurse should be prepared to describe his or her education, experience, and sexual assault training. The nurse may need to explain the SART process to the jury. Attire in the courtroom should be professional and businesslike. It is generally not acceptable to wear a nursing uniform in the courtroom. In most cases the nurse will be excluded from the courtroom until he or she is called in for actual testimony. When on the witness stand, act as follows:

- Answer questions in a calm, confident manner.
- Listen to the complete question before answering.
- Be prepared to spell and define medical terms.
- Answer only the question you are asked.
- Ask for clarification of any questions you do not understand.
- Face the jury when you respond to questions.
- Avoid becoming angry or defensive.
- Wait to answer a question until the judge has ruled on an objection by one of the attorneys.

SUMMARY

In an expanded role, emergency nurses are uniquely suited to act as sexual assault nurse examiners or as coordinators of care for a sexual assault survivor. However, if this role is not identified in the nurse's institution or state, it is still vital that the emergency nurse be knowledgeable about local or state protocol. The emergency nurse should care for the patient in a supportive, nonthreatening, nonjudgmental manner. The ED visit can significantly affect the emotional recovery of the sexual assault survivor.

REFERENCES

1. Amir M: *Patterns of forcible rape,* Chicago, 1971, University of Chicago Press.
2. Antognoli-Toland P: Comprehensive program for examination of sexual assault victims by nurses: a hospital-based project in Texas, *J Emerg Nurs* 11(3):132, 1985.

3. Burgess AW, Holmstrom LL: Rape-trauma syndrome, *Am J Psychiatry* 131:981, 1974.

4. California Medical Training Center: *Training on the California medical protocol for the examination of sexual assault and child sexual abuse victims*, Sacramento, Calif, 2001, California Medical Training Center.

5. Centers for Disease Control and Prevention: *Sexually transmitted diseases: treatment guidelines,* 2006. Retrieved November 11, 2007, from http://www.cdc.gov/std/treatment/2006/sexual-asssault.htm

6. Ernoehazy W, Murphy-Lavoie H: Sexual assault, *eMedicine* 3(1), 2002. Retrieved November 11, 2007 http://emedicine.medscape.com/article/806120-overview.

7. Fahrenthold DA: Statistics show drop in U.S. rape cases, *Washington Post*, June 19, 2006.

8. Feldhaus KM: Lifetime sexual assault prevalence rates and reporting practices in an emergency department population, *Ann Emerg Med* 36(1):23, 2000.

9. Giardono AP: *Sexual assault: victimization across the life span*, Maryland Heights, Mo, 2002, GW Medical Publishing.

10. Girardin B, Faugno D, Senski P, et al: *Color atlas of sexual assault*, St. Louis, 1997, Mosby.

11. Groth AN: *Men who rape: the psychology of the offender*, New York, 1979, Plenum Press.

12. Ledray LE: *Sexual assault nurse examiner (SANE): development and operation guide*, Washington, DC, 1999, Office for Victims of Crime, U.S. Department of Justice.

13. Ledray LE: The clinical care and documentation for victims of drug-facilitated sexual assault, *J Emerg Nurs* 27(3):301, 2001.

14. Pinto NW, Meier RF: Gender differences in rape reporting, *Sex Roles: A Research Journal*, 40(11-12):979, 1999.

15. Rape, Abuse & Incest National Network (RAINN): Sexual Assault Statistics. Retrieved November 13, 2007, from http://www.rainn.org/statistics/index.html.

16. Sievers V, Murphy S, Miller J: Sexual assault evidence collection more accurate when completed by sexual assault nurse examiners: Colorado's experience, *J Emerg Nurs* 29(6):511, 2003.

17. U.S. Department of Justice: Rape and Sexual Violence. Retrieved September 2, 2007, from http://www.ojp.usdoj.gov/nij/topics/crime/rape-sexual-violence/welcome.htm.

18. U.S. Department of Justice. The Facts about the Office on Violence Against Women Focus Areas. Retrieved November 11, 2007, from http://www.usdoj.gov/ovw/sexassault.htm.

Nursing Diagnoses for Selected Emergency Conditions

NURSING DIAGNOSES FOR SURFACE TRAUMA (CHAPTER 11)

Fluid volume, Deficient
Infection, Risk for
Pain
Skin integrity, Impaired
Tissue perfusion, Ineffective

NURSING DIAGNOSES FOR HEAD INJURY (CHAPTER 21)

Airway clearance, Ineffective
Aspiration, Risk for
Gas exchange, Impaired
Injury, Risk for
Mobility, Impaired physical
Pain
Tissue perfusion, Ineffective

NURSING DIAGNOSES FOR SPINAL CORD INJURY (CHAPTER 22)

Airway clearance, Ineffective
Aspiration, Risk for
Breathing pattern, Ineffective
Coping, Ineffective
Fluid volume, Deficient
Gas exchange, Impaired
Injury, Risk for secondary injury of spinal cord
Skin integrity, Risk for impaired
Thermoregulation, Ineffective

NURSING DIAGNOSES FOR THORACIC TRAUMA (CHAPTER 23)

Airway clearance, Ineffective
Breathing pattern, Ineffective
Cardiac output, Decreased
Fluid volume, Deficient
Gas exchange, Impaired
Pain

NURSING DIAGNOSES FOR ABDOMINAL AND GENITOURINARY TRAUMA (CHAPTER 24)

Anxiety
Body image, Disturbed
Breathing pattern, Ineffective
Cardiac output, Decreased
Comfort, Impaired
Fear
Fluid volume, Deficient
Fluid volume, Risk for deficient
Infection, Risk for
Pain, Acute
Sexual dysfunction
Tissue perfusion, Ineffective
Tissue integrity, Impaired
Urinary elimination, Impaired

NURSING DIAGNOSES FOR ORTHOPEDIC OR SOFT-TISSUE INJURY (CHAPTER 25)

Fluid volume, Deficient
Infection, Risk for
Mobility, Impaired physical
Pain
Skin integrity, Impaired
Tissue perfusion, Ineffective

NURSING DIAGNOSES FOR BURN INJURY (CHAPTER 26)

Airway clearance, Ineffective
Body image, Disturbed
Family coping, Disabled
Fluid volume, Deficient
Gas exchange, Impaired
Hypothermia, Risk for
Infection, Risk for
Mobility, Impaired physical
Pain
Tissue perfusion, Ineffective

NURSING DIAGNOSES FOR FACIAL INJURY (CHAPTER 27)

Airway clearance, Ineffective
Infection, Risk for
Pain
Skin integrity, Impaired

NURSING DIAGNOSES FOR THE PEDIATRIC TRAUMA PATIENT (CHAPTER 28)

Airway clearance, Ineffective
Anxiety
Breathing pattern, Ineffective
Cardiac output, Decreased
Family processes, Interrupted
Fear
Fluid volume, Deficient
Gas exchange, Impaired
Pain

NURSING DIAGNOSES FOR THE PREGNANT TRAUMA PATIENT (CHAPTER 29)

Anxiety (patient and family)
Aspiration, Risk for
Fear (patient and family)
Fluid volume, Deficient
Gas exchange, Impaired
Grieving
Infection, Risk for
Pain
Tissue perfusion, Altered

NURSING DIAGNOSES FOR RESPIRATORY EMERGENCIES (CHAPTER 30)

Airway clearance, Ineffective
Fluid volume, Excess
Gas exchange, Impaired
Tissue perfusion, Altered

NURSING DIAGNOSES FOR CARDIOVASCULAR EMERGENCIES (CHAPTER 31)

Anxiety
Breathing pattern, Ineffective
Cardiac output, Decreased
Coping, Ineffective
Fear
Fluid volume, Deficient
Fluid volume, Excess
Gas exchange, Impaired
Pain
Tissue perfusion, Ineffective
Ventilation, Impaired spontaneous

NURSING DIAGNOSES RELATED TO SHOCK (CHAPTER 32)

Cardiac output, Decreased
Fluid volume, Deficient
Gas exchange, Impaired
Tissue perfusion, Ineffective

NURSING DIAGNOSES FOR NEUROLOGIC EMERGENCIES (CHAPTER 33)

Anxiety
Breathing pattern, Ineffective
Fear
Pain
Tissue perfusion, Ineffective
Verbal communication, Impaired

NURSING DIAGNOSES FOR GASTROINTESTINAL EMERGENCIES (CHAPTER 34)

Anxiety
Fluid volume, Deficient
Gas exchange, Impaired
Infection, Risk for
Knowledge, Deficient
Pain

NURSING DIAGNOSES FOR GENITOURINARY EMERGENCIES (CHAPTER 35)

Anxiety
Electrolyte imbalance
Fluid volume, Deficient
Fluid volume, Excess
Infection, Risk for
Knowledge, Deficient
Pain
Tissue perfusion, Ineffective
Urinary elimination, Impaired

NURSING DIAGNOSES FOR FLUID AND ELECTROLYTE ABNORMALITIES (CHAPTER 36)

Bowel incontinence
Breathing pattern, Ineffective
Cardiac output, Decreased
Constipation
Fluid volume, Deficient
Fluid volume, Excess
Gas exchange, Impaired
Nutrition, Imbalanced
Urinary elimination, Impaired

NURSING DIAGNOSES FOR ENDOCRINE EMERGENCIES (CHAPTER 37)

Cardiac output, Decreased
Fluid volume, Deficient
Fluid volume, Excess
Gas exchange, Impaired
Hyperthermia
Tissue perfusion, Ineffective

NURSING DIAGNOSES FOR INFECTIOUS AND COMMUNICABLE DISEASES (CHAPTER 38)

Breathing pattern, Ineffective
Fluid volume, Deficient (active loss)
Fluid volume, Deficient (regulatory failure)
Fluid volume, Risk for deficient
Gas exchange, Impaired
Infection, Risk for
Nutrition, Imbalanced: less than body requirements
Skin integrity, Risk for impaired
Tissue integrity, Impaired
Ventilation, Impaired spontaneous

NURSING DIAGNOSES FOR INFLUENZA (CHAPTER 39)

Infection, Risk for
Coping, Ineffective
Powerlessness

NURSING DIAGNOSES FOR ENVIRONMENTAL EMERGENCIES (CHAPTER 40)

Airway clearance, Ineffective
Fluid volume, Deficient
Gas exchange, Impaired
Knowledge, Deficient
Skin integrity, Impaired
Thermoregulation, Ineffective
Tissue perfusion, Ineffective

NURSING DIAGNOSES FOR HEMATOLOGIC AND ONCOLOGIC EMERGENCIES (CHAPTER 41)

Anxiety
Fluid volume, Deficient
Infection, Risk for
Injury, Risk for
Knowledge, Deficient
Pain
Tissue perfusion, Ineffective

NURSING DIAGNOSES FOR TOXICOLOGIC EMERGENCIES (CHAPTER 42)

Airway clearance, Ineffective
Breathing pattern, Ineffective
Cardiac output, Decreased
Coping, Ineffective
Family processes, Interrupted
Fluid volume, Deficient
Fluid volume, Excess
Gas exchange, Impaired
Injury, Risk for
Thermoregulation, Ineffective
Tissue perfusion, Ineffective
Violence, Risk for

NURSING DIAGNOSES FOR GYNECOLOGIC EMERGENCIES (CHAPTER 43)

Anxiety
Body image, Disturbed
Cardiac output, Decreased
Fear
Fluid volume, Risk for deficient
Infection, Risk for
Knowledge, Deficient
Pain
Self-esteem, Situational low

NURSING DIAGNOSES FOR DENTAL, EAR, NOSE, THROAT, AND FACIAL EMERGENCIES (CHAPTER 44)

Airway clearance, Ineffective
Anxiety
Breathing pattern, Ineffective
Gas exchange, Impaired
Hypovolemia
Infection, Risk for
Pain

NURSING DIAGNOSES FOR OCULAR EMERGENCIES (CHAPTER 45)

Anxiety
Infection, Risk for
Injury, Risk for
Knowledge, Deficient
Pain
Sensory perception, Disturbed

NURSING DIAGNOSES ASSOCIATED WITH OBSTETRIC EMERGENCIES (CHAPTER 46)

Anxiety
Fear
Fetal risk
Fluid volume, Deficient
Knowledge, Deficient
Tissue perfusion, Ineffective

NURSING DIAGNOSES FOR THE PEDIATRIC PATIENT (CHAPTER 47)

Breathing pattern, Ineffective
Communication, Impaired verbal
Fluid volume, Risk for deficient
Nutrition, Imbalanced
Thermoregulation, Ineffective

NURSING DIAGNOSES FOR CHILD ABUSE AND NEGLECT (CHAPTER 48)

Anxiety
Communication, Impaired verbal
Coping, Ineffective (family)
Fear
Hopelessness
Injury, Risk for
Parenting, Impaired
Self-concept alteration

NURSING DIAGNOSES FOR ELDER ABUSE AND NEGLECT (CHAPTER 50)

Anxiety
Family processes, Interrupted
Fear
Injury, Risk for
Powerlessness
Self-concept alteration

NURSING DIAGNOSES FOR PSYCHOSOCIAL EMERGENCIES (CHAPTER 51)

Anxiety
Communication, Impaired verbal
Coping, Ineffective
Injury, Risk for
Thought processes, Disturbed
Violence, Risk for self-directed

NURSING DIAGNOSES FOR SUBSTANCE ABUSE (CHAPTER 52)

Anxiety
Fear
Injury, Risk for
Poisoning, Risk for
Sensory perception, Disturbed

NURSING DIAGNOSES FOR SEXUAL ASSAULT (CHAPTER 53)

Anxiety
Fear
Pain
Powerlessness
Rape-trauma syndrome

Index

Note: Pages followed by f indicated figures; t, tables; b, boxes.

Heroin, 692
  street name(s) and effects of, 696t
Herpes simplex genital infections
  in children, 659, 660f
  treatment regimen for, 487–489t, 584–585
Herpes simplex infection, of eye, 611
Herpes zoster ophthalmicus, 611
Hetastarch, 107t
HHS (Health and Human Services) Pandemic Influenza Plan,
    528–532
Hickman venous catheter, 103t
High frequency oscillatory ventilation (HFOV), 214
Hillcrest Baptist Med v Wade, 25|p0340
Hip dislocation, 333, 334f
Hip fractures, 327–328, 328f
HIPAA compliance officer, 18
History taking, during patient assessment, 77–78, 77t
Histoxic hypoxia, 91
HIV *See* Human immunodeficiency virus (HIV) infection.
Homeland Security Act, 187
Homeland Security All-Hazards Taxonomy, 192, 193f
  prevention (mission area one) in, 193f, 193–194t
  protection (mission area two) in, 193f, 194–195t
  recover (mission area four) in, 193f, 196–197t
  response (mission area three) in, 193f, 195–196t
Homeland Security Presidential Directive-5 (HSPD-5), 190
  credentialing of emergency responders under, 190
Hong Kong flu pandemic (1968), 526
Hordeolum, 610, 610f
Hornet sting emergencies, 551
HSV-1 (herpes simplex virus 1), in genital diseases, 584
HSV-2 (herpes simplex virus 2), 584–585 *See also* Genital herpes.
Huber needle, 102
Huffing, 691–692
Human bite wounds, 115–116
Human bites, 549
Human immunodeficiency virus (HIV) infection, 514, 518–519
  period of communicability of, 518–519
  postexposure prophylaxis for, 519
  stages of, and associated clinical syndromes, 519t
  transmission of, 518
Human papilloma virus (HPV), causing genital warts, 586
Human papilloma virus (HPV) infection, and treatment regimens,
    487–489t
Humeral shaft fracture, 323–325, 323f
Hydatidiform mole, 628
Hydrocarbon toxicity, 576
Hydrocodone, pediatric dosage, for moderate to severe pain,
    143t
Hydrocortisone, in sepsis management, 227
Hydromorphone, in pain management, 137
  pediatric dosage, 143t
  starting dose of, 137, 137t
Hymenopteran stings, 551
Hypemic hypoxia, 91
Hypercalcemia, 497
Hyperchloremia, 496
Hyperkalemia, 496
Hypermagnesemia, 497–498
Hypernatremia, 495
Hyperosmolar hyperglycemic state (HHS), 503–504
  and diabetic ketoacidosis, comparison of, 505t

Hyperosmolar hyperglycemic state (HHS) *(Continued)*
  differentiation of diabetic ketoacidosis and, 504, 504f
  fluid therapy in, 504
  onset of symptoms in, 503
Hyperosmolar therapy, in reducing intracranial pressure, 263
Hyperphosphatemia, 497
Hypertension, pregnancy induced, 621–622
Hypertensive crisis, 443
  patient management in, 443
Hyperthyroidism, 508
Hypertonic saline (7.5%), with dextran, 107t
Hypertonic saline (7.5%) solution, 107t
Hyperventilation, in traumatic brain injury, 261–262
Hyphema, 594, 596f
Hypocalcemia, 496–497
Hypochloremia, 496
Hypoglossal nerve (CN XII), 258t, 458t
Hypoglycemia, 504–505
  management of, 505
Hypokalemia, 496
Hypomagnesemia, 497
Hyponatremia, 495
Hypophosphatemia, 497
Hypotension, in positive pressure ventilation, 216–217
Hypothalamus, 256, 499
Hypothermia, 539–540
  cardiovascular response in, 539, 540f
  rewarming techniques in, 539, 540t
Hypovolemia, pediatric, 640–642
Hypovolemic shock, 448–449
Hypoxia, during patient transport, 91–92
Hypoxic hypoxia, 91

I

Ibuprofen, in pain management, pediatric dosage, 143t
Ibutilide fumarate (Corvert)
  in cardiovascular emergencies, 423–426t
  in dysrhythmia management, 440t
Ideal body weight (IBW), 212b
I:E ratio (inspiratory/expiratory ratio), 212b
  ventilator settings for, 215
Iliac artery trauma, 309–310
Immersion foot, 537–538
Immobilization, in orthopedic/neurovascular trauma,
    314–315
  casts for, 337
  scapular, sling and swath for, 323, 323f
Immobilization devices, in patient transport, 88b
Immobilization stress, during patient transport, 94
Immune thrombocytic purpura, 560
Immunomodulators, 400–403t
Impalement injury, 317
  mechanisms of, 247
Impetigo, 650
Implantable cardioverter-defibrillator (ICD), 419
In Re Estate of Allen, 20|p0200
Incarcerated hernia, 645
Incident Command System (ICS), 188–190
  for hospitals and practitioners, 190
  origin of, 189–190
Inderal *See* Propranolol HCl.
Induced emesis, 565